Elder Abuse

XinQi Dong
Editor

Elder Abuse

Research, Practice and Policy

Springer

Editor
XinQi Dong
Rush Institute for Healthy Aging
Rush University Medical Center
Chicago, IL
USA

ISBN 978-3-319-47502-8 ISBN 978-3-319-47504-2 (eBook)
DOI 10.1007/978-3-319-47504-2

Library of Congress Control Number: 2016953652

Printed on acid-free paper

This Springer imprint is published by Springer Nature
The registered company is Springer International Publishing AG
The registered company address is: Gewerbestrasse 11, 6330 Cham, Switzerland

Foreword

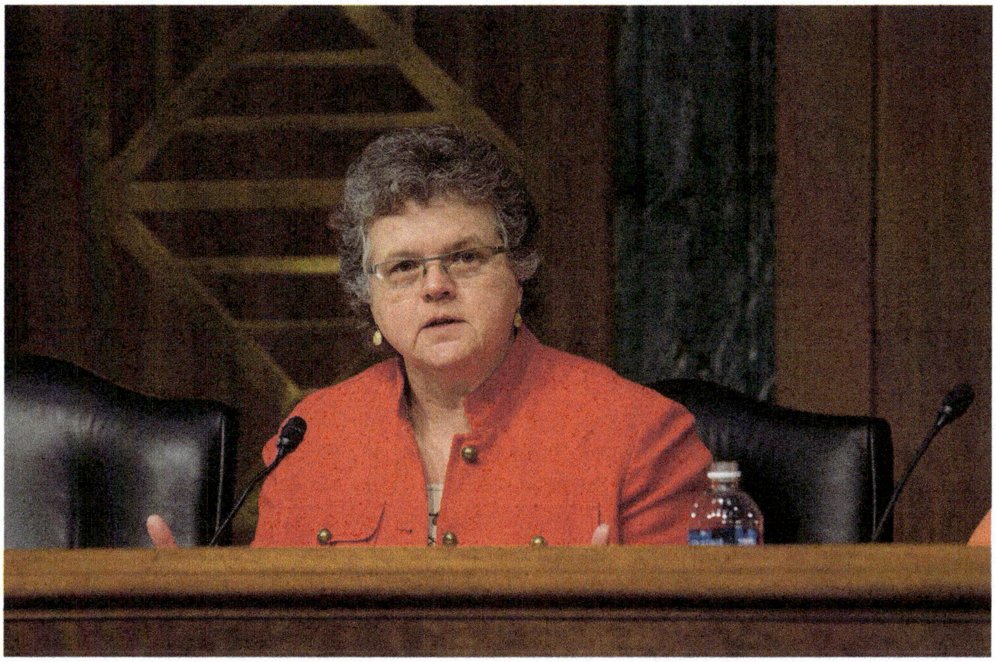

I often frame conversations about elder abuse with three questions: Do you know any older adults who are abused? Do you know who they are? Do you know what they need from you? The answer to the first questions is, yes—you always do. For many years, elder abuse has been a silent issue. Many older adults are afraid or embarrassed to bring their issues into the light. However, in recent decades, we have made tremendous strides on advancing recognition of interpersonal violence as a major public health concern, but not enough has been done to shed a light on abuse and neglect in older age. Despite the fact that elder abuse is less visible than other forms of abuse, we know that at least one in 10 adults over the age of 60 has experienced violence, neglect, or financial exploitation—usually by someone they know and trust—in the past month. Elder abuse is a public health and human rights problem of global concern. It erodes the humanity in all of us as we strive to reach old age and remain independent, with our dignity in place.

I am passionate about the issue of violence against older adults and their mistreatment. As Assistant Secretary for Aging in the U.S. Department of Health and Human Services, I have dedicated my leadership to forging and strengthening partnerships across federal government, with community partners and other expert stakeholders, to raise the visibility of elder abuse as a public health issue impacting, and impacted by, multiple areas of public policy.

The multifaceted nature of elder abuse has contributed, in part, to our insufficient knowledge of its prevalence and how best to respond. We need more comprehensive literature aimed at a broad constituency to address it. *Elder Abuse: Research, Practice and Policy* is an important step forward in the continuing effort to educate and challenge those in and out of the field of aging. By learning comprehensively where we are, we can begin to see where we need to be.

Part of the challenge that books such as this pose for all of us in the field is: How do we get the message out? This book may help professionals and policymakers alike to help reframe the public discussion and understanding about older adults; how they age, the challenges of abuse, and what do we need to learn from research to create effective policy. Aging experts already know that success in understanding and addressing elder abuse requires a multidisciplinary approach and success will only be measured through coordinated research and practice. We still have so much to learn.

As an advocate, I am heartened to see movement in the areas of aging policy, new interest in research and constant review in innovation in practice. This book will help raise questions, expand thinking of those in the field, and inspire additional research. In addition, I hope it spurs thinking about best approaches to addressing prevention and intervention for elder abuse. This book will shine a new light on the issues surrounding elder abuse, and thus the issue will find a new audience. What was once a very small field is expanding to include new minds and hearts. There are new voices in the field and they are invigorating it.

Learning what we know is essential to planning the next steps. This book is part of a foundation with others for us to think about where we are and where we need to go to bring the field of aging research, practice and policy in line with the very complex and growing needs of a demographic expanding by thousands every day.

We are mindful that our work has merely begun. The field of elder abuse remains far behind the fields of child abuse and intimate partner violence, but it is becoming more prominent. As we learn to articulate the needs of older victims and survivors, they will also be a voice to guide us. They will teach us what to research, how to practice and what policies are needed for a good, long life free from abuse.

With this book we have an important contribution to the field. With each new book focusing on elder abuse, the field grows in new and important ways. I am encouraged that this volume will find itself a catalyst for others, whose work we have yet to see.

Kathy Greenlee
Assistant Secretary for Aging
Administrator, Administration for Community Living
U.S. Department of Health and Human Services

Prologue

Elder abuse (EA) is a prevalent, identifiable, fatal and costly public health issue that affects populations living in both communities and institutional settings of all sociodemographic and socioeconomic strata. The problem is particularly disturbing given the estimated global population growth of people aged 65 from 2010 to 2050, is predicted to triple and reach 1.5 billion individuals or 16% of the world's population [35]. The field of elder justice has to take a vertical leap to understand and protect this vulnerable population through coordinated efforts across community, city/state, federal, and international organizations. This comprehensive volume aims to objectively provide the state of the science for the past, present, and future for the field of elder justice through systematic evaluations of research, practice, and policy.

Research

Defining EA

Definitions and typology of EA vary across nations, states, disciplines, organizations, and studies. For example, the World Health Organization, the National Center on Elder Abuse (NCEA), and the National Research Council (NRC) all define EA divergently regarding the terminology, subtypes, and case identification criteria [18, 25, 34]. Such methodological inconsistency has limited the ability of current research to systematically assess prevalence, incidence, correlates and severity of EA, further prohibiting translating the knowledge into intervention strategies and policy development. Recent studies showed great variations of EA prevalence estimates (e.g., 1.0–47.3% in North and South America; 0.1–61.1% in Europe; 0.22 per 1000–62% in Asia; 0.6, 30, and 64.3% in Africa) [4, 11, 36], which might be explained by the large methodological variations across studies. However, researchers should also be cautious of applying general definitions of EA to more specific populations because contextual factors (institutional, environmental, cultural, etc.) play essential roles in determining perceptions of acceptable and unacceptable behavior toward older adults. This might significantly influence the valuation of prevalence, incidence, severity, associated factors, and consequences, and efficacy of practices of EA. Hence, a balanced perspective asserting the importance of both a broad definition and specific definitions for particular populations and settings may better project directions for future actions on defining EA and subtypes. Additionally, while a variety of definitions for EA might still be used by different disciplines, the scholars should be more explicit concerning the terminology, typology, derivation of definitions, and process of refining definitions (if any) for EA and subtypes in their future publications.

Population Research

Large-scale representative longitudinal studies in diverse community and institutional settings are necessary to adequately examine the incidence of EA and subtypes. In the U.S., few studies have reached national representativeness, nor engaged longitudinal designs to detect the true incidence of EA through longitudinal studies [6, 9, 17]. While there exists no such national representative study and given the time and resources restraints, researchers and funders might consider integrate EA incidence measurement questions into the existing representative longitudinal aging studies in diverse settings [10].

It is also crucial to improving the validity, reliability, cultural sensitivity, appropriateness, and ability to capture multilevel factors of the screening instruments in population studies. Older persons might be presented with particular challenges to disclosing abusive events due to physical and cognitive impairment, medical conditions, recognition difficulties, and dependence on the perpetrators. Minority and marginalized older populations might have more cultural, linguistic, and literacy barriers in detection, reporting, and help-seeking behaviors. Hence, screening instruments should be rigorously tested and tailored to be appropriate considering individual traits, cultures, language, and literacy capacity. Second, best modes of administrating screening tools (e.g., phone, in person, computer-based) to certain populations should be examined. Third, despite victims and perpetrators traits, studies should design instruments with abilities to solicit contextual factors from multiple types of informants.

Risk Factors and Consequences of EA

Rigorously designed longitudinal studies measuring the incidence of EA and subtypes in both victims and potential perpetrators can enhance the knowledge of EA risk/protective factors, adverse health outcomes, and the effect size of these associations. Current knowledge remains rudimentary pertaining important sociodemographic and socioeconomic characteristics of EA victims as no consistent trend of associations has been found between these potential risk factors and abusive events [11, 15, 20]. However, several other characteristics of victims, perpetrators, social relationships, and environments have been linked to greater likelihood of different subtypes of EA including victim's cognitive impairment, physical function impairment, psychological distress; perpetrator's heavy burden as caregivers and psychological/psychiatric illness; poor social relationships; less supportive environments; and previous traumatic event exposure [1, 11, 17, 20, 22].

With respect to the consequences, EA has been linked to increased risk of morbidity and premature mortality, physical injuries, functional impairment and dependency, declined health status, psychological distress, and social isolation [8, 13, 14]. Furthermore, such adverse physical and psychological outcomes may lead to increased medical costs in the forms of healthcare utilization and nursing home placement [13, 14, 17]. Assessment of economic impact of EA and subtypes vary greatly across investigations—$2.9 billion estimated by MetLife Mature Market Institute (2011) and $36 billion projected by another organization (TrueLink) for the annual cost of elder financial abuse [30].

Understanding causal relationships and strengths between elder abuse with proximal and distal outcomes are vital for developing prevention and intervention strategies and measuring the impacts and magnitude of EA. To date, many EA studies are cross-sectional, making it impossible to draw the cause–effect inference between EA and potential risk/preventive factors and consequences. Sir Austin Bradford Hill's [19] groundbreaking criteria have shed light on examining causal associations between exposure variables and health outcomes in such longitudinal studies. The associated factors of EA should all be rigorously evaluated through longitudinal studies following the Branford Hill's Criteria. This also applies to the examination of the potential consequences of EA. The criteria (***strength, consistency, specificity, temporality, dose–response, plausibility, coherence, experimental evidence, and analogy***) can provide evidence for causality between a cause (e.g., victim's cognitive impairment) and effect (e.g., abusive events). Additionally, longitudinal studies may adopt theoretical frameworks to guide study design and situate abuse events in ecological contexts, accumulating life-course experiences, and intergenerational and family relationships.

Intervention

A number of proposed intervention and prevention strategies exist in public, community, clinical and policy arenas, but none has sufficient evidence for the long-term effectiveness on reducing occurrence or severity of EA. The strategies include public awareness campaigns, advocacy, clinical screening, educational programs for health professionals, counseling sessions, support groups, case management, and state statutes mandating abuse report to law enforcement officials or social services [11, 17, 26]. Each of the strategies ought to be tested rigorously for empirical evidence suggesting its intentional benefits and potential harms, since EA related practices may lead to adverse outcomes to the older adults [12]. A randomized clinical trial (RCT) by MacMillan and colleagues [23] shows insufficient evidence of both effectiveness and harm of IPV screening tools for a large cohort of women (n = 6743) in healthcare setting, which is nevertheless recommended by the U.S. Preventive Services Task Force. More evaluation research as such is needed to examine best practices for EA prevention and intervention.

Future EA intervention studies need improvements in several aspects. Findings of the Ploeg and colleagues [26] study reviewing current intervention studies of EA suggested common methodological limitations as follow: (a) lack of experimental designs; (b) poor presentation of research process such as randomization, assignment concealment, blinding researchers, and data analysis; (c) unrepresentative samples; (d) lack of psychometric outcome measures; (e) follow-up rates lower than 80%; (f) lack of adjustment of baseline differences between groups; (g) possible bias occurred in data collection by caseworkers.

Adherence to high ethical standards should be emphasized in future large-scale experimental designs and RCTs related to abuse, exploitation, and neglect. The investigators may follow the WHO recommendations for research in domestic violence against women to (a) paramount the safety of respondents and the research team; (b) hold participants' information and response to strict confidentiality; (c) carefully select, train, and support the research team; (d) design actions aimed at reducing any distress caused to the participants; (e) train fieldworkers to refer participants to available sources of assistance and support; (f) ensure findings are properly interpreted and used to advance policy and intervention development [27]. Also, researchers are well situated to leverage advocacy efforts by underscoring the importance of empirical evidence supporting effective intervention strategies in languages of stakeholders and the public, so that society is informed of where to best invest limited public resources.

Culture

Investigating cultural variations and their profound impact on beliefs, perceptions, and social norms should be prioritized in research since older adults from diverse racial/ethnic, gender, and sexual minority groups might be more susceptible to abuse, neglect, and exploitation. The pronounced demographic shift globally calls for extensive investigations to better understand EA surrounding prevalence, incidence in various populations, cultural variations in terms of the definitions, measurements, risk/preventive factors, and consequences, as well as culturally appropriate and effective intervention and prevention strategies. A few recent studies have enhanced the knowledge in diverse cultures such as African Americans, Latinos, and Chinese. For example, findings of the PINE study [16] surveying 3159 community-dwelling Chinese older adults in Chicago found a prevalence of 15.0% for abuse, and explored important correlates, potential risk factors, and consequences. Of note, it investigated possible cultural determinants for EA, such as the traditional practice of filial piety and its potential to influence the occurrence, perception, and response of abuse. The study also examined other possible confounding characteristics of U.S. minority populations, including acculturation, intergenerational differences, and the immigrant experience.

Innovative strategies should be used to better address EA in minority communities. The long-lasting and discriminatory system-level exclusion of the minorities, resources disparities, and cultural and linguistic barriers make it difficult to establish rapport between the communities and the research field. Community-Based Participatory Research (CBPR) has proved to be able to generate community-derived solutions that are culturally applicable throughout research initiation, implementation, results dissemination, and sustained development. Researchers have demonstrated that community health workers (CHWs) could boost community empowerment in CBPR intervention studies by translating intervention strategies designed by the academic institution into community practice and service [29]. The PINE study [10,15, 16] exemplified the success of the CBPR model employing bi-cultural and multilingual CHWs to untangle complicated cultural and linguistic barriers within large and diverse immigrant communities. The study also benefits from increased community engagement and commitment brought by the research-to-community shift of ownership, power, and resources by engaging CHWs. Furthermore, for complex research problems as culture-specific EA, it is valuable to combine quantitative and qualitative methods because their complimentary nature can result in a broader and deeper understanding of EA and its cultural context.

Interdisciplinary and Translational Research

Given the lack of empirical evidence for effective practices for EA, the merits of conducting multidirectional research from other disciplines is apparent. Researchers may be able to adapt screening measures and interventions that have proved promising within the areas of child abuse, youth violence, and IPV and test their efficacy for addressing EA. Several promising interventions worth examining are brief clinical interventions, bystander training, income supports, and environment modifications [32].

Many have recognized that a translational research framework might help fields including EA to integrate and translate multidisciplinary research findings (e.g., biomedical science, psychology, neuroscience, etiology, behavioral science, epidemiology, and political science) into improvements in public well being and health. Based on initial discussions, Rubio and colleagues [28] developed a translational model of multidirectional continuum, in which research investments and findings interact between basic research, patient-oriented research, and population-based research (e.g., epidemiology, social behavioral sciences, public health research). The model has thrown lights on promising translational research opportunities and partnerships among experts in the EA field and other disciplines. More support should be given to these areas of collaborative research such as biomarker and biology mechanism (e.g., relationship between vitamin D deficiency and EA), behavioral science techniques (e.g., motivational interview), neuroscience (e.g., human brains' influence on financial decision-making and exploitation), and technologies.

Practice

While rigorous and systematic evidence-based prevention and intervention strategies are not available, practical actions and systematic improvements can take place in communities, healthcare settings, and institutional facilities, where local organizations, staffs, and key personnel might be well situated to offer immediate response and protection to older adults susceptible to abuse.

Education and Training

We should leverage efforts to support worldwide and nationwide educational and training activities relating to EA for both workforce and the public. Research shows a lack of professional and public awareness of the prevalence and severity of abuse in community, institutional, and healthcare settings. Key workforce who are exposed regularly to older people have insufficient awareness, knowledge, skills, and confidence dealing with EA, and are unfamiliar with related case identification and report procedures, legislation, and referral agencies when confronted with suspected abuse occurrence [5, 21]. Educational activities should be tailored and incorporated into training of different personnel ranging from healthcare students and professionals, law enforcement, social services, community organization staffs, volunteers, and frontline health workers.

Community Settings

To date, 64.9 million older adults in the U.S. are living in a community setting. Adult Protective Services (APS) caseworkers are the first responders for abuse case report in each state, providing services including receiving reports of abuse, investigating cases, case planning, and service monitoring and evaluation [3]. Meanwhile, the National Aging Network, a government-funded services network, provides community-level resource and technical assistance for victims of EA. Within the network, 629 area agencies on aging, nearly 20,000 service providers, 244 tribal organizations, and 2 native Hawaiian organizations representing 400 Tribes serve communities with services that include, but not limited to information and referral, counseling, nutrition, social engagement and entertainment activities, legal services, personal/home care, instrumental service (e.g., transportation), and specific services for native populations [2].

Previous investigations [9, 17, 31] show major challenges confronted by the APS programs, which are (a) increasing numbers and complexity of cases that lead to heavier caseloads for staffs; (b) unstable and insufficient funding sources supporting APS programs and services; (c) the noted lack of empirical evidence suggesting best solutions for resolving EA; (d) lack of indispensable training and capacity to deal with complicated abusive cases; (e) lack of multidisciplinary collaborations among APS and other partners such as the medical, legal, criminal and financial fields to optimize the effects of the programs and services; (f) the varied data collection systems of the APS across states has resulted in missing opportunities for staff to use valid information from previous programming and intervening experience. In regard to APS practices and other federal-funded agencies addressing EA in communities, funding, personnel training and support, unified data system, and inter-agency collaborations should be given or developed to address these gaps in the ability to investigate and protect older adults from EA.

Institutional Settings

In addition to older adults living in community settings, abuse, neglect, and exploitation in long-term care settings are understudied and warrant further investigation. The Long-Term Care Ombudsman Program (LTCOP) resolves complaints, protects rights, and advocates change of policies and practice for long-term care residents. In many states, the APS caseworkers also address EA in institutional settings. Similar to APS, the LTCOP also face insufficient financial resources, and the National Association of State Long-Term Care Ombudsman Programs [33] has synthesized recommendations for future LTCOP activities such as to strengthen the autonomy of the ombudsman program to help individual residents, and to improve national reporting system that incorporate the rich information obtained from LTCOP data. More importantly, staff who care for long-term facility residents are likely to deal with more adverse health or medical conditions and declined function, such as chronic disease, dementia, and mental diseases. This urges efforts for more comprehensive education, training, supervision, support, and assessment for the LTCOP staff in terms of skills, values, and temperament.

Healthcare Settings

Professionals in healthcare settings (e.g., nurses, physicians, social workers, psychologists, discharge planners) can play important roles in detecting vulnerabilities and intervening suspected EA cases due to their regular interactions with older patients. Priority should be set to pursue evidence for the strategies in healthcare settings, as they have not been tested adequately through empirical research. But immediate field response and actions should be taken to avoid leaving tens of thousands of at-risk older adults unprotected. More guidance and support ought to be available for the professionals, and they may consider several brief screeners (e.g., HS-EAST, VASS, and EASI recommended by CMS) [12] and stepwise procedures for dealing with EA cases in healthcare settings developed by other experienced scholars.

Since most states in the U.S. mandate healthcare professionals to report EA cases to the APS caseworkers, the collaborations between the two parties might face specific challenges such as poor communications and health professionals' incompliance of reporting requirement. To optimize the efforts in healthcare settings to address EA, effective coordination and communication between professionals and APS, and culturally competent approaches and practices suit each healthcare facility might be appropriate [7].

Policy

Drafting and implementing policies must serve their purposes for protecting the rights of millions of older adults. Although steps have been taken in the legal system to protect the human rights of older adults globally (e.g., the International Plan of Action on Aging and the International Covenant on Economic, Social, and Cultural Rights), there is a lack of strength in policies to implement and enforce them at international and domestic levels [24]. Miller [24] called for a solution to developing a comprehensive and binding international treaty to set a standard of protection for the older people, by which, national governments would be accountable for protecting the human rights, addressing specific needs, ensuring safety and care quality in nursing homes and other institutional facilities, and supporting better EA public and professional education.

In the U.S., there are several major federal statutes addressing elder justice issues including the Older Americans Act (OAA), the Elder Justice Act (EJA) portion of the Affordable Care Act (ACA), the Violence against Women Act (VAWA), the Public Health Service Act, and the Social Security Act. Meanwhile, a number of federal agencies have been playing essential roles in protecting older adults from abuse such as the National Institutes of Health (NIH), the Center for Disease Control and Prevention (CDC), the Administration on Community Living (ACL), Department of Justice Civic Division, National Institute of Justice, Office of Victims of Crimes, and the Office on Violence Against Women [9, 17].

However, support for national activities protecting rights of older Americans have been scattered across the country, and there is a need for stronger federal leadership to prioritize EA in research, public advocacy, policy development, practice, and education. Second, there is insufficient coordination of these federal level agencies, legislation, and other efforts to provide most effective protection and treatment for older adults who are at risk of abuse, neglect, and exploitation [9, 17]. Most importantly, continuous funding support for the legislations is essential for implementation and service delivery. Federal spending on activities for EA ($11.9 million) was 54 times less than that for violence against women ($649 million) and 588 times less than that for child abuse ($7 billion) [11].

Conclusion

The world's rapidly growing population urges the needs for leveraged efforts and funding resources from global investigators and stakeholders within the realms of research, intervention, practice, education, and policy. Nationally representative longitudinal research is needed to better define the incidence, risk/protective factors, and consequences of EA in diverse racial/ethnic, gender, and sexual minority populations in each region globally, and methodological consensus has to be reached in related studies to generate systematic research results and knowledge. While we have incomplete empirical evidence for best intervention and prevention strategies to address EA, coordinated efforts are needed from governments, policymakers, global and national organizations, community stakeholders, frontline workforce, healthcare professionals, and law enforcement institutions to provide linguistically/culturally appropriate response for elder abuse, neglect, and exploitation and protect the rights of this extremely vulnerable population. As the editor for this comprehensive volume, I am forever indebted to the perspicacious contributors of this textbook. Their dedication, commitment, knowledge, and sage wisdom will continue to inspire the field of elder abuse and pave the road for the future global generations of researchers, educators, advocates, practitioners, and policymakers.

Chicago, IL, USA XinQi Dong

References

1. Acierno R, Hernandez MA, Amstadter AB, Resnick HS, Steve K, Muzzy W, Kilpatrick DG. Prevalence and correlates of emotional, physical, sexual, and financial abuse and potential neglect in the United States: the National Elder Mistreatment Study. Am J Public Health. 2010;100(2):292–97. doi:10.2105/AJPH.2009.163089.
2. Administration on Aging (AoA): Older Americans Act. 2014. Retrieved from http://www.aoa.gov/AoA_programs/OAA/Index.aspx.
3. Adult Protective Services. Intervention partners. 2016. Retrieved from https://ncea.acl.gov/Stop_Abuse/Partners/APS/index.aspx.
4. Bigala P, Ayiga N. Prevalence and predictors of elder abuse in Mafikeng Local Municipality in South Africa. Afr Popul Stud. 2014;28(1):463–74.
5. Cooper C, Selwood A, Livingston G. Knowledge, detection, and reporting of abuse by health and social care professionals: a systematic review. Am J Geriatr Psychiatry. 2009;17(10):826–38.
6. Daly JM, Merchant ML, Jogerst GJ. Elder abuse research: a systematic review. J Elder Abuse Negl. 2011;23(4):348–65. doi:10.1080/08946566.2011.608048.
7. DeLiema M, Navarro A, Enguidanos S, Wilber K. Voices from the frontlines: examining elder abuse from multiple professional perspectives. Health Soc Work. 2015;40(2):e15–24. doi:10.1093/hsw/hlv012.
8. Dong X. Consequences of elder abuse: the needs for social justice and policy implications. In: Social and economic costs of violence: workshop summary. Washington, D.C.: National Academies Press (US); 2011.
9. Dong X. Advancing the field of elder abuse: future directions and policy implications. J Am Geriatr Soc. 2012;60(11):2151–56. doi:10.1111/j.1532-5415.2012.04211.x.
10. Dong X. Elder abuse: research, practice, and health policy. The 2012 GSA Maxwell Pollack award lecture. Gerontologist. 2013;54(2):153–62. doi:10.1093/geront/gnt139.
11. Dong X. Elder abuse: systematic review and implications for practice. J Am Geriatr Soc. 2015a;63(6):1214–38. doi:10.1111/jgs.13454.
12. Dong X. Screening for elder abuse in healthcare settings: why should we care, and is it a missed quality indicator? J Am Geriatr Soc. 2015b;63(8):1686–88. doi:10.1111/jgs.13538.
13. Dong X, Simon M. Elder self-neglect: implications for health care professionals. CGS J CME. 2013;3(25–28).
14. Dong X, Simon MA, Fulmer T, Leon CFMd, Hebert LE, Beck T, … Evans DA. A prospective population-based study of differences in elder self-neglect and mortality between black and white older adults. J Gerontol A Biol Sci Med Sci. 2011;66(6):695–704. doi:10.1093/gerona/glr053.
15. Dong X, Chen R, Fulmer T, Simon MA. Prevalence and correlates of elder mistreatment in a community-dwelling population of U.S. Chinese older adults. J Aging Health. 2014a;26(7):1209–24. doi:10.1177/0898264314531617.
16. Dong X, Wong E, Simon MA. Study design and implementation of the PINE study. J Aging Health. 2014b;26(7):1085–99. doi:10.1177/0898264314526620.
17. Elder justice: stronger federal leadership could enhance national response to elder abuse. 2011. Retrieved from http://www.gao.gov/new.items/d11208.pdf.
18. Elder mistreatment: abuse, neglect, and exploitation in an aging America (0-309-08434-2). 2003. Retrieved from Washington, DC: http://www.nap.edu/read/10406/chapter/1.
19. Hill AB. The environment and disease: association or causation? J R Soc Med. 1965;108(1):32–7. doi:10.1177/0141076814562718.
20. Johannese M, LoGiudice D. Elder abuse: a systematic review of risk factors in community-dwelling elders. Age Ageing. 2013;42(3):292–98. doi:10.1093/ageing/afs195.
21. Kennedy RD. Elder abuse and neglect: the experience, knowledge, and attitudes of primary care physicians. Fam Med. 2005;37(7):481–85.
22. Laumann EO, Leitsch SA, Waite LJ. Elder mistreatment in the United States: prevalence estimates from a nationally representative study. J Gerontol B Psychol Sci Soc Sci. 2008;63(4):S248–54.
23. MacMillan HL, Wathen N, Jamieson E, Boyle MH, Shannon HS, Ford-Gilboe M, … McNutt L-A. Screening for intimate partner violence in health care settings: a randomized trial. JAMA. 2009;302(5):493–501. doi:10.1001/jama.2009.1089.
24. Miller JM. International human rights and the elderly. Marquette Elder's Advisor. 2010;11(2).

25. National Center on Elder Abuse: Frequently asked questions. 2016. Retrieved from https://ncea.acl.gov/faq/index.aspx.
26. Ploeg J, Fear J, Hutchison B, MacMillan H, Bolan G. A systematic review of interventions for elder abuse. J Elder Abuse Negl. 2009;21(3):187–210. doi:10.1080/08946560902997181.
27. Putting Women First: Ethical and Safety Recommendations for Research on Domestic Violence Against Women. 2001. WHO: Department of Gender, Women and Health. Retrieved from http://www.who.int/gender-equity-rights/knowledge/who_fch_gwh_01.1/en/.
28. Rubio DM, Schoenbaum EE, Lee LS, Schteingart DE, Marantz PR, Anderson KE, … Esposito K. Defining translational research: implications for training. Acad Med J Assoc Am Med Coll. 2010;85(3):470–75. doi:10.1097/ACM.0b013e3181ccd618.
29. Smith SA, Blumenthal DS. Community health workers support community-based participatory research ethics: lessons learned along the research-to-practice-to-community continuum. J Health Care Poor Underserved. 2012;23(4):77–87.
30. Stanger T. Financial elder abuse costs $3 billion a year. Or is it $36 billion? Consumer reports. 2015. Retrieved from http://www.consumerreports.org/cro/consumer-protection/financial-elder-abuse-costs-3-billion-or-is-it-30-billion.
31. Strasser SM, Kerr J, King PS, Payne B, Beddington S, Pendrick D, … McCarty F. A Survey of Georgia adult protective service staff: implications for older adult injury prevention and policy. W J Emerg Med. 2011. 12(3);357–64.
32. Sumner SA, Mercy JA, Dahlberg LL, Hillis SD, Klevens J, Houry D. Violence in the United States: status, challenges, and opportunities. JAMA. 2015;314(5):478–88. doi:10.1001/jama.2015.8371.
33. The long-term care ombudsman program: rethinking and retooling for the future: proceedings and recommendations. 2003. Retrieved from
34. WHO: Elder abuse. 2016. Retrieved from http://www.who.int/ageing/projects/elder_abuse/en/.
35. Why population aging matters: a global perspective. 2007. Retrieved from https://www.nia.nih.gov/sites/default/files/WPAM.pdf.
36. Yan E, Chan K-L, Tiwari A. A systematic review of prevalence and risk factors for elder abuse in Asia. Trauma Violence Abuse. 2015;16(2):199–219. doi:10.1177/1524838014555033.

Contents

Contributors

Ron Acierno College of Nursing, Medical University of South Carolina, Charleston, SC, USA; Ralph H. Johnson Veterans Affairs Medical Center, Charleston, SC, USA

Georgia J. Anetzberger Department of Medicine, Case Western Reserve University, South Euclid, OH, USA

Sophia Autrey Centers for Medicare and Medicaid Services, Baltimore, MD, USA

Scott R. Beach University Center for Social and Urban Research, University of Pittsburgh, Pittsburgh, PA, USA

Avital Benson The John A. Hartford Foundation, New York, NY, USA

William F. Benson National Adult Protective Services Association, Health Benefits ABCs, Silver Spring, MD, USA

Robert B. Blancato Elder Justice Coalition, Washington, DC, USA

E-Shien Chang Rush Institute for Healthy Aging, Rush University Medical Center, Chicago, IL 60612, USA

Ruijia Chen Department of Social and Behavioral Sciences, Harvard T.H. Chan School of Public Health, Cambridge, MA, USA

Kendon J. Conrad Department of Health Policy and Administration, University of Illinois at Chicago, Chicago, IL, USA

Loree Cook-Daniels FORGE, Inc, Milwaukee, WI, USA

Victoria L. Crabb Department of Epidemiology, University of Iowa College of Public Health, Iowa City, IA, USA

Jeanette Marie Daly Department of Family Medicine, University of Iowa Hospitals and Clinics, Iowa City, IA, USA

Margaret Davis Department of Psychiatry, VA Ann Arbor Health Care System/University of Michigan, Ann Arbor, MI, USA

Marguerite DeLiema Stanford Center on Longevity, Stanford University, Stanford, CA, USA

XinQi Dong Rush Institute for Healthy Aging, Rush University Medical Center, Chicago, IL, USA

Carmel B. Dyer Department of Internal Medicine, Division of Geriatric and Palliative Medicine, University of Texas Medical School, Houston, TX, USA; Texas Elder Abuse and Mistreatment Institute (TEAM), Houston, USA; Harris Health System, Houston, USA; UTHealth Consortium on Aging, Houston, USA

Gracy Fang Department of Social Work and Social Administration, University of Hong Kong, Hong Kong, Hong Kong

Terry Fulmer The John A. Hartford Foundation, New York, NY, USA

Jacqueline S. Gray Center for Rural Health, University of North Dakota School of Medicine and Health Sciences, Grand Forks, ND, USA

Kathy Greenlee Assistant Secretary for Aging and Administrator, Administration for Community Living, U.S. Department of Health and Human Services, Washington, DC, USA

Jeffrey E. Hall Division of Violence Prevention, Centers for Disease Control and Prevention, Atlanta, GA, USA

Candace J. Heisler Heisler and Associates, San Bruno, CA, USA

Shelly L. Jackson Department of Psychiatry and Neurobehavioral Sciences, Institute of Law, Psychiatry and Public Policy, University of Virginia, Charlottesville, VA, USA

Marshall B. Kapp Center for Innovative Collaboration in Medicine and Law, Florida State University, Tallahassee, FL, USA

Brian W. Lindberg Elder Justice Coalition, Washington, DC, USA

Jane Lucas Quality Insights of Pennsylvania, King of Prussia, PA, USA

Andy Mao United States Department of Justice, Washington, DC, USA

Meaghan McMahon Washington, DC, USA

Tara L. McMullen Centers for Medicare and Medicaid Services, Baltimore, MD, USA

Kylie Meyer Leonard Davis School of Gerontology, Los Angeles, CA, USA

Charles P. Mouton Family and Community Medicine, School of Medicine, Meharry Medical College, Nashville, TN, USA

Carrie F. Mulford National Institute of Justice, Office of Justice Programs, United States Department of Justice, Washington, DC, USA

Corey Nichols-Hadeed Department of Psychiatry, University of Rochester Medical Center, Rochester, NY, USA

Nora OBrien-Suric The John A. Hartford Foundation, New York, NY, USA

James G. O'Brien Institute on Sustainable Health and Optimal Aging, Louisville, KY, USA

Elizabeth Podnieks Department of English, Ryerson University, Toronto, ON, Canada

María D. Pérez-Cárceles Department of Legal Medicine, Institute of Research into Aging, Biomedical Research Institute (IMIB-Arrixaca), Regional Campus of International Excellence "Campus Mare Nostrum", School of Medicine, University of Murcia, Murcia, Spain

Mary Joy Quinn San Francisco Superior Court San Francisco, California, USA

Carlos A. Reyes-Ortiz Division of Geriatric and Palliative Medicine, Department of Internal Medicine, University of Texas Medical School, Houston, TX, USA; Texas Elder Abuse and Mistreatment Institute (TEAM), Houston, USA; Harris Health System, Houston, USA; UTHealth Consortium on Aging, Houston, USA

Gary Rezek Quality Insights of Pennsylvania, King of Prussia, PA, USA

Karen A. Roberto Center for Gerontology, Virginia Polytechnic Institute and State University, Blacksburg, VA, USA

Susan K. Roepke-Buehler Behavioral Sciences and Medicine, Rush University Medical Center, Chicago, IL, USA

Elizabeth J. Santos Department of Psychiatry, University of Rochester Medical Center, Rochester, NY, USA

Margot J. Schofield Department of Psychology and Counselling, School of Psychology and Public Health, La Trobe University, Melbourne, VIC, Australia

Kimberly Schwartz Centers for Medicare and Medicaid Services, Baltimore, MD, USA

Jeannette Shrift Quality Insights of Pennsylvania, King of Prussia, PA, USA

Joseph Snyder Philadelphia Corporation for Aging, Philadelphia, PA, USA

Anita Somplasky Quality Insights of Pennsylvania, King of Prussia, PA, USA

Janet H. Southerland Oral and Maxillofacial Surgery, School of Dentistry, Meharry Medical College, Nashville, TN, USA

Karen Stein School of Public Policy and Administration, University of Delaware, Newark, DE, USA

Lori A. Stiegel American Bar Association Commission on Law and Aging, Washington, DC, USA

Pamela B. Teaster Center for Gerontology, Virginia Tech, Blacksburg, VA, USA

Cynthia Thomas Committee on National Statistics, National Academies of Sciences, Engineering and Medicine, Rockville, MD, USA

Robert B. Wallace Department of Epidemiology, The University of Iowa Center on Aging, Iowa City, IA, USA

Kathleen H. Wilber Leonard Davis School of Gerontology, Los Angeles, CA, USA

Joah L. Williams Department of Psychology, University of Missouri—Kansas City, Kansas City, MO, USA

Erica Wood American Bar Association Commission on Law and Aging, Columbia, DC, USA

Elsie Yan Department of Applied Social Sciences, Hong Kong Polytechnic University, Hong Kong, Hong Kong

Jeanine Yonashiro-Cho Leonard Davis School of Gerontology, Los Angeles, CA, USA

Part I
Introduction

Toward Definitions of Elder Mistreatment

1

Robert B. Wallace and Victoria L. Crabb

1.1 Introduction

Definitions are important in understanding and using language. Various types of definition categories have their own typologies and uses. Importantly, most are relatively concise and serve to explain or illuminate in overview various concepts and ideas. Whether for elder mistreatment (EM) or any other term, they serve to improve and perhaps standardize the rhetorical use of defined terms. They bring new eyes and minds to the terms at hand, and inevitably shape subsequent thinking. However, as all languages evolve in structure and usage over time, so must definitions. In the case of definitions in the sciences, terms such as EM continuously change and evolve as knowledge and understanding are amassed. Further, changes in linguistic fashions that occur over time may result in shifting conceptualizations of terms.

This chapter addresses definitions for EM overall and for its major types. This is not an attempt to exhaustively catalog the terminology used in the past several decades. Nor will we provide the level of detail and description that helps understand the individual types of EM; these are discussed elsewhere in this book. Rather, our goals are to: (1) explore some of the reasons why it has been problematic to define EM; (2) identify various important types of definitions and their derivations and applications, such as syndromic taxonomy and nomenclature, diagnostic guidelines, administrative codes, and operational research designations and algorithms; (3) catalog several useful sources of overall EM definitions and relevant citations for them; (4) describe some definitional issues for each of the major types of EM; and (5) going forward, suggest opportunities to improve the crafting and use of definitions to enhance EM science and practice.

Two recent, important papers have addressed the general issues of complexity in EM definitions. Mysyuk et al. [1] reviewed the history of EM definitions for the past few decades, and suggested three types: (1) lexical—the existing meaning of an old word or term; (2) stipulative—a proposed meaning for a new word or term; and (3) explicatory—a combination of the other two. They describe the broadening of EM definitions and the tension between short, general definitions, useful for ease of understanding and application, and fuller definitions, which will apply to more specific EM subtypes [1]. Goergen and Beaulieu [2] suggest that difficulties in EM definitions result from lack of conceptual development in the area, and note the lack of clarity in the meaning of terms and concepts contained within EM definitions, such as vulnerability, trust, extent of actual harm, and the relation of abuse to neglect.

Thus, it is apparent why EM definitions vary and are difficult to construct and apply. They involve the depths of complex interpersonal human relationships, such as family and social dynamics, criminality, marriage, and community responsibility. They are promulgated by many scientific disciplines, such as legal, administrative, clinical, biological, social, and behavioral. Each discipline has its own interests, professional structures, social mandates, accumulated lore, intellectual traditions, observational methods, and dialectical processes. Each strives to understand and communicate its findings, and each suffers from environmental challenges such as limited resources, conceptual variability, and inadequate measurement methods, as well as, social challenges like great cultural variation among families, communities and populations, competing views of the role of government, protection from release of medical and other records and, in many instances, preserving individual autonomy in personal and political decision-making.

R.B. Wallace (✉)
Department of Epidemiology, The University of Iowa Center on Aging, S422 145 North Riverside Drive, Iowa City, IA 52241, USA
e-mail: robert-wallace@uiowa.edu

V.L. Crabb
Department of Epidemiology, University of Iowa College of Public Health, 145 N. Riverside Drive, S400 CPHB, Iowa City, IA 52242-2007, USA
e-mail: victoria-crabb@uiowa.edu

X. Dong (ed.), *Elder Abuse*, DOI 10.1007/978-3-319-47504-2_1

Despite this, there have been important EM definitions posited that most will find useful, particularly when newly approaching the EM arena. Many of these are offered in the beginning of research and clinical papers on EM, and some are derived from important reports or leadership bodies in the United States and elsewhere, such as from the World Health Organization [3]. EM definitions vary in length, coverage of behavioral phenomena, and other social dimensions. Table 1.1 shows some of the more salient, although not exhaustive, U.S. conferences, reports, and workshops providing further information relevant to definitions.

With this background and increasing experience in EM programs and research, one can further deduce reasons why EM definitions show variation. First, with important experience and observations from the justice, health, and public health systems, it is clear that in general there is substantial variation in the natural history of EM, both within and between individuals. Second, the nature and impact of EM usually evolve over time, with changes in severity and in health and social consequences. For example, with progressive exposure to mistreatment, new medical or psychiatric comorbidity may supervene. Definitions that attempt to define stable (static) states may lose utility as EM episodes unfold, including the effects of exposure to legal, social, and clinical interventions. Underlying risk factors, socioeconomic circumstances, and the clinical conditions of both victims and perpetrators may change. Third, definitions may lose their acuity because more than one type of mistreatment may be occurring concurrently within a particular social dyad or setting.

Fourth, in assessing definitions it is worth asking whose definition is being used, in terms of derivation of the wording. Different professional groups may use different approaches, and discipline-specific patient/victim definitions and jargon may be applied. Also, the concordance between a victim's situation and a particular definition may change or mature as more information about the subject and the behavioral circumstances is collected. This may occur, for example, during an Adult Protective Service (APS) evaluation or within a team-oriented multidisciplinary case review such as in an Elder Abuse Forensic Center [4]. Information on EM situations is known to be difficult to collect for many reasons, including absence of administrative records, victim fear of retribution due to the real or perceived lack of social and economic alternatives, or the progression of neurodegenerative illness.

Table 1.1 Selected U.S. national reports on elder abuse and mistreatment relevant to definitions

Elder mistreatment: abuse, neglect, and exploitation in an aging America (2003) [29] • Institute of Medicine and National Research Council • Comprehensive multidisciplinary work aimed at improving the understanding of the scope and nature of elder abuse – Discusses concepts, definitions and guidelines for measurement – Explores the theoretical model of elder mistreatment (EM) – Discusses the measurement of EM, including prevalence, risk factors and intervention evaluation – Examines U.S. laws addressing EM • http://www.nap.edu/catalog/10406/elder-mistreatment-abuse-neglect-and-exploitation-in-an-aging-america
Elder Abuse Workshop (2008) [172] • National Institute of Justice • Overview of current and recently completed research studies – Discusses research methodology and its challenges – Identifies short- and long-term research priorities, including critical priorities – Identifies potential partnerships with other federal agencies for purposes of increasing funding, planning, and communication of findings • https://www.ncjrs.gov/pdffiles1/nij/242211.pdf
Elder Abuse and its Prevention (2013) [100] • Institute of Medicine Forum on Global Violence Prevention and National Research Council • Explores the burden of elder abuse around the world with a focus on the impact of elder abuse on individuals, families, communities, and societies – Discusses the measurement of EM, including risk factors; potential adverse health outcomes; the role of culture; community; and other contextual factors along with evaluating intervention models – Discusses the screening and detection of EM – Proposes policy priorities for addressing EM – Identifies opportunities for prevention across sectors and settings • http://www.nationalacademies.org/hmd/Reports/2013/Elder-Abuse-and-Its-Prevention.aspx

(continued)

Table 1.1 (continued)

Understanding Elder Abuse: New Directions for Developing Theories of Elder Abuse Occurring in Domestic Settings (2013) [173]
- National Institute of Justice
- Explores the role of theory in EM
  - Critiques existing theories of EM
  - Reviews different theoretical frameworks of elder abuse
  - Facilitates the development of new theories to enhance our understanding of elder abuse
- http://papers.ssrn.com/sol3/papers.cfm?abstract_id=2277633

Elder Justice Roadmap Project (2014) [174]
- U.S. Department of Justice and Department of Health and Human Services
- Strategic planning resource by the field to advance the collective efforts to prevent and combat elder abuse
  - Identifies and ranks top priorities for addressing EM
  - Discusses six critically important topics, including diminished capacity/mental health, caregiving, diversity, prevention, screening and victim services
  - Identification of overarching themes
  - Compilation of a bibliography and a list of resources relevant to EM
- http://appleseednetwork.org/wp-content/uploads/2014/07/The-Elder-Justice-Report-07.07.14.pdf

Building Consensus on Research Priorities in Elder Mistreatment (2015) [175]
- U.S. Department of Justice
- Survey of 26 leading U.S. elder abuse researchers in the U.S. for the purpose of identifying and ranking research priorities in the field of EM
  - Provides a consensus of the top priorities for responding to EM as identified by leading researchers sorted by domains of direct services, education, policy and research
  - Identifies universal themes that arose during the project
- https://www.justice.gov/elderjustice/research/resources/Building_Consensus_On_Research_Priorities_In_Elder_Mistreatment.pdf

The 2015 White House Conference on Aging (2015) [176]
- White House Administration
- Describes public and private initiatives aimed at improving retirement security, promoting healthy aging, providing long-term services and supports, along with championing elder justice
- http://www.whitehouseconferenceonaging.gov/2015-WHCOA-Final-Report.pdf

Multiple Approaches to Understanding and Preventing Elder Abuse (2015) [177]
- National Institutes of Health
- Application of lessons learned across fields, common challenges and opportunities in elder abuse, child abuse, intimate partner violence and other related fields
  - Provides an overview of relevant reports and previously identified research priorities
  - Identifies challenges in the screening, standards, and detection of EM
  - Discusses dynamics of elder mistreatment across the lifespan with discussion of cultural implications and changes in cognitive and decisional capacity
  - Considers the bioethical and legal perspectives in EM research
  - Presents novel intervention and prevention strategies
- https://www.nia.nih.gov/about/events/2015/nih-workshop-multiple-approaches-understanding-and-preventing-elder-abuse

Elder Abuse: Systematic Review and Implications for Practice (2015) [31]
- Systematic review of studies examining the epidemiology of elder abuse including prevalence rates, major risk factors, and outcomes of EM
  - Suggestions for addressing EM
- http://www.ncbi.nlm.nih.gov/pubmed/26096395

Elder Abuse Surveillance: Uniform Definitions and Recommended Core Data Elements (2016) [178]
- Centers for Disease Control and Prevention and National Center for Injury Prevention and Control, Division of Violence Prevention
- Collaboration between CDC and EM experts for the purposes of
  - Provides uniform definitions and recommendations of core data elements for the surveillance and evaluation of interventions
- http://www.cdc.gov/violenceprevention/pdf/ea_book_revised_2016.pdf

Finally, it is also possible that at least the initial assessment and the preliminary designation of mistreatment type may depend on the circumstances that led to the potentially abused or neglected individual to a health or social system for evaluation and the types of professionals who participate in the initial evaluation. If the first notification or evidence of a problem is in a hospital emergency department, the initial evaluation and designations may be may be different than if the evaluation was first performed by a police officer or other first responder in the victim's residence, or if a patient is brought to a clinic by a relative or friend. In some circumstances, health, safety, and social professionals may have more immediate priorities than evaluating for mistreatment. If the presentation occurs in an acute or emergent setting, these may include bleeding cessation, repairing wounds or fractures, and the diagnosis and stabilization of progressive or life-threatening medical conditions may interfere with a rigorous and timely forensic examination of potential EM. In general, it is only when clinical stabilization occurs with a potential abuse/neglect victim, along with the provision and safe and helping environment that a thorough and rational EM evaluation can commence. This would be true regardless of the type of helping professionals or health care system, or conducted by Adult Protective Service agencies or within other community settings.

Often the content of definitions varies by the intended purpose, including: educating the reader on the nature of the term; providing a specific EM classification or taxonomy; predicting the course of a disease; and elucidating the terminology for purposes of clinical, administrative or legal codifications to aid in decision-making. Two additional EM characteristics add complexity to definition construction because they are so difficult to determine: ascertaining the presence and nature of "intent" in acts of mistreatment; and assessing causal mechanisms and pathways for various EM types. With regard to the latter, it is possible that psychological intimidation and stress earlier in life may lead self-neglect at later ages, which in turn may also result from financial abuse.

It is important to distinguish between definitions and alternative approaches to characterizing or categorizing EM, overall or for its major subtypes. Important examples of alternatives are classification and diagnostic criteria and the distinction between the two. In our view, each approach was developed for a useful purpose. Each takes a different form, and each may have greater or lesser effectiveness when applied to a substitute situation. These alternatives may end up informing basic definitions, but often only in hindsight. Classification criteria are basically standardized definitions, primarily intended for social, clinical or public health scientists to acquire uniform cohorts for research and evaluation [5]. Diagnostic criteria, on the other hand, are sets of clinical and behavioral phenomena in the form of guidelines and aids that help professionals identify diagnoses and direct treatments and other interventions. These latter "criteria" often take the form of elaborated, prose descriptions of clinical, social, and behavioral phenomena that may be enlightening and helpful but are not intended to offer unequivocal characterization for all of the diverse clinical situations that could arise. An important EM-relevant example is the Diagnostic and Statistical Manual for Mental Illnesses [6].

Another approach to EM definition and classification is the International Classification of Diseases (ICD), currently in its tenth revision. The ICD is "the standard diagnostic tool for epidemiology, health management and clinical purposes" [7]. The ICD has a companion formal nomenclature and other systems that can inform understanding of EM, such as "E-codes," designations of environmental injuries and poisonings clinical events (see the ICD-Clinical Modification guidelines for use), and a catalog of coded clinical interventions, the "Current Procedural Terminology," maintained by the American Medical Association. The ICD and ICD-derived codes appear to be underutilized as EM research and administrative tools, mainly because professionals are reticent to utilize these codes "because they have the potential to do more harm than good" due to issues such as breaches in confidentiality, discrimination by insurance companies, diagnostic uncertainties, and legal liability [8].

A final alternative approach to EM definition and classification is the body of laws and statutes promulgated mostly by state governments within the United States. As reviewed by Jirik and Sanders [9], among the states these statutes have broad areas of similarity and but in some respects, substantial differences. Most provide some EM-related definitions because they are central to applying and enforcing these laws and regulations, but in many instances definitional decisions are left to professional judgment or are implicit. In our view, review of statutes is of value in understanding definitional issues and the nature of professional behavior, including issues of personal and patient protections, the mechanisms of EM reporting, identifying various regulatory agencies and their investigational procedures, assessment of personal competence, and the extent of legal coverage, particularly with regard to long-term care institutions. Legal definitions are discussed in more detail below.

The next section addresses selected definitional issues for some of the major types of EM.

1.2 Elder Neglect

When considering the definition of elder neglect, many of the same issues that apply to EM in general also pertain to this type of mistreatment. Despite many attempts, research on defining elder neglect is limited [1]. There are sets of clinical and behavioral characteristics described for the "neglect" syndrome, but they vary by the type of study and the authors' orientation to the topic, and no particular cluster of risk factors is universally linked to each designated case. Similarly, understanding the causal origins of self-neglect can be extremely difficult. Pavlou and Lachs [10] identified more than ten definitions of this entity that have been employed in the self-neglect literature, and historically, elder neglect has raised several important and daunting philosophical issues [2, 4].

Elder "Neglect" is sometimes considered in two general forms: self-neglect and neglect by others. The National Centers on Elder Abuse [11] characterization of self-neglect as "...the behavior of an elderly person that threatens his/her health and safety." This places the causal responsibility on the individual and doesn't require the withholding of care by any "trusted other." A recent population study by Burnes et al. [12] defined neglect as, "the failure of a responsible caregiver to meet the elderly adult needs," these needs being defined by activities and instrumental activities of daily living [5]. Many neglect definitions include manifestations such as "refusal or failure to provide an elderly person with such life necessities as food, water, clothing, shelter, personal hygiene, medicine, comfort, personal safety, and other essentials included in an implied or agreed-upon responsibility to an elder" [11]. The focus on neglect, willful, or otherwise, by others, is common in definitions. In fact, the World Health Organization [3] defines elder abuse in part as a, "…single or repeated act or lack of appropriate action…" in a relationship where there is the expectation of trust.

Identifying those who are not fulfilling basic social needs for others may be difficult and has conceptual and philosophical connotations. Sometimes, there are household members or relatives where willful neglect is apparent, but if the caretaker is a spouse with cognitive impairment, a housekeeper who only cleans the apartment every 2 weeks, or a child who lives in the another part of the country, it may challenging to identify the source of willful neglect, if any. Can others in the trust relationship be unintentionally "complicit," including a primary care physician, or even a beleaguered APS staff member who has seen a client but is overwhelmed and unable to take full action? It is also possible that, other forms of active abuse are present but cryptic and fundamentally undetectable or that the neglected individual is incapable of reporting the problem, even if willing to do so. Understandably, recognition of the personal and environmental neglect manifestations by medical, social, health, or justice professionals is a challenging process due to lack of time and other investigative resources, and the critical tools to collect and evaluate historical events may not even exist, and thus useful definitions may often be unattainable.

In a qualitative study, Doron et al. [13] described three major themes of the personal and philosophical challenges to social workers who deal with elder neglect: (1) "How can you live like that?" self-neglect as an unsolved riddle; (2) "It's very difficult for me, I go outside and immediately start thinking about myself": the personal burden; and (3) "I keep trying": seeking intervention strategies following the refusal to accept assistance. As front line professionals struggle with these issues, more challenges to definition and classification will emerge.

Neither approach to defining neglect, with or without willful withholding of care and support, is necessarily correct or incorrect, but they point out the challenges and complexity of the neglect syndrome, and hence the definitional variation. Perhaps what is most important within the definitional content of neglect is whether it adversely alters the nature and intensity of client/patient evaluation and the optimal delivery of appropriate and optimal interventions. Speculatively, the conceptual unification of EM as encompassing both abuse and neglect may divert resources toward the identification of neglecting perpetrators and away from a more comprehensive psychological or psychiatric evaluation and subsequent management.

There may be value in borrowing from the experiences of other relevant social and health situations to improve the refinement of definitions and conceptualizations of elder neglect. Analogous historical precedents exist for child abuse and neglect, as suggested by Jackson [14], with regard to the nature of homelessness and severe physical disability. These issues can enlighten some of the conceptual dilemmas of elder neglect, having several societal problems in common: an overlay of mental illness in many individuals; mental illness among some members in the client/patient's social environment; inadequate fiscal, physical, or social resources; inadequate or ineffective treatment options; and various types of clinical and social vulnerability and dependency.

1.3 Physical Abuse

The conceptual definition of physical abuse by the National Center on Elder Abuse is "The intentional action of a person who stands in a position of trust to a vulnerable older adult (aged 65 or greater) that may result in bodily injury or physical pain of the older adult" [15]. First identified as "granny battering" by Baker in 1975 [16], the definition of physical abuse in older adults has evolved based on findings in the fields of child abuse and intimate partner violence [1, 14]. Although more closely aligned with intimate partner violence than child abuse, EM is further defined by the added vulnerability associated with aging and the identification of the abuser as a trusted caregiver [17]. According to Ziminski et al. [18], the "IPV (intimate partner violence) literature regarding injuries is fairly well advanced and pertinent to the study of elder abuse but rarely applied to elder abuse".

Based on a review of EM literature, three main types of physical abuse predominate: the intentional or reckless use of force to inflict pain or injury; the use of unnecessary force for the purpose of control or coercion; and the unlawful or excessive use of physical or chemical means to restrain or confine an elder [11, 15, 19–32]. Parallel to findings in the fields of IPV, the use of unnecessary physical force for the purpose of control or coercion as a means of physical abuse is widely recognized [17, 28, 32–38]. Although the appropriate use of restraints is intended to protect impaired elders, their misuse poses risks for injury and has been identified as a form of abuse [19, 25, 39, 40]. It is notable that the use of physical restraints in healthcare settings often fails to prevent falls [41]. Some authors have included force-feeding as an operational definition of abuse [11, 25, 27].

The aging process, as well as clinical disease and medical treatment, may impact the severity and presentation of injuries sustained in the older adult [42, 43]. Perhaps the most challenging aspect of differentiating physical abuse from accidental injury occurs when the elder is unable or unwilling to provide confirmation of abuse. It is important to note that evidence of injury is not considered necessary for proof of abuse. According to Langley and Brenner [44], "injuries, unlike most diseases must be defined simultaneously by the causative event and by the resulting pathology". Injuries to tissues may occur in the absence of mechanical insult, as seen with bruising brought on by non-traumatic processes such as sepsis or bleeding disorders [44]. Likewise, mechanical insults do not necessarily result in detectable injury. Diagnostic methods for detecting injuries vary in sensitivity and are unable to differentiate between accidental and intentional injury. Signs of physical abuse may not be obvious, even in fatal injuries [45]. Studies that rely on physical evidence of injury may not detect injuries due to modest forces. Improvements in medical diagnostics have increased the potential for detection of injury; however, studies indicate that clinicians often fail to consider physical abuse in their differential diagnosis [25, 39, 46, 47]. Biomarkers of physical abuse have been proposed; however, these tests are limited by their inability to differentiate accidental injury from intentional injury [18, 48]. In contrast, biomarkers reflecting inadequate hydration or malnutrition may be useful in determining the presence of neglect [49, 50]. As in child abuse and IPV, injury patterns suggestive of abuse have been identified [18, 51]. Although case reports of accidental injuries mimicking abuse are more frequently reported in child abuse, these types of injuries have also been reported in EM [52]. Since it is recognized that changes associated with aging predispose older adults to falls and other mishaps, injuries resulting from abuse may be incorrectly attributed to accidental causes [18, 49]. It is imperative that complete histories of the injury should be obtained, and screening of elders for abuse should be performed unless it is clear the injury was sustained accidentally [18]. Madden [39] noted that, "Awareness of the problem and a high index of suspicion are the most important elements in diagnosing elder abuse".

1.4 Financial Abuse

The conceptual definition of financial abuse or exploitation from the National Center on Elder Abuse [15] is: "improper taking, misuse, or concealment of a vulnerable older adult's (aged 65 or greater) resources, property or assets. The abuser is a person who stands in a position of trust with the older adult, acting for his or her own profit or benefit of a third party, by means of coercion, enticement, intimidation, deception or other forms of undue influence." Multiple terms have been used to describe the financial abuse of elders, including financial or material exploitation, fiduciary abuse, financial mistreatment or maltreatment, financial or economic victimization, and financial mismanagement. With the exception of economic victimization and fiduciary abuse, these terms are often used interchangeably. Prominent in intimate partner violence, economic victimization refers to coercive, controlling behaviors by the perpetrator for the purpose of limiting the victim's access to funds and resources, thus making the victim financially dependent on the perpetrator [53, 54]. Fiduciary abuse narrows the scope of trusted individuals to those who have a legal obligation to serve the financial interests of the elder through power of attorney, guardianship, and conservatorship [55–57].

Specific to financial abuse, vulnerability may be defined based on financial capacity of the older adult. Wood et al. [58] state that "memory, calculation and executive functioning" are fundamental to cognitive functioning relevant to financial capacity. Financial loss due to undue influence or misrepresentation has been demonstrated in older adults with no impairments in cognitive function [59, 60]. Problems with financial capacity may precede other decision-making difficulties [61, 62]. These impairments in decision-making may not be global but instead, limited to financial decisions [63]. Determination of impaired financial decision-making may require an assessment by a healthcare professional trained in assessing neurocognitive functioning in older adults [64].

The nature of the relationship between the older adult and the abuser is important in characterizing financial abuse. Conrad et al. [55] state the relationship should be evaluated as to the "extent to which the perpetrator is in a position of trust, the status inequality between perpetrator and victim, patterns of interactions over time and the extent to which there is a reciprocity versus highly skewed benefits and losses". The establishment of trust may occur within the context of a personal or professional relationship, new or existing [65]. A relationship of trust may be forged by an individual, perhaps a stranger or person not well known to the older person, with the intent to defraud [65, 66]. Often the elder has placed an unreasonable amount of trust in the alleged wrong-doer [65]. A trust relationship may have resulted "because the older person lacked alternatives" [65]. Identification of trusted others may add to the complexity of studies examining financial victimization targeted at older adults.

The type of influence utilized in the commission of financial abuse is important in distinguishing abuse from legitimate conduct [55, 63, 65]. Not all cases defined as financial abuse meet the criteria for criminal behavior, and these determinations may vary among states [67, 68]. Although an elder may consent to a transaction, if the consent was obtained by coercive or deceptive means, this would likely indicate abuse [69]. Unfortunately, establishing the presence of undue influence may be difficult [26, 55, 67]. Many times the victim is unaware that the abuse has taken place because the transactions are often conducted covertly [68, 70]. In distinguishing legitimate from non-legitimate transactions, adherence to standard, ethical practices is examined [65]. Cognitive evaluations may not have been performed prior to the transactions to determine if the elder possessed "sufficient mental capacity, self-determination and in the absence of undue influence" [65]. An older adult is assumed to be competent unless a qualified healthcare professional has determined otherwise [31]. Conrad et al. [55] report that illegitimate transactions may not be in accordance with the older adult's prior "beliefs, wishes or behaviors" [55]. As technology has expanded, there has been a concomitant increase in the variety of ways in which financial abuse and exploitation can occur [66].

One of the defining attributes of financial abuse is the incommensurate nature of the benefits realized by the perpetrator. The perpetrator acts in a manner to seek profit for themselves or a third party [15]. Although there may be some reciprocity between the perpetrator and elder, the proportion of benefits is skewed towards the abuser [55, 63].

1.5 Sexual Mistreatment

The conceptual definition of sexual abuse as defined by the National Center on Elder Abuse [15] is the "nonconsensual sexual contact or exposure with a vulnerable older adult (age 65 or greater) by a person who stands in a position of trust. It includes sexual contact with an older adult incapable of giving "informed consent". Although definitions of elder sexual mistreatment share the common element of nonconsensual sexual activity, ambiguity remains, particularly in the area of consent. Sexual abuse definitions should be broad enough to capture all instances of sexual abuse in the population but specific enough to facilitate unequivocal interpretation. Defining and characterizing elder sexual mistreatment can be challenging due to under reporting and "general theoretical difficulties, ethical dilemmas, and taxonomical inconsistencies that plague other forms of elder abuse" [71].

Elder sexual abuse is often characterized in part according to the setting in which the abuse occurs, the nature of the relationship between perpetrator and victim, the type of sexual abuse, the pattern of abuse, and the characteristics of the perpetrator. The location where the abuse takes place may be further characterized to include domestic, community or institutional settings, including assisted living. The setting often determines which entity is responsible for investigating the alleged mistreatment [72]. Although perpetrators in institutional settings are commonly identified as staff or other residents, perpetrators may also include family members of residents, visitors to the facility, or volunteers [73].

Teitelman [74] asserts that consent is "the key to differentiating between acceptable and abusive sexuality". An elder's refusal to participate in any sexual activity must be honored under any circumstance [71]. As with all adult sexual abuse, an older person may be unwilling to consent but specific to elder sexual abuse, the ability to consent may be impaired by cognitive or physical dysfunction [75]. However, defining incapacity and dysfunction can itself be difficult. Furthermore, the ability to consent may not be global with respect to the choice of partners and type of sexual activity proposed among elders experiencing cognitive changes [76]. Definitional as well as ethical and societal questions may arise when a partner caregiver who has "been in a loving and caring relationship for many decades make judgments about what is appropriate or inappropriate sexual behavior in relation to a partner who may lack capacity" [77]. Examination of changes in patterns of assent before dementia and after dementia may aid investigators in determining whether the sexual activity between partners constitutes mistreatment or not [71].

Perpetrators of sexual abuse may achieve compliance by means of: physical force, coercion, manipulation, threats, intimidation, or deception [31, 71, 74, 78–80]. Since sexual mistreatment definitions may not adequately address consent obtained by coercive means, it is important to note that compliance or submission gained by coercive means does not constitute consent [71]. Hanrahan et al. [75] suggest that the method of control used by the perpetrator should be a core element for surveillance of sexual abuse.

1.6 Psychological Mistreatment

The conceptual definition of psychological abuse as defined by the National Center on Elder Abuse [15] is "verbal or nonverbal act or acts of a person who stands in a position of trust to a vulnerable older adult (age 65 or greater) that result in mental pain, anguish, or distress in the older adult" [15]. Perhaps the most difficult type of abuse to define is that of psychological abuse. Unlike the other forms of abuse, this type of abuse seldom leaves physical scars or other tangible evidence. Although often more conspicuous than physical or sexual abuse, the likelihood of intervention to protect is victim from psychological mistreatment is lower [81, 82]. There are several terms that are used synonymous with psychological abuse, such as emotional abuse, mental abuse, mental anguish, psychological injury, and verbal abuse. However, commonalities between emotional and psychological abuse make differentiation between the two categories difficult [81]. In addition, the term verbal abuse can be problematic as it excludes nonverbal forms of psychological or emotional abuse. Although psychological abuse commonly occurs with other types of abuse or neglect, this classification is generally applied when psychological abuse is the exclusive or main type of abuse perpetrated [83].

Vulnerability to psychological and emotional mistreatment may be exacerbated by physical disability, cognitive changes, bereavement, and isolation and may affect the assessment of psychological abuse [15]. Most definitions of psychological and emotional abuse focus on the harm to victims, although other definitions concentrate on the perpetrator's behavior or the victim's response to the abuse [81]. The difficulty in differentiating poor interpersonal skills from intentional mistreatment of elders is parallel to differentiating poor parenting skills from intentional mistreatment in child abuse [84]. Definitions may not address the element of intent by the perpetrator to cause psychological duress in the victim [81]. Definitions may also differ based on the frequency of the abuse. Most characterizations of this type of abuse consider patterns of abuse while some definitions may contain isolated incidents [85]. Some studies limit their assessment to verbal abuse and may not capture all incidents of psychological or emotional abuse [86]. Often, emotional or psychological harm is sustained with other types of abuse, making estimates of prevalence of this type of abuse unreliable when singular or more easily measured types of abuse are identified [15, 86].

One of the largest obstacles faced in addressing elder psychological mistreatment is the challenge of measurement. Psychological abuse in elders is often assessed using screening instruments not specifically designed to measure psychological abuse nor developed for use in cognitively impaired adults [87, 88]. Screening tools may not adequately capture all forms of psychological abuse, and the reliability may differ depending on the setting of the alleged abuse [89].

1.7 Impact of Culture on Definitions

Among cultures, differences frequently exist in the identification, perception, and response to abuse; therefore, narrow definitions may not reflect the experience of the population under study [3, 77, 90–94]. In order to effectively address the problem of EM, definitions must reflect "cultural contexts" [3]. Numerous challenges exist in the definition of EM within cultural contexts [95]. According to Matsumoto [96], diversity among cultures exists "because of differences in the ecological contexts in which each group exists-the physical environment, resources available, social factors, history, and types and sizes of their families and communities." Cultural and social norms serve to guide the behaviors and attitudes for the members of a population. Yet, cultural and social mores may not always be reflected in an individual's attitudes or behavior [96–98]. The "existence of a given custom does not mean the custom is either adaptive, optimal, or consented to by the majority of its adherents" [99]. Broad assumptions about abuse within a cultural context should be avoided as they can hinder efforts to address EM [100]. Often these general characterizations do not account for variations that may occur due to other factors such as religion, family dynamics, and acculturation [101]. Although cultural dynamics have received more attention in addressing EM, gaps in knowledge persist [94, 102, 103].

According to Zechenter, "certain human rights are universal, fundamental, and inalienable, and thus they cannot and should not be overridden by cultural and religious traditions" [99]. Mistreatment of vulnerable elders has been identified by the World Health Organization as a violation of basic human rights [104]. Often regarded as a family problem, EM has broader implications for the health and well being of the older population and therefore should be regarded in a broader context as a societal problem [105]. Although cultural and societal norms may serve to protect others against abuse and exploitation, they can also play a role in perpetuating or promoting mistreatment [97]. Norms and practices perpetuate structural inequalities when used by specific groups to maintain an advantage or control over another group because of gender, race, ethnicity, social class, income, age, or religion.

Examining the role culture plays in the definition of EM is important because each culture uniquely identifies acceptable and unacceptable treatment of elders [106]. Although overall themes of elder care and respect, such as filial piety in Asian ethnic groups, may be a cultural value, studies have demonstrated that abuse still occurs [92, 107]. Abuse "encompasses an array of behaviors that falls along a continuum, ranging from serious offenses that almost everyone will agree constitute abuse to mild acts that very few will label as abusive [108]. Between these two ends of the continuum, lies a gray area in which agreement about abusive behavior is more difficult to establish" [108]. There is little doubt that certain practices are indeed harmful to the elder, such as the burning of "witches" in Kenya or widows (Sati) in India [109, 110]. Intuitively, the more severe forms of physical abuse will be uniformly characterized by different cultures. However, "low level" physically aggressive acts may not be regarded uniformly in different cultures [111]. Conrad et al. [88] suggest that "any definition of psychological abuse may reflect a cultural perspective". Differences in the identification of acts as abusive may be a result of differences in tolerance and thresholds of harm [94, 102, 112, 113]. What is perceived as abusive in one population may not be perceived as abusive in another.

In addition to what is likely true variation in the prevalence rates of EM in different populations, differences may also result from differing awareness of the scope of the problem. Although there has been growing recognition as an international problem, EM has not been uniformly addressed in all countries [93]. Numerous studies have demonstrated varying levels of awareness of EM among cultures [102, 107, 114]. Mitchel and Finkelhor [115] report that "greater awareness of abuse is correlated with lower tolerance for abusive behavior." The concept of "old age" is a social construct, based on societal expectations rather than on biological foundations [1]. Often categorized based on the standard age of retirement in developed countries, age may not be an accurate predictor of EM in resource poor developing countries with lower life expectancy [91, 116].

Cultural influences may affect how dementia is specifically viewed by a population [98]. Dementia may not be recognized as a neurologic illness but instead mistakenly considered by some groups to be a mental illness or as "possession by evil spirits" [3, 4]. Frequently, dementia has negative connotations that lack a true understanding of the disease process [114]. In some languages, there is no equivalent term for dementia, creating difficulties when performing cross-cultural research [114]. Furthermore, language used to identify dementia may vary from one social group to another [4]. Therefore, the use of the term dementia may pose problems in measurement.

Sociocultural values highly influence family roles and expectations. These values often define who is expected to provide care of the elder. Among Arabic-speaking immigrants in Australia, the son is expected to care for a widowed elderly parent unless the daughter is unmarried. The daughter, if married, is expected to care for both her parents and her husband's parents [114]. In contrast, the daughter-in-law is expected to care for aging parents in the Korean and Chinese cultures, even though the elder's spouse may be present in the household [117]. In many cultures, it is expected that families assume care for elders in their home, viewing formal long-term care as a form of abuse or as a last resort [114]. Legally, the expectation of care may be defined formally. In China, adult children have a legal responsibility to care for elder parents [118].

Moon and Williams [119] report that, elders "consider three major factors when deciding whether or not to define a given situation as abuse: the intentions of the person involved, circumstantial factors including the availability of alternative actions, and the nature of the act." Elders may tolerate abusive behavior because of perceived benefits or fear of reprisals [94]. In order to preserve family harmony, some cultures may tolerate intentional acts committed by family members more than other cultures [117].

Disconnection between the identification of abuse between professionals and researchers and the elder population has been identified [94]. Although these differences may result from a lack of awareness on the part of the elder, protective services and researchers may lack an understanding of legitimate cultural and familial practices. Some cultures place a higher value on interdependence among its members including sharing of resources [92]. Definitions of EM have relied heavily on research conducted in the United States and Great Britain reflecting "Westernized" values [116]. Perceptions of mistreatment of one culture by another culture reflect an ethnocentric view [120]. Often the screening tools utilized do not reflect cultural experiences in the populations under study [91]. Eguinados [94] suggests that "policy makers and practitioners looking to serve vulnerable populations may need to adopt a more inclusive framework that recognizes diverse and subtle forms of mistreatment."

Social acceptance or tolerance of abusive behaviors will affect its occurrence within a culture [121]. In traditional patriarchal societies, qualitative research suggests that rates of IPV "may be higher in settings where the behavior is normative" [121]. In an examination of spousal abuse in Ghana, Adjei [122] reports that males "have an implicit moral obligation to discipline their wives" and therefore, feel justified in using violence to control or discipline an "erring wife". Archer [111] notes that "As gender equality and individualism increased, the sex difference in partner violence moved in the direction of less female victimization and greater male victimization." In the area of sexual victimization, consent may be considered implicit within the context of a marital relationship therefore may not be viewed as rape [123, 124].

Certain acts of abuse are unique to some cultures or social groups. Threats of deportation in immigrant populations or threats of "outing" the victim in lesbian, gay, bisexual and transgender (LGBT) populations have been identified as special forms of abuse [109].

Homogeneity of the population within a given geographic region influences how strongly its members adhere to collective values of a culture [125]. Assimilation of immigrating individuals into new cultures may change how abuse is perceived; therefore, it may not be well characterized by traditional understanding of cultural dynamics [32, 92, 117, 126, 127]. In a comparative study of Chinese and Korean immigrants, Lee et al. [117] reported that recently immigrating Asian-Americans acculturate more slowly than other populations, adhering more closely to the traditional values of their native country. In addition to differences brought on by acculturation, Dong [128] asserts that generational differences exist due to "social changes brought about by modernization and industrialization", influencing "adherence to traditional cultural values and practices."

Differential identification of abuse may result from cultural and language barriers [26, 121, 128, 129]. For valid cross-cultural studies, difficulties arise in selecting terminology that allows for unambiguous translation. For example, there is no equivalent Mandarin term for "dependent" [3]. In a World Health Organization (WHO) study comparing prevalence rates of intimate partner violence (IPV) in different cultures, questions about sexual activity in unmarried Bangladeshi women are not considered appropriate, necessitating using a more culturally sensitive definition of "partner" [121]. Elders may demonstrate reluctance to use charged language in reporting abuse. Vietnamese may prefer "marital conflict" instead of "intimate partner violence" [109]. When examining immigrant populations, difficulties arise due to numerous dialects that may be spoken within a given ethnicity [114]. Studies examining EM may exclude populations that are unable to communicate in the languages determined by the investigator, resulting in selection bias.

Neglecting to adequately address sociocultural factors when defining abuse will impact EM detection and intervention. In making cross-cultural comparisons, it should be understood that various cultures may define mistreatment differently. These variations in definition may lead to inaccurate prevalence measures along with difficulties in developing effective interventions. Also important, commonly held stereotypes can negatively impact how EM is studied and addressed. Although culture often shapes an individual's attitudes and behaviors, it may not adequately explain an individual's actions.

1.8 Legal Dimensions of Elder Mistreatment

The diverse and complex nature of elder mistreatment (EM) requires a multidisciplinary approach from the healthcare, social services, ethics, and legal fields [14, 67, 130]. Initially conceived as a social services concern, the legal system plays a crucial role in addressing EM [131–134]. In addition to serving as a deterrent to abuse and establishing standards of care, laws frame how EM is defined and addressed by the legal system. To reduce ambiguity in the interpretation and application of laws, clear and unequivocal definitions are essential [135]. At the same time, overly specific definitions fail to adequately capture the scope of unacceptable behaviors [136]. When crafting laws, "lawmakers cannot effectively foresee all of the particular circumstances to which their laws could apply" [137]. Instead of characterizing all the behaviors associated with EM, laws reflect those behaviors lawmakers find most objectionable [136]. Laws are often a reflection of the social and political environments [138, 139]. The legal definitions used in legislation are derived from multiple sources and may not reflect the clinical understanding of EM [65]. There is a lack of consensus about the legal definitions that comprise laws addressing EM, and as a result, legal definitions tend to vary between and within countries.

Worldwide, there is significant variation in the laws governing EM, ranging from nonspecific guardianship laws to complex, elder abuse laws [139]. Most countries rely on "protection and criminal laws" to prevent or address EM [140]. Georgantz [141] reports the "legal protection of elder abuse is very much fragmented across EU (European Union) states." In a survey of 53 countries, Podnieks et al. found that not all countries had a definition of EM [140]. Although there are similarities in the definition of elder abuse globally, there is a lack of consensus on a "single definition" of elder mistreatment or abuse [140].

According to Policastro et al. [142] "elder abuse (laws) can be considered to fall within four broad categories: elder abuse, family violence, white-collar crime, or general crime". Although patterned off of child abuse and intimate partner violence (IPV) legislation, EM law shares more similarities with IPV [9, 14]. Domestic violence legislation often does not specifically address vulnerabilities associated with aging and as a result, domestic violence statutes may be inadequate for addressing mistreatment in older adults [143]. In the United States (US), EM may be handled by criminal, civil, family, or probate courts [144].

In legally addressing EM there are "four concepts critical to understanding abuse: autonomy, vulnerability, capacity, and undue influence" [145]. Determining the presence of abuse may require "assessing whether a person has capacity, gave consent, or was under the undue influence of trusted people in their lives" [146]. Laws and statutes often lack explicit characterization of capacity, consent and undue influence and instead rely on the assessment of a professional. The older adult is generally assumed to be competent unless determined otherwise by a qualified professional or the court [147–149]. The legal system is often faced with the challenge of balancing protection of the vulnerable adult against mistreatment with an older adult's right to autonomy and self-direction [9, 150]. As a result, "most (statutes) require that all inquiries and interventions be carried out in a manner least restrictive to the subject adult" [150]. Difficulties arise when a vulnerable adult at risk for mistreatment or neglect refuses protective services. An older adult's refusal of services may not serve as the sole reason to find the adult incompetent [63]. If the older individual is judged as incompetent and at risk of harm, the courts may appoint a guardian.

The terminology used to designate the target population in EM law includes adult in need of protective services, endangered adult, dependent adult, and vulnerable elder or older adult. Specific age thresholds for the classification of an older adult vary, generally between 60 and 65 years of age, although some countries may specify lower ages. Generally speaking, target populations identified for protection follow these three patterns: all adults who meet a specific age, regardless of vulnerability; all vulnerable adults regardless of age; or all vulnerable adults who have reached a specific age [150]. Each of these patterns pose challenges to addressing EM. Inclusion of all adults over a specified age threshold is problematic if the elder is physically and mentally competent. At the same time, identifying all vulnerable adults of any age does not capture those vulnerabilities associated with the aging process. In reality, "old age" is generally defined either by chronological age, traditional roles in society or deterioration in physical or mental functioning [151]. Although vulnerabilities generally increase with age, bias is introduced by the assumption that age is equivalent to vulnerability. Identification based solely on age does not address specific vulnerabilities that may be associated with the aging. Exclusion of independent older adults fails to recognize that this population may be targeted for mistreatment based on age [1].

Generally, legal definitions of vulnerability include the identification of an impairment that interferes or prevents an individual's ability to perform necessary activities for independent living. Cognitive impairments are more uniformly referenced than physical impairments, and impairments due to substance abuse or developmental disability may also be identified [152]. Vulnerability may be further specified to include the ability to protect oneself from exploitation or mistreatment or the inability to report mistreatment [139]. Likewise, an older adult may be classified as vulnerable if mistreatment has occurred previously. Some laws require "demonstrable physical, mental, or emotional dysfunction to the extent that the person is incapable of adequately providing for his or her own health or personal care" [152]. Some statutes include situational vulnerability due to incarceration [152]. Vulnerability may be assumed if the individual resides in an institutional setting although some statutes stipulate that older adults in outpatient chemical dependency treatment or "one who is committed as a sexual psychopathic personality or as a sexually dangerous person" does not automatically qualify as a vulnerable adult [152]. The lack of a responsible caretaker may be identified as vulnerability [152].

Vulnerability, in general, characterizes an older adult's susceptibility to EM whereas capacity centers on the adult's ability to avoid EM. In general, legal definitions of capacity vary from state to state and center on an individual's ability to understand the meaning of the proposed acts and recognition of any consequences of the acts [146, 153]. Definitions of capacity are usually broad and may not explicitly characterize circumstances in which the lack of capacity may apply. Further, determination of capacity is often not explicit in elder abuse laws [152]. Legally, "there are four conditions that impair capacity: cognitive capacity; severe mood disturbances (depression and anxiety); perceptual distortions (hallucinations); and thought processing defects (delusions)" [145]. Capacity is "not a fixed or static condition" [146]. As a result, it may be difficult to determine if the older adult had adequate capacity at the time of the alleged mistreatment. Capacity is often referenced in the provision of consent [152]. Incapacity may refer to mental or physical function [152]. A temporary lack of capacity may exist in instances where the older adult has experienced deterioration in health but is expected to regain capacity at some point during recovery [154]. Capacity is not an either/or situation. Individuals may exhibit adequate capacity to make judgments in some areas, such as providing sexual consent or consent for health care, but may be lack capacity to make complex financial decisions. This mirrors the clinical difficulties with establishing capacity, especially in mild to moderate impairment. The lack of capacity may only apply to certain areas such as financial or healthcare decision-making. In cases where the older individual lacks capacity, substitute decision-making in the form of directives, powers of attorney, trusts, and guardianships may be implemented. The application of substitute decision-making differs from one jurisdiction to another [57].

The determination of consent, an issue in individual refusal of protective services, sexual abuse, and financial exploitation, often varies from jurisdiction to jurisdiction [153]. The capacity to consent may not be explicitly defined in laws and statutes. Some laws may require that the perpetrator recognize that the victim was unable to provide consent [155]. Tactics such as misrepresentation or the use of undue influence may be identified in definitions, especially in financial exploitation and sexual abuse [152]. Quinn asserts, "undue influence takes place when one person uses his or her role and power to exploit the trust, dependency, or fear of another to gain psychologic control over the weaker person's decision-making, usually for financial gain" [59].

The relationship between the victim and the perpetrator is a core issue in EM. "One of the central questions is whether elder abuse is conceptually limited to a relationship of trust" [139]. Some legal definitions allow a broader range of perpetrators to include acquaintances and strangers. Some hold that mistreatment of an older person by a non-caregiver would qualify as a general crime while others identify those acts as EM. Legally determining who qualifies as a trusted caregiver may not be straightforward. According to Stiegel [156], "courts consider three different factors to determine who is a caregiver: caregiver relationship exists due to a contract; caregiver relationship is based on a statute; caregiver relationship exists due to the nature of the relationship or situation". Family relationships, friendships, or joint tenancy may be included as trust relationships [32, 139, 152].

Adult children may be held legally responsible for the care and protection of aging parents, depending on the jurisdiction [143]. These relationships generally involve "trust, dependency, or proximity" [139]. Some state definitions exclude law enforcement or correctional institutions, division of Medicaid, or long-term care facilities as caregivers [152].

A contract for care may exist between the older adult and an institution, a care provider agency or with another individual [156]. However, some legal definitions may limit EM to domestic settings only [141]. There may be legal obligation to continue to provide care for a vulnerable adult even if the caregiver has voluntarily assumed the role of caregiver [156]. Specific to sexual abuse, some definitions may not hold spouses accountable for abuse [30].

The demonstration of the intent to harm may be stated or implicit [30]. Unintentional harm may be considered when an actual or potential injury results from reckless behavior. Some may further stipulate that a reasonable individual should have recognized their actions might result in serious injury or harm. In addition, different investigating agencies require varying levels of evidence. Adult Protective Service agencies utilize a "preponderance of evidence" approach; whereas, the criminal justice system uses a "beyond a reasonable doubt" approach [73].

States often vary as to who is required to report suspected or witnessed acts of EM and follow these patterns: voluntary reporting, mandatory reporting by certain categories with voluntary reporting for other categories or mandatory reporting for all [150]. A main source of variation in legal definitions with regards to reporting is who may be required to report. In the U.S., banks are not considered mandatory reporters in all states [150]. Thresholds for mandatory reporting often vary from state to state with most states having "two different standards: a more stringent standard for individuals and agencies having contact with the elderly/disabled adult population in the professional capacity and a generic standard for everyone else" [150]. Penalties for failure to report in addition to protections offered to those who do report, can vary from state to state [157, 158].

Statutes may use umbrella terms such as abuse, maltreatment, or mistreatment that encompass different types of abuse instead of listing specific types of mistreatment [30]. The types of abuse identified by the National Center on Elder Abuse and the Centers for Disease Control include physical abuse, emotional or psychological abuse, exploitation, sexual abuse, neglect, and abandonment [15, 159]. The types of abuse identified in state Adult Protective Services laws may include abandonment, coercion, extortion, harassment, intimidation, isolation, physical injury, self-neglect, and unreasonable confinement [30]. The definitions of the subtypes range from broad references to more specific operational definitions. To illustrate, physical abuse may be referred to as physical injury or pain or may include operational definitions of behaviors (i.e., hitting, slapping) or physical outcomes (i.e., burns, subdural hematomas) [30]. There may be overlap between the identified types of mistreatment. For example, chemical or physical restraint may be captured under physical, emotional or psychological, or isolation types of abuse. Law enforcement and legal domains may use different terminology to identify physical abuse [30, 160]. In addition, the same manner of abuse may be identified as more than one type of abuse. For example, intimidation is considered both physically and emotionally abusive [160].

In financial exploitation, objectionable tactics such as use of "undue influence, harassment, deception, or fraud" to gain an advantage may be identified in some definitions [30]. Legal definitions may require evidence that the perpetrator demonstrate an intent to profit, use dishonest tactics, or demonstrate negligent, reckless conduct [155, 161]. In financial exploitation, the loss sustained by the older adult may be referred to as a loss of property, resources, or assets. Specific to exploitation, loss of the older adult's assets may not be required for determination of abuse, but rather the perpetrator received a substantial gain as a result of the transaction [30].

In an examination of legal statutes, all states within the US offer general protection against elder abuse; however, only a portion of states had statutes that specifically addressed elder sexual abuse [9]. Some states may not differentiate sexual abuse from physical abuse, making comparisons between states impossible [25, 35, 71, 74, 162, 163]. Teaster and Roberto [163] maintain that neglecting to differentiate sexual from physical mistreatment has "hindered systematic studies of sexual abuse". An added challenge to studying sexual abuse stems from inconsistencies in state laws. Not all forms of sexual abuse may be regarded as criminal [73, 79, 164]. State laws may require the act of penetration to qualify as a criminal act or require the victim to have demonstrated resistance to the abuse [74, 164]. Further, there is variation in statutes as to jurisdiction over investigation into sexual abuse within institutional settings [163].

As with other subtypes of EM, elder psychological or emotional abuse is not specifically defined in some state statutes but instead falls under the general category of abuse. Although all states have protections against physical, sexual, and financial abuse, not all states protect against psychological or emotional abuse [9]. Intimidation and isolation are defined separately from psychological abuse in some states [30]. Others include the use of restraints as a form of psychological abuse [30]. Evidence of intent to harm or reckless infliction of emotional harm by the perpetrator may be required by some states and may necessitate demonstration of severe mental harm or distress [30]. Most states do not attempt to quantify thresholds while a few states do require consistent patterns of abuse [30]. Legally, elder neglect is uniformly identified as a form of mistreatment although it is not uniformly identified as criminal [11]. In addressing elder neglect, laws focus on two issues: "whether there is a duty to care for an older person and whether such a duty has been breached" [11]. Some states may not provide a definition of caregiver requiring the court to determine if the alleged perpetrator may be held legally responsible [11]. Statute language may require that the perpetrator failed to provide the "degree of care that a reasonable person in a like position would exercise" [12]. Legal definitions of neglect may include the failure to address health problems, including neglecting to follow a prescribed treatment plan [12]. In New York, neglect is further dichotomized to active and passive neglect. In active neglect, the caregiver is "willful" in their failure to fulfill their responsibilities whereas, in passive neglect, the caregiver is "non-willful" [30].

The diversity demonstrated in legal definitions of EM reflects the challenges inherent in addressing EM. Although the legal system plays an important role, laws may not reflect the experience of mistreated dependent adults but instead, the acts that lawmakers find repugnant. The legal and law enforcement domains are primarily concerned with the violation of laws yet not all mistreatment may qualify as criminal. What is considered criminal by one state may not be considered criminal in another. When legal definitions vary between jurisdictions, it may be impossible to make comparisons [157].

1.9 Conclusions: The Future of Definitions for Elder Mistreatment

Definitions are important, but their value rests in succinctly informing the general meaning and appropriate use of the terms being defined. As more is understood about EM, its definitions will change with increasing knowledge and the general evolution of language styles. Definitions should not be substituted for or conflated with other, similar applications, such as diagnostic criteria or diagnostic manual descriptions, clinical guidelines, statutory stipulations, operational research criteria or administrative standards for management and reimbursement. Of course, all these applications will relate to each other, but in the end only more research on the behavioral and social measurement and mechanisms will improve knowledge and control of this critical societal problem.

The following are suggestions to help improve the development and use of enhanced EM definitions and related applications:

- Interested research and professional organizations should archive and make publicly available definitions generated by professional, legislative, and regulatory bodies and from administrative and research documents to allow more efficient perusal and research on the language and meanings of EM. Some of this has already been done by individual investigative groups, and the findings could be easily assembled. This might lead to a universally accepted EM dictionary to begin to tentatively standardize relevant terms.
- Quantitative studies should be pursued that detect clusters and groupings of the behavioral, social, and clinical phenomena of EM, in order to detect more homogeneous subgroups that may have more specific diagnostic, taxonomic, and intervention value. An example, cited above in the section on elder neglect, used latent class analysis to determine if subtypes of self-neglect could be identified [165]. The digital revolution has enabled the development of "phenomics," to expand understanding of the various patterns of phenotypes that accompany particular biological characteristics and processes [166].
- A greater exploration of the research applications of EM-related International Classification of Disease (ICD) codes in clinical practice is needed. This will not automatically improve definitional or nomenclature content, but it may help understand coding usage as well as how EM diagnosis and management fits into the fabric of general medical care, in all clinical settings. To the extent that diagnostic codes or computer-generated "suspicions" of possible EM can be captured for study, their application can be further evaluated in social and clinical practice using computerized decision support systems, to determine if outcomes can be improved [167].

In addition, several practices can support the provision of improved EM definitions in *data collection and research reporting*:

- Most obviously, report specification of definitions used in research should be explicit, with cited sources and administrative derivations. If new definitions are used, their structure and operational sources should be described.
- In developing new definitions or instruments, always consider that older populations are in general more likely to have lower educational attainment levels, different idiomatic usages than younger people in the same culture, and higher prevalence rates of cognitive impairment. All of these will challenge data quality. For new item development, use of the cognitive laboratory can improve instrument design [168].

- Search the literature for studies or commentary on the meanings and cultural understandings of definitions of EM when studying populations of mixed or varied nationalities or language groups. If items or instruments are translated from other languages, apply available procedures to best assure common definitions across language groups and nationalities [169].
- If legal definitions are used in research or related reports, be sure to use standard legal citations so the sources can be easily identified, recognizing there can be substantial variation across governmental jurisdictions within a state or country.
- When reporting observational or intervention studies of EM, attention to recommendations on formats and content of such reports is important, such as the "STROBE" and "CONSORT" protocols [170, 171]. These are useful approaches but may not always assign a high enough priority to case definition, and this should always be considered. The same attention is generally necessary for systematic reviews and meta-analyses, where definition consistency across studies would seem to be essential. This would be equally true for clinical studies attempting to identify biomarkers of EM, such as for screening or diagnosis.
- More research is being done on electronic medical records, which can provide increased detail on the clinical correlates and processes related to the diagnosis and management of EM. However, in general such records are less likely than structured research studies to offer standardized EM definitions. Thus, it will take explicit approaches to explain how definitions were derived in report analyses.

With regard to definitions, the goal is not per se to better define the presence and types of EM, but only to employ definitions to better understand the underlying processes, to mitigate the health and social harms and suffering that come with it.

Acknowledgments We wish to acknowledge the skillful assistance of Daniel Suh and Hayley J. Crabb in the creation of this chapter.

References

1. Mysyuk Y, Westendorp RG, Lindenberg J. Added value of elder abuse definitions: a review. Ageing Res Rev. 2013;12(1):50–7.
2. Goergen T, Beaulieu M. Critical concepts in elder abuse research. Int Psychogeriatr. 2013;25(8):1217–28.
3. A global response to elder abuse and neglect: building primary health care capacity to deal with the problem worldwide: main report. Geneva, Switzerland: WHO Press; 2008.
4. Navarro AE, Wysong J, DeLiema M, Schwartz EL, Nichol MB, Wilber KH. Inside the black box: the case review process of an elder abuse forensic center. Gerontologist. 2015;1–11.
5. Aggarwal R, Ringold S, Khanna D, Neogi T, Johnson SR, Miller A, et al. Distinctions between diagnostic and classification criteria? Arthritis Care Res (Hoboken). 2015;67(7):891–7.
6. American Psychiatric Association. Diagnostic and statistical manual of mental disorders (DSM-5®). American Psychiatric Pub; 2013 May 22.
7. World Health Organization. International classification of diseases (ICD).
8. Rovi S, Johnson M. More harm than good? Diagnostic codes for child and adult abuse. Violence Vict. 2003;18(5):491–502.
9. Jirik S, Sanders S. Analysis of elder abuse statutes across the United States, 2011–2012. J Gerontol Soc Work. 2014;57(5):478–97.
10. Pavlou MP, Lachs MS. Could self-neglect in older adults be a geriatric syndrome? J Am Geriatr Soc. 2006;54(5):831–42.
11. National center on elder abuse administration on aging department of health and human services. Types of abuse [internet] 2015. http://www.ncea.aoa.gov/FAQ/Type_Abuse/index.aspx. Accessed 21 Aug 2015.
12. Burnes D, Pillemer K, Caccamise PL, Mason A, Henderson CR Jr, Berman J, et al. Prevalence of and risk factors for elder abuse and neglect in the community: a population-based study. J Am Geriatr Soc. 2015;63(9):1906–12.
13. Doron I, Band-Winterstein T, Naim S. The meaning of elder self-neglect: social workers' perspective. Int J Aging Hum Dev. 2013;77(1):17–36.
14. Jackson SL. The shifting conceptualization of elder abuse in the United States: from social services, to criminal justice, and beyond. Int Psychogeriatr. 2015;1–8.
15. Center on elder abuse. Conceptual definitions and operational frameworks for five types of perpetrated elder mistreatment [internet] 2015. http://www.centeronelderabuse.org/files/elder_mistreatment_terms.pdf. Accessed 20 Aug 2015.
16. Baker AA. Granny battering. Nurs Mirror Midwives J. 1977;144(8):65–6.
17. Policastro C, Finn MA. Coercive control and physical violence in older adults: analysis using data from the National Elder Mistreatment Study. J Interpers Violence. 2015;1–20.
18. Ziminski CE, Wiglesworth A, Austin R, Phillips LR, Mosqueda L. Injury patterns and causal mechanisms of bruising in physical elder abuse. J Forensic Nurs. 2013;9(2):84–91 (quiz E1–E2).
19. Acierno R, Hernandez MA, Amstadter AB, Resnick HS, Steve K, Muzzy W, et al. Prevalence and correlates of emotional, physical, sexual, and financial abuse and potential neglect in the United States: the National Elder Mistreatment Study. Am J Public Health. 2010;100(2):292–7.
20. Young LM. Elder physical abuse. Clin Geriatr Med. 2014;30(4):761–8.
21. Bonnie RJ, Wallace RB, editors. Panel to review risk and prevalence of elder abuse. In: Elder mistreatment: abuse, neglect, and exploitation in an aging America. National Academies Press; 2003 Feb 6.
22. Taft LB, Barkin RL. Drug abuse? Use and misuse of psychotropic drugs in Alzheimer's care. J Gerontol Nurs. 1990;16(8):4–10.
23. Hughes CM, Lapane KL. Administrative initiatives for reducing inappropriate prescribing of psychotropic drugs in nursing homes: how successful have they been? Drugs Aging. 2005;22(4):339–51.
24. Capezuti E, Brush BL, Won RM, Wagner LM, Lawson WT. Least restrictive or least understood? Waist restraints, provider practices, and risk of harm. J Aging Soc Policy. 2008;20(3):305–22.

25. Aravanis SC, Adelman RD, Breckman R, Fulmer TT, Holder E, Lachs M, et al. Diagnostic and treatment guidelines on elder abuse and neglect. Arch Fam Med. 1993;2(4):371–88.
26. Nerenberg L. Communities respond to elder abuse. J Gerontol Soc Work. 2006;46(3–4):5–33.
27. Stiegel LA. Legal issues related to elder abuse: a desk guide for law enforcement [Internet]. American Bar Association Commission on Law and Aging 2015. http://www.americanbar.org/groups/law_aging/resources/elder_abuse/legal_issues_related_to_elder_abuse_guides.html. Accessed 16 Dec 2015.
28. Wolf RS, Daichman L, Bennett G. Abuse of the elderly. In: Krug BG, Dahlberg LL, Mercy JA, Zwi AB, Lozano R, editors. World report on violence and health. Geneva: World Health Organization; 2002. p. 148–71.
29. Taylor RM, editor. Elder abuse and its prevention: workshop summary. National Academies Press; 2014 Mar 18.
30. Stiegel LA, Klem EV. Types of abuse: provisions and citations in Adult Protective Services laws, by state: American Bar Association Commission on Law and Aging 2007. Available from: http://www.americanbar.org/content/dam/aba/migrated/aging/about/pdfs/Abuse_Types_Statutory_Provisions_by_State_Chart.authcheckdam.pdf.
31. Dong XQ. Elder abuse: systematic review and implications for practice. J Am Geriatr Soc. 2015;63(6):1214–38.
32. Kosberg JI. Rosalie Wolf Memorial Lecture: reconsidering assumptions regarding men as elder abuse perpetrators and as elder abuse victims. J Elder Abuse Negl. 2014;26(3):207–22.
33. Dutton MA, Goodman LA. Coercion in intimate partner violence: toward a new conceptualization. Sex Roles. 2005;52:743–56.
34. Schofield MJ, Mishra GD. Validity of self-report screening scale for elder abuse: Women's Health Australia Study. Gerontologist. 2003;43(1):110–20.
35. Crichton S, Bond JBJ, Harvey C, Ristock J. Elder abuse: feminist and ageist perspectives. J Elder Abuse Negl. 1999;10(3–4):115–30.
36. Tronetti P. Evaluating abuse in the patient with dementia. Clin Geriatr Med. 2014;30(4):825–38.
37. Hardesty JL, Crossman KA, Haselschwerdt ML, Raffaelli M, Ogolsky BG, Johnson MP. Toward a standard approach to operationalizing coercive control and classifying violence types. J Marriage Fam. 2015;77(4):833–43.
38. Schofield MJ, Powers JR, Loxton D. Mortality and disability outcomes of self-reported elder abuse: a 12-year prospective investigation. J Am Geriatr Soc. 2013;61(5):679–85.
39. Madden C. Elder abuse in the United States. J Clin Forensic Med. 1995;2(1):1–8.
40. Lindbloom EJ, Brandt J, Hough LD, Meadows SE. Elder mistreatment in the nursing home: a systematic review. J Am Med Dir Assoc. 2007;8(9):610–6.
41. Frank C, Hodgetts G, Puxty J. Safety and efficacy of physical restraints for the elderly. Review of the evidence. Can Fam Physician. 1996;42:2402–9.
42. Wiglesworth A, Austin R, Corona M, Schneider D, Liao S, Gibbs L, et al. Bruising as a marker of physical elder abuse. J Am Geriatr Soc. 2009;57(7):1191–6.
43. Paranitharan P, Pollanen MS. The interaction of injury and disease in the elderly: a case report of fatal elder abuse. J Forensic Leg Med. 2009;16(6):346–9.
44. Langley J, Brenner R. What is an injury? Inj Prev. 2004;10(2):69–71.
45. Hawley DA, McClane GE, Strack GB. A review of 300 attempted strangulation cases part III: injuries in fatal cases. J Emerg Med. 2001;21(3):317–22.
46. O'Brien JG. Screening for elder abuse and neglect. J Am Geriatr Soc. 2015 Aug;63(8):1689.
47. Rinker AG Jr. Recognition and perception of elder abuse by prehospital and hospital-based care providers. Arch Gerontol Geriatr. 2009;48(1):110–5.
48. Murphy K, Waa S, Jaffer H, Sauter A, Chan A. A literature review of findings in physical elder abuse. Can Assoc Radiol J. 2013;64(1):10–4.
49. Gibbs LM. Understanding the medical markers of elder abuse and neglect: physical examination findings. Clin Geriatr Med. 2014;30(4):687–712.
50. LoFaso VM, Rosen T. Medical and laboratory indicators of elder abuse and neglect. Clin Geriatr Med. 2014;30(4):713–28.
51. Ziminski CE, Phillips LR, Woods DL. Raising the index of suspicion for elder abuse: cognitive impairment, falls, and injury patterns in the emergency department. Geriatr Nurs. 2012;33(2):105–12.
52. Collins KA, Sellars K. Vertebral artery laceration mimicking elder abuse. Am J Forensic Med Pathol. 2005;26(2):150–4.
53. Adams AE, Sullivan CM, Bybee D, Greeson MR. Development of the scale of economic abuse. Violence Against Women. 2008;14(5):563–88.
54. Postmus JL, Plummer SB, McMahon S, Murshid NS, Kim MS. Understanding economic abuse in the lives of survivors. J Interpers Violence. 2012;27(3):411–30.
55. Conrad KJ, Iris M, Ridings JW, Fairman KP, Rosen A, Wilber KH. Conceptual model and map of financial exploitation of older adults. J Elder Abuse Negl. 2011;23(4):304–25.
56. Stiegel LA. Durable power of attorney abuse: it's a crime too [internet] 2008. http://www.americanbar.org/content/dam/aba/migrated/aging/about/pdfs/durable_poa_abuse_fact_sheet_consumers.authcheckdam.pdf. Accessed 20 Oct 2015.
57. Stiegel LA, Klemm EV. Power of attorney abuse: what states can do about it. Washington, DC: AARP Public Policy Institute; 2008. Available from: http://assets.aarp.org/rgcenter/consume/2008_17_poa.pdf.
58. Wood S, Rakela B, Liu PJ, Navarro AE, Bernatz S, Wilber KH, et al. Neuropsychological profiles of victims of financial elder exploitation at the Los Angeles County elder abuse forensic center. J Elder Abuse Negl. 2014;26(4):414–23.
59. Quinn MJ. Undue influence and elder abuse: recognition and intervention strategies. Geriatr Nurs. 2002;23(1):11–6.
60. James BD, Boyle PA, Bennett DA. Correlates of susceptibility to scams in older adults without dementia. J Elder Abuse Negl. 2014;26(2):107–22.
61. Griffith HR, Belue K, Sicola A, Krzywanski S, Zamrini E, Harrell L, et al. Impaired financial abilities in mild cognitive impairment: a direct assessment approach. Neurology. 2003;60(3):449–57.
62. Martin R, Griffith HR, Belue K, Harrell L, Zamrini E, Anderson B, et al. Declining financial capacity in patients with mild Alzheimer disease: a one-year longitudinal study. Am J Geriatr Psychiatry. 2008;16(3):209–19.
63. Wilber KH, Reynolds SL. Introducing a framework for defining financial abuse of the elderly. J Elder Abuse Negl. 1997;8(2):61–80.
64. Gassoumis ZD, Navarro AE, Wilber KH. Protecting victims of elder financial exploitation: the role of an Elder Abuse Forensic Center in referring victims for conservatorship. Aging Ment Health. 2015;19(9):790–8.
65. Kemp BJ, Mosqueda LA. Elder financial abuse: an evaluation framework and supporting evidence. J Am Geriatr Soc. 2005;53(7):1123–7.
66. Peterson JC, Burnes DP, Caccamise PL, Mason A, Henderson CR Jr, Wells MT, et al. Financial exploitation of older adults: a population-based prevalence study. J Gen Intern Med. 2014;29(12):1615–23.

67. Connolly MT. Where elder abuse and the justice system collide: police power, parens patriae, and 12 recommendations. J Elder Abuse Negl. 2010;22(1–2):37–93.
68. Payne BK, Strasser SM. Financial exploitation of older persons in adult care settings: comparisons to physical abuse and the justice system's response. J Elder Abuse Negl. 2012;24(3):231–50.
69. Conrad KJ, Iris M, Ridings JW, Langley K, Wilber KH. Self-report measure of financial exploitation of older adults. Gerontologist. 2010;50(6):758–73.
70. Choi N, Kulick DB, Mayer J. Financial exploitation of elders: Analysis of risk factors based on county Adult Protective Services data. J Elder Abuse Negl. 1999;10(3):39–63.
71. Lingler JH. Ethical issues in distinguishing sexual activity from sexual maltreatment among women with dementia. J Elder Abuse Negl. 2003;15(2):85–102.
72. Burgess AW, Ramsey-Klawsnik H, Gregorian SB. Comparing routes of reporting in elder sexual abuse cases. J Elder Abuse Negl. 2008;20(4):336–52.
73. Ramsey-Klawsnik H, Teaster PB, Mendiondo MS, Marcum JL, Abner EL. Sexual predators who target elders: findings from the first national study of sexual abuse in care facilities. J Elder Abuse Negl. 2008;20(4):353–76.
74. Teitelman J. Sexual abuse of older adults: appropriate responses for health and human services providers. J Health Hum Serv Adm. 2006;29(2):209–27.
75. Hanrahan NP, Burgess AW, Gerolamo AM. Core data elements tracking elder sexual abuse. Clin Geriatr Med. 2005;21 (2):413–27.
76. Rosen T, Lachs MS, Pillemer K. Sexual aggression between residents in nursing homes: literature synthesis of an underrecognized problem. J Am Geriatr Soc. 2010;58(10):1970–9.
77. Benbow SM, Beeston D. Sexuality, aging, and dementia. Int Psychogeriatr. 2012;24(7):1026–33.
78. Watts C, Zimmerman C. Violence against women: global scope and magnitude. Lancet. 2002;359(9313):1232–7.
79. Basile KC. Histories of violent victimization among women who reported unwanted sex in marriages and intimate relationships: findings from a qualitative study. Violence Against Women. 2008;14(1):29–52.
80. Gorbien MJ, Eisenstein AR. Elder abuse and neglect: an overview. Clin Geriatr Med. 2005;21(2):279–92.
81. Loue S. Redefining the emotional and psychological abuse and maltreatment of children: legal implications. J Leg Med. 2005;26 (3):311–37.
82. Behl LE, Conyngham HA, May PF. Trends in child maltreatment literature. Child Abuse Negl. 2003;27(2):215–29.
83. Creighton SJ. An epidemiological study of child abuse. Child Abuse Negl. 1979 Dec 31;3(2):601–5.
84. Trocme N, Fallon B, Maclaurin B, Chamberland C, Chabot M, Esposito T. Shifting definitions of emotional maltreatment: an analysis child welfare investigation laws and practices in Canada. Child Abuse Negl. 2011;35(10):831–40.
95. Cooper C, Selwood A, Blanchard M, Walker Z, Blizard R, Livingston G. The determinants of family carers' abusive behaviour to people with dementia: results of the CARD study. J Affect Disord. 2010;121(1–2):136–42.
86. Conrad KJ, Iris M, Ridings JW, Langley K, Anetzberger GJ. Self-report measure of psychological abuse of older adults. Gerontologist. 2011;51(3):354–66.
87. Wiglesworth A, Mosqueda L, Mulnard R, Liao S, Gibbs L, Fitzgerald W. Screening for abuse and neglect of people with dementia. J Am Geriatr Soc. 2010;58(3):493–500.
88. Conrad KJ, Iris M, Ridings JW, Rosen A, Fairman KP, Anetzberger GJ. Conceptual model and map of psychological abuse of older adults. J Elder Abuse Negl. 2011;23(2):147–68.
89. Castle N, Beach S. Elder abuse in assisted living. J Appl Gerontol. 2013;32(2):248–67.
90. Mihaljcic T, Lowndes G. Individual and community attitudes toward financial elder abuse. J Elder Abuse Negl. 2013;25 (2):183–203.
91. Sanchez YM. Distinguishing cultural expectations in assessment of financial exploitation. J Elder Abuse Negl. 1996;8(2):49–59.
92. Lee HY, Lee SE, Eaton CK. Exploring definitions of financial abuse in elderly Korean immigrants: the contribution of traditional cultural values. J Elder Abuse Negl. 2012;24(4):293–311.
93. Phelan A. International perspectives on elder abuse. Routledge; 2013 Mar 7.
94. Enguidanos S, DeLiema M, Aguilar I, Lambrinos J, Wilber K. Multicultural voices: attitudes of older adults in the United States about elder mistreatment. Ageing Soc. 2014;34(5):877–903.
95. Tomita SK. The consideration of cultural factors in the research of elder mistreatment with an in-depth look at the Japanese. J Cross Cult Gerontol. 1994;9(1):39–52.
96. Matsumoto D. Culture, context, and behavior. J Pers. 2007;75 (6):1285–319.
97. Violence prevention: the evidence. Geneva: World Health Organization; 2010.
98. Dilworth-Anderson P, Gibson BE. The cultural influence of values, norms, meanings, and perceptions in understanding dementia in ethnic minorities. Alzheimer Dis Assoc Disord. 2002;16(Suppl 2):S56–63.
99. Zechenter EM. In the name of culture: cultural relativism and the abuse of the individual. J Anthropol Res. 1997;53(3):319–47.
100. Leung J, Wong YC, editors. Community-based service for the frail elderly in China. Int soc work. 2002;45(2):205–216.
101. Kosberg JI, Lowenstein A, Garcia JL, Biggs S. Study of elder abuse within diverse cultures. J Elder Abuse Negl. 2003;15 (3):71–89.
102. Dong X. Culture diversity and elder abuse: implications for research, education and policy. J Am Soc Aging. 2012;36 (3):40–2.
103. Dong X. Advancing the field of elder abuse: future directions and policy implications. J Am Geriatr Soc. 2012;60(11):2151–6.
104. Krug EG, Mercy JA, Dahlberg LL, Zwi AB. The world report on violence and health. Lancet. 2002;360(9339):1083–8.
105. World Health Organization. Missing voices: views of older persons on elder abuse. In: Missing voices: views of older persons on elder abuse. 2002. p.23.
106. Jervis LL. Native elder mistreatment. Elder abuse and its prevention: workshop summary. Washington, DC: The National Academies Press; 2014.
107. Dong X, Simon MA, Gorbien M. Elder abuse and neglect in an urban Chinese population. J Elder Abuse Negl. 2007;19(3–4):79–96.
108. Ahn HN. Cultural diversity and the definition of child abuse. In: Barth RP, Berrick JD, Gilbert N, editors. Child welfare research review, vol. 1. New York: Columbia University Press; 1994.
109. Senturia K, Sullivan M, Ciske S, Shiu-Thornton S. Cultural issues affecting domestic violence service utilization in ethnic and hard to reach populations, final report. U.S. Department of Justice, 2000 98-WT-VX-0025.
110. Kenya 'witch' case mass arrests [televison broadcast]. Africa: BBC News; 2008. http://news.bbc.co.uk/2/hi/africa/7425386.stm. Accessed 29 May 2008.
111. Archer J. Cross-cultural differences in physical aggression between partners: a social-role analysis. Pers Soc Psychol Rev. 2006;10(2):133–53.
112. Anetzberger GJ, Korbin JE, Tomita SK. Defining elder mistreatment in four ethnic groups across two generations. J Cross Cult Gerontol. 1996;11(2):187–212.

113. Moon A, Tomita SK, Jung-Kamei S. Elder mistreatment among four Asian-American groups: an exploratory study on tolerance, victim blaming and attitudes toward third-party intervention. J Gerontol Soc Work. 2002;36(1–2):153–69.
114. Berisic M, Nesvadba N. Perceptions of dementia in ethnic communities. Project Report. Melbourne: Alzheimer's Australia Victoria. 2008. https://www.fightdementia.org.au/files/20101201-Nat-CALD-Perceptions-of-dementia-in-ethnic-communities-Oct08.pdf. Accessed 21 Feb 2016.
115. Mitchell KJ, Finkelhor D. Risk of crime victimization among youth exposed to domestic violence. J Interpers Violence. 2001;16:944–64.
116. Kosberg JI, Garcia JL. Elder abuse: international and cross-cultural perspectives. New York: Haworth Press; 1995.
117. Lee YS, Moon A, Gomez C. Elder mistreatment, culture, and help-seeking: a cross-cultural comparison of older Chinese and Korean immigrants. J Elder Abuse Negl. 2014;26(3):244–69.
118. Protection of the rights and interests of the elderly, 1996.
119. Moon A, Williams O. Perceptions of elder abuse and help-seeking patterns among African-American, Caucasian American, and Korean-American elderly women. Gerontologist. 1993;33(3):386–95.
120. Gellner E. Relativism and social sciences. New York: Cambridge University Press; 1985.
121. Garcia-Moreno C, Jansen HA, Ellsberg M, Heise L, Watts C. WHO multi-country study on women's health and domestic violence: initial results on prevalence, health outcomes and women's responses. Geneva: WHO Press; 2005.
122. Adjei SB. "Correcting an erring wife is normal": moral discourses of spousal violence in Ghana. J Interpers Violence. 2015 Dec 16. pii: 0886260515619751.
123. Ramsey-Klawsnik H. Elder sexual abuse within the family. J Elder Abuse Negl. 2004;15(1):43–58.
124. Jackson AL. State contexts and the criminalization of marital rape across the United States. Soc Sci Res. 2015;51:290–306.
125. Triandis HC. Collectivism and individualism as cultural syndromes. Cross-Cult Res. 1993;27(3–4):155–80.
126. Moon A. Perceptions of elder abuse among various cultural groups: similarities and differences. Generations. 2000;24 (2):75–80.
127. Dong X. Elder abuse in Chinese populations: a global review. J Elder Abuse Negl. 2015;27(3):196–232.
128. Dong X. Do the definitions of elder mistreatment subtypes matter? Findings from the PINE Study. J Gerontol A Biol Sci Med Sci. 2014;69(Suppl 2):S68–75.
129. Chang ES, Dong X. Understanding elder abuse in the Chinese community: the role of cultural, social, and community factors. Elder abuse and its prevention: Workshop summary. Washington, DC: The National Academies Press; 2014. p. 53–8.
130. Lowenstein A. Elder abuse and neglect—"old phenomenon": new directions for research, legislation, and service developments (2008 Rosalie S. Wolf Memorial Elder Abuse Prevention Award-International Category Lecture). J Elder Abuse Negl. 2009;21(3):278–87.
131. Heisler CJ. Elder abuse and the criminal justice system: new awareness, new responses. Generations. 2000;24(2):52–61.
132. Wolf RS, Hodge P, Roberts P. Elder abuse and neglect: prosecution and prevention. Crit Issues Aging. 1998;2:35–8.
133. Payne BK, Berg B. Perceptions about the criminalization of elder abuse. Crime Delinq. 2003;49(3):39–60.
134. Payne BK, Gainey RR. The criminal justice response to elder abuse in nursing homes: a routine activities perspective. West Criminol Rev. 2006;7(3):67–81.
135. Katz SN, Ambrosino L, McGrath M, Sawitsky K. Legal research on child abuse and neglect: past and future. Fam Law Q. 1977;11 (2):151–84.
136. Lynch MJ, Stretesky PB, Long MA. Defining crime: a critique of the concept and its implication. New York: Palgrave MacMillian; 2015.
137. Fon V, Parisi F. Codifications and the optimal specificity of legal rules. In: Law GMUSo, editor.George Mason University School of Law (VA). Available from: http://www.law.gmu.edu/assets/files/publications/working_papers/04-32.pdf.
138. Quinney R. The social reality of crime. Boston: Little; 1970.
139. Department of Justice, Government of Canada. Legal definitions of elder abuse and neglect. 2015 [Internet]. http://www.justice.gc.ca/eng/rp-pr/cj-jp/fv-vf/elder-aines/def/p1.html. Accessed 16 Jan 2016.
140. Podnieks E, Anetzberger GJ, Wilson SJ, Teaster PB, Wangmo T. WorldView environmental scan on elder abuse. J Elder Abuse Negl. 2010;22(1–2):164–79.
141. Georgantzi N. Elder abuse and neglect in the European Union. UN Open-ended Working Group on Ageing, 2012. Accessed 21-24 Aug 2012.
142. Policastro C, Gainey RR, Payne B. Conceptualizing crimes against older persons: elder abuse, domestic violence, white-collar offending or just regular "old" crime. J Crime Justice. 2015;38(1):27–41.
143. Moskowitz S. On Golden Pond: integrating legal issues of the elderly into family law. 30 Stetson Law Rev. 2001;1427:1453.
144. Elder abuse: basics: Centers for Elders and the Court [Internet]. 2016. http://www.eldersandcourts.org/Elder-Abuse/Basics/Elder-Abuse-Laws.aspx. Accessed 15 Jan 2016.
145. Olsen B, editor. Assessing vulnerability, capacity & undue influence in elder abuse. In: American judges association annual educational conference. Las Vegas, NV; 2009.
146. Center for Elders and the Courts. Elder abuse: key issues [Internet]. 2016. http://www.eldersandcourts.org/Elder-Abuse/Key-Issues/Capacity-consent-and-undue-influence.aspx. Accessed 15 Jan 2016.
147. Marson D. Loss of financial competency in dementia: conceptual and empirical approaches. Aging Neuropsychol Cognit. 2001;8 (3):164–81.
148. Moye J, Marson DC. Assessment of decision-making capacity in older adults: an emerging area of practice and research. J Gerontol B Psychol Sci Soc Sci. 2007;62(1):P3–11.
149. Moye J, Marson DC, Edelstein B. Assessment of capacity in an aging society. Am Psychol. 2013;68(3):158–71.
150. Roby JL, Sullivan R. Adult Protection Service laws: a comparison of state statutes from definition to case closure. J Elder Abuse Negl. 2000;12(3/4):17–51.
151. World Health Organization. Definition of an older or elderly person. 2013. Geneva, Switzerland. 2010.
152. Hamp LF. Appendix B analysis of elder abuse and neglect definitions under state law. In: Bonnie RJ, Wallace RB, editors. Elder mistreatment: abuse, neglect, and exploitation in an aging America. Washington, DC: National Academies Press; 2003.
153. Stiegel LA, Klem E. Capacity to consent/lacks capacity to consent definitions: provisions and citations in adult protective services laws, by state: American bar association commission on law and aging; 2007.
154. Mental Capacity Act. Code of Practice. United Kingdom: The Stationery Office; 2005. p. 2007.
155. Hafemeister TL. Financial abuse of the elderly in domestic setting National Research Council (US) panel to review risk and prevalence of Elder abuse and neglect. In: Bonnie RJWR, editor.

Elder mistreatment: abuse, neglect, and exploitation in an aging America. Washington, DC: National Academies Press; 2003.
156. Stiegel L, Klem E, Turner J. Neglect of Older Persons: An Introduction to Legal Issues Related to Caregiver Duty and Liability. 2007. Availabe from: http://www.americanbar.org/content/dam/aba/migrated/aging/about/pdfs/neglect_of_older_persons.authcheckdam.pdf.
157. Jogerst GJ, Daly JM, Brinig MF, Dawson JD, Schmuch GA, Ingram JG. Domestic elder abuse and the law. Am J Public Health. 2003;93(12):2131–6.
158. The Iowa Legislature. Chapter 235B dependent adult abuse services [internet]. https://www.legis.iowa.gov/docs/publications/IH/17112.pdf. Accessed 23 Nov 2015.
159. Centers for Disease Control. Understanding elder abuse. Atlanta, GA. 2016. Available from: https://www.cdc.gov/violenceprevention/pdf/em-factsheet-a.pdf.
160. Illinois Department on Aging. Protocol for law enforcement: responding to victims of elder abuse, neglect and exploitation. 2011. https://www.illinois.gov/aging/ProtectionAdvocacy/Documents/ea_lawenforcement.pdf. Accessed 15 Oct 2015.
161. Dessin C. Financial abuse of the elderly. Idaho Law Rev. 2000;36:203–26.
162. Hawks RA. Grandparent molesting: sexual abuse of elderly nursing home residents and its prevention. Marq Elder's Advisor. 2006;8:159.
163. Teaster PB, Roberto KA. Sexual abuse of older adults: APS cases and outcomes. Gerontologist. 2004;44(6):788–96.
164. Burgess AW. Elderly victims of sexual abuse and their offenders. U.S. Department of Justice, 2006 Contract No. 216550.
165. Burnett J, Dyer CB, Halphen JM, Achenbaum WA, Green CE, Booker JG, et al. Four subtypes of self-neglect in older adults: results of a latent class analysis. J Am Geriatr Soc. 2014;62(6):1127–32.
166. Sabb FW, Burggren AC, Higier RG, Fox J, He J, Parker DS, et al. Challenges in phenotype definition in the whole-genome era: multivariate models of memory and intelligence. Neuroscience. 2009;164(1):88–107.
167. Miller A, Moon B, Anders S, Walden R, Brown S, Montella D. Integrating computerized clinical decision support systems into clinical work: a meta-synthesis of qualitative research. Int J Med Inform. 2015;84(12):1009–18.
168. Jobe JB, Mingay DJ. Cognitive laboratory approach to designing questionnaires for surveys of the elderly. Public Health Rep. 1990;105(5):518–24.
169. Maneesriwongul W, Dixon JK. Instrument translation process: a methods review. J Adv Nurs. 2004;48(2):175–86.
170. Little J, Higgins JP, Ioannidis JP, Moher D, Gagnon F, von Elm E, et al. STrengthening the REporting of Genetic Association studies (STREGA)—an extension of the STROBE statement. Eur J Clin Investig. 2009;39(4):247–66.
171. Begg C, Cho M, Eastwood S, Horton R, Moher D, Olkin I, et al. Improving the quality of reporting of randomized controlled trials. The CONSORT statement. JAMA. 1996;276(8):637–9.
172. Elder Abuse Workshop. Washington, DC: National Institute of Justice; 2008. Available from: https://www.ncjrs.gov/pdffiles1/nij/242211.pdf.
173. Jackson SL, Hafemeister TL. Understanding elder abuse: new directions for developing theories of elder abuse occurring in domestic settings. Research in Brief, National Institute of Justice; 2013 Jun 11.
174. Connolly M, Brandl B, Breckman R. The elder Justice roadmap: a stakeholder initiative to respond to an emerging health, Justice, financial and social crisis. Department of Justice; 2014.
175. Stahl SM. Building consensus on research priorities in elder mistreatment. United States Department of Justice; 2015. Available from: https://www.justice.gov/file/852846/download.
176. 2015 White House Conference on Aging: final report; 2015. Washington, DC. Available from: https://whitehouseconferenceonaging.gov/2015-WHCOA-Final-Report.pdf.
177. Saylor KW. Multiple approaches to understanding and preventing elder abuse: introduction to the cross-disciplinary National Institutes of Health workshop. J Elder Abuse Negl. 2016 Sep 18.
178. Hall JE, Karch DL, Crosby AE. Elder abuse surveillance: uniform definitions and recommended core data elements for use in elder abuse surveillance, version 1.0. Atlanta, GA: National Center for Injury Prevention Centers for Disease Control and Prevention; 2016.

Theorizing Elder Abuse

2

Karen A. Roberto and Pamela B. Teaster

2.1 Theorizing Elder Abuse

Although tremendous growth has occurred in the breadth and depth of topics investigated within the elder abuse literature, identification of the theoretical underpinnings of elder abuse research, practice, and policy has lagged behind the empirical output. Many academicians as well as practitioners fail to acknowledge explicitly the influence of theory on their research, teaching, programmatic, and policy efforts. Reasons for the lack of theory guidance and interpretation include limited national attention and concern about elder abuse, little federal funding to support theory development, and over reliance on caregiver stress models [72]. To address the dearth of theory use within the field of elder abuse, experts were invited to a meeting coordinated by the National Institutes of Justice [106] to discuss the appropriateness of requiring research proposals and peer-reviewed manuscripts focused on elder abuse to have an underlying conceptual framework or theory. Opinion was mixed, with the support or lack thereof tending to fall along participants' disciplinary lines. As would be expected, investigators from academic disciplines that rely heavily on explicit theoretical foundations were highly supportive of the inclusion of theory, whereas investigators from research disciplines that more implicitly address theory regarded the requirement as an impediment to their work.

We contend that it is critical to the advancement of the field of elder abuse that theory development moves forward. In this chapter, we draw upon multiple literatures to inform theory within the context of elder abuse. We begin by discussing the importance of theory and theorizing in general, and for enhancing a nascent field of study like elder abuse in particular. Our argument for the importance of theory is followed by a historical overview of theories most often applied to the study of elder abuse and a depiction of theory use in scholarly articles. The next section provides an examination of key theories from the child abuse and intimate partner violence literature, as well as broader theoretical perspectives that have the potential to inform work on elder abuse. We then propose and explain a new approach for theorizing about elder abuse, *The Contextual Theory of Elder Abuse*. The final section presents opportunities for continued theory development and theorizing in future research and practice. Although scholars differentiate among theories, perspectives, conceptual models, and schools of thought, investigators frequently use the terms interchangeably. As we examine different theoretical lenses relevant to the study of elder abuse, we will use 'theory' to acknowledge all types and levels.

2.2 The Importance of Theory

Theories are at the heart of research and practice. They represent a systematic way of understanding behaviors, situations, and events. Observations of a phenomenon, often provided by individuals in professional and leadership roles (e.g., clinicians, service providers, educators, policymakers), lead to hunches or a personal theory about its causes and consequences. In order to fully intervene, professionals have to understand the issue under study, in all its complexity. Researchers rely on more formalized theoretical approaches and scientific methods to explore their guesses or test hypotheses. Theories provide powerful influences on how information is collected and analyzed, guiding description, explanation, prediction, or interpretation of the phenomenon under study. Findings that are consistent across studies provide practitioners and policymakers evidence to describe and understand complex phenomenon and act upon and change its course.

K.A. Roberto (✉) · P.B. Teaster
Center for Gerontology, Virginia Polytechnic Institute and State University, Blacksburg, VA 24061, USA
e-mail: kroberto@vt.edu

P.B. Teaster
e-mail: pteaster@vt.edu

X. Dong (ed.), *Elder Abuse*, DOI 10.1007/978-3-319-47504-2_2

Theories shape a field; influence the education, training, and socialization of its professionals; and define the scope of practice and policy. Sound research relies upon explicit theory use. Theory helps identify patterns and tendencies, and trajectories that in turn influence appropriate responses and strategies. Thus, recognizing the importance and contribution of theory and engaging in the process of theorizing is essential for promoting knowledge and advancing any field of study. To advance science, scholars must ask new questions and generate new hypothesis to test existing and emerging theories necessary for exploring and solving complex social concerns, both locally and globally. A lack of theory in research and practice leads to limited or spurious application of research findings that hinder building cumulative knowledge about an issue [16].

Theory also enhances students' and professionals' learning. Theory-driven knowledge is an essential platform of the curriculum for education and training programs and provides a platform upon which the expertise and skills of future leaders is built. In this realm, a healthy tension between theory and practice often develops. Many academics thrive on theoretical discussions with respect to both subject matter content and methodological advancements. Conversely, students may dismiss the importance of theory when presented in the classroom but often embrace their theoretical roots as they assume their professional roles and are faced with situations in the field that require substantive responses or opportunities to influence practice. Seasoned practitioners often minimize the importance of theory in service provision, or simply neglect to recognize the theoretical frameworks underpinning practice. For example, Bergeron [21] described how a family preservation framework, although not explicitly applied by elder protection service workers, provided an implicit guide for their decision-making processes. Bridging the dualisms between academic and professional knowledge, clinicians and practitioners can marshal the most appropriate theory and practice strategies for a given situation as they develop, implement, and test the effectiveness of treatments, services, and interventions.

Theory is critical not only for advancing science and practice, but also for the development of policy. Policy solutions and related decision making are not merely a technical function of legislators and government officials, but rather they are a complex interactive and iterative interplay of actions and actors influenced by the diverse nature of socio-political and other environmental forces. To create policy, leaders at the federal, state, and local levels must determine which issues merit attention, focus on those issues, and develop strategies to address them. As policy development processes unfold, informed decision makers make use of theoretically grounded, consistent, and coherent research to guide the policy prescription deemed most likely to solve the problem. Without sufficient evidence acquired from sound, theoretically-informed research and practice, policy planning and analysis is diffuse, limited, and often thwarted entirely because there is no clear avenue for problem resolution. Thus, the link between theory, practice, and policy is essential for diagnosing situations, explaining their causes, prescribing responses, and evaluating the impact of different solutions [163].

2.3 Theory and Theorizing

Responding to the importance of the call for more and better use of theory as an avenue for advancing the field of elder abuse requires researchers to address issues related to the definition of theory, stage of theory development, differences in theoretical presuppositions, and application of theory within study designs and professional writing. While definitions of theory vary by orientation (e.g., positivistic, interpretive, critical), nuances of varying disciplines (e.g., gerontology, family studies, psychology, law, medicine, social work, public health), and perspectives (e.g., micro, macro), a key element of any theory is a description or explanation of observed phenomena [19]. At its most basic level, a theory attempts to provide an explanation for and contribute meaning to the causes and consequences of beliefs and behaviors. To advance thinking about and understanding of an issue or event, such as elder abuse, theory needs to be viewed as a process and not as a static creation.

The process of theorizing draws attention to the explicit actions scholars and practitioners take in "developing ideas that allow us to understand and explain our data" ([17], p. 5). In other words, theorizing goes beyond what is observed to questioning the why and how a situation emerged. It is an ongoing, iterative, and engaging process. Theorizing begins with an awareness of ideas, followed by the development of hunches or beliefs about how the ideas are linked, empirical research, evidence-based associations, the creation of concepts, and an understanding of the complexity of the associations made. Finally, from this process, a theory emerges as a tool to help understand, explain, and give meaning to the data collected (see Fig. 2.1; [39]).

Ontological and epistemological considerations also influence theorizing. Ontology focuses on the nature and relationship of the object or occurrence of a phenomenon [144] and is critical for developing a more a sophisticated understanding of elder abuse. Implicitly, researchers and practitioners have focused on the ontological context of elder abuse for decades, particularly in establishing uniform and measureable definitions. Such a focus is essential for grasping the problem at the level of the individual as well as collecting reliable and valid data about other aspects of the problem. Ontological questions are definitional in nature;

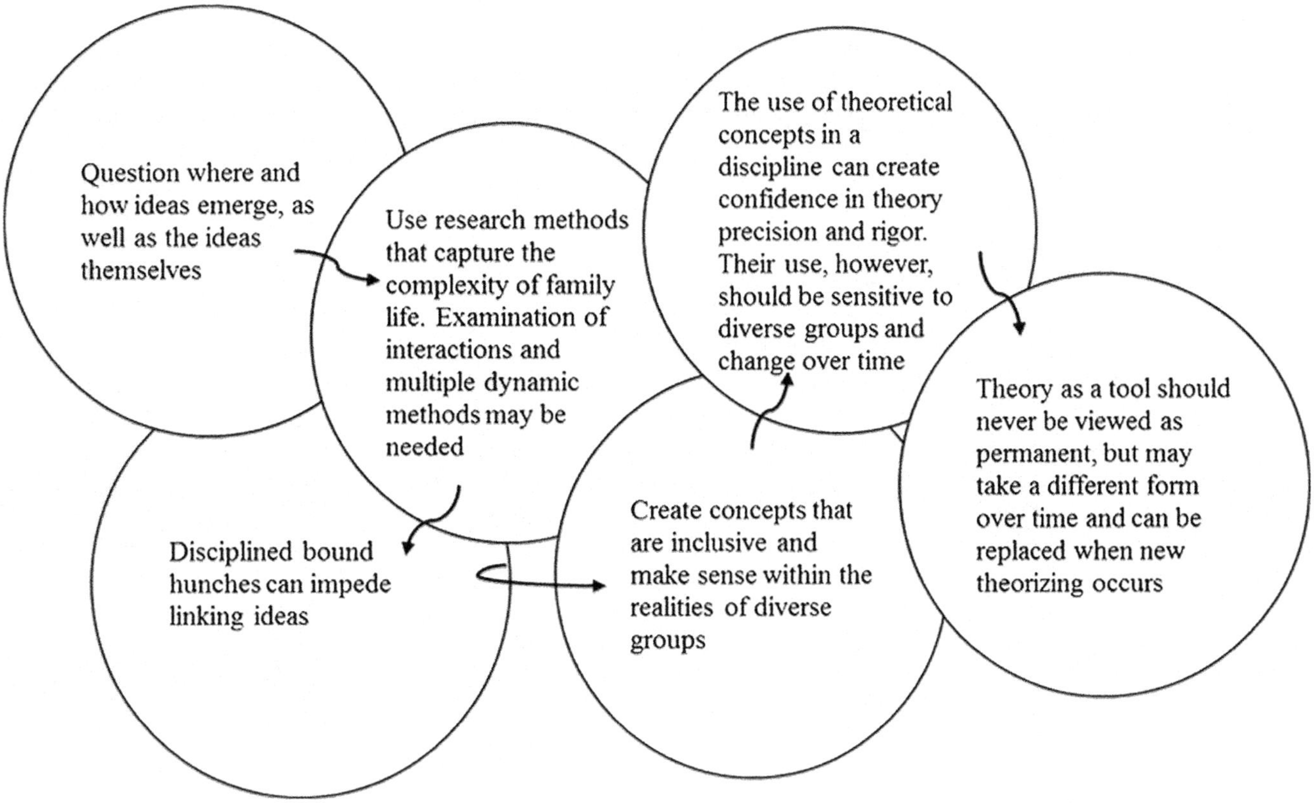

Fig. 2.1 The process of theorizing. Adapted from "My view: The process of theorizing," by [39]. Copyright 2008 by Sage Publications

they seek to explain the reality for the situation. Examples of questions frequently addressed in the literature include: What is elder abuse? What are subtypes of elder abuse? What is the relationship between various types of elder abuse? What does it mean to be a victim or perpetrator of elder abuse?

Epistemological considerations focus on the nature, origins, methods, and limits of knowledge [167]. While multiple epistemologies or ways of knowing exist (e.g., scientific view, interpretive perspective, critical perspective), no one approach is necessarily more useful or better than another. Rather, they provide different lenses from which to view and understand a phenomena. With respect to elder abuse, epistemological considerations address how investigators go about acquiring knowledge on the issue. For example, how is the occurrence of elder abuse confirmed? Is the perception that a victim was abused sufficient to indicate that elder abuse has occurred? Conversely, must the abuse be verified in order for it to have occurred? If yes, what entity or entities perform the verification (e.g., physician confirmation, court confirmation, agency confirmation)? By extension, at what level is the verification rigorous enough for the advancement of knowledge?

For elder abuse, as with any field of study, creating a knowledge base is a continuous process of discovery and confirmation that involves different methods of theorizing: deductive theorizing, inductive theorizing, combining, and borrowing [17]. *Deductive theorizing* involves drawing from an existing theory of larger scope and more generality to deduce a theory of smaller scope and less generality. A general theory, such as the life course perspective [48], allows investigators to infer logically a number of specific explanations about the nature of a phenomena, for example, elder self-neglect [8]. *Inductive theorizing* often starts with the data and induces logically a theory of larger scope and generality, such as a model developed from an analysis of barriers to help seeking for older women who experience intimate partner violence [15]. This approach also puts forth theory from confirmed empirical generalizations. A third approach of theorizing involves *combining*, either in totality or pulling together specific tenets or constructs from two or more theories relevant to the issue under study, as was used in theorizing about low levels of reporting of abuse by older immigrant women [135]. *Borrowing* promising theories and concepts from similar topics or other disciplines, such as the application of the stress process model to predict elder abuse by family caregivers [173], is common in emerging and multidisciplinary fields similar to elder abuse. To contribute stronger, theorized knowledge and demonstrate the usefulness of theory for understanding of elder abuse requires not only applying and testing existing theories but also constructing new ones. Although the latter approach is perhaps the most challenging, it also is likely to be the most fruitful, as it requires elder abuse scholars to be producers rather than just consumers of theory.

2.4 Theories Used to Advance Understanding of Elder Abuse

As elder abuse emerged as an area of scholarship, researchers often "borrowed" theories from other disciplines to guide their research [22, 72, 109]. This approach was entirely natural in the life course of a nascent area of inquiry concerning a complex societal problem. As scholars adopted and adapted these theories to inform their exploration of the many facets of elder abuse, their research contributed significantly to the quantity and quality of scholarship and informed the development of professional practices and policy addressing issues of elder abuse.

In this section, we present an overview of the conceptualization of early and predominant theories that have been used to explain elder abuse, highlighting their use with specific populations in particular settings, and with different types of abuse. When available, we include examples of the *explicit* application of each theory to empirical studies of elder abuse. Examples cited are by no means exhaustive of all theory-informed elder abuse research. We recognize that much of the published research is based upon *implicit* theoretical assumptions and explanations about various aspects of elder abuse; however, we chose not to include articles in which the authors provided neither a theoretical justification for the purpose and design of their studies nor included a theoretical explanation when discussing and interpreting their results.

2.5 Caregiver Stress and Elder Abuse

With roots in the gerontological literature, caregiver stress theory focuses on the response to stressors faced by family members and other individuals when providing care for an older person with functional and/or cognitive impairments [114]. Caregiving includes assuming new roles and responsibilities and involves recurrent redirection and reorganization of family life that leads to escalating dependencies that contribute to daily stressors and strains that challenge relatives providing care [5]. The nature of the care demands and the frequency, type, and the magnitude of the stress and strain experienced by caregivers associated both with their caregiving responsibilities and other aspects of their lives (e.g., work, relationships), as well as their use of coping strategies and reliance on others for support affect caregivers' abilities to provide effective care as well as their own physical and psychological well-being. Applied to the study of elder abuse, the *caregiver stress hypothesis* posited that the high levels of stress experienced by the caregiver resulted in abuse of dependent older adults. Thus, negative caregiver outcomes may have both direct and indirect effects on the caregiving process, the relationship between the caregiver and care receiver, and ultimately the welfare and well-being of the older person receiving care [107].

Early research in the late 1970s and early 1980s provided descriptive evidence in support of the relationship between caregiver stress and elder abuse (see review by [69]). As researchers attempted to disentangle the relationship of caregiver stress and elder abuse, evidence began to mount in support of the reverse of the caregiver stress hypothesis—rather than the stress of caring for a dependent older adult increasing the risk for elder abuse, it was the dependency of the abuser on the older adult that placed the elder at risk for abuse [120, 170]. The landmark study conducted by Pillemer and Finklehor [119], in which they compared non-abused elders to older adults who had experienced physical abuse, neglect, and chronic verbal aggression by a spouse or adult child, shed additional light on the relationship between caregiving and elder abuse. The authors found perpetrator characteristics (e.g., personality, deviant behaviors, dependence on the elder) to be more powerful predictors of abuse than victim characteristics (e.g., ill health; functional disabilities). Since then, the work of other investigators has confirmed that factors related to the need to depend on older family members for shelter, security, and support contribute to all types of elder abuse [3, 71, 72, 75].

Although scholars no longer consider caregiver stress the primary cause of elder abuse, researchers have continued to explore caregiving situations in which the behaviors of well-meaning caregivers may place older adults at risk for abuse. Analysis of data gathered for the *Family Relationships in Later Life Project*, which included caregivers of elderly relatives with whom they co-resided, identified a number of potentially harmful behaviors including handling the elder roughly, threatening the elder with abandonment or nursing home placement, and insulting, screaming at, or yelling at the elder [14, 142, 168, 169], that if not addressed, could lead to heightened incidences of abuse. Feelings of caregiver resentment [169], reliance on proactively aggressive caregiving strategies [142], and anger [95] were associated with caregiver self-reports of potentially harmful behaviors. Studies of family members of persons with dementia conducted outside the United States also found that caregivers often reported the use of potentially harmful caregiving tactics. Across studies, verbal aggression (e.g., shouting, insulting) was more commonly acknowledged by caregivers than the use of physically harmful actions (e.g., hitting). Predictors of the use of potentially abusive behaviors included care recipients' agitated behaviors and caregiver depersonalization [173], caregiver burden [35, 174], and care recipients' communication difficulties [33]. The relationship among stress, dependency, and elder abuse also has been examined in non-family care situations. For example, caregiver burden in conjunction with stress and conflict in the workplace were among factors contributing to abuse of residents by nursing home staff in Germany [57].

The problem of elder abuse within the context of family caregiving is not a consequence of a single event and cannot be explained by a single cause. Recognition of the complexity of caregiving situations has helped to refute the hypothesis that caregiver stress inevitably results in elder abuse. However, the effectiveness of stress-process theories for understanding elder abuse has been limited by researchers' focus on isolated components of the theory rather than testing such theories in their entirety. In addition, the focus of caregiver stress and abuse studies tend to focus primarily on outcomes for older adults with cognitive impairments and cover the range of abuse types indiscriminately. How well the theory will hold up for other populations of elders (e.g., older adults from different race or ethnic groups, physically frail elders) or in predicting caregiver risk for specific types of abusive has yet to be examined.

2.6 Ecological Theories of Abuse

Ecological theories of elder abuse have relied upon Bronfenbrenner's [26] *Ecological Model*, which suggests that individuals are embedded in a series of environmental systems that interact with one another and with the individual to influence personal development and life experiences. The innermost system, the microsystem, is the person's immediate surroundings and relationships. The next layer in the model is the mesosystem, where a person's microsystem structures interconnect and assert influence upon one another. The exosystem represents the third layer of the model, which is external to the individual, but affects him or her through interactions with structures in the microsystem. The outermost layer, the macrosystem, is comprised of cultural values, customs, and laws that have a cascading influence throughout interactions with all of the other systems.

Building on research that pointed to the importance of addressing the broader context in which elder abuse occurs [83, 138] combined tenets from ecological theory and the life course perspective to focus on the contextual risk factors for elder abuse by adult children as caregivers. Accordingly,

> The applied ecological model … posits the essential and crucial role of the intergenerational relationship between an adult child and an aging parent over the life course as a basis for both the understanding of elder abuse as well as the development of relevant prevention and intervention programs (p. 83)

They proposed a model that simultaneously focused on the adult child and aging parent [138, 139]. The development of both parties are given equal importance as is the context their relationship. They proposed a variety of variables or risk factors for abuse within each of the systems: (1) Aging Parent Microsystem—gender, marital status, chronological age, health, dementia/Alzheimer's disease, provocative/disruptive behavior, substance abuse, psychological factors (e.g., depression), and social isolation; (2) Adult Child Microsystem – substance abuse, mental/emotional illness, dementia, lack of caregiving experience, reluctance, stress and burden, personality traits (e.g., impatient behavior), and lack of social support; (3) Family Microsystem—dependency, living arrangements, history of abuse in the family, intergenerational transmission of violent behavior, and multigenerational demands; (4) Adult Child Mesosystem/Older Adult Exosystem: employment status and financial resources, social isolation, and lack of formal support; (5) Older Parent Mesosystem/Adult Child Exosystem—social isolation and lack of formal support; and (6) Macrosystem—cultural norms and public policy.

Parrra-Cardona et al. [111] expanded on Schiamberg and Gans' [138] model by identifying diverse factors and dynamics associated with elder abuse and neglect in Latino families. While many of the same risk factors identified in the applied ecological model are relevant to consider for elder abuse in Latino families, additional factors may come into play. For example, country of origin and language is viewed as a potential older adult microsystem risk factors. The authors also contend that within the family microsystem, cultural identity needs to be considered. At the Macrosystem, health care barriers can negatively impact the health of older Latino adults and subsequently place them at risk for abuse. In addition, Latino cultural values and gender roles need to be considered. Parrra-Cardona et al. [111] proposed the use of the model as an assessment and guide to clinical practice with Latino families.

The applied ecological model has also been adapted for informing the nature of elder abuse and neglect in African American families [68]. Unique risk factors added to the original model include (1) Caregiver Microsystem—limited caregiving skills; (2) Older Adult Microsystem—over identification with caregiver role and elder distrust of institutions; (3) Mesosytem—denial; (4) Exosystem—stressed family networks and caregivers' limited access to culturally relevant services; and (5) Macrosystem—legacy of slavery, internalized racism, poverty, and health disparities.

In one of the few studies to address elements of each of the ecological systems, Teaster et al. [149] used an ecological-community framework to organize and interpret the findings of their qualitative study of intimate partner violence of rural older women. Analysis of interviews with older women and focus groups with community service professionals revealed multiple interacting influences that perpetuated violence in the lives of the rural older women including their individual and family contexts (microsystem), the relationships between the women and their extended family, church, and others in her life (mesosystem), community support or lack thereof (exosystem), and rural culture (macrosystem).

Researchers continue to rely on variations of the ecological model as the foundation for studies of risk and vulnerability for elder abuse in general, specific types of elder abuse, and of elder abuse within specific cultural contexts. However, rather than embracing the model in its entirety, most authors introduced their work within the context of the ecological model and discussed the findings within one or more of the interacting or intersecting systems. For example, the study by Wangmo et al. [164] of Adult Protective Services focused on elder abuse broadly and formal relationships, formal supports, broader ideological values, norms, and institutional patterns of communities and states, whereas Mihaljcic and Lowndes [104] examined macro level factors in their exploration of individual and community attitudes toward financial elder abuse. Schiamberg et al. [140] identified individual, social, and contextual risk factors of physical abuse of nursing home residents. Similarly, Lee et al. [89] relied on the ecological model in combination with the cultural sensitivity model [128] to assess how cultural, social, and other contextual factors influenced perceptions of elder abuse among Korean and Chinese immigrants. Internationally, Walsh and Yon [162] used the ecological model to develop an empirical profile for elder abuse research in Canada, while Phelan [117] focused specifically on political changes in Ireland that directly affected individual and relation dynamics of elder abuse.

Ecological theories have helped facilitate an understanding of elder abuse as a complex problem requiring scientific understanding of the various systems in which older persons interact as well as coordinated responses from different levels of interventions and policies. While this is a strength of the theory, its multiplicity is also a limitation. In addition, variations in the application of ecological theory have emerged from a close-knit coterie of researchers and tend to be conceptual rather than empirically driven. Finally, while the theory stresses person-context interrelatedness, reasons associated with the development of the propensity for elder abuse (i.e., processes and behaviors) within and across the ecological systems have not been thoroughly addressed.

2.7 The Life Course Perspective

Often used in conjunction with another theory or framework, the *life course perspective* focuses on the changing contexts of lives and their consequences for human development. Central themes of the life course perspective include the interplay of human lives and historical times; the social meaning of age, age-norms, age-graded roles and events; the timing, sequencing and duration of life events; the linking and interdependence of lives; and human agency in choice making [47, 49]. A basic principle is that people experience sequences of transitions (i.e., a change in state or stage) and periods of stability throughout their lives that form distinctive trajectories in various life domains [49]. Both positive and adverse ontogenetic (i.e., individual), generational (i.e., family) and societal events, as well as the dynamic interactions among individual time (i.e., individual development), generational time (i.e., position within the family with associated roles and expectations), and historical time (i.e., events, periods, and eras dominated by seminal geopolitical or economic events) affect life trajectories [18]. The timing, sequencing, spacing, density, and duration of events also influence life transitions or turning points, which result in major directional changes or discontinuities in a trajectory [141]. Life course theorists acknowledge the importance of social bonds in life trajectories and transitions, specifically, the principle of "linked lives," which emphasizes relational interconnectedness [49]. Individual lives are at once embedded within relationships with family and other social network members and are influenced by them. Although the immediate relevance of social relationships may wax and wane over time, relationship stories are integral to how older adults make meaning of their lives. Individuals are active agents in interaction with social contexts and structures, with reciprocal influence on familial and social contexts.

Korbin et al. [81] used a life course framework as they explored the transmission of violence from one generation to another and its influence on elder abuse. They found that the experience of violence as children did not differ between elder abusing adult offspring and child abusing parents; however, child abusing parents were far more likely than elder abusing adult children to have experienced severe violence in their childhoods. Findings suggest that the intergenerational transmission of family violence is a more useful framework for explaining violence towards children rather than for violence towards elderly parents.

Similarly, Payne and Gainey [113] examined how the phenomenon of family violence varies over the course of one's life. They addressed elder abuse through a life course lens by placing abuse within the context of family violence, examining the intersection of macro-level characteristics that affect individuals' lives. Band-Winterstein and Eisikovits [9] examined how life-long intimate partner violence is experienced in old age and how age and violence interact and change throughout the life span. Their qualitative study explored the lived experiences of 40 persons who had lived for a signification time in violent situations, revealing four clusters of living situations, including living in violence and illness at the end of life.

In a recent application of the life course perspective, McDonald and Thomas [100] conducted a cross-sectional telephone survey measuring five types of elder abuse (neglect, physical, sexual, psychological, and financial) and its occurrence across the life course. When risk factors for abuse were considered simultaneously, including abuse during all three life stages of life, only a history of abuse during childhood retained its importance. Abuse in childhood increased the risk of experiencing one type of abuse relative to no abuse but was unrelated to experiencing two or more types of abuse as compared to no abuse.

The life course perspective provides a context for action and intervention into elder abuse, allowing multiple approaches to address the problem. Its limitations include its potential for misapplication of central tendency, confounding social change with social forces, confusing concepts of time and change, problematizing free exercise of choice, and neglect of inter-cohort variability.

2.8 Feminist Perspectives

Feminist frameworks offer an important lens for examining the complex intersection of social and historical context, age, gender, race, ethnicity, socioeconomics, and sexual orientation in the lives of an increasingly diverse and often marginalized population of victims of elder abuse [161]. Positioning old age and gender against a backdrop of inequality allows scholarly examination of the relationship between abuse and social and economic power [4, 62, 65]. In many cultures, women are economically and socially disadvantaged in comparison to men, thus making gender itself a risk factor for elder abuse. Without economic or social means, older women may elect to remain in unsafe relationships [80, 90].

The research and writings of Vinton [157, 158] provided some of the earliest applications of a feminist perspective to elder abuse. She identified the joint forces of ageism and sexism as affecting older females who experienced violent relationships. For example, her study of 25 women's shelters in Florida [159] revealed that shelters were inadequate for the needs of older women. In a state with one of the largest elderly populations, only two shelters offered special programming for older women at that time.

Scholars employing feminist perspectives to the study of elder abuse and violence typically have focused on relational inequities or power imbalance [64, 108, 115, 145]. Recently, for example, Yon et al. [175] identified differentials in age, education, and income contributions as risk factors for spousal abuse in mid-and old age, whereas Kalavar et al. [77] discussed societal changes in India and how perceived differential status within relationships created pathways to abuse, neglect, and abandonment of older adults by adult children. Harbison [60] used a critical feminist lens in her analysis of interviews with informal service providers in Canada to explore tensions between the domestic violence shelter movement and the predominant desires of older women to manage their abusive situations without leaving their homes.

The inclusion of principles of feminist theory in the study of elder abuse has helped to clarify the dynamics of intimate partner violence across the lifespan in particular, and elder abuse more generally. However, some authors critiqued the gender bias particularly in late life intimate partner violence research [126], as few investigations of issues relative to female on male or male on male violence in late life exist [131]. Methodologically, most studies that employ a feminist framework are qualitative in nature; researchers face the challenge of capturing concepts of values, power, and politics in quantitative terms that are meaningful to older study participants and that have universal recognition.

2.9 The National Academics of Science Elder Mistreatment Framework

Supporting the importance of relational factors is the internationally recognized framework for scholarship on elder mistreatment put forward by the National Academies of Sciences (NAS) [24]. Unlike any of the other theories discussed thus far, this framework was developed by members of the NAS panel, whose charge it was to elevate and guide scholarship specifically on the subject of elder mistreatment, defined as "(a) intentional actions that cause harm or create a serious risk of harm (whether or not harm is intended) to a vulnerable elder by a caregiver or other person who stands in a trust relationship to the elder or (b) failure by a caregiver to satisfy the elder's basic needs or to protect the elder from harm" ([24], p. 40). The NAS framework considers a variety of contributors to mistreatment and has as its premise elders in relationship with others. It is predicated on a conception of elder mistreatment as a series of transactions between the elder and a person(s) who has gained the older adult's trust and who is abusing, neglecting, and/or exploiting him or her. The framework also takes into account that the older adult and the abuser are embedded in a social context, one in which power and power exchanges exist and that there exits an inequality status of the older adult in relation to the abuser. Also, and importantly, the framework includes outcomes of the mistreatment for the elder and the abuser. The NAS framework is one of the few that positions mistreatment in a sociocultural context and takes into account quality of life and the continuation of elders in relationship with others.

Although the theory itself does not appear to have been empirically tested, the concepts from the framework have been adopted by many researchers in the field [2, 40, 73]. Disadvantages of this theoretical framework are its conceptualization of the "trusted other," placing primacy on the trust relationship but lacking specificity regarding when the trust relationship is established. It also does not address time in relationship to the abused person and the abuser or specific characteristics of the abuser. Notably, the framework excludes the major issue of elder self-neglect because there is no identified trusted other with this form of abuse.

2.10 Model of Self-Neglect

Self-neglect, or the inability of an individual to use goods and services to meet basic needs, is typically the most common form of abuse faced by Adult Protective Service agencies [146]. Using the charts of 538 patients referred by Texas Adult Protective Services, Dyer et al. [45] attempted to distinguish functional, cognitive, and social factors associated with self-neglect among older adults in order to identify etiologic models. Based on their findings, the authors contend that older adults who self-neglect have impairments in activities of daily living, lack critical support services, and fail to recognize the inherent danger of these deficits, thus losing their cognitive capacity to self-protect. Their model takes into account social issues, such as lack of family, lack of transportation, and inadequate funds by which to live to the extent that the elder is functionally impaired.

Dong et al. [41] built upon Dyer's self-neglect model to explore the association between elder self-neglect and mortality. Data were gathered from residents aged 65+ living in three adjacent neighborhoods in Chicago participating in the *Chicago Health and Aging Project*. Reported elder self-neglect was associated with a significantly increased risk of mortality after a year's time.

The self-neglect framework holds promise for evidence-based practices for intervention into and prevention of elder self-neglect. A limitation is that the model has not been fully tested and may not apply to all manifestations of self-neglect and its associated comorbidities.

2.11 International Perspectives

Like their counterparts in the US, international scholars have also grappled with the use of theory in elder abuse, stressing the need for its application cross-nationally and its sensitivity to diverse values and conceptualizations of the problem [22, 82, 121]. A human rights framework is emerging as an appropriate one for examining elder abuse internationally [23, 118]. A human rights perspective centers on issues of inequality and violence: dignity, respect for persons, and equality of social status, all conceptions that have a direct relationship with ageism [166].

The United Nations [153–155] defined human rights as a basic entitlement and first response of all governments. Drawing from a human rights perspective, The World Health Organization (WHO) places elder abuse within a context of world violence occurring across all age groups [84, 171]. Rights discourse has widened the recognition of disenfranchised groups to potentially include older adults [42], which expands the dialogue to embrace issues of justice and dignity [101]. A concept at the heart of human rights is that of ageism [29], a form of bigotry that explicitly and implicitly affects the treatment of older persons in such spheres as health care, economic security, decision making [37], and citizenship [118].

The human rights framework has not been explicitly applied to research on elder abuse, although a number of studies have examined its dimensions. For example, Doyle [43] explored the impact of power differentials on the care experiences of older people in South East Queensland and found active power inequality between the older adults as recipients of care and their caregivers, which affected their independence and autonomy. Keikelame and Ferreira [78] examined the treatment of older adults in Capetown, South Africa, and discovered abuse as well as dehumanizing treatment at health clinics, pension pay points, and government offices [44].

The human rights perspective for elder abuse holds much promise for elder abuse research on the world stage. Human rights foundations of dignity, justice, economic security, and safety are common concerns for both developed and developing countries. A limitation is inherent, however, in how expansive the issue is, as these core principles present difficulty in operationalization and empirical testing.

2.12 Challenges of Using Existing Theories in Research and Practice

The disparate use of the early and predominant theories presented above reveals that no one theory or set of theories has yet taken hold within the field. A number of reasons account for the lack of theoretical consensus. First, many studies, as mentioned earlier, do not use any theory or framework, either because researchers are unfamiliar with them or do not have a consensus regarding the most appropriate theory or set of theories to use. Second, theories may not be used because the research expressly confronts a problem and is conducted in reaction to a presenting problem rather than embedding a theory in the research *a priori*. Third, few cross-cutting theories have been embraced for various abuse typologies. For instance, a more holistic theory, such as the ecological model, is gaining acceptance, but in fact, only a handful of studies have applied it in its totality. Additionally, the framework suffers from the same problem as many of the others: that is was not intended for elder abuse but rather addressed child development. Fourth, theories continue to be discipline-specific, that is, the type of abuse and the remedy sought tends to drive the theory used (e.g., criminal justice theories, relational theories for family violence). Fifth, certain models, frameworks, and theories also fail to pass the test of cultural embeddedness. That is, most of the theories discussed above may be difficult to apply to various cultures (e.g., African Americans, Native Americans, Latinos, Asians, Hindi) other than those that are Euro-centric. For example, in-depth focus groups with 30 participants revealed that older Korean participants were more influenced by hierarchy and cultural beliefs in family ties and less likely to disclose abuse than were their Chinese counterparts [89]. Finally, the very use of any type of theory in research has not yet been embraced by the field. Many scholars and practitioners alike contend that meaningful and informative research has been conducted without it and that requiring that research or practice is grounded in theory will impede their producing immediate and cutting-edge research.

2.13 Theoretical Insights from Other Disciplines

In addition to the theories identified in the current elder abuse literature, there are several other theories within and outside the realm of abuse that may prove helpful. We, along with others, contend that drawing from multiple disciplines and incorporating elements from multiple frameworks and paradigms is the most efficacious way of theorizing about the problem of elder abuse and its solutions ([28, 72, 129, 133, 151]). Although researchers often do not specifically apply theories of child abuse and intimate partner violence to older adult populations, these theories offer a way to think about factors that might be associated with elder abuse. In addition, more global theoretical perspectives emerging from public health and the social sciences provide insightful constructs that inform further theory construction within the field of elder abuse.

2.14 Child Abuse

A basic tenet of Bandura's [10] *social learning theory* is that behavior is learned by observing others. Children learn through the process of observation, imitation, and modeling their behaviors, attitudes, and emotional reactions of their parents. What they see as normative and acceptable behavior within their home influences their own behavior in future social situations [11]. With respect to abusive behavior, ample evidence exists linking experiences of abuse or exposure to family violence with perpetrating violence in adolescence and adulthood (see reviews by [55, 66]). Although no empirical evidence exists to either support or refute the intergenerational transmission of violence hypothesis with respect to elder abuse, (e.g., adult children abuse their elderly parents who abused them as young children), recent longitudinal findings showed that early exposure to abuse has lifelong relational consequences [100, 137].

One of the first comprehensive theories of the sexual abuse of children, Finkelhor's [51] *Precondition Model of Child Sexual Abuse* identified four preconditions for sexual abuse (motivation to sexually abuse, overcoming internal inhibitors, overcoming external inhibitors, and overcoming the resistance of the child) that operate on both individual and social levels and that can act as motivators or inhibitors to child sexual abuse perpetration. If the preconditions occur and the abuse is then perpetrated within families, despite its being socially taboo in the larger population, the abusive behavior becomes normative or ignored within a family unit and encoded by children who may later, as adolescents and adults, replicate the same learned behaviors [56]. With respect to older adults, a national study of sexual abuse in long term care facilities found that in some cases, staff members and residents substantiated for abuse had *a priori* criminal history, including sexual violence or a history of sexually inappropriate behavior [124, 148].

2.15 Intimate Partner Violence

The intimate partner literature also has identified an array of potential demographic, psychological, and sociological risk factors for violence against women perpetrated by their male intimate partners that may enhance elder abuse theory development. A recurrent theme across this substantial body of literature is that intimate partner violence occurs when one partner uses violence to secure power and control within the relationship. Two theoretical perspectives have been commonly used to explain the links between risk factors and the use of violence in intimate relationships: resource theories and feminist-informed theories [13].

Resource theories. Resource theories locate power in a relationship in the person who controls most of the resources (e.g., education, income, occupational prestige). In relationships where there is an absence or imbalance of material or cultural resources, violence against an intimate partner is likely to be used as the ultimate resource to gain and maintain power and control [54]. Although *resource theory* emphasizes men's absolute possession of structural resources [58], other scholars have proposed a *relative resource theory* that contends that it is not so much men's lack of overall resources that predicts wife abuse but rather lack of resources relative to their wives [99]. This theory combines the idea that social resource constraints and related social stress will increase risk for partner violence with the idea that traditional sex-role expectations (e.g., male as breadwinner) are violated by resource imbalances in favor of the female partner. While these theories have received wide support in the intimate partner violence literature, Atkinson et al. [6] argue that gender ideology (i.e., how one identifies oneself with regard to marital and family roles traditionally linked to gender) moderate the effect of husbands' relative resources on abuse by changing the meaning of relative resources. They found that the husband's relative resources are negatively associated with the likelihood of wife abuse for traditional husbands but are not necessarily associated for transitional or egalitarian husbands. Thus, a *gendered resource theory* advances understanding of the intersection of how social structure and culture creates a context under which wife abuse is a more or less likely event. Although intimate partner violence in late life has received much less attention in the research literature, the perceived resource and power imbalance identified within violent relationships is evident in older women's reluctance to seek services, which is often deeply rooted in personal shame and humiliation, fear of further abuse, lack of financial resources to live independently, guilt about abandoning an abuser in poor health, and the need to keep family problems private [132].

Feminist-informed theories. Feminist perspectives of intimate partner violence also focus primarily on issues of power and control. As discussed by Basile et al. [13], *feminist-informed perspectives* emphasize the importance of social context and purport that intimate partner violence is more likely to occur among men who have been socialized by their society, communities, families-of-origin, and peers to positively endorse the use of violence in close relationships, maintain hostile attitudes toward women, and adopt a traditional male (i.e., "macho") sex-role orientation. While there is a preponderance of research linking male intimate partner perpetration to witnessing or experiencing family-of-origin violence [55], peer group influences [30], negative attitudes toward women [134], a need for power and control [87], and positive views of violent attitudes and behavior [46], increasing attention has been given to a gender-inclusive approach to understanding intimate partner violence that thwarts preconceived notions that violence is primarily a male-to-female phenomenon [59]. This has not been the case in the late life violence literature, where women are most frequently identified as victims of intimate partner violence and men are most often the perpetrators of the violence [132].

Johnson [76] has argued that there are qualitatively distinct forms of intimate partner violence that have different effects on the victim. *Situational couple violence* involves low levels of violence perpetrated by both sexes in the absence of the control motive. It occurs when specific conflict situations escalate. *Intimate terrorism* involves coercive aggression by a man who is motivated by the need to maintain control over his partner. *Mutual violent control* is characterized by control and violence by both partners, and *violent resistance* is characterized by self-defense or retaliation by victims (mainly women).With the exception of self-defense, female perpetration of violence against male partners is more closely related to other forms of non-gender-specific unhealthy relationship behavior [125].

Recent research also suggests that a significant proportion of young adults are involved in acts of intimate partner violence that can be categorized as bidirectional with substantial overlap in victim and perpetrators roles [50, 127]. Although research on female-to-male and bidirectional violence may be considered a first step in bringing a more informed understanding of patterns of violence among young people, the gender-inclusive conceptualization has been controversial and criticized as undermining a gender analysis of intimate partner violence, directing the focus away from the burden on women [7] and ignoring the context surrounding the incidents of violence, such as the intent (e.g., to injure, threaten, or control; self-defense; or retaliation), sequence (which partner initiated violence), degree of physical harm, and emotional impact [110].

2.16 Public Health

Some researchers are asking how abusive behaviors can be transmitted among abusers, similar to a contagion of disease [112]. Contagions are phenomenon (e.g., information, warnings, influence) or behaviors (e.g. abuse, addictions) that can spread through a population. Contagion can also spread to an individual (e.g., some behavior is adopted) based on influences that he or she receives from peers, family, and environment. Much evidence exists for contagion (influence) processes in human populations, including general observations of social behaviors [32, 165] and specific studies of contagions and contagion-like influences for incarceration [94], propagating information on Twitter [136], stress [27], and emotions [61], among others. Intervention methods, based on social networks and contagion dynamics, have been shown to reduce the use of drugs [91] and control the spread of influenza [12]. A finding in obesity research [98]—that obesity causes social marginalization, and not the other way around—suggests new directions for interventions based on social network structure. Additional studies use models from the sociology and data mining communities to develop strategies that inhibit the spread of contagions (e.g., [85, 152]).

During a 2013 National Academies of Science workshop, participants provided evidence for a *Contagion of Violence Model* with respect to the abuse of young children and intimate partners [112]. For older adults, the symptom manifests itself as the physical abuse of an elder perpetrated by a family member. Violence may be transmitted either through direct victimization or by just witnessing abuse [52]; previous exposure to a traumatic event also creates susceptibility to elder abuse [2]. The contagion model suggests that the very fact of being an older adult may create susceptibilities to abuse, as in the situation of older adults in prison settings who are victimized by younger inmates [79]. Vulnerabilities that may increase as an individual ages may leave him or her susceptible to abuse by a younger family member.

2.17 Social Sciences

Social organization models represent how people in a community interrelate, cooperate, and provide mutual support. These models frequently make mention of social support norms, social controls that regulate behavior and interaction patterns and the networks that operate in a community [96]. Community members share norms that govern behaviors and expectations that permit both licit and illicit activities [53]. Certain communities may tolerate activities and behaviors that are considered unacceptable by the general population. These subgroups may be characterized by particular demographic characteristics (i.e., age, ethnicity) and attitudes about gender, sense of self, and attributes of others. The variation and complexity of a community is reflected in its structure and protective or risky processes and behaviors engaged in by its members. For example, an identified risk factor for intimate partner violence perpetration is living in violent or disadvantaged communities [36, 123, 172]. Benson et al. [20] theorized that residents of disadvantaged neighborhoods that are low on collective efficacy may be unwilling to report domestic disputes. Their unwillingness may arise out of their weak ties to their neighbors or their acceptance of a general community norm that people are expected to stay out of the personal affairs of others. Even if most residents personally disapprove of intimate partner violence, they may be reluctant to express their disapproval openly; thus, individuals may act aggressively against their partners because they have little to fear from either their neighbors or the police.

Conversely, community networks can also play a significant role in promoting the well-being of individual members and their families [96]. Informal relationship networks involve voluntary relationships (e.g., neighbors) whereas formal support networks involve obligatory relationships, such as those associated with agencies and organizations. These two networks often interact and are essential for providing support for community members. Because the lives of most victims and perpetrators of intimate partner violence intersect with the broader community and are therefore subject to community influence, prevention at the community level can influence what occurs within relationships [97].

2.18 The Contextual Theory of Elder Abuse

While we acknowledge the inherent challenges of theorizing, we emphasize that moving forward with theory development at this juncture in the progression of elder abuse scholarship is critical for the refinement of study design and subsequent interpretation of findings and explanations of their implications. Thus, we propose *The Contextual Theory of Elder Abuse*. Using this theory, the field stands to gain a more coherent, comprehensive, and applicable strand of research on elder abuse. The findings that emerge from studies informed by this theory will be relevant to both scholars and professionals, as the theory we advance has broad applicability for research, practice, and policy.

The Contextual Theory of Elder Abuse addresses the complexities of elder abuse. As gerontologists, we are aware of the often-discussed intersection of aging and abuse, which presents complications that are inherently difficult to address. When children are abused, they are victims of abuse with relatively short or no histories with the abuser(s). Importantly, their legal standing is that of a child. Alternately, older adults have lived long, and many share linked lives with their abusers. Unless determined legally incapacitated, they have the legal standing of an adult and thus the autonomy to make appropriate or inappropriate decisions (as determined by others) to either disentangle themselves from an abusive situation or remain enmeshed in one. Also, although many issues and relationships affect abused children, we argue that far more issues and relationships affect elders, consequently creating intricate problems to resolve when abuse occurs. By virtue of their age, most older adults have forged well-defined identities, influenced by distinct and often distant historical periods, have made a multiplicity of life choices, and usually have lives far more intertwined with others than their younger counterparts. Older adults' life pathways intersect with partners, children, friends, faith groups, private and governmental entities, informal and formal care systems, and so forth that are in turn shaped by pronounced attitudes and values woven throughout these relationships.

We acknowledge the important contribution of Bronfenbrenner's [26] ecological model for the study of human development and the Social-Ecological Model promulgated by the Centers for Disease Control [31] applied to violence in general for theorizing about elder abuse. Building upon these models, the Contextual Theory of Elder Abuse has at its center the victim, representing the first context that must be considered in any study of elder abuse. Placing the victim of abuse at the center is consistent with the "person-centered" approach currently applied to acute and long-term health care and essential to elder abuse prevention and intervention [93, 160].

Our theory, also informed by the insights and knowledge gained from theorizing presented within the child abuse and intimate partner violence literature, positions the phenomenon of elder abuse within a larger set of actors and behaviors found within relationships, communities, and societies. It recognizes the intersectionalities of individual identities (e.g., age, gender, race, sexuality) as well as the dynamic relationships of older individuals and establishes a foundation for exploration and examination of the breadth and depth of individual characteristics on the occurrence of elder abuse, how those occurrences are linked to the lives of others, the response of the communities in which older adults live, and the power and influence of societal norms and values for propagating or stopping elder abuse. Elder abuse is an individual, relational, and community problem situated in historical time, as time periods and cohorts may define acts as appropriate treatment that, in later generations, are regarded as abusive of an elder. Elder abuse is a public health problem for which both prevention and intervention efforts are necessitated, and, although it can be construed as an individual problem, it occurs in communities and societies worldwide.

Below, we present the four contexts that constitute our theory of elder abuse: the individual context, relational context, community context, and societal context. Within each context, we identify initial constructs and concepts, that is, abstractions or generalizations about an aspect of elder abuse that serves a building block of the theory [143]. In Table 2.1, we provide examples of constructs and concepts, propositions that denote the relations among the concepts,

Table 2.1 The contextual theory of elder abuse: example constructs, propositions, and hypotheses

Constructs/concepts	Propositions	Hypotheses
Individual context		
Personal characteristics Situational influences Past events	Negative life events contribute to the risk of being a victim or perpetrator of abuse in later life	H_1: Experiencing childhood or family trauma increases the likelihood of experiencing elder abuse H_2: Being abused as a child increases the likelihood of perpetrating elder abuse
Relational context		
Personal ties Social integration Dependency on others	Social relationships protect against elder abuse	H_1: Limited engagement with others increases an older adult's vulnerability to elder abuse H_2: Reliance on others contributes to the occurrence of elder abuse
Community context		
Community integration	High levels of community capacity reduce the occurrence and duration of elder abuse	H_1: Community priorities influence how formal and informal networks respond to elder abuse H_2: Adequate social capital increases the likelihood of focused and immediate intervention efforts for abuse victims, perpetrators, and others who are affected
Societal context		
Norms Values Policies	Societal attitudes about aging influence the level of resources devoted to the prevention of elder abuse	H_1: Societal values influence the adoption of policies that address elder abuse H_2: Societies in which women are disadvantaged have greater occurrences of elder abuse than those in which women have greater privilege

and hypotheses associated with each proposition. Because constructs and concepts have a variety of meanings, how they are operationalized, defined, and measured will depend upon the individual researchers and the methods used in their investigations [143] of elder abuse. Similarly, hypotheses will be generated from existing theory, existing literature, and logical reasoning, all of which will increase the explanatory power of the theory.

2.19 Individual Context

The *individual context* involves both biological and personal factors converging to influence how individuals behave, how risk factors increase the likelihood of becoming a victim or perpetrator, and how these factors, such as poor health or dementia, affect the individuals during and after an abusive situation. Within the individual context, variables of particular interest include personal characteristics (e.g., age, sex, gender, race/ethnicity) [2, 88], education, habilitation (e.g., community or long-term care setting; rural or urban geographic area), income level, physical health, mental health, and cognitive capacity [86]. Depending their definition, personal constructs situated within the individual context may heighten, moderate, or reduce the risk for elder abuse. Neither the contributions of individual characteristics nor the complex interactions between and among them are fully understood.

Along with the characteristics of the victim and abuser, it is equally important to understand the contribution of positive and adverse ontogenetic (i.e., individual), generational (i.e., family), and societal events, as well as the life trajectories [18] of victims and abusers. Timing, sequencing, spacing, density, and duration of key events influence life transitions or turning points, a backdrop against which abuse may occur when an adult is old [137].

2.20 Relational Context

Elder abuse occurs within the context of relationships. The *relational context* focuses on the interactions and dynamics between older adults and other individuals they encounter as a means of (1) understanding the role social networks play in lessening the risk for elder abuse and (2) identifying the types of relationships between elder abuse victims and perpetrators. Within this context, it is important to keep in mind that relationships are not formulaic; rather, they are variable and dynamic, occurring between and among individuals and over time.

Social engagement is a protective factor against the risk of elder abuse. Findings from both national [1] and international [102] surveys have shown that older adults who were actively involved with members of their social network were less likely to experience abuse. Having social ties within dense networks (i.e., connections among network members) also lessens older persons' risk for abuse. However, unless older adults are forthright about how they are being treated, they may dismiss concerns raised about the nature and intent of a relationship. Such is the case in the classic scam whereby a seemingly romantic or caring relationship is established with an older person for the sheer intent of financial gain [103]. Conversely, family members, friends, and neighbors may perceive alleged perpetrators as the older adult's primary source of support rather than as an individual who is causing him or her harm.

Attention also needs to be given to the characteristics of the current relationship and the history of the relationship between victims and perpetrators. To illustrate the dynamics and variation within the context of abusive relationships, we focus on a common situation in which an older adult is reliant upon an adult child for care. Although the overwhelming majority of adult children provide appropriate care and a supportive environment for their older parents, it is important to recognize family care dynamics that foster abusive situations in order to disentangle the interdependencies of caregivers and care recipients in late life. Changes in roles and the nature of the parent-children relationship affect both caregivers and care recipients. Adult child caregivers may experience distress in the provision of care for which they may be ill-equipped, in turn leading to a range of often escalating, potentially abusive behaviors ranging from verbally assaulting their elderly relatives to depriving them of daily essentials, care, and services [3, 14]. Family members' reactions to the stress of caregiving may be compounded by factors present in the individual context, such as dependencies on alcohol, drugs, or other mental health problems [34]. Conversely, while an adult child may be the designated provider of care, s/he may also be reliant upon an elderly parent for housing, finances, and emotional support [71, 151]. If the availability of these resources are threatened, the adult child may attempt to take control of the situation by physically, psychologically, or financially abusing the elderly parent.

2.21 Community Context

The *community context* sheds light on people's sense of place and how members relate to one another within the space in which they live, work, worship, and so forth. Although the structure and culture of communities may shield elders from abuse, they may also inadvertently conceal and facilitate elder abuse. From this context, questions raised about elder abuse include how characteristics of settings affect the prevalence of elder abuse, what are the community's short term responses and long-term supports for older persons who experience abuse, and how does the community respond to perpetrators of elder abuse.

Most communities have an array of formal programs and services aimed at older adults. They are designed to enhance personal and social well-being (e.g., information and referral/assistance, senior centers, employment and income programs), assist older adults in maintaining their level of functioning (e.g., nutrition and meal programs, transportation services, mental health services), and provide long-term care to meet the needs of more dependent elders (e.g., case management services, home care services, respite services). Participation in community programs and use of available supportive services can help assuage some of the vulnerability and risk associated with elder abuse [63, 116].

Formal support networks also involve obligatory relationships, such as those with agencies and organizations tasked with addressing the problem of elder abuse. In the United States, Adult Protective Services (APS) is the principle public agency responsible for investigating the situation occurring in the community. In addition to, and often in conjunction with APS, members of the criminal justice system (e.g., police officers, detectives, lawyers, elder focused courts), social workers, mental health counselors, primary care physicians, emergency healthcare providers (e.g., emergency medical technicians, forensic nurses, emergency room physicians) and aging services professionals (e.g., home and community-based service providers, nursing home providers, Agency on Aging staff, Long-Term Care Ombudsman) work to either prevent or intervene when elder abuse is reported or otherwise recognized or alleged. Many communities have created multidisciplinary teams comprised of local professional (e.g., physicians, social workers, law enforcement, APS workers) to work with or on behalf of older victims [147, 150]. Such teams offer an integrative and holistic approach to elder abuse by having multiple professional disciplines involved in the development of interventions. The response of formal networks, individually and collectively, can reflect powerful and public attempts to address the problem; however, each is constrained by local statute and regulation, funding, public scrutiny, and workforce preparation.

Informal relationship networks are also part of the community context. These networks are voluntary relationships, such as those with church members, friends, and neighbors and are characterized by mutual exchanges and reciprocal responsibility. Community networks provide a strong influence over interactions with and treatment of older adults that is accepted, for example, caring for older adults in the community through parish nurses or home visitation [122] or through establishing behaviors that are under scrutiny, such as Neighborhood Watch programs.

Informal and formal networks usually intersect. The degree to which they demonstrate community capacity, or a sense of shared responsibility for the welfare of the community and its individual members [25] is essential for stopping the spread of abuse and providing support for older adults who experience abuse or for those who abuse. Efforts to reduce and treat elder abuse must include multiple, responsive, interrelated primary, secondary, and tertiary intervention strategies that addresses issues over the long term. For example, within one Native American community, members developed the Family Care Conference, a community-based intervention strategy for preventing and mitigating elder abuse [67]. Participants, with a facilitator and service providers, presented their views on the needs of the elders, designed a plan to address their needs, and identified strategies for its implementation.

2.22 Societal Context

The societal context involves overarching ideological values and norms that can foster a climate in which abuse is either normative or non-normative, encouraged or discouraged. Concepts emanating from the societal contact include large-scale changes in power and control dynamics such as age-related changes in social positions and financial resources that may escalate the experience of late life abuse or the propensity to abuse [145]. More generally, ageism is pervasive throughout the United States and elsewhere, leading to prejudiced attitudes, actions, and societal marginalization. It follows that societal tolerance of the abuse of older adults is a reflection of such ageism.

Many state governments are enacting laws or enhancing penalties for cases in which elders have been exploited, another reflection of a growing societal intolerance for mistreating older adults by taking their assets. Such is the case in Alabama where increased attention to elder abuse and legislative changes to law has resulted in increased public support for criminalization of elder abuse and endorsement of felony offense categorizations for acts of elder abuse and longer prison sentences for perpetrators [105].

Implementation of federal laws often results in less variability across state statutes on elder abuse. In 2004, the Centers for Medicare and Medicaid Services (CMS) implemented a federal complaint/incident system that provided the first national database of mistreatment in the nursing home setting. Although state nursing home licensure and certification statutes guide investigations of nursing home abuse allegations and deficiencies, with the implementation of this system, categories for these deficiencies became uniform across the United States. While substantial differences in reporting rates across states remain, differences can no longer attributed to variations in the laws, reflecting a movement toward a national consensus promoting the health, safety, and welfare of older adults [74].

Large scale actions of government are emblematic of the societal context. Enactment of the Elder Justice Act in 2010 reflects a societal acknowledgement that the welfare and safety of older adults is important and worthy of national focus and funding, so much so that it is necessary to mount a concerted, national effort to protect them. A part of the larger Affordable Care, the Elder Justice Act includes provisions for federal resources to address elder abuse, neglect, and exploitation. Within the Department of Health and Human Services, the act provides for the establishment of the Elder Justice Coordinating Council, an advisory board, and forensic centers. Funding is also provided for improving long-term care, Adult Protective Services, and the long-term care ombudsman program. The Act charges the Department of Justice with examining existing laws, changing them as appropriate, and enhancing the investigation and prosecution of cases involving elder abuse [156]. Advocates, practitioners, researchers and supportive legislators worked diligently for many years to give elder abuse the legislative attention it deserves. Passage of the Elder Justice Act significantly raised national awareness of elder abuse.

2.23 Challenges and Opportunities for Advancing the Contextual Theory of Elder Abuse

Like most theories, the Contextual Theory of Elder Abuse is a work in process that will evolve with use. A limitation, as with any newly proposed theory, is that it has yet to be empirically tested or critiqued. Establishing its validity and reliability is a critical next step in the theory development process. Specifically, the extent to which hypotheses generated by the Contextual Theory of Elder Abuse match empirical observations and are replicable over time and across studies [72] as well as for the study of all types of elder abuse will be vital to its acceptance and use among researchers and practitioners. As part of this process, key concepts must be agreed upon, operationally defined, and be capable of being measured.

While the underlying assumption of the Contextual Theory of Elder Abuse is that each context exerts an influence on elder abuse, whether readily apparent or not, we stress that the theory does not have to be used in its totality. Currently, many prevention and intervention efforts and methodological approaches focus solely on one or two of the identified contexts. For example, while elder abuse may occur because an older person lives alone or has dementia (individual context), the designated family care provider may not have inadequate skills or resources to meet the older person's care needs and may be dependent upon the older relative for material support (relational context). The abuse may escalate because organizational resources are inadequate for prevention and intervention (community context) or because older adults are not viewed as a population deserving of public attention (societal context). Though most studies of elder abuse would over-extend available data if research questions and hypotheses were posed for each context, we encourage researchers and practitioners to broaden the lens from which they approach their work and acknowledge the influence of the multiple contexts of elder abuse regardless of where they focus their emphasis and expertise.

As a global approach for the study of elder abuse, the Contextual Theory of Elder Abuse emphasizes that elder abuse is not "just a family problem," but rather that abuse occurs against a backdrop and interplay of larger contextual issues, including why older adults are abused by trusted others as well as why they are the target of abuse by complete strangers. Regardless of the type of abuse, the location of the abuse, or the population of elders under study, we maintain that without an awareness of context, the understanding of elder abuse will remain incomplete.

2.24 Next Steps in Theorizing Elder Abuse Research and Practice

To move the field forward necessitates a course correction in the ways in which elder abuse research is conducted, published, and integrated into practice and policy. As highlighted in this chapter, independent efforts by a handful of researchers have put forth a number of perspectives for advancing theoretically informed elder abuse research. We argue for greater intentionality with the theorizing of elder abuse research and practice.

2.25 Directions for Theory Use in Research

Often, research on elder abuse has been problem rather than theory driven. That is, the work of pioneering elder abuse scholars and others from a variety of disciplines, many whom have more recently turned their attention to the study of elder abuse, has been pushed by a set of problems or concerns (e.g., fraud, violence, eldercare) in search of a solution rather than testing why some older adults experience actual or threats of abuse and others do not. Dynamic theories are powerful tools in identifying and understanding the complexities of elder abuse. Ignoring theory when planning studies and interpreting findings conceals gaps in research and knowledge that would be more apparent if investigators operated from a theory-based stance [130]. With well-articulated, constant development and testing of theories, the processes and dynamics of elder abuse and the influence that outcomes of abuse have on the quality of older adults' lives and the lives of affected others can be explored and explained more adequately.

The field is ripe for the development and adoption of theory to more precisely predict what formal community intervention strategies will be acceptable to older adults and under which circumstances and conditions. Theory-driven research in the U.S. and elsewhere that accounts for social and political differences across nations will enhance a global understanding of elder abuse. Only by grounding research in theoretical principles of human nature and behavior will scholars and practitioners achieve a full understanding of what empirical findings reveal about the complexity of elder abuse and be able to apply and share this information widely. With their guidance, editors of peer-reviewed journals in which studies on elder abuse are published can increase their emphasis that studies be grounded in a framework or theory. Likewise, when research studies funded by either public or private dollars are proposed, an expectation of reviewers that theoretical frameworks undergird the study will also serve to influence the direction of research and its influence on practice.

2.26 Directions for the Use of Theory in Practice

Sound theories will also guide practice. Findings from research grounded in theoretical constructs can have a critical impact on a field that has received mixed guidance on how to intervene in "boots on the ground" problems. The exchange of research findings and best practice strategies among researchers, practitioners, and policymakers is critical for understanding the growing phenomena of elder abuse and the development and implementation of services and interventions. Studies of elder abuse have often been guided by real life experiences encountered by entities confronting the problem. Importantly, scholars must continue to refine methodologies that cross-link the increasingly sophisticated data from APS with aggregated information from cross-sectional longitudinal datasets, particularly those that include reliable measures of health and health outcomes. Additionally, data mining of already conducted studies is another source of rich information that can guide policy and practice. Large, population-based studies such as those conducted by Acierno et al. [2] and Lifespan of Greater Rochester [92] have been exceptionally useful in influencing public policy.

The major piece of legislation on the topic, The Elder Justice Act ([156]; Public Law 111–148) has the potential to play an important role in the expansion of theory, especially concerning prevention and intervention efforts. Major tenets of the Act, such as the provision for state demonstration grants to test a variety of methods to improve APS, the development of forensic centers, and the improvement of data collection and dissemination by the Department of Health and Human can shape the field by grounding such efforts in suitable frameworks and theories. These initiatives can unify the field and provide much-needed evidence for promising prevention and intervention practices. Employing theory on a federal level will also have a trickle-down effect to initiatives at state and local levels as well.

Theoretical development is needed to more precisely predict the acceptability of formal community interventions for older adults and under what circumstances and conditions. Theory-driven research that accounts for social and political differences across nations also is required to enhance the global understanding of elder abuse. Only by grounding research in theoretical principles of human nature and behavior will scholars and practitioners achieve a full understanding of what empirical findings reveal about the complexity of elder abuse and be able to apply this information widely. Thus, the exchange of research findings and best practice strategies among researchers, practitioners, and policymakers is critical for understanding the growing phenomena of elder abuse and the development, implementation, and evaluation of services and evidence-based interventions.

A promising approach to formalizing relationships among theory, research, and practice is implementing community-based participatory research (CBPR) strategies to address issues and concerns of elder abuse within communities. CBPR is a collaborative process of research involving investigators and community representatives [70]. In both the process and products of research, CBRP encourages active exchange between community members (i.e., service providers, educators, and consumers) and researchers, employs local knowledge in the understanding of issues of concern, invests community professionals in both the study design and evaluation of outcomes and the dissemination and use of research findings, and reflects prevailing societal norms. Although examples of studies using principles of CBRP can be found in the elder abuse literature (e.g., [38, 40, 73]), elder abuse scholars must bring theoretically grounded information to discussions with practitioners and policy makers in order to ensure that future initiatives recognize and address the contexts affecting older adults who experience abuse. Conversely, discussions of the realities and complexities of 'real-world' experiences, as perceived by practitioners, provide scholars with new theoretical insight and questions to explore.

Although prevention and intervention services for elder abuse have their unique nuances, a theoretical explanation and meaning that is transferable will lead to greater sustainability. We view the connections among theory, research, and practice as a dynamic and ongoing interchange among professionals and propose the Contextual Theory of Elder Abuse as a bridge to make these connections.

References

1. Acierno R, Hernandez-Tejada M, Muzzy W, Steve K. National elder mistreatment study (2007-WG-BX-0009). Retrieved from Rockville, MD. 2009. https://www.ncjrs.gov/pdffiles1/nij/grants/226456.pdf.
2. Acierno R, Hernandez MA, Amstadter AB, Resnick HS, Steve K, Muzzy W, Kilpatrick DG. Prevalence and correlates of emotional, physical, sexual, and financial abuse and potential neglect in the United States: The National Elder Mistreatment Study. Am J Public Health. 2010;100:292–7. doi:10.2105/ajph.2009.163089.
3. Amstadter AB, Cisler JM, McCauley JL, Hernandez MA, Muzzy W, Acierno R. Do incident and perpetrator characteristics of elder mistreatment differ by gender of the victim? Results from the National Elder Mistreatment Study. J Elder Abuse Negl. 2011;23:42–57. doi:10.1080/08946566.2011.534707.
4. Anderson KL. Conflict, power, and violence in families. J Marriage Fam. 2010;72:726–42. doi:10.1111/j.1741-3737.2010.00727.
5. Aneshensel CS, Pearlin LI, Mullan JT, Zarit SH, Whitlatch CJ. Profiles in caregiving: the unexpected career. New York: Academic Press; 1995.
6. Atkinson MP, Greenstein TN, Lang MM. For women, breadwinning can be dangerous: gendered resource theory and wife abuse. J Marriage Fam. 2005;67:1137–48. doi:10.1111/j.1741-3737.2005.00206.x.
7. Bates EA, Graham-Kevan N, Archer J. Testing predictions from the male control theory of men's partner violence. Aggress Behav. 2014;40:42–55. doi:10.1002/ab.21499.
8. Band-Winterstein T, Doron II, Naim S. Elder self neglect: a geriatric syndrome or a life course story? J Aging Stud. 2012;26:109–18. doi:10.1016/j.jaging.2011.10.001.
9. Band-Winterstein T, Eisikovits Z. "Aging out" of violence: the multiple faces of intimate violence over the life span. Qual Health Res. 2009;19(2):164–80. doi:10.1177/1049732308329305.
10. Bandura A. Social learning theory. New York: General Learning Press; 1977.
11. Bandura A, Huston AC. Identification as a process of incidental learning. J Abnorm Soc Psychol. 1961;63:311–8. doi:10.1037/h0040351.
12. Barrett C, Bisset K, Leidig J, Marathe A, Marathe M. Economic and social impact of influenza mitigation strategies by demographic class. Epidemics. 2011;3:19–31. doi:10.1016/j.epidem.2010.11.002.
13. Basile KC, Hall JE, Walters ML. Expanding resource theory and feminist-informed theory to explain intimate partner violence perpetration by court-ordered men. Violence Against Women. 2013;19:848–80. doi:10.1177/1077801213497105.
14. Beach SR, Schulz R, Williamson GM, Miller LS, Weiner MF, Lance CE. Risk factors for potentially harmful informal caregiver behavior. J Am Geriatr Soc. 2005;53(2):255–61. doi:10.1111/j.1532-5415.2005.53111.x.
15. Beaulaurier RL, Seff LR, Newman FL. Barriers to help-seeking for older women who experience intimate partner violence: a descriptive model. J Women Aging. 2008;20(3–4):231–48. doi:10.1080/08952840801984543.
16. Bengtson V. My view: theory as puzzle-building. In: Bengtson VL, Acock AC, Allen KR, Dilworth-Anderson P, Klein D, editors. Sourcebook of family theory and research. Thousand Oaks, CA: Sage; 2005. p. 5.
17. Bengtson VL, Acock AC, Allen KR, Dilworth-Anderson P, Klein D. Theory and theorizing in family research: puzzle building and puzzle solving. In: Bengtson VL, Acock AC, Allen KR, Dilworth-Anderson P, Klein D, editors. Sourcebook of family theory and research. Thousand Oaks, CA: Sage; 2005. p. 3–22.
18. Bengtson VL, Allen KA. The life course perspective applied to families over time. In: Boss PG, Doherty WJ, LaRossa R, Schumm WR, Steinmertz SK, editors. Sourcebook of family theories and methods: a contextual approach. New York: Plenum Press; 1993. p. 469–99.
19. Bengtson VL, Gans D, Putney NM, Silverstein M. Theories about age and aging. In: Bengtson VL, Gans D, Putney NM, Silverstein M, editors. Handbook of theories of aging. 2nd ed. New York: Springer Publishing Company; 2009. p. 23.
20. Benson ML, Wooldredge J, Thistlethwaite AB, Fox GL. The correlation between race and domestic violence is confounded with community context. Soc Probl. 2004;51:326–42. doi:10.1525/sp.2004.51.3.326.
21. Bergeron LR. Family preservation: An unidentified approach in elder abuse protection. J Contemp Human Serv. 2002;83:547–56. doi:10.1606/1044-3894.48.
22. Biggs S, Goergen T. Theoretical development in elder abuse and neglect. Ageing Int. 2010;35(3):167–70. doi:10.1007/s12126-010-9066-z.
23. Biggs S, Haapala I. Elder mistreatment, ageism, and human rights. Int Psychogeriatr. 2013;25(08):1299–306. doi:10.1017/S1041610212002372.
24. Bonnie RJ, Wallace RB, editors. Elder mistreatment: abuse, neglect, and exploitation in an aging America. Washington, DC: National Academies Press; 2003.
25. Bowen GL, Martin JA, Mancini JA, Nelson JP. Community capacity: antecedents and consequences. J Commun Pract. 2000;8(2):1–21. doi:10.1300/J125v08n02_01.
26. Bronfenbrenner U. Ecology of the family as a context for human development: research perspectives. Dev Psychol. 1986;22:723–42. doi:10.1037/0012-1649.22.6.723.
27. Bulger N, DeLongis A, Kessler R, Wethington E. The contagion of stress across multiple roles. J Marriage Family. 1989;51:175–83. doi:10.2307/352378.
28. Burnight K, Mosqueda L. Theoretical model development in elder mistreatment. U.S. Department of Justice. 2011. https://www.ncjrs.gov/pdffiles1/nij/grants/234488.pdf.
29. Butler RN. Ageism: another form of bigotry. Gerontologist 1969;9(4 Part 1):243–6. doi:10.1093/geront/9.4_Part_1.243.
30. Casey EA, Beadnell B. The structure of male adolescent peer networks and risk for intimate partner violence perpetration: findings from a national sample. J Youth Adolesc. 2010;39(6):620–33. doi:10.1007/s10964-009-9423-y.
31. Centers for Disease Control. The social-ecological model: a framework for prevention. 2015. http://www.cdc.gov/violenceprevention/overview/social-ecologicalmodel.html.
32. Centola D, Macy M. Complex contagions and the weakness of long ties. Am J Sociol. 2007;113:702–34. doi:10.11745/2482540.2482550.
33. Cooney C, Howard R, Lawlor B. Abuse of vulnerable people with dementia by their carers: can we identify those most at risk? Int J Geriatr Psychiatry. 2006;21(6):564–71. doi:10.1002/gps.1525.

34. Cooper C, Livingston G. Mental health/psychiatric issues in elder abuse and neglect. Clin Geriatr Med. 2014;30:839–50. doi:10.1016/j.cger.2014.08.011.
35. Cooper C, Selwood A, Blanchard M, Walker Z, Blizard R, Livingston G. Abuse of people with dementia by family carers: representative cross sectional survey. BMJ 2009; 338. doi:10.1136/bmj.b155.
36. Cunradi CB. Intimate partner violence among Hispanic men and women: the role of drinking, neighborhood disorder, and acculturation-related factors. Violence Vict. 2009;24:83–97. doi:10.1891/0886-6708.24.1.83.
37. Daly G. Citizenship, public accountability and older people: user involvement in community care provision. Educ Aging. 2001;16:55–74.
38. DeLiema M, Gassoumis ZD, Homeier DC, Wilber KH. Determining prevalence and correlates of elder abuse using promotores: low-income immigrant Latinos report high rates of abuse and neglect. J Am Geriatr Soc. 2012;60:1333–9. doi:10.1111/j.1532-5415.2012.04025.x.
39. Dilworth-Anderson P. My view: the process of theorizing. In: Bengtson VL, Acock AC, Allen KR, Dilworth-Anderson P, Klein, editors. Sourcebook of family theory and research. Thousand Oaks, CA: Sage; 2005. p. 7–8.
40. Dong XQ, Chang E, Wong E, Wong B, Skarupski KA, Simon MA. How do U.S. Chinese older adults view elder mistreatment? Findings from a community-based participatory research study. J Aging Health. 2011;23:289–312. doi:10.1177/0898264310385931.
41. Dong X, Simon M, de Leon CM, Fulmer T, Beck T, Hebert L, Dyer C, Paveza G, Evans D. Elder self-neglect and abuse and mortality risk in a community-dwelling population. JAMA. 2009;302(5):517–26. doi:10.1001/jama.2009.1109.
42. Doron I, Apter I. The debate around the need for an international convention on the rights of older persons. Gerontologist. 2010;50(5):586–93. doi:10.1093/geront/gnq016.
43. Doyle S. The impact of power differentials on the care experiences of older people. J Elder Abuse Negl. 2014;26:319–32. doi:10.1080/08946566.2013.875970.
44. DPhil MF, Lindgren P. Elder abuse and neglect in South Africa: a case of marginalization, disrespect, exploitation and violence. J Elder Abuse Negl. 2008;20(2):91–107. doi:10.1080/08946560801974497.
45. Dyer CB, Goodwin JS, Pickens-Pace S, Burnett J, Kelly PA. Self-neglect among the elderly: a model based on more than 500 patients seen by a geriatric medicine team. Am J Public Health. 2007;97(9):1671. doi:10.2105/AJPH.2006.097113.
46. Eckhardt CI, Samper R, Suhr L, Holtzworth-Munroe A. Implicit attitudes toward violence among male perpetrators of intimate partner violence: a preliminary investigation. J Interpers Violence. 2012;27:471–91. doi:10.1177/0886260511421677.
47. Elder G. Family history and the life course. J Family Hist. 1977;2:279–304. doi:10.1177/036319907700200402.
48. Elder G. Life course dynamics: trajectories and transitions, 1968–1980. Ithaca, NY: Cornell University Press; 1985.
49. Elder G. The life course and human development. In: Lerner RM, editor. Handbook of child psychology: vol: 1. Theoretical models of human development. 5th ed. New York: Wiley; 1998. p. 939–91.
50. Fass DF, Benson RI, Leggett DG. Assessing prevalence and awareness of violent behaviors in the intimate partner relationships of college students using internet sampling. J College Stud Psychother. 2008;22(4):66–75. doi:10.1080/87568220801952248.
51. Finkelhor D. Child sexual abuse. New York: Free Press; 1984.
52. Flannery DJ, Singer MI, Van Dulmen MM, Kretschmar J, Belliston LM. Exposure to violence, mental health and violent behavior. In: Flannery DJ, Vazsonyi AT, Waldman I, editors. The Cambridge handbook of violent behavior and aggression. Cambridge, UK: Cambridge University Press; 2007. p. 306–21.
53. Furstenberg FF, Hughes ME. The influence of neighborhoods on children's development: a theoretical perspective and research agenda. In: Brooks-Gunn J, Duncan GJ, Aber JL, editors. Neighborhood poverty: policy implications in studying neighborhoods. New York: Russell Sage Foundation; 1997. p. 22–47.
54. Gelles R. Family violence. In: Flannery DJ, Vazsonyi AT, Waldman ID, editors. The Cambridge handbook of violent behavior and aggression. Cambridge, UK: Cambridge University Press; 2007. p. 403–17.
55. Gil-Gonzalez D, Vives-Cases C, Ruiz M, Carrasco-Portino M, Alvarez- Dardet C. Childhood experiences of violence in perpetrators as a risk factor for intimate partner violence: a systematic review. J Public Health. 2008;30(1):14–22. doi:10.1093/pubmed/fdm071.
56. Glasser M, Kolvin I, Campbell D, Glasser A, Leitch I, Farrelly S. Cycle of child sexual abuse: links between being a victim and becoming a perpetrator. Br J Psychiatry. 2001;179:482–94. doi:10.1192/bjp.179.6.482.
57. Goergen T. Stress, conflict, elder abuse and neglect in German nursing homes: a pilot study among professional caregivers. J Elder Abuse Neglect. 2001;13(1):1–26. doi:10.1300/J084v13n01_01.
58. Goode WJ. Force and violence in family. J Marriage Family. 1971;33:624–36. doi:10.2307/349435.
59. Hamel J. Toward a gender-inclusive conception of intimate partner violence research and theory: part 1—traditional perspectives. Int J Men's Health. 2007;6:36–53. doi:10.3149/jmh.0601.36.
60. Harbison J. Stoic heroines or collaborators: ageism, feminism and the provision of assistance to abused old women. J Social Work Pract. 2008;22(2):221–34. doi:10.1080/02650530802099890.
61. Hatfield E, Cacioppo JT, Rapson RL. Emotional contagion. New York, NY: Cambridge University Press; 1994.
62. Held V. The ethics of care: personal, political, and global. Oxford: Oxford University Press. 2006.
63. Henderson D, Buchanan JA, Fisher JE. Violence and the elderly population: issues for prevention. In: Schewe PA, editor. Preventing violence in relationships: interventions across the life span. Washington: American Psychological Association; 2002. p. 223–45. doi:10.1037/10455-009.
64. Hightower J, Smith MJ, Hightower HC. Hearing the voices of abused older women. J Gerontol Soc Work. 2006;4(3–4):205–27. doi:10.1300/J083v46n03_12.
65. Holstein M, Parks J, Waymack M. Ethics, aging, and society: the critical turn. New York: Springer; 2011.
66. Holt S, Buckley H, Whelan S. The impact of exposure to domestic violence on children and young people: a review of the literature. Child Abuse Negl. 2008;32:797–810. doi:10.1016/j.chiabu.2008.02.004.
67. Holkup PA, Salois EM, Tripp-Reimer T, Weinert C. Drawing on wisdom from the past: an elder abuse intervention with tribal communities. Gerontologist. 2007;47:248–54. doi:10.1093/geront/47.2.248.
68. Horsford SR, Parra-Cardona JR, Post LA, Schiamberg L. Elder abuse and neglect in African American families: informing practice based on ecological and cultural frameworks. J Elder Abuse Neglect. 2010;23:75–88. doi:10.1080/08946566.2011.534709.

69. Hudson MF. Elder neglect and abuse: current research. In: Pillemer KA, Wolf RS, editors. Elder abuse: conflict in the family. Dover, MA: Auburn House; 1986.
70. Israel BA, Schulz AJ, Parker EA, Becker AB, Allen AJ, Guzman JR. Critical issues in developing and following community based participatory research principles. In: Minkler M, Wallerstein N, editors. Community based participatory research for health. San Francisco: Jossey-Bass; 2003. p. 53–76.
71. Jackson SL, Hafemeister TL. Pure financial exploitation versus hybrid financial exploitation co-occurring with physical abuse and/or neglect of elderly persons. Psychol Violence. 2012;2:285–96. doi:10.1037/a0027273.
72. Jackson SL, Hafemeister TL. Understanding elder abuse: new directions for developing theories of elder abuse occurring in domestic settings. 2013. https://www.ncjrs.gov/pdffiles1/nij/241731.pdf.
73. Jervis LL, Fichenscher A, Beals J. Assessment of elder mistreatment in two American Indian samples: psychometric characteristics of the HS-EAST and the native elder life-financial exploitation and neglect measures. J Appl Gerontol. 2014; 33 (3):336–56. doi:10.1177/0733464812470748.
74. Jogerst GJ, Daly JM, Hartz AJ. State policies and nursing home characteristics associated with rates of resident mistreatment. J Am Med Dir Assoc. 2008;9:648–56. doi:10.1016/j.jamda.2008.05.005.
75. Jogerst GL, Daly JM, Galloway BA, Zheng S, Xu Y. Substance abuse associated with elder abuse in the United States. Am J Drug Alcohol Abuse. 2012;38(1):63–9. doi:10.3109/00952990.2011.600390.
76. Johnson MP. A typology of domestic violence: intimate terrorism, violent resistance, and situational couple violence. Lebanon, NH: Northeastern University Press; 2010.
77. Kalavar JM, Jamuna D, Ejaz FK. Elder abuse in India: extrapolating from the experiences of seniors in India's "Pay and Stay" homes. J Elder Abuse Negl. 2013;25(1):3–18. doi:10.1080/08946566.2012.661686.
78. Keikelame MJ, Ferreira M. *Mpathekombi, ya bantu abadala. Elder abuse in black townships on the Cape Flats*. Cape Town, University of Cape Town, Institute of Ageing in Africa. 2000. www.instituteofageing.uct.ac.za.
79. Kerbs JJ, Jolley JM. Inmate-on-inmate victimization among older male prisoners. Crime Delinq. 2007;53:187–218. doi:10.1177/0011128706294119.
80. Koenig TS, Rinfrette ES, Lutz WA. Female caregivers' reflections on ethical decision-making: the intersection of domestic violence and elder care. Clin Soc Work J. 2006;34:361–72. doi:10.1007/s10615-005-0023-3.
81. Korbin JE, Anetzberger GJ, Austin C. The intergenerational cycle of violence in child and elder abuse. J Elder Abuse Negl. 1995;7 (1):1–15. doi:10.1300/J084v07n01_01.
82. Kosberg JI, Lowenstein A, Garcia JL, Biggs S. Study of elder abuse within diverse cultures. J Elder Abuse Negl. 2003;15(3–4):71–89. doi:10.1300/J084v15n03_05.
83. Kosberg JI, Nahmiash D. Characteristics of victims and perpetrators and milieus of abuse and neglect. In: Baumhover LA, Ball SC, editors. Abuse, neglect and exploitation of older persons: strategies for assessment and intervention. London: Jessica Kingsley; 1996. p. 31–50.
84. Krug EG, Mercy JA, Dahlberg LL, Zwi AB. The world report on violence and health. Lancet. 2002;360(9339):1083–8. doi:10.1016/S0140-6736(02)11133-0.
85. Kuhlman CJ, Kumar AVS, Marathe MV, Ravi SS, Rosenkrantz DJ. Inhibiting diffusion of complex contagions in social networks: theoretical and experimental results. J Data Mining Knowl Discov. 2015;29:423–65. doi:10.1007/s10618-014-0351-4.
86. Lachs MS, Williams C, O'Brien S, Hurst L, Horwitz R. Risk factors for reported elder abuse and neglect: a nine-year observational cohort study. Gerontologist. 1997;37:469–74. doi:10.1093/geront/37.4.469.
87. Langhinrichsen-Rohling J, McCullars A, Misra TA. Motivations for men and women's intimate partner violence perpetration: a comprehensive review. Partner Abuse. 2012;3(4):429–68. doi:10.1891/1946-6560.3.4.429.
88. Laumann EO, Leitsch SA, Waite LJ. Elder mistreatment in the United States: prevalence estimates from a nationally representative study. J Gerontol B Psychol Sci Soc Sci. 2008;63:S248–54.
89. Lee Y, Moon A, Gomez C. Elder mistreatment, culture, and help-seeking: a cross-cultural comparison of older Chinese and Korean immigrants. J Elder Abuse Negl. 2014;26(3):244–69. doi:10.1080/08946566.2013.820656.
90. Lev-Wiesel R, Kleinberg B. Elderly battered wives' perceptions of the spousal relationship as reflected in the drawings of the couple. Arts Psychother. 2002;29:13–7. doi:10.1016/S0197-4556(01)00122-8.
91. Li J, Weeks MR, Borgatti SP, Clair A, Dickson-Gomez J. A social network approach to demonstrate the diffusion and change process of intervention from peer health advocates to the drug using community. Subst Use Misuse. 2012;47:474–90. doi:10.3109/10826084.2012.644097.
92. Lifespan of Greater Rochester I, University WCMCOC, Aging NYCDFT. Under the radar: New York state elder abuse prevalence study—Self-reported prevalence and documented case surveys. 2011. http://www.lifespan-roch.org/documents/UndertheRadar051211.pdf.
93. Lithwick M, Beaulieu M, Gravel S, Straka SM. The mistreatment of older adults: perpetrator-victim relationships and interventions. J Elder Abuse Negl. 2000;11(4):95–112. doi:10.1300/J084v11n04_07.
94. Lum K, Swarup S, Eubank S, Hawdon J. The contagious nature of imprisonment: an agent-based model to explain racial disparities in incarceration rates. Interface. 2014;11(98):20140409. doi:10.1098/rsif.2014.0409.
95. MacNeil G, Kosberg JI, Durkin DW, Dooley WK, DeCoster J, Williamson GM. Caregiver mental health and potentially harmful caregiving behavior: the central role of caregiver anger. Gerontologist. 2010;50(1):76–86. doi:10.1093/geront/gnp099.
96. Mancini JA, Bowen GL. Families and communities: a social organization theory of action and change. In: Peterson GW, Bush KR, editors. Handbook of marriage and the family. 3rd ed. New York, NY: Springer; 2013. p. 781–813.
97. Mancini JA, Nelson JP, Bowen GL, Martin JA. Preventing intimate partner violence. J Aggress Maltreatment Trauma. 2006;13(3–4):203–27. doi:10.1300/J146v13n03_08.
98. Marathe A, Pan Z, Apolloni A. Analysis of friendship network and its role in explaining obesity. ACM Trans Intell Syst Technol. 2013;4(3):56. doi:10.1145/2483669.2483689.
99. McCloskey L. Socioeconomic and coercive power within the family. Gender Soc. 1996;10:449–63. doi:10.1177/089124396010004006.
100. McDonald L, Thomas C. Elder abuse through a life course lens. Int Psychogeriatr. 2013;25(8):235–43. doi:10.1017/S104161021300015X.
101. Mégret F. The human rights of older persons: a growing challenge. Human Rights Law Review. 2011;11(1):37–66. doi:10.1093/hrlr/ngq050.
102. Melchiorre MG, Chiatti C, Lamura G, Torres-Gonzales F, Stankunas M, Lindert J, Ioannidi-Kapolou E, Barros H, Macassa G,

Soares JFJ. Social support, socio-economic status, health and abuse among older people in seven European countries. PLoS ONE. 2013;8(1):e54856. doi:10.1371/journal.pone.0054856.
103. MetLife Mature Market Institute. Broken trust: elders, family, and finances. 2009. http://www.gerontology.vt.edu/docs/mmi-studies-broken-trust.pdf.
104. Mihaljcic T, Lowndes G. Individual and community attitudes toward financial elder abuse. J Elder Abuse Negl. 2013;25(2):183–203. doi:10.1080/08946566.2012.712867.
105. Morgan E, Johnson I, Sigler R. Public definitions and endorsement of the criminalization of elder abuse. J Crim Justice. 2006;34(3):275–83. doi:10.1016/j.jcrimjus.2006.03.004.
106. National Institute of Justice. Elder mistreatment: using theory in research. 2014. http://www.nij.gov/topics/crime/elder-abuse/Documents/elder-mistreatment-theory-meeting-summary.pdf.
107. Navaie-Waliser M, Spriggs A, Feldman PH. Informal caregiving: differential experiences by gender. Med Care. 2002;40(12):1249–59.
108. Nerenberg L. A feminist perspective on gender and elder abuse: a review of the literature. National Committee for the Prevention of Elder Abuse. 2002. http://www.ncea.aoa.gov/Resources/Publication/docs/finalgenderissuesinelderabuse030924.pdf.
109. Nerenberg L. Elder abuse prevention: emerging trends and promising practices. New York: Springer; 2008.
110. Palmetto N, Davidson LL, Breitbart V, Rickert VI. Predictors of physical intimate partner violence in the lives of young women: victimization, perpetration, and bidirectional violence. Violence Vict. 2013;28:103–21. doi:10.1891/0886-6708.28.1.103.
111. Parra-Cardona JR, Meyer E, Schiamberg L, Post L. Elder abuse and neglect in Latino families: an ecological and culturally relevant theoretical framework for clinical practice. Fam Process. 2007;46(4):451–70. doi:10.1111/j.1545-5300.2007.00225.x.
112. Patel DM, Simon MA, Taylor RM. Contagion of violence: workshop summary. National Academies Press. 2013. http://www.nap.edu/catalog/13489/contagion-of-violence-workshop-summary.
113. Payne BJ, Gainey RR. Family violence and criminal justice: a life-course approach. 3rd ed. New Providence, NJ: Routledge; 2010.
114. Pearlin LI, Mullan JT, Semple SJ, Skaff MM. Caregiving and the stress process: an overview of concepts and their measures. Gerontologist. 1990;30:583–94. doi:10.1093/geront/30.5.583.
115. Penhale B. Older women, domestic violence, and elder abuse: a review of commonalities, differences, and shared approaches. J Elder Abuse Negl. 2003;15(3–4):163–83.
116. Penhale B. Responding and intervening in elder abuse and neglect. Ageing Int. 2010;35:235–52. doi:10.1007/s12126-010-9065-0.
117. Phelan A. Elder abuse: a review of progress in Ireland. J Elder Abuse Negl. 2014;26(2):172–88. doi:10.1080/08946566.2013.784088.
118. Phelan A. Elder abuse, ageism, human rights and citizenship: implications for nursing discourse. Nurs Inq. 2008;15(4):320–9. doi:10.1111/j.1440-1800.2008.00423.x.
119. Pillemer K, Finkelhor D. Causes of elder abuse: caregiver stress versus problem relatives. Am J Orthopsychiatry. 1989;59(2):179–87. doi:10.1111/j.1939-0025.1989.tb01649.x.
120. Pillemer KA, Wolf RS. Elder abuse: conflict in the family. Santa Barbara: Greenwood Publishing Group; 1986.
121. Podnieks E, Anetzberger GJ, Wilson SJ, Teaster PB, Wangmo T. WorldView environmental scan on elder abuse. J Elder Abuse Negl. 2010;22(1–2):164–79. doi:10.1080/08946560903445974.
122. Podnieks E, Wilson S. An exploratory study of responses to elder abuse in faith communities. J Elder Abuse Negl. 2003;15(3–4):137–62. doi:10.1300/J084v15n03_09.
123. Raghavan C, Rajah V, Gentile K, Collado L, Kavanagh AM. Community violence, social support networks, ethnic group differences, and male perpetration of intimate partner violence. J Interpers Violence. 2009;12:1132–49. doi:10.1177/0886260509331489.
124. Ramsey-Klawsnik H, Teaster PB, Mendiondo MS, Marcum JL, Abner EL. Sexual predators who target elders: findings from the first national study of sexual abuse in care facilities. J Elder Abuse Negl. 2008;20(4):353–76. doi:10.1080/08946560802359375.
125. Reed E. Intimate partner violence: a gender-based issue? Am J Public Health. 2008;98:197–8. doi:10.2105/AJPH.2007.125765.
126. Reeves KA, Desmarais SL, Nicholls TL, Douglas KS. Intimate partner abuse of older men: considerations for the assessment of risk. J Elder Abuse Negl. 2007;19(1–2):7–27. doi:10.1300/J084v19n01_02.
127. Renner LM, Whitney SD. Risk factors for unidirectional and bidirectional intimate partner violence among young adults. Child Abuse Negl. 2012;36:40–52. doi:10.1016/j.chiabu.2011.07.007.
128. Resnicow K, Braithwaite R, Ahluwalia J, Baranowski T. Cultural sensitivity in public health: defined and demystified. Ethn Dis. 1999;9:10–21.
129. Roberto KA. Abusive relationships in late life. In: George LK, Ferraro KF, editors. Handbook of aging and the social sciences. 8th ed. New York: Elsevier/Academic; 2016. p. 337–56.
130. Roberto KA, Blieszner R, Allen KR. Theorizing in family gerontology: new opportunities for research and practice. Fam Relat. 2006;55:513–25. doi:10.1111/j.1741-3729.2006.00422.x.
131. Roberto KA, McPherson MC, Brossoie N. Intimate partner violence in late life: a review of the empirical literature. Violence Against Women. 2014;19:1538–58. doi:10.1177/1077801213517564.
132. Roberto KA, McPherson M, Brossoie N. Intimate partner violence in late life: a review of the empirical literature. Violence Against Women. 2013;19:1538–58. doi:10.1177/1077801213517564.
133. Roberto KA, Teaster PT, McPherson M. Abuse in late life: unsuspecting elders and trusted others. In: Arditti J, editor. Family problems: stress, risk, and resilience. Hoboken, NJ: Wiley; 2015. p. 228–48.
134. Robertson K, Murachver T. Correlates of partner violence for incarcerated women and men. J Interpers Violence. 2007;22:639–55. doi:10.1177/0886260506298835.
135. Roger KS, Brownridge DA, Ursel J. Theorizing low levels of reporting of abuse of older immigrant women. Violence Against Women. 2015;21:632–51. doi:10.1177/1077801214545021.
136. Romero D, Meeder B, Kleinberg J. Differences in the mechanics of information diffusion across topics: Idioms, political hashtags, and complex contagion on twitter. The 20th International World Wide Web Conference (WWW), Hyderabad, India. 2011.
137. Savla J, Roberto KA, Jaramillo AL, Gambrel LE, Karimi H, Butner LM. Childhood abuse affects emotional closeness with family in mid and later life. Child Abuse Negl. 2013;37:388–99. doi:10.1016/j.chiabu.2012.12.009.
138. Schiamberg LB, Gans D. An ecological framework for contextual risk factors in elder abuse by adult children. J Elder Abuse Negl. 1999;11(1):79–103. doi:10.1300/J084v11n01_05.
139. Schiamberg LB, Gans D. Elder abuse by adult children: an applied ecological framework for understanding contextual risk factors and the intergenerational character of quality of life. Int J Aging Hum Dev. 2000;50(4):329–59. doi:10.2190/DXAX-8TJ9-RG5K-MPU5.
140. Schiamberg LB, Oehmke J, Zhang Z, Barboza GE, Griffore RK, Von Heydrich L, Post LA, Weatherill RP, Mastin T. Physical abuse of older adults in nursing homes: a random sample survey

of adults with an elderly family member in a nursing home. J Elder Abuse Negl. 2012;24(1):65–83. doi:10.1080/08946566.2011.608056.

141. Settersten RA, editor. Invitation to the life course: toward new understandings of later life. Amityville, NY: Baywood; 2003.
142. Shaffer DR, Dooley WK, Williamson GM. Endorsement of proactively aggressive caregiving strategies moderates the relation between caregiver mental health and potentially harmful caregiving behavior. Psychol Aging. 2007;22(3):494–504. doi:10.1037/0882-7974.22.3.494.
143. Shoemaker PJ, Tankard JW, Lasorsa DL. How to build social science theories. Thousand Oaks, CA: Sage; 2004.
144. Smith B. Objects and their environments: From Aristotle to ecological ontology. In: Frank A, Raper J, Cheylan J, editors. The life and motion of socioeconomic units (GISDATA 8). London: Taylor and Francis; 2001. p. 79–97.
145. Straka SM, Montminy L. Responding to the needs of older women experiencing domestic violence. Violence Against Women. 2006;12(3):251–67. doi:10.1177/1077801206286221.
146. Teaster PB, Otto JM, Dugar TD, Mendiondo MS, Abner EL, Cecil KA. The 2004 survey of state Adult Protective Services: Abuse of adults 60 years of age and older. Report to the National Center on Elder Abuse, Administration on Aging, Washington. 2006. http://www.ncea.aoa.gov/Resources/Publication/docs/2-14-06_FINAL_60_REPORT.pdf.
147. Teaster PB, Nerenberg L, Stansbury K. A national study of multidisciplinary teams. J Elder Abuse Negl. 2003;15(3/4):91–108. doi:10.1300/J084v15n03_06.
148. Teaster PB, Ramsey-Klawsnik H, Abner EL, Kim S. The sexual victimization of older women living in nursing homes. J Elder Abuse Negl. 2015;. doi:10.1080/08946566.2015.1082453.
149. Teaster PB, Roberto KA, Dugar TA. Intimate partner violence of rural aging women. Fam Relat. 2006;55:636–48. doi:10.1111/j.1741-3729.2006.00432.x.
150. Teaster PB, Wangmo T. Kentucky's local elder abuse coordinating councils: a model for other states. J Elder Abuse Negl. 2010;22(1/2):191–206. doi:10.1080/08946560903446063.
151. Teaster PB, Wangmo T, Vorsky F. Abuse in aging families. In: Blieszner R, Bedford V, editors. Handbook of families and aging. 2nd ed. Denver, CO: Praeger; 2012. p. 409–30.
152. Tong H, Prakash BA, Eliassi-Rad T, Faloutsos M, Faloutsos C. Gelling and melting large graphs by edge manipulation. 21st ACM international conference on information and knowledge management (CIKM), Maui, HI. 2012.
153. United Nations. Universal declaration of human rights. 1948. http://www.un.org/en/universal-declaration-human-rights/.
154. United Nations. Vienna declaration and programme for action. World conference on human rights, (14–25 June 1993, Vienna). Geneva: United Nations General Assembly 1993.
155. United Nations. Abuse of older persons; recognising and responding to abuse of older persons in a global context. New York: United Nations Economic and Social Council. United Nations/International Association of Gerontology; 2002.
156. United States Government Printing Office. Public law 111-148-MAR. 23, 2010. Retrieved from http://www.gpo.gov/fdsys/pkg/PLAW-111publ148/pdf/PLAW-111publ148.pdf.
157. Vinton L. Abused older women: battered women or abused elders? J Women Aging. 1991;3(3):5–19. doi:10.1300/J074v03n03_03.
158. Vinton L. Working with abused older women from a feminist perspective. J Women Aging. 1999;11(2–3):85–100. doi:10.1300/J074v11n02_07.
159. Vinton L. Battered women's shelters and older women: The Florida experience. J Family Violence. 1992;7(1):63–72. doi:10.1007/BF00978725.
160. Vladescu D, Eveleigh K, Ploeg J, Patterson C. An evaluation of a client-centered case management program for elder abuse. J Elder Abuse Negl. 2000;11(4):5–22. doi:10.1300/J084v11n04_02.
161. Walsh CA, Olson JL, Ploeg J, Lohfeld L, MacMillan HL. Elder abuse and oppression: voices of marginalized elders. J Elder Abuse Negl. 2010;23(1):17–42. doi:10.1080/08946566.2011.534705.
162. Walsh CA, Yon Y. Developing an empirical profile for elder abuse research in Canada. J Elder Abuse Negl. 2012;24(2):104–19. doi:10.1080/08946566.2011.644088.
163. Walt SM. The relationship between theory and policy in international relations. Annu Rev Polit Sci. 2005;8:23–48. doi:10.1146/annurev.polisci.7.012003.104904.
164. Wangmo T, Teaster PB, Mendiondo M, Grace J, Blandford C, Fisher S, Wong W, Fardo D. An ecological systems examination of elder abuse: a week in the life of adult protective services. J Elder Abuse Negl. 2014;26(5):440–57. doi:10.1080/08946566.2013.800463.
165. Watts D. A simple model of global cascades on random networks. Proc Natl Acad Sci, 2002;99:5766–71. http://www.jstor.org/stable/3058573.
166. Wilkinson R. Linking social structure and individual vulnerability. J Commun Work Dev. 2004;5:31–47.
167. Williams M. Problems of knowledge: a critical introduction to epistemology. New York: Oxford University Press; 2001.
168. Williamson GM, Shaffer DR. Relationship quality and potentially harmful behaviors by spousal caregivers: how we were then, how we are now. Psychol Aging. 2001;16:217–26. doi:10.1037/e323142004-005.
169. Williamson GM, Martin-Cook K, Weiner MF, Svetlik DA, Saine K, Hynan LS, Dooley WK, Schulz R. Caregiver resentment: explaining why care recipients exhibit problem behavior. Rehabil Psychol. 2005;50:215–23. doi:10.1037/0090-5550.50.3.215.
170. Wolf RS, Strugnell C, Godkin M. Preliminary findings from the three models project on elderly abuse. Worcester, MA: University of Massachusetts, University Center of Aging; 1982.
171. World Health Organization. The Toronto declaration on the global prevention of elder abuse. Geneva: WHO; 2002.
172. Wright EM, Benson ML. Clarifying the effects of neighborhood context on violence "behind closed doors". Justice Q. 2011;28:775–98. doi:10.1080/07418825.2010.533687.
173. Yan E. Abuse of older persons with dementia by family caregivers: Results of a 6-month prospective study in Hong Kong. Int J Geriatr Psychiatry. 2014;29:1018–27. doi:10.1002/gps.4092.
174. Yan E, Kwok T. Abuse of older Chinese with dementia by family caregivers: an inquiry into the role of caregiver burden. Int J Geriatr Psychiatry. 2011;26(5):527–35. doi:10.1002/gps.2561.
175. Yon Y, Wister AV, Mitchell B, Gutman G. A national comparison of spousal abuse in mid- and old age. J Elder Abuse Negl. 2014;26(1):80–105. doi:10.1080/08946566.2013.784085.

Part II
Epidemiology of the Issue

Global Prevalence of Elder Abuse in the Community

3

Joah L. Williams, Margaret Davis, and Ron Acierno

The number of people aged 65 or older will triple to well over one billion, or 16 % of the world's population, by 2050 [67]. The majority of these older adults will, of course, continue to reside independently in the community, albeit with relatively increased health and care needs, requiring families and societies to determine how to best provide support to these elders. Failure to provide such care, however, particularly insofar as care includes social support and connection, is reflected in high rates of elder abuse. Despite cross-cultural reverence, at least in principle, for older adults, as many as 6 % of community-residing elders worldwide have experienced significant abuse *in the past month*, with rates of abuse varying widely across general population studies, ranging from 3.2 to 27.5 % [21]. Therefore, prevalence of elder abuse around the world likely varies significantly across cultures and nations, both with respect to specific acts of abuse, as well as culturally derived definitions of those acts as abusive. This chapter reports on the global prevalence of elder abuse, focusing primarily on general population-based studies from around the world to highlight the scope of the problem. While trying to minimize overlapping content with other chapters, we will begin briefly with definitions central to the study and evaluation of elder abuse.

J.L. Williams
Department of Psychology, University of Missouri—Kansas City, Kansas City, MO, USA
e-mail: williamsjoah@umkc.edu

M. Davis
Department of Psychiatry, VA Ann Arbor Health Care System/University of Michigan, Ann Arbor, MI, USA

R. Acierno
College of Nursing, Medical University of South Carolina, 99 Jonathan Lucas Street, MSC 160, Charleston, SC 29425, USA

R. Acierno (✉)
Ralph H. Johnson Veterans Affairs Medical Center, Charleston, SC, USA
e-mail: acierno@musc.edu

3.1 Concept Definitions

Given that the focus of this chapter is on the prevalence of elder abuse in the community, we will begin by orienting the reader to the basic definition of prevalence. Prevalence is here defined as the proportion of persons in a given population (i.e., older adults) who have a particular attribute (i.e., has experienced elder abuse) over a specified period of time [66]. Turning to definitions of elder abuse, most widely accepted taxonomies of elder abuse include five categories of mistreatment: emotional/psychological/verbal abuse, financial exploitation, neglect, physical abuse, and sexual abuse. While categories of mistreatment are generally consistent across taxonomies, one point of divergence is whether elder abuse should only include those violent acts that occur in the context of a "trust relationship" or can include violent acts perpetrated by strangers [12]. These trust relationships can include relationships with family members, friends, or other caregivers—essentially anyone the older adult knows and trusts to help care for them and offer support. Historically, nonfamilial perpetrated criminal violence has been classified as assault, while violence perpetrated by those in trust relationships with the older adult has been classified as abuse. We assert that from the perspective of the victim, and from the perspective of the health care provider, being hit, threatened, or sexually assaulted are acts of violence demanding remedy, irrespective of the perpetrator relationship to the victim. Moreover, as both the outcomes (e.g., injury, depression, isolation) and the remedies (e.g., social support and connection, reporting to authorities, referral for services) are similarly independent of "trust relationship," excluding assaults perpetrated by strangers and others outside of a trust relationship may grossly underestimate the true prevalence of the problem. Additionally, both types of violence may share overlapping risk and protective factors, so that neglecting to study one may impede progress in the other. Finally, the definition of a "trust relationship" is a moving target (e.g., is such a

X. Dong (ed.), *Elder Abuse*, DOI 10.1007/978-3-319-47504-2_3

relationship defined by legal fiduciary duty, cohabitation or proximity, bidirectional expectations of service for payment, etc.). Therefore, we here provide definitions of each category of elder abuse used in the National Elder Mistreatment Study (NEMS; [4]), the largest United States epidemiological (i.e., nationwide random sampling) study to date of mistreatment against community-residing older adults age 60 and over perpetrated by individuals both known and unknown to the older adult. For the purposes of this chapter, we use the terms abuse and mistreatment interchangeably, although others also may use terms such as maltreatment, domestic violence, family assault, and intimate partner violence to capture some of the same events.

The category of mistreatment called emotional or psychological abuse includes events such as being yelled at, verbally attacked, threatened, or scolded in such a way that an older adult feels threatened or concerned about their safety. Emotional abuse can also include repeated acts of verbal humiliation or embarrassment like calling an older adult stupid or ignoring them for days at a time. Financial abuse or exploitation is defined as acts including spending or stealing an older adult's money without their consent, withholding documents or other important financial information, or forcing older adults to sign financial documents against their will. Note that this is different from stranger fraud in which an older adult is "scammed," as in cases of insurance fraud or investment schemes. Neglect involves instances in which an older adult has one or more unmet needs of daily living *and* an identified individual responsible for meeting those needs repeatedly refuses to do so. Note that neglect is differentiated from emotional abuse-related neglect, in which attention is withdrawn. Neglect is also differentiated from the related phenomenon of elder self-neglect, which is not typically included in the category of neglect as elder abuse [2]. Self-neglect refers to situations where an older adult refuses to meet his or her own health, nutritional, or hygienic needs. Elder physical abuse can include being hit, restrained, or otherwise injured (e.g., being struck by someone or threatened with a weapon). Elder sexual abuse includes acts of forced, unwanted touching, viewing, intercourse, being forced to undress or to be photographed in states of undress, and molestation.

3.2 Methodological Issues in Assessing Elder Abuse Prevalence in the Community: Specific Lessons Learned

Population estimates of elder mistreatment may be obtained through multiple methods of varying reliability, cost, and accuracy, including agency record reviews, sentinel (e.g., healthcare provider) reports, translation of criminal justice statistics, caretaker and family member interviews, and interviews of elderly respondents themselves. Choosing the means by which elder mistreatment is measured in epidemiological studies will be determined in large part by the cognitive status of the participants and the budget of investigators. Quite simply, interview and self-report survey assessment methods with excellent reliability, validity, and supporting empirical literatures that are used effectively with cognitively intact individuals are not applicable to some groups, such as very young children, or individuals with dementia, a disorder characterizing a small proportion of the older adult community population. That is, in the small minority of community-residing older adults (about 5–8 %) who suffer from *significant* dementia, there is no real means by which to directly obtain information regarding mistreatment. By contrast, methods by which to assess mistreatment against demented or otherwise cognitively impaired older adults in nursing homes or other residential settings have been validated, such as ecological momentary analysis via video recording in situ [63]. However, this population is not the focus of this chapter.

For older adults without cognitive impairment, we suggest that the most feasible, sensitive, and cost-effective means of assessing mistreatment will be to directly interview older adults themselves using either in-person (preferably with a computer or tablet interface to enhance anonymity while maintaining social presence, see [9, 10]) or telephone survey methodology, although telephone survey methodology is probably far more cost-effective than in-person interviewing [3]. Telephone-based interviewing also appears to be a valid alternative to in-person interviewing, with both methods producing comparable rates of lifetime and recent elder abuse [5]. Regardless of the methodology chosen (e.g., in-person vs. telephone), prevalence estimates for criminal victimization, including sexual assault, physical assault, and domestic violence will vary widely according to parameters of assessment methodology, including assessment context, assessment structure, assessor characteristics, and trauma definition [13, 31, 35, 38, 56, 57]. For example, contextual cues may prime respondents to respond in a particular manner. That is, assessment by medical doctors conducted in a primary care facility may be less likely to detect victimization than assessment by criminal justice system epidemiologists.

In addition to definitional problems, mistreatment, particularly that type of mistreatment associated with interpersonal, psychological, or cultural stigma (e.g., sexual abuse), is not readily reported by all victims. Indeed, many victims of assault or abuse do not openly identify themselves as such. Reasons that older adults may be reluctant to report episodes of abusive violence include blaming oneself for the abuse (e.g., an older adult blames his/her parenting style for an adult child's abusive behavior), embarrassment, and fear of retribution or more violence if the disclosure were discovered [3]. In light of these barriers to disclosure, a victim must: (1) recall the abuse event, (2) label the abuse as such, (3) be queried by an investigator who is using a similar label/definition, (4) be willing and psychologically able to disclose the abuse, and (5) be able to safely disclose the abuse (e.g., when the perpetrator lives with the respondent) in order to report to an investigator that a particular type of elder mistreatment has occurred. While straightforward, these factors must not be overlooked. Many respondents do not label mistreatment as such when the perpetrator is a relative or spouse, or when there was only limited force or *threat* of force used, or when the psychological effects of such a label are too distressing.

Given that the aforementioned factors combine to minimize disclosure of elder abuse by its victims, certain procedural aspects of assessment can be used to improve sensitivity, and two components appear crucial: (1) contextually orienting, empathetic preface statements, and (2) behavioral descriptions of index events that elicit closed-ended responses, as opposed to culturally laden terms that reference index events. Preface statements must provide contextual orientation along three lines: first, they must inform the respondent that the assessor is interested in abuse that happened at any time, not just in the past month or year. Second, preface statements must clarify that the assessor is interested in abuse perpetrated by any person, not just one class (e.g., spouse, stranger, children). Finally, preface statements should clarify that the assessor is interested in events irrespective of whether or not they were reported to authorities, as there is some indication that individuals may be less likely to disclose events they did not report.

After the preface statement orients a respondent contextually (e.g., "please report any mistreatment by any person occurring at any time"), it is essential to use detailed, behaviorally specific, closed-ended descriptions of abuse events under investigation. Early surveys employed "gateway" screening questions characterized by very limited behavioral specificity (e.g., "have you ever been sexually assaulted?"). If respondents endorsed the gateway question, further questions about assault followed. Unfortunately, gateway questions without preface statements lack specificity and do not adequately orient respondents to the type of responses the examiner is interested in evaluating and are extremely subject to an individual respondent's subjective interpretation of queries [38]. By contrast, behaviorally specific descriptions of abuse events minimize variance associated with cultural differences, personal differences in intellect, psychological stability, general willingness to disclose, or understanding of criminal justice terminology (e.g., "rape," "aggravated assault"). Another advantage of using behaviorally specific descriptions of abuse events is that using multiple, behaviorally specific questions helps to capture the considerable heterogeneity in events that constitute specific categories of abusive violence (e.g., physical abuse may involve being restrained or threatened with a weapon). These questions are highly detailed and require only "yes" or "no" answers. In addition to removing definitional and cultural variance, closed-ended "yes" or "no" questions simplify the role of respondent and minimize the risk that anyone will overhear disclosure of highly personal events, particularly during telephone interviews, where queries are unintelligible to others not on the phone. Examples of preface statements and behaviorally specific responses used in our National Elder Mistreatment Study for sexual abuse are given below. You will note that they give very little room for error of interpretation:

Sexual Mistreatment: Sexual mistreatment was defined as an affirmative answer to any one of the following three questions. After it was determined that such an event had occurred, the timing and characteristics of the event (e.g., since age 60, past year, perpetrator status, reporting to police, time frame) were defined.

1. "I am going to ask you questions about unwanted sexual advances that you may have experienced over your lifetime. People do not always report such experiences to the police or discuss them with family or friends. The person making the unwanted advances isn't always a stranger, but can be a friend, romantic partner, or even a family member or someone you trust to help you or help take care of you. Such experiences can occur anytime in a person's life. Regardless of how long ago it happened or who made the advances, has anyone ever made you have sex or oral sex by using force or threatening to harm you or someone close to you?"

2a. "Has anyone ever touched your breasts or pubic area or made you touch his penis by using force or threat of force?"

2b. "Has anyone ever touched your pubic area or made you touch their pubic area by using force or threat of force?"

3a. "Has anyone ever forced you to undress or expose your breasts or pubic area when you didn't want to?"

3b. "Has anyone ever forced you to undress or expose your pubic area when you didn't want to?"

3.3 Methods

To provide a comprehensive review of the global prevalence of elder abuse in the community, we searched the global literature in PubMed and CINAHL using search terms *prevalence*, *elder abuse*, and *elder mistreatment*. We also searched the reference lists of review articles to identify relevant studies. For the purposes of this chapter, we chose to include primary research on the prevalence of elder abuse

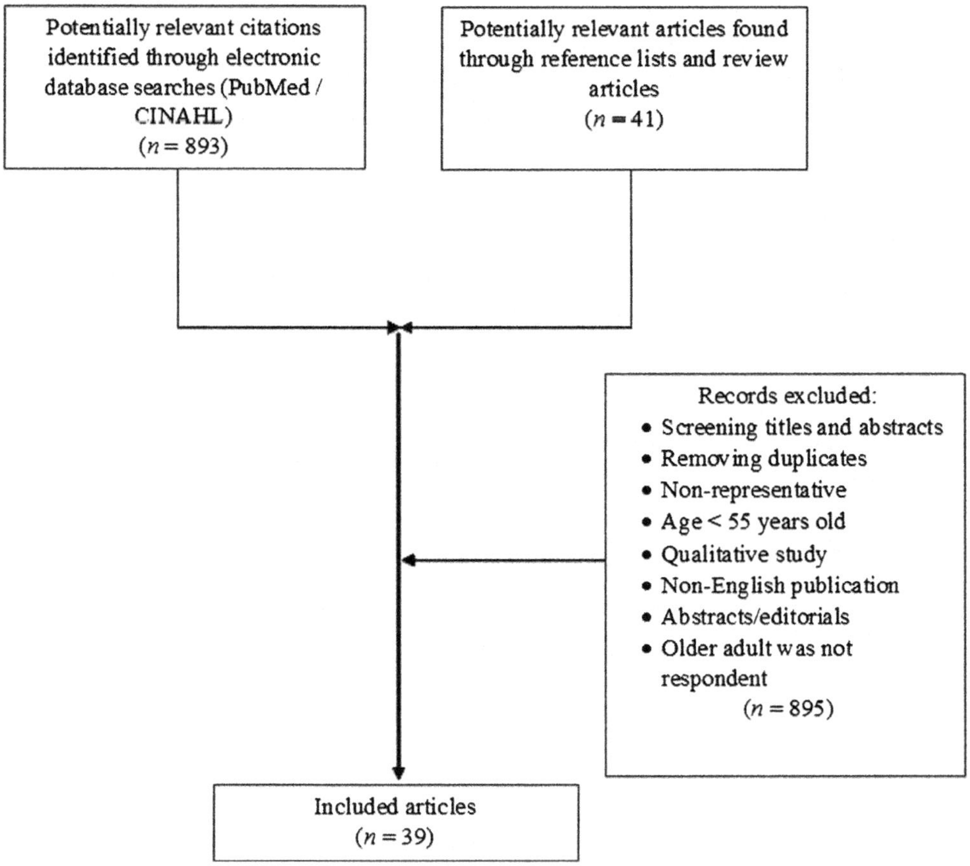

Fig. 3.1 Logic chart depicting review process for global prevalence studies

among community-residing adults (age 55 and older), where older adults were directly asked about their abusive experiences given that this is the recommended method of assessment with cognitively intact older adults. Therefore, we did not include studies where prevalence estimates were based on reports of caregivers or other persons in close contact with the older adult. Other exclusion criteria included studies of older adults living in nursing homes or residential care settings, qualitative studies, and studies that recruited individuals younger than 55 years of age. We also excluded studies that appeared only as editorials, meeting abstracts, and non-English publications (see Fig. 3.1). The studies selected for inclusion are listed in Table 3.1.

3.4 Global Prevalence of Elder Abuse in the Community

Rather than discuss each study listed in Table 3.1, our goal in this section is to highlight the variability in methodology across elder abuse prevalence studies and illustrate common challenges in assessing the community prevalence of elder abuse by discussing select studies in detail. We begin close to home by discussing the methodology and associated findings from the first large-scale studies of domestic elder abuse prevalence based directly on reports from nationally representative samples of older adults across the U.S. The first major attempt was conducted as part of the National Social Life, Health and Aging Project (NSHAP; [40]). The NSHAP included a nationally representative probability sample of 3005 community-residing adults aged 57–85 years who were asked a series of single item questions assessing the past year prevalence of specific forms of abuse, including verbal abuse ("Is there anyone who insults you or puts you down?"), financial exploitation ("Is there anyone who has taken your money or belongings without your OK or prevented you from getting them even when you ask?"), and physical mistreatment ("Is there anyone who hits, kicks, slaps, or throws things at you?"). The overall weighted response rate for the study was 75.5 %. Participants were asked about potential abusive events during in-home interviews completed by field interviewers, while 33 % of the sample completed elder abuse screening questions on mail-in self-report questionnaires left by the interviewer during in-home interviews. As discussed earlier in this chapter, contextual factors such as assessment context and assessor characteristics can influence response patterns, and another individual was present in approximately one-third of the in-home interviews. Overall, 9 % of these older adults reported past year verbal abuse, 3.5 % endorsed past year

Table 3.1 Prevalence of elder abuse in the community

References	Population	Age, sex and race/ethnicity	Survey methods	Participation rate	Measure	Alpha	Elder abuse types	# item	Cut-off points	Prevalence
North America										
Pillemer and Finkelhor [52]	2020 older adults in Boston	65 or older; 65 % women; 94 % white	Telephone and in person	72 %	Modified CTS, OARS	N/A	Verbal	N/A	≥10 times	1-year 1.1 %
							Physical	10	≥1 item	Since 65 2.0 %
							Neglect	10	≥10 times/serious problem	1-year 0.4 %
							Overall	N/A	[a]	3.2 %
Podnieks [53]	2008 Canadian older adults	65–100 years old; 67 % women	Telephone	N/A	Modified CTS, OARS, Own items	N/A	Financial	6	≥1 item	Since 65 2.5 %
							Verbal	2	≥10 times	1-year 1.4 %
							Physical	N/A	N/A	1-year 0.5 %
							Neglect	N/A	2–10 times/serious problem	1-year 0.4 %
							Overall	N/A	[a]	4.0 %; ≥2 types: 0.8 %
Buri et al. [14]	498 older adults in the Iowa Medicaid Waiver Program	65–101; 70.9 % women; 96 % white and 3 % AA	Mail survey	49 %	Elder abuse screen	N/A	Psych	1	≥1 item	1.0 %
							Physical	1	≥1 item	2.0 %
							Financial	2	≥1 item	17.5 %
							Neglect	1	≥1 item	6.8 %
							Overall	5	≥1 item	20.9 %; 1 type:15.8 %; 2 types: 4.0 %; 3 types:1.0 %
Laumann et al. [40]	3005 older adults in the National, Social Life, Health and Aging project	57–85 years old; 51.2 % women; 80.7 % white, 10.0 % AA; 6.8 % Latino; 2.5 % other	In person and mail survey	75.5 %	H–S/EAST and the VASS	N/A	Verbal	1	≥1 item	1-year 9 %
							Financial	1	≥1 item	1-year 3.5 %
							Physical	1	≥1 item	1-year 0.2 %
							Overall	3	[a]	N/A

(continued)

Table 3.1 (continued)

References	Population	Age, sex and race/ethnicity	Survey methods	Participation rate	Measure	Alpha	Elder abuse types	# item	Cut-off points	Prevalence
Acierno et al. [4]	5777 cognitively intact US community population	60–97 years; 60 % women, 88 % white, 7 % AA, 4 % Latino, 2 % Am Indian, 1 % Asian	Random digit dialing and computer-assisted interview	69 %	Interpersonal violence measure and Acierno EM measure	N/A	Emotional	4	≥1 item	1-year 4.6 %; Since 60: 13.5 %
							Physical	3	≥1 item	1-year 1.6 %; Since 60: 1.8 %
							Sexual	3	≥1 item	1-year 0.6 %; Since 60: 0.3 %
							Neglect	6	≥1 item	1-year 5.1 %
							Financial	6	≥1 item	1-year 5.2 %
							Overall	22	≥1 item	Any abuse (exclude financial): 10 %
Beach et al. [9] [10]	903 U.S. community person with landline phone, English-speaking, no severe cognitive impairment	60 or older; 73.3 % female; 23.3 % AA, 72.8 % white, 3.9 % other	Random digit dialing, and in-person, self-administered CAIVR	37.7 %	Modified CTS	N/A	Financial	4	≥1 item	6-month 3.5 %, AA 12.9 %, white 2.4 %
							Psych	8	≥3 items or any yes to threats items	6-month all 8.2 %, AA 16.1 %, white 7.2 %
							Overall	12	[a]	N/A
Amstadter et al. [7]	902 cognitively intact South Carolina community population	60–97 years; 59.9 % women, 77 % white, 17.3 % AA, 1.9 % Am Indian, 0.1 % Pac Islander	Random digit dialing and computer-assisted interview	82 %	Interpersonal violence measure and Acierno EM measure	N/A	Emotional	4	≥1 item	1-year 5.1 %; Since 60 12.9 %
							Physical	3	≥1 item	1-year 1.8 %; Since 60 2.1 %
							Sexual	3	≥1 item	1-year 0.3 %; Since 60 0.3 %
							Neglect	6	≥1 item	1-year 5.4 %
							Financial	6	≥1 item	1-year 6.6 %
							Overall	22	[a]	N/A
DeLiema et al. [22]	198 Latinos in low-income, minority areas in Los Angeles	66 years or older; 56 % women	In person interview	65 %	The USC-OACS	Psy: 0.80; Phy: 0.85; Sex: 0.65; Fin: 0.49	Psych	9	≥1 item	1-year 24.8 %;
							Physical	15	≥1 item	1-year 10.7 %
							Sexual	4	≥1 item	1-year 9.0 %
							Financial	14	≥1 item	1-year 16.7 %
							Neglect	12	≥1 item	1-year 11.7 %
							Overall	54	≥1 item	1-year 40.4 %; multiple: 21 %

(continued)

Table 3.1 (continued)

References	Population	Age, sex and race/ethnicity	Survey methods	Participation rate	Measure	Alpha	Elder abuse types	# item	Cut-off points	Prevalence
Dong et al. [26]	4627 adults Chicago Health and Aging project	65 and older; 64.4 % women	In person interview	N/A	The Chicago elder self-neglect scale	0.97–0.98	Self-neglect	21	≥1 item	AA: men: 13.2 %, women: 10.9 % white: men: 2.4 %, women: 2.6 %
Dong et al. [25]	3159 Chinese elderly in Chicago	60 and older; 58.9 % women	In person interview	91.9 %	H–S/EAST and VASS	0.80	Overall	10	≥1 item	Since 60 15.0 %
Dong [23]	3159 Chinese elderly in Chicago	60 and older; 58.9 % women	In person interview	91.9 %	CTS; caregiver neglect assessment; Financial abuse assessment	N/A	Psych	8	≥1 item ≥2 items ≥3 items Beach Def Pillemer Def	Since 60 1.1–9.8 %
							Physical	10	≥1 item	Since 60 1.1 %
							Sexual	1	≥1 item	Since 60 0.2 %
							Financial	17	≥1 item of the 17 items; ≥1 item of the 14 items	Since 60 8.8–9.3 %
							Neglect	20	Least restrictive; More restrictive	Since 60 4.6–11.1 %
							Overall	56	Most restrictive; Moderate restrictive; Least restrictive	Since 60 13.9–25.8 %
Peterson et al. [51]	4156 English or Spanish speaking community cognitive intact older New Yorkers	60–101 years; 64.5 % women; 19.0 % AA, 75.5 % Caucasian, 6.0 % Latino, 0.8 % AI, 1.2 % Asian	Random digit dialing	75.2 %	Built on prior measures and expert consensus	N/A	Financial	5	≥1 item	1-year 2.7 %
Burnes et al. [15]	4156 English or Spanish speaking community cognitive intact older New Yorkers	60–101 years; 64.5 % women; 19.0 % AA, 75.5 % Caucasian, 6.0 % Latino, 0.8 % AI, 1.2 % Asian	Random digit dialing	75.2 %	Modified CTS, OARS	N/A	Emotional	N/A	≥10 times and rated "very serious"	1-year 1.9 %
							Physical	N/A	≥1 item	1-year 1.8 %
							Neglect	N/A	2–10 times/serious problem	1-year 10.8 %
							Overall	N/A	[a]	1-year 4.6 %

(continued)

Table 3.1 (continued)

References	Population	Age, sex and race/ethnicity	Survey methods	Participation rate	Measure	Alpha	Elder abuse types	# item	Cut-off points	Prevalence
South America										
Carmona-Torres et al. [17]	210 cognitively intact older adults in the Health Insurance for Elderly Care of Santa Cruz de la Sierra (Bolivia)	60 and older; 57.6 % women	Interview	N/A	EASI, Social Work Evaluation Form	N/A	Psych	N/A	N/A	1-year 32.4 %
							Physical	N/A	N/A	1-year 7.1 %
							Financial	N/A	N/A	1-year 6.7 %
							Neglect	N/A	N/A	1-year 21.9 %
							Overall	N/A	N/A	1-year 39 %
Europe										
Kivelä et al. [37]	1086 older adults from a semi-industrialized town in Finland	65 and older	Interview and mail survey	89 %	Own items	N/A	Overall	N/A	≥ 1 time	Since retirement excluding stranger and institutional abuse 5.4 %; men: 2.5 %, women: 7.0 %
Comijs et al. [19]	1797 older people living independently in Amsterdam, the Netherlands	69–89 years; 62.8 % women	Interview	44 %	CTS, Measure of Wife Abuse, Violence Against Man Scale	N/A	Verbal	N/A	≥ 10 times	1-year 3.2 %
							Physical	N/A	≥ 1 time	1-year 1.2 % Since 65, 3.9 %
							Financial	N/A	≥ 1 time	1-year 1.4 % Since 65 4.8 %
							Neglect	N/A	≥ 10 times	1-year 0.2 %
							Overall	N/A	[a]	1-year 5.6 %, ≥ 2 types 0.4 %
Puchkov [54]	2881 older adults known to Social Services in four districts of Saratov, Russia	60 or older; 85.4 % women	Self-administered questionnaire or structured interview	N/A	Not specified	N/A	Overall	N/A	N/A	28.6 %
Pérez-Cárceles et al. [55]	460 older patients visiting several different health centers in Spain	65 years and older; 53.3 % women	In person interview	N/A	The Canadian Task Force and the AMA	N/A	Psych	4	≥ 1 item	20.7 %
							Physical	1	≥ 1 item	2.4 %
							Sexual	1	≥ 1 item	1.3 %
							Financial	3	≥ 1 item	7.2 %
							Neglect	9	≥ 1 item	24 %
							Withhold	1	≥ 1 item	31.1 %
							Overall	19	≥ 1 item	44.6 %

(continued)

Table 3.1 (continued)

References	Population	Age, sex and race/ethnicity	Survey methods	Participation rate	Measure	Alpha	Elder abuse types	# item	Cut-off points	Prevalence
Ajdukovic et al. [6]	303 older adults in Croatia	65–97 years; 76.6 % women	In person interview	N/A	Elder Abuse in the Family Questionnaire	Overall: 0.97; phy: 0.93; psy: 0.87; sex: 0.91; fin: 0.91	Psych	8	N/A	1-year 24.1 %
							Physical	7	N/A	1-year 4.4 %
							Sexual	2	N/A	1-year 2.1 %
							Financial	3	N/A	1-year 6.4 %
							Overall	20	N/A	1-year 61.1 %
Biggs et al. [11]	2111 older adults in the community in U.K.	66 and older	In person interview	N/A	Built on literature	N/A	Psych	6	≥10 times	1-year 0.4 %
							Physical	10	≥1 time	1-year 0.4 %
							Sexual	7	≥1 time	1-year 0.2 %
							Financial	8	≥1 time	1-year 0.7 %
							Neglect	3	≥10 or ≤10 but serious	1-year 1.1 %
							Overall	34	[a]	2.6 % with neglect 1.6 % without neglect
Garre-Olmo et al. [28]	676 community-dwelling older adults in Girona, Spain	75 years and older; 58.2 % women	In person interview	82 %	The AMA	N/A	Psych	3	≥1 item	1-year 15.2 %
							Physical	2	≥1 item	1-year 0.1 %
							Financial	2	≥1 item	1-year 4.7 %
							Neglect	2	≥1 item	1-year 16.0 %
							Overall	9	≥1 item	1-year 29.3 %; 2 types: 3.6 %; 3 types: 0.1 %
Kissal and Beşer [36]	331 older adults in a population offering care by a primary health care center in Izmir, Turkey	65 years and above; 56.8 % women	In person interview	N/A	The investigator decided whether abuse and neglect	N/A	Psych	1	≥2/month	6-month 9.4 %
							Physical	1	≥2/month	6-month 4.2 %
							Sexual	1	Any	6-month 0.9 %
							Financial	1	Any	6-month 2.1 %
							Neglect	1	≥2/month	6-month 8.2 %
							Overall	5	[a]	6-month 13.3 %
Naughton et al. [46]	2021 community-dwelling older people in Ireland	65 years and older; 55 % women	In person interview	83 %	CTS and questions from the U.K. and NY prevalence studies	N/A	Psych	N/A	≥10 items or serious	1-year 1.2 %
							Physical	N/A	≥1 item	1-year 0.5 %
							Sexual	N/A	≥1 item	1-year 0.05 %
							Financial	N/A	≥1 item	1-year 1.3 %
							Neglect	N/A	≥10 items or serious	1-year 0.3 %
							Overall	N/A	[a]	1-year 2.2 %

(continued)

Table 3.1 (continued)

References	Population	Age, sex and race/ethnicity	Survey methods	Participation rate	Measure	Alpha	Elder abuse types	# item	Cut-off points	Prevalence
Lindert et al. [42]	4467 older adults in seven cities from seven countries in Europe	60–84; 57.3 % women	In person interview and mail questionnaire	45.2 %	Modified CTS	N/A	Psych	11	≥ 1 item	1-year 10.4–24.6 %
							Physical	17	≥ 1 item	1-year 1.4–4.0 %
							Sexual	8	≥ 1 item	1-year 0.3–1.5 %
							Financial	9	≥ 1 item	1-year 1.8–7.8 %
							Neglect	13	≥ 1 item	1-year 0.6–3.7 %
							Overall	52	≥ 1 item	1-year 12.7–30.8 %
Gil et al. [29]	1123 older adults living in private households in Portugal	60 and older; 56.4 % women	Random digit dialing and computer-assisted interview	74 %	Own items	N/A	Psych	3	≥ 10 times	1-year 6.3 %
							Physical	3	≥ 1 time	1-year 2.3 %
							Sexual	1	≥ 1 time	1-year 0.2 %
							Financial	4	≥ 1 time	1-year 6.3 %
							Neglect	1	≥ 10 times	1-year 0.4 %
							Overall	12	[a]	1-year 15.0 %; ≥ 2 types 3.4 %
Africa and the Middle East										
Lowenstein et al. [44]	1045 community older adults from the first national survey in Israel	65 or older; 62.5 % women	In person interview	75 %	CTS2, short situational descriptions, and the IRTA	N/A	Verbal	N/A	N/A	1-year 13.9 %
							Phy/sex	N/A	N/A	1-year 2 %
							Financial	9	N/A	1-year 6.6 %
							Neglect	5	N/A	1-year 24.2 %
							Limitation freedom	N/A	N/A	1-year 2.7 %
							Overall	N/A	[a]	1-year 35.0 %
Abdel Rahman and El Gaafary [1]	1106 older adults living at their homes in the rural area of Mansoura city, Dakahilia Governrate, Egypt	60 and older; 53.2 % women	In person interview	95.3 %	Actual abuse tool, questionnaire to elicit EA, EM instrument, risk for abuse tool	N/A	Psych	5	N/A	1-year 5.1 %
							Phy/sex	3	N/A	1-year 5.7 %
							Financial	2	N/A	1-year 3.8 %
							Neglect	5	N/A	1-year 42.4 %
							Overall	15	N/A	1-year 43.7 %; 1 type 35.4 %; 2 types 3.8 %; 3 types 3.8 %; 4 types 0.6 %

(continued)

Table 3.1 (continued)

References	Population	Age, sex and race/ethnicity	Survey methods	Participation rate	Measure	Alpha	Elder abuse types	# item	Cut-off points	Prevalence
Cadmus and Owoaje [16]	404 elderly women in Oyo state, south western Nigeria	60 or older; 100 % women; All Yoruba ethnicity	Semi-structured questionnaires	N/A	Standardized questionnaire developed by the WHO	N/A	Emotional	6	Score ≥1	1-year 11.1 %
							Physical	6	Score ≥1	1-year 14.6 %
							Sexual	2	Score ≥1	1-year 0.04 %
							Financial	3	Score ≥1	1-year 13.1 %
							Neglect	1	Score ≥1	1-year 1.2 %
							Overall	18	As above	1-year 30 %
Oveisi et al. [48]	600 community-residing older adults in Qazin, Iran	60 and older; 53 % women	Self-administered questionnaire	N/A	Not specified	N/A	Psych	N/A	N/A	2-month 100 %
							Phy/sex	N/A	N/A	2-month <1 %
							Financial	N/A	N/A	2-month 41 %
							Neglect	N/A	N/A	2-month 66 %
							Overall	N/A	[a]	N/A
Asia and the Western Pacific										
Yan and Tang [71]	355 community-dwelling older adults in Hong Kong, China	60 or older; 62 % women	Self-administered survey	N/A	CTS2	Phy: 0.82; verbal: 0.81; social: 0.71	Verbal	8	≥1 item	1-year 20.8 %
							Physical	12	≥1 item	1-year 2 %
							Social	5	≥1 item	1-year 2.5 %
							Overall	25	≥1 item	1-year 21.4 %; multiple types 17.1 %
Chokkanathan and Lee [18]	400 community dwelling cognitive intact older adults in Chennai, India	65 or older; 49.5 % women	In person interview	80 %	CTS	Overall: 0.94; verbal: 0.91; phy: 0.88; fin: 0.75; neglect: 0.98	Verbal	8	≥10 times	1-year 10.8 %
							Physical	6	≥1 time	1-year 4.3 %
							Financial	2	≥1 time	1-year 5 %
							Neglect	2	≥10 times	1-year 4.3 %
							Overall	18	[a]	1-year 14 %
Oh et al. [47]	15,230 older adults in Seoul, Korea	65 or older; 65.3 % women	In person interview	N/A	Compiled through literature	0.92	Emotional	5	≥2 times	1-month 4.2 %
							Verbal	5	≥2 times	1-month 3.6 %
							Physical	5	≥2 times	1-month 1.9 %
							Financial	5	≥2 times	1-month 4.1 %
							Neglect	5	≥2 times	1-month 2.4 %
							Overall	25	≥2 times	1-month 6.3 %

(continued)

Table 3.1 (continued)

References	Population	Age, sex and race/ethnicity	Survey methods	Participation rate	Measure	Alpha	Elder abuse types	# item	Cut-off points	Prevalence
Dong et al. [27]	412 cognitively intact community persons from general medical clinics in China	60 or older; 34 % women	Self-administered survey	82.4 %	H–S/EAST and the VASS	N/A	Psych	3	≥1 item	Since 60 11.4 %
							Physical	3	≥1 item	Since 60 5.8 %
							Sexual	1	≥1 item	Since 60 1.2 %
							Financial	4	≥1 item	Since 60 13.6 %
							Neglect	1	≥1 item	Since 60 16.9 %
							Abandon	1	≥1 item	Since 60 0.7 %
							Overall	13	≥1 item	Since 60 35.2 %;
Somjinda Chompunud et al. [62]	233 cognitively functioning older adults in Thailand	60–90 years old; 73.4 % women	In person interview	73.3 %	IGSEA	N/A	Psych	3	≥1 item	1-year 3.0 %
							Physical	1	≥1 item	1-year 0.4 %
							Financial	1	≥1 item	1-year 6.0 %
							Neglect	1	≥1 item	1-year 0.4 %
							Overall	6	≥1 item	1-year 14.6 %; 1 time 9.9 %; 2 or more times 4.7 %
Wu et al. [70]	2039 Chinese older adults in rural communities in Hubei, China	60 or older; 59.9 % women	In person interview	90.8 %	H–S/EAST and the VASS	0.75	Psych	N/A	≥1 item	1-year 27.3 %
							Physical	N/A	≥1 item	1-year 4.9 %
							Financial	N/A	≥1 item	1-year 2.0 %
							Neglect	N/A	≥1 item	1-year 15.8 %
							Overall	N/A	≥1 item	1-year 36.2 %; >2 types 10.5 %
Lee and Kim [41]	1023 older adults living alone in the community in South Korea	65–100 years old; 82.8 % women	In person interview	N/A	Screen-ing Scale for Elder Abuse	0.76	Self-neglect	5	≥1 item experienced often or always	1-year 23 %
Saikia et al. [58]	331 community-dwelling older adults from Guwahati City, India	60 and older; 46.8 % women	In person interview	N/A	H–S/EAST	N/A	Overall	N/A	N/A	9.4 %; men: 5.1 %, women: 14.2 %

(continued)

Table 3.1 (continued)

References	Population	Age, sex and race/ethnicity	Survey methods	Participation rate	Measure	Alpha	Elder abuse types	# item	Cut-off points	Prevalence
Tareque et al. [64]	896 elderly in Rajshahi district, Bangladesh	60 and older; 54.1 % female	In person interview	N/A	The investigator decided using NCEA definition and types	N/A	Emotional	N/A	N/A	5.1 %; rich: 1.6 %, poor: 6.1 %
							Physical	N/A	N/A	1.9 %; rich: 0.8 %, poor: 3.1 %
							Sexual	N/A	N/A	0.0 %
							Financial	N/A	N/A	0.7 %; rich: 1.6 %, poor: 1.1 %
							Neglect	N/A	N/A	32.6 %; rich: 3.2 %, poor: 60.0 %
							Abandon	N/A	N/A	3.2 %; rich: 0.0 %, poor: 6.7 %
							Overall	N/A	N/A	34.6 %; rich: 5.6 %, poor: 62.2 %
Trans-regional										
Guedes et al. [30]	1995 community-dwelling older adults in Canada, Colombia, Brazil, and Albania	65–74 years	In person interview	28 % in Canadato ~100 % in Columbia and Brazil	HITS	0.73–0.89	Psych	3	≥1 time	6-month 14.8 %
							Physical	1	≥1 time	6-month 0.9 %
							Overall	N/A	[a]	N/A

Table adapted from Dong [24]

EM elder mistreatment, *EA* elder abuse, *AA* Africa American, *Phy* physical, *Psy* psychological, *sex* sexual, fin financial, *RDD* random digit dialing, *CAIVR* computer and interactive voice response, *CTS* Conflict Tactics Scale, *OARS* Older Americans Resources and Services instrument, *USC-OACS* University of Southern California Older Adult Conflict Scale, *EASI* Elder Abuse Suspicion Index, *H–S/EAST* Hwalek–Sengstok elder abuse screening test, *VASS* Vulnerability to Abuse Screening Scale, *IRTA* the respondents' reactions to aggression, *AMA* The American Medical Association Screen, *IGSEA* interview guideline for screening elder abuse, *WHO* World Health Organization, *NCEA* National Center on Elder Abuse, ≥1 item: any positive response to one or more items

[a] The cut-off point varies by the subtype of abuse. NA: The information was not clearly indicated in the study

financial exploitation, and 0.2 % reported past year physical mistreatment. While there were no group differences in reports of financial or physical mistreatment by mode of question administration (i.e., in-person interview or self-report questionnaires), older adults using the self-administered questionnaire reported higher rates of verbal abuse (11.8 %) than those who completed in-person interviews (8.0 %). Interestingly, there were no differences in reports of verbal abuse and financial exploitation among older adults with or without another individual present during the interviews, and all but one individual who reported physical mistreatment during an in-person interview did so in the presence of another person besides the interviewer. In terms of limitations, the NSHAP did not assess for less common forms of abuse such as sexual abuse and neglect, and abuse questions that were asked were relatively circumscribed.

To address these gaps in the literature, Acierno et al. [4] conducted the National Elder Mistreatment Study (NEMS) with 5777 cognitively intact, community-residing adults aged 60 years and older. Respondents were identified using stratified random digit dialing, with interviews conducted over the telephone in either English or Spanish depending on the participant's preference. Unlike the NSHAP, the NEMS interview included multiple behaviorally defined questions for each category of abuse (see Sect. 3.2) and asked respondents about both past year abuse and prevalence of abusive events since turning age 60 (e.g., abuse experienced during any time as an older adult). The overall participation rate (69 %) was comparable to that reported in the NSHAP. Cases of potential elder abuse were identified if a respondent gave a positive response to any of the questions for each category of abuse. Over 11 % of respondents reported experiencing at least one category of abuse in the past year. The most frequently endorsed form of mistreatment was financial exploitation by family members (5.2 %). Note that the NEMS did not assess for stranger fraud in evaluating prevalence of financial mistreatment. Approximately 5.1 % of respondents reported past year neglect. Slightly fewer respondents (4.6 %) reported past year verbal or emotional abuse including harassment, humiliation, or being ignored. Physical abuse was also more prevalent in the NEMS than indicated in other studies on elder abuse in the community at 1.6 % past year prevalence. Lastly, the NEMS provided the first national prevalence estimates of elder sexual abuse. Just under 1 % of older adults reported being sexually abused in the past year. While sexual abuse appears relatively less common than other forms of abuse, these numbers are still alarmingly high when considering the total size of the older adult population. Not surprisingly, rates of abuse since turning age 60 were much higher, with a staggering 13.5 % of older adults reporting being verbally or emotionally abused in some form since turning age 60. Rates of physical abuse since turning age 60 were only incrementally higher than past year prevalence estimates at 1.8 %. Prevalence estimates for sexual abuse since turning age 60, however, were lower than past year prevalence estimates at 0.3 %, perhaps because some respondents were more confident in stating whether an event occurred in the past year than whether it occurred before or after turning age 60.

While prevalence estimates from both the NSHAP and NEMS were based on the "yes/no" endorsement of any abusive experience during the designated time frame (i.e., past year or since turning age 60), many researchers use frequency and intensity criteria in determining "caseness." This is especially true for verbal/psychological/emotional mistreatment and neglect. For example, in a nationally representative sample of adults age 65 and older in Ireland, Naughton et al. [46] adopted criteria used by other elder abuse prevalence researchers (e.g., [39, 49]) to define cases of psychological abuse and neglect as those where 10 or more episodes of abuse had occurred during the past year or cases where the psychological abuse or neglect were deemed to have a "serious impact" on the older person. As with the NEMS, past year physical and sexual abuse and financial exploitation were defined as any episode of abuse. In contrast to the NEMS, however, abuse was restricted to those cases where an older adult was abused by someone in a position of trust (i.e., family, close friends, care workers). In-person interviews were conducted in participants' homes, with an overall participation rate of 83 %. Categories of abuse, namely psychological, physical, and sexual abuse, were assessed using the Conflict Tactics Scale, a valid, reliable measure of abusive violence commonly used in epidemiological studies of elder abuse (e.g., [11, 52]). Questions assessing financial exploitation and neglect were derived from those used by Lachs and Berman and O'Keefee and colleagues in elder abuse prevalence studies in New York State and the U.K. (see [15, 51], in Table 3.1). Using these criteria, the past year prevalence rates for financial exploitation and psychological abuse were 1.3 and 1.2 %, respectively—much lower than those rates reported by the NSHAP and NEMS. Past year prevalence of physical abuse was 0.5 %, neglect was 0.3 %, and sexual abuse was 0.05 %. Compare these past year rates of neglect to those reported in the NEMS (5.1 %) where neglect was defined as cases where an older adult has unmet needs of daily living and an identified individual responsible for meeting those needs refuses to do so, regardless of whether a trust relationship exists between that person and the neglected older adult.

Perhaps one of the most ambitious studies to date to assess the prevalence of elder abuse, the Abuse of the

Elderly in the European Region, or ABUEL, project [42, 43, 61], also used a modified version of the Conflict Tactics Scale to assess the past year prevalence of elder abuse. Unlike other regional prevalence studies, ABUEL aimed to compare differences in prevalence estimates between countries in the E.U. using operational definitions of elder abuse derived from the UK Study of Abuse and Neglect of Older People [49]. ABUEL used three sampling methods, including randomized sampling of city population registries, random route sampling, and cluster sampling, to obtain a sample of 4467 older adults aged 60–84 years living in urban centers of seven countries (Germany, Greece, Italy, Lithuania, Portugal, Spain, and Sweden). Administration procedures were performed according to national requirements where the data was collected, and, thus, interview methodology varied across sites. Two primary methods of data collection consisted of (a) in-person interviews and (b) in-person interviews combined with mailed questionnaires (in Germany and Sweden only). Across countries, 19.4 % of older adults reported experiencing some form of verbal or psychological abuse such as being insulted in the past year, with the highest prevalence of psychological abuse in Sweden (29.7 %) and Germany (27.1 %). Of course, these extremely high numbers may call into question either or both the definitions or methods of data collection, in that the 'bar' above which an interpersonal interaction was considered abusive may have been set relatively too low and included many instances of interpersonally negative, but not necessarily *abusive* behaviors. Indeed, there were 11 questions related to psychological abuse used in ABUEL in contrast to the four questions used in the NEMS in the United States. This interpretation of the data may also be applied to the estimates discussed in other countries and continents throughout this volume and speaks to the common problem across studies, which is individual level interpretation of behaviors by others toward themselves as abusive.

Approximately 4.8 % of older adults across countries reported past year financial exploitation, with prevalence reaching as high as 7.8 % in Portugal. Prevalence of physical abuse ranged from 4 % in Sweden to 1 % in Italy, with an overall prevalence across countries of 2.7 %. Lastly, prevalence of sexual abuse ranged from 1.5 % in Greece to 0.3 % in Lithuania and Spain. The overall prevalence of sexual abuse in the study sample was 0.7 %. Prevalence of neglect was not assessed as part of ABUEL. Given the nature of the study design, findings from the ABUEL project must be interpreted with caution in that these older adults resided in urban centers and may not be representative of the general population of older adults across the E.U.

In discussing these studies, we have pointed out problems associated with definitional inconsistencies used across different studies, and this problem was empirically demonstrated by Dong [23] in a community-residing sample of 3159 Chinese older adults in Chicago age 60 and over. In this sample, in-person interview methodology was used to assess the prevalence of elder abuse, with an overall response rate of 91.9 %. In this sample, psychological and physical abuse were both assessed using items from the Conflict Tactics Scale, sexual abuse was assessed using one gateway item where a positive response cued follow-up questions, and neglect and financial exploitation were assessed using multi-item needs and financial abuse assessments. Prevalence estimates of psychological abuse were derived using five definitional criteria applied in other prevalence studies. These criteria required (a) endorsement of at least one CTS psychological abuse item, (b) endorsement of at least two CTS psychological abuse items, (c) endorsement of three or more CTS psychological abuse items, (d) endorsement of three or more items or threats of nursing home placement or abandonment (Beach criteria; [10, 9]), and (e) occurrence of 10 or more times for the CTS items (Pillemer criteria; [52]). Both physical and sexual abuse were defined as a positive response to any of the physical/sexual abuse items. Prevalence estimates of financial exploitation were derived using two definitional criteria: (a) endorsement of at least one item on the financial abuse assessment and (b) endorsement of at least one item on the financial abuse measure except someone felt entitled to use your money, someone prevented you from spending your money, and someone tricked or pressured you into buying something (items that may be less likely to be considered financial exploitation). Lastly, estimates of neglect were also derived using two definitional criteria: (a) caregiver neglect that was defined as having identified unmet needs and living with a family member and (b) caregiver neglect defined as having moderate or severe unmet needs and living with a caregiver. Applying different definitional criteria, prevalence of psychological abuse ranged from 1.1 % (Pillemer criteria) to 9.8 % (one or more items endorsed on the Conflict Tactics Scale). There was also considerable variability in the prevalence of elder neglect using different definitional criteria, with estimates ranging from 4.6 % (individuals identifying moderate/severe unmet needs and living with a caregiver) to 11.1 % (individuals identifying any unmet needs and living with a caregiver). Prevalence of financial exploitation was less variable, ranging from 8.8 to 9.3 %. Approximately 1.1 % of Chinese older adults in this sample reported physical abuse and 0.2 % reported sexual abuse, estimates that are in line with other studies using similar criteria. Readers are referred to Table 3.1 for a more detailed comparison of prevalence rates derived using different methodology and abuse definitions.

3.5 Research Challenges

A number of conceptual and methodological issues complicate collection of accurate data concerning both prevalence and incidence of elder abuse. Broadly, these issues fall into two categories: definitional and practical. Definitional issues confounding the accurate collection of elder abuse rates concern how "abuse" is defined and what measures are used to establish whether or not this established definition is met. Definitions of abstract constructs such as elder abuse are necessarily culturally bound. That is, while it may be relatively straightforward to define the act of physical assault, emotional abuse is a moving target, and what may be rudeness in one culture may well be severe emotional abuse in another. Thus, cultural norms and values at multiple levels (from government policy to individual family dynamics) shape how such constructs are defined. For example, expectations and beliefs concerning the point at which adult children ought to assume caretaking responsibilities for parents are different in the U.S. compared to China. Beliefs concerning family boundaries and the cultural requirements of family privacy regarding challenging situations also differ widely [8]. Thus, while one culture may view disrespect of one's elders as abusive, that same culture may also frown on disclosure or intervention. Moon and Williams [45] illustrated this point by presenting Korean American and African American women with identical scenarios containing indicators of possible elder abuse and comparing their reactions and appraisals. Meaningful differences in both perceptions of the presence of abuse and openness to reporting perceived abuse were observed; Korean-American women were less willing to define a scenario as "abusive," and less willing to assert that it was appropriate for those involved to seek outside help. Variability in the family structure and rigidity of expectations concerning living arrangements can also influence both how elder abuse is defined, and how it most commonly occurs. In an international examination of elder abuse, the World Health Organization [69] observed that mother-in-law abuse—specifically verbal abuse and neglect—occurs disproportionately in India, Austria, and Lebanon, countries in which the mother-in-law role commonly overlaps for a time with that of the daughter-in-law, leading to conflict and potential retributive neglect.

The problem with establishing a widely accepted definition of elder abuse is compounded by variability in accepted definitions of specific subtypes (i.e., physical, verbal, sexual, neglect, financial exploitation). In the case of financial exploitation, for example, some might consider serious mismanagement of an elderly dependent's money abusive, where others would draw the line closer to outright theft. Decisions concerning where to set the threshold for each individual subtype of abuse must be made before combined, general elder abuse estimates can be established. Adopting a "loose" definition (e.g., financial mismanagement in the case of financial abuse) would arguably maximize sensitivity, and by extension improve researchers and policy-makers' ability to detect and intervene. Given that elder abuse is widely acknowledged to be the most underreported form of domestic abuse [34], the ability to capture as many potential cases as possible is appealing. However, available resources for addressing elder abuse are limited [33], and casting too wide a net risks overwhelming adult protective service workers. Likewise, establishing too broad a definition risks grouping widely different cases of "abuse" into a single category, potentially obscuring meaningful differences and undermining intervention efforts that may necessarily vary by abuse subtype. Decisions concerning the establishment of definitional boundaries for both elder abuse and its subtypes must be made with care.

In addition to the noted definitional challenges a number of practical considerations complicate examination of elder abuse. First, a variety of factors impede elder abuse reporting leading to chronic underestimation of the phenomenon. Characteristics of the elderly population, including frailty and functional impairment resulting in dependence (in some cases, on abusers), may limit both opportunity and willingness to report abuse. Further, lack of clarity in legal guidelines regarding compelled reporters, coupled with inadequate education concerning identification of warning signs for elder abuse discourages health professionals from reporting a number of incidents [33]. Another challenge to the formulation of universal guidelines for elder abuse is the need to make such guidelines relevant, practical, and applicable for a broad group of professionals (e.g., healthcare providers, financial officials who might be in a position to detect exploitation) with widely different training, and different levels of exposure to reporting practices.

Even in the event that abuse is reported, resources for investigating and addressing it in most countries are limited [69]. When social service resources are already strained, prompt, thorough investigation is not always feasible [60]. Cross-national research must also account for national variability in rates of abuse over the course of the year. For example, the rate of family "abandonment" of dependent elders at medical facilities rises markedly during Carnival in Brazil and during the harvest season in agrarian countries [50]. Failure to appreciate such patterns could lead to widely different prevalence estimates where data is collected at different times of year. Both definitional and practical barriers to the detection and confirmation of abuse impede accurate estimation of the prevalence, and to an even greater degree the incidence of elder abuse, which is discussed next.

3.6 Global Incidence Studies

So far in this chapter, we have reviewed the global literature on prevalence and discussed important challenges in conducting prevalence research. In contrast to prevalence, which is concerned with the number of older adults affected by elder abuse at a specific point in time or over a specified period of time, incidence refers to the occurrence of new cases over a specified period of time [66]. Incidence and prevalence are similar constructs, and past year prevalence is often used to estimate incidence in elder abuse research. For conceptual and methodological purposes, however, we assert that data derived directly from older adult respondents about episodes of past year abuse better captures period prevalence, or the number of people who were abused during a given period of time, rather than incidence. Operating on this assumption, it is certainly the case that the global literature on elder abuse incidence is considerably less developed than the global literature on prevalence. In this section, our goal is to briefly illustrate the kinds of methodology used in capturing global elder abuse incidence, or the occurrence of new cases of elder abuse. Because of the dearth of incidence literature available, this discussion includes original research not published in scientific journals and data not derived directly from older adult self-report. Thus, it represents a departure from our previous section on global prevalence.

In the 1990s, the National Elder Abuse Incidence Study (NEAIS; [65]) conducted by the American Public Health Services Association's National Center on Elder Abuse sought to provide the first national incidence data in the U.S. on domestic elder abuse and neglect by collecting data from Adult Protective Service (APS) records and sentinel reports of abuse from 20 nationally representative counties in 15 states. For study purposes, data collection began in January 1996 and was spread over 12 months. A contact person at each APS site was called approximately every 10 days to determine the number of new reports made, and similar data collection procedures were used for sentinels. Results of this study found that an estimated 449,924 older adults in the U. S. aged 60 and over were victims of abuse or neglect in 1996, a number that increases to an estimated 551,011 older adults when self-neglect is included. Of note, these numbers are well below the estimates extrapolated from Pillemer and Finkelhor's [52] Boston prevalence study, which indicated that approximately 1,000,000 U.S. adults had experienced abuse since reaching age 60. The NEAIS was based on a review of records from sentinel agencies and sentinels, though, and not from reports directly solicited from older adults, and, so, it is likely that these numbers underestimated the actual incidence of elder abuse in that many new incidents of abuse are never reported to authorities.

Iecovich et al. [32] used similar procedures to report on the incidence of elder abuse in Beer-Sheva, Israel. In a two-phase project, professional and paraprofessional workers in contact with elderly persons were asked to complete a short questionnaire and submit it to the municipal department of Social Services if they suspected that the older adult was being abused or neglected. In phase two, trained social workers would follow-up on these reports by visiting the older adult directly in their home and completing a structured questionnaire to identify actual cases of abuse. Data was collected from December 2001 to December 2002. During this period of time, a total of 120 new cases of abuse and neglect were confirmed, yielding a citywide incidence rate of 0.5 % (based on a citywide elderly population of 24,800). As with the NEAIS in the United States, these results are based on new cases detected by professionals and paraprofessionals and are not directly based on new reports of abuse made by older adults themselves.

3.7 Discussion

In this chapter, we reviewed studies reporting on the global prevalence of elder abuse among community-residing older adults. Across studies, overall community prevalence ranged from as low as 2.2 % in Ireland to as high as 44.6 % among older adults visiting health centers in Spain. Estimates clearly vary across regions, and, while abusive violence against older adults is certainly influenced by sociopolitical factors within regions, methodological inconsistencies across studies generally preclude comparisons within and across regions and cultures. To minimize such methodological inconsistencies, we restricted our review of global prevalence studies to those where community-residing older adults were directly asked about their abusive experiences. Consequently, studies discussed herein may not generalize to the subset of community-residing older adults with dementia or other physical and/or cognitive disabilities that limit reporting. Indeed, attempts to study elder abuse among older adults with dementia, whether in community or in residential care settings, must rely on reports from caregivers, sentinels, or other individuals or agencies with close contact with those adults, and it is important to mention that some researchers have used these approaches to estimate community prevalence of elder abuse among older adults with dementia. For example, Wiglesworth et al. [68] utilized reports from older adults with dementia and their caregivers to estimate the prevalence of elder abuse among community-residing older adults with dementia. Results of in-person surveys revealed that fully 47.3 % of these older adults had been mistreated in the past year, of whom 88.5 % experienced psychological abuse and 19.7 % experienced physical abuse. Just over a quarter of the sample (29.5 %) experienced neglect over the past year. Together, these findings suggest that, relative to their cognitively intact peers, older adults living with dementia may be at increased risk for elder abuse and mistreatment. As with studies utilizing reports of family caregivers in the United States, the prevalence of abusive violence appeared to be much higher for those community-residing older adults with dementia relative to general community-based samples of older adults in the U.K. where 52 % of caregivers reported some abusive behavior in the past 3 months [20]. Past 3 month prevalence of psychological abuse was 33 %, while 1 % of caregivers reported some form of physical abuse against older adult care recipients. Similar results were also found in a study of disabled older adults and their caregivers in Japan, with more than 30 % of caregivers admitting potentially harmful behaviors toward their older adult care recipients [59].

In sum, prevalence estimates vary wildly across region, culture, sociopolitical, and domestic situation. However, it is very likely that most of the variability in estimates results from differences in assessment methodology and elder mistreatment definition. And this makes sense, because that which is considered rudeness in one culture may well be considered severe emotional abusiveness in another culture where reverence for one's elders is more socially lauded and defines the social role of the older adult. Indeed, even within cultures it has been extraordinarily difficult to arrive at consensus definitions of elder abuse or mistreatment. In fact, it has been difficult to even agree on a name for the event, with arguments made in favor of mistreatment vs. maltreatment vs. abuse vs. assault, etc. This inability to specify a metric, or basis of measurement, has significantly delayed research in this area, for any scientific inquiry depends, at its start, on a commonly agreed upon system of measurement. Where then, are we to start so that we may have some common ground across which to compare elder mistreatment in different locations, cultures, and sociopolitical spheres? We believe the first step should be reductionistic. That is, starting with the specific definitions of specific perpetration behaviors, and whether or not these specific behaviors occurred. By breaking mistreatment into its smallest, culturally independent, behaviorally specific common denominators, different perspectives can be brought to bear to recombine or aggregate these events into the definition of mistreatment most consistent with a given researcher's culture, while at the same time publishing this algorithm of precisely which parts of the aforementioned questions do and do not constitute their abuse definition. Until this is done, it is of little use to review and compare prevalence rates from across the world. However, the fact that this work has begun is reassuring, and it is the intention of this chapter to illustrate the emerging recognition of the problem and the initial estimates of its scope.

3.8 Recommendations and Future Directions

Deriving an accurate and detailed understanding of the scope and nature of elder abuse is essential to its prevention. With that in mind, there are a number of steps both researchers and policy-makers can and should take moving forward. Establishing standardized screening procedures for elder abuse is a crucial first step. Ideally, screening data would both facilitate identification and prevention of abuse, and be compiled into a database for use in both research and program/intervention assessment efforts. At present estimates of the prevalence, and especially incidence, of elder abuse are compromised by considerable variability in the nature and quality of data collection efforts across care-systems. Progress toward understanding the antecedents of various forms of elderly abuse requires access to detailed, longitudinal data, and unfortunately, such large-scale epidemiological studies have not been funded. Design and implementation of screening procedures should be undertaken with the simultaneous goal of generating a minimum dataset on elderly abuse to fuel research and inform policy. In addition to strategic allocation of resources to high-risk areas where screening is both most essential and arguably least likely to occur, training targeted at increasing professionals' 'buy-in' by emphasizing the importance of accurate data collection to understanding and reducing elder abuse, and subsequently improving health and quality of life is recommended.

Of note, successful integration of elder abuse screening procedures into standard practice will require substantial cross-professional cooperation. First, cross-disciplinary standards for screening and reporting should be developed with consideration for the varied needs, experience, and knowledge base of professionals who will be asked to use it. Guidelines should ideally be flexible, but comprehensive enough to facilitate screening and reporting across the wide variety of contexts in which abuse can occur. Collaboration across disciplines and systems is essential to ensure that often limited resources both for intervention and data collection are being used to maximal effect. While screening practices will necessarily vary across countries and cultures, all should be designed to allow for the collection of sufficient data to inform accurate estimates of prevalence and incidence. Second, professionals in a position to identify and report potential elder abuse should be given information concerning potential risk factors and warning signs for abuse. Such training should, where possible, include information designed to increase professionals' ability to obtain accurate reports (e.g., being mindful of care-takers' efforts to dominate the conversation during appointments). Finally, efforts should be made to ensure that the perspectives of the abused population, older adults, are being taken into account by both researchers and policy-makers seeking to understand this phenomenon. Elder abuse is already a significant, if under-appreciated public health issue. With advances in medical technology, the elderly population will continue to grow, as will rates of elder abuse [8]. That considered, institution of standard screening and data collection practices to inform advocacy efforts and policy changes must be prioritized.

References

1. Abdel Rahman TT, El Gaafary MM. Elder mistreatment in a rural area in Egypt. Geriatr Gerontol Int. 2012;12:532–7.
2. Abrams RC, Lachs M, McAvay G, Keohane DJ, Bruce ML. Predictors of self-neglect in community-dwelling elders. Am J Psychiatry. 2002;159:1724–30.
3. Acierno R. Elder mistreatment: Epidemiological assessment methodology. In: Bonnie RJ, Wallace RB, editors. Elder mistreatment: abuse, neglect, and exploitation in an aging America. Washington: National Academies Press; 2003. p. 261–302.
4. Acierno R, Hernandez MA, Amstadter AB, Resnick HS, Steve K, Muzzy W, Kilpatrick DG. Prevalence and correlates of emotional, physical, sexual, and financial abuse and potential neglect in the United States: the national elder mistreatment study. Am J Public Health. 2010;100:292–7.
5. Acierno R, Resnick H, Kilpatrick D, Stark-Riemer W. Assessing elder victimization: demonstration of a methodology. Soc Psychiatry Psychiatr Epidemiol. 2003;38:644–53.
6. Ajdukovic M, Ogresta J, Rusac S. Family violence and health among elderly in Croatia. J Aggress Maltreat Trauma. 2009;18:261–79.
7. Amstadter AB, Zajac K, Strachan M, Hernandez MA, Kilpatrick DG, Acierno R. Prevalence and correlates of elder mistreatment in South Carolina: the South Carolina elder mistreatment study. J Interpers Violence. 2011;26:2947–72.
8. Anthony EK, Lehning AJ, Austin MJ, Peck MD. Assessing elder mistreatment: instrument development and implications for adult protective services. J Gerontol Soc Work. 2009;52(8):815–36.
9. Beach SR, Schulz R, Castle NG, Rosen J. Financial exploitation and psychological mistreatment among older adults: differences between African Americans and non-African Americans in a population-based survey. The Gerontologist. 2010;50:744–57.
10. Beach SR, Schulz R, Degenholtz HB, Castle NG, Rosen J, Fox AR, Morycz RK. Using audio computer-assisted self-interviewing and interactive voice response to measure elder mistreatment in older adults: feasibility and effects on prevalence estimates. J Off Stat. 2010;26(3):507.
11. Biggs S, Manthorpe J, Tinker A, Doyle M, Erens B. Mistreatment of older people in the United Kingdom: findings from the first national prevalence study. J Elder Abuse Negl. 2009;21:1–14.
12. Bonnie RJ, Wallace RB, editors. Elder mistreatment: abuse, neglect, and exploitation in an aging America. Washington: National Academies Press; 2003.
13. Breslau N, Davis GC, Andreski P, Petersen E. Traumatic events and posttraumatic stress disorder in an urban population of young adults. Arch Gen Psychiatry. 1991;48:216–22.
14. Buri H, Daly JM, Hartz AJ, Jogerst GJ. Factors associated with self-reported elder mistreatment in Iowa's frailest elders. Res Aging. 2006;28:562–81.
15. Burnes D, Pillemer K, Caccamise PL, Mason A, Henderson CR, Berman J, et al. Prevalence of and risk factors for elder abuse and neglect in the community: a population-based study. J Am Geriatr Soc. 2015;63:1906–12.
16. Cadmus EO, Owoaje ET. Prevalence and correlates of elder abuse among older women in rural and urban communities in south western Nigeria. Health Care Women Int. 2012;33:973–84.
17. Carmona-Torres JM, López-Soto PJ, Coimbra-Roca AI, Gálvez--Rioja RM, Goergen T, Rodríguez-Borrego MA (2015) Elder abuse in a developing area in Bolivia. J Interpers Violence (advance online publication).
18. Chokkanathan S, Lee AEY. Elder mistreatment in urban India: a community based study. J Elder Abuse Negl. 2005;17:45–61.
19. Comijs HC, Pot AM, Smit JH, Bouter LM, Jonker C. Elder abuse in the community: prevalence and consequences. J Am Geriatr Soc. 1998;46:885–8.
20. Cooper C, Selwood A, Blanchard M, Walker Z, Blizard R, Livingston G. Abuse of people with dementia by family carers: representative cross sectional survey. BMJ. 2009;338:b155.
21. Cooper C, Selwood A, Livingston G. The prevalence of elder abuse and neglect: a systematic review. Age Ageing. 2008;37:151–60.
22. DeLiema M, Gassoumis ZD, Homeier DC, Wilber KH. Determining prevalence and correlates of elder abuse using promoters: low income immigrant Latinos report high rates of abuse and neglect. J Am Geriatr Soc. 2012;60:1333–9.
23. Dong X. Do the definitions of elder mistreatment subtypes matter? Findings from the PINE study. J Gerontol Ser A. 2014;69:S68–75.
24. Dong X. Elder abuse: systematic review and implications for practice. J Am Geriatr Soc. 2015;63:1214–38.
25. Dong X, Chen R, Fulmer T, Simon MA. Prevalence and correlates of elder mistreatment in a community-dwelling population of U.S. Chinese older adults. J Aging Health. 2014;26:1209–24.
26. Dong X, Simon MA, Evans DA. Prevalence of self-neglect across gender, race, and socioeconomic status: findings from the Chicago Health and Aging Project. Gerontology. 2012;58:258–68.
27. Dong X, Simon MA, Gorbien M. Elder abuse and neglect in an urban Chinese population. J Elder Abuse Negl. 2007;19:79–96.
28. Garre-Olmo J, Planas-Pujol X, López-Pousa S, Juvinyà D, Vilà A, Vilalta-Franch J, the Frailty and Dependence in Girona Study Group. Prevalence and risk factors of suspected elder abuse subtypes in people aged 75 and older. J Am Geriatr Soc. 2009;57:815–22.
29. Gil AP, Kislaya I, Santos AJ, Nunes B, Nicolau R, Fernandes AA. Elder abuse in Portugal: findings from the first national prevalence study. J Elder Abuse Negl. 2015;27:174–95.

30. Guedes DT, Alvarado BE, Phillips SP, Curcio CL, Zunzunegui MV, Guerra RO. Socioeconomic status, social relations, and domestic violence (DV) against elderly people in Canada, Albania, Colombia, and Brazil. Arch Gerontol Geriatr. 2015;60:492–500.
31. Hanson RF, Kilpatrick DG, Falsetti SA, Resnick HS. Violent crime and mental health. In: Freedy JR, Hobfoll SE, editors. Traumatic stress: from theory to practice. New York: Plenum Press; 1995. p. 129–61.
32. Iecovich E, Lankri M, Drori D. Elder abuse and neglect—a pilot incidence study in Israel. J Elder Abuse Negl. 2004;16:45–63.
33. Jogerst GJ, Daly JM, Brinig MF, Dawson JD, Schmuch GA, Ingram JG. Domestic elder abuse and the law. Am J Public Health. 2003;93(12):2131–6.
34. Kennedy RD. Elder abuse and neglect: the experience, knowledge, and attitudes of primary care physicians. FAMILY MEDICINE-KANSAS CITY-. 2005 Jul 1;37(7):481–485.
35. Kilpatrick DG, Saunders BE, Amick-McMullan A, Best CL, Veronen LJ, Resnick HS. Victim and crime factors associated with the development of crime-related post-traumatic stress disorder. Behav Ther. 1989;20:199–214.
36. Kissal A, Beşer A. Elder abuse and neglect in a population offering care by a primary health care center in Izmir, Turkey. Soc Work Health Care. 2011;50:158–75.
37. Kivelä SL, Köngäs-Saviaro P, Kesti E, Pahkala K, Ijäs ML. Abuse in old age—epidemiological data from Finland. J Elder Abuse Negl. 1992;4:1–18.
38. Koss MP, Goodman LA, Browne A, Fitzgerald LF, et al (1993) No safe haven: violence against women at home, at work, and in the community. Final report of the American Psychological Association Women's Programs Office Task Force on Violence Against Women.
39. Lachs M, Berman J. Under the radar: New York State Elder Abuse Prevalence Study. Final report prepared by Lifespan of Greater Rochester, Inc., Weill Cornell Medical Center of Cornell University, and New York City Department for the Aging. 2011.
40. Laumann EO, Leitsch SA, Waite LJ. Elder mistreatment in the United States: prevalence estimates from a nationally representative study. J Gerontol Ser B. 2008;63:S248–54.
41. Lee M, Kim K. Prevalence and risk factors for self-neglect among older adults living alone in South Korea. Int J Aging Hum Dev. 2014;78:115–31.
42. Lindert J, Luna J, Torres-Gonzalez F, Barros H, Ioannidi-Kapolou E, Melchiorre MG, et al. Abuse and neglect of older persons in seven cities in seven countries in Europe: a cross-sectional community study. Int J Public Health. 2013;58:121–32.
43. Lindert J, Luna J, Torres-Gonzalez F, Barros H, Ioannidi-Kapolou E, Quattrini S, et al. Study design, sampling and assessment methods of the European study 'abuse of the elderly in the European region'. Eur J Pub Health. 2012;22:662–6.
44. Lowenstein A, Eisikovits Z, Band-Winterstein T, Enosh J. Is elder abuse and neglect a social phenomenon? Data from the First National Prevalence Survey in Israel. J Elder Abuse Negl. 2009;21:253–77.
45. Moon A, Williams O. Perceptions of elder abuse and help-seeking patterns among African-American, Caucasian American, and Korean-American elderly women. The Gerontologist. 1993;33 (3):386–95.
46. Naughton C, Drennan J, Lyons I, Lafferty A, Treacy M, Phelan A, Delaney L. Elder abuse and neglect in Ireland: results from a national prevalence survey. Age Ageing. 2011;41:98–103.
47. Oh J, Kim HS, Martins D, Kim H. A study of elder abuse in Korea. Int J Nurs Stud. 2006;43:203–14.
48. Oveisi S, Karimi R, Mahram M. Note from Iran: self-reported elder abuse in Qazvin, 2012. J Elder Abuse Negl. 2014;26:337–40.
49. O'Keeffe M, Hills A, Doyle M, McCreadie C, Scholes S, Constantine R, Erens B. UK study of abuse and neglect of older people: prevalence survey report. London, UK: National Centre for Social Research; 2007.
50. Perel-Levin S. Discussing screening for elder abuse at primary health care level. Geneva: World Health Organization; 2008.
51. Peterson JC, Burnes DPR, Caccamise PL, Henderson CR, Wells MT, Berman J, Lachs MS. Financial exploitation of older adults: a population-based prevalence study. J Gen Intern Med. 2014;29:1615–23.
52. Pillemer K, Finkelhor D. The prevalence of elder abuse: a random sample survey. Gerontologist. 1988;28:51–7.
53. Podnieks E. National survey on abuse of the elderly in Canada. J Elder Abuse Negl. 1993;41:5–58.
54. Puchkov PV. Elder abuse: current research in the Russian Federation (2004–2006). J Adult Prot. 2006;8:4–12.
55. Pérez-Cárceles MD, Rubio L, Pereniguez JE, Pérez-Flores D, Osuna E, Luna A. Suspicion of elder abuse in South Eastern Spain: the extent and risk factors. Arch Gerontol Geriatr. 2009;49:132–7.
56. Resnick HS, Falsetti SA, Kilpatrick DG, Freedy JR. Assessment of rape and other civilian trauma-related PTSD: emphasis on assessment of potentially traumatic events. In: Miller TW, editor. Theory and assessment of stressful life events. Madison: International Universities Press; 1996. p. 235–71.
57. Resnick HS, Kilpatrick DG, Dansky BS, Saunders BE, Best CL. Prevalence of civilian trauma and PTSD in a representative national sample of women. J Consult Clin Psychol. 1993;61:984–91.
58. Saikia AM, Mahanta N, Mahanta A, Deka AJ, Kakati A. Prevalence and risk factors of abuse among community dwelling elderly of Guwahati City, Assam. Indian J Community Med. 2015;40:279–81.
59. Sasaki M, Arai Y, Kumamoto K, Abe K, Arai A, Mizuno Y. Factors related to potentially harmful behaviors towards disabled older people by family caregivers in Japan. Int J Geriatr Psychiatry. 2007;22:250–7.
60. Schofield MJ, Mishra GD. Validity of self-report screening scale for elder abuse: Women's Health Australia Study. The Gerontologist. 2003;43(1):110–20.
61. Soares JJF, Barros H, Torres-Gonzales F, Ioannidi-Kapolou E, Lamua G, Lindert J, Stankunas M. Abuse and health among elderly in Europe. Kaunas: Lithuanian University of Health Sciences Press; 2010.
62. Somjinda Chompunud ML, Charoenyooth C, Palmer MH, Pongthavornkamol K, Vorapongsathorn T, Jitapunkul S. Prevalence, associated factors and predictors of elder abuse in Thailand. Pac Rim Int J Nurs Res. 2010;14:283–96.
63. Stevens S, Bharucha A, Christel M, Hauptmann A, Wactlar H, Chen D. Automatic collection, analysis, access, and archiving of individual and group psycho-social behavior. In: Proceedings of the 3rd ACM workshop on continuous archival and retrieval of personal experiences. ACM; 2006, p. 27–34.
64. Tareque MI, Islam TM, Koshio A, Kawahara K. Economic well-being and elder abuse in Rajshahi district of Bangladesh. Res Aging. 2015;37:200–24.
65. Tatara T. The national elder abuse incidence study: executive summary. New York: Human Services Press; 1997.

66. U.S. Department of Health and Human Services, Centers for Disease Control and Prevention. Principles of epidemiology in public health practice. 3rd ed. Atlanta: U.S. Department of Health and Human Services, Centers for Disease Control and Prevention; 2012.
67. U.S. Department of Health and Human Services, National Institutes of Health, National Institute on Aging. Global health and aging (NIH Publication No. 11-7737); 2011. Retrieved from http://www.who.int/ageing/publications/global_health.pdf.
68. Wiglesworth A, Mosqueda L, Mulnard R, Liao S, Gibbs L, Fitzgerald W. Screening for abuse and neglect of people with dementia. J Am Geriatr Soc. 2010;58:493–500.
69. World Health Organization and International Network for the Prevention of Elder Abuse. Missing voices: views of older persons on elder abuse. Geneva: World Health Organization and International Network for the Prevention of Elder Abuse; 2002.
70. Wu L, Chen H, Hu Y, Xiang H, Yu X, Zhang T, Wang Y. Prevalence and associated factors of elder mistreatment in a rural community in People's Republic of China: a cross-sectional study. PLoS ONE. 2012;7:e33857.
71. Yan E, Tang CS. Prevalence and psychological impact of Chinese elder abuse. J Interpers Violence. 2001;16:1158–74.

Elder Abuse in Long Term Care and Assisted Living Settings

4

Jeanette Marie Daly

In long term care and assisted living settings, abuse, neglect, and exploitation take on a different meaning than in the community setting [1, 2]. Nursing homes, nursing facilities, skilled nursing, residential care facilities, and assisted living facilities are collectively known as *long term care facilities,* with each providing a myriad of services governed through the Centers for Medicare and Medicaid Services (CMS) and state agencies [3, 4]. Wierucka and Goodridge describe "the collective nature of institutions means there is greater potential for abuse/neglect to occur, as there are more people and more interactions than in community settings. The nature of the interactions may create very strong tensions among administrators, staff and residents. The client and his/her family are more physically and psychologically vulnerable than in other settings" [5]. One of the main services provided in these long term care settings is protection of residents against abuse, neglect, and exploitation.

CMS provides the administrative structure and oversight for long term care and its services in the United States. Nursing homes can be certified by either Medicare and/or Medicaid and must comply with the applicable laws and regulations. Another term used in lieu of nursing home is *nursing facility* (NF), which implies that a nursing home is certified by the state survey agency to provide services to Medicaid recipients. *Skilled nursing facility* (SNF) is yet another term denoting nursing home but specifically referring to a facility or section of a facility that provides rehabilitative services to Medicare beneficiaries. Many nursing homes are dually certified as both NFs and SNFs.

No federal oversight is provided for assisted living facilities in the United States, while licensure of assisted living facilities is required by most states. An *assisted living facility* is housing for residents who receive supportive services because they cannot live independently but generally do not require a nursing home level of care [3]. Various terms are used to connote assisted living facilities, such as *assisted care living facility, personal care home,* or *residential care home,* and each state has its own definition of assisted living [6].

The latest national figures on certified nursing homes in the United States for 2013 indicated there were 15,663 with 1,697,484 nursing home beds. Occupancy rate for that year averaged 81 % with 1,371,926 residents [7]. The latest national figures for residential care/assisted living facilities for 2012 indicated there were 713,300 residents in 22,200 residential care communities [8, 9].

4.1 History of Nursing Home Abuse

In the early nineteenth century, nursing homes began to be established in lieu of almshouses when women's and church groups began to form special homes for the elderly. Prior to that, states were responsible for their poor and provided for them through the county system, whereby each county's officials provided for the poor through housing built and paid for by taxpayers. Different terms used for this housing were *poorhouses, poor farms, almshouses, county infirmaries,* and *county homes.* States supported the poor and those in need.

In 1935 with the passage of the Social Security Act, the government began to get involved with the care of the poor and those in need because they were receiving substandard care in the almshouses; the act made persons residing in the almshouse ineligible to receive a social security check. Older persons began to seek other institutions for residence such as county homes or sanitariums. Later, in the 1950s, the Social Security Act was amended to allow individuals to receive federal support while residing in public facilities. The Medical Facilities Survey and Construction Act of 1954

J.M. Daly (✉)
Department of Family Medicine, University of Iowa Hospitals and Clinics, 01290-F PFP, 200 Hawkins Drive, Iowa City, IA 52242, USA
e-mail: jeanette-daly@uiowa.edu

X. Dong (ed.), *Elder Abuse*, DOI 10.1007/978-3-319-47504-2_4

allowed for the development of public institutions for persons in need.

In 1959, the Senate Committee on Labor and Public Welfare established a Subcommittee on Problems of the Aged and Aging, authorizing a complete study of any and all matters pertaining to the problem of aging [10]. From this subcommittee's work in 1961, a Special Committee on Aging was established, which later established a Subcommittee on Long-Term Care. One of the reports from this subcommittee was the 1974 Nursing Home Care in the United States: Failure in Public Policy. Fifteen years of fact finding preceded this report with supporting paper number 1 entitled "The Litany and Dimensions of Nursing Home Abuses." Content in this paper included negligence leading to death and injury; unsanitary conditions; poor food or poor preparation; hazards to life or limb; lack of dental care, eye care, or podiatry; misappropriation and theft; inadequate control of drugs; reprisals against those who complain; assault on human dignity; and profiteering and "cheating the system." Some excerpts from the report demonstrate the monstrosities occurring in our nursing homes at that time:

- One patient was found by a family member tied to a chair running a 106-degree temperature. She died the next day [11].
- In 1970, the Detroit Health Department reported that a dead body was allegedly kept for 2 days near the center's food handling area [11].
- "On occasion … food was taken from one patient's plate by help (that worked for you) and moved over to another person's plate to use up, to fill that plate or put the portion on it and sometimes it was moved even a third time" [11].
- "On the second day that my husband was in the home after I had brought these clothes in, all the dress shirts were gone; all the slack were gone; all the pajamas were gone; all the socks were gone; and all the handkerchiefs were gone" [11].
- The facility was short 300 medication doses during 1 weekend [11].
- Medication and narcotics storage containers were not locked, contrary to law [11].
- Employees regularly take food and groceries from the home [11].
- "I returned the next morning to find her tied, without clothes, in bed in the midst of her own wastes…it's seared into my memory, seeing her struggling to free herself, crying out for someone to help her" [11].
- "We have only two people who need to be constantly restrained in geriatric chairs all day. The amount of time they are under restraint is not logged" [11].
- "I complained to the head nurse about the other meals. Because I complained, the head nurse stopped helping my mother" [11].
- "In the treatment room we have a big box of dentures. When we can't find a patient's teeth, we just go into this box and get him some other ones" [11].

Long term care reform has improved the care provided to those living in long term care and assisted living settings. However, abuse, neglect, and exploitation are still threats and realities today. Federal and state legislation have facilitated the improvement of care in long term settings.

4.2 Legislation Regarding Long Term Care Settings

4.2.1 Nursing Home

Laws pertaining to elder abuse have been enacted by all states. Some laws regulate domestic and institutional elder abuse; other laws solely regulate institutional elder abuse while other laws regulate domestic elder abuse, with many of the laws covering dependent/vulnerable adults 18 years and older as well as the elderly [12]. Additional laws pertaining to elder abuse include the Elder Justice Act (Subtitle H in Title VI of ACA, P.L. 111-148) enacted as part of the Patient Protection and Affordable Care Act in 2010 (42 U.S. Code §18001) the State Long-Term Care Ombudsman program (42 U.S. Code §3058g), the Older Americans Act (42 U.S. Code §3011), the Omnibus Budget Reconciliation Act (OBRA) (42 U.S. Code §1396r) of 1987, state licensing laws for different eldercare institutions and facilities, and laws of criminal prosecution [12, 13].

State licensing and re-certification legislation sets forth provisions for the development, establishment, and enforcement of basic standards for the health, care, and treatment of persons residing in long term care settings. These laws provide for the maintenance and operation of those institutions that ensure safe, adequate, and appropriate care, treatment, and health for their residents [14]. All states have legislation for the licensing and re-certification of nursing homes and 14 states (CA, DE, FL, GA, IL, KS, MA, NV, NH, NY, OH, OR, TN, TX) have specific language in the statute addressing abuse reports and investigations [15]. Those specific statutes also have definitions of mistreatment in the nursing home setting [16].

Each statute provides different definitions for abuse in the nursing homes. Georgia Code 31-8-81 minimally defines abuse and exploitation; abuse as "any intentional or grossly negligent act or series of acts or intentional or grossly negligent omission to act which causes injury to a resident, including, but not limited to, assault or battery, failure to provide treatment or care, or sexual harassment of the resident;" exploitation as "the illegal or improper use of a resident or the resident's resources through undue influence, coercion, harassment, duress, deception, false representation, false pretense, or other similar means for one's own or another's profit or advantage." The Florida code 415.102 provides definitions for abuse and exploitation, and in addition definitions for intimidation, neglect, psychological injury, and sexual abuse. Intimidation is defined as the "communication by word or act to a vulnerable adult that person will be deprived of food, nutrition, clothing shelter, supervision, medicine, medical services, money, or financial support or will suffer physical violence".

The Nursing Home Reform Act, part of OBRA '87 (Public Law 100-203, Subtitle C) provided for specific requirements for establishing skilled nursing facilities, the comprehensive minimum resident assessment, and the survey and certification process for nursing homes to maintain certification. This reform established the basics of the residents' rights: free choice, free from restraint, privacy, accommodation of needs, and grievances. The description for free from restraint was "the right to be free from physical or mental abuse, corporal punishment, involuntary seclusion, and any physical or chemical restraints imposed for purposes of discipline or convenience and not required to treat the resident's medical symptoms" (100-203 STAT. §1330-165).

The standard survey process set forth in OBRA '87 allowed for each state to designate the agency responsible for conducting the unannounced survey. Components of the survey included quality of care furnished as measured by indicators of medical, nursing, and rehabilitative care, dietary and nutrition services, activities and social participation, and sanitation, infection control, and the physical environment (100-203 STAT. §1330-175). In addition, the designated agency would also be responsible for the receipt, review, and investigation of allegations of neglect, abuse, and misappropriation of resident property.

4.2.2 Assisted Living

Laws governing assisted living facilities are enacted by each state. A link to each states legislation and agency responsible for regulations can be found on the Assisted Living Federation of America's website at www.alfa.org/alfa/State_Regulations_and_Licensing_Informat.asp.

An example of such legislation from the Alabama code defines an assisted living facility as "an individual, individuals, corporation, partnership, limited partnership, limited liability company or any other entity that provides, or offers to provide, residence and personal care to two or more individuals who are in need of assistance with activities of daily living" (Chap. 420-5-4-.01). The Alabama State Board of Health licenses assisted living facilities, and that license can be revoked or downgraded if the owner or administrator of a facility is convicted of any crime involving the physical, sexual, mental, or verbal abuse on an individual or a resident. In addition, assisted living facilities must have policies that cover how allegations of abuse, neglect, and exploitation will be handled, may not hire an individual who is on the state's Public Health Nurse Aide Abuse Registry, and must provide initial training and refresher training on identifying and reporting abuse, neglect, and exploitation. The law is specific that when an incident of suspected abuse, neglect, or exploitation is evident then it shall be reported immediately to the Department of Human Resource or to law enforcement. The facility must conduct an investigation immediately, and within 24 h it has to be reported to the Department of Public Health. The legislation specifies the content to be included in the report, which needs to be maintained for at least 3 years.

Content in the state laws for assisted living may include definitions of abuse. Alabama's definitions of abuse in its assisted living facilities code include the following:

1. Abuse means the willful infliction of injury, confinement, intimidation, or punishment with resulting physical harm, pain, or mental anguish. Abuse shall also include verbal abuse, sexual abuse, physical abuse, and mental abuse, as defined below.
2. Verbal abuse means the use of oral, written, or gestured language that willfully includes disparaging or derogatory terms to residents or their families, or that is used or uttered within the hearing distance of residents or their families, regardless of their age, ability to comprehend, or disability. Examples of verbal abuse include threats of harm, or saying things to frighten a resident, such as telling a resident that the resident will never see his or her family again.
3. Sexual abuse means any sexually oriented behavior directed at a resident by a staff member, any sexually oriented behavior between residents that is not fully and freely consented to by both residents involved, or any sexually oriented behavior between residents when either or both residents are incapable of consenting to the behavior because of cognitive impairment.
4. Physical abuse means any willful act directed at a resident that is intended to result in or that is likely to result

in injury or pain. Physical abuse includes slapping, pinching, kicking, shoving, and corporal punishment of any kind.
5. Mental abuse means any willful act directed at a resident that is intended to result in or that is likely to result in mental distress or mental anguish. It includes humiliation, harassment, threats of punishment, and threats of deprivation.
6. Neglect means the failure to provide goods and services necessary to avoid physical harm or mental distress or anguish.
7. Exploitation means the deliberate misplacement or wrongful temporary or permanent use of a resident's belongings, money, or property without the resident's consent (Chap. 420-5-4-.05).

4.3 Nursing Home Elder Abuse Prevalence

The actual overall prevalence of elder abuse in nursing home settings is not known, and the specific types of emotional/psychological abuse, physical abuse, financial exploitation, neglect, and sexual abuse are not known. Estimates of elder abuse prevalence in nursing homes have been described through interviews/surveys with long term care setting employees, family members, and other relatives [17–23], and the prevalence is difficult to estimate and compare.

Reports of elder abuse in nursing homes are also available from a variety of sources, such as Adult Protective Services programs [24, 25], Medicaid Fraud Control Unit reports [26–29], the National Ombudsman Reporting System [30–33], the On-line Survey and Certification and Reporting System (OSCAR) [34, 35], agencies responsible for Licensure and Re-certification (i.e., Facility and Provider Compliance Division, Minnesota Department of Health or Division of Licensing and Certification, Maine Department of Health and Human Services) [36, 37], and the Long Term Care Minimum Data Set (MDS) [38–40]. These databanks are available nationwide and measure nursing home quality. They are unique to each agency, and the extent to which the data crosses agencies is unknown. Other abuse atrocities in long term care settings are even more difficult to discern and are not necessarily tracked in national databases; these include seclusion, withholding medication, overmedicating, resident-to-resident aggression [41, 42], under-treating pain [43], chemical or physical restraint [44, 45], poor hygiene, skin lesions, dehydration, malnutrition, pressure ulcers, urine burns and excoriation, contractures, delirium, vermin infestation, and accelerated functional decline [46–53].

The multitude of various studies depicting elder abuse prevalence from healthcare professionals, caregivers and family, medical record review, and agency reports represents the wide variation in different research methods employed. Inherent distinctions in these studies include differences in abuse definitions, the types of abuse studied, the definition of incidence or prevalence, sample sizes, sampling methods, the age of subjects, the variety of settings studied, and method of data collection used.

In one of the first studies providing reliable information regarding nursing home abuse, investigators randomly called 30 % of nurses and nurse aides from 31 nursing homes in New Hampshire inviting them to participate in a telephone interview [21]. Of the 691 potential subjects, 577 (85 %) participated. Rates of witnessed abuse by others were reported, with 36 % of respondents seeing physical abuse and 81 % psychological abuse [21]. Ten percent of the respondents reported they had committed physical abuse and 40 % had committed psychological abuse [21]. Situational characteristics of staff burnout and level of staff–patient conflict are strongly associated with engaging in resident abuse [18].

In a survey of all nursing home administrators and directors of nursing, 285 (54 %) of the 594 respondents reported they had seen an incident of abuse or that one or more incidents had been reported to them in the last year [17]. From 90 % of the 409 Iowa nursing home administrators responding, the mean rate of abuse incidents was 17.9 per 1000 nursing home residents, of which 15.9 reports were made and 4.5 were substantiated [17]. In determining the association of reported nursing home abuse with nursing home characteristics, lower percentage occupancy was significantly associated with higher incident and report rates [19].

A few studies have interviewed relatives of residents residing in nursing homes. These studies are able to determine the percentage of subjects with a specific type of abuse. In a random-digit dial survey of 718 relatives of persons receiving care in nursing homes, assisted living, or paid at home care, 72 % of the respondents indicated no abuse had occurred in the previous 12 months. Of the other 28 %, neglect was the most common type of abuse reported at 17 %, followed by emotional abuse at 13 %, verbal abuse at 12 %, material abuse at 9 %, physical abuse at 4 %, and sexual abuse at 0.6 %. Findings from this study indicate that nursing homes have the worst abuse records compared to assisted living or paid at home care [23]. From this same random-digit dial survey, 452 respondents were relatives of persons 65 years and older living in nursing homes and reported that 110 (24 %) residents were subjected to physical abuse by nursing home staff [20]. Residents who were younger in age were associated with more staff physical abuse [20]. Higher incidences of neglect were associated with residents who had functional impairments in activities of daily living, previous resident-to-resident victimization, and behavior problems [22].

4.4 Agency Reports of Long Term Care Setting Elder Abuse Prevalence

4.4.1 Medicaid Fraud Control Unit

The Medicaid Fraud Control Unit investigates and prosecutes Medicaid provider fraud and patient abuse and neglect in health care facilities or board and care facilities. The fiscal year 2014 report indicated there were 362 (27 %) cases of patient abuse and neglect which includes aggravated assaults, injury to elderly or disabled persons, and theft of patient funds [27]. The number of criminal and civil convictions for abuse and neglect was 285 with a recovery amount of $913,642 [27]. The number of criminal and civil convictions for theft of patient funds was 115 with a recovery amount of $2,644,990 [27]. Cases brought forward to the Medicaid Fraud Control Unit are only those brought to the attention of the criminal justice system.

Data from 42 states through the 1987 through 1992 Medicaid Fraud Control Unit Reports indicated there were 488 cases of nursing home abuse ranging from simple assault to homicide [28]. Of the 488 cases, 411 were reported physical abuse [28]. Nurse aides were the main perpetrators of abuse in these cases. However, they have the most frequent contact with the residents [28]. Of the 488 cases, 335 (69 %) were convicted, of which 68 (23 %) of the offenders were jailed or imprisoned [28].

From the Medicaid Fraud Control Unit Reports between January 1997 and May 2002, 801 patient abuse cases were content analyzed [29]. From the review, 63 % of the offenders were female and 73 % were nurse aides, and 48 % were classified as serial abusers [29]. Physical abuse, 68 %, was the predominant type of abuse found in the reports, followed by 10 % sexual abuse and 10 % duty-related (failing to perform some job duties) [29]. Of the 801 cases reviewed, 467 had information about the sanctions of the offense [29]. Findings indicate that sexual offenses are sentenced more severely than physical abuse cases. Sentencing practices were similar across states regardless if mandatory reporting was required.

From Medicaid Fraud Control Unit Reports, between 1993 and 2003, 242 cases of elder financial abuse were identified for residents of long term care settings [26]. Mean age of the victims was 82 years; where gender was known about two-thirds were female. Perpetrators were mainly employees of the facilities including aides, directors, bookkeepers, laundry workers, and other caregivers. Their crimes usually extended over a period of time. Witnesses were available for seven cases. Penalties for the perpetrators were mainly fines, with an average amount of $26,592, with probation the next most common penalty. In 32 cases the perpetrators were jailed and in 29 cases the perpetrators were imprisoned [26]. Using Medicaid Fraud Control Unit Reports may not provide a representative sample of abuse cases.

4.4.2 State Long-Term Care Ombudsman Program

The State Long-Term Care Ombudsman Program was mandated in 1978 under the Older Americans Act to provide a consumer advocacy program that aims to maintain or improve the quality of life for residents in long term care settings [54]. The program operates in each state, with both paid and volunteer ombudsmen available to investigate complaints. The Administration on Aging houses the National Ombudsman Reporting System (NORS), which provides data on abuse in long term care settings.

The latest report from the NORS indicates there were 9701 complaints of abuse, gross neglect, and exploitation in 2013. Of those complaints, physical abuse was the most frequent at 27 % and has been the main complaint since 2008 (see Table 4.1) [55].

Table 4.1 2013 NORS complaints of abuse, gross neglect, and exploitation

Year	Physical abuse (corporal punishment)	Sexual abuse	Verbal/psychological abuse (punishment and seclusion)	Financial exploitation	Gross neglect	Resident-to-resident physical or sexual abuse	Total abuse, gross neglect, exploitation
2013	2657	767	1883	766	1488	2140	9701
2012	2858	775	2113	806	1544	1903	9999
2011	2955	785	2197	756	1721	2068	10,482
2010	3245	817	2345	810	1560	2507	11,284
2009	3305	817	2588	859	1746	2313	11,628
2008	3702	788	2881	887	1865	2793	12,916

The long term care ombudsman program provides a source of information that is different from complaints in unannounced surveys. Ombudsmen are in contact with residents and families in long term care settings on an ongoing basis, whereas surveys may occur about every 15 months.

In a 1989–1990 report of ombudsman data, total abuse and neglect complaints were 134,612, of which 28 % were for resident care [33]. Examining the 1997 through 2000 NORS data on abuse, gross neglect, and exploitation category (with the following complaints investigated: physical abuse, sexual abuse, verbal/psychological abuse, financial exploitation, gross neglect, resident-to-resident sexual abuse, and other), a mean of 17.4 complaints per 1000 beds was found [32]. In a recent NORS report describing national trends in reporting of abuse and neglect in nursing facilities from 2006 to 2013, it was found that complaints trended down from 7.5 to 5.6 reports per 1000 beds [31]. Both studies investigated the same complaint and reported physical abuse as the most frequently reported type of abuse [31, 32]. The NORS database has improved tremendously with standardizing data reported over the years.

Matching NORS data for all 261 nursing homes in Connecticut with a comprehensive nursing home file, findings indicated that 47 % of the nursing homes had one or more accounts of abuse, of which 87 % were substantiated [30]. By matching the two datasets, the investigators were able to interpret the NORS data by nursing home [30]. Physical abuse explained 41 % of the abuse, followed by gross neglect and verbal abuse each at 19 %. Organizational facility characteristics associated with significantly higher abuse complaints included larger nursing homes, homes with unionized staff, and semi-private rooms [30]. Matching the same sets of data and including the MDS Quality Indicators, findings indicated a higher volume of complaints to the state agency 3 months before an inspection is associated with more deficiencies at an inspection. No association was found between MDS Quality Indicators and complaints [56].

In a survey of 642 certified volunteer ombudsmen in Texas, 361 (56 %) responded and they were primarily white women with a mean age of 65 years with some postsecondary education [57]. These ombudsmen visited their facilities weekly with 2-h visits. They perceived their greatest role as being an advocate for residents [57]. While being an advocate for residents, ombudsmen face challenges as reported in a separate survey to 408 paid ombudsmen in 26 states, where 203 (51 %) respondents described their most common problem as lack of support from state and local agencies. Other problems included difficulty in fact gathering, lack of witnesses for the allegation, family denial of abuse, and lack of authority for what they do [58]. More than half of the respondents reported allegations of abuse to adult protectives services or another appropriate state agency [58].

4.4.3 On-Line Survey and Certification and Reporting System (OSCAR)

All data collected during unannounced state nursing home inspection surveys are compiled in OSCAR for the purpose of certification or re-certification of nursing homes for participation in Medicare and Medicaid programs. OSCAR is a national and uniform database maintained by the CMS in cooperation with the state nursing home surveying agencies. Standardized information about the facility characteristics, e.g., number of beds, affiliation, resident characteristics, census, and staffing levels, are entered in OSCAR. Deficiency findings, complaint investigations, and other information from interim surveys are also recorded in OSCAR. OSCAR data are available for download from the Nursing Home Compare website at www.medicare.gov/nhcompare/.

Individual nursing home and assisted living survey results can also be found on each state's respective agency website. The state survey agencies are housed in different agencies depending on the state. For example, in Hawaii the Department of Health Office of Health Care Assurance is the monitoring agency and in Idaho the Department of Health and Welfare Bureau of Facility Standards in the monitoring agency, whereas in Delaware, it is the Division of Long Term Care Residents Protection, Health and Social Services (see "Appendix 1"). On the agency websites, the reports of deficiencies found during survey and complaints are displayed categorized as Life Safety Code Deficiencies, Clinical Deficiencies, Complaints, and Complaint Follow Up. Examples of deficiencies found during survey include making sure that a working call system is available in each resident's room/bathroom; store, cook, and serve food in a safe and clean way; provide routine and emergency drugs through a licensed pharmacist and only under the general supervision of a licensed nurse; try to resolve each resident's complaints quickly; hire only people with no legal history of abusing, neglecting, or mistreating residents; report any acts or reports of abuse, neglect, or mistreatment of residents [35].

Deficiencies are cited by surveyors when a nursing home fails to meet one or more of the federal requirements. In years 2005 through 2007, 91 % of surveyed nursing homes were cited for deficiencies, with a greater percent occurring at for-profit nursing homes compared to not-for-profit [34]. There are more than 190 possible deficiencies that fall into 13 categories. Deficiency categories include the following:

- Resident Rights
- Admission, Transfer, and Discharge Rights
- Resident Behavior and Facility Practices
- Quality of Life
- Nursing Services
- Dietary Services

- Physician Services
- Specialized Rehabilitative Services
- Dental Services
- Pharmacy Services
- Infection Control
- Physical Environment
- Administration [35]

The Resident Behavior and Facility Practices deficiency category houses the abuse categories of restraints, abuse, and staff treatment of residents. In 2012, 9.5 % of nursing homes were deficiency-free, while those with deficiencies had a mean number of 5.9 [35]. The inappropriate use of restraints deficiency has declined from 10 % in 2008 to 5.6 % in 2012 [35]. Likewise, nursing homes who received a citation for failure to treat/prevent pressure ulcers declined from 17.5 % in 2008 to 13.9 % in 2012 [35].

When a facility receives a deficiency, the deficiency is denoted as an *F-Tag*. The "F" preceding the term indicates that it pertains to long term care facilities. Six F-Tags are designated for restraints, abuse, and staff treatment of residents (see Table 4.2).

In addition to deficiencies, complaints in the OSCAR system are "allegations of noncompliance with Federal and/or State requirements" and are investigated by state surveyors [59]. Complaints can be lodged by nursing home residents, family members, facility employees, and others in which the state survey agency has to investigate them all. Complaint categories include the following:

- Resident Abuse
- Resident Neglect
- Resident Rights
- Patient Dumping
- Environment
- Care or Services
- Dietary
- Misuse of Funds/Property
- Certification/Unauthorized Testing
- Proficiency Testing
- Falsification of Records/Reports
- Unqualified Personnel
- Quality Control
- Specimen Handling
- Diagnostic Discrepancy/Erroneous Test Results
- Fraud/False Billing
- Fatality/Transfusion Fatality
- Other [60]

The CMS Nursing Home Compare website's datasets pages (https://data.medicare.gov/data/nursing-home-compare) provide detailed information about every nursing home that is

Table 4.2 Deficiency F-tags denoting restraints, abuse, and staff treatment of residents in nursing facilities

F-Tag	Definition
F221 and F222	(a) Restraints. The resident has the right to be free from any physical or chemical restraints imposed for purposes of discipline or convenience, and not required to treat the resident's medical symptoms
F223	(b) Abuse. The resident has the right to be free from verbal, sexual, physical, and mental abuse, corporal punishment, and involuntary seclusion
F224 and F226	(c) Staff treatment of residents. The facility must develop and implement written policies and procedures that prohibit mistreatment, neglect, and abuse of residents and misappropriation of resident property
	(1) The facility must—
	(i) Not use verbal, mental, sexual, or physical abuse, corporal punishment, or involuntary seclusion;
F225	(ii) Not employ individuals who have been—
	(A) Found guilty of abusing, neglecting, or mistreating residents by a court of law; or
	(B) Have had a finding entered into the State nurse aide registry concerning abuse, neglect, mistreatment of residents or misappropriation of their property; and
	Other
	(iii) Report any knowledge it has of actions by a court of law against an employee, which would indicate unfitness for service as a nurse aide or other facility staff to the State nurse aide registry or licensing authorities
	(2) The facility must ensure that all alleged violations involving mistreatment, neglect, or abuse, including injuries of unknown source, and misappropriation of resident property are reported immediately to the administrator of the facility and to other officials in accordance with State law through established procedures (including to the State survey and certification agency)
	(3) The facility must have evidence that all alleged violations are thoroughly investigated, and must prevent further potential abuse while the investigation is in progress
	(4) The results of all investigations must be reported to the administrator or his designated representative and to other officials in accordance with State law (including to the State survey and certification agency) within 5 working days of the incident, and if the alleged violation is verified appropriate corrective action must be taken [14]

certified. The site allows for comparison of different nursing homes.

4.4.4 Adult Protective Services Programs

Adult Protective Services (APS) programs were established in 1965 with the passage of the Older Americans Act (42 U. S. Code §3001 et seq.) and are administered through each state. The purpose of the programs is to provide services to those in need of assistance. APS workers are frequently the first responders in cases of elder abuse. In some states APS conducts domestic abuse investigations only, and in other states APS conducts both domestic and institutional abuse investigations.

Early attempts to compile data from APS have provided domestic reports, investigations, and substantiations of elder abuse, while no information was provided on abuse in long term care settings [61–63]. A more recent report expanded the data collection of these national reports to include abuse reports in institutional settings such as nursing homes, but very meager data are provided. In the 2000 survey report, 38 states reported there were 31,277 reports/investigations of abuse in long term care facilities. Ten states reported substantiation numbers from institutional setting; 5072 were substantiated [24]. In the 2004 survey report from 13 states, there were 9823 substantiated cases of abuse in long term care facilities [25].

4.4.5 Agencies Responsible for Licensure and Re-Certification

Nursing homes with residents receiving Medicare or Medicaid receive federal payments for their services. In doing so, they have unannounced survey visits approximately every 15 months to determine if the nursing homes are meeting the requirements for licensure and re-certification. Components of the survey process include review of resident rights; admission, transfer, and discharge rights; resident behavior and facility practices; quality of life; resident assessment; quality of care; nursing services; dietary services; physician services; specialized rehabilitative services; dental services; pharmacy services; infection control; physical environment; and administration.

Concerned that these announced surveys were not ensuring nursing home residents' health and safety, complaint investigations in 14 states were examined [64]. Findings included the following problems: certain procedures or practices may limit the filing of complaints, the seriousness of the complaint itself is understated, and there is a failure to investigate serious complaints promptly [64]. An example of a serious complaint was understaffing, where 64 residents were attended by only 3 or 4 aides. This complaint wasn't investigated for 123 days [64]. In another complaint, a resident received no medications for 10 days and family was not notified. This complaint wasn't investigated for 137 days [64]. As a result of this report, stronger federal requirements were created to require states to promptly investigate serious complaints where situations may harm a residents [64].

In 2004, nursing facilities were mandated to use the Automated Survey Processing Environment (ASPEN) Complaints/Incidents Tracking System (ACTS) established by CMS to comply with completion and submission of each complaint/incident [59]. The system was implemented to "protect Medicare/Medicaid beneficiaries from abuse, neglect, exploitation, inadequate care or supervision" [59]. The goals of this system are to provide protective oversight and prevention, and to promote efficiency and quality for residents within the health care delivery system. Complaints and incidents are entered into the national database with content that is standardized across states.

Until ACTS was implemented, no reliable source of data on the reported incidence or prevalence of elder abuse in nursing homes was available [18, 65, 66]. In ACTS, a complaint is a report made to the state agency or regional office by anyone other than the administrator or authorized official for a provider or supplier that alleges noncompliance with federal and/or state laws and regulations [59]. An incident is an official notification to the state agency or regional office from a provider or supplier of services (i.e., the administrator or authorized official for the provider or supplier) and results in an onsite survey [37, 59]. A report of an allegation of abuse is either an incident or a complaint, not both [37, 59]. Allegation categories for incidents and complaints in ACTS are comprehensive; some examples include resident abuse, resident neglect, injury of unknown source, misappropriation of property, restraints, seclusion, or death. Definitions of injuries of unknown source and misappropriation of resident property are provided:

- *Injuries of unknown source*—An injury should be classified as an "injury of unknown source" when both of the following conditions are met:
  - The source of the injury was not observed by any person or the source of the injury could not be explained by the resident; and,
  - The injury is suspicious because of the extent of the injury or the location of the injury (e.g., the injury is

located in an area not generally vulnerable to trauma) or the number of injuries observed at one particular point in time or the incidence of injuries over time (42 C.F.R. §488.301).
- *Misappropriation of resident property*—the deliberate misplacement, exploitation, or wrongful, temporary, or permanent use of a resident's belongings or money without the resident's consent (42 C.F.R. §488.301).

Nursing home employees are required to report alleged violations of mistreatment, neglect, abuse, including injuries of unknown source, and misappropriation of resident property in accordance with their state law (42 C.F.R. §483.13). When an allegation of abuse is made in long term care settings, the appropriate agency must be notified within 24 h (varies by state). After notification, a written report is submitted to the agency, which is followed by an agency investigation (see "Appendix 2").

Through a Freedom of Information Act request, CMS 2004 complaints and incidents were a rate of 16 reports, 9 investigations, and 4 substantiations of mistreatment per 1000 nursing home residents for the US [37]. While analyzing the nursing home complaint/incident reports, it was evident there is a variation in the rates of abuse by state [37]. Complaint report rates ranged from 0.42 (Hawaii) to 52 (New Mexico), complaint investigation rates ranged from 0.42 (Hawaii) to 39 (Nevada), and complaint substantiation rates ranged from 0 (Hawaii, Montana, North Dakota, South Carolina, and the District of Columbia) to 16 (Nevada) per 1000 nursing home residents. Incident report rates ranged from 0.04 (Virginia) to 46 (Alabama), incident investigation rates ranged from 0.6 (Colorado) to 41 (Rhode Island), and incident substantiation rates ranged from 0 (Arizona) to 19 (Alaska) [37]. In 2009 state survey agencies received 53,313 complaints about nursing homes, which equated to 38 complaints per 1000 nursing home residents ranging from less than 1/1000 in South Dakota to about 137/1000 in Washington [36].

4.4.6 Long Term Care Minimum Data Set

With the passage of OBRA '87, completion of the Long Term Care Minimum Data Set (MDS) is required for all residents of certified nursing facilities. The MDS is a quality of care measure, a primary screening and assessment tool of health status and it provides a comprehensive assessment. The MDS consists of more than 400 items and has the following categories including identification information; hearing, speech, and vision; cognitive patterns; mood; behavior; preferences for customary routine and activities; functional status; bladder and bowel; active diagnosis; health conditions; swallowing/nutritional status; oral/dental status; skin conditions; medications; special treatments, procedures, and programs; restraints; and participation in assessment and goal setting. The Research Data Assistance Center, a CMS contractor, at the University of Michigan provides assistance for research and requests for MDS data [67].

Abuse and neglect may be discerned from various data points collected on the MDS. For example, in the health conditions section, there are three questions regarding pain management (medication regimen, receipt of when needed (PRN) pain medications, and receipt of non-medication intervention for pain) and four questions on pain assessment (pain presence, frequency, effect on sleep, and effect on activity) that can be indicators of quality of care. Analyzing MDS pain data of 8094 residents from 1382 nursing homes, findings revealed 66 % of nursing home residents with cancer experience pain, and 18 % of those residents with daily pain did not receive medication treatment for pain in their first week of admission to the nursing home [39]. Using MDS pain data and Medicare Current Beneficiary annual survey data, findings indicate that annual prevalence of moderate-to-severe pain in nursing homes declined from 29 % in 2006 to 22 % in 2009, but that moderate-to-severe pain is still a problem for residents [40]. With a CMS revision to F-Tag 309 for nursing homes to meet compliance in the evaluation and management of pain in nursing home residents, MDS pain data were compared prior to and after the F-Tag 309 changes. Findings indicated there was improved documentation of pain and increases in scheduled analgesic prescription after implementation of F-Tag 309 changes [38].

Each of the agencies accumulating and providing information on abuse, neglect, and exploitation has unique data that isn't really comparable. An overview of the most recent reports of abuse from the agencies is depicted in Table 4.3. It is difficult to obtain information from the same time period or to obtain complete information. Since there are multiple agencies responsible for investigating elder abuse in long term care settings, reports of elder abuse may be made to one or many of those agencies; thus cross-over of reports is difficult to discern. To ascertain the F-Tags for abuse, the Nursing Home Compare dataset was downloaded from the Internet and had to be manipulated to include only standard surveys conducted in 2014 which may have missed some nursing homes as unannounced surveys are approximately every 15 months. Of the 10,477 nursing homes having a standard survey in 2014, 2774 (27 %) had abuse F-Tags.

Table 4.3 Agencies' latest available nursing home abuse report data

Agency	Year	Definition	Number of cases
Automated Survey Processing Environment Complaints/Incidents Tracking System	2009	Complaint is a report made to the state agency or regional office by anyone other than the administrator or authorized official for a provider or supplier that alleges noncompliance with federal and/or state laws and regulations	53,313 (of which 5.6 % were resident abuse and 1.3 % were misappropriation of property)
		Incident is an official notification to the state agency or regional office from a provider or supplier of services (i.e., the administrator or authorized official for the provider or supplier) and results in an onsite survey[c]	
Medicaid Fraud Control Unit[a]	2014	Patient abuse & neglect = aggravated assaults, injury to persons, & theft of patient funds	362
National Ombudsman Reporting System	2013	Physical abuse	2657
		Sexual abuse	767
		Verbal abuse	1883
		Financial exploitation	766
		Gross neglect	1488
		Resident-to-residents physical or sexual abuse	2140
		Total	12,916
On-line Survey and Certification and Reporting System[b]	Last 15 months	Survey F tag	
	Data pulled 6/23/15	221—keep each resident free from physical restraints, unless needed for medical treatment	435
		222—keep each resident free from drugs that restrain them, unless needed for medical treatment	15
		223—protect each resident from all abuse, physical punishment, and involuntary separation from others	46
		224—protect each resident from mistreatment, neglect and misappropriation of personal property	65
		225—(1) hire only people with no legal history of abusing, neglecting or mistreating residents; or (2) report and investigate any acts or reports of abuse, neglect or mistreatment of residents	753
		226—develop and implement policies for (1) screening and training employees; and the (2) prevention, identification, investigation, and reporting of any abuse, neglect, mistreatment and misappropriation of property	1460

[a]Cases brought forward are only those brought to the attention of the criminal justice system
[b]Only for providers that had an abuse F-tag in their last standard survey in 2014
[c]Only complaint data was available

4.5 Elder Abuse Research in Long Term Care Settings

A systematic review of original abuse research in nursing homes, intermediate care facilities, and skilled nursing facilities found that completed research focused on neglect and poor care quality (pressure sores, nutrition/hydration issue), physical abuse and the staff–resident dynamic, sexual abuse, psychological abuse, and violation of personal rights and financial/material issues [41]. Other important areas of research include inappropriate use of antipsychotic medication/chemical restraint, staff education and nursing home theft. Research involving these areas will be reviewed.

4.5.1 Resident-to-Resident Aggression

Various terms, such as *non-staff abuse* [68], *resident-to-resident abuse* [69], *resident-to-resident aggression* [42, 70], *resident-to-resident relational aggression* [71], *resident-to-resident violence* [72], and *resident-to-resident violent incidents* [73] have been used in the literature. Through a consensus-building workshop using a modified Delphi approach, expert participants agreed on the term *resident-to-resident aggression* with the following definition: a "negative, aggressive and intrusive verbal, physical, sexual, and material interactions between long term care residents that in a community setting would likely be unwelcome and potentially cause physical or psychological distress or harm to the recipient" [74].

In the latest National Ombudsman Reporting System (NORS) report, 22 % of the complaints lodged were resident-to-resident physical or sexual complaints [55]. Thirty-five different types of resident-to-resident aggression have been identified, with verbal and physical aggression the most common; some specific types are taking another's food, kicking, room invasion, and ramming another with a wheelchair [42]. Different factors that may be attributed to triggering this type of abuse are resident's wandering into another resident's room, residents being unable to speak, and just the mere fact of commingling of residents with and without dementia [42]. In these situations both residents, the perpetrator and victim, can be harmed. Recently a consensus meeting was hosted to identify a research agenda for resident-to-resident aggression. The top five priorities were "(a) developing/assessing resident-to-resident aggression environmental interventions; (b) identification of the environmental factors triggering resident-to-resident aggression; (c) incidence/prevalence of resident-to-resident aggression; (d) developing/assessing staff resident-to-resident aggression education interventions; and (e) identification of resident-to-resident aggression perpetrator and victim characteristics" [74].

One of the earliest studies on resident-to-resident aggression was to assess risk factors for violent injury in nursing homes [73]. Retrospectively using the MDS files from CMS and merging them with the Massachusetts Department of Public Health's Complaint and Incident Reporting System data for a year comparing 294 residents with incidents and those without incidents, the most frequent type of injury was lacerations (n = 113), followed by bruises or hematomas (n = 105), fractures (n = 39), reddened areas (n = 31), and dislocations (n = 6) [73]. Residents who had greater cognitive impairment were associated with greater risk of being injured [73]. In another study from 1985 to 1995, determining police involvement with episodes of resident-to-resident elder mistreatment of 42 subjects in the Established Population for Epidemiological Studies in Elderly residing in nursing homes, 79 police involvement incidents occurred, with simple assault the main complaint [75]. It was noted that cohort members were more likely to interact with police in the community setting than after being a resident in the nursing home. Validating the prevalence of resident-to-resident aggression, Castle surveyed 6606 nurse aides from 249 nursing homes in 10 states and found from the 4451 (67 %) respondents that 91–97 % of the respondents reported residents yelling at each other; residents pushing, grabbing, or pinching each other; and aggressive behavior toward each other. Sixty-nine percent of the respondents reported intervening when one resident took another resident's belonging [69].

To determine nursing home staff responses to resident-to-resident aggression, 282 certified nursing assistants were interviewed from five nursing homes and it was found that 97 reported their actions as physically intervening/separating residents, talking calmly to settle residents down, no intervention, and verbally intervening to defuse the situation [76]. Seldom did they report the behavior to a nurse or document it in the residents' behavior record. In an effort to train nursing staff about resident-to-resident aggression, recognition, and reporting, 47 units of five New York nursing homes were involved in a prospective, cluster-randomized, controlled trial. Data collected at three time periods over 12 months revealed that training increased knowledge and reporting of resident-to-resident aggression [77].

As front-line caregivers in long term care setting, nursing assistants can enhance the residents living environment by predicting and preventing resident violence. Putting the resident first is a major strategy for preventing violence [78]. To implement this strategy, three key concepts are important: knowing the residents, keeping the residents safe, and spending quality times with the residents [78].

4.5.2 Resident-to-Staff Aggression

Resident-to-staff aggression involves verbal aggression, physical intimidation/physical assault, and/or sexual harassment [79, 80]. Common forms of verbal aggression are bossiness, profanity, racial slurring, screaming, and trying to scare with words [81]. Frequent physical aggressions include biting, destroying property, grabbing, hitting, kicking, pinching, pushing, scratching, shoving, spitting, throwing things, and threatening gestures [82, 83]. The occurrences of resident-to-staff aggressions occur most frequently during the provision of hygienic cares [80, 84, 85]. The actual prevalence of resident-to-staff aggression is unknown; it is difficult to compare the prevalence studies of resident-to-staff aggression because the measurement methods vary.

Seventy percent of 126 nursing assistants in a 350-bed Winnipeg nursing home reported physical aggression from residents in the previous month [86]. Being pushed, grabbed, shoved, or pinched by residents was the most common type of physical aggression, with conflicts being provoked by residents not wanting to get dressed and by wanting to go outside the facility [86]. A slight correlation between burn-out and aggression from residents was noted [86]. Findings indicated a nurse assistant in this facility may expect to be verbally assaulted 11.3 times per month and physically assaulted 9.3 times per month by residents [86]. From a study of 21 nursing homes in Switzerland, 81 % of 804 employees experienced aggressive behavior in the previous 12 months, while 77 % experienced verbal aggression, 54 % physical aggressions, and 28 % threats [79]. Lower education levels, being female, being younger than 30 years of age, and being confident in managing physical aggression were associated with resident-to-staff physical aggression [79].

Studying the number of residents who are aggressive towards staff in five New York City nursing homes, 282 staff member participated in interviews regarding 1552 residents (80 % of the nursing home population) [80]. Staff reported 15.6 % of residents had directed aggressive behaviors toward them in the previous 2 weeks, with verbal aggression 7.5 % of the time, physical aggression 2.8 % of the time, sexual aggression 0.5 % of the time, and a combination of verbal and physical aggression 4.8 % of the time [80]. Factors associated with resident-to-staff aggression were need for activities of daily living in the morning, greater disordered behavior, and affective disturbance [80].

Unfortunately, resident-to-staff aggression may precipitate staff-to-resident aggression as retaliation against the resident. Abuse of residents can be considered reactionary/reflex or sadistic [87]. Thirty-two percent of staff in 24 community-based facilities in Sweden reported feelings of aggression as a consequence of resident's aggression [88]. In 10 Philadelphia nursing homes, 108 nurse aides self-reported they had yelled at residents in anger and 49 had excessively restrained residents [89]. Consequences of staff-to-resident aggression for the resident have involved forceful holding, pharmacological treatment, isolation, ignoring requests for help, no response to questions, reprimands, and relocation to another residence [85, 88].

4.5.3 Sexual Abuse/Resident-to-Resident Sexual Aggression

The definition of sexual abuse is "non-consensual sexual contact of any kind, coercing an elder to witness sexual behaviors" [90]. However, in long term care settings, the connotation of sexual abuse is expanded and also includes resident-to-resident sexual aggression defined as "sexual interaction between long-term care residents that in a community setting would likely be construed as unwelcome by at least one of the recipients and have high potential to cause physical or psychological distress in one or both of the involved" [91].

Actual prevalence studies of elder sexual abuse or resident-to-resident sexual abuse in long term care settings have not been conducted [92]. The NORS latest report has 767 sexual abuse complaints lodged, which are 8 % of all complaints [55]. Other reports on sexual abuse occurring in nursing homes or assisted living facilities are found in research publications. Six research publications focus solely on sexual abuse in long term care settings [92]. Otherwise, sexual abuse findings in nursing homes are usually found in studies that have collected information on all types of abuse. It is evident from the few studies available that sexual abuse occurs in long term care settings and that both men and women are victims, with perpetrators being both male and female.

From Ann Burgess's own cases, a convenience sample of 20 sexual assault cases of residents in nursing homes were reviewed; data was abstracted to gather demographic, dynamics of the offense, and forensics for each case [66, 93]. Eighteen of the residents were female, 16 were white, 14 widowed, 16 were 70 years or older, and all resided in long term care and needed skilled nursing interventions. Eighteen of the residents had cognitive disabilities and the other 2 had amyotrophic lateral sclerosis (ALS) and major depression. None of the victims reported his or her abuse to nursing home administrators; 10 informed family or staff, 7 incidents were witnessed, and the remaining was detected by family or staff. The incidents are horrific; the resident who had ALS used her keyboard and eye-blink sign to spell out that the respiratory therapist had abused her. Clues in these cases were not always instantly obvious and might take time to present, such as pelvic bruising, venereal warts, and discharge of pelvic fluid [66]. Eighteen offenders were known, 15 were nursing home employees (nurse aides, respiratory therapist, and a maintenance worker), and 3 were residents [93]. Some residents were able to provide a full description of the perpetrators [66]. Eleven of the employees were arrested and 5 were convicted [93]. These perpetrators victimized residents who were incapacitated, had dementia, and were frail.

Experts in the field of elder sexual abuse, who brought their own nursing home cases of elder sexual abuse, were convened to analyze the 125 cases. Their review highlights the issues in managing alleged elder sexual abuse and includes trauma masquerading as accidental bruising, communication difficulties, denial or recanting of the act, unwitnessed events, signs and symptoms as evidence, inadequate evidentiary examination, sexually transmitted disease, and resident-on-resident sexual abuse [94]. Evident from these case reviews is not only the physical abuse of the sexual act but the psychological impact on the victim as demonstrated in behavior changes that include agitation, depression, fearfulness, being withdrawn, refusing care, and wanting a gun to "shoot someone" [94].

Staff from state adult protective service's investigating agencies across five states (NH, OR, TN, TX, WI) voluntarily completed a Sex Abuse Survey providing details of sexual abuse in various institutional settings. From the forms completed, there were 177 investigations and 52 substantiations of sexual abuse for persons 50 years and older. Tweaking this information for just men residing in nursing homes, there were 26 alleged male victims of which 6 cases were substantiated. Victims had cognitive and physical impairment, and were predominantly white, with fondling as the main substantiated type of sexual abuse. Perpetrators were either staff or other residents [95].

In a similar study of adult protective case reports from Virginia for a 5-year period, 50 cases of sexual abuse for women in nursing homes were reviewed. The most common form of sexual abuse was sexualized kissing and fondling (76 %), followed by unwelcome sexual interest in the women's body (38 %). Most incidents were isolated (82 %) but 10 % were ongoing over time. The main witnesses of the abuse were staff members and other residents. Most of the perpetrators were residents of the nursing home. In three cases, the alleged perpetrator was prosecuted [96].

Data-driven investigations of sexual abuse in nursing homes are difficult to conduct. As noted from the current research, investigators in the field having access to the allegation and investigation files have attempted to describe the assaults, the victims and perpetrators, and the outcomes of the cases. Types of sexual abuse described were anal and vaginal penetration [66], digital penetration of anus [95], exposure to embarrass or humiliate [95], sexualized kissing [96], fondling [96], oral genital contact [95], verbal sexual abuse, sexual interest in the victim's body [95], and showing victim pornography [95].

4.5.4 Exploitation/Nursing Home Theft

A definition of *exploitation* is "illegal taking, misuse, or concealment of funds, property, or assets of a vulnerable elder" [90]. For those in long term care settings, other known types of exploitation include misuse of power of attorney, illegal property transfers, fraud, and theft [97]. In long term care settings, exploitation is expanded and also comprises resident-to-resident theft. The fiscal year 2014 Medicaid Fraud Control Unit Report indicated that there were 115 criminal and civil convictions for theft of patient funds with a recovery of $2,644,990 [27].

Estimates of exploitation in long term care settings are difficult to obtain. In a mailed survey to all 925 employees of 6 nursing homes in Tennessee and Virginia, 59 % of the 281 (30 %) returned useable questionnaires were from nursing [98]. Eleven (4 %) respondents reported they had taken something from a resident, with the main item being money [98]. While 105 (37 %) employees had seen someone else take from a resident, the thefts witnessed were perpetuated by staff members or other residents [98]. The self-reported thieves had a mean age of 33 years were male, non-white, and never married [98]. They were less satisfied with their jobs than the non-thieves [98]. Fifty-eight percent of these respondents reported the theft occurred on the day shift, with the remainder on the evening shift [98].

Conducting a survey of employees and family members of 47 nursing homes in ten states, completed questionnaires were returned from 1116 (22 %) employees [99]. Seventeen employees reported they had stolen at the nursing home for a rate of 1.53 %, and 58 (6 %) reported they had seen a coworker steal from a patient [99]. Four hundred seventeen (47 %) of the family members reported that items were missing from their relatives room [99].

In an attempt to determine the difference between elder financial exploitation cases and physical abuse cases, 242 cases of elder financial abuse and 314 cases of elder physical abuse were reviewed from the 1993 through 2003 Medicaid Fraud Control Unit reports and from other case information (offender identity, occupation, and gender, type of crime, and stage of criminal justice processing, and sentence) [26]. Gender of offender and victim were similar between the elder financial abuse and physical abuse cases. For the elder financial abuse cases, the victims tended to be older and the offenders were from a broad range of occupations, including nurse aides, directors, bookkeepers, laundry workers, and others [26]. However, for the elder physical abuse cases, 90 % of the abusers were nurse aides [26]. The criminal penalties for financial abuse cases applied in corresponding highest order were fines, probation, jail, and prison. Physical abusers were more likely to be jailed than financial abusers, who were more likely to be imprisoned [26]. As well, the physical abusers had longer prison sanctions, shorter probations sentences, and lower fines [26].

4.5.5 Pressure Ulcers

Pressure ulcers are "localized injury to the skin and/or underlying tissue usually over a bony prominence, as a result of pressure, or pressure in combination with shear" [100].

They can be a result of neglect in long term care settings. The National Pressure Ulcer Advisory Panel reached a consensus statement that "unavoidable pressure ulcers do occur" [101]. However, the panel noted in the vast majority of cases, pressure ulcers are avoidable.

A mailed survey entitled "Are Pressure Ulcers Preventable in Nursing Homes?" was returned by 65 (71 %) pressure ulcer experts [102]. One-third of the respondents indicated all pressure ulcers are preventable. Only 5 % agreed that nursing homes have sufficient resources to prevent pressure ulcers, while the majority agreed more staff or specialized beds would help reduce pressure ulcer development [102]. Fifteen percent of the experts agreed a stage II pressure ulcer, 38 % agreed stage III pressure ulcer, and 42 % stage IV pressure ulcer were evidence of neglect, indicating the more complex pressure ulcer was likely to poor care [102]. Some studies indicate that more registered nurse staff, licensed practicing nurse staff, and nurse aide staff in the nursing home are associated with fewer pressure ulcers [103, 104].

In a secondary data analysis of the MDS 3.0 for comprehensive assessments completed between January and March 2012 on all 843,616 nursing home residents, 41,680 (5 %) residents had pressure ulcers [105]. Twenty-nine percent of the pressure ulcers were stage I, 44 % were stage II, 8 % were stage III, 4 % were stage IV, and 14 % were deep tissue injury [105]. Seventy-seven percent had pain associated with the pressure ulcer, with 7 % having excruciating pain [105]. Greater bodily pain was associated with advanced stages of pressure ulcers.

4.5.6 Assisted Living Research

Elder abuse research in assisted living settings is sparse [106, 107]. Research available describes abuse allegations and findings from a state database, a mailed survey regarding elder abuse to nursing assistants, interview of assisted living residents, and an assessment of public programs investigating elder abuse in assisted living facilities [107–112].

From the online Arizona Department of Health Surveys (ADHS) complaint surveys of 2007–2008, 239 (53 %) of the 454 assisted living facilities had a total of 978 allegations of abuse for 708 unique residents [107]. Neglect was the most frequent allegation at 65 % followed by physical and psychological abuse at 7 %, financial exploitation at 5 %, verbal abuse at 4 %, and medication and sexual abuse at 3 % [107]. Significantly more allegations were associated with facilities owned by nationwide corporations and facilities 51 beds and larger [107]. Substantiations of the various types of abuse ranged from 26–67 % [107]. Continuing to explore assisted living complaints through the ADHS, complaints investigated from the 165 assisted living facilities having them from 2001 through 2009 were reviewed [110]. From the 165 facilities, there were 616 complaints with 1196 total allegations involving 526 residents [110]. Personal neglect, failure to provide goods or services necessary to avoid physical harm, mental anguish, or mental illness, was the most frequent complaint by 132 residents. Five hundred and thirty-five (45 %) of the allegations were substantiated [110]. Exploring this data in another analysis from 2006 to 2008, among 1710 assisted living facilities, 63 (4 %) were cited for inflicting abuse, and 18 (1 %) were cited for failure to report abuse [111]. Forty-eight of the inflictions of abuse were physical restraints [111].

From a selected sample of 27 assisted living residents in three different facilities, the residents were unable to describe external resources for support for allegations of abuse. Of 17 abuse scenario videotapes shown to the participants, only 54 % could identify the abuse and 50 % could describe how they would handle the situation [108]. From a mailed survey to 832 nurse aides, who had recently worked in assisted living facilities, reported observing all types of abuse with cursing observed the most frequently at 59 % [109]. Other high observations of abuse were being argumentative with a resident at 51 %, pulling resident's hair at 49 %, aggressive behavior at 29 %, and destroying resident's belongings at 26 % [109].

In a final report to the U.S. Department of Justice, Hawes and Kimball summarized their investigation of the detection, investigation, and prevention of elder abuse in assisted living facilities [112]. Conclusions were states are extremely variable in their respective regulations for assisted living facilities with similarities across states with a tremendous shortage of resources within adult protective services, ombudsman, and licensing agencies [112]. Another main conclusion was that significant training is need in all sectors, that includes training on one's authority to involve law enforcement, investigative techniques and use of forensics, and how to write reports and gather data that are useful for law enforcement and prosecutors [112].

4.6 Inappropriate Use of Antipsychotic Medication/Chemical Restraint

A chemical restraint is "the use of a drug to control an individual's behavior and is legally appropriate only if used to ensure the physical safety of residents or other individuals [113]. A component of OBRA '87 legislation focused on the overuse of psychoactive medications mandating nursing homes be sanctioned for unnecessary drug use. Approximately, 50 % of nursing home residents have a dementia diagnosis with 60–98 % of these residents with dementia having neuropsychiatric disturbances which place them in the nursing home and trigger the use of antipsychotic

Table 4.4 List of conventional and atypical antipsychotic drugs

Conventional antipsychotic drugs	Atypical antipsychotics
Compazine (prochlorperazine)	Abilify (aripiprazole)
Haldol (haloperidol)	Clozaril (clozapine)
Loxitane (loxapine)	FazaClo (clozapine)
Mellaril (thioridazine)	Geodon (ziprasidone)
Moban (molindrone)	Invega (paliperidone)
Navane (thithixene)	Risperdal (risperidone)
Orap (pimozide)	Seroquel (quetiapine)
Prolixin (fluphenazine)	Zyprexa (olanzapine)
Stelazine (trifluoperazine)	Symbyax (olanzapine and fluoxetine)
Thorazine (chlorpromazine)	
Trilafon (perphenazine)	

treatment [114–116]. In April 2005, the Food and Drug Administration issued a black box warning for atypical antipsychotic drugs (see Table 4.4) and again in June 2008 issued the same warning for the "conventional" antipsychotic drugs (see Table 4.4) because of an increased risk of mortality when they are administered for the treatment of behavioral disorders in elderly patients with dementia [117].

In a report regarding psychotropic drug use in nursing homes, findings indicated that 85 % of residents receive psychotropic drugs medically appropriately and 8 % received them inappropriately [113]. In the second quarter of 2014, 19.4 % of nursing home residents in the United States received antipsychotic drugs, compared to 23.2 % 2 years earlier [118]. Those antipsychotic drugs that are used sub optimally are based on lack of appropriate indications, inappropriate dosing, and high variability in usage rates across facilities [119, 120].

In a systematic review of intervention studies designed to reduce inappropriate prescribing of antipsychotic drugs in nursing homes, finding indicate that intervention, such as educational programs, in-reach services, medication review, and multicomponent interventions are effective short-term but not longer-term [121]. Interventions that sustain the outcome of reducing antipsychotic drug prescribing are warranted as many adverse outcomes are associated with the use of antipsychotic drugs that include increased risk of hospitalization, hip fractures, cardiovascular events, and mortality [122].

4.7 Education Programs to Prevent Abuse

Education programs with specialized training in abuse prevention are important to prevent abuse occurrence, learn new skills, and expand ones' knowledge base. Research has demonstrated that attendance at an educational course is superior to printed material in increasing knowledge on how to deal with elder abuse [123]. Iowa is the only state that requires education for its mandatory reporters [124]. Such education includes a 2-h course every 5 years on dependent adult abuse identification and reporting [124].

A well-planned, 8-module abuse prevention curriculum was developed and provided for nursing home employees to increase awareness of abuse, prevent and reduce incidents of abuse, and provide conflict intervention strategies [125]. In a pre-test/post-test designed study, 211 nurse aides from 10 nursing homes were provided an 8-module abuse prevention curriculum in 6–8 h [89]. Prior to participating in the education program, 51 % of participating nurse aides self-reported abusive behaviors of yelling at residents, and 17 % had restrained residents. The self-reported abusive acts by staff significantly declined after the training [89]. The participating nurse aides found it to be beneficial to express their concerns throughout the program and felt that on-going stress management training is necessary [125].

Training materials on elder abuse and neglect prevention were developed by and for native Hawaiians with the involvement of nursing home nurse aides [126]. During work on the training material, it was evident that nurse aides felt ill-prepared to deal with challenging resident behaviors and that handling stressful situations in the workplace was difficult [126].

4.8 Challenges of Conducting Research in Long Term Care Settings

In long term care facilities, all residents have guaranteed rights under Federal and State laws, one of which is the right to decline experimental research. The CMS State Operations Manual notes, "A resident being considered for participation in experimental research must be fully informed of the nature of the experimental research (e.g., medication, other treatment) and the possible consequences of participating.

The resident must give informed consent in order to participate" [35]. Ownership of following this directive is placed on the facility staff. Staff and investigators must be responsible for determining a resident's capacity to consent and if a resident is unable, a proxy consent must be properly obtained. The guidance states that "a facility participating in any experimental research involving residents must have a process for committee (e.g., an Institutional Review Board) approval of this research [35].

Elder abuse research itself raises two main ethical issues; that is, if abuse is discovered during the research process the investigator by most state laws has to report the allegation and how to gain informed consent from persons whose decisional capacity is impaired [65]. Furthermore, conducting elder abuse research in long term care settings adds other challenges, such as the health problems of the residents, obtaining informed consent, the routines of the living setting and physical environment, and facility administrators/governing boards.

To reside in a nursing home, a person must meet certain eligibility criteria to be approved; that is they have to need medical, nursing or rehabilitative services on a regular basis because their mental or physical condition requires that which is above the level of room and board and which can only be provided by institutional facilities and is not primarily for the care and treatment of mental diseases [35]. An estimated 50–60 % of nursing home residents have a diagnosis of dementia while 13 % of those have a primary diagnosis of Alzheimer's disease [114, 115, 127, 128]. Sixty-one percent of residents need assistance with bathing, 54 % with walking, 45 % with dressing, 37 % with toileting, 26 % with transferring in or out of bed, and 18 % with eating [9]. Older residents also have hearing and/or vision problems, pain, fatigue, and incontinence that can severely impact a resident's recruitment, informed consent, and participation in the research process [129].

Residents in long term care settings are considered vulnerable populations and as such Institutional Review Boards provide specific protections determining if the population is adequately justified and safeguards are in place to minimize risks. Consideration is also taken for persons with impaired decision-making capacity. Four elements are necessary for making a meaningful decision: understanding of information provided, appreciation of how the information applies to their situation, reasoning, and the ability to express choice [130]. One method for measuring capacity is to ask a resident a series of questions regarding the research that assess the four elements and assign criteria to answers as 2 = adequate answer, 1 = marginal answer, and 0 = inadequate answer. Summing the scores for each element provides a range of possible scores from 0 to 8 [131].

The layout of most nursing homes is typically that of hospitals with multiple rooms located on long corridors with a central location for the nurse's station, dining and activity rooms. The resident rooms are designed as singles, doubles, or even larger to hold 4–8 residents. In this confined space there are more people and interactions than in a single family household. Safety regulations are imposed in the facility by mandating railings, fire-retardant material, heavy fire doors, and wide corridors [132]. Along with the different living environment, the routines of the facility are imposed on the resident, that is the early morning breakfast, group or individual activities in the morning and afternoon, shower every few days, and to bed after dinner with staff hurriedly accomplishing this for numerous residents. Amidst all the activity are residents with varying degrees of cooperation and staff with fluctuating moods. In this tenuous situation, a researcher can face the following challenges: allowing for special events, conflict and jealousy among the residents, continuous background noise, unexpected interruptions, looking out for confused residents, negotiating the nursing home routines, participating resident's death or hospitalization, and privacy [133].

A particular problem noted in nursing home research impacting the sampling challenge is the turnover of administrators and study site coordinators. In one study comparing the nursing home completers of a study to the non-completers, the turnover rate for the administrators and site coordinators for the non-completers was 100 % higher for administrators and 86 % higher for site coordinators than the completers [134]. Also, survey deficiencies were 75 % higher, mean of 14 for non-completer nursing homes than completer nursing homes [134].

4.9 Future Directions

Noting there is a paucity in high quality nursing home research, an expert panel from the International Association of Gerontology and Geriatrics was convened and ranked the most important research questions needing to be explored in the nursing home setting which included dementia care, psychosocial interventions for behavioral and psychological symptoms of dementia, advanced care planning, improving nutrition, and polypharmacy [135]. Restraint free was the one elder abuse topic mentioned by the experts for research exploration [135]. Two top reasons for lack of good research in nursing homes deemed by the experts was inadequate research support from funding agencies and nursing home administrators lack of enthusiasm for research [135].

Unfortunately, no expert group or advocates for residents in assisted living settings have worked to develop a research agenda regarding elder abuse. In the 1990s, a cadre of researchers in different fields began studying assisted living facilities; describing the industry, delegation of authority in nurse practice acts, quality issues, privacy, state regulations, payment policies, resident characteristics, medication management, and risk management [136]. In 2003, the Agency for Healthcare Quality and Research funded a conference for assisted living researchers and federal officials to identify knowledge gaps, research questions, and methodological issues for assisted living. Suggestions for future research included topics on consumers and their families, facilities and services, and values and policy with no specific mention of elder abuse [136]. One question in the values and policy section explored an issue close to elder abuse, that was, is assisted living safe compared to nursing homes and life at home for similar populations [136].

Problems inherit in both nursing home and assisted living elder abuse research include the very basics: (1) no standardized terminology/language; (2) data across settings is not interchangeable; (3) lack of elder abuse research funding; (4) lack of multitude of researchers focusing on elder abuse [136, 137].

An elder abuse standardized language would be a common language, readily understood by all professionals working in the field of elder abuse to describe its phenomenon. In this way, social workers from different adult protective service agencies or nurses from intensive care or police officers in the field anywhere in the country would be able to use commonly understood terminology to identify the specific problem, intervention, or outcome related to their specific documentation. A standardized elder abuse language should be defined so the professional can communicate accurately among themselves. The increased use of electronic data entry in the practice settings has accelerated the need for standardized language.

In 1990, guidelines for gathering and compiling domestic elder abuse data were recommended for the purpose of ensuring greater comparability among state-level data [138]. A proposed data set was suggested to ensure comparability across states, and in doing so the credibility of aggregate elder abuse statistics would be improved. Four elements were proposed for the date set: elder abuse incidence flow data (counts of elder abuse reports), types and frequencies of elder abuse, characteristics of elder abuse perpetrators, and characteristics of elder abuse victims [138]. This suggested data set is the bare minimum of essential data elements needed for the science of elder abuse. Each distinct component of an elder abuse report needs standardized terminology. For example, 27 states and the District of Columbia's adult protective service's annual reports list 248 different terms for reporters of abuse with diverse terms as employer, housemate, building manager, medical examiner, caretaker, educator, circuit judge, and clergy [139]. The term elder abuse should mean the same to everyone regardless of where it occurs or what discipline is working with the allegation. The term sexual abuse should stand alone and not be imbedded in physical abuse. Implications for not having a standardized language are many and hold back the science of elder abuse. "If we cannot name it, we cannot control it, practice it, teach it, finance it, or put it into public policy" [140].

In addition to standardized language, the data needs to be consistently defined and used across agencies. Every set of approved data elements need to have the same meaning across agencies, which will improve data quality. In 2014, the Digital Accountability and Transparency Act (DATA ACT), Public Law No. 113-101 was signed into law to establish common standards for financial data provided by all government agencies. Established by the Elder Justice Act, the elder justice coordinating council meets twice yearly to coordinate activities related to elder abuse across the federal government. The coordinating council has developed a recommendation to develop a national adult protective services system based upon standardized data collection and a core set of service provision standards and best practices. This system, National Adult Maltreatment Reporting System, is being developed along with data specifications [141]. At this time, the draft case component data specifications has a data element named, report source, with the following choices: guardian/conservator, community based services, education, financial, law enforcement/judicial/legal, medical/health, mental health, residential care community, social service/rehabilitative services, other professional, self, family member, non-family member, and anonymous [141]. It is evident from this list that it is very different from the adult protective services reporter source but making it standardized is important. The coordinating council should make this same recommendation, a system for data collection, across all agencies that collect elder abuse data especially agencies involved in long term care settings abuse investigations.

Research funding for elder abuse can be found from public and private institutions. The problem is that there are few private foundations that focus on elder abuse research and few federal dollars are allocated for elder abuse research with fewer resources then geared to research in long term care settings.

Through the National Institute of Justice, the U.S. Department of Justice provides for research, development and evaluation. For the past 11 years, NIJ has solicited and funded research on elder abuse, neglect, and exploitation usually making 3–4 awards per year totaling about $1 million. Of the awards since 2004, two have been dedicated to research in long term care settings: an examination of resident abuse in assisted living facilities by the University of Pittsburgh and physician documentation of resident to resident mistreatment in residential care facilities from Cornell University.

In 2012, the U.S. Department of Health and Human Services Administration for Community Living had a one-time call to test and evaluate comprehensive approaches to preventing elder abuse. None of the six funded proposals were geared to research regarding elder abuse in long term care settings.

The National Institute on Aging in 2005 and 2006 issued a Request for Applications with a focus on methodological issues related to elder mistreatment. Nine projects were awarded with none having a focus on elder abuse research in long term care settings. Since that time no specific solicitations for elder abuse research has been issued but unsolicited applications have been funded based on merit.

Some of the private foundations that have funded elder abuse research are the Archstone Foundation of Long Beach, CA, The Fan Fox and Leslie R. Samuels Foundation, Inc. of New York, NY, The Harry and Jeanette Weinberg Foundation of Owings Mills, MA, and the Retirement Research Foundation of Chicago, IL. The funding doesn't necessarily apply to long term care settings. Each of the foundations has their specific requirements with some being territorial.

Funding for elder abuse research in long term care has been bleak along with the cadre of researchers in the field. The 43 frequently published elder abuse researchers are mainly from the fields of criminology, medicine, nursing, political science, psychology, public administration and public affairs, public health, social welfare policy, sociology, and social work [142]. When combining the fields of elder abuse and long term care settings, the number of researchers dwindles to very few. In the coordinating councils report to congress, it was suggested to increase the researchers in the field, consider target funding in the field [137].

In the future, it would be ideal for law enforcement to accompany case workers investigating all allegations of abuse in long term care settings. It is essential that police officers know the signs of elder abuse and take the time to investigate. Having a dual investigative team will allow the two team members to accomplish more than as individuals working alone. The dual team may provide higher quality outcomes for the alleged victim with a more efficient and thoughtful investigation. Each person, the case worker and the police officer, bring different information and knowledge to their work which may result in a more thorough forensic investigation. By bringing this duo together the benefits to the field of elder abuse will explode.

Screened out allegations of abuse in long term care settings may need investigating [112]. Investigating agencies should routinely randomly investigate screened out allegations of elder abuse. If the results of such exploring result in further investigation and substantiation of an allegation, then the screened out process needs to be reviewed, revised, and potentially omitted.

Despite the extensive achievements in investigating and prosecuting nursing home abuse, additional national initiatives need to occur. The following initiatives are critical:

- States should have a clearly defined statute that designates various forms of patient abuse, neglect, and exploitation in long term care settings (including nursing facilities and assisted living)
- Federal legislation is needed to provide oversight for all assisted living facilities
- A national directory of all caregivers convicted of abuse, neglect, and exploitation should be accessible to employers
- Agencies housing the abuse data should have provisions for easy access to the raw data
- Larger number of advocates for the prevention of abuse in long term care settings are needed.

4.10 Conclusions

Each state has its respective long term care licensure agency, adult protective services agency, Medicaid Fraud Control Unit, and long term care ombudsman—yet with all these various agencies and their respective legislation, abuse is still rampant and in many forms. Musing about the 1974 report "The Litany and Dimensions of Nursing Home Abuses" and its horrendous descriptions of abuse in nursing homes, the truth is that similar acts are still happening today [11].

In the practice setting, the following incidents of abuse, neglect, and exploitation have been observed by this author:

- Instead of taking a resident's weekly blood pressure, a new blood pressure recording was documented adjusting the previous week's recording by 2 mm Hg
- The toothbrush was dipped in a glass of water to indicate it had been used in lieu of brushing the resident's teeth
- Tylenol #3 was stolen from the residents, resulting in pain being uncontrolled
- Water was flicked on the resident's head to give the appearance of dampness to indicate a shower had been given
- Duragesic patches were removed from the residents
- An antique picture and frame were taken from the resident's wall
- A resident eloped and was found 3 h later sleeping in daylilies behind a garage
- A female resident took off her upper clothes and taunted a male resident with her breasts.

Unfortunately, these incidents are recent, were abusive to residents, and had repercussions. For example, it took 8 months of investigation to determine the registered nurse who was stealing the Tylenol #3. She was terminated from her job and lost her nursing license. In another situation, the nursing home was cited for poor quality of care for a resident's dirty finger nails—it was the same resident who had been sprinkled with water. A state surveyor was standing outside the shower room during the supposed shower.

The results of this review indicate there is no definitive evidence about prevalence of abuse, neglect, and exploitation in long term care settings, but such abuse, neglect, and exploitation is still widespread. The Elder Justice Roadmap notes in the research section that "standards and data collection methods used by various entities (such as surveyors, adult protective services, long term ombudsman, and others) are variable" [143]. And the recommendation is made that "researchers should assist in developing the parameters and methods used to build an evidence base system designed to collect accurate data and show the impact of effective practices" [143].

Appendix 1: Institutional Reporting Abuse Agencies Web Address and Hotline Number by State (Current as of 6/19/2015)

State	Report nursing home abuse
Alabama	Alabama Department of Senior Services
	Tel: (800) 356-9596
	http://www.adph.org/HEALTHCAREFACILITIES/Default.asp?id=688
Alaska	Alaska Health Facilities Licensing and Certification
	Tel: (888) 387-9387 or (907) 334-2482
	http://dhss.alaska.gov/dhcs/Pages/hflc/contact.aspx
Arizona	Arizona Division of Public Health Services Licensing Services
	Tel: (877) 767-2385
	http://www.azdhs.gov/als/index.htm
Arkansas	Arkansas Office of Long Term Care
	Tel: (800) 582-4887
	http://humanservices.arkansas.gov/dms/pages/oltchome.aspx/
California	Licensing and Certification Division, Department of Public Health
	(Contact local Licensing and Certification District Office)
	Tel: Bakersfield: (866) 222-1903
	Chico: (800) 554-0350
	East Bay: (866) 247-9100
	Fresno: (800) 554-0351
	Los Angeles: (800) 228-1019
	Orange County: (800) 228-5234
	Riverside: (888) 354-9203
	Sacramento: (800) 554-0354
	San Bernardino: (800) 344-2896
	San Diego (North): (800) 824-0613
	San Diego (South): (866) 706-0759
	San Francisco: (800) 554-0353
	San Jose: (800) 554-0348
	Santa Rosa: (866) 784-0703
	Ventura: (800) 547-8267
	http://www.cdph.ca.gov/programs/LnC/Pages/LnCContact.aspx
Colorado	Health Facilities Division, Department of Public Health & Environment
	Tel: (303) 692-2442 or (800) 886-7689 ext. 2442
	https://www.colorado.gov/pacific/cdphe/health-facilities-complaint-and-occurence-contacts
Connecticut	Facility Licensing and Investigation Section, Department of Public Health
	Tel: (860) 509-7400
	http://www.ct.gov/dph/cwp/view.asp?a=3121&q=387678&dphNav=%7C&dphNav_GID=1821
Delaware	Division of Long Term Care Residents Protection, Health and Social Services
	Tel: (877) 453-0012
	http://www.dhss.delaware.gov/dhss/dltcrp/contact.html
Florida	Division of Health Quality Assurance, Agency for Health Care Administration
	1-888-419-3456
	http://www.fdhc.state.fl.us/Contact/call_center.shtml
Georgia	Division of Healthcare Facility Regulation, Department of Community Health
	Tel: (404) 657-5726 or (404) 657-5728
	http://dch.georgia.gov/hfr-file-complaint
Hawaii	State Department of Health, Office of Health Care Assurance
	Tel: (808) 234-5380 or (877) 236-5380
	http://health.hawaii.gov/ohca/
Idaho	Bureau of Facility Standards, Department of Health and Welfare
	Tel: (208) 364-1899
	http://www.healthandwelfare.idaho.gov/Medical/LicensingCertification/FacilityStandards/NursingFacilities/tabid/281/Default.aspx
Illinois	Office of Health Care Regulation, Department of Public Health
	Tel: (800) 252-4343
	http://www.idph.state.il.us/about/ohcr.htm
Indiana	Health Care Quality and Regulatory Commission, State Department of Health
	Tel: (317) 233-7709 or (800) 246-8909
	http://www.state.in.us/isdh/25766.htm
Iowa	Tel: (877) 686-0027
	https://dia-hfd.iowa.gov/DIA_HFD/Process.do;jsessionid
	=8FA05CC384F58F4FC3394522EE0EDFB7.worker1
	Iowa Department of Inspections and Appeals

(continued)

State	Report nursing home abuse
Kansas	Bureau of Community Health Systems, Department of Health and Environment
	Tel: (800) 842-0078
	http://www.kdheks.gov/bhfr/elder_abuse_hotlines.html
Kentucky	Division of Health Care, Cabinet for Health and Family Services
	Tel: Western Enforcement Branch: (270) 889-6052
	Northern Enforcement Branch: (502) 595-4958
	Southern Enforcement Branch: (606) 330-2030
	Eastern Enforcement Branch: (859) 246-2301
	http://chfs.ky.gov/os/oig/dhcfs.htm
Louisiana	Health Standards, Department of Health & Hospitals
	Tel: (888) 810-1819
	http://new.dhh.louisiana.gov/index.cfm/page/254
Maine	Division of Licensing and Regulatory Services, Medical Facilities Unit
	Tel: (800) 624-8404
	http://www.maine.gov/dhhs/dlrs/medical_facilities/nursing.html
Maryland	Office of Health Care Quality, Department of Health and Mental Hygiene
	Tel: (877) 402-8219 or (410) 402-8201
	http://dhmh.maryland.gov/ohcq/LTC/default.aspx
Massachusetts	Division of Health Care Facility Licensure and Certification, Health and Human Services
	Tel: (800) 462-5540 or (617) 753-8150
	http://www.mass.gov/eohhs/gov/departments/dph/programs/hcq/healthcare-quality/healthcare-facility-complaints/complaints-for-nursing-homes-health-care-facilities.html
Minnesota	Office of Health Facility Complaints, Department of Health
	1-800-369-7994
	http://www.health.state.mn.us/divs/fpc/ohfcinfo/contohfc.htm
Mississippi	Mississippi Department of Health, Health Facilities Licensure & Certification
	Tel: (800) 227-7308
	http://msdh.ms.gov/msdhsite/_static/30,0,83.html
Missouri	Missouri Department of Health and Senior Services, Licensing & Regulations
	Tel: (800) 392-0210
	http://www.dhss.mo.gov/ElderAbuse/
Montana	Montana Department of Public Health and Human Services, Quality Assurance Division
	Tel: (406) 444-2037
	http://www.dphhs.mt.gov/qad/index.shtml
Nebraska	Nebraska Health Care Facilities and Services Complaints, Department of Health and Human Services
	Tel: (402) 471-0316
	http://dhhs.ne.gov/publichealth/Pages/crl_invest_invest.aspx
Nevada	State Health Division, Department of Health and Human Services
	Tel: (775) 687-4475 Carson City or (702) 486-6515 Las Vegas
	http://dhhs.nv.gov/Health/HCQC_HealthFacilities.htm
New Hampshire	Health Facilities Administration, Office of Operations Support, Department of Health & Human Services
	Tel: (603) 271-9039
	http://www.dhhs.nh.gov/oos/bhfa/complaint.htm
New Jersey	Division of Health Facilities Evaluation and Licensing, Department of Health
	Tel: (800) 792-9770
	http://www.state.nj.us/health/healthfacilities/hotlines.shtml
New Mexico	Bureau of Health Facility Licensing & Certification, Department of Health
	Tel: (800) 752-8649
	http://dhi.health.state.nm.us/hflc/index.php
New York	Hospitals, Nursing Homes & Other Health Care Facilities, Department of Health
	Tel: (888) 201-4563
	http://www.health.ny.gov/facilities/nursing/complaints.htm
North Carolina	Complaint Intake, Division of Health Service Regulation
	Tel: (800) 624-3004 or (919) 855-4500
	http://www.ncdhhs.gov/dhsr/ciu/filecomplaint.html
North Dakota	Health Facilities, Health Resources Section, Department of Health
	Tel: (701) 328-2352 http://www.health.state.nd.us/hf/North_Dakota_Basic_Care_Facilities.htm
Ohio	Nursing Homes/Facilities, Department of Health
	Tel: (800) 342-0553 http://www.odh.ohio.gov/odhprograms/ltc/nurhome/nurhome1.aspx
Oklahoma	State Department of Health, Long Term Care Programs
	Tel: (800) 747-8419, then press 3
	http://www.ok.gov/health/Oklahoma_State_Department_of_Health_Hotlines.html
Oregon	Health Care Licensure & Certification, Department of Human Services
	Tel: (800) 282-8096
	http://www.oregon.gov/dhs/spwpd/Pages/ltc/licensing/index.aspx
Pennsylvania	Bureau of Facility Licensure and Certification, Bureau of Quality Assurance, Department of Health
	Tel: (800) 254-5164 or (877) 401-8835
	http://www.portal.health.state.pa.us/portal/server.pt/community/nursing_home_care/14152/nursing_home_complaints/558484
Rhode Island	Division of Health Services Regulation, Department of Health
	Tel: (401) 222-5200 or (401) 272-5952 after hours
	http://www.health.ri.gov/complaints/

(continued)

State	Report nursing home abuse
South Carolina	Division of Nursing Homes, Department of Health & Environmental Control
	Tel: (800) 922-6735
	http://www.scdhec.gov/Health/FHPF/HealthFacilityRegulationsLicensing/MedicareMedicaidCertification/NursingHomes/
South Dakota	South Dakota Department of Health, Health Care Facility Complaints
	Tel: (605) 773-3497
	https://doh.sd.gov/providers/licensure/Complaints.aspx
Tennessee	Division of Health Care Facilities, Department of Health
	Tel: (877) 287-0010
	http://tn.gov/health/article/hcf-complaint
Texas	Health Facilities Program, Department of State Health Services
	Tel: (888) 973-0022
	http://www.dshs.state.tx.us/facilities/complaints.aspx
Utah	Department of Health, Bureau of Health Facility Licensing, Certification and Resident Assessment
	Tel: (800) 662-4157
	http://health.utah.gov/hflcra/
Vermont	Division of Licensing and Protection, Department of Aging and Disabilities
	Tel: (800) 564-1612 (in state toll free) or (802) 871-3326 (outside of Vermont)
	http://www.dlp.vermont.gov/abuse-reporting-form
Virginia	Office of Licensure & Certification, Department of Health
	Tel: (800) 955-1819
	http://www.vdh.virginia.gov/OLC/Complaint/
Washington	Facilities and Services Licensing, Department of Health
	Tel: (800) 633-6828
	http://www.doh.wa.gov/LicensesPermitsandCertificates/FileComplaintAboutProviderorFacility/FacilityComplaintProcess
Washington, DC	Health Regulation Administration, Department of Health
	Tel: (877) 672-2174
	http://doh.dc.gov/node/181312
West Virginia	Office of Health Facility Licensure & Certification, Department of Health & Human Resources
	Tel: (800) 352-6513 or (304) 558-0050
	https://ohflac.wv.gov/complaint.html
Wisconsin	Division of Quality Assurance, Department of Health
	Tel: (800) 642-6552 http://dhfs.wisconsin.gov/bqaconsumer/HealthCareComplaints.htm
Wyoming	Wyoming Office of Health Licensing and Survey, Department of Health
	Tel: (307) 777-7123
	http://www.health.wyo.gov/ohls/complaint.html

Appendix 2: Case Study Reporting an Allegation of Nursing Home Abuse

On a Friday afternoon at 16:30, the evening charge nurse walked into the director of nursing's office in a 48-bed nursing home and said, "All of the nurses are mad at you!" The director asked why they were mad as she had no idea. The charge nurse replied because you didn't report the physical abuse allegation for Mary to the state authorities. The director responded that no one had told her about such an allegation. The charge nurse responded that she reported it to the assistant director of nursing a week ago and expected her to relay the message.

Iowa legislation mandates that, "a person who, in the course of employment, examines, attends, counsels, or treats a dependent adult and reasonably believes the dependent adult has suffered abuse, shall report the suspected dependent adult abuse to the department. Persons required to report include all of the following: A health practitioner, as defined in section 232.68 (Iowa Code Ann. §235B.3). The definition of health practitioner "includes a licensed physician and surgeon, osteopathic physician and surgeon, dentist, optometrist, podiatric physician, or chiropractor; a resident or intern in any of such professions; a licensed dental hygienist, a registered nurse or licensed practical nurse; a physician assistant; and an emergency medical care provider (Iowa Code Ann. §232.68). Any of the 16 employed registered and licensed practical nurses were obligated to report the allegation, but did not and the responsibility defaulted to the director of nursing.

The director of nursing immediately went to the administrator's office and told her of the allegation and that she was going to report it to the Iowa Department of Inspections and Appeals. The administrator asked that she not report the incident, that it would not be founded and that it would make the nursing home look bad. She also said if you report the allegation, I will terminate your employment. The director of nursing then went to the assistant administrator's office and conveyed the entire event to the assistant administrator. She said it was time for her to go home for the day; she got up from her chair, put her coat on, and left the office.

The director of nursing went back to her office and called the Iowa Department of Inspections and Appeals. She attempted to give the respondent a hypothetical scenario. The respondent wouldn't accept that and said you have an allegation to report and if you don't report it now, you could lose your license. The director of nursing said the administrator threatened to terminate her employment if she made the report. That of course didn't matter. The director of nursing proceeded to report the allegation and the next day mailed the agency a written report.

Upon receipt of the allegation made, the department made a preliminary review of the complaint and determined an on-site inspection of the nursing home should be completed. The department determined the allegation was a non-immediate jeopardy situation and had twenty working days to complete the investigation (Iowa Code Ann. §135C.38). During the onsite visit, it was determined the allegation of abuse was not founded. The director of nursing wasn't terminated.

References

1. Livengood M. A group-process approach to resident and staff abuse. J Am Health Care Assoc. 1980;6(1):29–30, 35.
2. Pillemer K, Moore DW. Highlights from a study of abuse of patients in nursing homes. J Elder Abuse Negl. 1990;2(1–2):5–30.
3. Caffrey C, Sengupta M, Park-Lee E, Moss A, Rosenoff E, Harris-Kojetin L. Residents living in residential care facilities: United States, 2010. National Center for Health Statistics data brief, No. 91 [Internet] Hyattsville, MD: National Center for Health Statistics; 2012 [cited 2015 May 20]. http://www.cdc.gov/nchs/data/databriefs/db91.pdf.
4. Centers for Disease Control and Prevention. Nursing homes and assisted living (long-term care facilities [LTCFs]) [Internet] Altanta, GA: Centers for Disease Control and Prevention; [updated 2015 Jan 27; cited 2015 May 20]. http://www.cdc.gov/longtermcare/.
5. Wierucka D, Goodridge D. Vulnerable in a safe place: institutional elder abuse. Can J Nurs Adm. 1996;9(3):82–104.
6. Mollica RL. Residential care and assisted living: state oversight practices and state information available to consumers. AHRQ publication no. 06-M051-EF. [Internet] Rockville, MD: Agency for Healthcare Research and Quality; 2006 [cited 2015 May 18]. http://www.ahcancal.org/ncal/resources/Documents/AHRQ_study_2006r.pdf.
7. Centers for Disease Control and Prevention. Health, United States, 2014: with special feature on adults aged 55-64 Atlanta, GA: Centers for Disease Control and Prevention; 2015 [updated May 6, 2015; cited 2015 August 2]. http://www.cdc.gov/nchs/hus.htm.
8. Caffrey C, Harris-Kojetin L, Rome V, Sengupta M. Operating characteristics of residential care communities, by community bed size: United States, 2012. National Center for Health Statistics data brief, no. 170. [Internet] Hyattsville, MD: National Center for Health Statistics; 2014 [cited 2015 Jun 5]. http://www.cdc.gov/nchs/data/databriefs/db170.htm.
9. Caffrey C, Harris-Kojetin L, Rome V, Sengupta M. Characteristics of residents living in residential care communities, by community bed size: United States, 2012. National Center for Health Statistics data brief, no. 171. [Internet] Hyattsville, MD: National Center for Health Statistics; 2014 [cited 2015 Jun 5]. http://www.cdc.gov/nchs/data/databriefs/db171.htm.
10. Hill L. Memorandum. S. Res. 65, Authorizing a comprehensive study of the problems of the aging 1959 [cited 2015 June 2]. http://www.aging.senate.gov/imo/media/doc/publications/1959SubcommitteeOnTheProblemsOfTheAgingAndAged.pdf.
11. Subcommittee on Long-Term Care of the Special Committee on Aging United States Senate. Nursing home care in the United States: failure in public policy; Supporting Paper No. 1. The litany of nursing homes abuses and an examination of the roots of controversy (Report No. 93). Washington, DC: U.S. Government Printing Office; 1974. p. 163–241.
12. Tatara T. An analysis of state laws addressing elder abuse, neglect, and exploitation. Washington, DC: National Center on Elder Abuse; 1995.
13. Alford DM. The elder justice act. J Gerontol Nurs. 2011;37(8):14–6.
14. American Health Care Association. The long term care survey [Internet]. Washington, DC: American Health Care Association; 2014 [cited 2015 Jun 5]. http://www.ahcancal.org/Pages/LTC-Survey.aspx.
15. Daly JM, Jogerst GJ. Nursing home abuse report and investigation legislation. J Elder Abuse Negl. 2007;19(3–4):119–31.
16. Daly JM, Jogerst GJ. Nursing home statutes: mistreatment definitions. J Elder Abuse Negl. 2006;18(1):19–39.
17. Daly JM, Jogerst GJ. Association of knowledge of adult protective services legislation with rates of reporting of abuse in Iowa nursing homes. J Am Med Dir Assoc. 2005;6(2):113–20.
18. Pillemer K, Bachman-Prehn R. Helping and hurting: predictors of maltreatment of patients in nursing homes. Res Aging. 1991;13(1):74–95.
19. Jogerst GJ, Daly JM, Dawson JD, Peek-Asa C, Schmuch G. Iowa nursing home characteristics associated with reported abuse. J Am Med Dir Assoc. 2006;7(4):203–7.
20. Schiamberg LB, Oehmke J, Zhang Z, Barboza GE, Griffore RJ, Von Heydrich L, et al. Physical abuse of older adults in nursing homes: a random sample survey of adults with an elderly family member in a nursing home. J Elder Abuse Negl. 2011;24(1):65–83.
21. Pillemer K, Moore DW. Abuse of patients in nursing homes: findings from a survey of staff. Gerontologist. 1989;29(3):314–20.
22. Zhang Z, Schiamberg LB, Oehmke J, Barboza GE, Griffore RJ, Post LA, et al. Neglect of older adults in Michigan nursing homes. J Elder Abuse Negl. 2010;23(1):58–74.
23. Page C, Conner T, Prokhorov A, Fang Y, Post L. The effect of care setting on elder abuse: results from a Michigan survey. J Elder Abuse Negl. 2009;21(3):239–52.
24. Teaster PB, The National Center on Elder Abuse, National Committee for the Prevention of Elder Abuse, The National Association of Adult Protective Services Administrators, and the National Center on Elder Abuse. A response to the abuse of vulnerable adults: the 2000 survey of State Adult Protective Services. Washington, DC: National Center on Elder Abuse; 2003.
25. Teaster PB, Dugar TD, Otto JM, Mendiondo MS, Abner EL, Cecil KA, et al. The 2004 survey of state Adult Protective Services: abuse of vulnerable adults 18 years of age and older. A report of the National Center on Elder Abuse. Washington, DC: The National Committee for the Prevention of Elder Abuse and The National Adult Protective Services Association; 2007.
26. Payne BK, Strasser SM. Financial exploitation of older persons in adult care settings: comparisons to physical abuse and the justice system's response. J Elder Abuse Negl. 2012;24(3):231–50.
27. U.S. Department of Health and Human Services Office of Inspector General. Medicaid Fraud Control Units fiscal year 2014 annual report [Internet]. 2015 [cited 2015 May 28]. http://oig.hhs.gov/oei/reports/oei-06-15-00010.pdf.
28. Payne BK, Cikovic R. An empirical examination of the characteristics, consequences, and causes of elder abuse in nursing homes. J Elder Abuse Negl. 1996;7(4):61–74.

29. Payne BK, Gainey RR. The criminal justice response to elder abuse in nursing homes: a routine activities perspective. West Criminol Rev. 2006;7(3):67–81.
30. Allen PD, Kellett K, Gruman C. Elder abuse in Connecticut's nursing homes. J Elder Abuse Negl. 2004;15(1):19–42.
31. Bloemen EM, Rosen T, Clark S, Nash D, Mielenz TJ. Trends in reporting of abuse and neglect to long term care ombudsmen: data from the National Ombudsman Reporting System from 2006 to 2013. Geriatr Nurs. 2015;36(4):281–3.
32. Jogerst GJ, Daly J, Hartz A. Ombudsman program characteristics related to nursing home abuse reporting. J Gerontol Soc Work. 2005;46(1):85–98.
33. Paton RN, Huber R, Netting FE. The long-term care ombudsman program and complaints of abuse and neglect. J Elder Abuse Negl. 1994;6(1):97–115.
34. Department of Health & Human Services Office of Inspector General. Memorandum report: trends in nursing home deficiencies and complaints, OEI-02-08-00140. [Internet] Washington, DC: Department of Health & Human Services, Office of Inspector General; 2008 [cited 2015 June 12]. http://oig.hhs.gov/oei/reports/oei-02-08-00140.pdf.
35. Centers for Medicare & Medicaid Services (CMS). State Operations Manual Appendix PP—Guidance to surveyors for long term care facilities [Internet] 2015 [cited 2015 June 12]. https://www.cms.gov/Regulations-and-Guidance/Guidance/Manuals/downloads/som107ap_pp_guidelines_ltcf.pdf.
36. U.S. Government Accountability Office. Nursing homes: more reliable data and consistent guidance would improve CMS oversight of state complaint investigations [Internet] April 2011 [cited 2015 June 5]. http://www.gao.gov/new.items/d11280.pdf.
37. Jogerst GJ, Daly JM, Hartz AJ. State policies and nursing home characteristics associated with rates of resident mistreatment. J Am Med Dir Assoc. 2008;9(9):648–56.
38. Lapane KL, Quilliam BJ, Chow W, Kim MS. Impact of revisions to the F-Tag 309 surveyors' interpretive guidelines on pain management among nursing home residents. Drugs Aging. 2012;29(5):385–93.
39. Pimentel CB, Briesacher BA, Gurwitz JH, Rosen AB, Pimentel MT, Lapane KL. Pain management in nursing home residents with cancer. J Am Geriatr Soc. 2015;63(4):633–41.
40. Shen X, Zuckerman IH, Palmer JB, Stuart B. Trends in prevalence for moderate-to-severe pain and persistent pain among Medicare beneficiaries in nursing homes, 2006–2009. J Gerontol A Biol Sci Med Sci. 2015;70(5):598–603.
41. Lindbloom EJ, Brandt J, Hough LD, Meadows SE. Elder mistreatment in the nursing home: a systematic review. J Am Med Dir Assoc. 2007;8(9):610–6.
42. Rosen T, Lachs MS, Bharucha AJ, Stevens SM, Teresi JA, Nebres F, et al. Resident-to-resident aggression in long-term care facilities: insights from focus groups of nursing home residents and staff. J Am Geriatr Soc. 2008;56(8):1398–408.
43. Rich BA. Thinking the unthinkable: the clinician as perpetrator of elder abuse in patients in pain. J Pain Palliat Care Pharmacother. 2004;18(3):63–74.
44. Bell J. The use of restraint in the care of elderly patients. Br J Nurs. 1997;6(9):504–8.
45. Thurmond JA. Nurses' perceptions of chemical restraint use in long-term care. Appl Nurs Res. 1999;12(3):159–62.
46. Aziz SJ, Campbell-Taylor I. Neglect and abuse associated with undernutrition in long-term care in North America: causes and solutions. J Elder Abuse Negl. 1999;10(1–2):91–117.
47. Fulmer T, Ashley J. Clinical indicators of elder neglect. Appl Nurs Res. 1989;2(4):161–7.
48. Glendenning F. Elder abuse and neglect in residential settings: the need for inclusiveness in elder abuse research. J Elder Abuse Negl. 1999;10(1–2):1–11.
49. Gold MF. Regulators crack down on abuse. Provider. 2000;26(4):24–6, 29–30, 33–7.
50. Hawes C. Elder abuse in residential long-term care settings: what is known and what information is needed. In: Bonnie RJ, Wallace RB, editors. Elder mistreatment, abuse, neglect, and exploitation in an aging America. Washington, DC: National Research Council of the National Academies; 2003. p. 446–500.
51. Kimsey LR, Tarbox AR, Bragg DF. Abuse of the elderly—the hidden agenda. I. The caretakers and the categories of abuse. J Am Geriatr Soc. 1981;29(10):465–72.
52. MacLean DS. Abuse and neglect of elderly persons. N Engl J Med. 1995;333(1):70.
53. Tammelleo AD. 'Reckless' neglect of elders violates Elder Abuse Act. Regan Rep Nurs Law. 1999;39(11):1.
54. Colello KJ. Older Americans Act: long-term care Ombudsman program [Internet] Washington, DC: Congressional Research Service; 2012 [cited 2015 May 19]. http://www.law.umaryland.edu/marshall/crsreports/crsdocuments/RS21297_02152012.pdf.
55. U.S. Department of Health and Human Services. Administration for Community Living. Administration on Aging. 2013 National Ombudsman Reporting System data tables [Internet] 2014 [cited 2015 May 19]. http://www.aoa.acl.gov/AoA_Programs/Elder_Rights/Ombudsman/National_State_Data/2013/Index.aspx.
56. Troyer JL, Sause W. Association between traditional nursing home quality measures and two sources of nursing home complaints. Health Serv Res. 2013;48(4):1256–78.
57. Ostwald SK, Runge A, Lees EJ, Patterson GD. Texas certified volunteer long-term care ombudsmen: perspectives of role and effectiveness. J Am Med Dir Assoc. 2003;4(6):323–8.
58. Payne BK, Gray C. Theoretical orientation and responses to abuse in nursing homes. J Soc Work in Long-Term Care. 2002;1(4):31–54.
59. Centers for Medicare & Medicaid Services (CMS). State Operations Manual Chapter 5—Complaint Procedures [Internet] 2014 [cited 2015 May 22]. https://www.cms.gov/Regulations-and-Guidance/Guidance/Manuals/downloads/som107c05.pdf.
60. Forms Workflow. Medicare-Medicaid-CLIA complaint form CMS-562-official federal form [Internet] 2006 [cited 2015 June 12]. http://www.formsworkflow.com/d69564.aspx.
61. Tatara T. A comprehensive analysis of state policy and practice related to elder abuse. Washington, DC: National Association of State Units on Aging and the American Public Welfare Association; 1986.
62. Tatara T, Blumerman LM. Summaries of the statistical data on elder abuse in domestic settings: an exploratory study of state statistics for FY 93 and FY 94. Washington, DC: National Center on Elder Abuse; 1996.
63. Tatara T, Kusmeskus LB. Summaries of the statistical data on elder abuse in domestic settings for FY 95 and FY 96. Washington, DC: National Center on Elder Abuse; 1997.
64. U.S. General Accounting Office. Nursing homes: complaint investigation processes often inadequate to protect residents [Internet] March 1999 [cited 2015 July 14]. http://www.gao.gov/assets/230/227108.pdf.
65. National Research Council. Elder mistreatment: abuse, neglect, and exploitation in an Aging America. Panel to Review Risk and Prevalence of Elder Abuse and Neglect. In: Bonnie RJ, Wallace RB, editors. Washington, DC: The National Academies Press; 2003.

66. Burgess AW, Dowdell EB, Prentky RA. Sexual abuse of nursing home residents. J Psychosoc Nurs Ment Health Serv. 2000;38 (6):10–8.
67. Research Data Assistance Center. Research identifiable files (RIF) requests [Internet] Minneapolis, MN: University of Minnesota School of Public Health; 2013 [cited 2015 August 6]. http://www.resdac.org/cms-data/request/research-identifiable-files.
68. Zhang Z, Page C, Conner T, Post LA. Family members' reports of non-staff abuse in Michigan nursing homes. J Elder Abuse Negl. 2012;24(4):357–69.
69. Castle NG. Resident-to-resident abuse in nursing homes as reported by nurse aides. J Elder Abuse Negl. 2012;24(4):340–56.
70. Pillemer K, Chen EK, Van Haitsma KS, Teresi J, Ramirez M, Silver S, et al. Resident-to-resident aggression in nursing homes: results from a qualitative event reconstruction study. Gerontologist. 2012;52(1):24–33.
71. Trompetter H, Scholte R, Westerhof G. Resident-to-resident relational aggression and subjective well-being in assisted living facilities. Aging Ment Health. 2011;15(1):59–67.
72. Snellgrove S, Beck C, Green A, McSweeney JC. Resident-to-resident violence triggers in nursing homes. Clin Nurs Res. 2013;22(4):461–74.
73. Shinoda-Tagawa T, Leonard R, Pontikas J, McDonough JE, Allen D, Dreyer PI. Resident-to-resident violent incidents in nursing homes. JAMA. 2004;291(5):591–8.
74. McDonald L, Hitzig SL, Pillemer KA, Lachs MS, Beaulieu M, Brownell P, et al. Developing a research agenda on resident-to-resident aggression: recommendations from a consensus conference. J Elder Abuse Negl. 2015;27(2):146–67.
75. Lachs M, Bachman R, Williams CS, O'Leary JR. Resident-to-resident elder mistreatment and police contact in nursing homes: findings from a population-based cohort. J Am Geriatr Soc. 2007;55(6):840–5.
76. Rosen T, Lachs MS, Teresi J, Eimicke J, Van Haitsma K, Pillemer K. Staff-reported strategies for prevention and management of resident-to-resident elder mistreatment in long-term care facilities. J Elder Abuse Negl. 2015;28(1):1–13.
77. Teresi JA, Ramirez M, Ellis J, Silver S, Boratgis G, Kong J, et al. A staff intervention targeting resident-to-resident elder mistreatment (R-REM) in long-term care increased staff knowledge, recognition and reporting: results from a cluster randomized trial. Int J Nurs Stud. 2013;50(5):644–56.
78. Snellgrove S, Beck C, Green A, McSweeney JC. Putting residents first: strategies developed by CNAs to prevent and manage resident-to-resident violence in nursing homes. Gerontologist. 2015;55(Suppl 1):S99–S107.
79. Zeller A, Dassen T, Kok G, Needham I, Halfens RJ. Factors associated with resident aggression toward caregivers in nursing homes. J Nurs Scholarsh. 2012;44(3):249–57.
80. Lachs MS, Rosen T, Teresi JA, Eimicke JP, Ramirez M, Silver S, et al. Verbal and physical aggression directed at nursing home staff by residents. J Gen Intern Med. 2013;28(5):660–7.
81. Bowie CR, Moriarty PJ, Harvey PD, Parrella M, White L, Davis KL. Aggression in elderly schizophrenia patients: a comparison of nursing home and state hospital residents. J Neuropsychiatry Clin Neurosci. 2001;13(3):357–66.
82. Gates D, Fitzwater E, Succop P. Relationships of stressors, strain, and anger to caregiver assaults. Issues Ment Health Nurs. 2003;24(8):775–93.
83. Gruber-Baldini AL, Boustani M, Sloane PD, Zimmerman S. Behavioral symptoms in residential care/assisted living facilities: prevalence, risk factors, and medication management. J Am Geriatr Soc. 2004;52(10):1610–7.
84. Gates DM, Fitzwater E, Meyer U. Violence against caregivers in nursing homes. Expected, tolerated, and accepted. J Gerontol Nurs. 1999;25(4):12–22.
85. Zeller A, Hahn S, Needham I, Kok G, Dassen T, Halfens RJ. Aggressive behavior of nursing home residents toward caregivers: a systematic literature review. Geriatr Nurs. 2009;30(3):174–87.
86. Goodridge DM, Johnston P, Thomson M. Conflict and aggression as stressors in the work environment of nursing assistants. J Elder Abuse Negl. 1996;8(1):49–67.
87. Shaw MMC. Nursing home resident abuse by staff: exploring the dynamics. J Elder Abuse Negl. 1999;9(4):1–21.
88. Aström S, Karlsson S, Sandvide A, Bucht G, Eisemann M, Norberg A, et al. Staff's experience of and the management of violent incidents in elderly care. Scand J Caring Sci. 2004;18 (4):410–6.
89. Pillemer K, Hudson B. A model abuse prevention program for nursing assistants. Gerontologist. 1993;33(1):128–32.
90. National Center on Elder Abuse Administration on Aging. Frequently asked questions 2015 [cited 2015 May 26]. http://www.ncea.aoa.gov/faq/index.aspx.
91. Rosen T, Lachs MS, Pillemer K. Sexual aggression between residents in nursing homes: literature synthesis of an underrecognized problem. J Am Geriatr Soc. 2010;58(10):1970–9.
92. Malmedal W, Iversen MH, Kilvik A. Sexual abuse of older nursing home residents: A literature review. Nurs Res Pract. 2015;2015. Article ID 902515.
93. Burgess AW, Prentky RA, Dowdell EB. Sexual predators in nursing homes. J Psychosoc Nurs Ment Health Serv. 2000;38 (8):26–35.
94. Burgess AW, Hanrahan NP. Issues in elder sexual abuse in nursing homes. Nurs Health Policy Rev. 2004;3(1):5–17.
95. Teaster PB, Ramsey-Klawsnik H, Mendiondo MS, Abner E, Cecil K, Tooms M. From behind the shadows: a profile of the sexual abuse of older men residing in nursing homes. J Elder Abuse Negl. 2007;19(1–2):29–45.
96. Teaster PB, Roberto KA. Chapter 7 sexual abuse of older women living in nursing homes. J Gerontol Soc Work. 2004;40(4):105–19.
97. Rabiner DJ, Brown D, O'Keeffe J. Financial exploitation of older persons: policy issues and recommendations for addressing them. J Elder Abuse Negl. 2004;16(1):65–84.
98. Harris DK, Benson ML. Nursing home theft: the hidden problem. J Aging Stud. 1998;12(1):57–67.
99. Harris DK, Benson ML. Theft in nursing homes: an overlooked form of elder abuse. J Elder Abuse Negl. 2000;11(3):73–90.
100. National Pressure Ulcer Advisory Panel EPUAPaPPPIA. Prevention and treatment of pressure ulcers: quick reference guide. Osborne Park, Western Australia: Cambridge Media; 2014 [cited 2015 August 25]. http://www.epuap.org/wp-content/uploads/2010/10/Quick-Reference-Guide-DIGITAL-NPUAP-EPUAP-PPPIA-16Oct2014.pdf.
101. Edsberg LE, Langemo D, Baharestani MM, Posthauer ME, Goldberg M. Unavoidable pressure injury: state of the science and consensus outcomes. J Wound Ostomy Cont Nurs. 2014;41 (4):313–34.
102. Brandeis GH, Berlowitz DR, Katz P. Are pressure ulcers preventable? A survey of experts. Adv Skin Wound Care. 2001;14(5):244 (5–8).
103. Castle NG, Anderson RA. Caregiver staffing in nursing homes and their influence on quality of care: using dynamic panel estimation methods. Med Care. 2011;49(6):545–52.
104. Horn SD, Buerhaus P, Bergstrom N, Smout RJ. RN staffing time and outcomes of long-stay nursing home residents: pressure ulcers and other adverse outcomes are less likely as RNs spend

more time on direct patient care. Am J Nurs. 2005;105(11):58–70 (quiz 1).
105. Ahn H, Stechmiller J, Fillingim R, Lyon D, Garvan C. Bodily pain intensity in nursing home residents with pressure ulcers: analysis of national minimum data set 3.0. Res Nurs Health. 2015;38(3):207–12.
106. Castle N, Ferguson-Rome JC, Teresi JA. Elder abuse in residential long-term care: an update to the 2003 National Research Council report. J Appl Gerontol. 2015;34(4):407–43.
107. Phillips LR, Guo G. Mistreatment in assisted living facilities: complaints, substantiations, and risk factors. Gerontologist. 2011;51(3):343–53.
108. Wood S, Stephens M. Vulnerability to elder abuse and neglect in assisted living facilities. Gerontologist. 2003;43(5):753–7.
109. Castle N, Beach S. Elder abuse in assisted living. J Appl Gerontol. 2013;32(2):248–67.
110. Phillips LR, Ziminski C. The public health nursing role in elder neglect in assisted living facilities. Public Health Nurs. 2012;29 (6):499–509.
111. Phillips LR, Guo G, Kim H. Elder mistreatment in U.S. residential care facilities: the scope of the problem. J Elder Abuse Negl. 2013;25(1):19–39.
112. Hawes C, Kimbell A. Detecting, addressing and preventing elder abuse in residential care facilities College Station, TX: The Program on Aging & Long-Term Care Policy, The School of Rural Public Health, Texas A&M Health Science Center; 2010. https://www.ncjrs.gov/pdffiles1/nij/grants/229299.pdf.
113. Office of Inspector General. Psychotropic drug use in nursing homes. Washington, DC: Department of Health & Human Services; 2001.
114. Barton C, Miller B, Yaffe K. Improved evaluation and management of cognitive impairment: results of a comprehensive intervention in long-term care. J Am Med Dir Assoc. 2006;7 (2):84–9.
115. Magaziner J, German P, Zimmerman SI, Hebel JR, Burton L, Gruber-Baldini AL, et al. The prevalence of dementia in a statewide sample of new nursing home admissions aged 65 and older: diagnosis by expert panel. Epidemiology of Dementia in Nursing Homes Research Group. Gerontologist. 2000;40(6):663–72.
116. Sink KM, Holden KF, Yaffe K. Pharmacological treatment of neuropsychiatric symptoms of dementia: a review of the evidence. JAMA. 2005;293(5):596–608.
117. U.S. Food and Drug Administration. FDA requests boxed warnings on older class of antipsychotic drugs. 2008 June 16.
118. Centers for Medicare & Medicaid Services (CMS). Partnership to improve dementia care in nursing homes: antipsychotic drug use in nursing homes trend update: quarterly prevalence of antipsychotic use for long-stay nursing home residents 2011Q2 to 2014Q2 [cited 2015 September 29]. http://www.cms.gov/Outreach-and-Education/Outreach/NPC/Downloads/2014-10-27-Trends.pdf.
119. Briesacher BA, Limcangco MR, Simoni-Wastila L, Doshi JA, Levens SR, Shea DG, et al. The quality of antipsychotic drug prescribing in nursing homes. Arch Intern Med. 2005;165 (11):1280–5.
120. Rochon PA, Stukel TA, Bronskill SE, Gomes T, Sykora K, Wodchis WP, et al. Variation in nursing home antipsychotic prescribing rates. Arch Intern Med. 2007;167(7):676–83.
121. Thompson Coon J, Abbott R, Rogers M, Whear R, Pearson S, Lang I, et al. Interventions to reduce inappropriate prescribing of antipsychotic medications in people with dementia resident in care homes: a systematic review. J Am Med Dir Assoc. 2014;15 (10):706–18.
122. Chiu Y, Bero L, Hessol NA, Lexchin J, Harrington C. A literature review of clinical outcomes associated with antipsychotic medication use in North American nursing home residents. Health Policy. 2015;119(6):802–13.
123. Richardson B, Kitchen G, Livingston G. The effect of education on knowledge and management of elder abuse: a randomized controlled trial. Age Ageing. 2002;31(5):335–41.
124. Jogerst GJ, Daly JM, Dawson JD, Brinig MF, Schmuch GA. Required elder abuse education for Iowa mandatory reporters. J Elder Abuse Negl. 2004;15(1):59–73.
125. Hudson B. Ensuring an abuse-free environment. J Elder Abuse Negl. 1993;4(4):25–36.
126. Braun KL, Suzuki KM, Cusick CE, Howard-Carhart K. Developing and testing training materials on elder abuse and neglect for nurse aides. J Elder Abuse Negl. 1997;9(1):1–15.
127. Jones AL, Dwyer LL, Bercovitz AR, Strahan GW. The National Nursing Home Survey: 2004 overview. Vital Health Stat. 2009;167:1–155.
128. Alzheimer's Association. Special care units Chicago, IL: Alzheimer's Association; 2015 [cited 2015 October 1]. http://www.alz.org/join_the_cause_special_care_units.asp.
129. Hall S, Longhurst S, Higginson IJ. Challenges to conducting research with older people living in nursing homes. BMC Geriatr. 2009;9:38.
130. Tunzi M. Can the patient decide? Evaluating patient capacity in practice. Am Fam Phys. 2001;64(2):299–306.
131. Karlawish J. Measuring decision-making capacity in cognitively impaired individuals. Neurosignals. 2008;16(1):91–8.
132. Cutler LJ, Kane RA, Degenholtz HB, Miller MJ, Grant L. Assessing and comparing physical environments for nursing home residents: using new tools for greater research specificity. Gerontologist. 2006;46(1):42–51.
133. Higgins I. Reflections on conducting qualitative research with elderly people. Qual Health Res. 1998;8(6):858–66.
134. Tilden VP, Thompson SA, Gajewski BJ, Buescher CM, Bott MJ. Sampling challenges in nursing home research. J Am Med Dir Assoc. 2013;14(1):25–8.
135. Morley JE, Caplan G, Cesari M, Dong B, Flaherty JH, Grossberg GT, et al. International survey of nursing home research priorities. J Am Med Dir Assoc. 2014;15(5):309–12.
136. Kane RA, Wilson KB, Spector W. Developing a research agenda for assisted living. Gerontologist. 2007;47 Spec No 3:141–54.
137. Elder Justice Coordinating Council. Elder justice coordinating council 2014 report to Congress 2014 [cited 2015 October 5]. http://www.aoa.acl.gov/AoA_Programs/Elder_Rights/EJCC/index.aspx.
138. National Aging Resource Center on Elder Abuse. NARCEA's suggested state guidelines for gathering and reporting domestic elder abuse statistics for compiling national data. Washington: National Agine Resource Center on Elder Abuse; 1990.
139. Daly JM, Gaskill KJ, Jogerst GJ. Essential data elements for reporters of elder abuse. J Elder Abuse Negl. 2011;23(3):234–45.
140. Clark J, Lang N. Nursing's next advance: an internal classification for nursing practice. Int Nurs Rev. 1992;39(4):109–11.
141. Walter R. McDonald & Associates I. Development of a national adult protective services (APS) data system Rockville, MD: Walter R. McDonald & Associates, Inc.; 2015 [cited 2015 October 5]. http://www.aoa.acl.gov/AoA_Programs/Elder_Rights/ NAMRS/index.aspx.
142. Daly JM, Merchant ML, Jogerst GJ. Elder abuse research: a systematic review. J Elder Abuse Negl. 2011;23(4):348–65.
143. U.S. Department of Justice. The elder justice roadmap [Internet] Jul 2014 [cited 2015 July 10]. http://ncea.acl.gov/library/gov_report/docs/ejrp_roadmap.pdf.

Risk Factors of Elder Abuse

5

Ruijia Chen and XinQi Dong

Elder abuse is a growing and emergent global public health concern. According to the estimates from World Health Organization, approximately one in ten older adults globally has experienced abuse each month, and the prevalence is expected to increase due to the rapid growth of aging populations in many countries [1]. Being a victim of elder abuse has been associated with a variety of psychological, social, and physical impacts. Existing literature has suggested that elder abuse may lead to increased risk of depression [2], suicidal ideation [3], medical morbidity, and even mortality [4, 5].

Recently, attention has been focused on understanding the etiology of elder abuse. Although a growing number of studies and comprehensive reviews on elder abuse risk factors have been published [2, 6–8], evidence on risk factors of elder abuse is still not very well established, mainly due to inconsistent methodologies used across studies, difficulties of collecting data from perpetrators, as well as insufficient attentions on risk factors across different cultural and racial/ethnic groups. Another major issue in studying risk factors of elder abuse is that efforts tend to focus on understanding who has a higher likelihood of being abused, rather than the characteristics of perpetrators. Yet, victim risk factors alone are insufficient for explaining one's likelihood of committing or victimized by elder abuse. Indeed, perpetrator's characteristics as well as the relationship between victims and perpetrators play substantial roles in elder abuse occurrence. Research on elder abuse risk factors should take both victim and perpetrator characteristics into consideration.

A better understanding of risk factors of elder abuse could help us develop effective screening methods to identify individuals who are at risk of elder abuse, allocate resources and services to those who are in need of help, and develop preventions and interventions to address the issue. This chapter provides a review of theories for explaining risk factors of elder abuse, describes victim and perpetrator risk factors contributing to elder abuse, and proposes implications to improve future research on risk factors of elder abuse. In particular, to offer a more comprehensive review on risk factors of the issues, this chapter discusses studies on victim and perpetrator characteristics separately.

5.1 Methods

We defined "risk factors" as attributes, characteristics, or exposure that may increase an individual's likelihood of experiencing elder abuse or increase a perpetrator's likelihood of directing abusive behavior. We conducted a search of the most up-to-date global literature on risk factors of elder abuse in PubMed, MEDLINE, PsycINFO, BIOSIS, Science Direct, and Cochrane Central. The search was limited to studies published in English. Search terms included elder abuse, elder mistreatment, elder maltreatment, risk factors, and protective factors. Review studies were identified, and their reference lists examined for relevant articles. Studies existing only as abstracts, case series, or case reports or that recruited individuals younger than 60; qualitative studies; and non-English publications were excluded. Only studies in which elder abuse was the primary dependent variable and confounding factors were used were included. Studies in which primary analyses were bivariate in nature were not included, articles identified using the search methods were independently reviewed, and studies were selected according to the criteria.

R. Chen (✉)
Department of Social and Behavioral Sciences, Harvard T.H. Chan School of Public Health, 900 Memorial Drive, 2#711, Cambridge, MA 02138, USA
e-mail: ruijia.chen@mail.harvard.edu

X. Dong
Rush Institute for Healthy Aging, Rush University Medical Center, 1645 W. Jackson Blvd, Suite 675, Chicago, IL 60612, USA

X. Dong (ed.), *Elder Abuse*, DOI 10.1007/978-3-319-47504-2_5

5.2 Theoretical Framework for Understanding Risk Factors of Elder Abuse

5.2.1 Social Exchange Theory

The social exchange theory is rooted in psychology and posits that individuals develop relationship and interactions based on the cost and reward of the relationship. In the context of elder abuse, older adults are often frailer and do not have enough exchange possibilities. Caregivers who contribute most to the relationship often have the power advantage and may perceive the caregiver–recipient relationship as unequal [9]. In particular, older victim's increased dependence on the caregivers resulting from declines in physical and cognitive abilities may exacerbate the imbalanced relationship and lead to violent behavior by the perpetrators.

5.2.2 Situational Theory

The situational theory posits that the dependence and frailty of older adults may create a stressful environment for caregivers who may not be able to cope with stress and thus result in elder abuse. Studies that used the situational theory to explain elder abuse often look at caregiver stress or burden as well as factors that lead to dependence of the older adults such as poor physical and cognitive health.

5.2.3 The Psychopathology of the Caregiver Theory

The psychopathology of the caregiver theory focuses on abuser's characteristics and posits that caregivers' psychological problems may decrease the quality of care and give rise to abusive behavior. Applied to elder abuse, substance abuse and depression affect the relationship between caregiver and care recipients, affect the quality of caregiving, and elicit abusive behavior.

5.2.4 Life Course Framework

The life course theoretical framework posits that an individual's health is attributable to lifelong accumulation of advantage and disadvantage experiences. Prior traumatic experience may contribute to the risk of abuse in late life. As applied to elder abuse, traumatic childhood experiences, immigration, prior victimization, and perpetrator relationship may account for elder abuse in late life. Similarly, perpetrators who experienced previous traumatic stress and abuse experience may be more likely to resort to violent revenge.

5.2.5 Ecological Theory

Built on the Bronfenbrenner's human ecological theory as well as the life course perspective [10], Schiamberg and Gans proposed the use of the applied ecological model as the foundation of explaining elder abuse [11]. Instead of focusing on individual risk factors of elder abuse, the ecological theoretical framework places emphasis on the broader context in which elder abuse occurs. Research that applies the applied ecological theory focuses on contextual risk factors, especially the social and cultural context as well as the relationship between individuals and the context.

5.3 Risk Factors Contributing to Elder Abuse

5.3.1 Victim Characteristics (Fig. 5.1a–c)

5.3.1.1 Sociodemographic Characteristics

Age

There has been inconsistent evidence regarding the association between age and elder abuse. In a study of 1089 older Mexican adults with long-term disabilities, age 80 years and older is associated with a higher risk of elder abuse of any kinds [12]. In another study of 676 inhabitants aged 75 and older in Girona, Spain, financial abuse is associated with aged 85 and older [13]. These studies argued that compared with younger elderly, older elderly may be frailer and have more physical and cognitive disabilities, and thus are more likely to experience elder abuse. However, there is also evidence suggesting that younger age is associated with increased risk for elder abuse in that younger age groups have a higher likelihood of engaging in abusive situations that may threat their health and safety [14–16]. A telephone survey of 82 community-dwelling caregivers reported that younger demented patients have a higher possibility of suffering from verbal abuse [14].

Gender

Women comprise the majority of elder abuse victims [17]. Compared to men, women tend to suffer from larger socioeconomic and health disadvantages, which may increase their risk of elder abuse. Also, women may be less likely to cope with stress, which may put themselves in a situation that is more susceptible to elder abuse [18]. Further, women tend to have longer life expectancy and often live alone, increasing their vulnerability to abuse. The majority of studies demonstrate that being women is a risk factor for experience elder abuse [15, 18, 19]. A case-control study of 41 elder abuse cases and 123 controls in Chicago found that victims of severe traumatic elder abuse were more likely to be

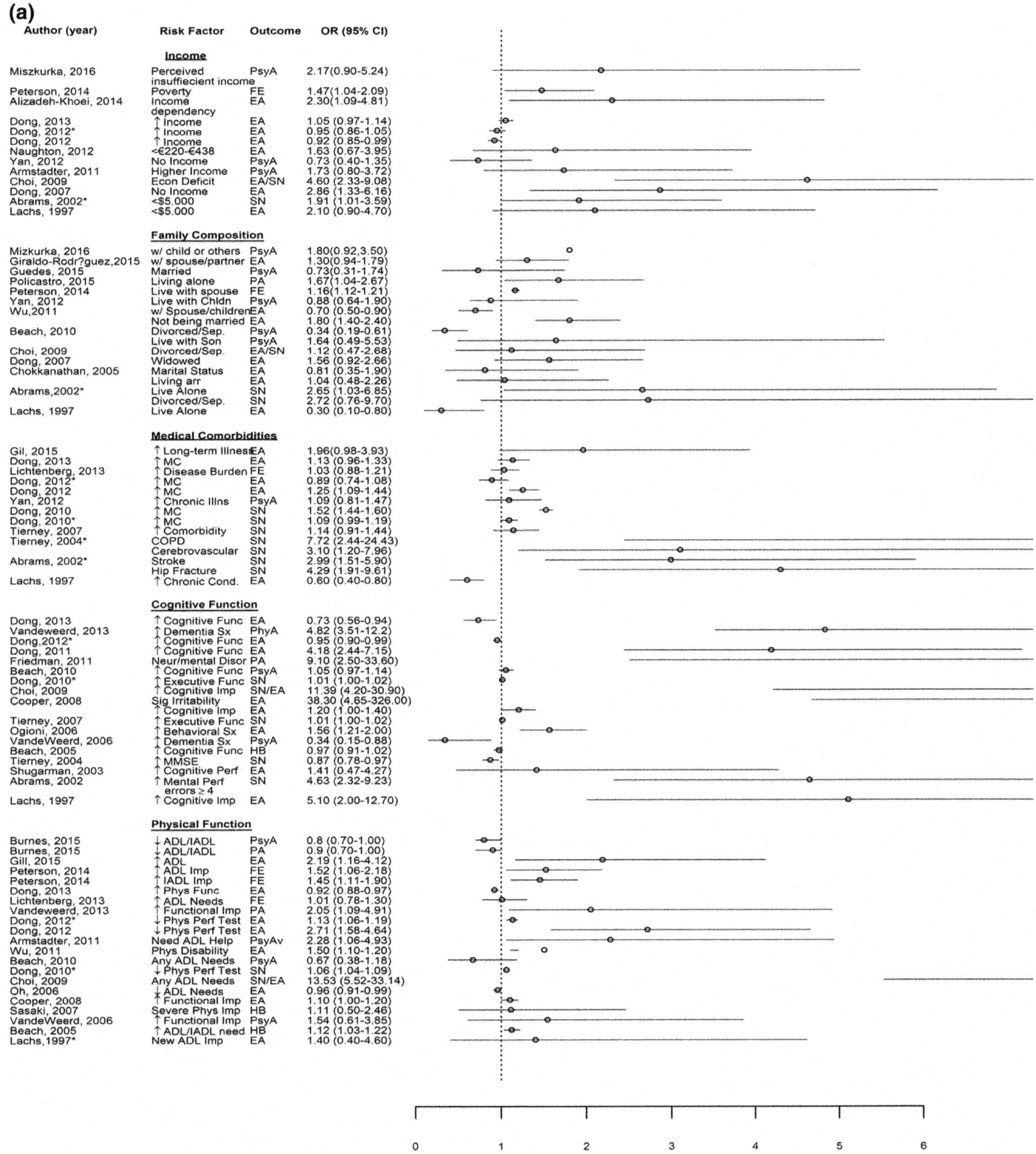

Fig. 5.1 a–c Victim risk factors

female (OR 3.5, 95 % CI 1.4–8.8, p = 0.008) [19]. In another study of 400 community-dwelling older adults aged 65 and above in Chennai, India, being women is a significant risk factor for elder abuse [18]. However, in a study of 112 older adults aged 60 and older who seek legal assistant services in five metro Atlanta community centers, males were 5.5 times more likely to have a positive screen for elder abuse than females (OR 5.54, 95 % CI 1.85–16.57, p = 0.002) [20].

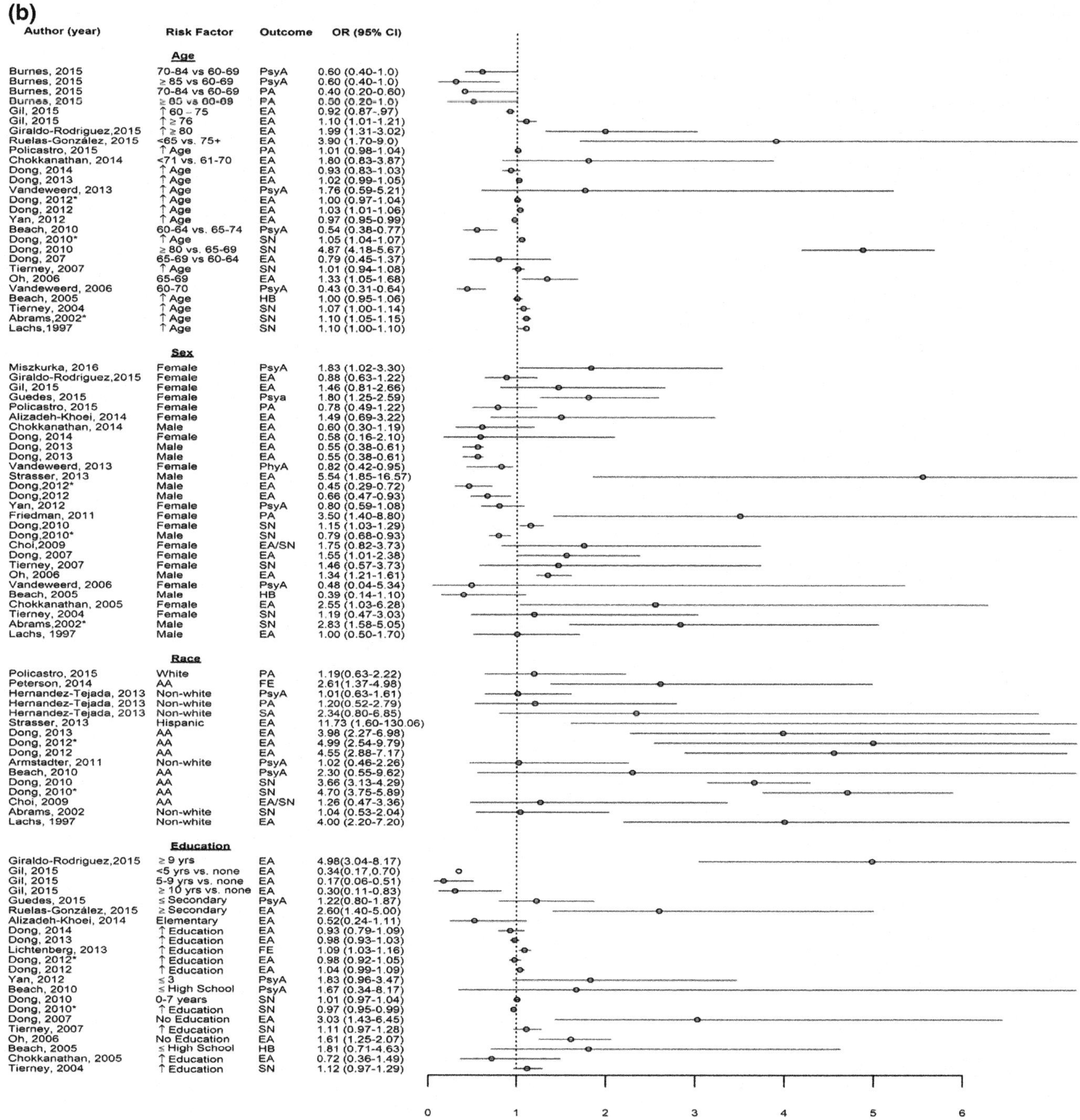

Fig. 5.1 (continued)

Race and Ethnicity

The National Research Council proposed a model that included race to be a broad social status factor that may relate to elder abuse. Different racial ethnic groups may confront with different levels of social disadvantages, which may lead to different risks of elder abuse. Some studies posited that the emphasis of family in Asian and Latino culture might protect minority older adults from experiencing elder abuse. In the National Elder Mistreatment Study, non-white status was not associated with increase risk of any form of elder abuse, after adjusting for income, social support, and health status [21]. Others, however, believe that life stressors such as immigration and discrimination that are associated with minority status may increase the probability of elder abuse in racial/ethnic groups. Beach et al. [22] explicitly considered race as a risk factor and found

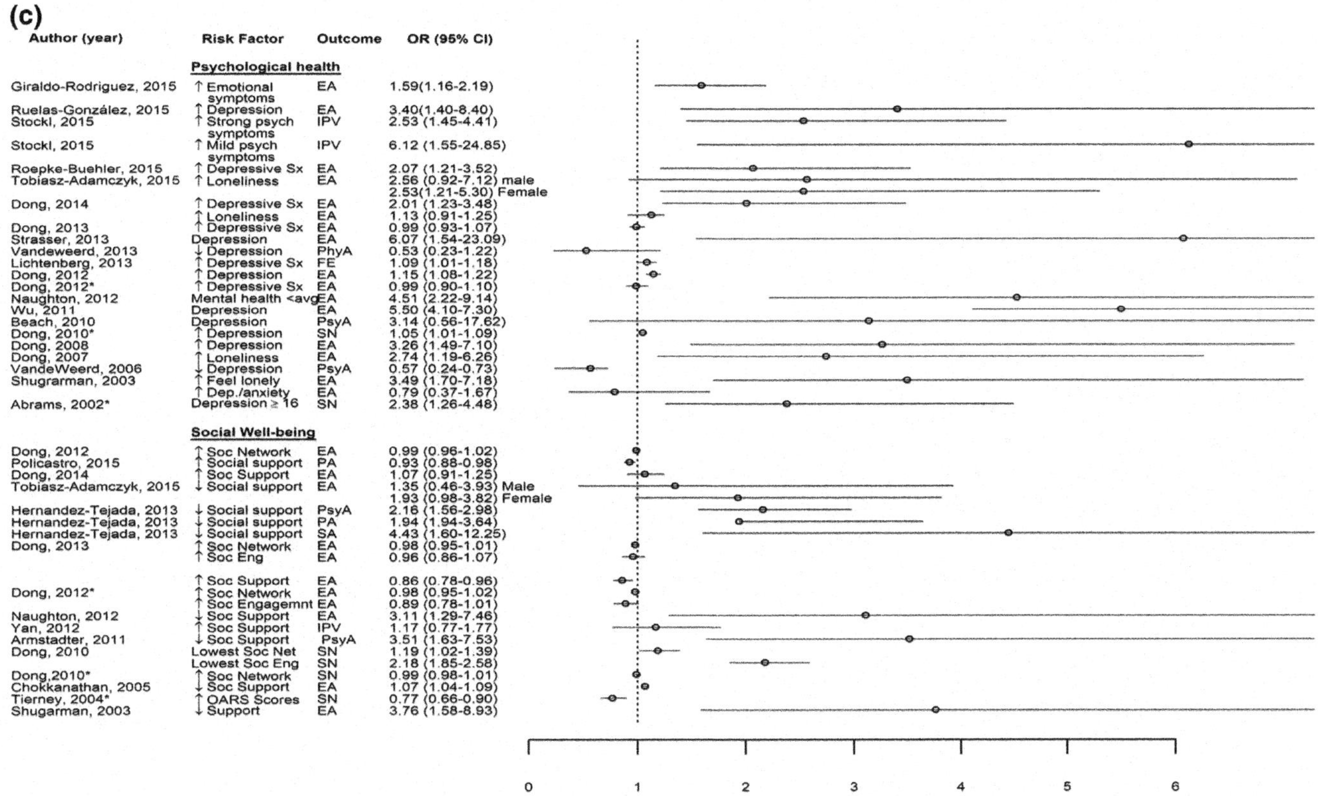

Fig. 5.1 (continued)

significant racial difference in prevalence of financial exploitation and psychological abuse. There are also studies suggesting that the association between race and elder abuse may vary by types of abuse. A study examining the association between race and types of abuse showed that whites are more likely to be associated with self-neglect, while blacks are more likely to be associated with neglect by others. In addition, the study found no association between race and physical and material abuse [23].

Marital Status

Being married may improve the levels of social support to the older adults, and thus reduce the risk of being abused. Yet, being married may also increase the opportunities for conflicts and abuse. Existing studies show quite divergent findings on marital status and elder abuse. In China, a study conducted among 2039 adults aged 60 and older in three rural communities found that not being married was associated with increased risk of psychological abuse (OR 2.1, 95 % CI 1.5–2.8) [24]. In the New York Elder Abuse Prevalence Study, being divorced or being separated was associated with increased risk of emotional (OR 2.7, 95 % CI 1.5–5.0) and physical abuse (OR 2.0, 95 % CI 1.0–3.7) [25]. Because most of the studies on marital status and elder abuse are cross-sectional, it is hard to differentiate whether the changes in marital status occur before or after the abuse.

5.3.1.2 Socioeconomic Characteristics

Income

Income is one of the major social determinants that are associated with elder abuse. Some studies have used individual income to measure the socioeconomic status, while others used the household-level income. A cross-sectional study 4156 English or Spanish-speaking, community-dwelling, cognitively intact individuals aged 60 years and older in the New York State Elder Mistreatment Prevalence Study, living in a low income household was associated with increased risk of emotional abuse (OR 2.69, 95 % CI 1.45–4.99) and physical abuse (OR 2.16, 95 % CI 1.24–3.77), but not with elder neglect [25]. In addition to objective income, many studies also examined subjective income and elder abuse. For example, a study of 960 adults aged 65 years and older from eight statistical regions participated in the Macedonian study, dissatisfaction with household income was associated with higher risk for elder abuse (OR 1.3) [26]. Similar findings were detected for individual income and elder abuse. Dong et al. [27] surveyed 412 older adults in Nanjing, China and found that lower income was associated with elder abuse.

In addition to income, a growing number of studies have focused on macro-level factors such as economic inequality or income disparity and how they contribute to different rates of elder abuse in various populations. Fraga et al. conducted the project on abuse of elderly in Europe and the findings showed that countries with higher Gini coefficient have a higher prevalence of financial abuse and a lower prevalence of psychological abuse when compared to those with a lower Gini coefficient.

In addition, the Gini coefficient seemed to explain country difference in elder abuse, suggesting the role of income inequality and the occurrence of elder abuse [28]. In another study that examined the distribution of wealth and elder abuse in Rajshahi district of Bangladesh, older adults from the rich and middle-income households were less likely to be abused than those in poor households [29].

Education

Education is a controversial risk factor of elder abuse in the literature. Most studies have demonstrated that education levels protect older adults from experiencing elder abuse, as older adults with higher educational levels tend to receive more respect from others and thus, are less likely to be abused [30, 31]. However, recently, an increased number of studies have found a higher risk of elder abuse among high-educated individuals. A study conducted among Latino older adults aged 66 and older found that higher educational levels are associated with increased risk for elder abuse [32]. In another study of 3159 Chinese older adults in Chicago, Chinese older adults with higher educational levels are also more likely to report elder abuse [32]. This may be due to the fact that high-educated older adults are more likely to be aware of elder abuse, and thus are more prone to report elder abuse. Similar to the association between income and elder abuse, the relationship between education and elder abuse also vary by types of abuse. Compared with other types of abuse, financial exploitation is more commonly found among high-educated older adults. For instance, a study of 4400 older participants from a Health and Retirement Study shows that more education is associated with fraud among older adults [33].

Living Arrangement

A shared living arrangement may increase the possibility of conflicts and elder abuse [34]. In a study of 676 inhabitants aged 75 and older in eight rural villages in Girona, Spain, living with other people were associated with increased risk for elder abuse (OR 5.29, 95 % CI 2.65–10.56) [13]. Types of abuse should be taken into account when examining the effects of living arrangement on elder abuse. A study of 1797 older adults in Amsterdam, The Netherlands showed that living with someone else was associated with chronic verbal aggression and physical aggression, whereas living alone was associated with financial abuse [35]. In another study of 2812 community older adults from New Haven ESPESE cohort, living alone (OR 2.83, 95 % CI 1.58–5.05) was associated with increased risk for elder self-neglect among community-dwelling older adults.

5.3.1.3 Psychosocial Factors

Depression

The positive association between depression and elder abuse has been well established in a wide range of studies [14, 19, 36–40]. Research has further demonstrated that the association between elder abuse and depression may vary by the dimensions of depression such that higher levels of depressed affect, somatic complaints, and interpersonal problems are significantly associated with elder abuse, whereas positive affect does not show a significant association with elder abuse [40]. Age and education may moderate the association between depression and elder abuse. A study of the urban Chinese population found that among older adults with depressive distress, those who were older and had lower education levels may have an increased risk of elder abuse. In addition, after adjusting socioeconomic variables and adding social support into the logistic regression model, depression is associated with increased risk among women but not among men [38]. One major issue with studying elder abuse and depression is that many studies have utilized the cross-sectional design and it is hard to clarify the causal inference. Despite the strong association between depression and elder abuse established in many cross-sectional studies, it is challenging to rule out the possibilities that elder abuse victims are more likely to develop depression.

Loneliness

Older adults are particularly venerable to loneliness, which can lead to elder abuse. Feeling of loneliness may increase dependency and vulnerability, which may give rise to increased risk of elder abuse. In addition, loneliness is very likely to be associated with social isolation and a lack of social support, which may put these older adults at abusive situation. Dong et al. conducted a study among 412 older adults aged 60 and older in a general medical clinic in Nanjing, China and found that feeling of lacking companionship (OR 4.06, 95 % CI 1.49–11.10) and feeling of sometimes being left out of life (OR 1.69, 95 % CI 1.01–2.84) [41]. Tobiasz-Adamczyk, 2014 studied emotional loneliness and social loneliness separately and found that older women with higher emotional loneliness were more likely to experience elder abuse, whereas the association was not detected among older men [42]. Yet it is worth noting that the association between loneliness and elder abuse has not been well addressed in existing literature. There remained large unknown with respect to how loneliness may lead to elder abuse.

Substance Abuse

Substance abuse may increase the risk of elder abuse through multiple mechanisms. First, substance abuse may lead to impairment such as cognitive loss and physical disabilities, which may increase the frailty of the older adults and reduce their abilities to detect elder abuse. Second, older adults with long-standing substance abuse problems tend to have poor relationships with caregivers, which may reduce caregiver's motivation to provide good care and increase the risk of neglect. Furthermore, older adults who abuse alcohol may be more likely to self-neglect [43]. In a clinical case-control study of 41 cases resulting in severe traumatic injury and 123 controls randomly selected from the list of elderly patients in the trauma registry, after controlling for injury severity, hospital, length of stay, and age, victims of severe traumatic elder abuse were more likely to report drug or alcohol abuse [19].

Social Support and Isolation

Social isolation and lower levels of social support may facilitate a potential violent environment and may decrease an older person's self-esteem, and thus increase the risk of elder abuse [21, 44–46]. Extant studies have consistently demonstrated the positive association between social isolation/lower social support and elder abuse [13, 21]. A cross-sectional study of 203 older adults from the Midlife development in the United States study showed that the social isolation of the older adults was a strong risk factor for physical abuse [47]. In cross-sectional community-dwelling older adults in Ireland, poor social support (OR 4.91, 95 % CI 2.1–11.5) was independently associated with increased risk for elder abuse [46]. As social support can be categorized into positive and negative social support, the association between social support and elder abuse may vary by the types of social support. A study on 2744 older adults aged 57–85 in the United States from the National Social Life, Health, and Aging Project found that negative social support, such as criticism from close relationships (OR 3.35, $p < 0.001$) was associated with increased risk of elder abuse. On the contrary, positive social support (OR 0.69, $p < 0.01$) was associated with decreased risk of elder abuse [45].

5.3.1.4 Physical Function

Older adults with physical impairments are frailer and have higher dependence on the caregivers, which may lead to higher risk for elder abuse [30]. Dong et al. examined the association between physical function and elder abuse among 8932 older adults in the Chicago and found that lower risk of physical performance, Nagi impairment, and Rosow impairment were associated with increased risk for elder abuse [34]. In the same cohort, researchers found that every point decline in physical performance was associated with increased risk of elder self-neglect. In another study of 2005 samples of reported APS for self-neglect, Choi found that any ADL impairment was associated with 2.08 increased risk of elder self-neglect [48]. A recent large-scale prospective study of 154,902 Women's Health Initiative participants showed that women aged 50 and above who experienced verbal and physical abuse had 1.33 times greater odds of baseline significant physical impairment than who did not experience abuse, indicating that physical impairment may be a significant risk factor for elder abuse. Interestingly, the study also found that trajectories of decline in physical function did not meaningfully differ by abuse experience [49].

5.3.1.5 Cognitive Function and Dementia

The prevalence and severity of elder abuse are associated with older adults' cognitive functional status. Studies have consistently shown that lower cognitive functional status is associated with increased risk for elder abuse. In a population-based study of 238 community-dwelling older adults with elder abuse experience, Dong et al. found that lower global cognitive function level (OR 4.18, 95 % CI 2.44–7.15), MMSE (OR 2.97, 95 % CI 1.93–4.57), episodic memory (OR 2.27, 95 % CI 1.49–3.43), and perceptual speeds (OR 2.37, 95 % CI 1.51–3.73) are associated with increased risks of elder abuse [50]. A longitudinal study follows up 2688 older adults over 9 years and found that after adjusting for age, sex, race, and income, older adults who began an interval cognitively intact and became subsequently impaired had a high risk (OR 5.1, 95 % CI 2.0–12.7) of elder abuse than older adults without any cognitive impairment [34].

Older adults with dementia are particularly vulnerable to abuse [2]. In particular, older adults with dementia often have psychological or behavioral symptoms such as agitation and aggression, which may intensify caregiver–recipient conflicts and result in elder abuse [51]. In addition, older adults with dementia may experience a higher burden of chronic illness and physical impairment, which further increases their risk of abuse, compared to older adults without dementia [2].

5.3.2 Perpetrator Characteristics (Fig. 5.2)

5.3.2.1 Sociodemographic and Socioeconomic Characteristics

Studies on the relationship between perpetrators' sociodemographic characteristics and elder abuse have yielded divergent results. Caregivers with lower educational levels may lack awareness of the consequences of delaying seeking healthcare, resulting in a high risk of caregiver neglect toward older adults [52]. One study suggests that being a male caregiver, lacking adequate economic resources, and sharing living arrangements with a care recipient may be associated with an increased risk of exhibiting abusive behavior toward older adults [53]. However, there is also evidence that shows no significant difference between abusive and nonabusive individuals regarding sociodemographic characteristics [14].

5.3.2.2 Psychosocial Factors

Caregiver Burden and Stress

Taking care of an older adult, especially a demented older adult, could be challenging and burdensome. Caregivers of older adults, especially those with dementia, experience a higher level of burden because of great physical and time demands. Bearing a higher level of burden is associated with an increased incidence of abusive behaviors toward care recipients. Being a caregiver for more years, providing more hours' care per day and caring for patients with higher levels of impairment are likely to increase the occurrence of abusive behaviors [54]. In a survey of 86 caregivers of people with dementia, caregiver burden (OR 1.1, 95 % CI 1.0–1.1) was significantly associated with increased risk for elder abuse [53]. Caregiver burden and strain could come from other sources, in addition to the task of taking care of older adults. In a survey of 902 older adults aged 61 years and older in rural Tamil Nadu, caregivers reflecting role strain related to taking care of children and other parents are 2.06 times more likely to exhibit abuse toward older adults [55].

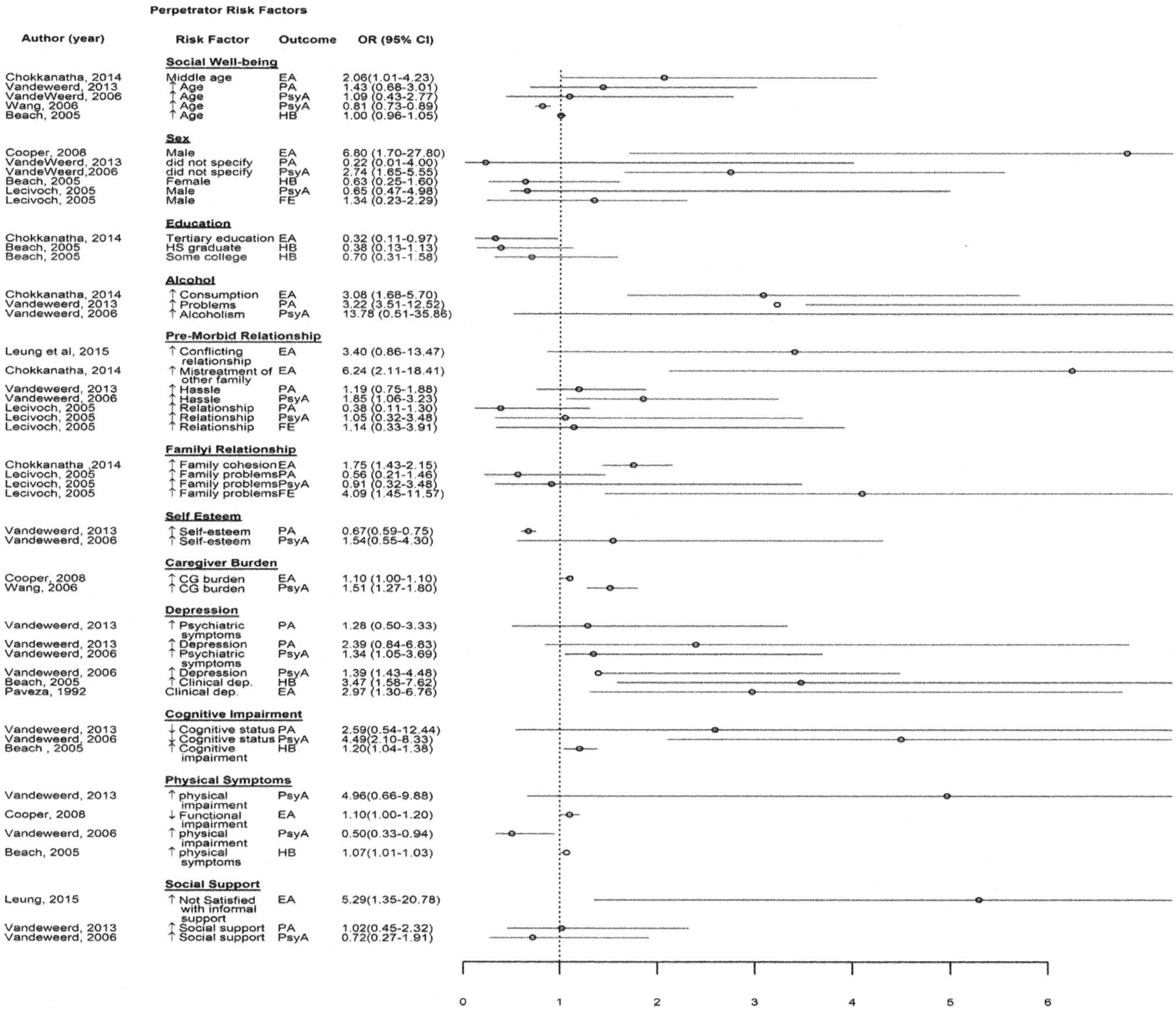

Fig. 5.2 Perpetrator risk factors

Caregivers' objective and subjective burdens are both associated with elder abuse. Compared with objective caregiver burdens, subjective burdens—including the perception of stress, caregivers' responses to the situation and the nature of the caregiver–recipient relationship—play a more crucial role in explaining abusive behaviors. Caregiver stress mainly stems from an overwhelming burden and ineffective coping strategies and is likely to cause significant health issues [56, 57]. Higher levels of stress in turn reduce caregivers' coping abilities and trigger potential elder abuse.

Depression

Depression often results in a lack of confidence in caregiving ability and/or caregiving skills and thus potentially increases the use of abusive acts to manage these difficulties. After controlling for demographics, interpersonal relationship, and illness severity, care recipients were still more likely to experience abuse when caregivers were at risk of clinical depression in the previous week [58]. In terms of subtypes of abuse, a study on caregiver risk factors of abuse of older adults with dementia showed that lower levels of psychological health in caregivers were associated with physically abusive behavior, but not associated with verbal abuse and neglect [59]. The association between caregiver depression and elder abuse may be further complicated by physical health and cognitive impairment, but unfortunately none of the existing studies have been conducted to examine the issue.

Social Support

Social support reduces elder abuse occurrence through improving caregiver self-efficacy—the caregiver's belief in his or her ability to manage difficult tasks and deal with care recipients' behavior problems. Increasing the availability and accessibility of social support is likely to improve caregivers' confidence in stressful caregiving situations, and thus reduce the chance of abuse. Social support also buffers the burden and stress on caregivers' well-being and reduces the incidence of elder abuse. Social support could be categorized into formal and informal support, which may have different effects on elder abuse. For instance, a study of 1000 primary family caregivers from the Comprehensive Study for the Elderly Welfare Policy in Seoul found that formal social support significantly buffered the severity of elder abuse, while informal social support was associated with less abuse by caregivers [60]. Social isolation, on the contrary, increases the likelihood of caregivers directing abuse toward demented older adults [59]. Caregivers of frail adults are limited in their personal and social activities, which may exacerbate the sense of helplessness and loneliness and increase the possibility of admitting to abuse.

Substance Abuse

Substance abuse also emerges as an important predictor of elder abuse. Under the influence of alcohol or drugs, caregivers are more likely to use violence as a conflict resolution strategy [62]. A study of 254 caregivers and 76 elders with Alzheimer's disease supports this view by showing that caregivers who abused alcohol are three times more likely to exhibit physically abusive behaviors toward dementia patients [63]. In addition, dependent caregivers with substance abuse problems may be more likely to be involved in financial abuse to provide money for drug or alcohol consumption. In another study of 254 caregivers and 76 older adults with dementia, Vandeweed found that caregivers with alcohol problems were three times as likely to be violent for whom they were providing care. Interestingly, the study also found additive effects of dementia and alcohol abuse such that caregivers who abused alcohol and who were providing care to violent elderly with high levels of dementia symptoms were six times as likely to engage in violent behavior as those who did not.

5.3.2.3 Cognitive Function and Dementia

Current elder abuse literature tends to exclusively focus on the cognitive function of victims, but cognitive impairment among perpetrator may lead to violent behavior. Beach et al. showed that higher levels of cognitive impairment among caregiver were associated with increased risk of elder abuse [58]. As dementia often accompanies with aggressive behaviors, perpetrators with dementia may display abusive behaviors, although sometimes may not be related to power or control. In a study of elder abuse and dementia, 35 % of 82 caregivers of patients with dementia reported experiencing mutual verbal abuse with the care recipients, and 6 % reported experiencing mutual physical abuse with the recipients [14], In another of 184 Alzheimer patient–caregiver dyads, 15.8 % of the patients directed abusive behavior toward caregivers and mutual violence reported in 3.8 % of the families, suggesting that elder abuse may also be initiated by older adults with dementia [61].

5.3.2.4 Victim–Perpetrator Relationships

The quality of premorbid relationships between perpetrators and victims also influences the likelihood of elder abuse occurrence. High premorbid relationship satisfaction reduces the care burden and enhances the quality of care, whereas a problematic premorbid relationship may lead to negative moods and abusive behaviors. Elder abuse in community-dwelling populations could be the consequence of long-term family violence. The experience of child abuse or domestic abuse may affect caregivers' reactions toward the problem behaviors of demented patients, increase caregiver burden, and decrease communication efficiency and coping skills [64]. A study with a cohort from a psychiatry of old age service in rural Ireland has demonstrated that abusers had significantly poorer premorbid relationships with the patients than nonabusers [65].

5.4 Discussion

Existing literature has demonstrated a wide range of sociodemographic, socioeconomic, and psychosocial factors that are associated with elder abuse. However, the inconsistent findings yielded from these studies make it hard to draw conclusions on risk factors and translate the research findings into policy and practices.

5.4.1 Methodological Issues

5.4.1.1 Definitions of Elder Abuse

Although a large number of studies have examined risk factors of elder abuse, methodological limitations in many studies make it hard to interpret and generalize the findings. Such imitations also result in inconsistency in findings across studies. While many studies have used an "any positive EM item" approach, other studies have more systematically considered the heterogeneity of the definitions and have been stricter in the categorization of EM cases. Recently, Dong et al. used different definitions of elder abuse and examined their associated characteristics. The findings suggested that risk factors of elder abuse differed by definitions, implying the importance of a unified definition to understand the risk factors of elder abuse [66]. Future studies should expand the effort to develop a more consistent instrument to understand elder abuse and its risk factors.

5.4.1.2 Issues in Defining and Measuring Risk Factors

Although literature on the association between socioeconomic status and elder abuse has been well established, the majority of these studies used income and educational levels as proxies. However, income and educational levels may be associated with reporting bias. Respondents may not report income sources apart from labor market earnings, such as transfer program or assets income. Similarly, measures of educational attainment rarely take into account differing quality of education offered by different institutions. Future studies that examined risk factors of elder abuse may need to consider other important sociodemographic characteristics such as caregiver's occupational status.

5.4.1.3 Applying Bradford Hill's Criteria for Causation to Elder Abuse

Unlike many other areas of studies, it is almost impossible and unethical to understand the causality of elder abuse through using experimental designs, and thus, most of the risk factors studies on elder abuse are nonexperimental and observational. Yet this does not suggest that we are not able to establish causality in the studies of elder abuse, we can still use causal criteria to elucidate causation. The Branford Hill's Criteria, for example, has been widely used in epidemiologic studies to identify the causal relationship. Sir Austin Bradford Hill proposed nine criteria for evidence of causality. These criteria are: (1) strength of the association; (2) consistency; (3) specificity; (4) temporality; (5) biology gradient; (6) plausibility; (7) coherence; (8) experiment; and (9) analogy. However, the application of the criteria to evaluate causality of studies on elder abuse should be cautious (Table 5.1).

Strength of the association Bradford Hill argued that the stronger the association is, the more likely the causal association can be drawn. Say, for example, a 20-fold increase in elder abuse may have more credence than a 2-fold increase in the outcome. However, in the studies of elder abuse, the association is often weak, and residual confounding is commonly present, making it challenging to use this criterion to justify causal relationship.

Consistency of the study findings This criterion proposes that consistent findings across different populations in different settings may imply causal relationship. The findings of the review show that findings on risk factors of elder abuse vary significantly across studies such that some studies found older age was associated with increased elder abuse, whereas others showed that younger adults were at higher risk of abuse. Differences in methodological designs may partly explain discrepancies in these study findings. Given there is no consistent definition of elder abuse; methodological variations across studies may limit the validity of this criterion in the field of elder abuse.

Specificity This criterion requires that any exposure may lead to only one outcome. This is especially hard to implement in social and behavioral sciences where exposures tend to have multiple outcomes and the outcomes are often caused by the interplay of different exposures. In particular, it is hard to identify a single factor that causes elder abuse. Risk factors such as depression may also lead to other health outcomes such as declines in physical or cognitive functions.

Temporal Sequence This criterion requires that risk factors should occur prior to outcomes. Currently, many studies in elder abuse are cross-sectional, making it difficult to

Table 5.1 Bradford Hill's criteria of causation applied to elder abuse

Strength	The stronger the relationship between risk factors and elder abuse, the less likely that the relationship is due to a third factor
Consistency	Multiple studies across different populations in different settings should find similar relationship between risk factors and elder abuse
Specificity	If a risk factor is only associated with elder abuse but not with other outcomes, then the relationship is more likely to be causal
Temporality	Risk factors should occur prior to the occurrence of elder abuse
Biology gradient	An increasing level of risk factors (in amount and/or frequency) should increase the risk of elder abuse
Plausibility	The association between risk factors and elder abuse should have biological rationale
Coherence	The association between risk factors and elder abuse should be consistent with existing knowledge or theory
Experiment	Causation is more likely if evidence on risk factors and elder abuse is based on randomized experimental studies
Analogy	If a risk factor is found to have causal relationship with elder abuse, then other factors analogous to that particular risk factor may also potentially cause elder abuse

determine the direction of the relationship. For example, although some cross-sectional studies found significant associations between depression and elder abuse, we are not able to draw causal inference between depression and elder abuse, as it is likely that elder abuse may lead to increased risk of depression. Prospective study designs are important to establish temporal relationship for elder abuse studies. Unfortunately, only a small proportion of studies has utilized longitudinal designs to understand factors associated with elder abuse.

Biology gradient There is strong evidence for causal relationship if biology gradient or dose–response relationship is present. For example, if depression is a cause of elder abuse, then an increase in risk of depression should result in increased severity of elder abuse. However, such quantitative relationship may be very hard to establish, as in some situations greater exposure to the factors such as physical or cognitive impairments may not necessarily increase the risk of elder abuse.

Plausibility This criterion suggests that the association between a factor and outcome should have biological rationale. For example, research may find random factors that are associated with elder abuse. Yet, it is hard to draw causal inference if we are not able to find out any potential mechanisms that may link that random factor to elder abuse.

Coherence The association between factors and outcomes should be consistent with existing knowledge or theory. However, this criterion also depends on how much we know in the field of elder abuse. Giving very few studies has been done in the field of elder abuse as compared to other areas, it may be risky to easily preclude the possibilities of causation simply based on existing knowledge. On the contrary, controversy findings warrant more attention and further studies, as our existing knowledge is limited and could be misleading.

Experiment Experimental designs, such as randomized clinical trials, may provide the strongest evidence for causation. Such designs allow investigators to minimize confounding and bias that are not able to achieve by other study designs or statistical techniques. However, often these studies can only be done in a small group of populations, which may limit the representativeness of the studies and lower the study power. In the case of elder abuse, randomized studies often encounter fundamental ethnic issues involving the process of informed consents, study participant assignment, etc.

Analogy This criterion suggests that if a risk factor is found to have causal relationship with the outcome, then other factors analogous to that particular risk factor may also potentially cause the outcome. For example, if we can establish the causal relationship between depression and elder abuse, we may conclude that anxiety, which shares a lot in common in depression, may have potential causation association with elder abuse. However, this criterion should be taken with caution because even minor differences in risk factors may cause sustainably different outcomes.

5.4.2 Understanding Risk Factors of Incidence of Elder Abuse in Prospective Studies

Much of what is known about risk factors of elder abuse is based on cross-sectional study designs, which are relatively inexpensive and avoid the risk of loss-to-follow-up issues that may occur in longitudinal designs. However, simultaneously assessing psychosocial determinants and elder abuse may restrict an understanding of the temporal relationship between changes in psychosocial determinants and elder abuse. It is also impossible to draw causal inference in cross-sectional studies, as reverse causations may occur. Consider, for example, older adults who have experienced elder abuse may have lower self-esteem and are more likely to be social isolated. Under this scenario, it is difficult to know whether social isolation leads to elder abuse or elder abuse contributes to social isolation.

In addition, due to lack of prospective studies, we are unable to understand risk factors associated with incidence of elder abuse. With cross-sectional designs, studies on risk factors of elder abuse only manage to measure elder abuse at one time. However, in many situations, elder abuse that the participants report may occur a long time ago, while risk factors (e.g., social support and depression) measured are under current status. Different time periods of the variables may produce biased estimates of the relationship between risk factors and elder abuse. Therefore, future studies should use the prospective design to elucidate risk factors associated incidence of elder abuse. Special attention should be given to risk factors of recurrent elder abuse because victims who experience elder abuse multiple times may be most vulnerable and are most in need of help.

5.4.3 Studies on Elder Abuse Among People with Dementia

Abuse of older adults with dementia is understudied because the detection of abuse is often complicated by various biological, pathological, ethnic, and cultural factors. For example, dementia is associated with a high level of dependence. Thus, older adults may be reluctant to disclose abuse because they fear retaliation or losing support [67]. In addition, common physical signs of and reactions to abuse, such as withdrawal from communication or increased dependence, may be difficult to distinguish from dementia symptoms [68]. Ethical issues such as challenges in obtaining informed consent from patients with dementia may impede research on elder abuse [69]. Moreover, cultural nuances increase the difficulty of understanding the abuse of older adults with dementia.

Elder abuse among people with dementia is a pressing issue. A recent review just found that approximately 27.9–62.3 % of the older adults with dementia have experienced elder abuse (7). Elder abuse in demented older adults may cause serious short-term and long-term health issues, including physical impairment, psychological distress, and increased intervention and medical cost. There is an urgent need to improve our understanding of elder abuse among people with dementia.

Although elder abuse in the demented population may vary by the subtypes and/or multiple forms of abuse, the majority of studies have examined the association between physical abuse or psychological abuse and dementia. As the number of financial abuse and sexual abuse cases reported has been increasing in recent years, the risk factors of these subtypes of abuse in the demented population should be assessed in future research. Because studies also found that mutual abuse is common among older adults with dementia, future studies may also need to examine risk factors associated with mutual abuse and multiple types of abuse among older adults with dementia.

5.4.4 Understanding Risk Factors of Elder Abuse from an Intergenerational Perspective and Within the Family Settings

Elder abuse often occurs in family settings, and research has shown that adult children are the most common perpetrators of elder abuse [70]. However, current studies on risk factors of elder abuse tend to collect data from older adults, while overlooking the adult children's perspectives. As intergenerational conflicts and caregiver stress take a significant toll on elder abuse occurrence, it is necessary to investigate risk factors of elder abuse from adult children's perspectives. In particular, in minority communities and immigrant families, adulteration levels may vary significantly across generations, which often lead to intergenerational conflicts and elder abuse. In addition, because of stigma attached to reporting elder abuse as well as memory loss due to cognitive impairment, older adults tend to underreport elder abuse. A recent study conducted by Dong et al. found that prevalence of elder abuse reported by adult children is higher than that was reported by older adults [71]. Understanding risk factors of elder abuse through collecting data from adult children may enable us to fully capture factors that are associated with elder abuse.

5.4.5 Contextual Risk Factors Associated with Elder Abuse

Multilevel thinking is crucial for researchers to understand risk factors of elder abuse and future studies should take the social context in which study participants function into account. Currently, the majority of studies on risk factors of elder abuse tends to consider individual-level factors and do not take group-level factors such as state or neighborhood characteristics into consideration, even though this type of broader social environment influences individual's likelihood of being abused. For example, neighborhood disorders may reduce the access of better transportation and community activities, increasing the risk of social isolation and elder abuse. Without family- and neighborhood-level data, the studies cannot address whether community and neighborhood environment influences elder abuse. To the best of our knowledge, only two recent studies have examined family-level risk factors of elder abuse. Peshevska et al. explored community risk factors for elder abuse and neglect among aged 65 years and above in private households and found that living with close relatives, dissatisfaction with the household income, less equipped households, lacking property of house/flat, living in the northeast, southeast, and Polog region are associated with elder abuse [26].

In addition, very few studies have linked elder abuse with broader social factors such as sexism and ageism. Discrimination against older adults or stereotype of older adults as physically or mentally disable may induce inappropriate behavior toward older adults. Future studies may need to document how broader social factors contribute to elder abuse.

5.4.6 Understanding Risk Factors of Elder Abuse Through a Life Course Perspective

A life course theoretical framework, which posits that an individual's health is attributable to lifelong accumulation of advantage and disadvantage experiences, may support an understanding of how prior life events and past socioeconomic status account for elder abuse. The life course perspective posits that elder abuse was related to prior life circumstances such as child abuse and immigration. Older victims who suffer from negative life events may be more likely to report elder abuse. Similarly, caregivers who have experienced child abuse or domestic violence by the older adults may present the older victims by abusing them physically, emotionally, or financially, especially under the situations where the victims are frail. Unfortunately, very few studies have explored risk factors of elder abuse using the life course approach. There is a need to investigate prior life events as risk factors for elder abuse from both the victim and perpetrator perspectives.

5.4.7 Cross-Cultural Studies on Risk Factors of Elder Abuse

This review also identifies major gaps in understanding the cultural complexities of abuse among minority older adults. Although elder abuse affects older adults in every culture, risk factors associated with elder abuse may differ significantly. Insufficient data are available to understand risk factors of elder abuse in certain minority groups. The majority of studies on risk factors of elder abuse were conducted among white older adults, African American, and Latino older adults, whereas there is a relative dearth of data on Asian Americans and Pacific Islanders, a rapidly growing minority population in the United States. Even within Asian Americans, great variations persist with respect to culture, socioeconomic status, and acculturation levels among subgroups of Asian Americans such as Chinese, Vietnamese, and Indian Asian Americans. However, existing studies on risk factors of elder abuse tend to lump Asian Americans into one category. Likewise, it is important to disaggregate Asian American and Native Hawaiian/Pacific Islander Data to obtain a better understanding of how racial/ethnic status and cultural factors may associate with elder abuse in different ethnic/minority populations.

The community-based participatory research (CBPR) approach could be a potential model to explore risk factors of elder abuse in different racial/ethnic communities. CBPR necessitates equal partnerships between academic institutions, community organizations, and key stakeholders to examine the relevant issues. These partnerships require reciprocal transfer of expertise and need to build infrastructure toward sustainability. Recent elder abuse research in the Chicago Chinese community has demonstrated success and has enhanced infrastructure and networks for community-engaged research and community–academic partnerships. CBPR could be a novel model for conducting systematic and culturally appropriate research in diverse populations.

5.5 Conclusion

Elder abuse is associated with various sociodemographic, socioeconomic, and psychosocial risk factors from both the victim and perpetrator perspectives. Future studies should address methodological limitations and expand the research in minority populations. More longitudinal studies are necessary for us to understand the mechanisms through which risk factors relate to elder abuse.

References

1. Organization WH. Elder abuse fact sheet 2015. http://www.who.int/mediacentre/factsheets/fs357/en/.
2. Dong X, Chen R, Chang E-S, Simon M. Elder abuse and psychological well-being: a systematic review and implications for research and policy—a mini review. Gerontology. 2012;59 (2):132–42.
3. Dong X, Chen R, Wu B, Zhang N, Mui A-S, Chi I. Association between elder mistreatment and suicidal ideation among community-dwelling Chinese older adults in the USA. Gerontology. 2015;62(1):71–80.
4. Dong X, Simon M, de Leon CM, Fulmer T, Beck T, Hebert L, et al. Elder self-neglect and abuse and mortality risk in a community-dwelling population. JAMA. 2009;302(5):517–26.
5. Dong X. Medical implications of elder abuse and neglect. Clin Geriatr Med. 2005;21(2):293–313.

6. Cooper C, Selwood A, Livingston G. The prevalence of elder abuse and neglect: a systematic review. Age Ageing. 2008;37 (2):151–60.
7. Dong X, Chen R, Simon MA. Elder abuse and dementia: a review of the research and health policy. Health Aff. 2014;33(4):642–9.
8. Johannesen M, LoGiudice D. Elder abuse: a systematic review of risk factors in community-dwelling elders. Age Ageing. 2013;0:1–7.
9. Burnight K, Mosqueda L. Theoretical model development in elder mistreatment. US Department of Justice; No: 234488, 2011.
10. Bronfenbrenner U, Bronfenbrenner U. The ecology of human development: experiments by nature and design. Harvard University Press; 2009.
11. Schiamberg LB, Gans D. Elder abuse by adult children: an applied ecological framework for understanding contextual risk factors and the intergenerational character of quality of life. Int J Aging Hum Dev. 2000;50(4):329–59.
12. Giraldo-Rodríguez L, Rosas-Carrasco O, Mino-León D. Abuse in Mexican older adults with long-term disability: national prevalence and associated factors. J Am Geriatr Soc. 2015;63(8):1594–600.
13. Garre-Olmo J, Planas-Pujol X, López-Pousa S, Juvinyà D, Vilà A, Vilalta-Franch J. Prevalence and risk factors of suspected elder abuse subtypes in people aged 75 and older. J Am Geriatr Soc. 2009;57(5):815–22.
14. Cooney C, Howard R, Lawlor B. Abuse of vulnerable people with dementia by their carers: can we identify those most at risk? Int J Geriatr Psychiatry. 2006;21(6):564–71.
15. Buchwald D, Tomita S, Hartman S, Furman R, Dudden M, Manson SM. Physical abuse of urban native Americans. J Gen Intern Med. 2000;15(8):562–4.
16. Ruelas-González MG, Duarte-Gómez MB, Flores-Hernández S, Ortega-Altamirano DV, Cortés-Gil JD, Taboada A, et al. Prevalence and factors associated with violence and abuse of older adults in Mexico's 2012 National Health and Nutrition Survey. Int J Equity Health. 2016;15(1):1.
17. Lachs M, Berman J. Under the radar: New York State elder abuse prevalence study. Prepared by Lifespan of Greater Rochester, Inc, Weill Cornell Medical Center of Cornell University, and New York City Department for the Aging; 2011.
18. Chokkanathan S, Lee AE. Elder mistreatment in urban India: a community based study. J Elder Abuse Negl. 2006;17(2):45–61.
19. Friedman LS, Avila S, Tanouye K, Joseph K. A case–control study of severe physical abuse of older adults. J Am Geriatr Soc. 2011;59(3):417–22.
20. Strasser SM, Smith M, Weaver S, Zheng S, Cao Y. Screening for elder mistreatment among older adults seeking legal assistance services. West J Emerg Med. 2013;14(4).
21. Alexandra Hernandez-Tejada M, Amstadter A, Muzzy W, Acierno R. The national elder mistreatment study: race and ethnicity findings. J Elder Abuse Negl. 2013;25(4):281–93.
22. Beach SR, Schulz R, Castle NG, Rosen J. Financial exploitation and psychological mistreatment among older adults: differences between African Americans and non-African Americans in a population-based survey. Gerontol. 2010; doi:10.1093/geront/gnq053.
23. Longres JF. Race and type of maltreatment in an elder abuse system. J Elder Abuse Negl. 1993;4(3):61–84.
24. Wu L, Chen H, Hu Y, Xiang H, Yu X, Zhang T, et al. Prevalence and associated factors of elder mistreatment in a rural community in People's Republic of China: a cross-sectional study. PLoS ONE. 2012;7(3):e33857.
25. Burnes D, Pillemer K, Caccamise PL, Mason A, Henderson CR, Berman J, et al. Prevalence of and risk factors for elder abuse and neglect in the community: a population based study. J Am Geriatr Soc. 2015;63(9):1902–12.
26. Jordanova Peshevska D, Markovik M, Sethi D, Serafimovska E. Relationships and community risk factors for elder abuse and neglect: findings from the First National Prevalence Study on elder maltreatment. Maced J Med Sci. 2014;7(2):369–74.
27. Dong X, Simon MA, Gorbien M. Elder abuse and neglect in an urban Chinese population. J Elder Abuse Negl. 2007;19(3–4):79–96.
28. Fraga S, Lindert J, Barros H, Torres-González F, Ioannidi-Kapolou E, Melchiorre MG, et al. Elder abuse and socioeconomic inequalities: a multilevel study in 7 European countries. Prev Med. 2014;61:42–7.
29. Tareque MI, Islam TM, Koshio A, Kawahara K. Economic well-being and elder abuse in Rajshahi District of Bangladesh. Res Aging. 2015;37(2):200–24.
30. Gil APM, Kislaya I, Santos AJ, Nunes B, Nicolau R, Fernandes AA. Elder abuse in Portugal: findings from the First National Prevalence Study. J Elder Abuse Negl. 2014;1–22.
31. Skirbekk V, James K. Abuse against elderly in India—the role of education. BMC Public Health. 2014;14(1):1.
32. Dong X, Chen R, Fulmer T, Simon MA. Prevalence and correlates of elder mistreatment in a community-dwelling population of US Chinese older adults. J Aging Health. 2014;26(7):1209–24.
33. Lichtenberg PA, Stickney L, Paulson D. Is psychological vulnerability related to the experience of fraud in older adults? Clin Gerontol. 2013;36(2):132–46.
34. Lachs MS, Williams C, O'Brien S, Hurst L, Horwitz R. Risk factors for reported elder abuse and neglect: a nine-year observational cohort study. Gerontol. 1997;37(4):469–74.
35. Comijs HC, Smit JH, Pot AM, Bouter LM, Jonker C. Risk indicators of elder mistreatment in the community. J Elder Abuse Negl. 1999;9(4):67–76.
36. Abrams RC, Lachs M, McAvay G, Keohane DJ, Bruce ML. Predictors of self-neglect in community-dwelling elders. American Journal of Psychiatry. 2002 Oct 1;159(10):1724–30.
37. Cooper C, Katona C, Finne-Soveri H, Topinková E, Carpenter GI, Livingston G. Indicators of elder abuse: a crossnational comparison of psychiatric morbidity and other determinants in the Ad-HOC study. Am J Geriatr Psychiatry. 2006;14(6):489–97.
38. Dong X, Beck T, Simon MA. The associations of gender, depression and elder mistreatment in a community-dwelling Chinese population: the modifying effect of social support. Arch Gerontol Geriatr. 2010;50(2):202–8.
39. Dyer CB, Pavlik VN, Murphy KP, Hyman DJ. The high prevalence of depression and dementia in elder abuse or neglect. J Am Geriatr Soc. 2000;48(2):205–8.
40. Roepke-Buehler SK, Simon M, Dong X. Association between depressive symptoms, multiple dimensions of depression, and elder abuse a cross-sectional, population-based analysis of older adults in urban Chicago. J Aging Health. 2015; doi:10.1177/0898264315571106.
41. Dong X, Simon MA, Gorbien M, Percak J, Golden R. Loneliness in older Chinese adults: a risk factor for elder mistreatment. J Am Geriatr Soc. 2007;55(11):1831–5.
42. Tobiasz-Adamczyk B. Relation between medical sociology and sociology of ageing or later life. A new challenges, social expectations and dilemmas. Anthropol Rev. 2015;78(3):233–42.
43. Abuse NCftPoE. Elder abuse and substance abuse. 2003. http://www.preventelderabuse.org/issues/substance.html.
44. Melchiorre MG, Chiatti C, Lamura G, Torres-Gonzales F, Stankunas M, Lindert J, et al. Social support, socio-economic status, health and abuse among older people in seven European countries. PLoS ONE. 2013;8(1):e54856.
45. Luo Y, Waite LJ. Mistreatment and psychological well-being among older adults: exploring the role of psychosocial resources

and deficits. J Gerontol Ser B Psychol Sci Soc Sci. 2011;66 (2):217–29.
46. Naughton C, Drennan J, Lyons I, Lafferty A, Treacy M, Phelan A, et al. Elder abuse and neglect in Ireland: results from a national prevalence survey. Age Ageing. 2011; doi:10.1093/ageing/afr107.
47. Von Heydrich L, Schiamberg LB, Chee G. Social-relational risk factors for predicting elder physical abuse: an ecological bi-focal model. Int J Aging Hum Dev. 2012;75(1):71–94.
48. Choi NG, Kim J, Asseff J. Self-neglect and neglect of vulnerable older adults: reexamination of etiology. J Gerontol Soc Work. 2009;52(2):171–87.
49. Cannell MB, Weitlauf JC, Garcia L, Andresen EM, Margolis KL, Manini TM. Cross-sectional and longitudinal risk of physical impairment in a cohort of postmenopausal women who experience physical and verbal abuse. BMC Women's Health. 2015;15(1):1.
50. Dong X, Simon M, Rajan K, Evans DA. Association of cognitive function and risk for elder abuse in a community-dwelling population. Dement Geriatr Cogn Disord. 2011;32(3):209–15.
51. Yan E, Kwok T. Abuse of older Chinese with dementia by family caregivers: an inquiry into the role of caregiver burden. Int J Geriatr Psychiatry. 2011;26(5):527–35.
52. Cohen M. Research assessment of elder neglect and its risk factors in a hospital setting. Intern Med J. 2008;38(9):704–7.
53. Cooper C, Manela M, Katona C, Livingston G. Screening for elder abuse in dementia in the LASER-AD study: prevalence, correlates and validation of instruments. Int J Geriatr Psychiatry. 2008;23 (3):283–8.
54. Abuse E. The relationship between dementia and elder abuse. Am J Psychiatry. 1993;150:643–6.
55. Chokkanathan S. Factors associated with elder mistreatment in rural Tamil Nadu, India: a cross-sectional survey. Int J Geriatr Psychiatry. 2014;29(8):863–9.
56. Son J, Erno A, Shea DG, Femia EE, Zarit SH, Stephens MAP. The caregiver stress process and health outcomes. J Aging Health. 2007;19(6):871–87.
57. Schulz R, Martire LM. Family caregiving of persons with dementia: prevalence, health effects, and support strategies. Am J Geriatr Psychiatry. 2004;12(3):240–9.
58. Beach SR, Schulz R, Williamson GM, Miller LS, Weiner MF, Lance CE. Risk factors for potentially harmful informal caregiver behavior. J Am Geriatr Soc. 2005;53(2):255–61.
59. Cooney C, Mortimer A. Elder abuse and dementia—a pilot study. Int J Soc Psychiatry. 1995;41(4):276–83.
60. Lee M. Caregiver stress and elder abuse among Korean family caregivers of older adults with disabilities. J Fam Violence. 2008;23(8):707–12.
61. Paveza GJ, Cohen D, Eisdorfer C, Freels S, Semla T, Ashford JW, et al. Severe family violence and Alzheimer's disease: prevalence and risk factors. Gerontol. 1992;32(4):493–7.
62. Choi NG, Mayer J. Elder abuse, neglect, and exploitation: risk factors and prevention strategies. J Gerontol Soc Work. 2000;33 (2):5–25.
63. VandeWeerd C, Paveza GJ, Fulmer T. Abuse and neglect in older adults with Alzheimer's disease. Nurs Clin N Am. 2006;41(1):43–55.
64. Steadman PL, Tremont G, Davis JD. Premorbid relationship satisfaction and caregiver burden in dementia caregivers. J Geriatr Psychiatry Neurol. 2007;20(2):115–9.
65. Compton S, Flanagan P, Gregg W. Elder abuse in people with dementia in Northern Ireland: prevalence and predictors in cases referred to a psychiatry of old age service. Int J Geriatr Psychiatry. 1997;12(6):632–5.
66. Dong X, Chen R, Roepke-Buehler SK. Characteristics associated with psychological, physical, sexual abuse, caregiver neglect and financial exploitation in US Chinese older adults: findings from the population-based cohort study in the greater Chicago area. 2014.
67. Burgess AW, Phillips SL. Sexual abuse, trauma and dementia in the elderly: a retrospective study of 284 cases. Vict Offenders. 2006;1(2):193–204.
68. Paris B, Meier D, Goldstein T, Weiss M, Fein E. Elder abuse and neglect: how to recognize warning signs and intervene. Geriatrics. 1995;50(4):47–51 (quiz 2–3).
69. Wallace RB, Bonnie RJ. Elder mistreatment: abuse, neglect, and exploitation in an Aging America: National Academies Press; 2003.
70. Yan E, Tang CS-K. Prevalence and psychological impact of Chinese elder abuse. J Interpers Violence. 2001;16(11):1158–74.
71. Dong XQ, Li G. Caregiver Abuse of Chicago Chinese Older Adults in a Community-Dwelling Population. Journal of geriatric medicine and gerontology. 2015;1(1):1–19.

6 The Consequences of Elder Abuse

Elizabeth Podnieks and Cynthia Thomas

6.1 Introduction

Major demographic changes over the past 70 years have brought attention to the problems and concerns of older adults. Increased life expectancy has resulted in a growing number of persons over age 65, and this number continues to escalate. The increasing population of older people has led to the prediction that aging is accompanied by greater physical and mental problems that result in dependency—and also lead to situations in which elders may be mistreated. This chapter explores the consequences of elder abuse and neglects using a lived experience and social determinants of health framework.

While the prevalence rates of elder abuse have been investigated, the serious, often irreversible, and long-term consequences of abuse on older persons, on the health system and on society, are not well understood and have not been fully explored or documented. An increasing global prevalence of elder abuse requires an examination of its significant consequences in order to advance research, policy, and practice in the field.

Definitions of elder abuse remain unclear and confusing. Some researchers refer to the entire range of problems the elderly can experience as "abuse," including lack of proper housing, untreated medical conditions and inadequate social services. In this chapter "'abuse" means any physical, mental, or sexual injury inflicted on an older adult by a trusted person, including exploitation of an adult's financial resources. Harm also may come about through neglect by a responsible person. Elder abuse may also result from the interventions of well-meaning professionals and family members who paternalistically believe they "know what is best" for the older person.

The purpose of this chapter is to demonstrate that the consequences of elder abuse, a complex multifaceted problem, is best examined through a social determinants of health (SDH) framework, with an additional focus on lived experiences to add greater depth to our understanding of the problem. A framework that incorporates a human rights context and lived experiences facilitates comparisons at population and individual levels, and, most importantly, places the older person at the center of the analysis. Since individuals bear the full impact of the abuse, the authors believe an examination of consequences must originate with the older person. A contextual analysis of consequences on the health system and society at large is then properly anchored. As we use older individuals as research subjects, as we plan services for them, as we explain their behavior through a multitude of theories, we need to pause and consider who is at the center of this profusion of activity—the older person—the focus of this chapter. In tapping into elder's psyches to reveal their inner strength, a fuller picture may emerge. In addition to focusing on experiences of specific persons, the chapter, using evidence from large data bases, first shows that abused elders suffer over the long term in multiple ways.

6.2 Demonstrated Consequences of Elder Abuse

Before exploring the personal experiences of individual older adults victimized by abuse, we consider the harmful impact of abuse overall. While many studies of elder abuse have been persuasive and heartrending in their depictions of the effects of abuse on older vulnerable adults, until fairly recently, most studies have been based on small numbers of people, and often have only provided examples in the form of case studies. Over 20 articles, sixteen of which were based on studies conducted after 2000, have demonstrated a

E. Podnieks (✉)
Department of English, Ryerson University, 350 Victoria Street, JOR-1040, Toronto, ON M5B 2K3, Canada
e-mail: elizabeth.podnieks@utoronto.ca

C. Thomas
Committee on National Statistics, National Academies of Sciences, Engineering and Medicine, 5802 Nicholson Lane, Rockville, MD 20852, USA
e-mail: cynthiathomas101@gmail.com

X. Dong (ed.), *Elder Abuse*, DOI 10.1007/978-3-319-47504-2_6

connection between elder abuse and three categories of tragic outcomes. Some of the studies on which the articles were based found that elders' experiences of abuse or neglect resulted in more than one type of harmful consequence or outcome. These studies are summarized in Table 6.1.

The outcomes include actual loss of life, the most visible and alarming, and extreme physical deterioration, injury or long-term emotional illness. Victims of abuse also may experience less extreme but lingering health consequences or may end up in a hospital or other institution. Adverse outcomes often are connected to sociodemographic characteristics of the victims, and often result when people are extremely frail or suffering from some form of mental deterioration.

Mortality—Five of the articles cited data that show that elder abuse can lead to mortality. All five were based on studies with substantial sample sizes, ranging from some 1200 respondents (in a study of Australian women) to over 160,000 respondents (selected from the Women's Health Initiative.) The articles all were based on prospective studies, which measured abuse at baseline and then followed respondents for 7 years or more. Although three of the five studies focused solely on women, substantial numbers of men were included in the other two. Results did not differ between men and women.

People with poor physical or mental health, including physical frailty and limitations in cognitive and physical functioning, are more likely than others who are healthier to die at some point but not necessarily immediately following abusive experiences. In two of the studies, the victims' experiences of abuse were self-reported to the investigators. In the other three studies, adult protective service agencies (APS) had identified and verified the reports of abuse. The types of abuse measured in these studies included multiple or unspecified forms of abuse; neglect; exploitation; and self-neglect. These studies did not specifically focus on physical or psychological abuse.

Two studies examined the relationship between so-called self-neglect and mortality (reported to APS and verified) where study participants were followed for up to 13 years. Self-neglect is often excluded from definitions of elder abuse since there is no alleged perpetrator; although the potential consequences are often severe enough to merit the attention of social service providers. Self-neglect can encompass a wide range of behaviors, including those with less immediately harmful results such as eccentricity or hoarding, or lack of personal hygiene and cleanliness. More drastic examples include failure to maintain health by not seeking medical care for injuries or serious illnesses, misusing prescribed medications, or neglecting to eat adequate meals or drink liquids. Self-neglect has been shown to be associated with dementia or other forms of mental illness. These two studies, however, find that the importance of a prior diagnosis of self-neglect is independently associated with shorter survival time, even when controlling for various sociodemographic characteristics as well as cognitive status and depressive symptomatology.

Serious physical or emotional consequences—Still harmful but short of death are outcomes related either to severe physical consequences or emotional suffering. Serious physical and emotional results of abuse measured in these studies include poor physical health, becoming disabled, anxious, depressed, or suffering from other mental health consequences. Five articles documented one or more such serious consequences of abuse. All five studies were based on cross-sectional data, relying on respondents' recollections of past experiences of abuse reported at the same time as their assessments of their current health status. While the cross-sectional nature of the studies may be a limitation, the studies were consistent in their findings and were based on a diverse range of samples, including a rural population in South Carolina, a national survey in Sweden, and 40 sites around the US as part of the Women's Health Initiative.

According to the Centers for Disease Control (CDC), approximately 20 % of adults ages 60 and older have some form of mental or emotional illness. The most common illnesses are anxiety, severe cognitive impairment, and mood disorders such as depression and bipolar disorder. Emotional consequences of various forms of abuse, especially physical and psychological abuse, were specifically documented in all five articles. Two of the articles focused exclusively on women. The consequences of abuse include poor emotional health, according to standard measures, such as higher rates of anxiety, depression, or irritability compared to the rates reported for those who reported no prior abuse. Two of the articles also documented more physical health problems in those who reported experiencing abuse in contrast to those claiming not to have suffered abuse in the past. These physical problems include general physical malaise in one study and a variety of more specific symptoms including bone or joint problems, digestive problems, chronic pain, high blood pressure, or heart problems in the other studies.

Hospital visits and institutionalizations—Five articles showed a connection between abuses and visiting an emergency department, being hospitalized, entering hospice care, or being admitted to a nursing home. Four of the articles were based on participants in the Chicago Health and Aging Study (CHAP). Self-neglect was associated with a greater risk of entering a hospice program, visiting a hospital emergency department, or being admitted to a hospital for an overnight stay among CHAP respondents. Adults who were served by APS and especially those referred to APS as suffering from self-neglect, had a significant risk of being placed in a nursing home. Whether such placement was a "good" outcome or could have been avoided under other circumstances is unknown. In addition to self-neglect, other

Table 6.1 Consequences of elder abuse and self-neglect

Author/year	Sample	Study design	Measures of abuse	Variables (dependent/other)
Consequence: mortality				
Dong et al. [11]	9318 men and women in the Chicago Aging Project (CHAP)	Prospective Study:	Reports to social service agencies	Dependent: mortality
	ages 65 and over	in person interviews		Other/controls: cognition, physical functioning
		Followup:		
		6, 9 years median		
Schofield et al. [49]	12,066 Australian women ages 70–75 at baseline	Prospective Study	12 item vulnerability to abuse screening scale (VASS)	Dependent: mortality
		Followup: 12 years		Other/controls: demographic characteristics, social support, health behavior, chronic conditions
Dong XQ et al. [9]	7841 men and women from CHAP	Prospective Study	Reports to social service agencies	Dependent: mortality
	ages 65 and over	in person interviews		Other/controls: Depression, social networks, social engagement
		Followup: in the home		
		7.6 years		
Baker et al. [2]	160,600 women from the Women's Health Initiative	Retrospective Study	Participants' reports of prior year physical or verbal abuse	Dependent: mortality
		prior year abuse		Other/controls: age, education, ethnicity, health status
Lachs et al. [26]	2812 men and women (New Haven EPESE)	Prospective Study	Reports to Adult Protective Services on abuse, neglect, or exploitation or self-neglect	Dependent: mortality
	aged 65 and over in 1982	Followup: 13 years		Other/controls: demographic, chronic conditions, functional status, social networks, cognitive status, symptoms of depression
Consequence: physical and mental health				
Begle et al. [3]	90South Carolina	Cross sectional telephone interviews	Respondents' reports of emotional, physical and sexual mistreatment	Dependent: mental and physical health status
	ages 60–97	(CAT1)	since age 60	Other/controls: race/ethnicity, employment status, income, gender, social support
Mouton et al. [38]	93,676 women at 40 clinical sites nationwide	Cross sectional observational cohort study	Self reports of exposure to physical or verbal abuse over past 3 years	Dependent: mental component summary (MCS) score of RAND medical outcomes study
	ages 50–79			Other/controls: sociodemographic characteristics
Olofsson et al. [40]	9360 Swedish men and women from nationwide public health survey	Cross sectional national survey	Self reports of psychological and physical abuse	Dependent: self-reported physical and psychological health
	ages 65–84			
Mouton et al. [37]	257 women from the Women's Health Initiative in Newark ages 50–79	Cross sectional survey	27 item questionnaire on domestic violence at some point in respondent's life	Dependent: health measures from medical outcomes survey (short form)
Fisher and Regan [22]	842 community dwelling women from a clinical sample	Cross sectional telephone interviews	Questions on psychological control, threat, physical or sexual abuse since age 55	Dependent: mental and physical health problems (e,g., depression, anxiety, chronic pain, high blood pressure)
	ages 60 and over			Other controls: demographic characteristics

(continued)

Table 6.1 (continued)

Author/year	Sample	Study design	Measures of abuse	Variables (dependent/other)
Consequence: hospital visits and institutionalization				
Dong and Simon [14]	6674 community dwelling men and women in CHAP	Prospective population based study: in person interviews in the home	Confirmed reports to social services agencies for elder abuse	Dependent: Annual rate of hospitalization obtained from the Centers for Medicare and Medical Services (CMS)
				Other/controls: sociodemographic and socioeconomic variables, measures of cognitive and functional impairment, psychosocial distress, medical comorbidities
Lachs et al. [27]	2812 community dwelling men and women in New Haven EPESE study ages 65 + in 1982	Prospective population based study	Referrals to Adult Protective Services over a 9 year period	Dependent: Nursing home placement
		9 year followup		Other/controls: Demographics, medical, functional and social characteristics
Dong et al. [15]	6864 community dwelling men and women in CHAP	Prospective population based study: in person interviews in the home	Incidents of self-neglect reported to social service agencies	Dependent: Annual rate of emergency department utilization obtained from CMS
				Other/controls: sociodemographic variables and socioeconomic characteristics, medical conditions, cognitive and physical function
Dong Xin Qi et al. [8]	6864 community dwelling men and women in CHAP	Prospective population based study: in person interviews in the home	Level of severity of self-neglect, scored from 1 to 45, as rated by case workers from social service agencies	Dependent: hospitalization
				Other/controls: demographic variables income, self-reported medical conditions, cognitive and physical; function
Dong and Simon [16]	6864 community dwelling men and women in CHAP	Prospective population based study: in person interviews in the home	Level of severity of self-neglect, scored from 1 to 45, as rated by case workers from social service agencies	Hospice utilization obtained from CMS

Source Adapted from [7], Table 3, pp. 1228–1231)

forms of abuse were also associated with increased rates of hospitalization, including physical abuse, care giver neglect, and even financial exploitation.

Societal as well as individual consequences of abuse— These articles suggest that, depending on the type of abuse an older person experiences, some consequences are more likely than others, although additional research is needed to test these possible connections more directly. Self-neglect was the form of abuse most often associated with mortality in the particular studies cited here, although other forms of abuse were implicated as well. Self-neglect also seemed to result in a greater likelihood that elders would be admitted to a hospital or enter a nursing home or hospice care, in contrast to the experiences of other forms of abuse, or no prior abuse. On the other hand, poor physical health, disability, and depression and anxiety, were apparently more often preceded by such types of abuses as physical assaults or threats of assault, emotional or psychological abuse, or sexual abuse.

These large data-based studies present a broad brush picture of the overall consequences of various forms of abuse on large populations of older adults. There are consequences for both victims and for society. For society as a whole, there are costs associated with designing and providing services, medical treatments, and placing victims in long-term care facilities or hospitalizing them. The details of the suffering and resiliency of many older adults are revealed not only from examining collective bodies of data, but also from reports of lived experiences at the individual level.

6.3 Lived Experiences

Before engaging in a discussion of the appropriateness of SDH approach, we explore the lived experiences of older adults to better understand the elder abuse phenomenon and why it is critical for voices to be heard, respected, and acknowledged. It is through the actual articulation of harmful situations that interveners can help mistreated older persons to navigate their own journeys. A study completed in Tehran identified four themes: "being deprived of human rights and dignities," "smashed up integrity," "silent suffering," and "painful ending." [50] Older individuals experienced elder abuse as a deprivation of their human rights and dignity resulting in negative physical, psychological, and socioeconomic consequences, decreased quality of life, and painful endings.

A startling gap in the literature is the absence of voices of older individuals telling their experiences of elder mistreatment. Listening to older people describe their experiences illuminates the dramatic lasting and long-term effects. By using ethnographic material, it is possible to some extent to enter their lives and to understand the meanings older people give to abusive situations. The voices of the abused older people reveal the long-lasting effects of violent experiences and the devastating consequences this violence has on the way older people live their lives [34]. Research has positioned the idea of lived experiences within an empirical scientific paradigm. The social sciences have long accepted the value of lived experiences, but now there is growing recognition of its power to enhance understanding in the "harder" fields.

A pioneering early Canadian survey of 2008 randomly selected seniors living in private dwellings revealed that at least 4 % had recently experienced serious maltreatment at the hands of a partner, relative, or other close contact. Material abuse accounted for the largest number of cases, followed by chronic verbal aggression, physical abuse, and neglect. Nearly 19 % of victims experienced multiple forms of maltreatment [42]. Subsequently 28 interviews with older women who had been identified as abused in the initial prevalence survey were conducted. Because at the time there was little written on the lived experiences of elder abuse victims, the main goal was to ask older people to look back over the years and tell the story of their main life events. The in-depth interviews allowed people to share their insights, perceptions and fears, including their experiences with mistreatment. It became apparent that this particular group of older people was anything but powerless or helpless. The informants talked about personal and subjective experiences. They described how they had worked through life's events (e.g., the Depression); they talked about coping and surviving.

The elder abuse literature abounds with references to the impact of stress in all forms of family violence, especially in dysfunctional families. Stressors have been mentioned by abused older women and referred to as hardship and hard times. They also referred to stress as a causative factor in abusive circumstances. At times it appears as if they are excusing or possibly forgiving their abuser:

> There were many ways he [the husband] treated me roughly and humiliated me. But he has had a very stressful life and I think this was something to do with the way he mistreated me and took it all out on me. (Age 72, victim of physical and verbal abuse. Husband died after the first interview.)

The lived experiences of elders who have been mistreated provide important insights into the way older people negotiate their way through tragedy, change and the ability to cope with hardship; they talk about their mistreatment and for some it may be very therapeutic. Through qualitative research, we are able to obtain more data about the lives of older people as perceived *by them.*

Mysyuk et al. [39] have explored the perceptions of individuals as potential victims, witnesses, and reporters of abuse. In listening to people's experiences, we can learn how they are impacted and how they cope with abuse….what supports, activities or comforts helped them to survive the most difficult and challenging parts of their experience. Everyone has a different story, about the systems meant to support them as victims or survivors, about community resource centers or about the criminal justice system. It is important to consider the knowledge and perspectives of professionals when developing policy and practice for elder abuse but it is even more critical to ask older survivors of abuse what they believe would help them and others in similar situations. Could it be that surviving abusive behaviors actually make a person stronger? More empowered, more self-reliant? There is so much to be explored about the consequences of elder abuse, especially based on the perceptions of the victims.

Abuse flourishes when respect is missing. For older people, ageism is experienced in many forms, but elder abuse is arguably the most visible. It has a devastating impact on the physical, mental, emotional, and financial health of the older person. The impact is also carried by the broader community through the costs of services and the victim's diminished engagement with society in general. From preventative programs, to early interventions and later responses, we can pay attention to the rights of older people, which include identifying and meeting their wishes as well as ensuring their safety, while listening to their voices. Some voices are strong and resonant and we respond to them; some are so soft—barely a whisper; these are the ones that need to be amplified.

6.4 Coping Skills: Resilience

Psychologists have long recognized the ability of people to adapt to and overcome risk and adversity. Many individuals and communities are able to rebuild lives even after indescribable tragedy. This trait of resiliency can be seen in older people as they respond to situations of elder mistreatment. Resilience is the ability to withstand stress and catastrophe. Everyone experiences adversity often beginning with daily challenges that sometimes result in serious losses. Fortunately many people are able to adapt. There are many ways of overcoming adversity. Resilience allows people to adapt successfully in the face of harm or threats. It has been shown that people can improve their capacity for resilience at any time in life.

Most lives involve several phases, while experience is accumulated along the way: childhood; adolescence and coming of age; and gradually aging. Old age has usually been associated with vulnerabilities, which can be mitigated when modern societies respond appropriately. Older individuals do not suddenly become vulnerable; there is clear evidence that their vulnerability bears the long-term markings of experiences. There is a need for specific interventions that either mitigate the adverse impacts, or amplify the positive effects of early life experiences. Life cycle transitions can have an impact on the vulnerabilities and resilience of old age. All older people are not at risk and all older people are not vulnerable. Resilience can play a part in this dynamic. Personal resilience can be fostered by providing age-friendly enabling environments. Society has been slow to appreciate the advantages of longevity. Lifelong learning, access to information and communication technology, social connectedness, physical safety, civic freedom, and access to key public services such as transport, are critical to enhancing the ability of older adults to achieve maximum benefits from greater longevity [54].

In many ways, the concept of resilience is the opposite of the well-known concept of vulnerability. Victims of elder mistreatment identified in the Canadian study appear to be characterized by resiliency. They seemed to have a basic strength through which they were able to cope or adapt, and this skill has emerged over the life course. Their resilience has been described in their own words: "I have been strong," "I was always able to manage." The study did not permit a comparison of the hardiness of these older people and other nonabused elders. Perhaps it is inconsistent to label individuals who have been victims of elder abuse as resilient but, on reviewing the life experiences of many adults, it was abundantly clear that they had a realistic perspective on life and have been able to cope with "the hand dealt to them"—even when this meant enduring mistreatment.

Being resilient does not mean going through life without experiencing stress and pain. People feel grief, sadness, and a wide range of emotions after adversity and loss. The key to resilience lies in working through the emotions and the effects of stressful and painful events. Resilience is not something someone is born with or without; it develops as people grow and acquire better self-management skills and more knowledge. Resilience comes from supported relationships with parents, peers and others, as well as cultural beliefs and traditions that help people cope with the inevitable ups and downs in life. Resilience is present in a variety of behaviors, thoughts and actions; it can be developed across a lifespan.

Factors that contribute to resilience:

- Close relationships with families, friends, and neighbors
- Confidence in one's own strength and abilities
- Feeling in control
- Ability to seek help and resources
- Good problem-solving and communication skills
- Viewing oneself as resilient rather than as a victim
- Coping with stress in healthy ways; avoiding harmful coping strategies such as substance abuse
- Ability to find a positive meaning in life despite difficult or traumatic events (PBS online 2009).

Research has emphasized the importance of early childhood as a time to promote resilience [31]. Children need high-quality care and opportunities for developing and maintaining relationships as well as adequate nutrition and support from family, educators, and communities. When these and other protective factors are in place, children can expect to acquire the internal adaptive resources to cope with trauma and stress. Thus resilience developed early on can be reserved and used throughout life [4].

6.5 Social Determinants of Health

The factors that shape health around the world are not only medical treatments or lifestyle choices but rather the physical and social circumstances that people experience over and above their genetic makeup. Genetic endowment predisposes people to certain diseases and health conditions, the social environment can dominate its influence on health.

The World Health Organization notes the damage to health resulting from "a toxic combination of poor social policies and programs, unfair economic arrangements, and bad politics." The interrelationships among these factors determine the health of individuals and populations at large. Because of these interrelationships, interventions that target multiple health-related factors all at once are most likely to be effective. As demonstrated above, physical, psychological, or financial abuse or neglect can be a risk to health and well-being. Strong health status affects the sense of control that people have over their lives which in turn may protect them from abusive and neglectful situations. The social and economic environment and personal income, education and social status all contribute to the sense of control people have over their lives and their capacity to cope with stressful situations. The sense of control that people has over their lives can be enhanced or inhibited, depending on physical and social environments.

In addition, health and well-being are influenced by income and wealth. Well-being is further affected by available health and social services and the ability to obtain quality education, food, and housing, along with other factors. People do not always have personal control over the quality of their communities, housing, work settings, health and social service agencies, and educational institutions with which they interact. The quality of living conditions is strongly determined by decisions that governments make in a range of different public policy domains. These different levels of government pass laws, establish policies, and promulgate regulations that impact income, employment, social assistance, family benefits, housing, health and social services, transportation, and recreational opportunities. All of these situations contribute to the social determinants of health.

Personal health and coping skills also affect how well older people are able to deal with difficult situations in positive way. Gender and culture affect how older people maintain their personal and group identities, status and traditions, and contribute to their sense of control. Health services and resources are critical in an older person's ability to participate in activities of daily living and remain involved in their communities. The quality of the living environment is an important influence on the quality of older person's life. Table 6.2 summaries these social determinants of health.

Table 6.2 Summary: social determinants of health

Biology and Genetic Endowment	Genetic endowment provides a predisposition to a large number of individual responses that affect health status. Genetic endowment appears to predispose some people to certain diseases or health problems
Healthy Child Development	Early child development is a powerful determinant of health. Experiences from conception to age six have the most important influence in the life cycle on the connecting and sculpting of the brain's neurons. Positive stimulation early in life improves learning, behavior and health into adulthood
Gender	Gender norms influence the health system's practices. Many health issues are a function of gender-based social status or roles. Although women live longer than men, they more frequently suffer depression, stress overload, chronic conditions and family violence
Culture	Some individuals or groups may experience health risks due to a socioeconomic environment which is mainly determined by dominant cultural values that contribute to the perpetuation of conditions such as marginalization, stigmatization, loss or devaluation of language and culture and a lack of access culturally appropriate health care and services (5)
Personal Practices and Coping Skills: Resiliency	Actions by which individuals can prevent diseases and promote self-care, cope with challenges, and develop self-reliance, solve problems and make choices will enhance their health. Personal life choices are influenced by the socioeconomic environments in which people, work, learn and play
Health Services and the Role of Physicians	Health services maintain and promote health, prevent disease, and contribute to a continuum that includes treatment and secondary prevention
Social Support Networks	Support from families, friends, neighbors and community is associated with better health. Help people solve problems, deal with adversity: provide a sense of mastery and control over life circumstances
Education and Literacy	Health status improves with the level of education. Closely tied to socioeconomic status. Effective education for children and lifelong learning for adults contribute to health and prosperity for individuals and the country
Employment and Working Conditions	Unemployment, stressful or unsafe work conditions are associated with poorer health. People who have control over their work and less stress-related demands of the job are healthier
Social Environments	The importance of social support extends to the broader community. It is reflected in the organizations, institutions and informal giving practices that people create to share resources and build relationships and attachments with each other
Physical Environment: Housing	The physical environment is an important determinant of health. In the built environment factors related to housing, indoor air quality, and the design of communities and transportation systems all influence our physical and psychological well-being
Legal and Judicial Systems	Legislation supports programs to prevent, detect, and intervene in elder abuse. Programs of restorative justice help victims to reconcile with perpetrators

6.6 Healthy Child Development

Early childhood experiences have strong immediate and long lasting biological, psychological, and social effects upon health. "Latency effects" refer to how early childhood experiences predispose children to either good or poor health regardless of later life circumstances. For example, low birthweight babies living in disadvantaged conditions are generally more susceptible to health problems than babies of advantaged populations. These latency effects result from biological processes during pregnancy associated with poor maternal diet, parental risk behaviors, and the experience of stress.

Health effects may also result from early psychological experiences that create a sense of control or self-efficacy. "Pathway effects" refer to a situation when children's exposures to risk factors at one point do not have immediate health effects but later lead to situations that do have health consequences. For instance, it is not an immediate health issue if young children lack readiness to learn as they enter school. But limited learning abilities can lead to experiences that are harmful to health in later life such as lower educational attainment. One way to weaken the relationship between parents' socioeconomic status and children's developmental outcomes is by providing high-quality early child education regardless of parents' wealth.

"Cumulative effects" suggest that the longer children live under conditions of material and social deprivation, the more likely they are to show adverse health and developmental outcomes. Accumulated disadvantage can lead to cognitive and emotional deficits such as incompetence and emotional immaturity. In addition, adverse childhood experiences can create a sense of inefficacy—or learned helplessness—which is a strong determinant of poor health. The state of early child development is cause for concern. The most obvious indicator of the situation is whether children are living under conditions of material and social deprivation. The quality of early childhood development is shaped by the economic and social resources available to parents. Government can provide a range of supports and benefits to children through family friendly public policies.

Public support and benefits to families form a base for healthy childhood development. Providing higher wages and social assistance benefits would reduce child poverty and be one of the best means to improve early childhood development. The effects of early childhood development on later abusive behavior toward older persons are an evolving topic of research. Some studies indicate that children raised in abusive families go on to become "bullies" in school and later perpetrators of elder mistreatment. Do abused children become abusers themselves?

6.7 Gender and Culture

It is acknowledged that culture and gender have crosscutting, influential effects on the other health determinants. Gender refers to the many different roles, personality traits, attitudes, behaviors, relative powers, and influences which society assigns to the two sexes [55]. Culture comes from both a personal history and wider situational, social, political, geographic, and economic factors. Gender can have a profound effect on such factors as social status, how older individuals access health care, meaningful work, and leisure/recreational opportunities and other resources. Gender and cultural characteristics affect how older individuals maintain their personal and group identity, status, and traditions, all of which contribute to the health of individuals and populations. While many studies have found that older women are more likely than men to be victims of abuse, the type of abuse may also differ by gender [43]. Material abuse is equally common among men and women living alone, and although men are more likely to be physically abused, physical abuse by men toward women tends to be more violent [46]. Vulnerability can make it more difficult for either a man or a woman to escape or report abuse. However, ageist social attitudes toward older people are probably greater factors in the underdetection and underreporting of abuse. Ageist attitudes reinforce and perpetuate an increased vulnerability to abuse and neglect in older individuals.

It is important to emphasize the special and unique needs of abused older women. Older women should be represented on staff, boards of directors and in volunteer agencies so that their experiences, perspectives, and struggles are recognized and validated. It would be helpful for women's organizations to assume much greater responsibility in addressing the plight of older women in abusive situations.

Culture is considered a key determinant of health, since some individuals or groups may face additional health risks due to their socioeconomic circumstances, which are influenced by dominant cultural values. The social environment, influenced by mainstream culture, may perpetuate conditions such as marginalization, stigmatization, loss or devaluation of language, and lack of access to culturally appropriate health care and services, all resulting in social exclusion [17, 43]. There is little question that these factors can severely impact the degree of social isolation and subsequent mistreatment experienced by older people. Negative societal attitudes and ignorance of the aging process may result in a climate that is favorable to abusive situations. There needs to be an understanding of the barriers that discourage and prevent older individuals and their families from seeking help or disclosing information to service providers.

6.8 Personal Practices and Coping Skills: Resilience

Personal health practices and coping skills are imperative for maintaining good health. Older persons who are physically active report a greater sense of subjective well-being, and control over their lives, and are therefore better equipped to cope with life stresses [24]. Active older adults are more likely to be capable of defending themselves from abusive situations both physically and psychologically. Such adults are often more independent, and if threatened, can leave abusive situations.

Social environments that enable and support healthy choices and lifestyles, as well as people's knowledge, intentions, behaviors, and coping skills for dealing with life in healthy ways, are key influences on health. It is critical that we consider the impact of various chronic conditions and disabilities that people develop as they age on the person's coping strategy and style, body image, self-perception, and self-efficacy. Coping styles influence a person's attitudes and perceptions of the ability to manage the challenges and stressors. Older individuals who develop resilient traits and attitudes may experience increased sense of control over their lives, thus protecting them from abusive and neglectful situations. Low self-esteem and stress among older individuals reduces coping skills and often places them at risk for abuse and neglect [43].

6.9 Health Services and the Role of Physicians

Physicians and other health service providers can be an important source for detecting elder abuse, and stopping it. In some locations, hospital employees and physicians are mandated reporters of elder abuse. A new model for care under the Patient Protection and Affordable Care Act (P.L. 111-148), may lead to improvements in detecting elder abuse and preventing it from continuing. The law, passed in 2010, requires Americans to obtain healthcare coverage, subsidizes premium costs for low-income persons, and fosters competition among providers across healthcare markets. The legislation also provides physicians, hospitals, and other providers with an opportunity to create so-called accountable care organizations, rewarding medical practices for saving costs by eliminating unnecessary medical procedures while at the same time increasing successful patient outcomes.

Any group of physicians or other healthcare providers with 5000 or more Medicare patients can contract with the federal government to create such an organization. Medical practices that save money receive bonuses based on a share of the savings. Early reports of the functioning of these organizations suggest that physicians are spending more time with patients, attending to their complaints, and paying attention to their symptoms. Physicians are achieving cost savings due to reductions in hospital and emergency room visits and unnecessary tests. Such practice settings have the potential for more careful observations of older patients and point to the possibility that these systems of care can lead to better detection of instances of elder abuse, and toward effect solutions for addressing it. Unfortunately, after the first year of the program, nearly a third of the participants left the program because the incentive payments they were to receive were not large enough to offset their investment costs. Despite this somewhat rocky start to the program, the model has promise and stronger medical practices are so far succeeding.

6.10 Social Support Networks

Strong social relationships make an important contribution to health. Social support from families, friends, and communities is associated with better health, equipping older individuals with the emotional and practical resources they need to cope with growing older. Belonging to social networks makes people feel cared for, loved, and valued, providing a powerful protective effect on mental and physical health [57]. Current social trends have weakened traditional family, friendships, neighborhood and community networks, leaving many families and individuals isolated from natural support systems. Older individuals who are isolated socially may have a wide range of health problems and risk factors, which further limit their social support networks, and those of their informal caregivers as well [30].

Lack of social support has been linked to abusive behavior [1]. Abused older individuals may be more socially isolated and have fewer social contacts than nonabused older individuals. Furthermore, when families are isolated from the support of friends and relatives, older members are at a greater risk for abusive behavior that may be undetected [43]. The absence of emotional and practical social support varies by social and economic status and places older individuals at an increased risk for abuse and neglect.

Social exclusion is a prime social determinant of health and the process of social exclusion negatively affects all other determinants. Social exclusion refers to specific groups being denied opportunity to participate in civil society. At special risk are persons of color, recent immigrants, women, and people with disabilities. Many people in today's society are marginalized and have limited access to social, cultural, and economic resources. Socially excluded people are more likely to be unemployed or earn lower wages, have less access to health and social services and to ways of furthering their education. These groups are increasingly being segregated into specific neighborhoods. Lacking power, excluded groups have little influence on governments or other institutions [35]. A critical concern relates to the effects of exclusion on the LBGT community. Not only is social support unavailable to many of these older people, but they tend to be actively excluded from mainstream society, adding to the shame and stigma they already experience.

Support networks can empower and liberate members to speak out about mistreatment. These networks can provide support for stories so they are more likely to be believed. "Help lies in listening, believing and helping people to take action as they choose it" [34]. Social exclusion is a major risk factor for elder abuse as older individuals and their circumstances may never come to the attention of advocates or concerned others. Simply put, "exclusion is the problem: inclusion is the solution" [18].

As we use older people as research subjects, as we plan services for them, as we explain their behavior through a multitude of theories, let us stop to consider who is at the center of this plethora of activity—the older individual. World Elder Abuse Awareness Day is an outstanding example of collective involvement—of all generations coming together to promote the prevention of elder abuse. This annual event addresses social isolation because it involves the entire community in implementing action plans on elder abuse.

6.11 Education and Literacy

Education is an important determinant of health. Health status increases with the level of education. Education increases opportunities for income and job security, equips people with problem-solving skills, and gives people a sense of mastery and control over their lives. Education and literacy also improve one's ability to access and understand information, which are key factors that influence health. Low literacy rates can make it more difficult for older individuals to care for their health, and to manage their finances [5]. When older individuals rely on social supports for help with reading and writing, dependency places them in a precarious situation in regard to abuse and neglect. It further inhibits their ability to respond to written care plans or directions.

Education has the potential to be a major factor in risk reduction for abuse but it must be accompanied by other interventions that are applied concurrently to help equalize the power between older individuals and those who interact with them. Training older individuals in strategies to arm themselves against abuse and to access help in abusive situations will enable them to develop "resiliency" to abuse. Training must include measures to change those administrative, legal, social, and cultural conditions that foster abuse. Educating children and youth to become aware of the abuse and neglect of older persons places them in a position to prevent it from happening [44]. Increased education benefits all ages.

Education should begin in early childhood and continue through professional school. Pre-retirement courses should be available and marketed by government organizations and through social media so that people will know early on that elder abuse exists and how to plan for their later lives accordingly. They need to assess whom they trust enough to carry out their wishes, and most importantly how to recognize and report mistreatment. All members of society need accurate information about older people and the aging process itself to overcome the effects of negative myths about old age and to foster a society in which violence against older adults will not be tolerated.

Victims of elder mistreatment have explained their reasons for remaining in abusive situations, often saying that they do not want any professional assistance. They often refuse to place criminal charges, particularly against loved ones. Seniors themselves should learn to become more assertive and aware of their rights. For current generations, pre-retirement courses can be directed toward educating middle-aged individuals and encouraging them to make early decisions, for example, how they want their assets distributed, whom they trust to receive power of attorney, and whether to complete a living will. Education also is needed for abusers. Society as a whole must relinquish the ageist attitudes that are so prevalent today.

6.12 Employment and Working Environments

Employment leads to economic stability which, combined with a healthy work environment, leads to good health. Unemployment, underemployment, and stressful work environments are associated with poor health. Older individuals who have control over their working circumstances and fewer stress-related demands on the job are healthier and often live longer than those with more stressful or riskier work demands [23]. Health is also increased through the effects of workplace supports. Employment and working conditions may have an impact on the behavior of the abuser. With regard to caretakers and close relatives of older adults, lack of control in the work environment, and presence of many stress-related demands, may lead to an escalation of abusive actions toward an older adult over whom they exert power.

6.13 Social and Physical Environments

Inequalities in resource allocation and service delivery are a reality that should not be accepted; as such discrimination only succeeds in marginalizing older populations. Older individuals may not receive health and social services or the services offered may be inadequate, unavailable, inaccessible, or not known to them. Furthermore, older adults may not meet the eligibility criteria, may have language difficulties, or lack transportation. There are a disproportionate number of services available for youth or younger adults in contrast to the older population. This discrepancy sends a message to society that as one ages one is not valuable, not worthy of the same health and social protections as younger age cohorts. These current political practices support ageist attitudes that behaviors that actually are abusive and neglectful are appropriate for "dealing" with older individuals [41].

Safe, accessible and affordable housing is an important aspect of the physical environment. The quality of housing is important to the health and well-being of older individuals who may increasingly spend more time at home. When older individuals are living in close quarters with family members, abusive and neglectful situations can accelerate. Crowding is a problem particularly for older people who are part of low-income families, including many immigrants. When older people are provided with adequate housing or shelter, they can regain a healthy sense of mental and physical well-being and create a life away from an abuser or potential abuser [23].

Transportation problems in both urban and rural communities can create major barriers to social contact, recreation, and active living for older individuals, especially those with disabilities. Lack of transportation is isolating and frustrating for many individuals, and can lead to an increase in health-damaging behaviors such as drug and alcohol dependency, both of which are positively correlated with incidents of abuse. Lack of transportation limits an older adult from accessing appropriate healthcare services, and limits participation in social events and religious activity [43].

Large proportions of the middle-aged residents of small towns age in place; however, as their children migrate to larger urban centers, they may face isolation, because of fewer social services in rural areas. Older people in urban areas have different social and physical environments. They may have poorer housing and be more susceptible to crime. Fear of crime, especially among those who are economically and socially disadvantaged, can be debilitating, also leading to isolation and increased risk of abuse and neglect [30].

6.14 Legal and Judicial Systems

Discussions of the SDH do not generally include the justice system. Elder abuse is a legal issue, a criminal issue, and Elder Law is a discrete and specialized area of the law. Unfortunately as the population of elderly increases, incidents of elder abuse are likely to increase. It is critical that attorneys fully understand the obligations imposed upon them, to act in the interests of older adults with impaired capacity. In other words, the legal profession itself must ensure that its members have the skills to act honestly and with reasonable diligence in situations of neglect or abuse [21]. As more knowledge is gained about the magnitude and consequences of abuse, neglect, and exploitation of older people, legislation can be introduced to strengthen the programs and services that help prevent, detect, and intervene.

Research shows that empowering individuals to actively participate in personal decision-making improves life outcomes and can reduce the risk of abuse and exploitation. There is a risk of abuse and exploitation in all forms of decision-making for people with differing abilities. An overly protective response to situations where people with limited capacities are at risk can stifle self-determination and empowerment. Protection needs to be carefully balanced with respect for human and constitutional rights. Adults have a basic right to make choices, good or bad, and determine the course of their lives. An overly aggressive or inappropriate protective response to limited capacity can itself be a form of abuse.

Restorative Justice—Interest in restorative justice, i.e., rehabilitating offenders by reconciling them with their victims and with the community at large, has been increasing since the early 1990s. Programs, studies and discussion groups on the subject have proliferated in many countries. The failure of the punitive justice model, excessive use of incarceration, and the alienation of victims and lack of response to their needs has generated support for this new way of thinking [48, 29].

In the 1980s, more than a hundred programs of mediation between victims and offenders were established, often by faith communities and volunteer groups. Most such efforts were part of diversion programs, although they were introduced at other stages of the criminal process as well. Family conferences also fall into the category of restorative justice practices. These conferences are aimed at young offenders and help engage family and friends of the victim and the offender in a dialogue in order to find the best ways of dealing with criminal behavior. In many Aboriginal communities, sentencing circles give victims, offenders, elders, and other community representatives the opportunity to examine the consequences of the offense, reparation for injuries to victims and reintegration of the offender into the community. Some of these sentencing circles operate within the formal justice system as alternatives to the conventional sentencing procedure and involve justice professionals [29]. In the past decade, practices have become more diverse but are still disparate in terms of philosophy, principles, and application.

Despite the progress that has been made, restorative justice is the subject of much criticism. Organizations that support victims and advocate for their rights have reservations and questions about the model [47, 48]. Compared with the traditional model of justice, restorative justice offers a more positive and constructive approach to restoring ties between the victim of an offense, the person who committed the offense, and the community as a whole. This approach does tend to make justice more compassionate and more sensitive to the suffering of the individuals and communities affected by crime [48]. Restorative justice promotes such values as healing for the offender and the victim, community input, respectful dialogue between the parties involved, forgiveness and accountability. It is an alternative to the adversarial system of justice and an antidote to punitive policies [48].

The aim of restorative justice is to provide a larger role for victims; meet their needs for information about the reasons for and circumstances of the offense; allow them to be heard and to obtain tangible or symbolic compensation; and regain the independence and power that the crime took away from them [28, 29]. Restorative justice is also meant to have a positive impact on offenders by confronting them with the consequences of their actions and their responsibilities, giving them the opportunity to repair the damage caused to the victim and having them work on finding a solution to their problems [53, 20]. The concept of restorative justice is especially promising in cases of elder abuse, where strong social ties often provide an underpinning to an abusive situation, making possible reconciliation and reform.

6.15 The Capacity to Forgive

Psychologist Michael McCullough has written extensively on forgiveness: who tends to forgive and the psychological processes that may foster or hinder forgiveness for specific transgressions [32]. Forgiveness is a suite of prosocial motivational changes that occurs after a transgression.

Researchers have found that the disposition to forgive is correlated (positively or negatively) with a broad array of variables, including several personality traits, psychological symptoms, moral emotions, hope, and self-esteem [51]. Research has shown that people who are more agreeable, more emotionally stable, and (possibly) more spiritual, or religious have a stronger disposition to forgive than do their less agreeable, less emotionally stable, and less spiritually, and religiously inclined counterparts. Moreover, research has shown that empathizing with the transgressor, making generous attributions and appraisals regarding the transgressor and transgression and refraining from focusing obsessively about the transgression are associated with the extent to which a victim forgives a specific person [32].

Interesting questions in relation to forgiveness which have not been posed by McCullough relate to older individuals and their perceptions of experienced mistreatment either in their earlier lives or their later years. Have lived experiences contributed to the capacity to accept and forgive? Under what circumstances do older people move on from abusive situations? What is the relationship between traits of empathy, generosity, spirituality, faith, and kindness, and to what extent have these traits been present over the life span of the victim of the abuse?

6.16 The Ethical Dimension

Ethical dilemmas widely vary in different cultures; it is essential to respect the cultural norms that shape certain behaviors. Ethical dilemmas occur when there is a conflict of values between individuals. The challenge is to identify and explore the nature of the conflict [10]. Dr. Xin Q. Dong has summarized relevant terminology and basic principles of ethics while providing an overview of the legal history of elder abuse. The basic goals of ethics related to elder abuse are to prevent unnecessary suffering and to maintain quality of life. Dr. Dong encourages healthcare workers and other service providers to examine their own values more closely, including attitudes toward aging and toward professional versus family responsibilities. What are the most important guiding principles? Why do physicians have low rates of reporting elder abuse when most municipalities have mandatory reporting laws? What is "good" for older people? According to many, we should promote autonomy, use the least restrictive approach to dealing with problematic situations, and work across disciplines [56]. In the field of elder abuse, ethical questions have been raised concerning individual rights. Accusations of ageism and excessive paternalism have been made concerning services provided by communities as they redesign projects due to shrinking resources [36].

Older individuals can be affected by important ethical issues, just as the lives of other adults are. Among the questions that professionals struggle with include:

- Breaches of confidence and trust
- Compromising the relationship with patients and families
- Fear that the patient will be abandoned when the physician is not there
- Concern that a patient's quality of life will be compromised
- Worry that a patient will be harmed by a report [19].

6.17 Innovative Interventions

At the Institute of Medicine's forum on global violence prevention, it was suggested that instead of placing the responsibility for violence prevention on the government, responsibility could be placed on individuals to allow them to engage directly with the issues behind the violence, so that everyone is a part of the solution. This framing shifts the paradigm away from victims and perpetrators into a paradigm about collective and shared responsibility and reimagining a community [25].

Innovation in gaming can be used as a tool for helping older individuals overcome the distress of elder abuse. Internationally renowned game designer Jane McGonigal, following a serious concussion, turned her recovery process into a resilience-building game. What started as a simple motivational exercise quickly became a set of rules for "post-traumatic growth" that she shared on her blog. These rules led to the digital game "SuperBetter" and a major research study with the National Institute of Health. Today nearly half a million people have played SuperBetter to get stronger, happier, and healthier. But the life-changing ideas behind SuperBetter are much larger than just one game. McGonigal reveals a decade's worth of scientific research into the way all games—including video games, sports, and puzzles—can change how we respond to stress, challenge, and pain. She explains how we can cultivate new powers of recovery and resilience in everyday life simply by adopting a more "gameful" mindset. Being gameful means bringing the same psychological strengths naturally displayed when playing games—such as optimism, creativity, courage, and determination—to real-world goals [33].

Older individuals enjoy and participate in many levels of gaming. The authors of this chapter propose that this recreational activity could well be applied in empowering older people and victims of elder mistreatment. The game framework and its application to interventions in elder mistreatment could be incorporated into elder abuse awareness programs for youth and younger people. Building on young people's digital culture or simply adopting a "gameful" mindset can possibly cultivate new powers of recovery and resilience in everyday life.

6.18 Can Body Language Lead to Empowerment?

Psychologist Amy Cuddy has used images from everyone from Oprah and Mick Jagger to world leaders and athletes to talk about the relationship between posture and power. "We make sweeping judgments and inferences from body language, and those judgments can predict really meaningful life outcomes." In other words when people pretend to be powerful they are more likely to feel powerful. This concept can be applied to victims, enabling them to portray confidence and an ability to stand up to an abuser and abusive situations. Cuddy's studies show that if someone stands like a superhero privately before going into a stressful situation, there actually will be hormonal changes in body chemistry that can cause someone to be more confident and in-command. Her work is grounded in science and her theories have been applied extensively in university studies. If elders can apply this concept, they may gain confidence and decisiveness in the presence of potential abusers and even combat ageism when doctors, lawyers, and others intimidate them by their posture or language [6].

6.19 Forging a New Vision

The consequences of elder abuse are a major source of pain and stress and can have long-term effects on the health and well-being of older people. The physical effects have been well documented and include problems with all major systems. Abuse has a huge impact on people of all ages but there is a special vulnerability attached to an older person because of frailty, or the presence of disabilities or other impairments. Abused older people may be isolated and thus not attract the attention needed for appropriate intervention. Hidden, often subtle consequences may be overlooked. It is important to understand the feelings and perceptions of people who have been abused, namely, their lived experiences.

This chapter has focused on examining the consequences of elder abuse through a social determinant of health lens. It advocates for working with older people to determine their own preferred course of action, reflecting their reasoning and their sense of reality. A recent report by the Frame Works Institute [55] extends this concept by analyzing how the public feels about elder abuse in relation to the patterns of thinking of experts. By understanding the public's attitudes toward elder abuse, researchers can compare the different perceptions and explanations, note gaps, and overlaps and lay the groundwork for future research by identifying areas where messages need to be changed and strategies developed. The Frame Works Report describes the public's struggle to see elder abuse as a collective problem that can and must be addressed through collective action and public policy. The authors here argue that older people, experts, and the public must work together to understand their roles and responsibilities to recognize elder abuse as a societal problem needing to be addressed through action at the systemic level. Older persons not only must be listened to but also involved in the planning, research, and evaluation of all aspects of interventions [55]. A world-wide project is needed to examine how such a framework could become universally accepted as a viable and realistic methodology for addressing elder abuse and its consequences. This chapter asks that we listen to older people: their voices can move us and change us.

References

1. Anetzberger J. editor. The clinical management of elder abuse. Binghamton, NY: The Haworth Press, Inc.; 2005.
2. Baker MW, et al. Mortality risk associated with physical and verbal abuse in women aged 50 to 79. J Am Geriatr Soc. 2009; 57:1799–809.
3. Begle AM, et al. Elder mistreatment and emotional symptoms among older adults in a largely rural population: the South Carolina elder mistreatment study. J Interpers Violence. 2011;26:2321–32.
4. Benard B. Fostering resiliency in kids: Protective factors in the family, school, and community. www.wested.org/wp-content/files_mf/1373568312resource93.pdf 1991.
5. Commission on Social Determinants of Health. Final report of the commission on the social determinants of health. Geneva: World Health Organization; 2002.
6. Cuddy A. Your body language shapes who you are. Ted Talks. 2012 Oct.
7. Dong XQ. Elder abuse: systematic review and implications for practice. J Am Geriatr Soc. 2015;63:1214–38.
8. Dong XQ, et al. Elder self neglect and hospitalization: findings from the Chicago health and aging project. Am Geriatr Soc. 2012;60(2):201–9.
9. Dong, XQ, et al. Elder abuse and mortality: the role of psychological and social wellbeing. Gerontology. 2011;57 (6):549–58.
10. Dong X. Medical implications of elder abuse and neglect. Clinics in geriatric medicine. 2007;21:293–313.
11. Dong X, Simon M, et al. Elder self-neglect and abuse and mortality risk in a community-dwelling population. JAMA. 2009;302:517–26.
12. Dong X, Simon MA, et al. Decline in cognitive function and risk of elder self neglect: finding from the Chicago Health and Aging Project. J Am Geriatr Soc. 2010;58:2292–9.
13. Dong X, Simon M, et al. Association of cognitive function and risk for elder abuse in a community-dwelling population. Dement Geriatr Cogn Disord. 2011;32:209–15.
14. Dong X, Simon MA. Elder abuse as a risk factor for hospitalization in older persons. JAMA Intern Med. 2013a;173:911–7.
15. Dong X, Simon MA, et al. Prospective study of the elder self neglect and ED use in a community population. Am J Emerg Med. 2012;30:553–61.
16. Dong X, Simon MA. Association between elder self-neglect and hospice utilization in a community population. Arch Gerontol Geriatr. 2013b;56:192–8.
17. Dow Pittaway E. Collaboration and inclusion leading to a prevalence study of abuse. In: Paper presented at linking ontario to the broader elder abuse community. Toronto, Canada. 3 March 1998.
18. Guildford J. Making the case for social and economic inclusion. Population & public health branch, Atlantic Regional Office, Health Canada, Halifax; 2000.
19. Faith K, Wagner F. Elder abuse: ethical decision-making and communities of practice. Toronto Central CCAC Workshop, Nov 2007.
20. Fattah E. A critical assessment of two paradigms: contrasting restorative and retributive justice models. In: Fattah E., Peters T., editors. Support for crime victims in a comparative perspective. Leuven: Leuven University Press, 1998. p. 99–110.
21. Fine art of balancing protection with self determination. Webinar. National Legal Resource Center, 22 Sep 2015.
22. Fisher BS, Regan SL. The extent and frequency of abuse in the lives of older women and their relationship with health outcomes. Gerontologist. 2006;46:200–9.
23. Health Canada. Population health approach: key determinants of health. Ottawa Charter for Health Promotion; 1994.
24. Health Canada. A Discussion paper towards a common understanding. July 1996.
25. Institute of Medicine. Open session of the educating health professionals to address the social determinants of health: a consensus study. National Academy of Sciences. 15 Sept 2015. p. 38.
26. Lachs MS, et al. The mortality of elder mistreatment. JAMA. 1998;280(5):428–32.
27. Lachs MS, et al. Adult protective service use and nursing home placement. Gerontologist. 2002;42(6):734–9.
28. Law Commission of Canada. Discussion paper: from restorative justice to transformative justice. Ottawa Government Services; 1999.
29. Law Commission of Canada. Transforming relationships through participative justice. Ottawa Government Services; 2003.
30. MacLeod L. Toward healthy-aging communities: a population health approach. Prepare for Division of Aging and Seniors, Population Health Directorate, Health Promotion Branch, Health Canada; 1997
31. Masten AS, Gewirtz AH. Resilience in development: the importance of early childhood. In: Tremblay R.E., Dev Peters R., Boivin M., Barr R.G., editors. Encyclopedia on early childhood development; 2006.
32. McCullough ME. Forgiveness: Who does it and how do they do it?. Current Directions in Psychological Science. Dec 2001; 10(6).
33. McGonigal J. Super Better. Penguin: Random House; 15 Sept 2015.
34. Mears J. It's my life now: older women speak up about violence: understanding the complexities of violence against women. University of Sydney, Feb. 18–22, 2002.
35. Mikkonen J, Raphael D. Social determinants of health: the Canadian facts. Toronto: York University, School of Health Policy and Management; 2010
36. Mixson PM. How adult protective services evolved, and the obstacles to ethical casework. Aging. 1996;367:14–8.

37. Mouton CP, et al. The associations between health and domestic violence in older women: results of a pilot study. J Women's Health Gend Based Med. 1999;8:1173–9.
38. Mouton CP, Rodabough, et al. Psychosocial effects of physical and verbal abuse in postmenopausal women. Ann Fam Med. 2010;8:206–13.
39. Mysyuk Y, Westendorp RGJ, Lindenberg J. Perspectives on the etiology of violence in later life. J Interpers Violence. 2015.
40. Olofsson N, Lindqvist K, et al. Fear of crime and psychological and physical abuse associated with ill health in a Swedish population aged 65–84 years. Public Health. 2012;126:358–64.
41. Podnieks E. Determinants of active aging. In: Paper presented at the second world assembly on aging. Madrid, Spain; April 2002.
42. Podnieks E, Pillemer KN, Phillip J, Shillington T, Frizzel A. National survey on abuse of the elderly in Canada: The Ryerson university. Toronto, Canada; 1990.
43. Podnieks E. Relationship of health determinants of abuse and neglect of older canadians. In: Presented at the 16th world congress on gerontology Adelaide, Australia; 1997.
44. Podnieks E, Baillie F. Education as the key to prevention of elder abuse and neglect. In: McLean M, editor. Abuse and neglect of older Canadians: strategies for change. Toronto: Thompson Educational Publishing; 1995.
45. Podnieks E. Emerging themes from a follow-up study of Canadian victims of elder abuse. J Elder Abuse Neglect. 1992;4(1)2:59–111.
46. Podnieks E, Pillemer K. National survey on abuse of the elderly in Canada. Toronto, Ontario, Canada: Ryerson University; 1990.
47. Reeves H. The Victim Support Perspective In Wright M., Galaway B., editors, Mediation and Criminal Justice: Victims, Offenders and Community. Sage Publications, 44–56.
48. Roach K. Changing punishment at the turn of the century: Restorative justice on the rise. Criminol. 2000; 42(3):250–80.
49. Schofield MJ, et al. Mortality and disability outcomes of self-reported elder abuse: a 12 Year Prospective Investigation. J Am Geriatr Soc. 2013; 61:679–85.
50. Sheykhi MT. Safety and security of older persons in Tehran, Iran: a sociological appraisal of elder abuse. J Aging Hum Dev. 2010 Sep;71(2):139–52.
51. Tangney J. Assessing individual differences in the propensity to forgive. Paper presented at the annual meeting of the American Psychological Association. Boston MA; August 1999.
52. Umbreit M. Victims meet offender: The impact of restorative justice and mediation. Monsey: Criminal Justice Press; 1994.
53. UN Human Development Report. 24 July 2014.
54. Volmert A, Lindland E. You only pray that somebody would step in. Frame Works Institute; 2016.
55. Williams, E. Ethical Challenges of Elder Abuse. Medscape Internal Medicine, LLC; 2006.
56. Wilkinson RG, Marmot MG. Social determinants of health: the solid facts. Health Canada, Healthy Cities; 2002.
57. World Health Organization. Health and aging: a discussion paper. Department of Health Promotion, Non-Communicable Disease Prevention and Surveillance. Geneva, Switzerland; 2001.

Epidemiology of Elder Self-neglect

7

Carmel B. Dyer and Carlos A. Reyes-Ortiz

7.1 Background

While the more sensational cases of physical abuse are described in the public press, self-neglect (SN) among the elderly is the most common allegation reported to Adult Protective Services (APS) nationwide [1]. In fact, SN is three times more common than physical abuse or caregiver neglect [2]. SN occurs in older adults who have deficits in several domains such as social, functional, mental and physical, and who often live in squalor conditions [3]. These individuals are often socially isolated with poor health and unkempt appearance. Their living environments often include overwhelming amounts of garbage (e.g., used food containers, newspapers); numerous animals and insect or rodent infestations, and their homes may be without working utilities [4]. Yet, alarmingly, these persons have a laissez-faire attitude, are often comfortable in their surroundings, and refuse any intervention [5, 6].

A drive through any neighborhood in the US, regardless of socioeconomic status, will reveal homes with obvious evidence of personal and/or domestic squalor. These have been used extensively in the literature as the key characteristics of SN since the early 1960s. These include equivalent terms such as "the aged recluse" [7], "senile breakdown" [8], "lack of cleanliness" [9, 10], "Diogenes syndrome" [5, 11], "social breakdown in the elderly" [12, 13], "squalor syndrome" [14, 15], "gross self-neglect" [16], "hoarding" [17, 18], "collectionism" [19], "animal hoarding" [20], or "Noah syndrome" [21] (Table 7.1).

Although there is slight variation in definition by state, SN is defined by the National Committee for the Prevention of Elder Abuse and the National Adult Protective Services Association as "an adult's inability, due to physical or mental impairment or diminished capacity, to perform essential self-care tasks including (a) obtaining essential food, clothing, shelter, and medical care; (b) obtaining goods and services necessary to maintain physical health, mental health, or general safety; and/or (c) managing one's own financial affairs" [1].

Self-neglecting elders have been defined as persons who exhibit at least one of the following: (1) Persistent inattention to personal hygiene and/or environment; (2) Repeated refusal of some/all indicated services which can reasonably be expected to improve quality of life; and (3) Self-endangerment through the manifestation of unsafe behaviors (e.g., persistent refusal to care a disease) [22] (Table 7.2). Recently, in a cohort study using archived data of APS substantiated cases of elder SN, including 5686 individuals aged 65 and older, four subtypes of elder SN were identified, with approximately 50 % of individuals manifesting physical and medical neglect problems. Other subtypes included environmental neglect (22 %), global neglect (21 %), and financial neglect (9 %) [23]. The global neglect subtype is characterized by individuals presenting with high probabilities of a problem in four domains (physical, medical, environmental, and financial) rather than in a single domain.

Hoarding, also called Diogenes Syndrome, has received more attention in recent years due to reality television shows that highlight both young and old persons. Hoarding is the accumulation of rubbish or syllogomania and is considered an important clinical characteristic of the SN syndrome [4, 5, 17, 18, 24, 25]. Hoarding behavior results in stacks of trash, and other objects which significantly reduce the total living space and present falls risk, and fire and safety risks.

C.B. Dyer (✉) · C.A. Reyes-Ortiz
Internal Medicine, Division of Geriatric and Palliative Medicine, University of Texas Health Science Center at Houston, 6431 Fannin Street, MSB 5.111, Houston, TX 77030, USA
e-mail: carmel.b.dyer@uth.tmc.edu

C.A. Reyes-Ortiz
e-mail: carlos.a.reyesortiz@uth.tmc.edu

C.B. Dyer · C.A. Reyes-Ortiz
Texas Elder Abuse and Mistreatment Institute (TEAM), Houston, USA

C.B. Dyer · C.A. Reyes-Ortiz
Harris Health System, Houston, USA

C.B. Dyer · C.A. Reyes-Ortiz
UTHealth Consortium on Aging, Houston, USA

X. Dong (ed.), *Elder Abuse*, DOI 10.1007/978-3-319-47504-2_7

Table 7.1 Summary of terms used for the self-neglecting elderly

• The aged recluse
• Senile breakdown
• Lack of cleanliness
• Diogenes syndrome
• Social breakdown of the elderly
• Squalor syndrome
• Gross self-neglect
• Hoarding
• Collectionism
• Animal hoarding
• Noah syndrome

Table 7.2 Key characteristics for self-neglect

• Neglected personal hygiene or self-care
• Environmental neglect or domestic squalor
• Financial neglect
• Unsafe behaviors
• Refusal of care or help

Hoarding becomes more severe when it extends beyond simple clutter or collecting and interferes with daily tasks such as cleaning, cooking, sleeping, and socialization [6, 26].

In order to characterize the severity of SN, three domains of indicators have been identified: (1) Personal hygiene (e.g., dirty hair and clothing, poor condition of nails and skin); (2) Impaired function (e.g., decline in cognitive function and activities of daily living); and (3) Environment neglect (e.g., evidence of subject's inability to clean the house and yard, and manage material goods acquired over the years) [27]. This Self-neglect Severity Scale developed by Houston researchers is scored from 0 to 4, with 0 meaning "no problem" to 4 meaning "among the worst," or dichotomously as 0 or 4, plus N/A for not applicable; examples of variables items and domains are provided in Fig. 7.1 [27]. The scale has been used for research. The scale is completed through observation and could easily be used in clinical settings after minimal training.

American society is characterized by a strong affinity for self-determination. Some social scientists have questioned whether or not SN is a choice made by elders who are fiercely independent. Most experts feel that SN occurs in those who lack mental capacity and is not a choice. Confusion occurs because lack of mental capacity can be due to

Domain	Sub-domain	Items related
Personal hygiene		Hair Nails Skin Clothing Insect infestation
Functioning		Clock score Evidence of delusional state Response to emergency Untreated conditions Time since last MD visit
Environment	Condition of exterior	Yard Roof Windows Walls
	Interior Cleanliness Clutter Structure	Odor Kitchen Bathroom Bedroom Living room
	Condition of pets Utilities	

Fig. 7.1 Self-neglect severity scale

memory impairment alone, executive dysfunction alone, or both. Purists believe that SN can only exist in the setting of diminished capacity. Choices, even poor choices, are the prerogative of autonomous adults with full mental capacity.

The development of executive dysfunction, a condition in which an individual is unable to translate simple tasks into complex, goal-directed behaviors such as cooking, dressing oneself, and performing basic housework, has been proposed as an important etiologic factor of elder SN [28, 29]. Related to this, some cases of severe domestic squalor or SN have been found to have frontal lobe dysfunction or frontal lobe dementia [25, 30]. However, others may have Alzheimer's disease, other types of dementia, mental illness, and alcohol or drug abuse [31]. Recently, a cross-sectional study, including 50 adults aged 65 and older were recruited from APS with confirmed SN, was found that those individuals had impairments consistent with executive dysfunction: "concept generation," "planning," "inhibition," and "spatial working memory" [32].

7.1.1 Methods for the Epidemiology of the Elder Self-neglect

A systematic review approach was used to provide research references for this chapter. The solution paradigm is described in Fig. 7.2. The global literature in PubMed, MEDLINE, PsycINFO, BIOSIS, Science Direct and Cochrane Central was searched. Search terms included elder SN, prevalence, incidence, risk factors, and outcomes. Review and case studies were identified and their reference lists examined for relevant research articles. Studies existing only as abstracts, qualitative studies or focused on age <60 years old, non-English publications, without a clear definition of SN or non-representative (e.g., elder abuse but not SN) were excluded. We wanted to show the heterogeneity of SN definitions and epidemiology on the major continents: North America, South America, Europe, Asia, and Africa. Due to the limited number of studies around the world, no distinction was made by the type of analysis used (e.g., bivariate vs. multivariate) or restriction on data reported.

7.2 Prevalence and Incidence of the Elder Self-neglect

Results of estimate research on the prevalence and incidence of SN of older adults are difficult to compare due to the lack of uniformity in the definition of it and different methods of assessment. The systematic selection of the main studies included in Table 7.3 is depicted in Fig. 7.2. The selected studies characteristics for prevalence and incidence for elder SN are described in Table 7.3 [8, 33–43]. Not like elder abuse where there is a plenty number of studies, there is a limited number of studies around the world on the epidemiology of SN. According to the search most of the studies are located in the US (North America). The prevalence has a broad range since it is related to different populations such as (1) at study population level (in general or stratified by subgroups or characteristics); (2) among cases of SN reported to APS or similar agencies; and (3) in particular populations (e.g., hospitalized elders, living alone elders). In addition, the prevalence could be not compared across the globe since different definitions or study designs

Fig. 7.2 Flowchart describing review process for identification of eligible studies. *Note* additional studies were described into the manuscript text

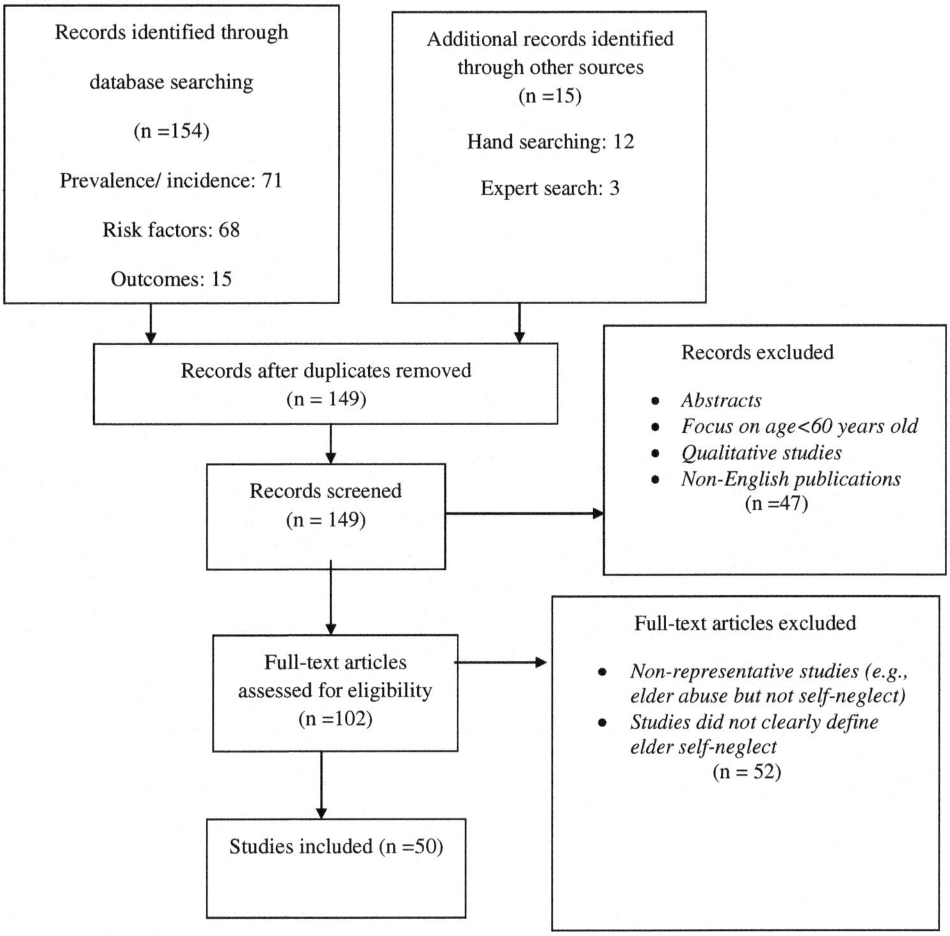

Table 7.3 Prevalence and incidence estimates of elder self-neglect by population, survey methods, and definitions

Author, year	Population	Age, sex	Methods and design	SN Measure	Prevalence or incidence of SN	Comments
North/South America						
Dong and Simon [33]	3159 Chinese elderly in Chicago, 2011–2013	60 and older; 58.9 % women	Cohort	The Chicago elder self-neglect scale—27 items	Moderate-severe-SN 19.6 % for poor health status; 8.6 % for fair, and 9.7 % for good–very good[a]	Prevalence at population level
Dong [34]	3159 Chinese elderly in Chicago, 2011–2013	60 and older; 58.9 % women	Cohort	The Chicago elder self-neglect scale—27 items	Prevalence of SN was 18.2 % for mild SN and 10.9 % for moderate to severe SN. Prevalence of SN according to quality of life measure were 33.8 % for poor/fair, 22.6 % for good, and 16.7 % for very good[a]	Prevalence at population level
Dong et al. [35]	4627 elders Chicago Health and Aging project, 2007–2010	65 and older; 64.4 % women	Cohort	The Chicago elder self-neglect scale	SN: Black men 13.2 %, black women 10.9 %; white men 2.4 %, white women 2.6 %. Among those with < high school education: 14.7 % in men and 10.9 % in women; among those with annual income <$15000: 21.7 % in men, and 15.3 % in women	Prevalence at population level
Dong et al. [36]	4627 elders Chicago Health and Aging project, 2007–2010	65 and older; 64.4 % women	Cohort	The Chicago elder self-neglect scale	SN: For men: 4.7 % for very good/excellent health, 7.9 % in good health, 14.9 % in fair/poor health; for women: 4.5 % for very good/excellent health, 7.9 % in good health, 10.6 % in fair/poor health. Those with ≥3 Katz impairments: 12.8 % in men and 13.8 % in women. For those with MMSE ≤20, 18.8 % in men and 13.6 % in women	Prevalence at population level
Thomson et al. [31]	3384 cases of elder abuse, 2006–2009	60 and older	Cross-sectional analysis	Milwaukee County Department of Aging definition	Prevalence of SN was 26 %	Prevalence among records for cases of elder abuse
Moon et al. [37]	575 veterans, 3-year period	65 and older	Retrospective medical records review	O'Brien et al. (1999) definition	Prevalence of SN was 2.1 %	Prevalence among outpatient elders
Abrams et al. [38]	2812 elders, 9 years follow-up	65 and older, 65.4 % women	Cohort	SN defined by state's ombudsman	Incidence of SN was 7 per 1000 person-years	Incidence at population level
Otiniano and Herrera [39]	16,677 Hispanic elders	65 and older	Analysis of APS records	APS SN definition	63.2 % of abuse cases were SN	Prevalence among records for cases of elder abuse
Lachs et al. [40]	2812 older adults, 11-year follow-up	65 and older	Cohort	APS SN definition	Prevalence of SN was 73 % of APS use	Prevalence among those referred to the Ombudsman

(continued)

Table 7.3 (continued)

Author, year	Population	Age, sex	Methods and design	SN Measure	Prevalence or incidence of SN	Comments
Europe						
Luzny and Jurickova [41]	203 in hospitalized in mental ward and 103 in medical ward	65 and older	Cross-sectional, convenience sample	Mosqueda and Dong (2011) definition	Prevalence of SN was 41.7 % in the mentally ill; 33.3 % in the somatically ill	Prevalence among hospitalized patients
Macmillan and Shaw [8]	72 SN cases collected	60 and older	Prospective, referral cases during 3 years	Personal and environmental uncleanliness criteria	Incidence of SN was 0.5 per 1000 persons aged 60 and older	Incidence at the general population
Asia-Australia						
Lee and Kim [42]	1023 older adults, South Korea, in 2012	65 and older who live alone, 82.8 % women	Stratified random sampling	SN was measured by a subscale of the screening scale for elder abuse (SSEA) (Kim et al. 2006)	Prevalence of SN was 22.8 %	Prevalence among those who live alone
Snowdon and Halliday [43]	173 cases referred to an old age psychiatry service	65 and older, 35.8 % women	Cases of domestic squalor referred to psychiatry service in Central Sydney	Living conditions rating scale (LCRS) (Samios 1996)	Prevalence was 1 per 1000 elderly people (1.35 per 1000 males, 0.63 per 1000 females) in the catchment area- Central Sydney, Australia	Incidence of referrals at the general population

Note SN Self-neglect; *APS* Adult protective services
[a]Prevalence calculated as at least one form of elder SN

make difficult a reliable comparison. The estimation of incidence based in prevalence is not possible for now until more uniformity in prevalence is reached across diverse populations. Based on few studies, the incidence of SN tends to be low, between 0.5 and 7 per 1000 elders per year.

7.3 Risk Factors for Elder Self-neglect

Due to the lack of uniformity in the definition of it and different methods of assessment, the data on risk factors have a lot of variation. Despite of those limitations, data show common risk factors across different studies. The systematic selection of the main studies included in Table 7.4 is depicted in Fig. 7.2. A summary of the main selected studies characteristics for risk factors for elder SN is described in Table 7.4 [11, 24, 29, 31, 33, 37, 38, 44–60]. Studies also report that extreme SN occurs along an age continuum. SN cases include younger adults but in the early studies, the average age for severe SN was over 75 years [8, 11, 62]. Recent studies showed also that age is an increased risk for developing SN [23, 45, 46, 61–63]. In a cross-sectional study among 201 community persons aged 60 and older living in the state of Selangor in Malaysia, the percentage of SN increased by age (60–74 years = 30.9 %; 75–79 years = 40.9 %, 80–90 years = 66.7 %) [59].

Socioeconomic status has variation in its association with elder SN. Severe SN was found by authors of the early literature to exist only within the wealthy or among professionals [8, 11]. In the Chicago Health and Aging Project (CHAP) study, in multivariate analyses, lower income was associated with increased risk for SN [46]. Further evidence showed that severe SN is seen in persons from every education level and economic class [59, 64].

Gender is not a consistent risk factor for SN. Some researchers have shown that men are at higher risk for SN than women [38]. However, others found that women were at higher risk than men [46].

The majority of affected SN elders lived alone in their own home or apartment [8, 11, 31, 61]. Interestingly, some case reports describe a condition called 'Diogenes a deux' or Diogenes by Proxy in which two or more persons living

Table 7.4 Risk factors for elder self-neglect by population, survey methods, and definitions

Author, year	Population	Age, sex	Methods and design	SN measure	Risk/associated factors
North/South America					
Dong and Simon [33]	3159 Chinese elderly in Chicago	60 and older; 58.9 % women	Cohort	The Chicago elder self-neglect scale—27 items	Poor health status, lower physical function, lower cognitive function, more depressive symptoms
Thomson et al. [31]	3384 cases of elder abuse, 875 SN cases, 2006–2009	60 and older	Cross-sectional analysis	Milwaukee County Department of Aging definition	65 % Frail (vs. 71 % among those abused by perpetrator), 20 % dementia (vs. 26 % among those abused by perpetrator)
Ernst and Smith [44]	210 SN older adults	65 and older, 53.8 % women	Retrospective record-based study	Code of Maryland regulations 2011 SN definition	Nutritional deficiency, frailty, arthritis, incontinence
Dong et al. [45]	9056 elders Chicago Health and Aging project, 1812 cases of SN	65 and older; 66.8 % of SN were women	Cohort	The Chicago elder self-neglect scale	Elder SN was associated with age, female gender, African American ethnicity, lower education/income, lower levels of cognitive and physical function, nutritional status, psychosocial f\unction and higher number of medical comorbidities
Dong et al. [46]	5519 elders Chicago Health and Aging project, 1017 cases of SN	65 and older; 67 % women	Cohort	The Chicago elder self-neglect scale	Decline in executive function and global cognitive function were associated with increased risk for elder SN
Dong et al. [47]	5570 elders Chicago Health and Aging project, 1068 cases of SN	65 and older; 67 % women	Cohort	The Chicago elder self-neglect scale	Physical performance decline (Katz and Rosow-Breslau scales) was associated with increased risk for elder SN
Franzini and Dyer [48]	131 cases, 131 controls	65 and older, 69.5 % women	Case–control	APS SN definition	Higher % of mental disorders
Spensley [49]	704 APS SN cases	65 and older; 55.4 % women	Secondary data analysis of chart review, APS SN cases	Recidivism risk of SN	Less recidivism with Cognitive deficits [OR 0.62 p = 0.017]; more recidivism with substance/alcohol abuse [OR 1.66 p = 0.033]
Naik et al. [50]	100 cases, 100 controls	65 and older, women 66 %	Cross-sectional	APS SN definition	IADLs functional impairment (Kohlman evaluation of living skills scale) was associated with elder SN
Dyer et al. [29]	500 cases of SN elderly	65 and older, 70 % women	Cross-sectional chart review	APS SN definition	50 % had abnormal MMSE; 15 % abnormal geriatric depression scores; 95 % had moderate to poor social support; 76 % had abnormal physical performance scores
Tierney et al. [51]	139 cognitively impaired seniors who live alone	65 and older	Inception cohort, 18 months follow-up	APS SN definition	Incident harm as result of SN was associated with memory recognition, executive function, conceptualization
Aung et al. [52]	44 SN cases	65 and older, 75 % women	Secondary data analysis of APS SN cases	APS SN definition	Vitamin D deficiency was detected in 36 % of SN cases; SN cases with vitamin D deficiency had lower scores in the Physical Performance Test and higher scores in the Kohlman Evaluation of Living Skills

(continued)

Table 7.4 (continued)

Author, year	Population	Age, sex	Methods and design	SN measure	Risk/associated factors
Burnett et al. [53]	91 SN cases, 91 controls	65 and older, 67 % women	Case–control	APS SN definition	Higher depression score ($p = 0.001$); decreased social resources (family, friends, religious affiliation- all $p < 0.05$)
Burnett et al. [54]	50 SN cases, 50 controls	65 and older, 64 % women	Case–control	APS SN definition	Higher depression scores ($p = 0.019$); untreated medical conditions (among depressed—OR 4.84 95 % CI 1.37–17.09)
Moon et al. [37]	575 veterans	65 and older	Retrospective medical records review	SN O'Brien et al. (1999) definition	Depression, dementia
Pickens [55]	80 SN cases, 80 controls	65 and older, 66.2 % women	Case–control	APS SN definition	Higher levels of pain ($p = 0.014$)
Smith et al. [56]	40 SN cases, 40 controls	65 and older	Case–control	APS SN definition	Greater homocysteine, lower folate, lower b-carotene and alpha-tocopherol, lower vitamin D (all $p < 0.05$)
Tierney et al. [57]	139 cognitively impaired seniors who live alone	65 and older	Inception cohort, 18 months follow-up	APS SN definition	Incident harm as result of SN was associated with perception fewer social resources, poor MMSE, COPD, cerebrovascular disease
Abrams et al. [38]	2812 elders, 9 years follow-up	65 and older, 65.4 % women	Cohort	SN corroborated by State's Ombudsman	Age, poverty, living alone, separated/divorced or widowed, stroke, hip fracture, diabetes, cognitive impairment (≥4 errors in Pfeifer), depression (CESD ≥16)
Dyer et al. [58]	45 cases (37 were SN), 97 controls	65 and older	Case–control	APS SN definition	Depression was present in 62 % and dementia in 51 % of SN elders
Europe					
Halliday et al. [24]	81 community dwelling elders	40 subjects were 65 and older	Cross-sectional	Living conditions rating scale [measuring domestic squalor and SN]	Mental disordered 70 %; physical health problem 26 %
Clark et al. [11]	30 hospitalized elders	66 and older, 53 % women	Cases—hospitalized	Domestic squalor, extreme personal SN	Living alone; wealthier; high IQ, deficiencies (iron, folate, vitamin B12, vitamin C, calcium, vitamin D, albumin)
Asia-Australia					
Lee and Kim [42]	1023 older adults, South Korea, in 2012	65 and older who live alone, 82.8 % women	Stratified random sampling	SN was measured by a subscale of the Screening Scale for Elder Abuse (SSEA) (Kim et al. 2006)	Higher education, higher cognitive abilities, more children, lower number of medical conditions
Mardan et al. [59]	201 older adults, Malaysia	60 and older	Cross-sectional survey design with cluster sampling	New SN scale with 16 items	Older age, primary education, and lower self-care skills score were associated with SN
Snowdon [60]	83 subjects living in unclean conditions	68 subjects were 60 and older	Survey sent to community health centers	Uncleanliness was considered equivalent to SN	64 % had memory impairment, 40 % had history of heavy drinkers

Note SN Self-neglect; *APS* Adult protective services
[a]Prevalence calculated as at least one form of elder SN

together displayed signs of extreme SN [65, 66]; while cases were also reported for elders living in their own home with others [31, 67]. For example, more than 96 % of SN cases in Milwaukee County occurred in an elder's place of residence, and 29.9 % were living in their own home with others [31].

Psychological maladaptation as a risk factor for SN has not been well established. Most data are based on case reports and show that SN may be associated with premorbid personality traits (with poor interpersonal relationships; being aloof, detached, suspicious, quarrelsome, unfriendly) [11, 24, 61, 68], behaviors (reclusive, hoarding), or disorders (obsessive–compulsive, paranoid, schizoid, delusional disorders, substance abuse) [5, 11, 12, 24, 25]. In one population-based study, personality traits (neuroticism, extraversion, information processing, and rigidity) were significantly associated with increased risk of elder SN; however, after adjusting for confounding factors, the associations were no longer significant [69]. On the other hand, hoarding has been linked to obsessive–compulsive disorder [6, 26, 70, 71]. Hoarding occurred in up to 72 % of the severe SN cases in these studies [6, 25]. One study of PET scanning supported this observation [70].

Mental disorders are commonly described in elders with severe SN. These include schizophrenia, dementia, alcohol abuse, and psychosis with dementia being the most common [3, 8, 11, 25, 58, 64]. In a community study of people living in squalor was found that 70 % of the individuals were classified as having a mental disorder. Identifiable psychiatric illnesses are more common among younger individuals who manifest SN [10, 24, 64].

A summary of main risk factors and disorders associated with elder SN are listed in Table 7.5.

Functional impairment has been associated with elder SN. Some studies described physical disability in 17–44 % of subjects [8, 61]. In a study including elderly SN victims in Milwaukee County, 64.8 % of them tended to be described as frail [31]. In the CHAP study, declines in physical performance, in Katz index, or in Rosow-Breslau mobility index were associated with increased risk of reported elder SN [47]. In the Consortium for Research in Elder SN of Texas study, elder SN was associated with impairments in instrumental activities of daily living [50].

Individuals with severe SN were often described as having sensory impairment along with other medical conditions [8, 11, 61]. MacMillan and Shaw [8] reported sensory impairment in approximately one-half of the subjects in their case series.

Multi-morbidity including cognitive impairment, depression, delirium, medical illness (stroke, hip fracture), functional and social dependence, stressful events (e.g., bereavement), history of social isolation, and alcohol and substance abuse is seen in self-neglecting elders [29, 38, 50, 68, 72]. For example, in a cohort study, the New Haven Established Population for Epidemiologic Studies in the Elderly (EPESE), cognitive impairment (odds ratio = OR 4.63, 95 % confidence interval = CI 2.32–9.23), and clinically significant depressive symptoms (OR 2.38, 95 % CI 1.26–4.48) were independent predictors of SN after 9 years of follow-up [38]. In a longitudinal follow-up in the CHAP study (1993–2005), decline in executive function was associated with increased risk of reported and confirmed elder SN. Also, decline in global cognitive function was associated with increased risk of greater SN severity [46].

A summary of health outcomes associated with SN is listed in Table 7.7. SN, like other geriatric syndromes, is associated with significant comorbidity. These include hypertension, dementia, diabetes mellitus, arthritis, stroke, depression, urinary incontinence, or delirium [3, 29].

Table 7.5 Summarized risk factors and associated disorders for self-neglect

• Older age
• Isolation
• Lack of social support
• Poverty
• Personality disorders
• Hoarding
• Mental disorders: dementia, depression, substance abuse
• Physical illness: stroke, diabetes, nutritional deficiency
• Functional impairment

7.4 Health Outcomes Associated with Elder Self-neglect

The systematic selection of the main studies included in Table 7.6 is depicted in Fig. 7.2. A summary of the selected studies characteristics for health outcomes associated with elder SN is described in Table 7.6 [72–82].

SN is an independent risk factor for death. Indeed, in the New Haven EPESE, SN elders had increased risk of 3-year all-cause mortality (OR 1.7; 95 % CI 1.2–2.5), when compared with other members of the cohort [72]. Also, in the CHAP study, self-neglecting elders had an increased risk of 1-year mortality (hazard ratio = HR 5.82; 95 % CI 5.20–6.51) which remained significant over the entire 9-year follow-up period, but was greatly reduced starting in year 2 (HR 1.88; 95 % CI 1.67–2.14) [80].

Probably, due to the severity of SN and accompanied comorbidity or health complications, self-neglecters may have increased health services use. These include increased risk for nursing home placement (HR 5.23; 95 % CI 4.07–6.72) [81], hospice utilization (HR 2.34, 95 % CI 2.10–2.81)

Table 7.6 Outcomes for elder self-neglect by population, survey methods, and definitions

Author, year	Population	Age, sex	Methods and design	Measure of SN	Outcomes for SN
North/South America					
Dong and Simon [73]	7219 elders Chicago Health and Aging project, 1228 reported for SN	65 and older; 56.6 % women	Cohort	The Chicago elder self-neglect scale (score ≥1)	Increased 30-day hospital readmission (HR 2.50, 95 % CI 2.02–3.10). Greater SN severity was associated with increased rates of 30-day hospital readmission
Charles et al. [74]	224 cognitively impaired seniors who live alone	65 and older, 84.8 % women	12 month period follow-up	APS SN definition	Incident harm due to SN, 10.3 % by GDS ≥10 h 3.54 (95 % CI 1.34–9.40; $p = 0.01$) and s-rated fair/poor health HR 3.36 (95 % CI 1.30–8.67; $p = 0.01$)
Dong and Simon [75]	8669 elders Chicago Health and Aging project, 1438 reported for SN	65 and older; 65.5 % of SN were women	Cohort	The Chicago elder self-neglect scale (score ≥1)	Increased hospice utilization (HR 2.34, 95 % CI 2.10–2.81). Greater SN severity was associated with increased risk for hospice utilization
Dong and Simon [76]	10,333 elders Chicago Health and Aging project, 1460 reported for SN, 180 for elder abuse	65 and older	Cohort	The Chicago elder self-neglect scale (score ≥1)	Elder SN was associated with increased risk for subsequent elder abuse (HR 1.75, 95 % CI 1.18–2.59). It was also associated with increased risk for caregiver neglect, financial exploitation, and multiple forms of elder abuse
Dong et al. [77]	6864 elders Chicago Health and Aging project, 1165 reported for SN	65 and older; 65.7 % women	Cohort	The Chicago elder self-neglect scale (score ≥1)	Hospital utilization (rate ratio = RR 1.47, 95 % CI 1.39–1.55). Greater SN severity was associated with increased annual rates of hospital use
Dong and Simon [78]	6864 elders Chicago Health and Aging project, 1165 reported for SN	65 and older; 65.7 % women	Cohort	The Chicago elder self-neglect scale (score ≥1)	Increased emergency department utilization (RR 1.42, 95 % CI 1.29–1.58). Greater SN severity was associated with increased ED use
Turner et al. [79]	100 SN elders	65 and older	Cross-sectional	APS SN definition	90 % of elder self-neglecters were non-adherent to at least one medication
Dong et al. [80]	9318 elders, 1993–2005	65 and older	Prospective cohort	The Chicago elder self-neglect scale	SN elders had an increased risk of 1-year mortality (hazard ratio = HR 5.82; 95 % CI 5.20–6.51), confirmed SN have HR 5.76, 95 % CI 5.11–6.49). Severe SN had greater mortality than moderate or mild SN
Tierney et al. [51]	139 cognitively impaired seniors who live alone	65 and older	Inception cohort, 18 months follow-up	APS SN definition	Incident harm as result of SN, 20.6 %
Tierney et al. [57]	139 cognitively impaired seniors who live alone	65 and older	Inception cohort, 18 months follow-up	APS SN definition	Incident harm as result of SN, 21.6 %
Lachs et al. [81]	2812 older adults, 9-year follow-up	65 and older	Prospective cohort	APS SN definition	Self-neglect elders had increased risk for nursing home placement (HR 5.23; 95 % CI 4.07–6.72)
Lachs et al. [72]	2812 older adults, 9-year follow-up	65 and older	Prospective cohort	APS SN definition	self-neglect elders had increased risk of 3-year all-cause mortality (OR 1.7; 95 % CI 1.2–2.5), when compared with other members of the cohort
Europe					
Cotton et al. [82]	358 cases of psychiatric initial crisis	65 and older, 49 % women	Cohort recruited over 9-month period	SN definition as part of threshold assessment grid for severity of mental illness	SN at risk of psychiatric hospital admission (within 8 weeks of initial crisis) OR 2.93 1.42–6.05
Asia-Australia					

Note SN Self-neglect; *APS* Adult protective services
[a]Prevalence calculated as at least one form of elder SN

[75], hospital utilization (rate ratio = RR 1.47, 95 % CI 1.39–1.55) [77], and emergency department utilization (RR 1.42, 95 % CI 1.29–1.58) [78]. However, once self-neglecters are brought into the healthcare system, they are no more expensive than other similar patients [48]. In a recent report of the CHAP study, elder SN was associated with increased risk for 30-day hospital readmission (HR 2.50, 95 % CI 2.02–3.10) [73].

Interestingly, interventions that include acute hospitalization of patients who SN often resulted in worse outcomes compared with patients treated in the outpatient setting for the same conditions [8, 11, 61]. This was described by MacMillan and Shaw in the 1960s, where hoarders that were admitted had a higher monthly rate than those left in their environments [8].

In addition, non-adherence to medical treatment has been studied in the elder SN population. Turner et al. [79] reported that 90 % of 100 elder self-neglecters were non-adherent to at least one medication and the majorities were non-adherent on approximately four medications. Non-adherence was associated with the number of prescribed medications as well as lower objective physical function. A summary of main outcomes associated with elder SN is listed in Table 7.7.

As a consequence of living in squalor conditions, self-neglecting elders may have altered nutritional status. These include multiple nutritional deficiencies such as iron, folate, vitamin B12, vitamin C, β-carotene, α-tocopherol, serum proteins/albumin, calcium, and vitamin D [11, 56].

Table 7.7 Summary of health outcomes associated with elder self-neglect

• Higher mortality
• Functional decline
• Poor nutritional status
• Non-compliance of medical treatment
• Increased hospitalization
• Increased hospital readmission
• Higher number of emergency room visits
• Increased hospice utilization
• Increased nursing home placement

7.5 The Need for a Self-neglect Model

Dyer et al. [29] developed a biopsychosocial path model proposing causal links between health conditions and the development of elder SN. The TEAM model depicted in Fig. 7.3 illustrates the path from certain illnesses to SN within specific social contexts [29]. This model proposes elders who are those with medical syndromes or diagnoses leading to executive dysfunction and resulting in impairment of activities of daily living. The syndromes or diagnoses included in the top box may be due to a variety of reasons including poor self-management skills, limited or fragmented health care, reduce resources, psychiatric illnesses, delusional disorders, and substance abuse [6, 22, 83]. These individuals lack the needed support services and fail to

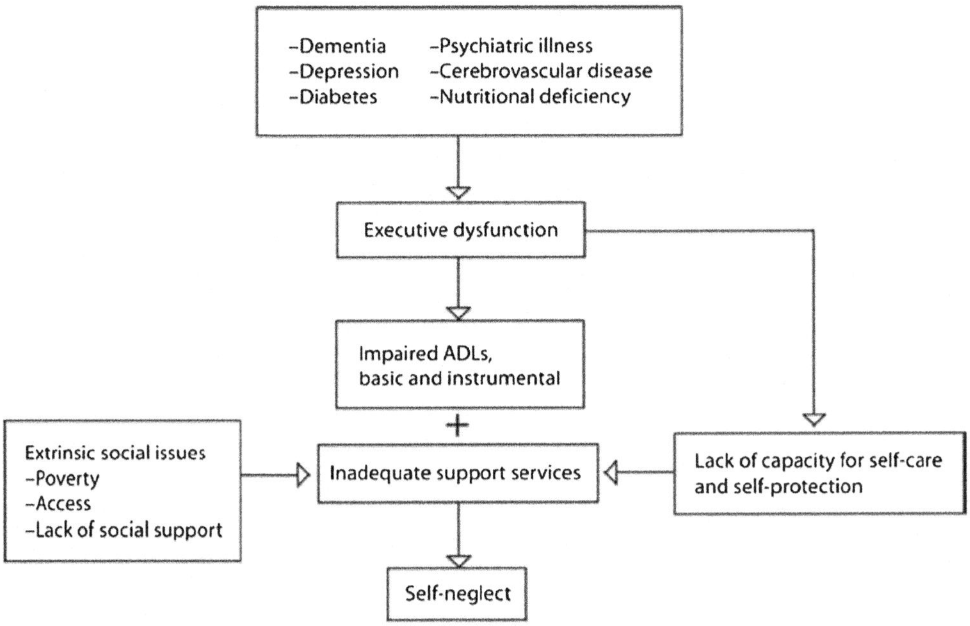

Fig. 7.3 Model of self-neglect among the elderly. ADLs, activities of daily living. (From Dyer CB, Goodwin JS, Vogel M, et al. Characterizing self-neglect: a report of over 500 cases of self-neglect seen by a geriatric medicine team. Am J Public Health 2007;97:1675; with permission.)

recognize the danger of their health or living conditions. These older persons lose the cognitive capacity for self-protection. However, there are social issues beyond access to support such as lack of family, lack of transportation, social isolation, homeless, and insufficient funds that likely also impact SN [6, 22, 24, 83].

For example, a qualitative study, among 60 cases of suicidal attempts and ideations among elderly people from 13 Brazilian municipalities, showed that SN is reduced when there is family support, care, and bonds of unit [84]. In a study involving a shelter-based convalescence care facility in Amsterdam, a cohort of homeless adults was followed for about 7 years. Over the years, significantly more SN persons were admitted to the center [85]. In the CHAP study, lower levels of social network (OR 1.02, 95 % CI 1.01–1.04) and social engagements (OR 1.15, 95 % CI 1.09–1.22) were associated with increased risk of elder SN [45]. Multiple subsequent studies have supported this model [45–47, 50, 86–90] which can serve as springboard for intervention and prevention studies. Other models, for example, the sociological and psychological theories of SN, suggest that SN is the failure to maintain a socially acceptable standard of personal and household hygiene and/or the failure to adequately care for one's own health [91]. Spensley has proposed a model for recidivism of SN cases including (1) social isolation, (2) mental illness, (3) cognitive deficits, and (4) substance/alcohol abuse. In her research, she has been demonstrated that only substance and alcohol abuse was significantly associated with recidivism of SN [49].

7.5.1 Discussion

First described in medical literature in NYC in the 1960s, SN is a complex construct with social, medical, psychological, and legal dimensions. SN has likely always existed, as long as disease and/or aging have resulted in the inability to perform basic activities of daily living.

The construct of SN is muddled amidst hoarding, mental illness, and degenerative mental and physical disease. There is much debate about whether SN is primarily a social issue versus psychological versus medical. But like so many geriatric syndromes, SN is multidimensional. There is much debate about whether social, psychological, or medical issues are risk factors, associated factors or etiologies. Regardless of the complexity, researchers in nursing, social work and medicine have struggled to characterize a study SN. While social scientists and nursing researchers embraced this field of study, medicine was a bit late to recognize this field of study, but over the last 10–15 years there has been much more interest.

SN has suffered as a subject of study because medical researchers believe strongly that it is not elder abuse. Simply put elder abuse requires a perpetrator and there is a victim; these features garner the attentions of legislators, law enforcement, prosecutors, and funders. SN is considered "victim-less," simply a social problem, or even worse, individual choice. Research has shown that many self-neglectors and abused victims suffer from the same disorders of aging such as dementia depression. More research has been done to show the interrelations and that SN is a risk factor for abuse. And is the same way that the CDC and other public health organizations measure homicide and suicide, so too is SN worthy of attention by researchers, clinicians, the legal system, and government policy makers.

In the mid 1990s Dr. Mark Lacks, in a landmark study, demonstrated that elder abuse was an independent risk factor for death, also showed the same for SN. Many epidemiologic studies showed that SN is the most common report made to APS despite the fact that not all states require reporting of SN. Thus the interest of medical researchers in SN was sparked.

Following that study, in 2000, Dyer and members of the Texas Elder Abuse and Mistreatment Institute (TEAM) showed a relationship between dementia and depression with SN. Subsequent studies by others supported these associated disorders and SN. TEAM researchers continued to characterize key elements of SN. In 2004, the TEAM Institute was awarded a grant as part of the NIH Roadmap initiative for a retrospective cohort study of elder self-neglectors and controls. This study was conducted by a subsidiary of TEAM called CREST—Consortium for Research in Elder Self-neglect of Texas. Multiple analyses resulted.

The CREST team showed relationships between SN and nutritional deficiencies, dementia, depression, and executive dysfunction. They characterized phenotypes, developed the Self-neglect Severity Scale, and demonstrated a high prevalence of non-adherence and studied health care utilization. As a part of the CREST studies, a national conference or Elder SN, funded by the NIA-NCRR, was held in Houston with experts from the fields of protective service, nursing, epidemiology, social worker, and multiple medical disciplines. At the time several issues were raised and challenges put forth, these included

1. The need for further evaluations of executive function and SN.
2. Was SN associated with other forms of abuse?
3. The need for more rigorous screening tools.
4. Health care utilization and other economic analyses.
5. The need for longitudinal studies to better study outcomes.

Following these events Dong and colleagues embarked on a very deliberate prospective, population-based cohort study. They conducted database analyses of residents living in Chicago neighborhoods. These were seniors who had been followed in the CHAP. The strengths of these studies were that they were prospective, population-based, and longitudinal. Criterion for elder SN was a report to social services agencies. These studies provided further evidence for several epidemiologic aspects of SN including the relationship between elder SN and executive dysfunction, depression, dementia, other forms of elder abuse, and failure to perform activities of daily living. They have also done a great deal of work in ethnically diverse populations, especially Chinese-Americans.

Perhaps, the greatest contributions to the literature from this group have been in the realms of mortality and health care utilization. Dong et al. study on the mortality of SN was stunning. One-year mortality for CHAP participants with confirmed SN was significantly associated with increased risk of mortality. The risk for death remains high after one year as well. This risk increased with increasing severity before and after one year. They also looked at hospice utilization and self-neglector had shorter lengths of stay in hospice care and there was a shorter time from hospice admission to death. These studies underscored the urgency and secured the place of elder SN as a highly priority public health problem for seniors.

Further fascinating data addressed health care utilization. Hospitals and health care entities must look at these issues more closely with each and every year as payment reforms hinge around these metrics. Dong et al. found that elder SN was associated with increased rates of 30-day hospital readmissions, irrespective of associated medical conditions. In fact the higher the severity of SN, the more likely was readmission.

7.5.2 Future Directions in Research

Despite the challenges, the future for work in self-neglectors is brighter; now an accepted topic at national scientific meetings, with funding support increasing, and receiving more attention by clinicians. There are a few frontiers to be traversed.

The first of these frontiers is definitions and case identification. These include (1) Different definitions across the world; although in the US, we have tried to do an effort to standardize the usual APS definition. Changing this may help to get a more comparable data across several populations. (2) Different methods of referral of cases or sources for referral that may affect the detection of cases across the world (most of them no mandatory reporters). Modifying this may help to find the real number of cases into communities since many times elder SN is underreported. (3) Few data on SN subtypes (e.g., physical, medical, environmental, and financial) or phenotypes (e.g., personal hygiene, lack of health maintenance, and environmental neglect) that may help to focus potential efforts on prevention or management of cases.

Another frontier is the dearth of intervention trials. While Adult Protective Service agencies have been interceding for their self-neglecting clients for years, there has been limited scientific research. Dyer et al. (1R21AG033261-01A1—Feasibility of Vitamin D Replacement in Self-Neglecting Elders) performed the first medical intervention clinical trial. Funded by the NIA, this feasibility study demonstrated that with in-home interventions, vitamin D levels can be successfully raised in self-neglectors. The best methods for intervening in self-neglecting elders are yet unknown. Currently, research through house calls is expensive, and require quite a bit of time. Would phone calls or telehealth approaches be useful? Could community health workers be useful in implementing interventions or even in research? The methodology for social versus medical intervention will likely differ. These interventions will need to include economic analyses. While it is important to understand the economic benefit of SN interventions is important, the actual costs of the SN syndrome on the community and state is much less the human toll. Comparative effectiveness research on the various state interventions has the potential to provide useful data.

While a great deal of work has been done in the area of capacity assessment, there is still a need for a streamlined screening that is feasible for use in the field by APS and other community social service agencies, as well as hospitalists, emergency medicine physicians, and police officers. Any capacity tool must be coupled with common sense approach to interpret the range of human behavior, yet apply a reasonable person standard. This is necessary to be certain that we do not abandon a vulnerable elder and intervene before a crisis occurs.

Another frontier that is being explored is GIS mapping. Kao and other members of the TEAM Institute have begun to look at GIS mapping to study the impact of community resources or the lack there of. The goal would be to study areas in communities where the reports of SN are the highest. This mapping technique can look at items such as day-care centers, grocery stores, medical supply houses, physician offices, etc. These data could be the beginning of the design of service (i.e., intervention) centers that would be community—based and tailored to the specific needs of the respective residents/locales.

There is also some preliminary work being done on poly-victimization. Poly-victimization is a term that describes individuals who have experienced multiple victimizations of different kinds. This has been studied in child abuse populations [92, 93]. With the association of SN with other forms of mistreatment, poly-victimization may be seen with elder SN as well.

7.5.3 Challenges in Research

There has been a paucity of funded research in SN that has changed of late. In 2006, the National Institute on Aging funded the consortium for research in SN. Since then, the Administration for Community Living, the Agency for Healthcare Research and Quality, and the National Institute of Aging have supported to conduct multiple studies of elders who seriously neglect themselves. Various foundations such as Borchard, Archstone, Bailey Family, and Greenwall have also supported SN research. Behind the funding concerns, the methodological challenges loom large. Unlike many geriatric syndromes, there is not gold standard for SN. Dong has used the CHAP scales, and Dyer, APS report. However, these are convenience samples and most cases of SN are never reported. This makes state databases less than perfect for comprehensive study. There are screening tools such as Kohlman Evaluation of Living Skills (KELS), Clox 2, Self-Neglect Severity Scale, and the Delis–Kaplan Card Sort Test (D–KEFS), but there has not been the funding for the rigorous evaluation that is needed [27, 28, 32, 87].

Moreover, it is always challenging to study vulnerable populations. Some institutional review boards are uncertain about including these subjects in studies. The very nature of SN is that some reject intercession in their daily lives. And the most impaired among those would never be able to consent to research. These problems are further magnified when intervention research is considered. Due to the nature of SN, these interventions often have to be done at the subject's home.

Further, with multidimensional syndrome, what are the appropriate outcomes? Should they be social or medical? Perhaps quality of life measure would be best. And especially among the cognitively impaired, it would be difficult to know when the desired outcome is achieved, and this hinders rigorous research.

It appears that the approach being taken to "unpack" and describe well the many facets of SN is an approach that provides bite-sized pieces that permit progress to be made in this field.

7.6 Conclusion

Unlike elder abuse where there are more systematic and consensual definitions, the results of research on the prevalence, incidence, associated risk factors, and outcomes of SN of older adults are difficult to compare due to the lack of uniformity in the definition of SN and different methods of assessment. There are several variations in data for prevalence and incidence in very specific populations, but still we need data at the general population level. However, there are common risk factors worthy to highlight such as executive dysfunction, comorbidity, cognitive decline, depression, functional decline, and social factors such as isolation or lack of social support. Regarding the outcomes, there are more uniform data as a consequence of SN including higher mortality and use of health services for the elderly.

References

1. Teaster PB, Dugar TA, Mendiondo MS, Abner EL, Cecil KA, Otto JM. The 2004 survey of state adult protective services: abuse of adults 60 years of age and older. The National Center on Elder Abuse, 2007. http://www.ncea.aoa.gov/Resources/Publication/docs/APS_2004NCEASurvey.pdf. Accessed 24 Jan 2014.
2. Pavlik VN, Hyman DJ, Festa NA, Bitondo Dyer C. Quantifying the problem of abuse and neglect in adults—analysis of a statewide database. J Am Geriatr Soc. 2001;49:45–8.
3. Pavlou MP, Lachs MS. Could self-neglect in older adults be a geriatric syndrome? J Am Geriatr Soc. 2006;54:831–42.
4. Reyes-Ortiz CA, Burnett J, Flores DV, Halphen JM, Dyer CB. Medical implications of elder abuse: self-neglect. Clin Geriatr Med. 2014;30:807–23.
5. Reyes-Ortiz CA. Diogenes syndrome: the self-neglect elderly. Compreh Therapy. 2001;27:117–21.
6. Poythress EL, Burnett J, Naik AD, Pickens S, Dyer CB. Severe self-neglect: an epidemiological and historical perspective. J Elder Abuse Negl. 2006;18:5–12.
7. Granick R, Zeman FD. The aged recluse—an exploratory study with particular reference to community responsibility. J Chron Dis. 1960;12:639–53.
8. Macmillan D, Shaw P. Senile breakdown in standards of personal and environmental cleanliness. BMJ. 1966;i:1032–7.
9. Leake CD. Senile lack of cleanliness. Geriatrics. 1967;22(7):76.
10. Snowdon J. Uncleanliness among persons seen by community health workers. Hosp Community Psychiatry. 1987;38:491–4.
11. Clark AN, Mankikar GD, Gray I. Diogenes syndrome: a clinical study of gross neglect in old age. Lancet. 1975;i:366–8.
12. Ungvari GS, Hantz PM. Social breakdown in the elderly. I. Case studies and management. Compr Psychiatry. 1991;32:440–4.
13. Radebaugh TS, Hooper FJ, Gruenberg EM. The social breakdown syndrome in the elderly population living in the community: the helping study. Br J Psychiatry. 1987;151:341–6.
14. Shah AK. Senile squalor syndrome. What to expect and how to treat it. Geriatr Med. 1990;20(10):26.

15. Snowdon J. Squalor syndrome. J Am Geriatr Soc. 1997;45: 1539–40.
16. Cybulska E, Rucinski J. Gross self-neglect. Br J Hospital Med. 1986;36:21–5.
17. Kim HJ, Steketee G, Frost RO. Hoarding by elderly people. Health Soc Work. 2001;26:176–84.
18. Rosenthal M, Stelian J, Wagner J, Berkman P. Diogenes syndrome and hoarding in the elderly: case reports. Isr J Psychiatry Relat Sci. 1999;36(1):29–34.
19. Montero-Odasso M, Schapira M, Duque G, Chercovsky M, Fernández-Otero L, Kaplan R, et al. Is collectionism a diagnostic clue for diogenes syndrome? Int J Geriatr Psychiatry. 2005;20:709–11.
20. Nathanson JN. Animal hoarding: slipping into the darkness of comorbid animal and self-neglect. J Elder Abuse Negl. 2009;21:307–24.
21. Saldarriaga-Cantillo A, Rivas Nieto JC. Noah syndrome: a variant of diogenes syndrome accompanied by animal hoarding practices. J Elder Abuse Negl. 2015;27:270–5.
22. Pavlou MP, Lachs MS. Self-neglect in older adults: a primer for clinicians. J Gen Intern Med. 2008;23:1841–6.
23. Burnett J, Dyer CB, Halphen JM, Achenbaum WA, Green CE, Booker JG, Diamond PM. Four subtypes of self-neglect in older adults: results of a latent class analysis. J Am Geriatr Soc. 2014;62:1127–32.
24. Halliday G, Banerjee S, Philpot M, Macdonald A. Community study of people who live in squalor. Lancet. 2000;355:882–6.
25. Snowdon J, Shah A, Halliday G. Severe domestic squalor: a review. Int Psychogeriatrics. 2007;19:37–51.
26. Rasmussen JL, Steketee G, Frost RO, Tolin DF, Brown TA. Assessing squalor in hoarding: the home environment index. Community Ment Health J. 2014;50:591–6.
27. Kelly PA, Dyer CB, Pavlik V, Doodey R, Jogerst G. Exploring self-neglect in older adults: preliminary findings of the self-neglect severity scale and next steps. J Am Geriatr Soc. 2008;56(Suppl 2):253–60.
28. Royall DR, Palmer R, Chiodo LK, Polk MJ. Declining executive control in normal aging predicts change in functional status: the freedom house study. J Am Geriatr Soc. 2004;52:346–52.
29. Dyer CB, Goodwin JS, Vogel M, Pickens-Pace S, Burnett J, Kelly PA. Self-neglect among the elderly: a model based on more than 500 cases seen by a geriatric medicine team. Am J Public Health. 2007;97:1671–6.
30. Naik AD, Pickens S, Burnett J, Lai JM, Dyer CB. Assessing capacity in the setting of self-neglect: development of a novel screening tool for decision-making capacity. J Elder Abuse Negl. 2006;18:79–91.
31. Thomson MJ, Lietzau LK, Doty MM, Cieslik L, Williams R, Meurer LN. An analysis of elder abuse rates in Milwaukee County. WMJ. 2011;110:271–6.
32. Pickens S, Ostwald SK, Pace KM, Diamond P, Burnett J, Dyer CB. Assessing dimensions of executive function in community-dwelling older adults with self-neglect. Clin Nurs Stud. 2014;2:17–29.
33. Dong X, Simon M. Prevalence of elder self-neglect in a Chicago Chinese population: the role of cognitive physical and mental health. Geriatr Gerontol Int. 2015. Doi:10.1111/ggi.12598.
34. Dong X. Self-neglect in an elderly community-dwelling U.S. Chinese population: findings from the population study of Chinese elderly in Chicago study. J Am Geriatr Soc. 2014;62(12):2391–7.
35. Dong X, Simon MA, Evans DA. Prevalence of self-neglect across gender, race, and socioeconomic status: findings from the Chicago Health and Aging Project. Gerontology. 2012;58(3):258–68.
36. Dong X, Simon MA, Mosqueda L, Evans DA. The prevalence of elder self-neglect in a community-dwelling population: hoarding, hygiene, and environmental hazards. J Aging Health. 2012;24(3):507–24.
37. Moon A, Lawson K, Carpiac M, Spaziano E. Elder abuse and neglect among veterans in Greater Los Angeles: prevalence, types, and intervention outcomes. J Gerontol Soc Work. 2006;46(3 4):187–204.
38. Abrams RC, Lachs M, McAvay G, Keohane DJ, Bruce ML. Predictors of self-neglect in community-dwelling elders. Am J Psychiatry. 2002;159:1724–30.
39. Otiniano ME, Herrera CR. Abuse of Hispanic elders. Tex Med. 1999;95(3):68–71.
40. Lachs MS, Williams C, O'Brien S, Hurst L, Horwitz R. Older adults. An 11-year longitudinal study of adult protective service use. Arch Intern Med. 1996;156(4):449–53.
41. Luzny J, Jurickova L. Prevalence of elder abuse and neglect in seniors with psychiatric morbidity—example from central Moravia, Czech Republic. Iran J Public Health. 2012;41(8):27–32.
42. Lee M, Kim K. Prevalence and risk factors for self-neglect among older adults living alone in South Korea. Int J Aging Hum Dev. 2014;78(2):115–31.
43. Snowdon J, Halliday G. A study of severe domestic squalor: 173 cases referred to an old age psychiatry service. Int Psychogeriatr. 2011;23(2):308–14.
44. Ernst JS, Smith CA. Adult protective services clients confirmed for self-neglect: characteristics and service use. J Elder Abuse Negl. 2011;23(4):289–303.
45. Dong XQ, Simon M, Evans D. Cross-sectional study of the characteristics of reported elder self-neglect in a community-dwelling population: findings from a population-based cohort. Gerontology. 2010;56:325–34.
46. Dong X, Simon MA, Wilson RS, Mendes de Leon CF, Rajan KB, Evans DA. Decline in cognitive function and risk of elder self-neglect: finding from the Chicago Health Aging Project. J Am Geriatr Soc. 2010;58:2292–9.
47. Dong X, Simon M, Fulmer T, Mendes de Leon C, Rajan B, Evans DA. Physical function decline and the risk of elder self-neglect in a community-dwelling population. Gerontologist. 2010;50:316–26.
48. Franzini L, Dyer CB. Healthcare costs and utilization of vulnerable elderly people reported to Adult Protective Services for self-neglect. J Am Geriatr Soc. 2008;56:667–76.
49. Spensley C. The role of social isolation of elders in recidivism of self-neglect cases at San Francisco Adult Protective Services. J Elder Abuse Negl. 2008;20(1):43–61.
50. Naik AD, Burnett J, Pickens-Pace S, Dyer CB. Impairment in activities of daily living and the geriatric syndrome of self-neglect. Gerontologist. 2008;48:388–93.
51. Tierney MC, Snow WG, Charles J, Moineddin R, Kiss A. Neuropsychological predictors of self-neglect in cognitively impaired older people who live alone. Am J Geriatr Psychiatry. 2007;15(2):140–8.
52. Aung K, Burnett J, Smith SM, Dyer CB. Vitamin D deficiency associated with self-neglect in the elderly. J Elder Abuse Negl. 2006;18(4):63–78.
53. Burnett J, Regev T, Pickens S, Prati LL, Aung K, Moore J, Dyer CB. Social networks: a profile of the elderly who self-neglect. J Elder Abuse Negl. 2006;18(4):35–49.
54. Burnett J, Coverdale JH, Pickens S, Dyer CB. What is the association between self-neglect, depressive symptoms and untreated medical conditions? J Elder Abuse Negl. 2006;18(4):25–34.
55. Pickens S, Burnett J, Naik AD, Holmes HM, Dyer CB. Is pain a significant factor in elder self-neglect? J Elder Abuse Negl. 2006;18(4):51–61.

56. Smith SM, Mathews Oliver SA, Zwart SR, Kala G, Kelly PA, Goodwin JS. Nutritional status is altered in the self-neglecting elderly. J Nutr. 2006;136:2534–41.
57. Tierney MC, Charles J, Naglie G, Jaglal S, Kiss A, Fisher RH. Risk factors for harm in cognitively impaired seniors who live alone: a prospective study. J Am Geriatr Soc. 2004;52(9):1435–41.
58. Dyer CB, Pavlik VN, Murphy KP, Hyman DJ. The high prevalence of depression and dementia in elder neglect. J Am Geriatr Soc. 2000;48:205–8.
59. Mardan H, Hamid T, Redzuan M, Ibrahim R. Correlate of self-care and self-neglect among community-dwelling older adults. Iran J Nurs Midwifery Res. 2014;19(7 Suppl 1):71–6.
60. Snowdon J. Uncleanliness among persons seen by community health workers. Hosp Community Psychiatry. 1987;38(5):491–4.
61. Wrigley M, Cooney C. Diogenes syndrome: an Irish series. Irish J Psychol Med. 1992;9:37–41.
62. Garre-Olmo J, Planas-Pujol X, López-Pousa S, Juvinya D, Vilà A, Vilalta-Franch J. Frailty and dependence in Girona Study Group. Prevalence and risk factors of suspected elder abuse subtypes in people aged 75 and Older. J Am Geriatr Soc. 2009;57:815–22.
63. Stephens C, Alpass F, Towers A, Stevenson B. The effects of types of social networks, perceived social support, and loneliness on the health of older people: accounting for the social context. J Aging Health. 2011;23:887–911.
64. Hurley M, Scallen E, Johnson H, De La Harpe D. Adult service refusers in the greater Dublin. Ir Med J. 2000;93:208–11.
65. Cole AJ, Gillet TP, Fairbairn A. A case of senile self-neglect in a married couple: 'Diogenes a deux'. Int J Geriatr Psychiatry. 1992;7:839–41.
66. O'Mahoney D, Evans JG. Diogenes syndrome by proxy. Br J Psychiatry. 1994;164:705–6.
67. Reyes-Ortiz CA, Mulligan T. A case of diogenes syndrome. J Am Geriatr Soc. 1996;44:1486.
68. Reyes-Ortiz CA. Self-neglect as a geriatric syndrome. J Am Geriatr Soc. 2006;54:1945–6.
69. Dong X, Simon M, Wilson R, Beck T, McKinell K, Evans D. Association of personality traits with elder self-neglect in a community-dwelling population. Am J Geriatr Psychiatry. 2011;19:743–51.
70. Saxena S, Brody AL, Maidment KM, Smith EC, Zohrabi N, Katz E, Baker SK, Baxter LR Jr. Cerebral glucose metabolism in obsessive-compulsive hoarding. Am J Psychiatry. 2004;161(6):1038.
71. Grignon S, Bassiri D, Bartoli JL, Calvet P. Association of diogenes syndrome with a compulsive disorder. Can J Psychiatry. 1999;44:91–2.
72. Lachs MS, Williams CS, O'Brien S, Pillemer KA, Charlson ME. The mortality of elder mistreatment. JAMA. 1998;280:428–32.
73. Dong X, Simon MA. Elder self-neglect is associated with an increased rate of 30-day hospital readmission: findings from the Chicago Health and Aging Project. Gerontology. 2015;61:41–50.
74. Charles J, Naglie G, Lee J, Moineddin R, Jaglal S, Tierney MC. Self-report measures of well-being predict incident harm due to self-neglect in cognitively impaired seniors who live alone. J Alzheimers Dis. 2015;44(2):425–30.
75. Dong X, Simon MA. Association between elder self-neglect and hospice utilization in a community population. Arch Gerontol Geriatr. 2013;56:192–8.
76. Dong X, Simon M, Evans D. Elder self-neglect is associated with increased risk for elder abuse in a community-dwelling population: findings from the Chicago Health and Aging Project. J Aging Health. 2013;25(1):80–96.
77. Dong X, Simon MA, Evans D. Elder self-neglect and hospitalization: findings from the Chicago Health and Aging Project. J Am Geriatr Soc. 2012;60:202–9.
78. Dong X, Simon MA, Evans D. Prospective study of the elder self-neglect and ED use in a community population. Am J Emerg Med. 2012;30:553–61.
79. Turner A, Hochschild A, Burnett J, Zulfiqar A, Dyer CB. High prevalence of medication non-adherence in a sample of community-dwelling older adults with adult protective services-validated self-neglect. Drugs Aging. 2012;29:741–9.
80. Dong X, Simon M, Mendes de Leon C, Fulmer T, Beck T, Hebert L, Dyer C, Paveza G, Evans D. Elder self-neglect and abuse and mortality risk in a community-dwelling population. JAMA. 2009;302:517–26.
81. Lachs MS, Williams CS, O'Brien S, Pillemer KA. Adult protective service use and nursing home placement. Gerontologist. 2002;42:734–9.
82. Cotton MA, Johnson S, Bindman J, Sandor A, White IR, Thornicroft G, Nolan F, Pilling S, Hoult J, McKenzie N, Bebbington P. An investigation of factors associated with psychiatric hospital admission despite the presence of crisis resolution teams. BMC Psychiatry. 2007;2(7):52.
83. Naik AD, Lai JM, Kunik ME, Dyer CB. Assessing capacity in suspected cases of self-neglect. Geriatrics. 2008;63:24–31.
84. Cavalcante FG, Minayo MC. Qualitative study on suicide attempts and ideations with 60 elderly in Brazil. Cien Saude Colet. 2015;20:1655–66.
85. Van Laere I, de Wit M, Klazinga N. Shelter-based convalescence for homeless adults in Amsterdam: a descriptive study. BMC Health Serv Res. 2009;18(9):208. Doi:10.1186/1472-6963-9-208.
86. Dong X, Wilson RS, Mendes de Leon CF, Evans DA. Self-neglect and cognitive function among community-dwelling older persons. Int J Geriatr Psychiatry. 2010;25:798–806.
87. Pickens S, Naik AD, Burnett J, Kelly PA, Gleason M, Dyer CB. The utility of the Kohlman evaluation of living skills test is associated with substantiated cases of elder self-neglect. J Am Acad Nurse Pract. 2007;19:137–42.
88. Schillerstrom JE, Salazar R, Regwan H, Bonugli RJ, Royall DR. Executive function in self-neglecting adult protective services referrals compared with elder psychiatric outpatients. Am J Geriatr Psychiatry. 2009;17:907–10.
89. McDermott S. The devil is in the details: self-neglect in Australia. J Elder Abuse Neglect. 2008;20:231–50.
90. Paveza G, Vandeweerd C, Laumann E. Elder self-neglect: a discussion of a social typology. J Am Geriatr Soc. 2008;56(Suppl 2):S271–5.
91. Lauder W, Anderson I, Barclay A. Sociological and psychological theories of self-neglect. J Adv Nurs. 2002;40(3):331–8.
92. Turner HA, Finkelhor D, Ormrod R. Poly-victimization in a national sample of children and youth. Am J Prev Med. 2010;38 (3):323–30.
93. National Institute of Justice. Evidence Integration: Children Exposed to Violence (CEV). https://www.crimesolutions.gov/OJPResearch.aspx?Research_id=7. Accessed on 6 Mar 2016.

Financial Exploitation of Older Adults

8

Marguerite DeLiema and Kendon J. Conrad

8.1 Introduction

The National Research Council [14] defines elder financial exploitation as "unjust, improper, and/or illegal use of another's resources, property, and/or assets" [14, p. 38]. Examples include: alleged perpetrator uses funds for own benefit and without permission; power of attorney or trustee misuses funds in a joint account; check forgery; unauthorized use of ATM/debit cards; theft of income (social security, pension); and illegal transfer of property. Exploitation may also involve coercion, enticement, intimidation, and/or undue influence for one's own profit or benefit. As distinct from fraud, financial abuse involves a breach of trust between a vulnerable older person and a family member, close friend, caregiver, or person in a position of trust, who misuses the elder's funds to serve his or her own needs at the elder's expense. Financial abuse is also called material abuse, fiduciary abuse, exploitation of resources, and economic victimization [93].

Another type of financial exploitation that targets older adults is fraud and scams. Seniors may be manipulated to send cash or checks, wire money, purchase prepaid cards, or disclose personal information like social security numbers, bank account, and credit card information to strangers. Although people of all ages and demographic groups can be defrauded, examples of fraud that commonly target seniors include bogus lottery scams, sweetheart swindles, grandparent scams, fake charities, home repair fraud, and IRS back taxes schemes (see Beals et al. [10] for a taxonomy of fraud and definition of sub-types). Fraud victims are intentionally deceived into complying with a perpetrator's demands after being promised goods, services, or other types of rewards that are either grossly misrepresented, never intended to be provided, or do not exist [88]. Fraud perpetrators may deliberately go after seniors based on assumptions that older adults are socially isolated, cognitively impaired, and have more money than people of younger ages, all factors that make them attractive targets.

Most perpetrators of elder fraud do not personally know their victims, whereas financial abuse perpetrators opportunistically take advantage of vulnerable adults within their existing social network. It is ironic that the stranger, who should not be trusted, is able to gain the elder's trust or confidence, i.e., confidence game; while the person already in a position of trust takes advantage of that privilege in order to exploit the elder. For example, family members may feel entitled to the elder's money in exchange for providing care, or may justify their behavior as simply cashing in early on an inheritance. In this chapter, elder fraud and elder financial abuse are treated as distinct concepts, yet both are forms of elder financial exploitation.

Approximately 7.3 % of adults aged 65–74 and 6.5 % of adults aged 75 and older were victims of scams and fraud in the U.S. in 2011 [6]. This is slightly higher than past year prevalence of financial abuse by a family member: 5.2 % among community-residing adults 60 and older [1]. A few years earlier, Laumann et al. [60] found a prevalence of 3.5 % among adults of ages 57–85. More recently, Lachs and Berman [58] reported a prevalence of 4.1 % in a sample of over 4000 New York seniors. Although definitions and survey methods vary, reported risk factors include poor functional health, low social support, loneliness, self-neglect, and cognitive impairment [2, 8, 17, 32]. We note that prevalence studies tended to focus on victim risk factors and not those of perpetrators, and that they concentrate on financial abuse rather than elder fraud.

As with other forms of elder mistreatment, financial exploitation does not always occur in isolation. Other types

M. DeLiema
Stanford Center on Longevity, Stanford University, 365 Lausen St., Stanford, CA 94305, USA

K.J. Conrad (✉)
Department of Health Policy and Administration, University of Illinois at Chicago, 1603 West Taylor Street, Chicago, 60612, IL, USA
e-mail: kjconrad@uic.edu

X. Dong (ed.), *Elder Abuse*, DOI 10.1007/978-3-319-47504-2_8

of elder abuse may be financially motivated, such as isolating an elder in order to control his assets, or withholding care to avoid the high cost of medical treatment. In a meta-analysis of 28 studies from the U.S., Dong et al. [34] found that many older adults experienced multiple forms of abuse simultaneously. Jackson and Hafemeister [51, 52] found that compared to cases in which financial exploitation occurred alone (pure financial abuse), cases in which financial exploitation occurred in combination with neglect and/or physical abuse (hybrid financial exploitation) resulted in greater average losses: ~$80,000 compared to ~$185,500, although these differences were not statistically significant.

Hybrid financial exploitation cases were significantly more complex. In addition to experiencing other forms of elder abuse, victims had more forms of financial exploitation going on—e.g., theft, fraud, extortion, misappropriation of assets—and perpetrators were more likely to be chronically unemployed, be financially dependent on the victim, and be a relative. Interventions were also more extensive in these complex cases. Victims who suffered from multiple types of mistreatment were more likely to be separated from the abuser, usually their caregiver, and placed in a supervisory care setting where they have less autonomy.

8.1.1 Costs and Consequences

Deliema [26] found that fraud victims lost significantly more than financial abuse victims in a small sample of serious cases investigated by law enforcement—an average of nearly $619,000 compared to $200,000 per person. This supports the [22] finding that fraud is more serious than financial abuse, at least from a financial impact perspective. This difference may be explained by the fact that scam artists actively pursue targets with money and assets, and aim to take them for all they are worth. Financial abuse perpetrators, on the other hand, are more opportunistic; they exploit vulnerable older adults within their social networks who are most often older relatives who cover the entire spectrum of financial status from rich to poor. In support of this assumption, Stiegel [86] has noted that the incidence of financial abuse does not vary by income level. The National Elder Abuse Incidence Study [69] found that the likelihood of financial abuse did not increase with higher levels of income. In cases where adult protective services (APS) was able to estimate or determine the victim's income, 46 % had incomes between $5000 and $9,999; 29.8 % had incomes between $10,000 and $14,999; and 22.4 % had incomes of $15,000 or more (in fiscal years 1995 and 1996) [69].

Extrapolating from a small sample of financial exploitation cases substantiated by APS in Utah, Gunther [45] estimated that $4,766,196 was stolen from a total of 57 seniors. DeLiema [26] calculated a total loss of $19 million and 17 properties among 54 victims [26]. One explanation for these high dollar amounts is that victims who suffer significant financial losses are more likely to have their cases investigated by APS and law enforcement. Even if these cases are outliers, they suggest that the current $2.6 billion dollars per year calculation published by MetLife in 2009 underestimates the total losses suffered by elder financial exploitation victims in the U.S.

Middle-income seniors may experience the worst financial consequences of exploitation. Those who have modest retirement savings and who are no longer working have fewer chances to recoup losses and may become dependent on public nutrition, Medicaid, and housing programs after losing their life savings [64]. For elder abuse in general, research has shown that victims use 30 % more mental health and substance abuse services [82], and are hospitalized more often than non-victims [31]. These costs are borne by the government when the elder's savings are gone.

8.2 Theoretical Frameworks

Financial exploitation is often grouped with other forms of elder mistreatment in theories of elder abuse, but a number of models have been specifically proposed as explanations for elder financial exploitation (e.g., [23, 57, 77, 78, 94]), and others offer more general explanations of crime (e.g., [18]). Although these models vary, common among all of them is the vulnerable status of the older adult, the perpetrator's sense of entitlement, and the unequal balance of power between the two parties.

8.2.1 Financial Exploitation Models

Wilber and Reynolds proposed the first comprehensive framework for elder financial exploitation in 1996. They present four interacting criteria that distinguish financial exploitation from acceptable monetary exchange: (1) vulnerability characteristics of the elder, (2) the nature of the relationship between the elder and the perpetrator, (3) the interests served by the relationship, and (4) the type of influence used by the perpetrator. The second model by Rabiner et al. [77] presents an applied ecological perspective of financial exploitation in which the victim and perpetrator are embedded within a larger sociocultural and policy macrosystem. The macrosystem includes cultural perceptions of aging, public policies, state statutes, and interventions to protect elders from exploitation. Withing the macrosystem is the microsystem, which includes the victim-perpetrator dyad, the social networks of each person, and power and exchange dynamics underlying the relationship.

A third conceptual framework by Kemp and Mosqueda [57], which built on Wilber and Reynolds [94], was developed and validated with input from police detectives, district attorneys, and APS workers. The model lays out eight process-related features of exploitation describing how a vulnerable elder is persuaded to give money, property, or other assets to another person when it is not in the elder's best financial interests.

In the most recent conceptual framework by Conrad et al. [23], experts were recruited to generate a concept map of financial exploitation using a statement sorting procedure. This yielded six clusters ranked by seriousness: (1) theft and scams, (2) coercion, (3) financial victimization, (4) signs of possible financial abuse, (5) financial entitlement, and (6) money management difficulties. Of all clusters, statements pertaining to theft and scams were rated as the most severe. Least severe were money management difficulties, problems that are common to older persons on fixed incomes but that may make the older adult more vulnerable. Family involvement when an older adult faces declining health and cognition may help prevent more serious theft and scams by keeping financial predators at bay, but may open opportunities for caregivers to take advantage.

8.2.2 Health Model

The prevailing model in the health field views the victim as having mental or physical problems that cause him or her to mismanage money [80]. This perspective is stronger in the mental health context rather than in aging in particular, and is not referred to as financial exploitation but as money mismanagement. Therefore it puts most of the responsibility on the victim's vulnerabilities and disabilities, and it places responsibility on the healthcare system to prevent or remediate problems. It does not shoulder any of the blame on perpetrators as being the cause of exploitation. Pillemer [73] conducted a case-control study comparing abused elders with a matched group of non-abused elders. He found no significant differences in health status or impairments in activities of daily living between the two groups. In fact, abused elders were less impaired in a number of areas. Thus, the health model of financial exploitation has not received empirical support, at least not for older adults.

8.2.3 Undue Influence

Undue influence is the substitution of one person's will for the desires of another [75], often by using subtle threats or coercion. Undue influence models by Blum [13] and Bernatz [11] describe how susceptible targets are intentionally isolated by perpetrators who can be relatives, friends, or strangers who capitalize on an opportunity to control the elders' social environments, thereby creating a sense of powerlessness and increased dependency. Once isolated from others, these vulnerable elders begin to rely more and more on the perpetrator for functional and emotional support, thus becoming easier to manipulate. Undue influence models place more emphasis on the characteristics of perpetrators and how they act to control and isolate their victims and less on the vulnerabilities of the older adults.

8.2.4 Routine Activity Theory

Criminological theories add an additional perspective by focusing attention on perpetrators and the context of financial exploitation, especially the role of capable guardians or arrangements that prevent financial exploitation. According to Cohen and Felson's [18] *routine activity theory*, criminal acts require the convergence of three factors: (1) a motivated offender, (2) a suitable target, and (3) the absence of capable guardians. This theory focuses on how specific behavioral patterns and the intersection of people in time and space create opportunities for crime [44].

The first key component of routine activity theory is the presence of a motivated offender. In general, perpetrators are motivated by a desire for economic gain. Coleman [19] argues that this desire stems from a cultural emphasis on competition for higher economic status and the belief that wealth is an appropriate proxy for success. Perpetrators' may have robust rationalizations for engaging in the crime such as, "I need the money more than she does," "I will inherit the money anyway." Some perpetrators may feel a blinding sense of entitlement due to cultural and familial expectations.

The second component of routine activity theory is the presence of a suitable target. As stated before; older adults are likely targeted for reasons including greater economic resources (more remunerative targets), the perception that they are more susceptible to being deceived (easier targets), familial and other caregiving or trust relationships (religious, cultural, etc.), or the belief that they will not recognize and report the crime to law enforcement (low risk of detection). Routine activity theory asserts that the exploiter is the cause, while victims may have varying levels of vulnerability that make them better or worse targets. Some of these vulnerabilities have nothing to do with age, financial skills, health, etc. In other words, given a decent opportunity, a skilled exploiter, or scammer will find a way to get the money using appeals to greed, status, need for companionship or care, romance, and other desires the target might have.

The third factor, the absence of capable guardians, acknowledges that the action of financially exploiting an older person is contingent on an opportunity to do so. As many older people become increasingly vulnerable with age, benevolent family members, friends or institutions may step in, thereby preventing exploitation. A wide social network (more eyes and ears), trustworthy family members, financial professionals and legal documents that protect assets are all factors that act as capable guardians that protect against financial exploitation.

A strength *and* a weakness of the routine activity theory is its breadth. Although it focuses on victims, perpetrators, and the context that gives rise to crime, it does not seek to explain what motivates people to commit financial exploitation (A need to fund a drug addiction? A desire for power?); what factors make for a suitable target (Wealth? Impairment? Gullibility?), and who (or what) acts as a capable guardian (Law enforcement? Trusted family members? Legal safeguards protecting a person's assets?) It also does not account for the mechanisms of exploitation, or *how* money and assets are taken from victims.

A critique offered by Holtfreter et al. [48] is that the routine activity theory places too much emphasis on street crime involving deviant offenders, whereas fraud and financial abuse offenders are not inherently deviant. For one thing, fraudulent marketing relies on the same sales tactics and communication methods (e.g., Internet, mail, telephone, in-person) used by legitimate businesses to solicit customers. Another problem is that unlike street criminals who commit crimes such as rape, assault, and robbery, perpetrators of fraud and financial abuse often hold false beliefs that they are not breaking the law. Furthermore, elderly fraud victims are not "pure victims" [28, 51, 92]. There is some degree of complicity involved in agreeing to a perpetrator's demands or permitting a friend or family member to have access to one's finances (see [49]). Another critique of the theory is that it fails to explain exactly *why* elders are more vulnerable to financial exploitation compared to younger age groups [51]. Are older people actually easier to manipulate or just perceived to be by those who target them?

8.3 Cultural Differences in Perceptions of Financial Exploitation

Current definitions and theories of elder financial exploitation are largely based on White, middle-class perspectives [81]. Studies have shown that racial and ethnic minorities have different beliefs about what constitutes acceptable exchange of money and resources, particularly among relatives (e.g., [8, 67, 81]). For example, in a qualitative study on elder abuse, Sanchez [81] found that 92 % of the older Latinos who were interviewed stated that they share economic resources within their families. Through focus group discussions, Chang and Moon [16] found that compared to elders from other Asian countries, one-third of the Korean American cohort agreed that it is okay for adult children not to reimburse their elderly parents for money owed, even if the parents ask for the money. In another qualitative study on perceptions of elder mistreatment among Chinese Americans, psychological abuse was seen as the most severe, and that financial exploitation by adult children often happens in conjunction with emotional mistreatment. (Dong et al. [29]).

Abuse measures may not be culturally sensitive enough to capture differences in perceptions about what constitutes elder financial exploitation [27]. Using traditional assessments, cultural norms around resource sharing can lead to higher prevalence estimates in minority populations where it is often more acceptable to financially support younger relatives. Beach et al. [8] found that the rate of financial exploitation was nearly three times higher for African Americans (23.0 %) than non-African Americans (8.4 %). Among low-income Latino elders living in an urban environment, the prevalence of financial abuse was 16.7 % [27]. Dong et al. [35] reported rates of 8.8–9.3 % among urban Chinese. Therefore, future assessments used to determine prevalence and identify who is at risk need to accommodate unique cultural perspectives around what behaviors constitute fraud, theft, and misappropriation of assets.

8.4 Are Older Adults at Greater Risk for Financial Exploitation?

Spiegel [84] has noted that the lore that older adults are at greater risk of financial exploitation—e.g., Mickey Rooney's U.S. Senate testimony in [79], MetLife Mature Market Institute's [64] report of $2.9 billion annual loss—is not always supported by data. The Federal Trade Commission's (FTC) Consumer Sentinel Network reported that fraud-related complaints from persons over 60 were about proportional to the older adult population at 14 % in 2010 [25]. FTC fraud prevalence studies in 2004, 2007, and 2011 concluded that seniors were the least likely of any age groups to be victims of most forms of fraud [4–6].

One explanation for why the data does not support assumptions that older adults are more vulnerable is that older people are less likely to acknowledge victimization in a survey compared to people of younger ages, especially when the incident is framed in a criminal context [9]. There are also extremely low rates of self-reporting to APS and law enforcement agencies. In a study in New York State, Lachs and Berman [58] found that only 0.96 per 1000 cases of financial exploitation were reported to APS, law enforcement, etc., compared to a self-reported rate of 42.1 per 1000 (4.2 %). This implies that only 1 in 44 cases were being officially documented. A less conservative estimate is that one-in-four to one-in-five cases are reported to APS or law enforcement [57]. Reasons for not reporting may include feelings of embarrassment, failure to recall the incident due to cognitive impairment, desire to protect the perpetrator, fear of the perpetrator, dependency on the perpetrator, or denial of victimization [37]. Furthermore, victims are often intentionally isolated by perpetrators and are thus are not given opportunities to report. As such, elder financial abuse is largely a hidden crime.

8.5 The Role of Financial Capacity and Decision-Making

Financial capacity is a multidimensional concept defined as, "the capacity to manage money and financial assets in ways that meet a person's needs and which are consistent with his/her values and self-interest" [61]. Domains of financial capacity include the ability to carry out cash transactions, counting out change, writing checks, understanding bank statements and investment options, exercising sound financial judgment, and other money management behaviors [62]. According to the American Bar Association/American Psychological Association Assessment of Capacity in Older Adults Project Working Group [3], financial capacity varies across individuals according to their background and experiences. Every person has a different baseline of financial knowledge and skills, so a decline in one domain for a financially sophisticated person may equate to unimpaired functioning in another.

Declines in financial capacity are associated with age-related changes in the brain and cognitive disorders such as Alzheimer's disease and related dementias. Some of these conditions affect higher order cognitive tasks like executive functioning, which is necessary for sound financial planning and decision-making. Han et al. [46] found that the effect of mild cognitive impairment on financial and health-related decision-making was equivalent to the effect of being 10-years older, on average. This effect was driven largely by impairment in perceptual speed, an area that is often affected by the normal aging process [46]. Trouble managing money may place older adults at increased risk of exploitation. Indeed, poor cognitive functioning was significantly associated with elder financial abuse among older adults who had abuse reported to social services agencies [33].

Researchers and practitioners have suggested that elders may be most vulnerable to financial exploitation during these early stages of cognitive decline when deficits in financial capacity are hardest to recognize by the individuals themselves and by their family members [56, 63]. They may exhibit minor symptoms of impaired problem solving, trouble learning new information, difficulties making complex transactions, and changes in personality, yet function normally in other areas of cognition, like language and semantic knowledge, and need no assistance with personal care [68, 89]. The combination of subtle impairments in financial capacity and lack of oversight from family members provides a window of opportunity for perpetrators to take advantage of the elder. Therefore, if elder financial exploitation is suspected, documentation of financial capacity can provide needed evidence that the older person did not fully understand the financial arrangement or the risks of giving money or personal information to the suspected abuser. Cognitive domains that should be assessed by the examiner include memory, orientation, verbal fluency, numeracy, spatial reasoning, attention, and executive functioning [3]. Despite the importance of capacity evaluations, there are few experts to administer them who are trained to testify if the case is filed for prosecution [20].

One recommendation of the Elder Justice Coordinating Council [36] is to develop and test screening tools that can be used by APS to identify and document signs cognitive impairment when caseworkers are investigating a report. Similar tools need to be adapted for law enforcement and for financial services professionals. If Congress appropriates more funds to the Elder Justice Act that was enacted in March 2010, there will be more resources for APS to provide victim services and perhaps grants to test cognitive assessments that are easy to administer in the field. Yet as of 2015 Congress has appropriated only $4 million to implement the Elder Justice Act.

8.6 Impact of Social Isolation

A network of relationships, sometimes referred to as social embeddedness, can be a double-edged sword. While having many social connections increases the probability that one person in the network is a bad actor, social embeddedness has been found to prevent elder abuse in general [83]. This is likely because the actions of any one individual can be monitored by others if the social network is large. Low network density and social isolation may increase risk of financial exploitation [30, 40], particularly for fraud by strangers. Without meaningful and authentic social interactions, victims may become dependent on a financial predator who promises to fulfill their social and emotional needs. In a small sample of older fraud victims, DeLiema [26] found that nearly all were socially isolated, often following the loss of a spouse or becoming disabled, and over half of the fraud sample was intentionally isolated after the perpetrator became embedded in their lives.

By secluding the elder and restricting access to other friends and family, perpetrators can both hide the exploitation and use the power differential to force the victim to comply with their demands [11, 75]. For example, in one of the cases reviewed by DeLiema [26], the perpetrator changed the victim's locks and unplugged her telephones to prevent her son from communicating with her. By the time her son became aware of the abuse, the victim had already lost hundreds of thousands of dollars.

Whether a vulnerable person is victimized by strangers or trusted others may have less to do with his or her personal characteristics, and more to do with the size and connectedness of that person's social network (or lack thereof) [26]. Take for example an impaired widow who lives with her unemployed and drug-abusing son. This widow faces a high risk of financial abuse. However, if that same widow has no children and no close friends or relatives, she is more vulnerable to fraud by a stranger. In other words, the structure of the victim's social network determines whether s/he is more likely to be victimized by fraud or by financial abuse [26]. As the hypothetical scenario illustrates, the presence of adult children decreases risk of fraud because they protect their elderly parents from predatory strangers, yet increases the risk of financial abuse because adult children may take advantage of their parents' trust [26]. Adult children are the most common perpetrators of financial abuse [2]. This implies the importance of the elder's social network in predicting the risk of financial exploitation and how to intervene.

8.7 Building a Parsimonious, Testable Theory

Drawing upon the theoretical currents discussed above, Conrad et al. [24] tested a theory of financial exploitation. The scope was limited to immediate causal factors that would be actionable in community-based casework (i.e., not nursing homes or other long-term care facilities), measurable, and therefore, testable; more macro-factors such as sociocultural influences, social policies, broader community, and environment were not included. They also emphasized factors that could be remediated or improved. For example, gender, age, and other demographics were not included in the model [55] since they are not a focus of remediation and entering them would serve as unwanted "controls" that could obscure or confuse the influence of behavioral issues that are present in prevailing theories and that should have full capability to explain variance. To create a parsimonious and more readily testable theory to explain the factors that contribute to financial exploitation, they used the four factors most often cited in the literature: abuser characteristics, isolation/lack of support, victim vulnerabilities, and victim–abuser relationship. Additionally, they included factors that could ameliorate financial exploitation: exploiter–victim relationship strengths and intervention services to assess the situation and provide solutions that improve safety and access to care.

8.8 Causes of Financial Exploitation

Figure 8.1 presents this basic theory of the causes of financial exploitation and their remediation represented by directional arrows that can be tested with cross-sectional data. Hypotheses are represented by a plus or minus sign indicating the posited direction of the relationship. The plus signs (+) indicate factors that work to increase the risk of financial exploitation while minus signs (−) indicate factors that decrease it. While longitudinal data are needed to test causality if the temporal order is not clear, in this case such data are not needed, since reversing the order posited in Fig. 8.1 is not plausible. For example, financial exploitation of the alleged victim (AV) would not cause risk factors for abuse such as history of violence or mental illness in the alleged abuser (AA).

While this theory is parsimonious, it can be criticized for being too simplistic. However, the complexity of the model lies within the items measuring the constructs presented (please see Appendix for item descriptions). These measures include assessments of factors that increase exploitation: exploiter risk factors; relationship problems such as caregiver stress and burden and negative attitudes; lack of support and social isolation; and victim vulnerabilities. The factors that ameliorate or decrease exploitation are also measured: abuser strengths and use of services.

8.8.1 Abuser Risk Factors

The theoretical model represented by Fig. 8.1 posits that abuse starts with the *abuser* (a.k.a., exploiter, offender, perpetrator). A listing of all items used to measure abuser risk factors is available at www.eadss.org. Examples include difficulty keeping a job, a history of trouble with the law, being irresponsible, having drug or alcohol problems, and other negative characteristics and behaviors [7].

8.8.2 Relationship Problems

To test caregiver burden as a risk factor, Conrad et al. [22] included questions on this topic in the interview with the AA. They also included a variety of questions regarding negative attitudes of AAs toward AVs that would indicate a poor relationship.

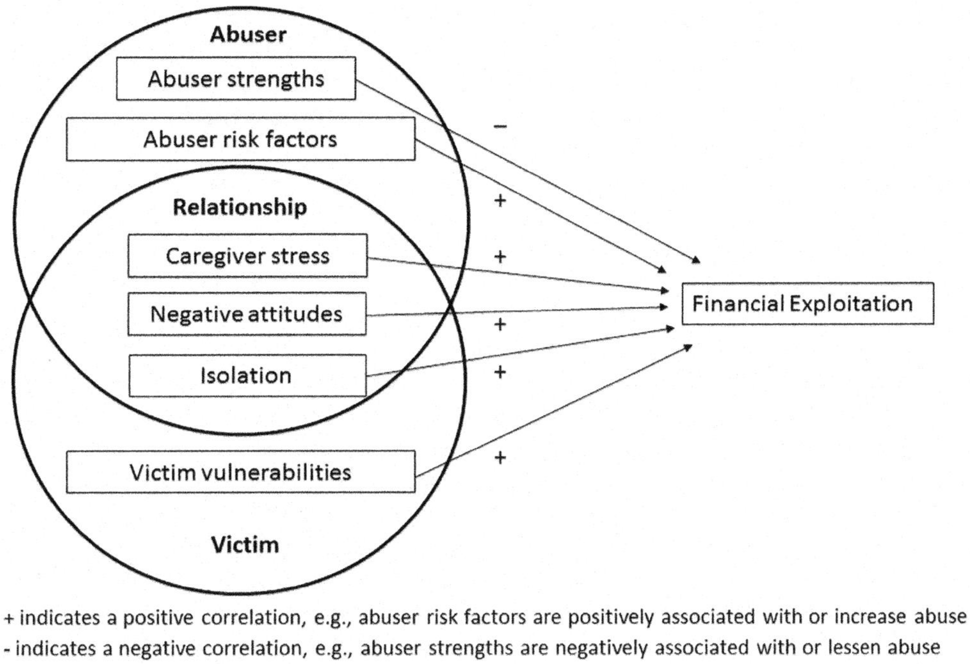

Fig. 8.1 Abuser, victim, and relationship risk/protective factors for elder financial exploitation

8.8.3 Isolation/Lack of Support

The exploitative aspects of a relationship generally develop in the context of isolation, away from potential support. This isolation creates an opportunity for financial exploitation to occur (lack of capable protectors/advocates).

8.8.4 Victim Vulnerability

Victim risk factors have received the most attention in previous elder abuse research [53–55]. Cognitive status, mental status, substance abuse, and functional limitations were assessed by the caseworkers during their interviews with AVs, through observation and reviews of records. The vulnerability of the victim (viable target) may create opportunities for the abuser, but we should recognize that perpetrators can prey on high functioning older adults as well as those who are cognitively and physically impaired. In other words, the elder's vulnerability is not a necessary nor sufficient condition for financial exploitation.

8.8.5 Outcome Variable—Financial Exploitation

The presence of financial exploitation can be determined by caseworkers, principally by interviewing the AV but also by interviewing collaterals (other persons with pertinent information) and through direct observation and review of financial records. The look-back period is 1 year using the Older Adult Financial Exploitation Measure [22].

8.9 Remediation

8.9.1 Relationship Strengths

Relationships may consist of positive exchanges and support between the AA and AV, as well as abusive, negative interactions. While we found no literature specific to the strengths or supportive behavior exhibited by alleged abusers in the context of elder abuse, our field research indicated that this is an important area to include, particularly because interventions for elder mistreatment should build on the abusers' strengths (e.g., [38, 87]). Unlike in domestic violence, elder abuse involves an older person who may be dependent on the abuser to meet their needs, so it is often less advisable to separate the abuser and the victim. Caseworkers note the importance of assessing the abusers' strengths to determine if it is possible to ameliorate the problems and improve the situation. Assessment of strengths may help to sort out the cause of the abuse, such as caregiver burden, financial stress, mental illness, or drug and alcohol dependency.

At this writing, tests of this model have been conducted [24]. Results have shown significant bivariate regression results of AA Risk and the Relationship subscales including

AA Strengths reported by the AA; AA Strengths reported by the AV; and Isolation. Higher AA Risk, lower AA Strengths, and Isolation were separate predictors of exploitation ($p < 0.001$). Neither Caregiver Burden nor Negative Attitudes were significantly related to financial exploitation. None of the vulnerability variables had a significant association in the predicted direction. In summary, this initial test of the theory supported criminological theory whereby the exploiter, lacking compensating strengths, is the chief risk factor with accompanying isolation of the victim. Neither victim vulnerabilities nor caregiver burden were significantly associated with financial exploitation. These findings add evidence to early findings by Pillemer [73], who found that victim functional impairment was less significant than abuser dependency in predicting elder abuse.

8.10 Assessment Models and Intervention Strategies

How do we assess the problems of elder financial exploitation and intervene effectively? There is surprisingly little information on the effectiveness of different interventions for elder financial exploitation [74]. To address this gap, Fig. 8.2 presents a model depicting the assessment of the causes of financial exploitation (inputs) from Fig. 8.1, the design of intervention programs and services (activities), the measurement of the intervention activities' success (output), and the actual outcomes of those inputs, activities, and outputs [85].

8.10.1 Input: Caseworker assessment of exploitation, victim isolation, vulnerability, and perpetrator risks and strengths

In the context of APS, when financial exploitation is reported to the agency, a caseworker must investigate the allegations and decide whether they should be substantiated. The first level of assessment involves interviewing the AV, the AA, if possible, and collaterals, i.e., others who might have pertinent information about abuse that was reported.

If the caseworker has obtained credible information that financial exploitation has taken or is taking place, the next phase is documenting the nature of the exploitation and how much was lost. This is the sticking point. APS caseworkers tend to be trained as social workers and behave as social workers in that their aim is to ensure that the older adult is safe and well cared for. They are not forensic accountants, police officers, or evidence technicians. If the case is cross-reported to law enforcement for further investigation, it may not be pursued. Law enforcement agencies do not always view financial abuse as a serious crime [91], and typically focus their efforts and limited resources on responding to violent crimes and life-threatening incidents such as assaults, robberies, burglaries, drugs, traffic accidents, and homicides. Few detectives are trained in forensic audits to validate allegations of financial exploitation, and there is insufficient departmental funding to hire a specialist in order to provide this expertise. Even if a case can be made, there is limited legal expertise to pursue it.

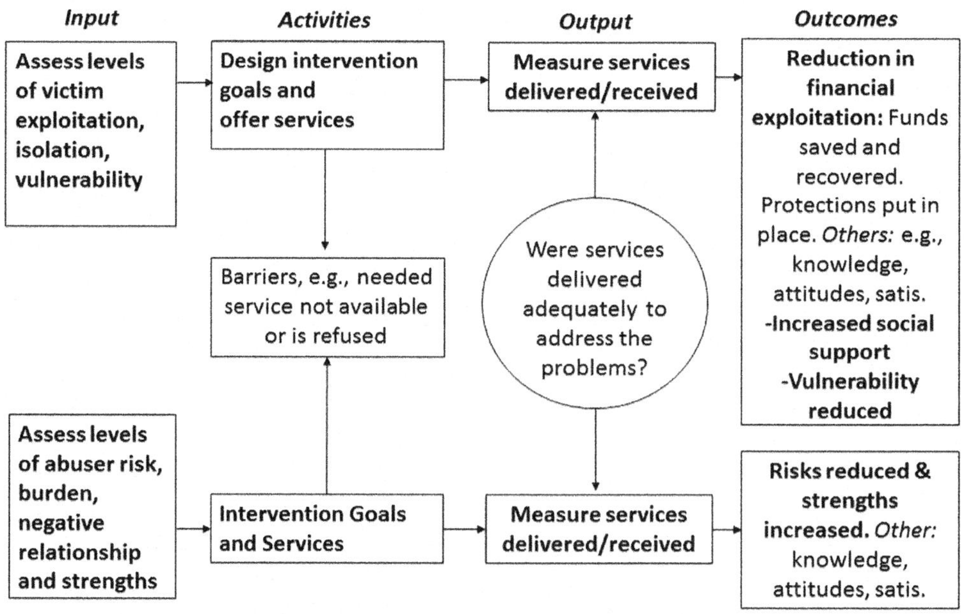

Fig. 8.2 Financial exploitation assessment and remediation model

Historically, there has been little interaction between APS and law enforcement agencies on elder abuse cases [53, 54]. The U.S. Department of Justice [91] reported that 65.8 % of elder financial exploitation cases were referred to APS while only 14.7 % were referred to law enforcement. Meirson [65] reported that APS in Rhode Island received 900 complaints of elder abuse in 1 year, with 85 % of them substantiated, but only 70 cases (7.7 %) were fully investigated by law enforcement. Criminal charges were filed in less than 20 cases (2.2 %), and few (if any) of these cases led to a conviction.

8.10.2 Activities, Services, Multidisciplinary Teams

While most cases go to either APS or law enforcement, victim service providers may also include: Long-term care ombudsmen, area agencies on aging, legal services, public guardians, fraud protection agencies, victim advocacy groups, domestic violence programs, financial services, mental health providers, neuropsychologists, forensic accountants, etc., but there is very little literature on the most effective ways to remediate financial exploitation. The U.S. Department of Justice [91] website reports that no studies are available on service offerings or service utilization exclusively for victims of financial exploitation.

Investigation of complex financial exploitation cases requires special training and teamwork between attorneys, trained fraud examiners (preferably with banking experience), APS caseworkers, and detectives that can investigate a range of financial crimes—from abuse by powers of attorney to telemarketing scams. Caseworkers do the best they can without law enforcement involvement in the majority of elder abuse investigations. They can have considerable influence if they separate the exploiter from the elder's funds by getting other friends or family members involved or by instituting representative payeeship or guardianship (also called "conservatorship" in some states). However, although these interventions protect what is left of the elder's assets, they do nothing to recover the funds that were already stolen and do nothing to hold the perpetrator accountable for exploitation. Part of the problem is the lack of coordination between APS, law enforcement, criminal justice, health care, and mental health providers.

To address the fragmentation in resolving elder financial exploitation, some communities have established elder abuse forensic centers and other multidisciplinary teams of professionals from health, finance, law enforcement, criminal justice, and social services. These teams coordinate efforts across agencies to deploy resources for investigation and response. For example, the Los Angeles County Elder Abuse Forensic Center will send trained clinicians to evaluate the victim's living environment, cognitive functioning, and financial decision-making capacity by administering a flexible battery of cognitive tests. Tests are selected based on the elder's perceived cognitive ability, mental status, financial capacity concerns, and the clinical judgment of the evaluator. The goal is to determine the elder's probable financial decision-making capacity at the time of exploitation and whether s/he reasonably understood the risks and benefits of the transaction to provide consent. If the elder is determined to have lacked financial capacity at that time, the findings may be presented to the District Attorney's Office and/or the Public Guardian's Office for prosecution of the abuser or conservatorship (guardianship) of the victim, assuming these outcomes are desirable to protect the victim's health, safety, and financial security [41].

Unfortunately, most communities do not have well-established multidisciplinary teams and must rely on other resources to investigate abuse. The Pennsylvania Department of Aging Institute on Protective Services at Temple University has developed a set of standardized procedures [42]. The following section draws heavily from a presentation by these authors. See the referenced link for examples of their forms. Standardized procedures that they have developed are

- Detailed investigative protocols and training for APS:
  - Financial investigation checklist—a detailed review of transactions
  - Standardized forms for recording credits and debits
  - Tips for working with law enforcement
  - Financial investigations using legal expertise at the state level
  - State-wide training for APS using webinar format
- Training and tools for law enforcement
- Training for bank employees
- Expansion of county-based multidisciplinary teams to assist where resources are not available
- Use of college interns to help with labor-intensive investigations

At the heart of the investigations are the procedures for documenting the exploitation such as reviewing financial records for unusual transactions, filing disputes with banks and credit card companies to recover funds, and protecting the remaining assets. Financial firms can share a client's personal financial information with state law enforcement agencies to aid in their investigations. There are procedures to learn to "follow the money" effectively. For example, it is important to obtain copies of the front and back of checks—deposits/withdrawals and offsets. "Offset" is a term used by the financial services industry to describe where the money came from or where it was deposited. Offsets provide information about whether the alleged perpetrator withdrew cash, transferred funds to another account, or purchased a bank check. Deposit slips can help determine if the alleged perpetrator was also making deposits and, rather than blatantly stealing, co-mingled funds.

Protecting assets may involve "clouding the title," i.e., disputing the claim of rights to the property by the alleged perpetrator if real estate was transferred when the older adult lacked the ability to consent. Caseworkers or family members may need to help the older adult write letters to the bank to request freezes on the accounts pending the outcome of the investigation, and to reimburse fraudulent charges. It is important to realize that the clock is ticking on many transactions such as unauthorized credit and debit card payments, so claims and freezes should be filed expeditiously.

Criminal referrals to the prosecutor's office should be made if a crime has been committed, however prosecution for financial exploitation remains uncommon [43, 47, 72]. According to APS workers, prosecution is the most difficult service to obtain from criminal justice professionals [12]. An American Prosecutor Research Institute (APRI) survey reported that the barriers to prosecution include a lack of dedicated staff; inadequate training in prosecuting cases where the victim is cognitively impaired, uncooperative, or deceased; limited funding for medical and forensic experts to evaluate victims and testify on their capacity; and disinterest among judges, law enforcement, and attorneys toward elder abuse [66].

Other concerns are deciding what is in the victim's best interest. For example, if the money was stolen by the elder's only beneficiary, it is still a crime, but is it worth the financial and emotional cost of a trial? Also, what if the perpetrator is the only family member available to provide care? If so, launching a criminal investigation and punishing this individual could be more disruptive and cause greater harm to the victim. For these and other reasons outlined above, elder abuse is very rarely prosecuted [76]. In a convenience sample of substantiated cases of financial exploitation alone or co-occurring with other types of elder abuse, Jackson and Hafemeister [53, 54] found that of 54 cases, only eight (15 %) were prosecuted. Navarro et al. [72] found that only 2.9 % of 239 APS financial exploitation cases were submitted to the district attorney's office for review in Los Angeles.

In summary, the primary goals in resolving financial exploitation are to advocate for the older adult, stop the loss of funds, and restore assets whenever possible. Claims against banks and credit card companies may be the best opportunity to do this, but there is limited time to file claims after funds are stolen. Sometimes the threat of arrest will motivate the perpetrator to return stolen assets if they are not already spent, but usually caseworkers and law enforcement detectives have to do significant investigative work to determine how much was stolen and how the funds were used. By the time the investigation is underway the perpetrator may have already spent the money and fled. Therefore, if the older adult still has substantial assets remaining, "stopping the bleeding" and pursuing civil action could be a viable option.

8.11 Assessing Case Resolution

Addressing the loss of funds is only one step in responding to financial exploitation. As shown in Fig. 8.1, the primary cause of financial exploitation is the perpetrator. Figure 8.2 illustrates that in order to prevent further exploitation, interventions and services (activities) are needed for both the perpetrator and victim. Since it may not be possible to sever ties between the perpetrator and the victim if that person is also a caregiver, addressing issues in their relationship or helping the perpetrator become financially independent may ameliorate much of the problem. Education could be especially effective when familial or cultural expectations are at odds with community norms.

8.11.1 Output: Measuring Service Delivery and Receipt

In order to determine the success of an intervention plan, it is necessary to assess how well the intended services were actually delivered and received. This is the output of the plan. Questions that should be answered include: How much money was lost, saved, and recovered? Did the victims receive the financial counseling, protective fiduciary arrangements and oversight they needed? Were the perpetrators removed from access to funds? Were they arrested and prosecuted? If abusers were key family supports, did they receive appropriate education and counseling? How well were these activities implemented and was the victim satisfied with the outcome?

8.11.2 Outcomes

In financial exploitation cases, the principal outcome is the safety and well-being of the older adult who was exploited. A comprehensive assessment procedure, the Elder Abuse Decision Support System (EADSS) with all measures included is available at www.eadss.org. The objective of most cases is to ensure that victims still have sufficient funds to remain safe and comfortable. Other positive outcomes include better social supports or an enhanced social network and close monitoring of finances to prevent abuse recurrence. This includes monitoring appointed guardians to ensure that inappropriate arrangements such as comingling funds and improper use of power of attorney or guardianship do not occur. As we noted, research about the effectiveness of available services to protect older persons is rare, but procedures to assess service delivery will be needed if we are to understand which approaches are effective and for which types of people. Evaluations should include measures of cost and length of services provided, amount of money that was recovered, if any, and long-term assessments of the victims' health, mental and emotional status, and satisfaction with outcomes.

8.12 Prevention

Elder abuse is a serious public health problem [15, 31, 59], and like most public health problems of the twenty-first century, the best course of action is prevention. The National Center on Elder Abuse website on prevention strategies [71] discusses four main foci for prevention: (1) abuse registries and criminal background checks; (2) addressing ageism; (3) advance planning tools; and (4) public awareness. We refer readers to this website for excellent discussion of these topics, and will comment as to how research and theory may inform these issues.

8.12.1 Abuse Registries and Criminal Background Checks

More effort is needed to identify inappropriate caregivers and to track scam artists. Some cases of elder financial exploitation involve paid caregivers who repeatedly target vulnerable older adults. To stop predatory individuals from being employed as caregivers, we need to standardize data collection systems on perpetrators and make this information available to law enforcement and potential employers. Standardization will enable investigators to track people who prey on the elderly from county to county and eventually from state to state, and ensure that people who have been convicted of elder abuse are not reemployed as elder caregivers or other professionals who provide senior services.

8.12.2 Addressing Ageism

Systematic stereotyping and marginalization of older adults lead to the sense of entitlement that enables perpetrators to justify exploitation [22]. Including measures to identify perpetrators' attitudes towards elders in abuse investigations using research tools may help to design educational programs to remediate ageist attitudes and reduce financial abuse. A look at the abuser measures in the Appendix will give a good (based on unpublished research in progress) and reasonably brief compendium of abuser risk factors, caregiver burden issues, and negative attitudes that may be predictive of financial exploitation and other forms of elder abuse.

8.12.3 Advance Planning Tools

Based on routine activity theory, capable guardians are keys to crime prevention. Upon reaching a certain age or life milestone, such as retirement, adults should have certain basic legal documents in place to designate a surrogate decision-maker in the event they no longer have capacity to make independent financial and health decisions. These legal safeguards can prevent against financial abuse and fraud and include:

- General Power of Attorney to name a person to make financial decisions when they no longer can
- Revocable Living Trust to name a trustee to make financial decisions when they no longer can and to specify the beneficiaries of the estate after death
- Healthcare Power of Attorney to appoint a person to make health care decisions when they no longer can
- Living Will or Advanced Directive to express end of life preferences, e.g., use of life supporting interventions or not
- HIPAA Authorization to authorize someone of their choice to be able to speak to the doctors when they no longer can
- Mental Health Power of Attorney for those with a psychiatric condition to authorize someone to help make decisions on their behalf if they are not making safe decisions for themselves, e.g., engaging in self-neglect, wandering out of the house, etc.

To ensure that checks and balances are in place, more than one family member or caregiver should be responsible for overseeing an older person's finances. Trusted family members or friends should make sure that beneficiary designations are as intended and that trust documents have not been altered without the older adult's permission. Bank statements should be viewed intermittently to ensure that bills are being paid on time, and that there are no unexpected expenditures. Medication use should be monitored frequently in addition to ensuring that the elder is keeping health care appointments. If there is any suspicion that someone is taking advantage of the elder or that the elder is mismanaging money, caregivers should ask questions such as those in the Older Adult Financial Exploitation Measure in the Appendix [22], and get multiple family members involved.

For caregivers, it is important to involve other family and community resources to avoid stress and isolation. For example, support from friends, relatives, and adult day health centers enable caregivers to take breaks. Even if only for a couple of hours, a temporary relief from caregiving duties can significantly reduce feelings of stress and improve psychological well-being [95].

8.12.4 Public Awareness

The rising threat of financial exploitation to an aging society has sparked the public's recognition of elder abuse as a serious problem, but most media coverage and research has focused on the victim. Logically, victims do not abuse themselves, except in cases of self-neglect. We believe the focus needs to shift on the logical cause of elder abuse: the perpetrator. Public service campaigns can be designed to educate law enforcement, family caregivers, APS, and the general public about perpetrator warning signs and risk factors that may be keys to prevention. To understand these warning signs we will need the aforementioned standardized data collection systems that include abuser measures (examples in the Appendix) so that ongoing research can be conducted.

The financial industry also has a critical role to play in the protection of older people. Exploitation of seniors is a growing concern in the financial services industry as banks and brokerages are now serving an aging client population. Firms have begun to train their employees to spot the red flags of exploitation, and have instituted procedures for how to escalate concerns so that the firm can contact local APS or law enforcement to investigate. There are also federal regulations that protect older investors. For example, the Financial Investor Regulatory Authority (FINRA) issued suitability rules that specify what investment products can be marketed and sold to older consumers given their age and investment risk profile. In addition to these regulations, FINRA issued a rulemaking item in October 2015 [39] that proposes allowing firms to place a temporary hold on the disbursement of funds or securities if a financial advisor has a reasonable belief that a client is being financially exploited. The rule also creates a duty for financial advisors to ask their new clients to specify one or more trusted "emergency contacts" upon account opening, or during the course of the firm's routine and customary business with existing clients. This gives the firm authorization to contact the specified individuals in situations where financial exploitation has occurred, is occurring, has been attempted, or will be attempted. FINRA's new rule would give firms safe harbor protection as long as they had reasonable suspicion of exploitation and were acting to protect the client. Comments on this new FINRA rule are forthcoming. If approved, the rule could potentially protect vulnerable adults, particularly those with investment assets whom perpetrators might preferentially target.

8.13 Needs for Future Research

8.13.1 Measurement

There are still significant methodological challenges impeding our understanding of elder financial exploitation. This chapter points in several directions for productive research. We noted that empirically validated measures now exist or are being developed for important constructs related to financial exploitation [22], such as abuser characteristics, social isolation, and so on (see Appendix and www.eadss.org), however there are still measurement issues that need to be addressed. For example, different racial and ethnic groups have distinct conceptualizations of what constitutes unacceptable exchange of money and other resources. Prevalence data needs to be based on culturally sensitive definitions of elder financial exploitation to ensure that underrepresented minority populations are accurately measured in national estimates. These figures will hopefully inform what interventions best respond their needs. We believe that good measurement is key and that further development will be fruitful in both clinical assessment and further theory testing.

It is important to note that existing definitions of elder financial exploitation do not differentiate between elder fraud and elder financial abuse, and in doing so they do not sufficiently account for differences between victims, perpetrators, and the context of exploitation [50]. This has important implications for determining the mechanisms and risk factors for fraud and financial abuse, and also for developing effective prevention and intervention programs. We have included abuser measures in the Appendix and are drafting papers on the quality of these measures.

Quantifying the cost of elder abuse, particularly financial exploitation, is one of the top five priorities documented in the Elder Justice Roadmap [70], a stakeholder initiative funded by the U.S. Department of Justice with support from the Department of Health and Human Services. We have yet to develop a standardized assessment of how much money is lost due to financial abuse and fraud. Estimates that are frequently cited are based of industry surveys (e.g., [64, 90]) and not rigorous scientific studies. Loss estimates should quantify the financial burden of exploitation on seniors and on society—e.g., the financial industry, Medicaid—and also show whether exploitation is becoming more or less prevalent from year to year. Validated cost figures can put a spotlight on the issue and motivate legislators to allocate more resources to prevent these types of crimes.

Longitudinal data on elder mistreatment will have a tremendous impact on the field by allowing researchers to differentiate the predictors of exploitation from the consequences. By following victims and non-victims over time, researchers can begin to answer questions such as: What are the exact changes in cognitive functioning that are precursors for financial exploitation? What are the most salient risk factors of perpetrators for each type of abuse? Why do some caregiving relationships result in exploitation whereas others do not? And what are the financial, physical, and mental health consequences of victimization? Answers to these questions will help practitioners identify and resolve areas of vulnerability before abuse occurs, and provide the right services when it does.

8.13.2 Standardized Assessment

Conrad et al. [21] work developing the Elder Abuse Decision Support System has employed standardized measures to obtain intimate and fine-grained detail for better clinical assessment, as well as valid data for empirical research (www.eadss.org). Further research is needed on how to deploy a standardized system within and across states so that data can be meaningfully compared. Once standardized systems are developed, how do caseworkers react to implementing them? If computerized, how do alleged victims react? How can data best be collected in the home setting, from financial records, and from institutions? Are computerized measures cost-effective? The resulting standardized data sets will provide large numbers of cases with great detail to enable ongoing research, and they could be immediately useful for states to evaluate the quality of their adult protection programs.

8.13.3 Services

As we noted, documentation of service delivery and receipt is essential to move the field forward in understanding what works to improve intervention for financial exploitation. Theory-based strategies such as forensic centers using multidisciplinary teams with investigation and documentation protocols should be formalized with program manuals and logic models so they can be faithfully implemented and tested in other regions. At this early point in the field, simple counts of interventions that are consistently delivered could begin to provide useful information for estimating effectiveness. The interventions could be put into a taxonomy with classification of types. Research is needed on how to train people to conduct investigations, assess service delivery and receipt, and to test whether more cases are adjudicated and more convictions obtained as a result.

8.14 Conclusion

We spent much of this chapter on theory, and we noted that recent work is pointing more to studying abuser characteristics that affect financial exploitation and other types of elder abuse. We believe that including the abuser in the APS assessment protocol is essential since this is overwhelmingly the source of the financial exploitation, but will be challenging in fraud cases where perpetrators orchestrate their schemes remotely, such as over the phone or online. The study of perpetrator characteristics is undeveloped, but it is key to understanding causation of various types of abuse. Generally, the development of standardized measures and procedures will lead to research that can clarify best practices and enable more effective prevention and intervention.

We presented only one theory about one area: financial exploitation. We must also test a myriad of theories on elder mistreatment including macro-perspectives on the ecology of elder mistreatment to micro theories that examine the motivations of abusers to commit various types of abuse. The key is obtaining the data like that presented here so as to enable theory development and testing by many researchers addressing various questions related to elder mistreatment.

Appendix: List of Measures and Brief Descriptions of Items

This appendix lists item numbers and brief descriptions of the constructs used to assess financial abuse by APS workers. Full questionnaires are available at www.eadss.org.

Abuser Risk Factor Item Numbers and Content

B1: AA history of trouble with the law, B2: AA history of violence, B3: AA history of previous abuse, B4: AA trouble keeping a job, B5: AA lack knowledge of the AV's needs, B6: AA unreliable in providing you with care and assistance, B7: AA too stressed to help you, B8: Relationship with AA drain you emotionally or wear you out, B9: AA ignore you, B10: AA seems irresponsible, B11: AA dependent on you for money, B12: AA have a drinking/alcohol problem, B13: AA abuse drugs, B14: AA have a problem with gambling, B15: AA have problems with mental illness, B19: AA have problems controlling his/her temper, B20: AA too pushy and demanding, B21: AA have a habit of telling lies, B22: AA sometimes seems out of control, B23: AA try to control your decisions too much, B24: AA complain about caring for you, B25: AA ever punish you, B26: AA expect too much of you, B27: AA live beyond his/her means, B28: AV been abusive to AA.

Victim Cognitive Status Item Numbers and Content

C4a: Disoriented to time, C4b: Disoriented to Place. C4c: Disoriented to Person, C4d: Incoherent, C4e: Poor Memory, C4f: Confused, C4g: Cannot follow conversation, C4h: Faulty judgment/reasoning.

Victim Mental Status Item Numbers and Content

C6a: Current Psychiatric DX, C6b: Bizarre behavior, C6c: Severely anxious, C6d: Unreasonably fearful, C6e: Unresponsive, C6f: Sees things that are not there, C6g: Hears voices, C6h: Compulsive behavior/hoarding, C6j: Appears depressed, C6k: Change in eating habits, C6m: Change in sleeping habits, C6n: Recent Loss, C6p: Decreased social interaction, C6q: Loss of Interest, C6r: Withdrawn, C6z: Other mental status indicators.

Victim Substance Abuse Item Numbers and Content

C9a: Substance abuse–alcohol, C9b: Substance abuse–drugs, C9c: Previous history SUD, C9d: Smells of alcohol, C9e: Slurred speech, C9f: Dilated pupils, C9g: Poor Coordination, C9h: Bottles and Cans present, C9j: Abuse of Rx or other medications, C9z: Other Substance abuse indicators.

Activities of Daily Living Item Numbers and Content

C10: Needs help with ADLs, C10a: Needs help doing housekeeping, laundry, C10b: Needs help with driving/arranging transportation, C10c: Needs help with using appliances safely, C10d: Needs help with using telephone, C10e: Needs help with seeking medical care, C10f: Self-administering medications, C10g: Needs help with Dressing and undressing self, C10h: Needs help with ADLs, C10j: Needs help with shopping for food, C10k: Needs help with Preparing Meals, C10m: Needs help with Eating, C10n: Needs help with Using Toilet, C10p: Needs help with transferring, e.g. bed to chair, C10z: Needs help with Other needs.

Alleged Abuser (AA) Strengths as Reported by Alleged Victim (AV)

C1: AA provide financial support for you, C2: AA take care of your personal needs well enough, C3: AA provide emotional support, C4: AA help you maintain activities outside the home, C5: AA do things that contribute to the well-being of your household, C7: AA is willing to work on the problem.

Alleged Abuser Strengths as Reported by Alleged Abuser

AQ2: Do you do things that show you care? AQ3: Do you provide personal care? AQ4: Do you provide financial support? AQ5: Do you provide non-monetary resources? AQ6: Do you help maintain activities outside the home?

Alleged Abuser Stress and Burden as Reported by the Alleged Abuser

AQ8: Do you feel that ___ expects too much from you? AQ9: Do you feel that you're being asked to do more than you can possibly do to care for _____? AQ10: Do you feel resentful of having to take care of _____? AQ11: Do you feel that _____ criticizes you unfairly? AQ12: Do you feel annoyed with _____? AQ13: Do you feel that because of the time you spend with _____ you don't have enough time to do things you would like to do? AQ14: Do you feel stressed between caring for your relative and trying to meet other responsibilities? AQ15: Are you fed up with taking care of _____? AQ17: Has ____ been abusive to you?

Alleged Abuser Negative Attitudes as Reported by the Alleged Abuser

AQ18: Do you feel that _____ is to blame for many of the bad things that happen to you? AQ19: Do you feel resentful of things _____ has done? AQ20: Do you feel that _____ is overly sensitive when you try to correct his/her behavior? AQ21: Do you criticize _____ a lot? AQ22: Are you angry with _____? AQ23: Do you feel bad about things you have said or done? AQ24: Do you feel like just leaving _____?

AQ25: Do you feel you have a right to AV's money and resources? AQ26: Have you felt like physically hurting _____?

Isolation as Reported by the Alleged Victim

P3OV: Have you been overmedicated, poisoned, or chemically restrained? P4CON: locked you up, tied you up, or confined you against your will, P4A: kept in a location unable to leave (for example, closet, room), P4BPHONE: not get to the phone due to physical restraints (like phone placed out of reach), P4DNOVIS: not allowed to have visitors, P4FRESTR; restrained without medical orders, N15: Does the older adult have any untreated sores, wounds, rashes, or other health conditions? N16: Is the older adult left alone without adequate supervision? E14: Has ____ abandoned or threatened to abandon you? E17: Has ____ prevented you from having contact with the outside world via telephone, newspapers, television, or radio, etc.?

Financial Exploitation

F1A: Has ____borrowed money from you but not paid it back? F2A: Has ____felt entitled to use your money for him/herself? F3A: Has ____used your money on their own behalf instead of for your benefit? F4: Have there been unexplained disappearances of your money or possessions? F5: Has ____ lied about how they were spending your money? F6: Has ____demanded money from you? F7: Did ____take advantage of you to get a hold of your resources such as a house, car, or money? F7A: Has______ lived with you, but refused to pay their share of expenses? F8: Has ____given unreasonable explanations for spending the older adult's money? F9: Has ____refused to give you an accounting of how your money was spent? F10: Has ____taken your money to do something for you but never did it? F11: Have there been unusual activities in your bank accounts, for example, large withdrawals, frequent transfers of funds? F12: Has ____said they were buying something for you, but it was really for their own use? F13: Has ____handled your money irresponsibly (for example, gambling, illegal activities)? F14: Have there been unauthorized withdrawals from your bank account? F15: Has ____taken advantage of cultural or family expectations to get your resources? F16: Has ____ persuaded you to sign any documents even though it was not in your best interest? F17: Has ____manipulated you to give him/her larger than usual gifts (money, cars, homes)? F18: Has ____ prevented you from spending your money in order to preserve their inheritance? F19: Has ____ promised care for you but then did not provide it? F20: Has ____ tricked or pressured you into buying something that you now regret buying? F21: Have your legal or financial documents been frequently changed? F22: Has ____become the payee on your benefit check and used the money for him/herself? F23: Has ____convinced you to turn the title of your home, property, farm, car, etc. over to them? F24: Has ____pressured you to modify your will? F25: Has ____ changed the direct deposit destination so as to benefit him/herself? F26: Other indicator (s) of FE.

References

1. Acierno R, Hernandez MA, Amstadter AB, Resnick HS, Steve K, Muzzy W, Kilpatrick DG. Prevalence and correlates of emotional, physical, sexual, and financial abuse and potential neglect in the United States: the national elder mistreatment study. Am J Public Health. 2010;100:292–7.
2. Acierno R, Hernandez MA, Muzzy W, Steve K. Final report: the national elder mistreatment study. Washington DC: National Institute of Justice; 2009.
3. American Bar Association (ABA)/American Psychological Association (APA) Assessment of Capacity in Older Adults Project Working Group. Assessment of older adults with diminished capacity: a handbook for psychologists. Washington: American Bar Association and American Psychological Association; 2008.
4. Anderson KB. Consumer fraud in the United States: an FTC survey. The Federal Trade Commission. 2004. http://www.ftc.gov/reports/consumer-fraud-us-ftc-survey-august-2004.
5. Anderson KB. Consumer fraud in the United States: the second FTC survey. The Federal Trade Commission. 2007. http://www.ftc.gov/reports/consumer-fraud-united-states-second-federal-trade-commission-survey.
6. Anderson KB. Consumer fraud in the United States, 2011: the third FTC survey. The Federal Trade Commission. 2013. http://www.ftc.gov/os/2013/04/130419fraudsurvey.pdf.
7. Anetzberger GJ. Elder abuse: risk. In: Jamieson A, Moenssens AA, editors. Wiley encyclopedia of forensic science. Chichester: Wiley; 2013. doi:10.1002/9780470061589.fsa480.
8. Beach SR, Schulz R, Castle NG, Rosen J. Financial exploitation and psychological mistreatment among older adults: differences between African Americans and non-African Americans in a population-based survey. Gerontologist. 2010;50(6):744–57.
9. Beals ME, Carr DC, Mottola GR, Deevy MJ, Carstensen LL, How does survey context impact self-reported fraud victimization? Gerontologist. 2015a; gnv082.
10. Beals ME, DeLiema M, Deevy MJ. A framework for a taxonomy of fraud. Report by the Stanford Center on Longevity. 2015b. http://longevity3.stanford.edu/framework-for-a-taxonomy-of-fraud/.
11. Bernatz S. Undue influence. In: Assessment of older adults with diminished capacity: a handbook for psychologists. Washington DC: American Bar Association Commission on Law and Aging and American Psychological Association; 2008. p. 114–17.
12. Blakely BE, Dolon R. Perceptions of adult protective services workers of the support provided by criminal justice professionals in a case of elder abuse. J Elder Abuse Negl. 2001;12(3–4):71–94.
13. Blum B. The "IDEAL" protocol for undue influence—an introduction. NCPJ Life Times. 2003;2(7):1–4.
14. Bonnie R, Wallace R. Elder mistreatment: abuse, neglect, and exploitation in an aging America. National Research Council (U. S.). Washington: National Academies Press; 2003.

15. Centers for Disease Control. Understanding elder abuse: fact sheet. National Center for Injury Prevention and Control Division of Violence Prevention. 2013. http://www.cdc.gov/features/elderabuse/.
16. Chang J, Moon A. Korean American elderly's knowledge and perceptions of elder abuse: a qualitative analysis of cultural factors'. J Multicult Soc Work. 1997;6(1/2):139–54.
17. Choi NG, Kulick DB, Mayer J. Financial exploitation of elders: analysis of risk factors based on county adult protective services data. J Elder Abuse Negl. 1999;10(3–4):39–62.
18. Cohen LE, Felson M. Social change and crime rate trends: a routine activity approach. Am Sociol Rev. 1979;52:170–83.
19. Coleman JW. Toward an integrated theory of white-collar crime. Am J Sociol. 1987;93:406–39.
20. Connolly MT. Where elder abuse and the justice system collide: police power, parens patriae, and 12 recommendations. J Elder Abuse Negl. 2010;22(1–2):37–93.
21. Conrad KJ, Iris M, Riley BB, Mensah E, Mazza J. Developing end-user criteria and a prototype for an elder abuse assessment system, document no. 241390. National Institute of Justice Grant #2009-IJ-CX-0202; 2013.
22. Conrad KJ, Iris M, Ridings JW, Langley K, Wilber KH. Self-report measure of financial exploitation of older adults. Gerontologist. 2010;50(6):758–73.
23. Conrad KJ, Iris M, Ridings JW, Fairman KP, Rosen A, Wilber KH. Conceptual model and map of financial exploitation of older adults. J Elder Abuse Negl. 2011;23(4):304–25.
24. Conrad KJ, Liu P, Beach S, Iris M. Testing a theory of financial exploitation of older adults. The Gerontol. 2015;55(Suppl 2):834.
25. Consumer Sentinel Network Data Book for January–December 2010. Federal Trade Commission. 2011. www.ftc.gov/sentinel/reports/sentinel-annual-reports/sentinel-cy2010.pdf. Accessed 25 July 2011.
26. DeLiema M. Using mixed methods to identify the characteristics of older fraud victims. Dissertation. University of Southern California; 2015.
27. DeLiema M, Gassoumis ZD, Homeier DC, Wilber KH. Determining prevalence and correlates of elder abuse using promotores: low-income immigrant Latinos report high rates of abuse and neglect. J Am Geriatr Soc. 2012;60(7):1333–9.
28. Doerner WG, Lab SP. Victimology. Newark: Lexis Nexis Matthew Bender; 2008.
29. Dong X, Chang ES, Wong E, Wong B, Simon MA. How do US Chinese older adults view elder mistreatment? Findings from a community-based participatory research study. J Aging Health 2010;23(2):289–312.
30. Dong X, Simon MA. Is greater social support a protective factor against elder mistreatment? Gerontology. 2008;54(6):381–8.
31. Dong X, Simon MA. Elder abuse as a risk factor for hospitalization in older persons. JAMA Intern Med. 2013;173(10):911–7.
32. Dong X, Simon M, Evans D. Elder self-neglect is associated with increased risk for elder abuse in a community-dwelling population findings from the Chicago Health and Aging Project. J Aging Health. 2013;25(1):80–96.
33. Dong X, Simon M, Rajan K, Evans DA. Association of cognitive function and risk for elder abuse in a community-dwelling population. Dement Geriatr Cogn Disord. 2011;32(3):209–315.
34. Dong X, Chen R, Simon MA. Elder abuse and dementia: a review of the research and health policy. Health Aff. 2014;33(4):642–9.
35. Dong X, Zhang M, Simon M. The expectation and perceived receipt of filial piety among Chinese older adults in the Greater Chicago area. J Aging Health. 2014;26(7):1225–47.
36. Elder Justice Coordinating Council. Eight recommendations from the elder justice coordinating council for increased federal involvement in addressing elder abuse, neglect, and exploitation. 2013. http://www.aoa.acl.gov/AoA_Programs/Elder_Rights/EJCC/index.aspx.
37. Enguidanos S, DeLiema M, Aguilar I, Lambrinos J, Wilber KH. Multicultural voices: attitudes of older adults in the United States about elder abuse. Ageing Soc. 2014;34:877–903.
38. Farran CJ. Theoretical perspectives concerning positive aspects of caring for elderly persons with dementia: stress/adaptation and existentialism. Gerontologist. 1997;37:250–7.
39. FINRA. Regulatory notice 15-37: financial exploitation of seniors and other vulnerable adults. 2015. http://www.finra.org/industry/notices/15-37.
40. Garre-Olmo J, Planas-Pujol X, López-Pousa S, Juvinyà D, Vilà A, Vilalta-Franch J. Prevalence and risk factors of suspected elder abuse subtypes in people aged 75 and older. J Am Geriatr Soc. 2009;57(5):815–22.
41. Gassoumis ZD, Navarro AE, Wilber KH. Protecting victims of elder financial exploitation: the role of an Elder Abuse Forensic Center in referring victims for conservatorship. Aging Ment Health. 2015;19(9):790–98.
42. Getgen D, Mill L. Financial exploitation investigation protocols for APS. Presentation at National Adult Protective Services Association Conference, 2013. 2013. http://www.napsa-now.org/wp-content/uploads/2013/10/Financial-Exploitation-Investigations-Protocols-for-APS.pdf. Downloaded 15 Sept 2015.
43. Gibson SC, Greene E. Assessing knowledge of elder financial abuse: a first step in enhancing prosecutions. J Elder Abuse Negl. 2013;25(2):162–82.
44. Goergen T, Beaulieu M. Criminological theory and elder abuse research—fruitful relationship or worlds apart? Ageing Int. 2010;35(3):185–201.
45. Gunther J. The Utah cost of financial exploitation. 2011. dhs.utah.gov/pdf/utah-financial-exploitation-study.pdf. Retrieved 10 Sept 2015.
46. Han SD, Boyle PA, James BD, Yu L, Bennett DA. Mild cognitive impairment is associated with poorer decision-making in community-based older persons. J Am Geriatr Soc. 2015; 63(4):676–83.
47. Heisler C, Stiegel LA. Enhancing the justice system's response to elder abuse: discussions and recommendations of the "Improving Prosecution" working group of the National Policy Summit on Elder Abuse. J Elder Abuse Negl. 2002;14(4):31–54.
48. Holtfreter K, Reisig MD, Pratt TC. Low self-control, routine activities, and fraud victimization. Criminology. 2008;46 (1):189–220.
49. Jackman MR. Violence in social life. Annu Rev Sociol. 2002;28:387–415.
50. Jackson SL. The vexing problem of defining financial exploitation. J Financ Crime. 2015;22(1):63–78.
51. Jackson SL, Hafemeister TL. Financial abuse of elderly people vs. other forms of elder abuse: assessing their dynamics, risk factors, and society's response. Final Report to U.S. Department of Justice (Document. No. 233613); 2011.
52. Jackson SL, Hafemeister TL. Pure financial exploitation vs. hybrid financial exploitation co-occurring with physical abuse and/or neglect of elderly persons. Psychol Violence. 2012;2(3):285–96.
53. Jackson SL, Hafemeister TL. Understanding elder abuse: new directions for developing theories of elder abuse occurring in domestic settings (June 11, 2013). Research in Brief, National Institute of Justice, June 2013. Available at SSRN: https://ssrn.com/abstract=2277633.
54. Jackson SL, Hafemeister TH. How do abused elderly persons and their adult protective services caseworkers view law enforcement involvement and criminal prosecution, and what impact do these views have on case processing? J Elder Abuse Negl. 2013b; 25(3):1–27.

55. Johannesen M, LoGiudice D. Elder abuse: a systematic review of risk factors in community-dwelling elders. Age Ageing. 2013;42:292–8.
56. Karp N. Protecting older investors: the challenge of diminished capacity. Generations. 2012;36(2):33–8.
57. Kemp BJ, Mosqueda LA. Elder financial abuse: an evaluation framework and supporting evidence. J Am Geriatr Soc. 2005; 53(7):1123–7.
58. Lachs M, Berman J. Under the radar: New York State elder abuse prevalence study, lifespan of greater Rochester, Inc.; Weill Cornell Medical Center of Cornell University; and New York City Department for the Aging. 2011. http://ocfs.ny.gov/main/reports/Under%20the%20Radar%2005%2012%2011%20final%20report.pdf.
59. Lachs MS, Williams CS, O'Brien S, Pillemer KA, Charlson ME. The mortality of elder mistreatment. J Am Med Assoc: JAMA. 1998;280(5):428–32.
60. Laumann EO, Leitsch SA, Waite LJ. Elder mistreatment in the United States: prevalence estimates from a nationally representative study. J Gerontol Ser B Psychol Sci Soc Sci. 2008;63(4): S248–54.
61. Marson DC, Hebert K, Solomon A. Assessing civil competencies in older adults with dementia: consent capacity, financial capacity, and testamentary capacity. In: Larrabee GJ, editor. Forensic neuropsychology: a scientific approach. 2nd ed. New York: Oxford University Press; 2011. p. 401–37.
62. Marson D, Sabatino C. Financial capacity in an aging society. Generations. 2012;36(2):6–11.
63. Martin RC, Okonkwo OC, Hill J, Griffith HR, Triebel K, Bartolucci A, Marson DC. Medical decision-making capacity in cognitively impaired Parkinson's disease patients without dementia. Mov Disord. 2008;23(13):1867–74.
64. MetLife Mature Market Institute. Broken trust: elders, family, and finances. 2009. https://www.metlife.com/mmi/research/broken-trust-elder-abuse.html#findings. Retrieved 18 Dec 2015.
65. Meirson A. Prosecuting elder abuse: setting the gold standard in the Golden State. Hastings Law J. 2008;60:431–52.
66. Miller ML, Johnson JL. Protecting America's seniors: what local prosecutors are doing to fight elder abuse. American Prosecutors Research Institute: Bureau of Justice Assistance, Office of Justice Programs, US Department of Justice; 2003.
67. Moon A, Williams O. Perceptions of elder abuse and help-seeking patterns among African-American, Caucasian American, and Korean-American elderly women. Gerontologist. 1993;33 (3):386–95.
68. Moye J, Marson DC. Assessment of decision-making capacity in older adults: an emerging area of practice and research. J Gerontol Ser B Psychol Sci Soc Sci. 2007;62(1):P3–11.
69. National Center on Elder Abuse. The national elder abuse incidence study. 1998. www.aoa.gov/AoARoot/AoA_Programs/Elder_Rights/Elder_Abuse/docs/ABuseReport_Full.pdf. Retrieved 10 Sept 2015.
70. National Center on Elder Abuse. Elder justice roadmap project report. 2014. http://www.ncea.aoa.gov/Library/Gov_Report/index.aspx. Retrieved 10 Dec 2015.
71. National Center on Elder Abuse. Prevention strategies. 2015. http://www.ncea.aoa.gov/Stop_Abuse/Prevention/Strategies/index.aspx. Retrieved 21 Sept 2015.
72. Navarro AE, Gassoumis ZD, Wilber KH. Holding abusers accountable: an elder abuse forensic center increases criminal prosecution of financial exploitation. Gerontologist. 2013;53 (2):303–12.
73. Pillemer K. The dangers of dependency: new findings on domestic violence against the elderly. Soc Probl. 1985;33(2):146–58.
74. Ploeg J, Fear J, Hutchison B, MacMillan H, Bolan G. A systematic review of interventions for elder abuse. J Elder Abuse Negl. 2009;21:187–210.
75. Quinn MJ. Undoing undue influence. Generations. 2000; 24(2):65–9.
76. Quinn MJ, Heisler CJ. The legal system: civil and criminal responses to elder abuse and neglect. Public Policy Aging Rep. 2002;12(2):8–14.
77. Rabiner DJ, O'Keeffe J, Brown D. A conceptual framework of financial exploitation of older persons. J Elder Abuse Negl. 2005;16(2):53–73.
78. Rabiner DJ, Brown D, O'Keeffe J. Financial exploitation of older persons: policy issues and recommendations for addressing them. J Elder Abuse Negl. 2005;16:65–84. doi:10.1300/J084v16n01_04.
79. Rooney M. Justice for all: ending elder abuse, neglect, and financial exploitation. Hearing before the U.S. Senate Special Committee on Aging, 112th Congress; 2011.
80. Rosen M, Rosenheck R, Shaner A. Payee relationships: institutional payees versus personal acquaintances. Psychiatr Rehabil J. 2003;26:262–9.
81. Sanchez YM. Distinguishing cultural expectations in assessment of financial exploitation. J Elder Abuse Negl. 1997;8(2):49–59.
82. Schonfeld L, Larsen RG, Stiles PG. Behavioral health services utilization among older adults identified within a state abuse hotline database. Gerontologist. 2006;46(2):193–9.
83. Schafer MH, Koltai J. Does embeddedness protect? Personal network density and vulnerability to mistreatment among older American adults. J Gerontol Ser B Psychol Sci Soc Sci. 2014;70 (4):597–606.
84. Spiegel DR. Financial exploitation of seniors. Washington: Washington Lawyer; 2011.
85. Stein K. A primer on outcomes-based evaluation for elder abuse projects, programs, and training. Washington: National Center on Elder Abuse; 2007.
86. Stiegel LA. An overview of elder financial exploitation. Generations. 2012;36(2):73–80.
87. Tarlow BJ, Wisniewski SR, Belle SH, Rubert M, Ory MG, Gallagher-Thompson D. Positive aspects of caregiving contributions of the REACH project to the development of new measures for Alzheimer's caregiving. Res Aging. 2004;26(4):429–53.
88. Titus RM, Heinzelmann F, Boyle JM. Victimization of persons by fraud. Crime Delinq. 1995;41:54–72.
89. Triebel KL, Marson DC. The warning signs of diminished financial capacity in older adults. Generations. 2012;36(2):39–45.
90. True Link. The True Link report on elder financial abuse 2015. 2015. https://www.truelinkfinancial.com/research.
91. U.S. Department of Justice. Society's response to financial exploitation. 2013. http://www.justice.gov/elderjustice/research/societys-response-to-financial-exploitation.html. Accessed 17 Sept 2015.
92. Wallace H. Victimology: legal, psychological, and social perspectives. Boston: Pearson A&B; 2007.
93. Wilber KW. Material abuse of the elderly: when is guardianship a solution? In: Dejowski E, editor. Protecting judgment-impaired adults: issues, interventions and policies. Binghamton: Haworth Press; 1990. p. 89–104.
94. Wilber KH, Reynolds SL. Introducing a framework for defining financial abuse of the elderly. J Elder Abuse Negl. 1997;8(2):61–80.
95. Zarit SH, Stephens MAP, Townsend A, Greene R. Stress reduction for family caregivers: effects of adult day care use. J Gerontol Ser B Psychol Sci Soc Sci. 1998;53B(5):S267–77.

Part III

Clinical Assessment and Management of Elder Abuse

9 Screening for Elder Abuse: Tools and Effectiveness

Margot J. Schofield

Elder abuse has been defined as "a single or repeated act or lack of appropriate action, occurring within any relationship where there is an expectation of trust which causes harm or distress to an older person" [162]. This consensus definition was adopted by the World Health Organization [168], and other key bodies such as the International Network for Prevention of Elder Abuse (INPEA). It highlights the complexity of this latent construct, which incorporates concepts of the multiple types of abuse, characteristics of the abuser and abuse victim, the nature of the relationship between abuser and person abused, whether suffering is experienced by the abuse victim, the intention of the behaviour, whether the abuse is an act of commission (abuse) or omission (neglect), and the context of the abuse [41].

Many have called for more comprehensive approaches to the measurement or screening of elder abuse and neglect that reflect this complexity [38, 35, 41], but many challenges remain to achieve this. This chapter undertakes a systematic review of research between 1995 and 2015 of screening measures for elder abuse or neglect that have been at least partially validated, and discusses methodological issues associated with the development of effective screening instruments in this challenging area. Others have proposed that there is inadequate research to support the effectiveness of screening [125, 126], and highlighted the need for more research to determine whether screening is indicated. Thus, the review will also examine the limited evidence that addresses the effectiveness of screening, and the research, policy and practice implications emerging from the review.

M.J. Schofield (✉)
Department of Psychology and Counselling, La Trobe University, Melbourne, VIC 3086, Australia
e-mail: m.schofield@latrobe.edu.au

M.J. Schofield
School of Psychology and Public Health, La Trobe University, Melbourne, VIC 3086, Australia

X. Dong (ed.), *Elder Abuse*, DOI 10.1007/978-3-319-47504-2_9

9.1 Screening for Elder Abuse

Screening for elder abuse is defined as a process of eliciting information about abusive experiences in a caring or family relationship from older or vulnerable adults who do not have obvious sign of abuse such as physical injuries [126]. The rationale for screening among non-symptomatic people, is that it may identify abuse not otherwise known, prevent future abuse, and reduce risk of future health impacts as a result of the elder abuse [126]. Screening is considered particularly important for problems with serious health implications, and where overall rates of identification are considered to be low. This is certainly the case for elder abuse and neglect [8, 144].

A cornerstone of effective screening is the development of valid and reliable screening measures with low measurement error. This has proved to be a challenging task, not only because of the methodological issues identified above, but because elder abuse, like other forms of family and interpersonal violence, is a largely hidden phenomenon, occurring in the home or institutions, usually without witnesses [93]. Victims are often reluctant to disclose the abuse [115, 137] because of shame or fear of being judged [22], failure to identify the behavior as abusive [132], dependence on the abuser, or feeling that the abuse is their fault [113]. Furthermore, elder abuse is poorly understood in the community and, as for domestic violence, there can a reluctance to question or interfere with what goes on within families.

The many faces of elder abuse add further complexity. While physical, sexual and, to some extent, financial forms of abuse are more readily measured and verified, other forms such as psychological, emotional, verbal, and coercive abuse, and neglect and abandonment are much more difficult to verify, or even for the elder to understand. Yet, these are the most prevalent forms of elder abuse [148]. In addition to the difficulties of measurement and identification of abuse, a number of other barriers have been noted by health professionals that impact on their ability to screen elders in their care. These include lack of time, lack of knowledge, lack of confidence that there are adequate resources and systems to address potential elder abuse, gaining sufficient privacy to ask the sensitive questions about abuse, and lack of skills in eliciting reports of abusive acts or situations [144].

There is a clear need for better measures of these more hidden forms of abuse since research has demonstrated considerable health impact of abuse and neglect [56, 50, 94, 109, 148]. In response, there has been growing interest over the past three decades in the development of valid and reliable screening instruments designed to detect risk of elder abuse and neglect in different contexts. Screening measures have been categorised in different ways. For instance, Cohen [25] categorised screening instruments into three groups based on both method and intention of the screening instrument. The first group comprised direct questioning tools that ask about the elders' experience, the second group were tools that assess signs of actual abuse, and the third group were measures designed to assess risk of abuse. Each of these have both strengths and limitations as screening measures, and Cohen has argued for a comprehensive screening model that incorporates all 3 forms of screening. The majority of screening instruments incorporate the direct questioning method, and assessment of risk of abuse. Those that assess signs of actual abuse tend to be used more in the phase of substantiating abuse [8] and are not the primary focus of this review on screening.

Direct questioning tools comprise a set of screening questions that are intended to be completed either by the elders themselves or by a health professional or researcher asking questions of the elder. Direct questioning tools tend to ask whether the elder has experienced a range of abusive behaviors by a caregiver or someone known to them, and they depend on the elders' willingness and ability to disclose abusive behaviors. Examples of direct questioning items about abuse include questions such as "Has anyone tried to hurt or harm you recently?", "Has anyone made you feel afraid?", or "Has anyone taken any of your belongings without your permission?". Direct questioning tools are useful to researchers who seek to establish prevalence and risk factors of abuse in certain populations, or who need to screen a larger population to identify those who have experienced potentially abusive actions. They are also used by clinicians to screen for abuse among elderly patients presenting in primary care or hospital settings to better understand the nature of care relationships and the possible contribution of abuse to the medical presentation.

Another common approach to screening are questions that probe for risk indicators for abuse. This has been justified because it can be difficult to get reliable answers to questions about direct abuse, and because risk factors have been demonstrated to reliably discriminate between abuse and non-abuse cases [26, 139]. Examples of the risk factor approach include checklists of risk factors assessed by professionals such as the Indicators of Abuse Screen (IOA) [139], and self-complete questionnaires about risk factors such as the Vulnerability to Abuse Screening Scale (VASS) [146]. Risk factors may include both client and care-giver factors associated with abuse, as well as characteristics of the situation. Many measures combine types of questions, including direct questions about specific behaviors, actual harm caused, and risk indicator.

Another way of categorising screening instruments is to consider the setting and purpose of the screening tool. One set of screening instruments have been designed for mass screening of elders and/or their caregivers at the community or population level. Another set of instruments has been designed for more targeted screening among elderly in health, welfare and institutional service settings. The following review of elder abuse and neglect screening instruments classifies them broadly into these two categories, primarily based on the intention when the scale was developed, and the context of the original validation studies. It is acknowledged however, that some instruments can potentially be used both ways. The chapter also separately reviews scales that have been developed to screen specifically for elder neglect and self-neglect, since these constructs pose additional measurement challenges as they seek to assess the absence of caring behaviour, rather than the presence of abusive behaviour.

9.2 Systematic Literature Search for Screening Measures for Elder Abuse and Neglect

A systematic literature search was undertaken to identify and review validated screening measures for elder abuse and neglect. A search was made of English language articles on two key electronic databases, Medline and Psych Info, from 1995 to 2015. The terms entered were: (exp Elder Abuse OR ["elder abuse" or "elder mistreatment" or "elder neglect" or "elder self neglect" or "elder financial abuse" or "elder financial mistreatment" or "elder sexual abuse"] AND (exp Screening [or exp Mass screening] OR [measurement or screening or survey* or questionnaire* or observation*). The Psych Info search produced 312 records and the Medline search produced 392 records, making a total of 704 records. An additional 65 records were identified using manual searches and reference lists of reviewed articles. After excluding 155 duplicate or irrelevant records, there were 614 records remaining. Abstracts were first reviewed, and then the full article for those deemed potentially relevant were assessed. After the review of abstracts, a further 274 were excluded: 39 not applicable, 50 books, and 116 non-empirical articles. The remaining 340 records were

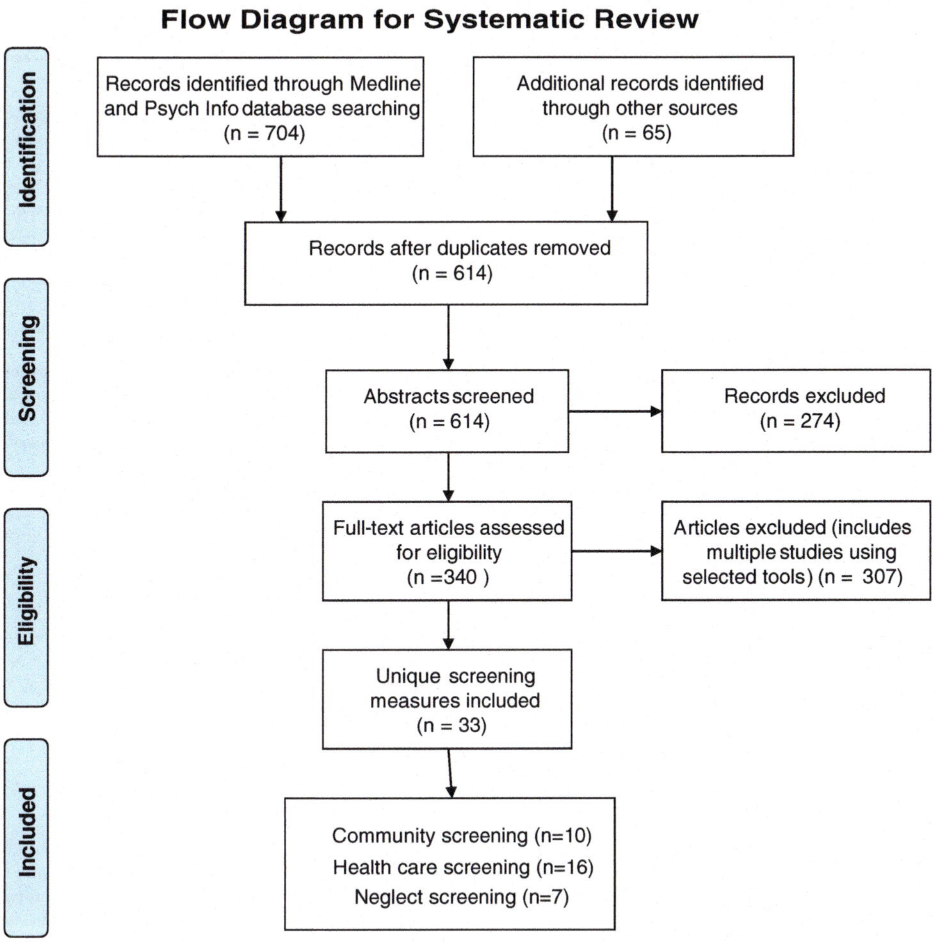

Fig. 9.1 Flow diagram for systematic review

retrieved and reviewed. From this more detailed review, a total of 33 screening tools met the minimum criteria of having detailed the development of the scale, reported items and scale structure, and some evidence of psychometric evaluation. A total of 10 scales were designed for use in community-based screening, 16 for screening in healthcare settings, and a further 7 scales are designed to screen specifically for neglect and self-neglect. These are reviewed in the following three sections (Fig. 9.1).

9.3 Measures for Community-Based Screening for Elder Abuse and Neglect

Community-based screening measures aim to identify the prevalence and determinants of elder abuse in the community. These measures are suitable for use in research (e.g., to assess prevalence and risk factors), as well as for screening older people who access services to determine who are at risk of abuse or neglect. They can be self-completed or administered via interview. Ten scales were identified that met the review criteria of being designed primarily for use in community-based studies, and including some reliability and validity evaluation. A critical review of these measures is described in the next section. Key characteristics of these measures are summarised in Table 9.1, with details related to the origin of the scale, the number of items and subscales, the intended respondent for the measures and the method of administration. In addition, details of the psychometric properties of each scale are provided along with the types of samples on which the validation was undertaken. A summary of strengths and limitations of each measure is also provided. It is noted that there are other large scale community studies published in the 1995–2015 period, but were not included due to inadequate description of the measure, or inadequate reporting of psychometrics.

9.3.1 Abuse of the Elderly in the European Region (ABUEL)

The Abuse of the Elderly in the European Region (ABUEL) study is one of the very few cross-cultural studies available that have used a common elder abuse scale [103, 108, 111,

Table 9.1 Validated measures for screening for elder abuse and neglect at population level

Screening measure	Authors (year)	Origin	Items/subscales	Respondent and method	Psychometric properties	Validation samples	Strengths and limitations	Studies using scale (whole or part)
Abuse of the Elderly in the European region (ABUEL)	Lindert et al. [103] Macassa et al. [108], [111]. Soares et al. [153]	Based on the CTS2 [156] and the UK study of abuse/neglect of older people [16]	52 items measuring severity and chronicity of abuse: Psychol. abuse (11; 6 severe, 5 minor); Physical abuse (17; 10 severe, 7 minor); Injuries (7; 4 severe, 3 minor); Sexual abuse (8; 5 severe, 3 minor); Financial abuse (9; 5 severe, 4 minor); frequency of abuse 8 pt. scale; Neglect-unmet needs (13); Perpetrator's main characteristics where abuse occurred	Elder interview or self-completed written questionnaire	Internal reliability Cronbach's α across countries: Psychological Abuse: = 0.85 Physical Abuse: = 0.80 Injury: = 0.72 Sexual Abuse: = 0.76 Financial Abuse: = 0.71; Validity: Associated with some hypothesized constructs such as gender and mental health	Representative community samples aged 60–84 years from cities in 7 European countries (N = 4467, 57 % women): Germany; Greece; Italy; Lithuania; Portugal; Spain, Sweden Varied sampling strategies used: registry, random, or cluster	Measures both chronicity and severity; Good reliability; No validity data; Measure used across 7 European countries, but varied sampling and modes of administration; sample restricted to large cities;	
Abuse and Violence against Older Women (AVOW)	De Donder et al. [40]; Lang et al. [96]	Based on WHO definition including 6 different types of abuse [168] and adaptation of CTS	34 indicators adapted from CTS: Neglect and emotional abuse 9 items each; financial, physical, sexual abuse and violation of personal rights —4 items each; Responses for last year on 4-point frequency scale. Validation reduced scale to 22 items	Elder self-report: postal survey, face-to-face interview, or telephone interview	Used item analysis to reduce items to 22 indicators that maximised reliability of prevalence estimates; Concurrent validity tested by examining relationship between abuse and quality of life	2880 home-dwelling older women aged 60 and over from 5 European countries	Large sample across 5 countries Relatively limited psychometrics undertaken. Did not test internal consistency reliability and validity tests limited	
Conflict Tactics Scale (CTS)	Straus [155]	Measures extent to which family members (e.g. Couples) engage in psychological and physical attacks on each other and use of negotiation to deal with conflicts; Items derived from conflict theory	19 item questionnaire; 3 subscales: • Violence: 9, • Verbal aggression: 6 • Reasoning: 3 Items range low-high coerciveness, rated frequency in past year: "Never" to "More than 20 times. Items summed	Developed for any family relationship. Items usually asked in pairs: whether respondent has enacted each behavior and whether the other party has (38 items). Can be completed by one or both parties	Cronbach α = 0.79–0.88 for Violence and Verbal Aggression, 0.50–0.76 for Reasoning, for different types of relationships	Nationally representative sample of 2143 couples in the US	Suitable for clinical settings; Easy to administer; Relatively brief; Not specific to elderly; Limited forms of abuse; Does not assess neglect, coercion, financial abuse; Violence scores very skewed, often dichotomised for analysis	Burnes et al. [17]; Chokkanathan and Lee [23]; Fulmer and Gurland [78]; Fulmer et al. [75]; Naughton et al. [122]

(continued)

Table 9.1 (continued)

Screening measure	Authors (year)	Origin	Items/subscales	Respondent and method	Psychometric properties	Validation samples	Strengths and limitations	Studies using scale (whole or part)
Conflict Tactics Scale version 2 (CTS2)	Straus et al. [156]	Modified from CTS, added Injury and Sexual Coercion scales	78 item questionnaire (2 × 39 items for abusive acts by partner and by self); 5 subscales: Phys. assault: 12, Psych Aggress: 8, Negotiation: 6, Injury: 6, Sexual coercion: 7	Elder self-report about self and partner's behaviour; Can also be completed by carer	Validated on sample of university students in relating to partners: Cronbach's $\alpha = 0.79–0.95$ for the subscales; Some construct and discriminant validity demonstrated	317 undergrad. US students	Suitable for clinical settings or research; Easy to administer; Lengthy; Not specific to elderly; Does not assess neglect, coercion, financial abuse	Beach et al. [14]; Biggs et al. [16]; Cooper et al. [36, 37]; Fraga et al. [68]; Lowenstein et al. [106]; Melchiorre et al. [111]; Yan and Tang [173, 174]
Modified Conflict Tactics Scale (MCTS)	Beach et al. [14]	Modified from the CTS: Caregivers and care recipients were asked how often (5-pt Likert scale from "never" to "most of the time")	10 items each for caregiver and elder; 5 items Psych. Mistreatment, 5 physical abuse	Interviews with carer and care-recipient dyads	Reliability on 10 items: $\alpha = 0.69$ elders, $\alpha = 0.67$ caregivers; Convergent and discriminant validity [38]	265 Family carers and care recipient dyads, Family Relationships in Late Life Project, multisite longitudinal study of informal care in 3 US communities	Brief, easily administered	Cooper et al. [35, 36]
Modified Caregiver Strain Index (MCSI)	Thornton and Travis [159]	Modified from CSI—changed yes/no response to 3 options: yes, sometimes, no	13 item questionnaire; Items cover Employment, Financial, Physical, Social, and Time strains	Non-professional care-giver	Reliability $\alpha = 0.90$; Test–retest rel $\alpha = 0.88$	158 family caregivers aged 53 and older in community, mean age 61	Effective in identifying families at risk; Easy and quick to administer No report from Elder	
Elder Mistreatment (own scale)	Dong [42]	Psychol/physical abuse items from CTS; Caregiver neglect from 2 measures of unmet needs—Katz Activities of Daily Living (1983) and Lawton and Brody IADL (1963); Financial Exploitation from Conrad et al. [33]	56 item self-report measure: Psychological abuse 8 items from CTS; Physical abuse 10 items from CTS; Sexual abuse 2 items (own); Care-giver neglect—20 items on unmet needs; Financial exploitation 17 items	Trained multicultural and multilingual interviewers conducted face-to-face interviews with elders in home	Not calculated for this study, relied on scales having been previously validated; Provided estimates for different restrictiveness criteria in defining overall elder mistreatment;	The Population Study of Chinese Elderly in Chicago N = 3159 aged 60+, living in community	Measured each of main types of elder abuse; Drew mainly on selection of validated scales; Clearly defined scoring system for determining caseness; No reliability or validity statistics for this study	
Native Elder Life Scale (NELS)	Jervis et al. [84]	Developed by Native American community elders and experts to fill perceived gap in financial exploitation and neglect items for Native people	NEL-Financial Exploitation (NELS-FE)—began with 26 items, reduced to 18 NEL-Neglect 12 items	Administered to elders by Native research staff	NELS-FE $\alpha = 0.65$ total, range 0.75–0.53 for Northern and SC communities; NELS-Neglect $\alpha = 0.78$ total, range 0.80–0.78 for Northern and SC communities	100 Native Americans aged 60 + recruited from tribal senior centre on Northern Plains reservation in USA ($n = 50$), and 2 protestant churches in urban South Central USA ($n = 50$)	Validation on 2 small communities of Native Americans;	
Vulnerability to Elder Abuse Scale (VASS)	Schofield and Mishra [146]	H-S/EAST + 2 additional questions: "Has anyone close to	12 item Likert Scale questionnaire; 4 subscales:	Elder—self-report research questionnaire	*Reliability* Dep $\alpha = 0.74$ Dej $\alpha = 0.44$ Vul $\alpha = 0.45$	10,421 women aged 73–78 from Australian	Very short, low cost, easy self-completion measure;	Schofield and Mishra [147]; Schofield et al. [148];

(continued)

Table 9.1 (continued)

Screening measure	Authors (year)	Origin	Items/subscales	Respondent and method	Psychometric properties	Validation samples	Strengths and limitations	Studies using scale (whole or part)
		you called you names or put you down or made you feel bad recently?" ([155]—CTS), and 'Are you afraid of anyone in your family?' (McFarland et al. [110])	Vulnerability, dependence, dejection, coercion		Coer $\alpha = 0.31$ Stable factor structure over time *Construct validity* Vulnerability and coercion factors related to relationship conflict or break up, physical and sexual abuse	Longitudinal Study on Women's Health	Vulnerabilty and coercion have face validity for abusive acts, dependence and dejection more closely related to neglect; Suitable for screening in research and clinical settings; Scale reliability adequate, modest construct validity Self-report—relies on recall and willingness to report abuse	*Modified VASS* Chang et al. [21]; Dong et al. [55, 56]; Laumann et al. [98]; Wu et al. [170]
					Predictive validity over 12 years; Coercion, dependence and dejection predict mortality; Vulnerability, coercion, and dejection predict disability (Schofield et al. [148])			
Own scale	Oh et al. [127]	Developed from literature review, reviewed by gerontological nurses, and pilot tested	Checklist of abuse in past month: 25 items, 5 for each of 5 abuse categories: emotional, verbal, economic, neglect, physical; Presence of abuse if 2 + times in last month; Total—sum of all incidents	Structured interview with elder in home	Internal reliabilities of subscales: $\alpha = 0.7–0.92$	Population based sample adults aged 65+ in one area of Seoul, Korea - N = 15,230 (52 % of population)	Population-based survey; Possible recall bias due to unwillingness to disclose; Sparse validation data	
Women's Health and Relationship Survey (WHRS)	Fisher and Regan [67]	Modified from Lachs and Pillemer [95]; and National Violence Against Women Survey [160]	15 item scale, abuse since 55 yrs, 5 factors: Psy/emot 3 items; Control 3 items; Threat 2 items; Physical 4 items; Sexual 3 items	Telephone interview with elder	Reliability of 5 subscales: $\alpha = 0.64$ $\alpha = 0.59$ $\alpha = 0.52$ $\alpha = 0.72$ $\alpha = 0.71$	842 community-dwelling women aged 60 and older	Assesses 5 types of abuse; Moderate reliability of 3 subscales; Self-report uncorroborated	

153]. It examined elder abuse among representative community samples aged 60–84 years from cities in 7 European countries (N = 4,467, 57 % women). These were: Stuttgart, Germany; Athens, Greece; Ancona, Italy; Kaunas, Lithuania; Porto, Portugal; Granada, Spain; and Stockholm, Sweden. Unfortunately varied sampling (registry, random community, cluster sampling) strategies and modes of administration (interview and self-complete written questionnaires) were used across countries. The scale was translated using recommended forward and backward translation, and some items were modified for cultural fit, although details of this are not reported.

The elder abuse questionnaire included 52 items based on the CTS2 [156] and the UK study of abuse/neglect of older people [16], although only examples of items are reported. It measured both the severity and chronicity of abuse in six domains. Psychological Abuse was assessed using 11 items (6 severe abuse, 5 minor abuse); Physical Abuse with 17 items (10 severe, 7 minor); Injuries with 7 items (4 severe, 3 minor); Sexual Abuse with 8 items (5 severe, 3 minor); Financial Abuse with 9 items (5 severe, 4 minor); Neglect—unmet needs (13). Chronicity was assessed by asking about the frequency of abuse on 8 point scale. Good internal reliability statistics are reported across countries, with Cronbach α of 0.85 for Psychological Abuse, 0.80 for Physical Abuse, 0.72 for Injury, 0.76 for Sexual Abuse, and 0.71 for Financial Abuse [153]. Validity was supported by associations with some hypothesized constructs such as gender and mental health.

9.3.2 Abuse and Violence Against Older Women (AVOW)

The Abuse and Violence against Older Women (AVOW) study undertook a formative evaluation of a newly developed elder abuse scale [96]. The scale was based on six different types of abuse defined by the World Health Organisation [168] and adaptation of items in the Conflict Tactics Scale (CTS) [155]. The original 34 items comprised domains of neglect and emotional abuse (9 items each), and financial abuse, physical abuse, sexual abuse and violation of personal rights (4 items each). Responses are provided by elders for the last year on a 4-point frequency scale. Three self-report methods of administration have been used in a large study of 2880 home-dwelling older women aged 60 and over from 5 European countries: postal survey, face-to-face interview, or telephone interview [96]. Relatively limited psychometrics have been reported, with no data available on internal consistency reliability. Rather, analysis of items with high missing data and low prevalence was used to reduce the 34 items to 22 indicators that maximised reliability of prevalence estimates. Concurrent validity was tested by examining relationships between abuse and quality of life.

9.3.3 Conflict Tactics Scale (CTS)

The Conflict Tactics Scale (CTS) was one of the earlier measures developed for assessing conflict and abusive behavior in close personal relationships [155]. It was originally designed to measure the extent to which partners in an intimate relationship engage in psychological and physical attacks on each other and their use of negotiation to deal with conflicts. The original CTS had 19 items with three validated subscales: Violence (9 items), Verbal Aggression (6 items), and Reasoning (3 items). The CTS was designed for self-completion by the couple, and is suitable for use in elder abuse research for completion by the older person and their care-giver, or simply by the elderly. Parallel forms of the scale are designed to be answered both in relation to one's own behavior towards a partner (carer) and one's experience of the partner's (carer) behavior towards the self (total 38 items).

The scale was developed based on theoretical principles derived from conflict theories [155]. It has face validity in terms of physical and psychological aggression but covers a very limited range of psychologically abusive behavior. It does not measure some important aspects of elder abuse such as coercive and intimidating behavior, sexual abuse and financial abuse. It has been found acceptable to family members, with reasonably good completion rates. There has been considerable research on the psychometric properties of the CTS, which have demonstrated moderate to high reliabilities for total scale and 3 subscales [155], and some construct and concurrent validity [155]. For instance, the internal consistency of the subscales ranged from Cronbach's alphas of 0.75–0.98, with a total scale alpha of 0.94. However, much of the early validation work has been on couples or student samples rather than on the elderly [155]. Criticisms of the CTS have included the limited range of abuse behaviors, the skewed nature of scale distributions, and limited validation. Studies using this scale have often modified the scale or used different criteria to establish elder abuse, making it difficult to compare across studies. In response to these criticisms, a revised and expanded version, the CTS2, was produced.

9.3.4 Conflict Tactics Scale V2 (CTS2)

The CTS2 represents a considerable expansion of the CTS and addressed some identified limitations [156]. It comprises a total of 78 items (2×39 pairs of items designed to measure acts by partner towards self and acts by self towards partner). The modified original scales were renamed as Physical

Assault (12 items), Psychological Aggression (8 items), and Negotiation (6 items), and two new scales were included: Injury (6 items), and Sexual Coercion (7 items). The validation sample comprised 371 undergraduate students from the US, with a mean age of 22 years, responding to the scale in relation to a dating, cohabiting or marital relationship. Reliabilities ranged from 0.79 to 0.95 for subscales and some construct and discriminant validity was demonstrated. None of the items were specific to the elderly or addressed unique forms of elder abuse. For instance, it does not address neglect, psychological coercion, or financial abuse. The CTS2, or particular subscales, have been used in a wide range of elder abuse studies, often supplemented by additional items or scales designed to tap into unique aspects of elder abuse and neglect (e.g., [14, 36, 37, 68, 106, 174]).

9.3.5 Modified Conflict Tactics Scale (MCTS)

The MCTS provides a further modification of the CTS designed more specifically for caring relationships, and with modified items suitable for elder abuse [14]. It comprises 10 items each for the elder person and 10 parallel items for their caregiver: 5 items each related to Psychological Mistreatment and 5 items for Physical Abuse, so each person answers 20 items in total. The MCTS has been validated on a sample of 265 family carer and care recipient dyads from three US cities, with moderate internal reliability on the 10 item scales ($\alpha = 0.69$ elder, 0.67 caregivers). Both convergent and discriminant validity has been established [38, 35]. The scale has been reported in further studies [36].

9.3.6 Modified Caregiver Strain Index (MCSI)

The MCSI [159] is a modification of the Caregiver Strain Index first developed by Robinson [140]. The MCSI is a 13 item questionnaire with items covering the domains of employment, financial, physical, social and time strains experienced by carers. It has been validated in a community sample of 158 family caregivers aged 53 and older, with a mean age of 61. High internal and 2-week test–retest reliabilities have been reported for the scale ($\alpha = 0.90$, 0.88, respectively). It is easy and quick to administer to those providing long-term care to a family member. Limitations of the scale are that it relies solely on the caregiver perspective, so does not take into account the elders' perspectives on possible abuse. As well, the scale does not target abuse behaviors specifically, but rather is a measure of general strain associated with the caregiving role. Its utility is most likely in identifying high strain caring dyads where more tailored assessment for elder abuse and neglect could be directed.

9.3.7 Native Elder Life Scale (NELS)

The Native Elder Life Scale (NELS) was developed by Native American community elders and experts to address unique cultural aspects of elder abuse in Native American communities [84]. In particular, it was designed to fill a perceived gap in financial exploitation and neglect items for this population. The scale is made up of two subscales: the NEL-Financial Exploitation (NELS-FE) comprised 18 items and the NELS-Neglect scales comprised 12 items. The scale is designed to be administered to elders by Native American research staff. Validation studies were undertaken in 2 small communities of Native Americans aged 60 and over ($N = 100$); a sample of 50 Native Americans were recruited from a tribal senior centre on Northern Plains reservation, and another 50 from two protestant churches in urban South Central USA. The scale demonstrated moderate reliability but with variation across the two communities for the NELS-FE. Internal consistency reliability of the NELS-FE was 0.65 total, with a range of 0.75–0.53 for the two communities. The low sample sizes may partially explain this less consistent reliability. The NELS-Neglect scale had a reliability of $\alpha = 0.78$ total, ranging from 0.80 to 0.78 for the two communities, suggesting this is the more reliable subscale. The NELS provides a useful starting point for screening Native American communities for elder abuse, but the lack of validity tests suggests much more work is needed.

9.3.8 Unnamed Korean Elder Abuse Scale

A Korean elder abuse scale contains a checklist of 25 items, 5 for each of 5 categories of abuse: emotional, verbal, economic, neglect, physical [127]. It was developed from literature reviews, then reviewed by gerontological nurses, pilot tested and refined. Respondents are asked the frequency of type of abuse in the past month. Abuse is considered present if it has occurred 2 or more times in last month, and total abuse is the sum of all incidents. Data were gathered by a structured interview in the home from a population based sample adults aged 65+ in one area of Seoul, Korea ($N = 15{,}230$, 52 % of population of area). The subscales have demonstrated internal consistency reliability with this Korean sample, with $\alpha = 0.70$–0.92. Some validation of the scale was demonstrated by expected associations with variables such as disability, sick days, cognitive function, living circumstances, economic level and family relationships. As for most elder abuse scales, validity is conditional on participant willingness to disclose abusive acts.

9.3.9 Vulnerability to Elder Abuse Scale (VASS)

The Vulnerability to Elder Abuse Scale (VASS) is a brief 12 item questionnaire designed to assess risk of elder abuse over past 12 months [146, 149]. It has 4 subscales of three items each with yes/no response options, and is supported by psychometric evaluation. The subscales are Vulnerability, Dependence, Dejection, and Coercion. Ten items were adapted from the Hwalek-Sengstock Elder Abuse Screening Test (H-S/EAST) [81, 123], with two additional questions: “Has anyone close to you called you names or put you down or made you feel bad recently?” from the CTS [155], and ‘Are you afraid of anyone in your family?’ [110]. The VASS is designed for self-completion by older adults and has been validated on a large population-based sample of 10,421 women aged 73–78 from Australian Longitudinal Study on Women’s Health [146, 149].

The four subscales were derived through factor analysis and have face and content validity. The vulnerability and coercion scales have greatest face validity for abuse as items ask direct questions about experience of abusive behavior, and have demonstrated moderate to good construct validity [146]. The dejection factor resembles a measure of depression, whereas the dependence factor seems to measure vulnerability to abuse, since frailty is a recognised risk factor [148]. Reliability of subscales is adequate only for the dependence subscale (α = 0.74), whereas the other subscales have alphas ranging from 0.45 for vulnerability to 0.31 for coercion. The factor structure has been found to be stable over time by analysis of repeated waves of the longitudinal study [146, 147, 149, 148]. Construct, convergent and discriminant validity was largely supported by correlations with hypothesized variables in the predicted direction and lack of correlations with those deemed unrelated. For instance, the vulnerability and coercion factors were correlated with relationship conflict or breakdown, and to coercive life events such as “major conflict with children”, or “being pushed, grabbed, shoved, kicked or hit” in the last 12 months but unrelated to variables such as height and body mass index [146].

The VASS has shown predictive validity for poor health outcomes over 3 years [147], and for mortality and disability outcomes over 12 years [148]. The measure is very short, easy to complete, and low cost, and is suitable for screening in research and clinical settings. Like most screening measures, the scale is based on self-report and relies on recall and willingness to report abuse. It is also limited by having only one item measuring neglect, and none specifically measuring sexual abuse. The scale has been used and validated in a range of other studies. For instance, Dong and colleagues have used a 10-item modified version of the VASS in studies of Chinese populations in both the USA and Mainland China and demonstrated good reliability of the modified scale with these populations [21, 47, 55, 45]. It has also been incorporated into a national survey of US elderly [98], and another Chinese study [170].

9.3.10 Women’s Health and Relationship Survey (WHRS)

Women’s Health and Relationship Survey (WHRS) measured five types of abuse via telephone interview among 842 community-dwelling women aged 60–90 years in the US [67]. Factor analysis of items yielded five subscales: Psychological/emotional (3 items), control (3 items), threat (2 items), physical (4 items), and sexual abuse (3 items). The items were adapted from two sources: the Abusive Behavior Inventory [151] and the National Violence Against Women Survey [160]. For each item, women responded about whether they had experienced the behavior “since you turned 55”. Abuse was scored in four different ways: any abuse, repeated abuse (more than one type within a subscale), multiple abuse (at least two different types of abuse), and frequency of each type rated on a 5-point Likert scale from “never” to “very frequently”. Moderate reliability was provided for psychological/emotional abuse, physical abuse, and sexual abuse with Cronbach alphas ranging from 0.64 to 0.71 for these 3 subscales. Alphas for the other two scales were less than adequate at 0.59 and 0.52 (see Table 9.1). Validity is partially supported by the factor analysis into five scales, the face validity, and relationships between abused and other constructs such as the number of self-reported chronic health conditions, and specific current health conditions, although limited psychometric evaluation has been reported. The self-report data are uncorroborated, and no predictive validity has been undertaken.

9.3.11 Summary of Community-Based Screening Measures

The CTS and later modifications provided an important impetus to the field of measuring abuse and conflict in close relationships and have been widely used, particularly for research on intimate relationships. However, it is a relatively long screening measure that wasn’t developed specifically for elder abuse and fails to measure some key aspects of elder abuse and neglect. Furthermore, although it is the most widely used scale, most studies have modified it, making comparisons across studies difficult. A useful screening measure for elder abuse and neglect must be brief, easily completed and targeted to specific types of abuse most common in the phenomenon of elder abuse and neglect. While there has been a growing body of research attempting to measure elder abuse and neglect, the field has suffered by the lack of a definitive gold standard and most scales seek to measure risk or vulnerability rather than abuse per se, or combine both direct and risk or vulnerability questions. Among the brief and partially validated scales designed for community-based screening, the VASS has a number of advantages, making it one of three screening measures recognised by the Centers for Medicare and Medicaid Services [19, 150]. It is very brief and easy to complete and score (sum or mean of responses), and has been shown to have moderate reliability, and construct, concurrent, discriminative, and predictive validity, albeit that further validation work is required. In particular, further work is needed to determine sexual and financial abuse among the elderly, and to strengthen the internal reliability of some scales. It would be useful to the field to develop some consensus on an appropriate scale for community screening, so that studies could be compared more readily.

9.4 Screening for Elder Abuse and Neglect in Healthcare and Institutional Settings: Review of Measures

Compared with the relatively limited research described above on community-based screening, considerably more effort has been expended on identifying those who have experienced abuse in settings where signs and indicators of abuse may be more readily assessed. The greatest body of research on screening for elder abuse and neglect occurs in healthcare and institutional settings. A review of methods for substantiating abuse when potential victims are reported to adult protective services is beyond the scope of this chapter. The review identified 16 scales used in the period 1995–2015 that report some psychometric evaluation. These scales are shown in Table 9.2 and reviewed below.

9.4.1 Brief Abuse Screen for the Elderly (BASE)

The Brief Abuse Screen for the Elderly (BASE) is a 5-item set of screening questions that trained health care professionals ask the elderly and their care-givers [138, 139]. The items address physical, psychosocial, and financial abuse or neglect by the caregiver. It takes only about 1 min, and is suitable for clinical settings. The health care professional requires some training in how to ask the questions and interpret the responses, as no scoring method is supplied. The internal consistency reliability was found to be 0.91; inter-rater reliability 90 % (using very small sample of raters), and predictive validity ranged around 0.89–0.91. However, the scale has essentially one item for each type of abuse, so it is not a scale in the full sense.

9.4.2 Caregiver Abuse Screen for the Elderly (CASE)

The Caregiver Abuse Screen for the Elderly (CASE) is an 8-item set of screening questions designed for trained health care professionals to ask care-givers to assess the risk of abuse [138, 139]. The items address physical, psychosocial, and financial abuse or neglect by the caregiver. It takes about 1 min, and is suitable for clinical settings. The health care professional requires some training in how to ask the questions and interpret the responses, as no scoring method is supplied. The internal consistency reliability was found to be 0.71.

9.4.3 Elder Abuse and Neglect Assessment Instrument (EAI)

The Elder Abuse and Neglect Assessment Instrument (EAI), a 41-item checklist, was designed for administration by health care providers to screen elderly patients in clinical settings [77, 72]. The measure assesses both objective signs and symptoms, and subjective complaints of abuse, neglect, exploitation, and abandonment across four domains: physical, level of independence, medical, and social. Sound psychometrics have been reported based on a random sample of 501 elder emergency department patients in the US. Psychometric results include an internal consistency reliability of 0.84, test–retest reliability of 0.83, content validity index of 0.83, and inter-rate agreement of 0.84. The scale has a sensitivity of 71 % and specificity of 93 %. The scale is considered easy to administer in clinical settings though it is longer than other screening options. There is no published scoring system so it relies on clinician judgement. The checklist has been used in a variety of studies (e.g., [71, 72, 73, 74]), and progressively refined. More recent studies have used either a 44-item scale designed to identify possible markers of EM over several domains: general assessment (4 items), neglect assessment, usual lifestyle, social assessment, medical assessment, emotional and/or psychological neglect, and a summary assessment [72] or a 51-item version, the EAI-R which includes four summary assessment items: evidence of abuse, evidence of neglect, evidence of psychological abuse, and evidence of financial abuse [76]. These are rated on four-point Likert scale ranging from no evidence, probably no evidence, probably evidence, and evidence.

Table 9.2 Validated measures for screening for elder abuse and neglect in health care and institutional settings

Screening measure	Authors (year)	Origin	Items/subscales	Respondent and method	Psychometric properties	Validation samples	Strengths and limitations	Studies using this scale
Brief Abuse Screen for the 'Elderly (BASE)	Reis and Nahmiash [138]; Reis and Nahmiash [139]		5 questions; Asks interviewer to make educated guess about presence or absence of physical, psychosocial, financial abuse or neglect by caregiver	Elder and Care-giver interviewed by health professional	Reliability: $\alpha = 0.91$ Team agreement on presence or absence of abuse 90 %; Predictive validity from 0.89 to 0.91		Easy to administer; Takes 1 min; Suitable for clinical settings; Assesses elder and care-giver; Training required to administer; Does not differentiate between types of abuse; No scoring method	
Caregiver Abuse Screen for the Elderly (CASE)	Reis and Nahmiash [138]	Developed to screen for physical, psychosocial or financial abuse, and neglect by primary or other unpaid caregivers; for senior abuse intervention and research project, PROJECT CARE	8-item screening questionnaire presented to caregivers Yes/No response options Reduced to 6 items to improve validity	Caregiver; Written questionnaire, used as part of community intervention study	Reliability: $\alpha = 0.71$ for 6-item version; Good construct, concurrent and convergent validity reported; discriminated abusing from non-abusing caregivers; 2 factors: general abuse and neglect/dependence	139 caregivers: 44 abusive and 45 non-abusive caregivers of clients of health and social services, and 50 non-abusive caregivers not receiving services	Brief valid tool, useful for research; No established scoring method; Only caregiver responses; Only two dimensions assessed; Financial abuse items deleted due to poor reliability	Perez-Rojo et al. [130]
Elder Abuse and Neglect Assessment Instrument (EAI)	Fulmer et al. [77]; Fulmer et al. [72]	EAI first published in 1984, progressively refined since; Designed to administer in clinical setting	44-item checklist—subjective and objective items measure signs, symptoms, and subjective complaints of abuse, neglect, exploitation and abandonment; across 4 domains: physical, level of independence, medical, and social	Elder interviewed by health care provider (nurses)	Reliability: $\alpha = 0.84$; Test–retest $\alpha = 0.83$; Content validity index $\alpha = 0.83$; Inter-rater agreement $\alpha = 0.84$; Sensitivity 71 %; Specificity 93 %	Random sample of 501 elder ED patients	Easy to administer; Available in Spanish; Assesses indicators in elder, not carer; No scoring system; Not clearly defined and validated subscales, though neglect seems to be primary construct assessed	Abdel Rahman and El Gaafary [1]; Fulmer et al. [73, 74]
Elder Abuse Questionnaire (EAQ)	Kottwitz and Bowling [92]	Designed for screening in institutional and home settings	25 item—Likert scale response; Single Factor	Long-term care providers; Family members	Mod. Reliability: $\alpha = 0.66$ Content validity assessed by experts	Very small sample of 29 long-term care providers and family members in rural Kansas ($n = 29$)	Report by carers—accuracy of abuse reports questionable; No construct or predictive validity	
Elder Abuse Suspicion Index (EASI)	Yaffe et al. [172]	Developed from literature, WHO definition, other scales, and taxonomies; Expert review,	5 patient items (types of abuse, general dependency) and 1 clinician item (observed indicators of abuse) yes/no response format	Clinician interviews elder; Elder self-administered version	Sensitivity 0.47 Specificity 0.75	Patients aged 65 + recruited by physicians at 2 Montreal family medicine centers and government community-based health social services center	Brief; Suitable for primary care setting; Scoring problematic—any abuse, but not all items measure abuse	Yaffe et al. [171]

(continued)

Table 9.2 (continued)

Screening measure	Authors (year)	Origin	Items/subscales	Respondent and method	Psychometric properties	Validation samples	Strengths and limitations	Studies using this scale
Detection Scales for the Risk of Domestic Abuse and Self-Negligent Behavior in Elderly Persons (EDMA)	Touza et al. [161]	Based on National Centre for Elder Abuse (2000) definitions. Scale measures quality of caregiver treatment of elder	2 scales: Elder Scale (33 items), Alleged Abuser Scale (21 items); Elder Scale comprised 3 subscales, Alleged Abuser Scale comprises 3 subscales; Items rated on 5-point Likert scale	Social Services professionals rate elders and caregivers	Total and subscale alphas were high, ranging from 0.93 for Total Elder Scale to 0.73 for self-neglect; Total Elder Scale discriminated abuse and neglect well, with good sensitivity and specificity (93 %, 88 %)	46 Social Services professionals from Majorca, Spain completed scale on 278 elders 65 and older, with 65 % women	First screening instrument to be validated in Spain; Good psychometric properties; Assesses both elder and caregiver risk; Small sample of professionals rating elders; Elders not representative;	
Elders' Psychological Abuse Scale (EPAS) Originally called: Psychological Elder Abuse Scale (PEAS)	Wang et al. [165]; Wang [164]	Developed in Taiwan originally in Chinese	32 item scale, yes/no format, sum of yes responses; Score of 10+ suggests possible abuse	Structured interview with elder in home/institution	Expert content validity index 0.92; Test–retest reliability (2 weeks), agreement between 2 raters 100 % for 7 indicators, and 79 % for 1 indicator; Int. consistency $\alpha = 0.82$; Construct validity: inverse relationships with SPMSQ [131], and Barthel's Index of physical functioning [39]	Taiwan 195 elderly Taiwanese 60 + years, partially dependent on caregiver	The scale is longer than many others, but includes both elder and caregiver subjective perspectives, and clinician observations	Cohen et al. [29]
Geriatric Mistreatment Scale (GMS)	Giraldo-Rodríguez and Rosas-Carrasco [79]	Items developed from literature, prior scales, review of complaints, and expert consensus panel, refined through psychometric evaluation	22-item scale physical, psychological, neglect, economic mistreatment and sexual abuse. Yes response to any item considered mistreatment	Interviews with elders in their home by trained professionals with previous experience in elder abuse	Internal consistency reliabilities = 0.83 for total scale, 0.82 psychological mistreatment, 0.72 physical mistreatment, 0.55 economic mistreatment, 0.80 neglect, and 0.87 sexual abuse; Content validity verified by experts; Construct validity—abuse related to depression, needing help with daily tasks, and cognitive impairment	Probabilistic sample of 613 Older Mexicans aged 60 years and older, mean age of 72, 60 % female	Well constructed and validated; Spanish and English versions; validation on Spanish speaking sample only; lower reliability of economic mistreatment scale; no predictive validity available	
Hwalek-Sengstock Elder Abuse Screening Test (H-S/EAST)	Neale et al. [123]	>100 items from various elder abuse screening instruments refined to best 15 items (Hwalek and Sengstock [81])	15 item questionnaire; measures 3 forms of abuse: violations of personal rights or direct abuse, characteristics of vulnerability, and potentially abusive situations	Elder—interview by Health Care Provider in clinical setting Clinician—review of case notes	Reliability poor: $\alpha = 0.29$; Discriminant function analysis correctly classified 74 % of abused cases; Yielded 9 and 6-item versions that best discriminated	Adult Protective Services (APS) patients—170 abused and 42 non-abused; Family practice controls—$n = 47$	Relies on elder recall and willingness to report abuse; limited to 3 types of abuse Debate about whether uni- or multi-dimensional scale High false negative rate	Edirisinghe et al. [63]; Fulmer et al. [72]; Jervis et al. [84]; Moody et al. [112]; Russell et al. [141], [142]; Schofield et al. [149]; Strasser et al. [154]

(continued)

Table 9.2 (continued)

Screening measure	Authors (year)	Origin	Items/subscales	Respondent and method	Psychometric properties	Validation samples	Strengths and limitations	Studies using this scale
Indicators of Abuse (IOA)	Reis and Nahmiash [139]	Checklist of problem indicators developed from theory and research that indicates both care giver and care recipient characteristics associated with risk of abuse (e.g., [91]	27-item checklist, 5 pt. response scale: care-recipient (12 items), care-giver (15 items), age and relation ship with care-giver (2 items); 3 domains: caregiver intrapersonal issues, caregiver interpersonal problems, and care receiver social support shortages, past abuse; Risk of abuse: any item present	Interviews by trained social worker or nurse with Elder and Care-giver, ratings by professionals	Reliability $\alpha = 0.92$ and 0.91 in 2 studies; *Divergent and concurrent validity:* 29-item IOA discriminated likely abuse from likely nonabuse in 96 % cases based on referent BASE tool, and with 16 % false negatives of abuse cases; IOA discriminated 89 % of confirmed abuse versus non-abused cases, with 22 % false negatives	Cohort sample, of 341 in PROJECT CARE Initiative in Canada—ages 55 or older and currently receiving health care and social service interventions and had caregiver	Time taken to administer	Cohen et al. [26]
Expanded-Indicators of Abuse (E-IOA)	Cohen et al. [26]	Based on IOA—break down 27 indicators into more specific questions, translated into Hebrew	46 items for elder and 44 items for care-giver; 5-pt. scale; Domains: behavior problems, social isolation, emotional/cog., developmental delay, alcohol abuse, drug abuse, financial dependence, unrealistic expectations, caregiver reluctance, marital/family conflicts, current relationships, blaming, emotional dependency, social support, and lacking understanding	Semi-structured interview of elders and carers by trained geriatric social workers (~2 h)	Reliability Inter-rater agreement 93 %; Inter-item reliability—α ranges from 0.78 to 0.91; Face and content validity found acceptable by experts; Discriminates confirmed abuse/non-abuse groups, and correctly classified 92 % of probably abused and 98 % of probably not abused, with low false positive and false negatives; Cutoff of 2.70—high risk of abuse	108 older hospital patients aged 65 and older in Israel, and their care-givers	Comprehensive set of indicators; good psychometrics; Caregiver characteristics (behavioural, emotional and family problems) found to be important indicators of abuse. Important indicators of elder abuse were blaming behavioural pattern, and own behavioural problems; Lengthy screen—part of 2 h assessment Validation on Hebrew version	Cohen et al. [28, 29]; Lindenbach et al. [102]
Minimum Dataset Home Care interview (MDS-HC)	Shugarman et al. [152]	Multidimensional assessment designed as community analog to the nationally mandated MDS for nursing homes (Morris et al. [117]	5-item elder abuse screen assessing: fear of family member, poor hygiene, unexplained injury, appears neglected or mistreated, signs of physical restraint; + other indicators such as physical and cog. functioning, and environmental assessment	Home-based interviews of elder by trained clinicians. Used all sources of information (client, care-givers, observation, medical records) to see each item	7-day inter-rater reliability, Kappa = 0.79 [117]; Good construct validity by associations with social functioning and support, memory problems, mental health, behavioural problems	701 older disabled people aged 60 + seeking long-term care services in Michigan, with at least 1 informal carer	Part of a comprehensive geriatric assessment process that allows for multiple sources of data to inform ratings; Limited information about reliability and validity of items; possible confounding of abuse by other versus neglect	Cooper et al. [34]

(continued)

Table 9.2 (continued)

Screening measure	Authors (year)	Origin	Items/subscales	Respondent and method	Psychometric properties	Validation samples	Strengths and limitations	Studies using this scale
Older Adult Financial Exploitation Measure (OAFEM)	Conrad et al. [33], Conrad et al. [32]	Developed in agreement with Illinois Department on Aging Review of theories and concept mapping, with severity ratings by expert panels to develop scale	79 items in 6 domains in descending severity (# items): theft and scams (22), financial victimization (16), financial entitlement (4), coercion (13) signs of financial exploitation (19), money management difficulties (5); 2 short forms, 54 and 30 items also validated [32]	Client and staff versions of scale; Client self-report in interview by APS staff; Staff complete a staff observation questionnaire on each of the clients they interviewed	Expert content validity; Scale met stringent Rasch analysis criteria for item fit, and unidimensionality; high internal consistency and item reliability for 79-, 54- and 30-item versions; supports a single hierarchy of severity levels; Rasch person reliability was very high at 0.92 ($\alpha = 0.96$) for 79 items, and 0.85 (α =0.93) for 30 item version. Rasch item reliability very high at 0.95 for 79 items and 0.96 for 30 items	16 experts rated severity of items for concept mapping; Client self-report measures of FE administered via interview by 22 APS staff in Illinois to 227 clients who were substantiated for at least one type of elder abuse	Strong theoretical base, use of expert wisdom; Large database of substantiated elder abuse clients, expert interviewers, modern measurement techniques; Limited to small geographic area of Illinois, USA; Groups and cut-points require further replication and validation using external criteria, and sensitivity–specificity analysis once a cut-point is defined	Dong [42] used 17 item version
Older Adult Psychological Abuse Measure (OAPAM)	Conrad et al. [31]	Developed in agreement with Illinois Department on Aging from literature review and expert panels	31 and 18 item forms; unidimensional, includes 4 types of Psych. Abuse (isolation, threats and intimidation, insensitivity and disrespect, and shaming and blaming), and risk factors	22 Elder abuse staff interviewed elders in their home	Reliability: $\alpha = 0.92$; Met stringent Rasch analysis fit and unidimensionality criteria; Suggested cut-off scores for abuse	226 clients of Illinois Department of Aging, with adequate cognitive capacity	Relatively large validation sample; Rasch analysis scale validation methods, items graded in severity, part of comprehensive assessment; Only validated in one area of Chicago	
Resident-to-Resident Elder Mistreatment- Staff version (R-REM-S)	Teresi et al. [158]	Modifications to some items from Cohen-Mansfield Agitation Instrument (CMAI; [27]) that measures behavioural disruption in nursing home residents, plus items	11-items measuring staff recollection of resident-to-resident mistreatment during past 2-week period. Items range from low to high aggressiveness	Certified nursing assistants were interviewed by researchers about their recollection of resident behaviours over past 2 weeks	Unidimensional 11-item scale with item factor loading ≥0.74 except for one item (0.51); Cronbach's $\alpha = 0.74$; Corrected item-total correlations from 0.30 to 0.61; Some support for verbal and physical subscales (4 items each) with Cronbach's $\alpha = 0.73$, 0.65 respectively	Aged residents of 5 long-term aged care facilities	Low prevalence of some items limits reliability estimates; distributions skewed with greater reliability at "caseness" end of distribution	

(continued)

Table 9.2 (continued)

Screening measure	Authors (year)	Origin	Items/subscales	Respondent and method	Psychometric properties	Validation samples	Strengths and limitations	Studies using this scale
		derived from staff focus groups						
Social Vulnerability Scale (SVS22)	Pinsker et al. [135]	Items from literature search and expert consultation, intended for cognitively impaired older adults; Measures susceptibility to financial exploitation, and social vulnerability	22 item scale measures gullible behaviors and credulity (cog. behaviours), thought to contribute to exploitation of older people; 5-pt Likert scale measures frequency of behaviour, higher score more vulnerable	Knowledgeable informant completes written questionnaire	IC Reliability: $\alpha = 0.92$; Test–retest $\alpha = 0.87$; Validity—distinguished between clinical and non-clinical samples	University undergraduate students completed scale in relation to a relative/friend 50 + years, with memory, stroke, dementia or other neuro condition (clinical sample) or health control	Good psychometric properties; 2 factors related. Clinical sample had varied neurological disorders, so some confounding between neurologic and social factors; Self-report bias; limited sample; Further validation needed with more diverse samples	
Social Vulnerability Scale (SVS15)	Pinsker et al. [134]	Shorter-form of SVS22 which measures informant report of older vulnerability to exploitation	15 items, 2-factors: • gullibility (8 items), • credulity (7 items); Gullibility factor relates to financial exploitation; Credulity factor relates to social vulnerability	Knowledgeable informant completes written questionnaire	Reliability: $\alpha = 0.90$ total scale $\alpha = 0.85$ Gullibility $\alpha = 0.86$ Credulity; discriminates clinical and non-clinical older adults on social vulnerability; CFA confirmed 15 item 2-factor solution; $\alpha = 0.88$ total scale $\alpha = 0.79$ Gullibility $\alpha = 0.85$ Credulity	266 informants—116 clinical, 150 non-clinical groups for exploratory FA; CFA conducted on new sample of 123 elders recruited by undergraduate students. Mean age 67 years	Suitable for cognitively impaired elders; Need larger samples; Informant-only ratings may be biased, especially if informant is abuser	

Note: Limited to measures used since 1995

9.4.4 Elder Abuse Questionnaire (EAQ)

The Elder Abuse Questionnaire (EAQ) is a 25-item single factor questionnaire [92]. The questionnaire is completed by long-term care providers or family members, using Likert scale response options. Only moderate reliability has been established with a Cronbach's alpha of 0.66 for internal consistency, although this involved a very small sample of 29 long-term care providers and family members in rural Kansas. A larger sample may provide greater reliability. The content validity was verified by experts. A limitation of the scale is that it elicits carers' reports only, and not the subjective experience of the elders, thus the accuracy of abuse reports is questionable.

9.4.5 Elder Abuse Suspicion Index (EASI)

The Elder Abuse Suspicion Index (EASI) was developed over 2002–2003 from literature searches, existing scales and taxonomies for elder abuse, and drew on the World Health Organisation (WHO) definition of elder abuse and family violence [172]. It comprises 5 interview questions for clinicians to ask of patients, and 1 item for completion by the clinician in relation to observed indicators of abuse. Compared with a gold standard elder abuse evaluation undertaken by trained social workers, moderate sensitivity has been reported as 0.47, and the specificity as 0.75. This validation was undertaken with a sample of 663 patients recruited by physicians at two Montreal family medicine centers and a government community-based health and social services center. A key advantage of the instrument is that it is very short and quick to administer, taking <2 min. It is available in French as well as English, and has been rated as having content validity in at least seven diverse countries [169]. There is also a self-administrable version for patients, the EASI-sa [171].

9.4.6 Detection Scales for the Risk of Domestic Abuse and Self-Negligent Behavior in Elderly Persons (EDMA)

The Detection Scales for the Risk of Domestic Abuse and Self-Negligent Behavior in Elderly Persons (EDMA) was developed in Spain by Touza et al. [161] for use by social services professionals to screen for elder abuse and self-neglect among social services clients. The EDMA comprises 2 separate scales: the Elder Scale (33 items), and Alleged Abuser Scale (21 items). The Elder Scale has 3 validated subscales: Abandonment, Neglect, and Self-Neglect (13 items); Domestic Abuse without Self-Neglect (17 items); Self-Neglect (3 items). The Alleged Abuser Scale has 3 validated subscales: Inflicted Inappropriate Treatment or Abuse (9 items); Restrictive Behaviors (6 items); and Inability to Offer Proper Treatment (6 items). All items are rated by the professional on a 5-point Likert scale. Good to excellent psychometric properties were demonstrated in this Spanish sample of 46 professionals who rated 278 elders. Alphas for total scale and subscale scores were high, ranging from 0.93 for Total Elder Scale to 0.73 for Self-Neglect. The Total Elder Scale discriminated abuse and neglect well, with good sensitivity and specificity (93 %, 88 %). An advantage of the scales is that they assess both the elder and caregiver risk indicators. However the results are based on ratings made by a relatively small sample of social service professionals who had prior knowledge of the older people and their caregivers. The method of administration would not work so effectively for larger groups who were less well known.

9.4.7 Elders' Psychological Abuse Scale (EPAS)

The Elders' Psychological Abuse Scale (EPAS), originally called the Psychological Elder Abuse Scale (PEAS), is a 32 item scale with yes/no response format [164, 165]. The scale was developed in Taiwan from focus groups and expert input to ensure it was consistent with community understandings. It was originally constructed in Chinese and translated into English. Screening takes place through a structured interview by clinicians of the elders in their home or institution (7 items), active observation (6 items), and questions to the elder person's caregiver (18 items). Positive responses are summed, with higher scores indicating higher risk of psychological abuse, and a cutoff of 10 was set to provide abuse versus non-abuse groups. The scale has demonstrated good reliability and validity in a sample of 195 elderly Taiwanese aged 60 years and older who lived in institutions (49 %) and private homes (51 %). Agreement between two raters was 100 % for 7 indicators, and 79 % for 1 indicator, and internal consistency reliability was 0.82. Construct validity was demonstrated by inverse relationships with SPMSQ [131], and Barthel's Index of physical functioning [39].

9.4.8 Geriatric Mistreatment Scale (GMS)

The Geriatric Mistreatment Scale (GMS) was developed and validated as a Spanish language scale by Giraldo-Rodríguez and Rosas-Carrasco [79]. Items were developed from the literature, prior scales, review of complaints made, and expert consensus panel, and refined through systematic psychometric evaluation. This resulted in a 22-item scale with subscales of physical, psychological, neglect, economic mistreatment and sexual abuse, with yes/no responses to each item. A positive response to any item was considered evidence of mistreatment. The scale was designed to be administered through interviews with elders in their home by trained professionals who had previous experience in elder abuse. The scale has demonstrated good psychometrics with a probabilistic sample of 613 older Mexicans aged 60 years and older, mean age of 72, 60 % female. Internal consistency reliabilities were 0.83 for the 22-item GMS, and 0.82, 0.72, 0.55, 0.80, and 0.87 respectively for the psychological mistreatment, physical mistreatment, economic mistreatment, neglect, and sexual abuse subscales. Content validity was established by expert ratings. Construct validity was founded on demonstrating hypothesised relationships between elder abuse and depression, needing help with daily tasks, and cognitive impairment. Overall, the scale was developed using sound psychometrics. Advantages include having Spanish and English versions, although it needs to be noted that the validation tests have been conducted on the Spanish version only. Less than acceptable reliability was found for the economic mistreatment scale, and no predictive validity is currently available.

9.4.9 Hwalek-Sengstock Elder Abuse Screening Test (H-S/EAST)

The Hwalek-Sengstock Elder Abuse Screening Test (H-S/EAST) is a 15 item questionnaire that measures three forms of elder abuse: violations of personal rights or direct abuse, characteristics of vulnerability, and potentially abusive situations [81, 123]. It was developed from a pool of over 100 items sourced from various elder abuse screening instruments and refined to best 15 items [81]. It is designed to be administered by interview of the elder person by health care providers in clinical settings, and by review of case notes. Internal consistency reliability of the scale is poor with Cronbach's alpha of 0.29. Nevertheless, discriminant function analysis correctly classified 74 % of abused cases in one validity study [123] and yielded 9 and 6-item versions that best discriminated between abused and non-abused elders. The scale relies on elder recall and willingness to report abuse, and is limited by rating only three types of abuse. There has been debate about whether the scale is uni- or multi-dimensional scale (e.g., [84]), and a high false negative rate has been reported [112]. Despite relatively low reliability, the scale has face validity and has been used in a number of studies and with different populations, either in whole, or in part [63, 76, 84, 112, 149, 154]. It has been found to discriminate abused and nonabused elders in a sample of 100 older people living in public housing [112], with evidence that a 9-item form was as valid as the 15 item form.

9.4.10 Indicators of Abuse (IOA)

The Indicators of Abuse (IOA) screen was validated as a 29-item checklist of abuse indicators related to both care giver and care recipient problems [139]. It was developed from theory and research (e.g., [91]). The validated scale comprises 27 problem indicators and 2 demographic indicators, rated on a 5-point Likert scale from non-existent to yes/severe). Of the 27 problem indicators, 12 relate to the care-giver, and 15 to the care recipient. Risk of abuse is determined if any problem indicator is present. The IOA is administered by trained professionals via an interview of both the elder and their care-giver in the context of a lengthy global home assessment.

Psychometric evaluation was undertaken with a cohort sample of 341 adults aged 55 and older who were currently receiving health care and social service interventions as part of the PROJECT CARE Initiative in Canada. The evaluation found excellent internal consistency reliability of 0.92 and 0.91 in 2 studies; and the scale was found to have divergent and concurrent validity, discriminating likely abuse from likely non-abuse in 96 % cases based on referent BASE tool, with 16 % false negatives of abuse cases. The IOA discriminated 89 % of confirmed abuse versus non-abused cases, with 22 % false negatives. Construct validation identified 3 problem domains: caregiver intrapersonal issues (e.g., mental health, behavioral); caregiver interpersonal problems (e.g., relationships generally and with care receiver); and care receiver social support shortages and past abuse. A limitation of the scale as a screening instrument is that it takes the health professional about 20 min to complete, but is part of a very long overall assessment over 2–3 h which helps to inform the clinician ratings of abuse. It is not clear how valid it is on its own.

9.4.11 Expanded-Indicators of Abuse (E-IOA)

The Expanded-Indicators of Abuse (E-IOA) screen is closely based on the IOA, but indicators are broken down into more specific indicators [26]. It comprises 46 indicators related to the care recipient and 44 indicators for care-givers. Screening occurs through semi-structured Interviews of elders and carers by trained geriatric social workers, part of an overall assessment that takes approximately 2 h, and ratings are completed by the professionals. The validation sample were 108 older hospital patients aged 65 and older in Israel, and their care-givers. Indicators cover a comprehensive range of behavior problems, social isolation, emotional/cognitive issues, developmental delay, alcohol abuse, drug abuse, financial dependence, unrealistic expectations, caregiver reluctance, marital/family conflicts, current relationships, blaming, emotional dependency, social support, and lacking understanding.

Psychometric evaluations report good reliability with an inter-rater agreement of 93 %, and inter-item reliabilities ranging from 0.78 to 0.91. Face and content validity was found acceptable by experts. The E-IOA was found to discriminate between confirmed abuse/non-abuse groups, and correctly classified 92 % of probably abused and 98 % of probably not abused, with low false positive and false negatives. A cut-off score of 2.70 was deemed to indicate high risk of abuse. Confirmatory factor analysis largely confirmed the hypothesized factor structure, and the main indicators for risk included behavioral, emotional and family problems of both caregiver and elder.

9.4.12 Minimum Dataset Home Care Interview (MDS-HC)

The Minimum Dataset Home Care interview (MDS-HC) is a multidimensional in-home geriatric assessment tool designed as a community analog to the nationally mandated MDS for nursing homes [117]. It involves home-based interviews of elders by trained clinicians, and use of multiple sources of information to rate each item (client, care-givers, observation, medical records). The original validation study reported good 7-day reliability for elder abuse items of 0.79 [117]. The brief 5-item elder abuse items related to fear of family member, poor hygiene, unexplained injury, observed neglect or mistreated, and signs of physical restraint; and assessment was enhanced by consideration of other indicators such as physical and cognitive functioning, environmental and caregiver assessment, and medical records.

The 5-item elder abuse screen was further validated by Shugarman, Fries, Wolf, and Morris [152]. Construct validity was supported by demonstrated associations with social functioning and support, memory problems, mental health, and behavioral problems. This was based on a study of 701 older people aged 60+ seeking long-term care services in Michigan, with at least one informal carer. A strength of the study is that the elder abuse assessment is embedded in a comprehensive geriatric assessment which allows for multiple sources of data to inform ratings, however, limited information is availability about reliability and validity of items, and there is a possible confounding of abuse and neglect. The MDS-HC has also been used in a large scale multisite, multinational European study of over 4000 people aged 65+ receiving health or social community services in 11 European countries [34]. It is worth noting that substantial variations in prevalence rates are reported across countries, as other cross-cultural studies have found, although it is difficult to determine to what extent this may be due to methodological issues such as question translation, sampling, interviewer training and judgement, or more purely cultural issues.

9.4.13 Older Adult Financial Exploitation Measure (OAFEM)

The Older Adult Financial Exploitation Measure (OAFEM) is the only measure identified that is specific to financial abuse [33, 32], although other scales tend to include one or more items which are scored as part of general elder abuse. The scale was developed in agreement with Illinois Department on Aging and involved several phases. The first phase involved reviewing theories of financial exploitation from literature review, generating a large pool of items, and expert panels to develop theoretically valid items. Then a panel of 16 experts rated the severity of items generated for the concept mapping; resulting in 79 items in 6 domains in descending order of severity (# items): (1) theft and scams (22), (2) financial victimization (16), (3) financial entitlement (4), (4) coercion (13), (5) signs of possible financial exploitation (19), and (6) money management difficulties (5). The scale was developed with both client and staff versions [33], and gained consensus content validation of items and key constructs by experts.

The next phase involved evaluating the scale in a study of APS clients. The FE was administered via interview by 22 APS staff to 227 clients who were substantiated for at least one type of elder abuse [32]. The APS staff completed a staff observation questionnaire on each of the clients they interviewed. The scale was found to meet stringent Rasch analysis criteria for item fit and uni-dimensionality, and with very high internal consistency and item reliability for 79-, 54- and 30-item versions. For instance, the Rasch person reliability ranged from 0.92 (alpha = 0.96) for 79 items, to 0.85 (alpha of 0.93) for 30 items. Similarly, Rasch item reliability was 0.95 for 79 items and 0.96 for 30 items. The analysis supported a conceptualisation of the scale as a single hierarchy of severity levels rather than distinct subdimensions, and authors suggest that the 30-item form is the most promising and parsimonious as a screening measure, although there are specific items in the longer version that may be useful for certain purposes.

Strengths of the scale include a strong theoretical base and use of expert wisdom, modern measurement techniques, well-targeted clients, expert interviewers, and a relatively large database of substantiated clients of elder abuse to test validity and suggest cut-points for judgments of severity. A limitation is that the validation sample is limited to a small geographic area of Illinois, USA, and Conrad suggests that the groups and cut-points will require further replication and validation against external criteria [32]. A sensitivity–specificity analysis can be applied once a suitable cut-point is more reliably established. A 17-item modified version was used by Dong [42, 43].

9.4.14 Older Adult Psychological Abuse Measure (OAPAM)

The Older Adult Psychological Abuse Measure (OAPAM) has 31 and 18 item forms [31]. It is a unidimensional scale and includes 4 types of psychological abuse: isolation, threats and intimidation, insensitivity and disrespect, and shaming and blaming, as well as risk factors. It was developed in agreement with the Illinois Department on Aging from a literature review and expert panels. The OAPAM is designed to be administered via interview by professionals. Validation involved data from 226 clients with adequate cognitive capacity who were interviewed in their homes by staff of the Illinois Department of Aging. A high internal consistency reliability of 0.92 was reported for the scale and it met stringent Rasch analysis fit and unidimensionality criteria. Analysis suggested a cut-off score for abuse. This is the only scale identified which used Rasch analysis scale validation methods, but further validation is needed, and it has been validated in one area of Chicago only.

9.4.15 Resident-to-Resident Elder Mistreatment: Staff Version (R-REM-S)

The Resident-to-Resident Elder Mistreatment- Staff version (R-REM-S) is an 11-item scale measuring staff recollection of resident-to-resident mistreatment over the past 2-weeks [158]. The items were modified from the Cohen-Mansfield Agitation Instrument (CMAI; [27]), plus items derived from staff focus groups. The CMAI is a tool that seeks to measure behavioral disruption in nursing home residents. The validation sample was based on ratings by certified nursing assistants on 1812 aged residents of 5 large long-term aged care facilities in New York. Psychometrics on the scale suggest that it has moderate reliability and validity. The 11-item scale had an internal consistency of $\alpha = 0.74$. There was some support for verbal and physical subscales (4 items each) with Cronbach's $\alpha = 0.73$, 0.65 respectively. Limitations to the robustness of the scale includes the low prevalence of some items that limits reliability estimates; and distributions are skewed with greater reliability at the "caseness" end of distribution. However, it provides a third-party assessment of potential abuse in long-term care facilities, where self-report may not be possible.

9.4.16 Social Vulnerability Scale (SVS)

Social Vulnerability Scale (SVS22). The Social Vulnerability Scale (SVS22) is a 22 item scale that measures gullible behaviors and credulity (cognitive behaviors) which are thought to contribute to exploitation of older people [135]. Gullibility items relate largely to financial exploitation while the credulity items relate to social vulnerability more generally. Because it seeks to assess vulnerability among cognitively impaired elders, knowledgeable informants complete the written questionnaire rather than self-completion by the elder themselves. Responses are provided on a 5-point Likert scale that measures frequency of behavior, with higher scores indicating greater vulnerability.

Sound psychometrics have been reported in terms of reliability, face and content validity. The scale has demonstrated excellent reliability among a small sample of informants, in this case, 167 University undergraduate students who completed the scale in relation to a relative/friend aged 50 years or older, with memory, stroke, dementia or other neurological condition (clinical sample) or a healthy control. The internal consistency reliability of the scale was $\alpha = 0.92$, with test–retest reliability at $\alpha = 0.87$. The scale was also found to distinguish between clinical and non-clinical samples, indicating good discriminant validity. A strength of the scale is its suitability for assessing vulnerability among the cognitively impaired, a high risk group for elder abuse. Limitations include no assessment of the subjective experience of the elders, potential bias of informants, a limited validation sample and few validation tests. Further validation is needed with more diverse and larger samples. Despite these limitations, the SVS22 seems useful as a measure of susceptibility to financial exploitation in particular, and social vulnerability more generally among this population that poses measurement challenges.

Social Vulnerability Scale (SVS15). The Social Vulnerability Scale has been further refined to a 15-item short form (SVS15) [134]. As for the SVS22, the SVS15 measures informant report of older vulnerability to exploitation. Validation tests support both the unidimensional scale and a two factor solution: gullibility (8 items), and credulity (7 items), making it a relatively brief and easily administered scale. Validation was undertaken with a sample of 266 informants, 116 in the clinical group and 150 in the non-clinical group. Reliability of the total scale and two subscales was good, range from 0.90 for the total scale to 0.85 and 0.86 for the gullibility and credulity subscales respectively. The scale was also found to discriminate between clinical and non-clinical older adults on social vulnerability. A confirmatory factor analysis confirmed the two factor solution with Cronbach alphas ranging from 0.79 to 0.88. Further validation is needed in terms of convergent, discriminant and predictive validity, along with larger samples.

9.4.17 Summary of Elder Abuse Screening Measures for Use in Healthcare Settings

The measures used to screen for elder abuse and neglect in healthcare and institutional settings range from general measures of abuse and conflict in relationships, such as the CTS and its derivatives, to increasingly more specific and differentiated measures of different forms of elder abuse and neglect. This trend has followed research and theory about different forms of abuse, especially in relation to psychological, emotional, and coercive abuse. This development in the understanding of forms of abuse also provides a challenge in terms of yielding measures that are brief enough to be useful in busy clinical settings, but specific enough to provide a reliable risk assessment. Further work is needed to meet this challenge and to improve the state of research on the validity of different screening instruments and types of abuse and neglect. In particular, little progress has been made in validating measures of sexual abuse, financial exploitation, or neglect by caregivers. As well, the complexity of caring relationship difficulties needs to be better captured. One aspect of elder abuse screening that has received some attention in recent years is the screening for elder neglect and approaches to screening for both care-giver neglect and self-neglect are reviewed in the following section.

9.5 Screening for Elder Neglect and Self-Neglect

The construct of elder neglect is complex and challenging to operationalise for the purposes of screening older people. It includes two distinct categories: care-giver neglect and self-neglect. Care-giver neglect has been defined as “the failure of an elderly person to receive essential services from a responsible caregiver” [2]. By contrast, elder self-neglect has been defined as the behaviors of an elderly person that threaten his/her own health or safety, and can involve an older person’s refusal or failure to provide himself or herself with adequate food, water, clothing, shelter, safety, personal hygiene, and medication (when indicated) [120]. Self-neglect is often considered in the context of elder abuse as a form of self-abuse, although, in many respects, it is conceptually quite distinct from usual definitions of interpersonal abuse, which imply abuse by another.

It needs to be noted that much has been written about assessment and substantiation of elder neglect but there are very few studies that report on the psychometric evaluation of screening instruments. A summary of seven screening measures for elder neglect and self-neglect, that are at least partially validated, are shown in Table 9.3. Unlike the measurement of other forms of elder abuse, the measurement of care-giver neglect and self-neglect largely involves measuring the absence of appropriate caring behaviors rather than the commission of specific acts of abuse. This review revealed only one study on the development of a specific screening measure for care-giver neglect and a small number of validated scales measuring self-neglect in the time period from 1995 to 2015, perhaps reflecting this challenge. Yet, the development of valid and reliable measures of neglect is important since neglect is thought to account for a majority of elder mistreatment cases, both reported and not reported [72]. For instance, the National Elder Abuse Incidence Study reported that 49 % of 70,942 elder mistreatment cases substantiated by Adult Protective Services (APS) were categorized as neglect [120].

The measurement of neglect is often embedded with more comprehensive or generic elder abuse scales and these have been reported in Tables 9.1 and 9.2. Table 9.3 presents scales that were designed specifically to measure care-giver neglect (n = 1) and self-neglect of the elderly (n = 6). Measurement of elder neglect draws heavily on two primary theoretical constructs related to risk or vulnerability factors rather than specific acts of neglect. One is the construct of unmet needs, as measured in scales of Activities of Daily Living (ADL) and Instrumental Activities of Daily Living (IADL). Another is the construct of self-care agency or self-care skills, as the hypothesised inverse of self-neglect. A third influence on the measurement of self-neglect is the importance of environmental assessment involving indirect and observational measure of the level of self-care and care of the home environment. Only one study was identified in the 1995–2015 period which reported on the reliability of a caregiver neglect screening scale [43, 46]. By contrast a growing number of studies have sought to validate measures of self-neglect.

9.5.1 Caregiver Neglect

The Caregiver Neglect scale was examined as a measure of unmet needs in the PINE Study of Chinese elders in Chicago [43]. The 20 item scale was modified from the Activities of Daily Living (ADL) scale (8 items) and the Instrumental

Table 9.3 Validated measures for screening for elder neglect

Screening measure	Authors (year)	Origin	Items/Subscales	Respondent and method	Psychometric properties	Validation samples	Strengths and limitations	Studies using scale (whole or part)
Caregiver Neglect	Dong [42, 43]; Dong et al. [60]	Modification of Katz [86] Index of Activities of Daily Living (ADL) and Lawton Instrumental Activities of Daily Living (IADL)	20 items; 8 ADL items measure physical function impairment in ability to perform basic self-care tasks on 4-point scale; 12 IADL items measure level of unmet need; Scored: any unmet need (none/some), and severity of unmet need on 4 point scale from none to severe)	Trained multicultural and multilingual interviewers conducted face-to-face interviews in home	ADL Cronbach $\alpha = 0.92$ IADL Cronbach $\alpha = 0.90$	Population Study of Chinese Elderly in Chicago (PINE)—3159 elders aged 60+ (59 % women) living in community	Demonstrates how definitions of abuse influence prevalence data; Limited psychometrics; Measures unmet needs rather than neglect per se; Provides data on any unmet needs + living with family member; and moderate/severe unmet needs + living with family member	
Elder Self-Neglect (Own scale)	Dong et al. [56]; Dong et al. [51, 52, 57, 53; Dong and Simon [49]	Developed for The Chicago Health and Aging Project (CHAP), a community study	21 items, 5 domains: Hoarding (4 items), Poor basic personal hygiene (4 items), Unsanitary conditions (5 items), House in need of repair (5 items), Inadequate utility (3 items); Ratings of severity on 4-point scale, with higher score being more severe self-neglect	In-home observational ratings by trained interviewers of severity of unmet needs in 5 domains	Int. consistency reliabilities were high $\alpha = 0.95$; Inter-rater reliability >0.70; Content validity via expert panel; Construct validity —correlated with impairments in: cognition ($r = 0.10$), phys. function ($r = 0.05$), and depressive symptoms ($r = 0.12$); External validity—predicts greater risk of mortality	1165 older people aged 65+ from the Chicago Health and Aging Project (CHAP), a community study, who were reported to social services agency for suspected elder self-neglect	Large sample of suspected elder self-neglect; High reliability and validity of observational ratings; Limitation is cost of in-home observational ratings	Dong [43]
Elder Self-Neglect Assessment (ESNA)	Iris et al. [82]	Designed as part of Illinois Comprehensive Care Assessment questionnaire for assessing elders for home and community services; Concept mapping by 50 professionals used to develop, sort and rate a list of self-neglect indicators for "likeness" and importance to concept of self-neglect	77-items, refined to 62 item long form and 25 item short form; Unidimensional measure with 2 key domains: Behavioral and Environmental; 7 conceptual areas: (1) personal endangerment, (2) environmental, (3) financial issues, (4) mental health, (5) personal living conditions, (6) physical health, (7) social network and culture	In-home interview and observational ratings by professionals based on 215 clients of 13 aged care agencies in Illinois, USA; Indicators rated on 5 pt. response scale: Yes (problem exists), No (problem doesn't exist), Suspected Problem, Don't Know, and Not Applicable	Both forms of ESNA met Rasch fit criteria with good personal internal consistency ($\alpha = 0.91$ for long form and 0.87 for short form), item reliability, and construct validity; Strong correlations between both forms and the 19-item Illinois Comprehensive Care Assessment, an environmental assessment in the home, and the Determination of Needs scale, a measure of ADL and IADL; Short form correlated 0.92 with long-form	Social workers, case managers, and APS providers from 13 Illinois agencies completed ESNA for 215 clients suspected of self-neglect	Rigorous Rasch analysis; Validation supports 2 broad categories of indicators: behavioral characteristics and environmental factors within a unidimensional structure; Supports hierarchy of items associated with severity of abuse by frequency of occurrence; 25-item short form recommended as more parsimonious, with comparable validity; Sample limited to those suspected of abuse, and limited diversity	

(continued)

Table 9.3 (continued)

Screening measure	Authors (year)	Origin	Items/Subscales	Respondent and method	Psychometric properties	Validation samples	Strengths and limitations	Studies using scale (whole or part)
Self-Care Agency Scale (ASA); Originally called Appraisal of Self-Care Agency Scale	Isenberg [83]; Lorensen [105]; Aish and Isenberg [3]	Scale derived from theory of self-agency, as the link between self-care need and action; Self-care agency comprises power components and self-care operations; Has 2 forms: A—Self B—Carer	24 items (15 positive and 9 negative statements); rated on 5-point Likert scale responses summed for total score with higher scores reflecting higher self-agency	Survey of elderly, administered by interview	Int. consistency 0.62 to 0.86 in different patient samples, (0.72 with elderly patients); 7-week stability 0.72 in Dutch elderly; 1week Test–retest reliability 0.71; Discriminated between clinical versus non-clinical sample; Concurrent Val.: associated with nutritional self-care	Has been validated in variety of patient samples, and samples of elderly	Theory-based; Validated across different patient groups; Limited use in context of elder abuse and neglect	Lauder [97]; Lorensen [105]
Screening Scale for Elder Abuse (SSEA)—Elder Self-Neglect subscale	Lee and Kim [100]	From the Screening Scale for Elder Abuse, a Korean language scale was developed for population survey	5 items measure frequency of elder self-neglect in past year, as part of the SSEA; Response options on 4 Pt scale with higher scores representing high self-neglect	Home-based interviews by trained interviewers	IC reliability $\alpha = 0.76$; Concurrent validity suggested through correlations with ADL and IADL scores	481 Korean professionals in social service agencies for elderly [89]; Then, random stratified sample of 1023 adults in 1 area of Metropolitan City, Sth Korea	Scale items available in English and Korean language; Limited validation data, not available in English	Kim et al. [89]
Self-Neglect Severity Scale (SSS)	Dyer et al. [61]; Kelly et al. [87]	Developed by the Consortium for Research in Elder Self-Neglect of Texas (CREST). Structured interviews of APS specialists [62], led to development of large item pool, reviewed by expert panel, refined, pilot-tested	Revised 2008 version—37 items, 3 domains: A.Personal hygiene (5 items); B.Impaired function (6); C. Environmental status (19); + APS comprehensive social history form, and physical exam; A global 0–10 risk assessment' item, and several summation scores	Observational assessment in home: 5–10 min; Sections A, C, and some of B rated on 4 pt. scale from none to severe self-neglect, others dichotomous; Scored: 3 domain totals, overall, and 4 composite summation scores	Inter-rater reliability high; Internal consistency acceptable for environment and composite scores; Discriminant val. —differences between self-neglect versus no neglect groups on 3 domain and composite scores, but clinical sig. of these differences not established; Poor sensitivity and specificity	23 older adults assessed in field test of scale	Objective observational screening measure for elder self-neglect; Limited in important area of self-neglect—no screen of food intake/nutrition due to poor validity; Scoring methods need further validation—unclear whether appropriate to sum across domains; Poor sensitivity and specificity	

(continued)

Table 9.3 (continued)

Screening measure	Authors (year)	Origin	Items/Subscales	Respondent and method	Psychometric properties	Validation samples	Strengths and limitations	Studies using scale (whole or part)
Self-neglect scale (unnamed)	Ayalon [11]	Measures unmet needs for services. Items developed from literature review, previous ADL/IADL tasks, expert panels, and pilot-testing [64]	7, 6 and 5-item versions; Final 5-item version found to be adequate; Ratings on 7-point scale, but dichotomised for analysis	Interviews in home, with some completing written questionnaire	Reliability $\alpha = 0.57–0.93$ across samples; Concurrent Val.: association with older adults' reports of loneliness, feelings of safety, and sense of overall neglect; lower financial status and satisfaction with caring relationship; 5-item measure has adequate configural, metric and scalar invariance across 3 informant groups	1045 community-dwelling older adults in Israeli national survey of elder mistreatment; convenience sample of 148 matched older adults in daycare centres ($n = 75$), family members, home care workers	5-item version identified as adequate to assess neglect from multiple perspectives: care recipient, care giver, family member, but in 5-item version excludes 2 key neglect indicators: nutrition and hygiene unmet needs	Ayalon [9, 10]; Lowenstein et al. [106]

Activities of Daily Living (IADL) scale [86, 99]. Internal consistency reliability was 0.93 for the 20 item scale (personal communication, [21], 0.92 for the eight ADL items, and 0.90 for the 12 IADL items [46]. The scale is administered by trained multicultural and multilingual interviewers in the elder's home. Severity of impairment and unmet need is rated on a 4 point scale from none to severe. There are limited psychometrics reported, although ADL and IADL have been used and validated by others as a surrogate measure of neglect (e.g. [11, 133]).

9.5.2 Elder Self-Neglect (Unnamed Scale)

The 21 item Elder Self-Neglect Scale was developed for the Chicago Health and Aging Project, a community study of elders who had been reported to social service agencies for suspected elder self-neglect [43, 49, 56, 54, 58, 59, 51, 52, 57, 53]. Conceptually it is based on identifying unmet needs for care and addresses five domains of self-neglect: hoarding (4 items), personal hygiene (4 items), unsanitary conditions (5 items), house disrepair (5 items), and inadequate utilities (3 items). The measure is completed by trained interviewers, mainly by observation, during in-home assessments. Each item is rated on a 4-point scale with a higher score indicating more severe self-neglect. The scale has demonstrated good to excellent reliability and some construct validity. Internal consistency reliability of 5 domains was 0.97–0.98, and inter-rater reliability >0.70. Content validity was supported by an expert panel review. Construct validity was supported by significant, though low, correlations with cognitive impairment (0.10), physical function impairment (0.05), and depressive symptoms (0.12). Predictive validity has also been supported by prediction of mortality [56], and hospital re-admissions [49].

9.5.3 Elder Self-Neglect Assessment (ESNA)

The Elder Self-Neglect Assessment (ESNA) comprises a 77 or 62-item assessment developed as part of the Illinois Comprehensive Care Assessment questionnaire for assessing elders for home and community-based services [82]. The items were developed through a concept mapping framework involving 50 professionals who developed, sorted and rated a list of self-neglect indicators for "likeness" and for their importance to the concept of self-neglect. This resulted in seven conceptual areas: personal endangerment, environmental, financial, mental health, personal living conditions, physical health, and social network and culture. These seven areas were grouped into two broad conceptual areas: environmental aspects, and physical and psychosocial aspects of self-neglect. Professionals completed the assessment through observation in the home on a 5-point response scale. The ESNA was found to meet RASCH fit criteria with good internal consistency, item reliability, and construct validity. A 25-item shorter version was also found to meet RASCH fit criteria. The ESNA is designed for assessment of those suspected of self-neglect, and the validation sample had limited diversity. Its strengths lies in the RASCH analysis of items, the involvement of 13 agencies in the validation phase, and the finding that both environmental and behavioural aspects are important to assess. The findings also supported a hierarchy of items associated with severity of abuse by frequency of occurrence, aspects of the validation process that other studies should pay attention to.

9.5.4 Self-Care Agency Scale (ASA)

The Self-Care Agency Scale (ASA) is a 24 item scale derived from the theory of self-agency which seeks to explain the link between self-care needs and action [3, 83]. Self-care agency is understood to comprise both power components and self-care actions. The 24 items are made up of 15 positive-worded items, and 9 negatively worded items, all rated on a 5-point Likert scale. Responses are summed for a total score, with higher scores reflecting higher self-agency. The scale is administered by interview and has demonstrated internal consistency reliabilities ranging from 0.71 to 0.86 for different patient samples [3, 83], with a reliability of 0.72 on one elderly Dutch sample [66]. The scale discriminates between elderly patients receiving institutional rehabilitation care versus those living at home [105], and was associated with nutritional self-care, providing some support for concurrent validity.

9.5.5 Screening Scale for Elder Abuse: Self-Neglect Subscale (SSEA-SN)

The Screening Scale for Elder Abuse (SSEA) was used in a population based survey in South Korea (Kim, Kwon, Lim, and Lee [89]. The full scale is not reported in this review as it had not been published in English. However, the 5-item Self-Neglect subscale is published in English and its inclusion here adds to the global picture of screening instrument development [100]. The scale was administered in home-based interviews by trained interviewers. It was first validated with a sample of 481 Koreans professionals who worked in social service agencies, then in a random stratified sample of 1023 adults in a metropolitan city of South Korea. The scale was found to have an internal consistency reliability of 0.76 in the population based sample and some concurrent validity was demonstrated through correlations with ADL and IADL scales [100]. The scale is available in Korean and English languages.

9.5.6 Self-Neglect Severity Scale (SSS)

The Self-Neglect Severity Scale (SSS) was developed by the Consortium for Research in Elder Self-Neglect of Texas (CREST) [87]. The item pool was developed through structured interviews with APS specialists and then reviewed and refined by an expert panel. It was further refined to comprise 30 items in three domains of personal hygiene (5 items), Impaired Function (6 items), and Environmental Status (19 items) [87]. The scale also includes social history questions and a physical examination, a global risk assessment item, and several summations scores. It is completed by observational assessment in the elder's home. Response options and scoring methods differ across items with some 4-point scale response and some dichotomous items. Inter-rater reliability has been found to be high, and internal consistency adequate for the environment and composite scores. Validation of the scale is at an early stage, with data provided from a field test on 23 older adults. The SSS has been found to discriminate between self-neglect and non-self-neglect groups on the three domains and composite scores, but the clinical significance of these differences has not been established, nor has the validity of the composite scores. The sensitivity and specificity of the scale was reported as poor. Like many neglect measures, it does not screen for nutrition issues.

9.5.7 Neglect Scale (Unnamed)

Ayalon [11] reports a validation study of a 7-item measure of unmet need for services, with items developed from the ADL and IADL literature, expert panels and pilot testing [64]. The scale was designed to be conducted via interview in the elder's home, though some elect to self-complete a written questionnaire. The scale was first validated in a study of over 1000 community-dwelling older adults taking part in an Israeli National Survey of Elder Mistreatment, and then in a convenience sample of 148 matched older adults in day-care centres, family members, and home care workers. The internal consistency reliabilities ranged from 0.57 to 0.93 for different samples. Concurrent validity was based on associations with the older adults' reports of loneliness, feelings of safety, and overall sense of neglect, as well as with lower financial status, and lower satisfaction with the caring relationship [11]. A 5-item version of the scale was determined to be a more adequate measure of neglect, as it demonstrated better configural, metric and scalar invariance across the three groups of informants.

9.5.8 Summary of Screening Measures for Elder Care-Giver Neglect and Self-Neglect

Screening for elder neglect and self-neglect requires further conceptual development. Only one study evaluated a screening tool for care-giver neglect, using ADL and IADL assessment of needs as the proxy measure [42, 46]. The six tools reviewed here for screening for elder self-neglect highlight the complexity and diversity of approaches in this area. There seems to be a growing consensus that effective screening needs to incorporate both behavioural/self-care skills as well as environmental assessments, although it could be argued that much of this investigation is perhaps more oriented towards substantiation of self-neglect rather than development of a simple screening measure. These two purposes could be better differentiated in future research, as there is room for both, given the potential expense of the environmental assessment aspects.

9.6 Development of Screening Tools for Elder Abuse and Neglect: Methodological Issues

A number of key methodological issues arise from the research reviewed and these are discussed in the following section to indicate some of the complex challenges associated with screening for elder abuse and neglect.

9.6.1 Conceptual Issues

Many have noted the complexity of the phenomenon of elder abuse (e.g., [16, 34, 41, 70]), which is generally understood to comprise one or more aspects of physical, psychological, emotional, verbal, financial, and sexual abuse, as well as neglect and (sometimes) self-neglect. Measurement of complex latent constructs such as elder abuse requires a formative measurement approach that seeks to identify indicators of abuse or vulnerability that are known to predict the phenomenon of interest [96]. Early measures tended to assess only limited aspects of these domains, and increasingly there has been recognition of the need for more differentiated measures. For instance, the original development of the CTS focused on physical assault and psychological aggression [155], whereas later developments have added in dimensions such as sexual coercion and injury in the CTS2 [156]. Others have expanded the forms of abuse to include financial exploitation [33, 32, 159], neglect [42, 43, 46] and self-neglect [56, 51, 52]. However, greater differentiation challenges the need for brevity and ease of completion in an effective screening instrument.

General measures of abuse include the EAQ [92], the EASI [172], and the IOA [139], but the constructs included vary and the relative weight of different constructs can influence any research that relies on such global measures of abuse. Measures differ in terms of whether they include one item per type of abuse or multiple items. The reliability and validity of measures for specific types of abuse has been at least partially demonstrated for the following: physical assault (e.g. Giraldo- Rodriguez and Rosas-Carrasco [79, 155, 156], psychological abuse (e.g., [31, 79, 155, 156, 164, 165]), sexual abuse (e.g.[79, 156]), financial abuse (e.g., [33, 32, 79]), neglect (e.g., [42, 79]), or self-neglect (e.g., [56, 51, 52, 57, 53, 82]). There are some conflicting findings in terms of whether scales such as the H-S/EAST [123] are unidimensional or multidimensional (e.g. [84]).

There is ample evidence of conceptual fuzziness in many attempts to measure abuse. For instance, neglect and self-neglect are often assessed using ADL and IADL tools which represent a very indirect way of assessing neglect. There may be many reasons why an older person's functioning is impaired and their care needs not met, which do not comfortably fit within the usual meaning of neglect [61]. Unfortunately many studies use poorly defined measurement tools and provide no information about reliability and validity. Even those measures that have received some level of validation, are frequently modified when taken up by other researchers, making it very difficult to build an evidence base for any particular measure [41].

Another aspect of conceptual fuzziness found throughout the research reviewed was the frequent conflating of the different purposes of an assessment instrument under the concept of screening for elder mistreatment. Some measures are designed to screen a large group of older people to identify those possibly at risk, who can then be referred for further evaluation. This purpose reflects the original definition of a screening measure [125, 128]. However, the term screening has also been applied to the purpose of investigating or substantiating abuse allegations, reflecting a more diagnostic evaluation. These are two different things, contributing to the very diverse approaches to measuring abuse.

Another conceptual issue is that the context of abusive behaviour is poorly understood and measured. For instance, most scales that assess caregiver characteristics seek to identify certain traits or behaviors associated with abuse, with little attention to contextualising the abuse. Family carers, for instance, may demonstrate no abusive behaviour over most of their caring experience, yet we know little about what specific circumstances or dyadic interactions may lead to abusive acts. Research on couple violence suggests that abusive behaviour can be interactive, reciprocal and retaliatory in specific circumstances, i.e., *situational violence* rather than an ongoing pattern of violence [88]. Future work needs to bring a greater understanding of relational dynamics, and context to better illuminate the phenomena. Such information can then inform more targeted interventions.

9.6.2 Item Generation

Most studies reviewed in this paper that set out to develop a new scale have used a methodologically sound approach to item generation, basing it on literature review, expert consensus, pilot testing and refinement through psychometric evaluation (e.g. [33, 32, 31, 79, 84, 123, 149, 164, 172]. However, a key issue affecting the reliability and validity of a measure is the number, breadth and appropriateness of items used to measure each construct. As elder abuse is a complex latent construct, reliable measurement requires more than a single item, and item generation needs to be guided by theory.

Much research has focused on the need for prevalence data, where the focus has been on generating a dichotomous variable of abuse: present or not. Thus, many studies, particularly in the medical literature, have relied on one item per type of abuse. This provides a very limited and potentially unreliable screen. Others have generated multiple items, and developed coherent reliable conceptual factors or scale. While this initially leads to a large number of items, progressive psychometric evaluation can be used to develop robust longer and shorter forms of scales with documented reliability and validity (e.g., [32]).

The use of multiple items to assess each type of abuse also allows for an exploration of more nuanced concepts of severity and chronicity of abuse. Elder abuse may occur as a one-off incident or an ongoing pattern of abusive behaviour, in single or multiple domains, and measures need to distinguish between these important characteristics. Abusive acts can also vary in severity from minor to severe, and the context in which it occurs can be an important component. Measures that define abuse on the basis of one incident, regardless of whether it is minor or severe, one-off or chronic, will have a large amount of variance in the data, and provide little guidance about what type of intervention may be required. As an example, the brief EASI measure has been criticised on face validity grounds, as the scoring method allows for a classification of abuse on the basis of any one item. This is problematic since four of the six items reflect a different type of abuse, one item measures a clinician's overall assessment of any sign, and one does not actually measure abuse, but rather functional impairment.

9.6.3 Response Options and Scoring

The construction of methodologically sound response options is a crucial aspect of scale construction (Schofield and Forrester-Knauss [145]). As already noted, questions on elder abuse often require a simple yes/no response option which provides limited and potentially inaccurate information—how does a person answer if they think neither option is accurate? The use of ordinal scaling methods allows for a more differentiated response which can provide useful information about issues such as severity, chronicity, importance and so on. Likert scales are a commonly used form of ordinal scaling in this type of research, but few studies are adequately informed by the psychometric theory, although recent research using Rasch analyses represents an advance in this area [33, 32, 31, 82]. Such analysis may lead to more robust methods of establishing appropriate cut-points on scales for identifying clinically relevant levels of elder abuse, in conjunction with use of better external criteria.

The review indicates a lack of consensus in how to score instruments for elder abuse. Some studies define "caseness" by any positive response to a single item (e.g. [108]), whereas others assess it in terms of the number of positive items (e.g., $\geq$10/32 items; [164], or number of times abuse is experienced (e.g., 10 or more times, [16]). Some researchers select a cutpoint on an ordinal or interval scale depending on how conservative they want to be. For instance, Cooper et al. [38] defined caseness as a score of $\geq$2 on a 5-point scale (sometimes occurs) for any item. Rasch analysis has also been used to define possible cutpoints based on a combination of severity and frequency data [32, 31]. Such differences will clearly produce very different results for prevalence and risk factor estimates and make comparisons across studies impossible.

Some researchers have evaluated the impact of using different combinations of elder abuse subtypes on prevalence rates. For instance, Dong [42] reports on variations to prevalence rates by applying criteria from least to most restrictive and demonstrates how this may account for some of the observed variation in prevalence rates across studies. Given the complex nature of elder abuse and the serious implications of identifying potential cases of abuse, this is an urgent challenge for the field. Most scales include both minor and severe forms of abuse, and research is needed to better encapsulate the severity and chronicity aspects of the phenomena in the scoring method.

9.6.4 Modes of Assessment

The most common modes of assessment are self-report questionnaires or interview by a health professional, either in the health setting or home environment. Self-report has the advantage of being more economical and better allowing for mass screening. It may also facilitate more honest answers when completed in private. Disadvantages include that it may be unsuitable for those who are cognitively impaired, do not have adequate language or reading ability, or who lack the time or motivation to complete. Another disadvantage of questionnaires administered to large samples such as national surveys is that there is often no strategy to follow up those who are identified as at risk of elder abuse.

Screening undertaken by health professionals has the advantage of optimising motivation, embedding the screen in a more comprehensive assessment, allowing for follow-up questions and elaborations if needed, and gathering of more information about context. It is also more likely than for questionnaire screening that appropriate referral pathways or interventions can be implemented by the health professional for those identified as at risk. Disadvantages include the lack of time for many busy clinicians, the resource intensive nature (especially for home interviews), potential lack of training and comfort in asking highly sensitive questions, potential bias in scoring and interpretation, and there may be a lack of known referral and intervention options in some cases.

Observational screening tools have been promoted, particularly for the assessment of neglect and self-neglect, when the older person may be unable or unwilling to reliably report on these aspects. Observational measures are viewed as more objective in some ways, but once again, can be subject to unreliable conclusions. For instance, many have noted that poor nutrition is a key feature of self-neglect, but attempts to validate an observational measure by methods such as pantry or refrigerator inventories have been repeatedly found to be unreliable (e.g., [61]). The amount and quality of food identified may vary dramatically depending on when the last shop was conducted, or the older person may have already prepared food brought in by others on a regular basis. Different diets will also make it difficult to develop a reliable scoring system.

Modes of administration using innovative technology such as hand held personal digital assistants (PDAs) for data collection are of emerging interest. PDAs have a number of advantages for use in research in healthcare settings such as efficiency of collection and entry of data, ease of use, portability, quick access to databases and use of information for intervention, and lower cost for large scale studies. However, it is not clear whether they are feasible and whether the data collected are comparable to more conventional methods. One research group has evaluated the use of PDAs in a multisite study of elder neglect in emergency department environments in the US [72, 80]. While thorough training of data collection staff led to competence in use of the devices to collect EAI data in the training environment, once collection began in busy emergency department settings, a number of difficulties were identified, which made them difficult to use in situ, both for technical as well as relational reasons [80]. This may be particularly problematic in research on sensitive issues such as elder abuse and neglect, where gaining good quality data depends on maintaining a good interpersonal relationship with the older person being interviewed. Many staff felt that the challenges of trying to enter data in the presence of the respondent was difficult and many resorted to writing responses and entering them later. Other challenges encountered were problems with uploading data due to an unreliable server connection, equipment loss or failure, concerns about security, battery failure, and problems associated with obsolence of both hardware and software over the course of a study. As technological innovations progress, some of these issues can be addressed, however, it is noted that technology will never be totally reliable and a number of recommendations are made to ensure there are back-up methods for optimising data collection under all conditions [80].

9.6.5 Multidimensional Assessment

To address the challenges of conceptual confusion, and provide a more comprehensive and rigorous screen, there has been a move towards using a multi-dimensional approach to assessment. An early trend was to include assessments of both the care-recipient and care-provider (e.g. [10, 14, 138, 139, 155, 156]). More recently, Fulmer and colleagues investigated the value of dyadic vulnerability and risk profiling among older people and their carers to see whether the dyadic profile provided a more thorough means of identifying elder neglect [73]. Their model was derived from an earlier risk-and-vulnerability model applied to elder abuse [69]. This involved measuring various proxy indicators such as: unmet needs using six ADL and nine IADL items; personal resources; childhood trauma; personality; and the Caregiver Hassles Scale [90]. Interestingly, their findings supported the inclusion of risk factors related to both caregiver and elder vulnerability as a means of screening more comprehensively for elder neglect. However, a limitation of this model is that contextual and relational dynamics are not included. Others have developed a more complex package of assessment tools such as the Ohio Elder Abuse and Domestic Violence in Late Life Screening Tools and Referral Protocol [65], but psychometric validation did not meet the eligibility criteria for this review.

Another interesting approach has been to develop a more comprehensive risk index by aggregating across various measures [48]. Dong and Simon found that a 9-item vulnerability index demonstrated good accuracy for reported and confirmed elder abuse outcomes in a community sample.

For instance, older adults with three or more risk factors were almost four times more likely to experience elder abuse as those with two or fewer risk factors. Those with five or more risk factors were 26 times more likely to experience elder abuse. The nine variables making up the index were: age, gender, race, income, medical conditions, cognitive function, physical function, depressive symptoms, and social network. To combine the variables into a risk index, cutpoints for each risk factor were examined for precision in detecting elder abuse, and the cutpoints with the strongest associations with elder abuse outcomes were applied in the combined index. Such studies address problems associated with using one risk indicator or one abusive behaviour as the basis for prevalence estimates and establishing 'caseness', and are potentially able to be applied in healthcare and statutory environments.

Environmental assessments have long been considered an important aspect of a comprehensive geriatric assessment [117] and have been used in a variety of elder abuse measures, particularly of neglect. Home-based assessment also allows for a higher level of contextual information to inform judgments about the level of abuse or neglect. Greater context is also required for accurate interpretation of relational dynamics that may contribute to abusive behaviour. While there is recognition that multiple perspectives are useful, what is of most interest is the interplay between perspectives. What does it mean if the elder person and their carer have very different responses to a question?

9.6.6 Culture and Language

A limited number of studies suggest that scales translated into other languages using established methods of forward and backward translation have shown adequate reliability. For instance, translated versions of the CTS and CTS2 have been reported to perform reliably for Chinese populations [20, 46, 173, 174], and for Tamil speakers [23]. Scales have been also translated and validated in Spanish such as the CASE [130], while the H-S/EAST and VASS have been validated in Chinese speaking populations [55, 170]. Others have used local expert input to develop or modify scales for specific cultural contexts, such as the development of the EDMA in Spain [161], the GMS in Mexico [79], the E-IOA in Israel [26], the PEAS/EPAS in Taiwan [164, 165], and a Korean language scale [127]. Nevertheless, there is a commonality across the content of major domains and items. Further work is needed to determine the effectiveness of translation and to better understand appropriate methods to measure elder abuse in difficult cultural context.

Few studies have administered screening measures in different cultural contexts or examined how they perform across cultures. The few multi-national studies identified in this review report different prevalence rates across countries (e.g., [40, 68, 108, 152]). The cause of these differences is not known, but could be partially explained by measurement error. Methodological issues could include translation problems, different meanings or values placed on certain behaviors or constructs in different cultures, different sampling strategies or modes of administration, differences in training and so on. However, there is some evidence that differences may also relate to community-level indicators of difference, as well as the individual characteristics of the elder or their caregiver. For instance, in the largest multi-national study identified, the ABUEL study [68, 111], a number of country and city level socioeconomic indicators helped to explain differences in elder abuse rates across seven European countries. More specifically, country-level indicators of economic inequality were significantly related to the prevalence of financial elder abuse, and the city mean tertiary education explained a significant amount of variation in the prevalence of psychological abuse among these elderly populations. This study provides valuable insight into the potential of additional community-based indicators to contribute to elder abuse, and provide a means of targeting higher risk groups for prevention, screening and intervention programs.

9.6.7 Cognitive Impairment

Most studies have not investigated the applicability of screening instruments for those with cognitive impairment, despite this being a risk factor for several forms of elder abuse and neglect [59]. This is partly due to the limited reliability of self-report data with this group, and potential bias arising from asking carers to report on their abusive behaviour towards the care-recipient. This is an area where alternative assessment methods need to be explored. One scale, the SVS22 and the SVS15 [134, 135], was designed specifically to assess vulnerability to exploitation among cognitively impaired older people. It has demonstrated good psychometrics for two subscales of gullibility and credulity, and discriminated well between clinical and non-clinical populations. However, it relies on care-givers as informants and doesn't not gain the elders' perspective. This is problematic for studying elder abuse by care-givers.

Another research group has explored the challenges of assessing cognitive capacity as an indicator of self-neglect. The Consortium for Research in Elder Self-Neglect of Texas (CREST) developed the COMP Screen to assess elders' capacity to make decisions relevant to safe and independent living [119]. The researchers argued that conceptualisation of self-neglect needed to distinguish between three forms of lack of self-care: that resulting from disability, an autonomous choice, or from a decline in decision-making capacity. They proposed that only this third group should be seen as suffering from self-neglect. Their COMP Screen was designed to test three cognitive domains (attention, expressive language, and delayed recall), and a fourth conceptual domain of awareness, which tests the ability to compare alternatives and articulate a choice between options. However, they failed to support this assessment as an adequate screening approach for self-neglect. One conclusion from this study is that a screening instrument for elder self-neglect needs to assess both the capacity to make decisions and the capacity to act on those decisions [119].

9.7 Effectiveness of Screening for Elder Abuse and Neglect

The USPSTF [163] criteria for the effectiveness of a screening test states that the test must be able to detect the target condition earlier than without screening and with sufficient accuracy to avoid producing large numbers of false-positive and false-negative results; and the screening and follow-up treatment should improve health outcomes compared with treating patients when they present with signs or symptoms of the disease. Whether screening for elder abuse meets these criteria has been the subject of some debate [129]. Some authoritative health bodies have recommended routine screening of older patients (American College of Emergency Physicians [5]; American Medical Association [AMA] [6, 7]; National Gerontological Nursing Association [NGNA] [121], while others suggest that research evidence fails to support this recommendation [126, 128, 166]. The most comprehensive systematic review of the effectiveness of screening for elder abuse and neglect has been undertaken by the US Preventive Services Task Force [126] for the years 2002–2012, extending their earlier review of studies from to 2002 [125]. This review examined the effect of screening asymptomatic elders or vulnerable adults in health care settings for elder abuse or neglect and found only a very small number of studies. Among these, the USPSTF found no adequate randomised control trials or controlled observational studies that examined whether screening reduced exposure to abuse and neglect, or reduced physical or mental health harm or mortality. The USPSTF concluded that there is insufficient evidence that screening or early detection reduces exposure of vulnerable elders to abuse or decreases any harm caused by the abuse [126].

The relative lack of evidence is a result of complex factors such as the nature of elder abuse itself, the difficulty in accurately measuring it, and the relatively early stage of development of valid and reliable measures. Furthermore, there have been few longitudinal studies that have examined the predictive validity of screening. Of course, lack of evidence is not proof that screening is ineffective, and there is broad agreement that efforts should be made to both identify elder abuse early and put in place measures to prevent or reduce its impact. Research related to specific questions about the effectiveness of screening are addressed next.

9.7.1 Does Screening for Elder Abuse and Neglect Identify Those at Most Risk of Elder Abuse and Neglect?

Because of a lack of a gold standard measure of elder abuse and neglect, it has been difficult to address the question of whether screening accurately identifies those at most risk of elder abuse and neglect. The 6-item EASI measure [172] was rated as of fair quality by the USPSTF in its most recent review and identified as the best validated measure suitable for screening for elder abuse in healthcare settings available at that time [126]. However, the scoring system is not clearly specified and the first item does not actually measure elder abuse.

Some studies of ADL and IADL measures have reported associations with confirmed elder abuse status, though sensitivity and specificity analysis is not available. For instance, a matched case–control study of abused and non-abused recipients of Israeli social welfare services found that the abused group was significantly more impaired [104]. This suggests that such a brief easily administered may be a useful measure of vulnerability to abuse, but the causal direction has not been established. Interestingly, while ADL measures are usually conceptualised as measures of neglect or self-neglect, functional impairment is related to elder abuse more broadly, not just neglect.

Some methodological issues that impact on this question include the representativeness of samples. Are those who take part in screening studies representative of all older people, or may those who are vulnerable to abuse be less likely to participate, leading to under-representation in studies? Item non-response is another methodological issue. Are older people willing to answer questions about abuse by a family member or carer? De Donder et al. [40] found that item non-response ranged from 1.8 % for neglect to 4.2 % for items such as excluding, ignoring, or destroying possessions. They found that different non-response patterns related to different types of abuse. For instance, response patterns for neglect and emotional abuse differed from those for more serious forms such as financial, physical, sexual abuse and violation of personal rights. Response patterns also differed by mode of administration—postal versus face-to-face interview versus telephone interview. Compared with postal survey, face-to-face interviews had less missing data. After taking into account individual characteristics and modes of administration—higher non-response was associated with higher age, lower income, lower education, and poorer mental health. Presence of another person (interviewer or family member/health care provider) was also associated with less missing data. Such issues have implications for the ability of screening measures to produce accurate identification of those at risk.

9.7.2 Does Screening for Elder Abuse and Neglect Predict Poor Health Outcomes and Mortality?

A very small number of studies have established that substantiated reports of elder abuse significantly predict shorter life spans after adjusting for other factors related to mortality in older adults. These include the New Haven Established Populations for Epidemiologic Studies in the Elderly [94], and the Chicago Health and Aging Project which found that reported and confirmed elder abuse and self-neglect predicted 1-year all-cause mortality [56]. Furthermore, mortality associated with reported and confirmed elder abuse was greatest for those with lowest levels of psychological and social well-being [50].

Of more relevance to this chapter are studies that have examined the long-term health outcomes for those identified by screening tools as at risk of abuse. These epidemiologic studies are based on self-report of abuse, not substantiated abuse. Two large community-based prospective studies have examined health outcomes associated with self-reported elder abuse. Analysis of data from the Australian Longitudinal Study on Women's Health (ALSWH) indicated that one of the four VASS subscales, dejection, predicted 3-year physical and mental health outcomes [146, 147, 149]. A longer-term follow-up study of this cohort found that the VASS subscale, coercion, significantly predicted mortality 12 years after screening. Disability was predicted by the vulnerability and dejection subscales, after controlling for other confounders. In the US, the Women's Health Initiative data of women aged 50–79, self-reported physical and verbal abuse independently predicted mortality over 7–8 years, with physical abuse having the highest predictive value [12].

Limitations of current research on health outcomes of elder abuse include the small number of studies, short-term follow-up in prospective studies [56, 147], a reliance on cross-sectional research [24, 30, 67], and a focus on cases of substantiated abuse only [50, 94], or on current symptomatology rather than longer-term serious health outcomes such as mortality and disability [30, 67]. Only one study was found that that examined long-term health outcomes over a decade or more [148], and few that examined disability as an outcome. Given the long-term costs of disability, this is an important outcome to investigate.

9.7.3 Does Screening Lead to Effective Referral and Treatment?

Screening practices are considered useful only if they lead to development, implementation and evaluation of effective preventive and early intervention programs. Very little research has addressed this question. Most studies of screening for elder abuse do not report on follow-up of those identified as at risk, except among studies of suspected cases reported to authorities such as Adult Protective Services (APS). One retrospective study of 575 elderly veterans (96 % male) aged 65–103 years in California, USA, identified those possibly exposed to abuse or neglect and referred them for social work interventions [114]. The actions taken to reduce exposure to abuse or neglect are reported, but actual health outcomes are not adequately measured.

9.7.4 Are There Effective Intervention Programs Available for Those at Risk?

A systematic review of the effectiveness of interventions for elder abuse found insufficient evidence to support any particular intervention [136]. In this review, only eight studies met inclusion criteria for the review, and many methodological weaknesses were identified in the studies. Of concern, intervention had no effect on abuse in most studies and may have even increased future abuse. The interventions were also found to have no positive effect on at-risk care-giver outcomes and behaviour, and mixed outcomes for professional knowledge and behaviour. This suggests that the pathway from identification of risk to successful improvement of outcomes is fraught with many difficulties, and will require more innovative approaches. The type of interventions available have also been reviewed by Alon and Berg-Warman [4]. Yet, those who work at the coalface, see a clear need for intervention programs, as a legal framework is insufficient on its own to address this complex social problem, and has potential to create harm as well as benefits, as has been found in the challenging area of child abuse.

9.7.5 Are There Adverse Outcomes from Screening?

Family violence research suggests that a major concern of screening is the potential for retaliation by the abuser should they find out about the screening, resulting in direct harm caused by the screening [107]. Given the added dependency between carers and elders, it may be that screening for elder abuse and neglect could put the older person at greater risk. For instance, postal surveys may be opened by abusive carers. The presence of carers may also make it difficult for screening to take place in the home or in the health care setting. Although no studies have specifically sought to examine this question, there is very little evidence available of actual harm caused by screening for elder abuse or neglect. The USPSTF systematic reviews suggested that the potential for harm is small, but may include shame, guilt, self-blame, fear of retaliation or abandonment by perpetrators, and distress caused by false-positive results [125, 126]. Further research is required to address this important question. A screening program needs to ensure that the questions are asked in a safe and private environment so that elders are not put in further harm.

9.8 Future Research

Despite a growing literature on screening tools for elder abuse, there is a need for further development and evaluation of brief reliable and valid screening instruments that can be widely used to screen for abuse in different screening contexts, as previously noted [35, 42]. A better distinction is needed between the three purposes of screening tools identified in the current research: population screening, screening as part of routine healthcare, and 'screening' whose primary purpose is to investigate suspected or reported elder abuse. Different tools are likely needed for these different purposes and each need to be validated within the context for which they are intended.

A need for greater specification and measurement of types of elder mistreatment has been identified [18, 42]. Some interesting research has been undertaken to explore the conceptual and theoretical framework underpinning elder mistreatment as a foundation for development of more differentiated screening instruments and this would seem to be a promising area for future research. For instance, Conrad and colleagues have undertaken concept mapping methodologies to identify expanded components of psychological abuse and financial exploitation, to inform the development of more robust screening measures [33, 32, 31]. In the area of elder self-neglect, Burnett and colleagues have used an analysis of APS data to define four unique subtypes of elder self-neglect: physical and medical neglect (50 %), environmental neglect (22 %), global neglect (21 %), and financial neglect (9 %) [18], paving the way for more differentiated methods of measurement. Others have identified potentially new constructs that have not been incorporated into most measures of elder abuse to date and these warrant further investigation. For instance, an observational study of staff-patient interactions in aged care settings identified infantilization of elders by their carers as a form of abuse in that it demeaned the older person and caused them distress [143], yet this behaviour is not adequately tapped by most existing measures. The field needs a clear consensus among researchers about a brief general measure of abuse suitable for widescale screening, as well as consensus about more differentiated measures of specific forms of abuse.

Clearly, there is a need for more robust psychometric evaluation of screening measures to progressively define conceptually clear, short versions that have adequate reliability and validity [35, 41, 96]. There is an ongoing tension between the thoroughness of longer forms, and the practical utility of more succinct but robust shorter forms of screening measures. Some examples are provided in this review of the progressive refinement of measures and ongoing validation (e.g., [33, 32, 31]). The Centers for Medicare and Medicaid Services [18, 150] used an expert technical panel to derive a consensus recommendation about screening tools that met a sufficient range of quality criteria to recommend for use for routine screening in healthcare settings. Three screening measures were commended: the H-S/EAST [124], the VASS [149], and the EASI [172]. Nevertheless, there is a clear need for more research into the reliability and validity of methods of data collection in this sensitive research area [41, 126].

Further research on the effect of modes of administration is needed to examine differences between the most commonly used modes of written questionnaire, face-to-face interview, and telephone interview. Observational measures also need further evaluation to determine optimal, reliable, valid and cost-effective methods. This is particularly so for assessing nutritional self-care, as no studies were identified that had successfully validated a method to assess this aspect of self-neglect. A relatively recent development in observational methods, particularly in nursing homes, is the use of electronic surveillance to monitor the wellbeing of residents. This offers interesting potential to assess staff-to-resident abuse, resident-to resident abuse, or even resident-to-staff abuse, but is fraught with ethical challenges [15].

Even less is known about the effectiveness of screening—what actions are taken with those who demonstrate higher risk on screening measures and how effective are those programs? What barriers are there to implementation of screening and interventions, and how can these barriers be overcome? These are fertile areas for multidisciplinary collaboration and further work could be undertaken to determine optimal team approaches to the detection and intervention for elder abuse risk. Research is also needed on the best ways of having screening embedded in routine care.

The majority of research on screening has been undertaken in either primary care or institutional care settings, or among higher risk individuals referred to adult protective services. Research on population based screening is sparse [96, 108, 148], and conclusions are difficult to draw given the wide range of measures and methods used. In addition to the need for further validation of screening instruments suitable for population studies, longitudinal studies are needed to determine the predictive power of the screening instruments for future abuse, for health and mortality outcomes and the effectiveness of appropriate intervention. Research is also needed on the impact of screening on care-giver and care-recipient dynamics.

Given the importance of familial care relationships to vulnerable elders, a valuable approach would be to examine the effectiveness of therapeutic interventions to ameliorate the triggers for abusive behavior and foster healthy caregiving dynamics. For instance, research evaluating interventions for other forms of family violence may be useful in developing appropriate therapeutic and supportive interventions for elder abuse and neglect. This would require development of appropriate measures to assess the impact of such interventions. The use of well-designed qualitative research could also provide a complement to the psychometric approach, as well as measurement of dyadic interactions.

Key recommendations for future research include:

- Further development of elder mistreatment theory and alignment of screening measures to better assess more clearly differentiated theoretical constructs and types of abuse.
- Greater clarity of screening purpose and alignment of measures to the purpose.
- More rigorous psychometric evaluation of instruments over different populations and cultures.
- Examination of modes of administration and adaptation to different cultural contexts.
- Refinement of existing instruments to produce shorter reliable and valid version.
- Well designed longitudinal research to examine the predictive validity of elder abuse screening measures for a range of outcomes including future abuse, substantiated abuse, mortality, and health outcomes.

9.9 Policy Implications

The value of screening is predicated historically on having reliable and valid measures of the phenomenon of interest, appropriate referral pathways, evidence of successful interventions for those found to be at risk on the screening measure, and evidence of improved outcomes [163]. Dong [44] notes, however, that screening for elder abuse is complex and can't be evaluated by the same criteria as for medical issues. Rather there is a need to consider the specific challenges associated with screening for elder abuse and determine whether the intended benefits of screening outweigh the potential harms. This review has highlighted some gaps between these criteria and available evidence, and raises a number of policy implications.

First, screening is necessary to raise awareness of the scope and nature of the elder abuse problem in society. It is only through accurate measurement, determination of prevalence and types of abuse, as well as risk factors, that appropriate policy planning can take place. Without a more thorough approach to screening, we will remain in a *catch-22* situation where it is argued that there is insufficient evidence to justify screening. As for all forms of family violence, accurate measurement of the phenomena will remain challenging, but it is only through such efforts that awareness of the scope of the problem and potential solutions can be articulated.

Second, a key policy debate relates to whether screening for elder abuse and neglect should be part of routine healthcare screening practice, or implemented for only higher risk groups, or where signs of abuse or suspected abuse reports are available. Some have argued that screening should occur routinely in healthcare settings [6, 7, 44, 121], while others have argued that there is insufficient evidence to support such a recommendation [125, 126, 128]. Dong [44] has made a strong case that elder abuse should not be subjected to the standard medical model criteria for implementation of screening programs, but rather that the contextual and often hidden nature of elder abuse requires a more proactive approach to identification, in order to prevent the significant negative health outcomes. This is more than a medical issue, it is also one of societal justice.

Third, to address these debates, coordinated multi-sector initiatives are needed to bring advances to the screening dilemmas currently facing the field. There are many examples of state-based systems working together to develop more comprehensive approaches to integrating screening, referral and interventions approaches (e.g., [13, 65]), but arguably there is an urgent need for better coordinated high-level national and international approaches. As an example, the CMS in the US convened a national symposium to examine the role of elder abuse screening as a Physician Quality Reporting System (PQRS) measure in Medicare beneficiaries [44]. The purpose was to review available evidence and make consensus recommendations about a comprehensive approach to screening, identifying and implementing appropriate follow pathways for those at risk of elder abuse [19].

The CMS Report of the Technical Expert Panel on Elder Maltreatment Screening documents agreement that screening should include screening for differentiated forms: physical abuse, emotional or psychological abuse, neglect (active or passive), sexual abuse, abandonment, financial or material exploitation, and unwarranted control [19]. The Panel recommended two scales as among the best available currently: The H-S/EAST and the VASS. Both measures have been tested in diverse populations, have shown adequate reliability and validity across cultures, and are relatively brief and suitable for both population screening and use by healthcare professionals. Self-neglect, while clearly important, was not included as a form of elder abuse per se as it is not perpetrated by a carer, but it is considered an important part of any geriatric assessment.

A fourth policy consideration is to need to further develop more differentiated pathways for referral and intervention when older people screen positive for elder abuse. Currently, the legal framework dominates, with reporting to authorities such as the APS in the US being legally mandated for suspected elder abuse. However, with advances in our knowledge of the range of types of abuse, and widely varying severity and chronicity, there is a need for more differentiated pathways following positive screens. The evidence base is accumulating about possible prevention and intervention strategies that may assist in reducing the risk of elder abuse and poor long-term outcomes. Policymakers need to work with researchers to define appropriate criteria to recognise a more differentiated understanding of suspected abuse, and develop more accessible and effective strategies. What non-legal options are there for follow-up screening and investigation, with potential implementation of effective intervention programs available for those identified as at risk of abuse?

9.10 Practice Implications

Research in the areas of child abuse and interpersonal violence suggests that it is possible to develop and implement effective interventions for complex societal issues such as family violence [157]. These include the use of home visits of potentially at risk families using a partnership model, carer training programs, school-based life skills training, public policy initiatives, and therapeutic approaches [118, 157]. While reporting of suspected abuse is mandatory in most jurisdictions, it may be necessary to find more appropriately tailored supportive interventions for all but the more severe end of the abuse continuum. An interesting alternative model for assessment and intervention that may be of value in this field comes from the family dispute/mediation area, where the traditional legal/family court approach to divorce disputes has increasingly been replaced by a model that puts the focus on a more supportive community-based family mediation/dispute resolution model [167]. Under this model, couples in dispute are required to attend family mediation to assess the extent of the problems and develop mediated solutions, prior to court attendance. Winkworth and McArthur outline a practice framework to guide screening and assessment throughout the period of contact, recognising that needs and safety concerns are likely to change over time. It proposes a more responsive and less reactive model than in may protection services. It may be that all but the more extreme end of elder abuse activity, could be better addressed in a more comprehensive community-based assessment and intervention centre as increasingly available for divorcing families, and partner violence. Demonstration projects to assess the effectiveness of such coordinated community-based approaches are needed.

Given that much elder abuse involves important familial relationships, and the majority of abuse involves psychological abuse and neglect, there is a need for greater development of psychological and therapeutic approaches to change potentially harmful relational dynamics. The burdens of caring can exacerbate long-standing relationship dynamics, as well as foster new problems, and there is a need to distinguish between these situations. While there has been considerable development of therapeutic approaches for intimate partner violence, there is little development of approaches to elder abuse that may help to preserve positive aspects of the carer relationship with victims. Approaches to date have largely focused on structural interventions such as placing the abused person in institutional care, or provision of nursing and home care services [118]. Community-level integration of elder services could potentially provide a more holistic approach to addressing the underlying issues and improve quality of life for older people, with less stigmatisation associated with APS referral.

Moracco and Cole [116] identified three types of interventions for intimate partner violence that may help reduce risk and improve outcomes, and it is worth considering how these approaches could be applied to elder abuse. The most common intervention is referral to community services such as counseling, legal services, alternative accommodation, and social welfare services, and empowerment strategies such as support groups, education, and volunteer advocates may be useful. The equivalent of dedicated domestic violence services is not readily available for those experiencing elder abuse, and their greater dependency makes it difficult to seek out support services. Yet, this is clearly an area that would benefit from a more supportive case management approach, especially for less severe forms of abuse, without the stigma and associated problems arising from official reporting to APS type bodies.

Second, home visits by professional staff could be expanded to provide more preventive and supportive interventions to assist those in the home. Social support is a critical element of any supportive care and needs to be provided in an ongoing way to be effective. A third approach to intervention is to offer programs to address risk factors of the abusive care-giver. These may include counselling, groups programs, provision of respite care, substance abuse therapeutic programs, and helpline support services. Individual supportive counseling may be useful to reduce anxiety, stress, and depression in the carer, and cognitive-behavioral methods can be used to educate the carer about the reasons for a dependent person's behavior, their needs, and developmental limitations. Such programs have been successful with abusive parents and could be adapted to elder abuse caregivers.

Drawing on evidence of successful parenting interventions for child abuse [85], it is suggested that supportive psychoeducational and therapeutic interventions that aim to support caregivers to undertake their demanding role would be useful for this population [157]. Both child and elder abuse occur in the context of a dependency relationship, where the needs of the dependent person (child or adult) need to take priority. These practices from the wider family violence field point to areas of potentially useful intervention and evaluation priorities.

9.11 Summary

This chapter has undertaken systematic review of elder abuse screening tools published in the 20-year period from 1995 to 2015. The review identified 33 measures that reported any psychometric evaluation in the period: 10 used primarily for population-based screening purposes, 16 for screening in health care settings, and a further 7 instruments developed to screen for elder neglect and self-neglect. Key issues related to screening for elder abuse are critically reviewed, and some future directions identified.

References

1. Abdel Rahman TT, El Gaagary MM. Elder mistreatment in a rural area in Egypt. Geriatr Gerontol Int. 2012;12:532–7. doi:10.1111/j.1447-0594.2011.00780.x.
2. Abrams RC, Lachs M, McAvay G, Keohane DJ, Bruce ML. Predictors of self-neglect in community-dwelling elders. Am J Psychiatry. 2002;159:1729–30. doi:10.1176/appi.ajp.159.10.1724.
3. Aish AE, Isenberg M. Effects of Oren-based nursing intervention on nutritional self-care of myocardial infarction patients. Int J Nurs Stud. 1996;33:259–70. doi:10.1016/0020-7489(95)00059-3.
4. Alon S, Berg-Warman A. Treatment and prevention of elder abuse and neglect—a model for intervention to prevent and treat elder abuse in Israel. J Elder Abuse Negl. 2014;26:150–71. doi:10.1080/08946566.2013.784087.
5. American College of Emergency Physicians (2016) Clinical and practice management: domestic family violence. American College of Emergency Physicians, Irving. Accessed 25 Oct 2016. http://www.acep.org/content.aspx?id=38378.
6. American Medical Association (AMA). Diagnostic and treatment guidelines on elder abuse and neglect. Chicago: Author; 1992.
7. American Medical Association (AMA) (2007) Amendment to Opinion E-2.02, "Physicians' obligations in preventing, identifying and treating violence and abuse". Report of the Council on Ethical and Judicial Affairs, CEJA Report 6-I-07. Accessed 15 Dec 2015. http://www.ama-assn.org/ama/pub/about-ama/our-people/ama-councils/council-ethical-judicial-affairs/ceja-reports.page.
8. Anthony EK, Lehning AJ, Austin MJ, Peck MD. Assessing elder mistreatment: instrument development and implications for adult protective services. J Gerontol Soc Work. 2009;52:815–36. doi:10.1080/01634370902918597.
9. Ayalon L. Evaluating the working conditions and exposure to abuse of Filipino home care workers in Israel: characteristics and clinical correlates. Int Psychogeriatr. 2009;21:40–9.
10. Ayalon L. Abuse is in the eyes of the beholder: using multiple perspectives to evaluate elder mistreatment under round-the-clock foreign home carers in Israel. Ageing Soc. 2011;31:499–520. doi:10.1017/S0144686X1000108X.
11. Ayalon L. Reports of elder neglect by older adults, their family caregivers, and their home care workers: a test of measurement invariance. J Gerontol Psychol Sci Soc Sci. 2015;70B:432–42. doi:10.1093/geronb/gbu051.
12. Baker MW, LaCroix AZ, Wu CY, Cochrane BB, Wallace R, Woods NF. Mortality risk associated with physical and verbal abuse in women aged 50–79. J Am Geriatr Soc. 2009;57:1799–809. doi:10.1111/j.1532-5415.2009.02429.x.
13. Bass DM, Anetzberger GJ, Ejaz FK. Nagpaul K. Screening tools and referral protocol for stopping abuse against older ohioans: a guide for service providers. J Elder Abuse Negl. 2001;13(2), 23–38. doi:10.1300/J084v13n02_03
14. Beach SR, Schulz R, Williamson GM, Miller LS, Weiner MF, Lance CE. Risk factors for potentially harmful informal caregiver behavior. J Am Geriatr Soc. 2005;53:255–61. doi:10.1111/j.1532-5415.2005.53111.x.
15. Bharucha AJ, London AJ, Barnard D, Wactlar H, Dew MA, Reynolds CF III. Ethical considerations in the conduct of electronic surveillance research. J Law Med Ethics. 2006;34:611–9. doi:10.1111/j.1748-720X.2006.00075.x.
16. Biggs S, Manthorpe J, Tinker A, Doyle M, Erens B. Mistreatment of older people in the United Kingdom: findings from the first national prevalence study. J Elder Abuse Negl. 2009;21:1–14. doi:10.1080/08946560802571870.
17. Burnes D, Pillemer K, Caccamise PL, Mason A, Henderson CR Jr, Berman J, et al. Prevalence of and risk factors for elder abuse and neglect in the community: a population-based study. J Am Geriatr Soc. 2015;63:1906–12. doi:10.1111/jgs.13601.
18. Burnett J, Dyer CB, Halphen JM, Achenbaum WA, Green CE, Booker JG, Diamond PM. Four subtypes of self-neglect in older adults: results of a latent class analysis. J Am Geriatr Soc. 2014;62:1127–32. doi:10.1111/jgs.12832.
19. Centers for Medicare and Medicaid Services (CMS) (2013) Technical expert panel (TEP) summary report: elder mistreatment screening and follow-up plan. Author. Accessed 30 Nov 2015. https://www.cms.gov/Medicare/Quality-Initiatives-Patient-Assessment-Instruments/MMS/Downloads/Elder-Maltreatment-Screening-and-Follow-Up-Plan.pdf.
20. Chan KL, Choi WMA, Fong DYT, Chow CB, Leung M, Ip P. Characteristics of family violence victims presenting to emergency departments in Hong Kong. J Emerg Med. 2013;44:249–58. doi:10.1016/j.jemermed.2012.01.061.
21. Chang E-S, Beck T, Simon MA, Dong X. A psychometric assessment of the psychological and social wellbeing indicators in the PINE study. J Aging Health. 2014;26:1116–36. doi:10.1077/0898264314543471.
22. Chang JC, Decker M, Moracco KE, Martin SL, Petersen R, Frasier PY. What happens when health care providers ask about intimate partner violence? A description of consequences from

the perspectives of female survivors. J Am Med Women's Assoc. 2003;58(2):76–81. doi:10.1016/j.pec.2004.10.008.

23. Chokkanathan S, Lee AE. Elder mistreatment in urban India: a community based study. J Elder Abuse Negl. 2005;17(2):45–61. doi:10.1300/J084v17n02_03.
24. Cisler JM, Begle AM, Amstadter AB, Acierno R. Mistreatment and self-reported emotional symptoms: results from the National Elder Mistreatment Study. J Elder Abuse Negl. 2012;24:216–30. doi:10.1080/08946566.2011.652923.
25. Cohen M. The process of validation of a three-dimensional model for the identification of abuse in older adults. Arch Gerontol Geriatr. 2013;57:243–9. doi:10.1016/j.archger.2013.06.009.
26. Cohen M, Halevi-Levin S, Gagin R, Friedman G. Development of a screening tool for identifying elderly people at risk of abuse by their caregivers. J Aging Health. 2006;18:660–85. doi:10.1177/0898264306293257.
27. Cohen-Mansfield J, Marx MS, Rosenthal AS. A description of agitation in a nursing home. J Gerontol Soc Sci. 1989;44:577–84.
28. Cohen M, Halevi-Levin S, Gagin R, Friedman G. Elder abuse: disparities between older people's disclosure of abuse, evident signs of abuse, and high risk of abuse. JAGS. 2007;55(8);1224–30. doi:10.1111/j.1532-5415.2007.01269.x
29. Cohen M, Halevi-Levin S, Gagin, R, Friedman G. Elder abuse in long-term care residences and the risk indicators. Ageing Soc. 2010;30:1027–40. doi:10.1017/S0144686X10000188
30. Comijs HC, Penninx BWJH, Knipscheer KPM, van Tilburg W. Psychological distress in victims of elder mistreatment: the effects of social support and coping. J Gerontol. 1999;54B:240–5. doi:10.1093/geronb/54B.4.P240.
31. Conrad KJ, Iris M, Ridings JW, Langley K, Anetzberger G. Self-report measure of psychological abuse of older adults. Gerontologist. 2011;51:354–66. doi:10.1093/geront/gnq103.
32. Conrad KJ, Iris M, Ridings JW, Langley K, Wilber KH. Self-report measure of financial exploitation of older adults. Gerontologist. 2010;50:758–73. doi:10.1093/geront/gnq054.
33. Conrad KJ, Iris M, Ridings JW, Fairman KP, Rosen A, Conceptualizing and measuring financial exploitation of older adults. In: Report to the National Institute of Justice. Grant #. 2006-MU-2004; 2009.
34. Cooper C, Katona C, Finne-Soveri H, Topinkova E, Carpenter GI, Livingston G. Indicators of elder abuse: a crossnational comparison of psychiatric morbidity and other determinants in the Ad-HOC study. Am J Geriatr Psychiatry. 2006;14:489–97. doi:10.1097/01.JGP.0000192498.18316.b6.
35. Cooper C, Manela M, Katona C, Livingston G. Screening for elder abuse in dementia in the LASER-AD study: prevalence, correlates and validation of instruments. Int J Geriatr Psychiatry. 2008;23:283–8. doi:10.1002/gps.1875.
36. Cooper C, Maxim K, Selwood A, Blanchard M, Livingston G. The sensitivity and specificity of the Modified Conflict Tactics Scale for detecting clinically significant elder abuse. Int Psychogeriatr. 2009;21:774–8. doi:10.1017/S1041610209009387.
37. Cooper C, Selwood A, Blanchard M, Walker Z, Blizard R, Livingston G. The determinants of family caregivers' abusive behaviour to people with dementia: results of the CARD study. J Affect Disord. 2010;121:136–42. doi:10.1016/j.jad.2009.05.001.
38. Cooper C, Selwood A, Livingston G. The prevalence of elder abuse and neglect: a systematic review. Age Ageing. 2008;37:151–60. doi:10.1093/ageing/afm194.
39. Dai Y, Yang C, Wang H, Cheng Y, Long-term care services functional classification system. In: National Science Council of Taiwan Report (in Chinese); 1995.
40. De Donder L, Lang G, Penhale B, Ferreira-Alves J, Tamutiene I, Verté D, Luoma M-L. Item non-response when measuring elder abuse: influence of methodological choices. Eur J Pub Health. 2013;23:1021–6. doi:10.1093/eurpub/cks172.
41. De Donder L, Luoma M-L, Penhale B, Lang G, Santos AJ, Tamutiene I, et al. European map of prevalence rates of elder abuse and its impact for future research. Eur J Aging. 2011;8:129–43. doi:10.1007/s10433-011-0187-3.
42. Dong X. Do the definitions of elder mistreatment subtypes matter? Findings from the PINE Study. J Gerontol A Med Sci. 2014a;69A(S2):S68–75. doi:10.1093/gerona/glu141.
43. Dong X. Self-neglect in an elderly community-dwelling U.S. Chinese population: findings from the Population Study of Chinese Elderly in Chicago Study. J Am Geriatr Soc. 2014b;62:2391–7. doi:10.1111/jgs.13140.
44. Dong X. Screening for elder abuse in healthcare settings: Why should we care, and is it a missed quality indicator? J Am Geriatr Soc. 2015;63:1686–92. doi:10.1111/jgs.1_13538.
45. Dong X, Beck T, Simon MA. The associations of gender, depression and elder mistreatment in a community-dwelling Chinese population: the modifying effect of social support. Arch Gerontol Geriatr. 2010a;50:202–8. doi:10.1016/j.archger.2009.03.011.
46. Dong X, Chang E-S, Simon MA. Physical function assessment in a community-dwelling population of U. S. Chinese older adults. J Gerontol A Med Sci. 2014e;62A:2391–7. doi:10.1093/gerona/glu205.
47. Dong X, Simon MA. Urban and rural variations in the characteristics associated with elder mistreatment in a community-dwelling Chinese population. J Elder Abuse Negl. 2013;25:97–125. doi:10.1080/08946566.2013.751811.
48. Dong X, Simon MA. Vulnerability risk index profile for elder abuse in a community-dwelling population. J Am Geriatr Soc. 2014;62:10–5. doi:10.1111/jgs.12621.
49. Dong XQ, Simon MA. Elder self-neglect is associated with an increased rate of 30-day hospital readmission: findings from the Chicago Health and Aging Project. Gerontology. 2015;61:41–50. doi:10.1159/000360698.
50. Dong XQ, Simon MA, Beck TT, Farran C, McCann JJ, Mendes de Leon CF, et al. Elder abuse and mortality: The role of psychological and social wellbeing. Gerontology. 2011;57:549–58. doi:10.1159/000321881.
51. Dong XQ, Simon MA, Evans DA. Prevalence of self-neglect across gender, race, and socioeconomic status: findings from the Chicago Health and Aging Project. Gerontology. 2012a;58:258–68. doi:10.1159/000334256.
52. Dong XQ, Simon MA, Evans DA. Elder self-neglect and hospitalization: findings from the Chicago Health and Aging Project. J Am Geriatr Soc. 2012b;60:202–9. doi:10.1111/j.1532-5415.2011.03821.
53. Dong XQ, Simon MA, Evans DA. Prospective study of the elder self-neglect and emergency department use in a community population. Am J Emerg Med. 2012d;30:553–61. doi:10.1016/j.ajem.2011.02.008.
54. Dong X, Simon M, Fulmer T, Mendes de Leon CF, Rajan B, Evans DA. Physical function decline and the risk of elder self-neglect in a community-dwelling population. Gerontologist. 2010b;50:316–26.
55. Dong X, Simon MA, Gorbien M. Elder abuse and neglect in an urban Chinese population. J Elder Abuse Negl. 2007;19(3–4):79–96.
56. Dong X, Simon M, Mendes de Leon C, Fulmer T, Beck T, Hebert L, et al. Elder self-neglect and abuse and mortality risk in a community-dwelling population. J Am Med Assoc. 2009;302:517–26. doi:10.1001/jama.2009.1109.
57. Dong XQ, Simon MA, Mosqueda L, Evans DA. The prevalence of self-neglect in a community-dwelling population: hoarding,

hygiene, and environmental hazards. J Aging Health. 2012c;24:507–24. doi:10.1177/0898264311425597.
58. Dong X, Wilson RS, Mendes de Leon CF, Evans DA. Self-neglect and cognitive function among community-dwelling older persons. Int J Geriatr Psychiatry. 2010c;25:798–806.
59. Dong X, Wilson RS, Simon MA, Rajan B, Evans DA. Cognitive decline and risk of elder self-neglect: the findings from the Chicago Health and Aging Project. J Am Geriatr Soc. 2010d;58:2292–9.
60. Dong X. Self-neglect in an elderly community-dwelling U.S. Chinese population: findings from the Population Study of Chinese Elderly in Chicago Study. JAGS. 2014b; 62:2391–7. doi:10.1111/jgs.13140
61. Dyer CB, Kelly PA, Pavlik VN, Lee J, Doody RS, Regev T, Smith SM. The making of a self-neglect severity scale. J Elder Abuse Negl. 2006;18:13–23. doi:10.1300/J084v18n04_03.
62. Dyer CB. Neglect assessment in elderly persons. J Gerontol: Med Sc. 2005;60A:1000–1. doi:10.1093/gerona/60.8.1000
63. Edirisinghe PAS, Paranitharn P, Perera WNS, Willams SS. Elder abuse among outpatient department attendees in a tertiary care hospital in Sri Lanka. Ceylon Med J. 2014;59(3):84–9. doi:10.4038/cmj.v59i3.6527.
64. Eisikovits Z, Winterstein T, Lowenstein A. The national survey on elder abuse and neglect in Israel. Haifa: University of Haifa and Eshel; 2004.
65. Ejaz FK, Bass DM, Anetzberger GJ, Nagpaul K. Evaluating the Ohio elder abuse and domestic violence in late life screening tools and referral protocol. J Elder Abuse Negl. 2001;13 (2):39–57. doi:10.1300/J084v13n02_04.
66. Evers GCM. Appraisal of Self-Care Agency. A.S.A.-scale. Assen, NL: Van Gorcum; 1989.
67. Fisher BS, Regan SL. The extent and frequency of abuse in the lives of older women and their relationship with health outcomes. Gerontologist. 2006;46:200–9. doi:10.1093/geront/46.2.200.
68. Fraga S, Lindert J, Barros H, Torres-Gonzales F, Ioannidi-Kapolou E, Melchiorre MG, Soares JF. Elder abuse and socioeconomic inequalities: a multilevel study in 7 European countries. Prev Med. 2014;61:42–7. doi:10.1016/j.ypmed.2014.01.008.
69. Frost MH, Willette K. Risk for abuse/neglect: documentation of assessment data and diagnoses. J Gerontol Nurs. 1994;20:37–45. doi:10.3928/0098-9134-19940801.
70. Fulmer T, Guadagno L, Paveza G, VandeWeerd C, Baglioni A, Abraham I. Profiles of older adults who screen positive for neglect during an emergency department visit. J Elder Abuse Negl. 2002;14:49–60. doi:10.1300/J084v14n01_03.
71. Fulmer T, McMahon DJ, Baer-Hines M, Forget B. Abuse, neglect, abandonment, violence, and exploitation: an analysis of all elderly patients seen in one emergency department during a six-month period. J Emerg Nurs. 1992;18:505–10. doi:10.1093/geront/45.4.525.
72. Fulmer T, Paveza G, Abraham I, Fairchild S. Elder neglect assessment in the emergency department. J Emerg Nurs. 2000;26 (5):436–43. doi:10.1067/men.2000.110621.
73. Fulmer T, Paveza G, VandeWeerd C, Fairchild S, Guadagno L, Bolton-Blatt M, Norman R. Dyadic vulnerability and risk profiling for elder neglect. Gerontologist. 2005a;45:525–34. doi:10.1093/geront/45.4.525.
74. Fulmer T, Paveza G, VandeWeerd C, Guadagno L, Fairchild S, Norman R, Bolton-Blatt M. Neglect assessment in urban emergency departments and confirmation by an expert clinical team. J Gerontol Med Sci. 2005b;60A:1002–6. doi:10.1093/gerona/60.8.1002.
75. Fulmer T, Rodgers RF, Pelger A. Verbal mistreatment of the elderly. J Elder Abuse Negl. 2014;26:351–64. doi:10.1080/08946566.2013.801817.
76. Fulmer T, Strauss S, Russell SL, Singh G, Blankenship J, Vermula R, Sutin D. Screening for elder mistreatment in dental and medical clinics. Gerondontology. 2012;29:96–105. doi:10.1111/j.1741-2358.2010.00405.x.
77. Fulmer T, Street S, Carr K. Abuse of the elderly: screening and detection. J Emerg Nurs. 1984;10:131–40. doi:10.1067/men.2000.110621.
78. Fulmer T, Gurland B. Restriction as elder mistreatment: differences between caregiver and elder perceptions. J Mental Health Aging. 1996;2:89–98.
79. Giraldo-Rodriguez L, Rosas-Carrasco S. Development and psychometric properties of the Geriatric Mistreatment Scale. Geriatr Gerontol Int. 2013;13:887–93. doi:10.1111/ggi.12024.
80. Guadagno L, VandeWeerd C, Stevens D, Abraham I, Paveza G, Fulmer T. Using PDAs for data collection. Appl Nurs Res. 2004;17:283–91. doi:10.1016/j.apnr.2004.09.008.
81. Hwalek M, Sengstock M. Assessing the probability of abuse of the elderly: toward the development of a clinical screening instrument. J Appl Gerontol. 1986;5:153–73. doi:10.1177/073346488600500205.
82. Iris M, Conrad KJ, Ridings J. Observational measure of elder self-neglect. J Elder Abuse Negl. 2014;26:365–97. doi:10.1080/08946566.2013.801818.
83. Isenberg M, International research project to test Orem's self-care deficit theory of nursing. In: Proceedings of scientific session of the 29th Biennial Convention of Sigma Theta Tau International. San Francisco: Sigma Theta Tau; 1987.
84. Jervis LL, Fickenscher A, Beals J, the Shielding American Indian Elders Project Team. Assessment of elder mistreatment in two American Indian samples: psychometric characteristics of the HS-EAST and the Native Elder Life-Financial Exploitation and -Neglect measures. J Appl Gerontol. 2014;33:336–56. doi:10.1177/0733464812470748.
85. Kaminski JW, Valle LA, Filene JH, Boyle CL. A meta-analytic review of components associated with parent training program effectiveness. J Abnorm Child Psychol. 2008;36:567–89.
86. Katz S. Assessing self-maintenance: activities of daily living, mobility, and instrumental activities of daily living. J Am Geriatr Soc. 1983;31:721–7.
87. Kelly P, Dyer C, Pavlik V, Doody R, Jogerst G. Exploring self-neglect in older adults: preliminary findings of the self-neglect severity scale and next steps. J Am Geriatr Soc. 2008;56:S253–60.
88. Kelly JB, Johnson MP. Differentiation among types of intimate partner violence: research update and implications for interventions. Fam Court Rev. 2008;46:476–99. doi:10.1111/j.1744-1617.2008.00215.x.
89. Kim MH, Kown K-J, Lim Y-O, Lee Y-H. Screening scale of elder abuse. J Korean Gerontol Soc. 2006;26:819–42.
90. Kinney JM, Stephens MA. Caregiving Hassles Scale: assessing the daily hassles of caring for a family member with dementia. The Gerontologist. 1989;29:328–32. doi:10.1093/geront/29.3.328.
91. Kosberg J. Preventing elder abuse: identification of high risk factors prior to placement decisions. The Gerontologist. 1988;28:43–50. doi:10.1093/geront/28.1.43.
92. Kottwitz D, Bowling S. A pilot study of the elder abuse questionnaire. Kansas Nurse. 2003;78(7):4–6.
93. Lachs MS, Pillemer K. Elder abuse. Lancet. 2004;364:1263–72. doi:10.1016/S0140-6736(04)17144-4.

94. Lachs MS, Williams C, O'Brien S, Pillemer K, Charlson M. The mortality of elder mistreatment. J Am Med Assoc. 1998;280:428–32. doi:10.1001/jama.280.5.428.
95. Lachs MS, Pillemer KA. Abuse and neglect of elderly persons. New England J Medicine. 1995;233:437–43. doi:10.1056/NEJM199502163320706
96. Lang G, De Donder L, Penhale B, Ferreira-Alves J, Tamutiene I, Luoma M-L. Measuring older adults' abuse: evaluation of formative indicators to promote brevity. Educ Gerontol. 2014;40:531–42. doi:10.1080/03601277.2013.857892.
97. Lauder W. A survey of self-neglect in patients living in the community. J Clin Nursing. 1999;8:95–102. doi:10.1046/j.1365-2702.1999.00231.x
98. Laumann EO, Leitsch SA, Waite LJ. Elder mistreatment in the United States: prevalence estimates from a nationally representative study. J Gerontol B Soc Sci. 2008;63B:S248–54. doi:10.1093/geronb/63.4.S248.
99. Lawton MP, Brody EM. Assessment of older people: self-maintaining and instrumental activities of daily living. Gerontologist. 1969;9:179–86. doi:10.2190/AG.78.2.b.
100. Lee M, Kim K. Prevalence and risk factors for self-neglect among older adults living alone in South Korea. Int J Aging Hum Dev. 2014;78:115–31.
101. Liamputtong P, editor. Research methods in health: Foundations for evidence-based practice. 2nd ed. Melbourne: Oxford University Press; 2013. ISBN 9780195520064.
102. Lindenbach JM, Larocque S, Lavoie A-M, Garceau M-L. Older adult mistreatment risk screening: contribution to the validation of a screening tool in a domestic setting. Can J Aging. 2012;31(2):235–52. doi:10.1017/S0714980812000153
103. Lindert J, Luna J, Torres-Gonzalez F, Barros H, Ioannidi-Kapolou E, Quattrini S, et al. Study design, sampling and assessment methods of the European study "Abuse of the Elderly in the European region". Eur J Pub Health. 2012;22:662–6.
104. Litwin H, Zoabi S. A multivariate examination of explanations for the occurrence of elder abuse. Soc Work Res. 2004;28:133–42.
105. Lorensen M, Halter IM, Evers G, Isenberg M, van Achterberg T. Cross-cultural testing of the "appraisal of self-care agency: ASA Scale" in Norway. Int J Nurs Stud. 1993;30:15–23. doi:10.1016/0020-7489(93)90089-D
106. Lowenstein A, Eisikovits Z, Band-Winterstein T, Enosh G. Is elder abuse and neglect a social phenomenon? Data from the first national prevalence survey in Israel. J Elder Abuse Negl. 2009;21:253–77. doi:10.1080/08946560902997637.
107. MacMillan HL, Wathen CN, Jamieson E, Boyle MH, Shannon HS, Ford-Gilboe M, Worster A, Lent B, Coben JH, Campbell JC, McNutt LA, McMaster Violence Against Women Research Group. Screening for intimate partner violence in health care settings: a randomized trial. J Am Med Assoc. 2009;302:493–501. doi:10.1001/jama.2009.1089.
108. Macassa G, Viitasara E, Sundin O, Barros H, Torres Gonzales F, Ioannidi-Kapolou E, et al. Psychological abuse among older persons in Europe: A cross-sectional study. J Aggress Confl Peace Res. 2013;5:16–34. doi:10.1108/17596591311290722.
109. Martin SL, Rentz ED, Chan RL, Givens J, Sanford C, Kupper LL, et al. Physical and sexual violence among North Carolina women: associations with physical health, mental health, and functional impairment. Women's Health Issues. 2008;18:130–40. doi:10.1016/j.whi.2007.12.008.
110. McFarlane J, Parker B, Soeken K, Bullock L. Assessing for abuse during pregnancy: severity and frequency of injuries and associated entry into prenatal-care. J Am Med Assoc. 1992;267:3176–8. doi:10.1001/jama.267.23.3176.
111. Melchiorre MG, Chiatti C, Lamura G, Torres-Gonzales F, Stankunas M, Lindert J, et al. Social support, socio-economic status, health and abuse among older people in seven European countries. PLoS One. 2013;8(1):e54856. doi:10.1371/journal.pone.0054856.
112. Moody LE, Voss A, Lengacher CA. Assessing abuse among the elderly living in public housing. J Nurs Meas. 2000;8:61–70.
113. Moon A, Benton D. Tolerance of elder abuse and attitudes toward third-party intervention among African American, Korean American, and white elderly. J Multic Soc Work. 2000;8:283–303. doi:10.1300/J285v08n03_05.
114. Moon A, Lawson K, Carpiac M, Spaziano E. Elder abuse and neglect among veterans in greater Los Angeles: prevalence, types, and intervention outcomes. J Gerontol Soc Work. 2006;46(3–4):187–204. doi:10.1300/J083v46n03_11.
115. Moon A, Williams O. Perceptions of elder abuse and help-seeking patterns among African-American, Caucasian American, and Korean-American elderly women. Gerontologist. 1993;33:386–95. doi:10.1093/geront/33.3.386.
116. Moracco KE, Cole KB. Preventing intimate partner violence is not enough. J Am Med Assoc. 2009;302:568–70. doi:10.1001/jama.2009.1135.
117. Morris JN, Fries BE, Steel K, Ikegami N, Bernabei R, Carpenter GI, Topinková E. Comprehensive clinical assessment in community setting: applicability of the MDSHC. J Am Geriatr Soc. 1997;45:1017–24. doi:10.1111/j.1532-5415.1997.tb02975.x.
118. Nahmiash D, Reis M. Most successful intervention strategies for abused older adults. J Elder Abuse Negl. 2000;12:53–70. doi:10.1300/J084v12n03_03.
119. Naik AD, Pickens S, Burnett J, Lai JM, Dyer CB. Assessing capacity in the setting of self-neglect: development of a novel screening tool for decision making capacity. J Elder Abuse Negl. 2006;18:79–91. doi:10.1080/08946566.2011.584049.
120. National Centre on Elder Abuse (NCEA) (1998) The national elder abuse incidence study: final report september 1998. Author. Accessed 10 Dec 2015. http://aoa.gov/AoA_Programs/Elder_Rights/Elder_Abuse/docs/ABuseReport_Full.pdf.
121. National Gerontological Nursing Association (NGNA) (2006) Position statement on elder abuse, neglect, and maltreatment. Accessed 26 Oct 2015. http://www.ngna.org/_resources/documentation/position_papers/ElderAbusePositionStatement.pdf.
122. Naughton C, Drennan J, Lyons I, Lafferty A, Treacy M, Phelan A, et al. Elder abuse and neglect in Ireland: results from a national prevalence survey. Age Ageing. 2012;41:98–103. doi:10.1093/ageing/afr107.
123. Neale AV, Hwalek MA, Scott RO, Sengstock MC, Stahl C. Validation of the Hwalek-Sengstock Elder Abuse screening test. J Appl Gerontol. 1991;10:406–18. doi:10.1177/073346489101000403.
124. Neale AV, Hwalek MA, Goodrich CS, Quinn KM. The illinois elder abuse system: program description and administrative findings. Gerontologist, 1996;36:502–11. doi:10.1093/geront/36.4.502
125. Nelson HD, Nygren P, McInerney Y, Klein J. Screening women and elderly adults for family and intimate partner violence: a review of the evidence for the U.S. Preventive Services Task Force. Ann Intern Med. 2004;140:387–96. doi:10.7326/0003-4819-140-5-200403020-00015.
126. Nelson HD, Bougatsos C, Blazina I (2012) Screening women for intimate partner violence and elderly and vulnerable adults for abuse: systematic review to update the 2004 U.S. Preventive Services Task Force Recommendation. Evidence Synthesis No. 92. AHRQ Publication No. 12-05167-EF-1. Rockville, MD: Agency for Healthcare Research and Quality; 2012.

127. Oh J, Kim HS, Martins D, Kim H. A study of elder abuse in Korea. Int J Nurs Stud. 2006;43:203–14. doi:10.1016/j.ijnurstu.2005.03.005.
128. O'Brien JG. Screening for elder abuse and neglect. J Am Geriatr Soc. 2015;63:1689–91. doi:10.1111/jgs.1_13538
129. Perel-Levin S. Discussing screening for elder abuse at primary health care level. Geneva: World Health Organization; 2008. Accessed 10 Nov 2015. http://www.who.int/iris/handle/10665/43523.
130. Perez-Rojo G, Nuevo E, Sancho M, Penhale B. Validity and reliability of the Spanish version of the Caregiver Abuse Screen (CASE). Res Aging. 2015;37:63–81. doi:10.1177/0164027514522275.
131. Pfeiffer E. A short portable mental status questionnaire for the assessment of organic brain deficit in elderly patients. J Am Geriatr Soc. 1975;23:433–41. doi:10.1111/j.1532-5415.1975.tb00927.x.
132. Phillips LR. Domestic violence and aging women. Geriatr Nurs. 2000;21(4):188–93. doi:10.1067/mgn.2000.109584.
133. Pickens S, Naik AD, Burnett J, Kelly PA, Gleeson M, Dyer CB. The utility of the Kohlman evaluation of living skills test is associated with substantiated cases of elder self-neglect. J Am Acad Nurse Pract. 2007;19:137–42.
134. Pinsker DM, McFarland K, Stone VE. The social vulnerability scale for older adults: an exploratory and confirmatory factor analytic study. J Elder Abuse Negl. 2011;23:246–72. doi:10.1080/08946566.2011.584049.
135. Pinsker DM, Stone VE, Pachana NA, Greenspan S. Social vulnerability scale for older adults: validation study. Clin Psychol. 2006;10:117–27. doi:10.1080/13284200600939918.
136. Ploeg J, Fear J, Hutchison B, MacMillan H, Bolan G. A systematic review of interventions for elder abuse. J Elder Abuse Negl. 2009;21:187–210. doi:10.1080/08946560902997181.
137. Podnieks E. National survey on abuse of the elderly in Canada. J Elder Abuse Negl. 1992;4:5–58. doi:10.1300/J084v04n01_02.
138. Reis M, Nahmiash D. Validation of the caregiver abuse screen (CASE). Can J Aging. 1995;14(Suppl. 2):45–61. doi:10.1017/S0714980800005584.
139. Reis M, Nahmiash D. Validation of the indicators of abuse (IOA) screen. Gerontologist. 1998;38:471–80. doi:10.1093/geront/38.4.471.
140. Robinson BC. Validation of a Caregiver Strain Index. J Gerontol. 1983;38:344–8.
141. Russell SL, Fulmer T, Singh G, Vermula R, Strauss S. Screening for elder mistreatment in a dental clinic population. J Elder Abuse Negl. 2012;24:326–39. doi:10.1080/08946566.2012.661683.
142. Saikia AM, Mahanta N, Mahanta A, Deka AJ, Kakati A. Prevalence and risk factors of abuse among community dwelling elderly of Guwahati City, Assam. Indian J Commun Med. 2015;40:279–91. doi:10.4103/0970-0218.164406.
143. Salari SM. Infantilization as elder mistreatment: evidence from five adult day centers. J Elder Abuse Negl. 2005;17(4):53–91. doi:10.1300/J084v04_04.
144. Schmeidel AN, Daly JM, Rosenbaum ME, Schmuch GA, Jogerst GJ. Health care professionals' perspectives on barriers to elder abuse detection and reporting in primary care settings. J Elder Abuse Negl. 2012;24:17–36. doi:10.1080/08946566.2011.608044.
145. Schofield MJ, Forrester-Knauss C. Surveys and questionnaires in health research. In: Liamputtong P, editor. Research methods in health: foundations for evidence-based practice. 2nd ed. Melbourne: Oxford University Press; 2013. pp. 198–218. ISBN 9780195520064.
146. Schofield MJ, Mishra G. Validity of self-report screening scale for elder abuse: Women's Health Australia. Gerontologist. 2003;43:110–20. doi:10.1093/geront/43.1.110.
147. Schofield MJ, Mishra G. Three year health outcomes among older women at risk of elder abuse: Women's Health Australia. Qual Life Res. 2004;13:1043–52. doi:10.1023/B:QURE.0000031343.15372.a5.
148. Schofield MJ, Powers JR, Loxton D. Mortality and disability outcomes of self-reported elder abuse: a 12-year prospective investigation. J Am Geriatr Soc. 2013;61:679–85. doi:10.1111/jgs.12212.
149. Schofield MJ, Reynolds R, Mishra GD, Powers JR, Dobson AJ. Screening for vulnerability to abuse among older women: Women's Health Australia study. J Appl Gerontol. 2002;21:24–39. doi:10.1177/0733464802021001002.
150. Schwartz K, McMullen T (2013) CMS elder mistreatment quality measurement initiative. Centers for Medicare and Medicaid Services. Accessed 5 Jan 2016. http://iom.nationalacademies.org/~/media/Files/Activity%20Files/Global/ViolenceForum/2013-APR-17/Presentations/02-07-McMullen.pdf.
151. Shepard M, Campbell J. The abusive behavior inventory: a measure of psychological and physical abuse. J Interpers Violence. 1992;7:291–305. doi:10.1177/088626092007003001.
152. Shugarman LR, Fries BE, Wolf RS, Morris JN. Identifying older people at risk of abuse during routine screening practices. J Am Geriatr Soc. 2003;51:24–31. doi:10.1034/j.1601-5215.2002.51005.x.
153. Soares JJF, Fraga D, Viitasara E, Stankunas M, Sundin O, Melchiorre MG, Barros H. The chronicity and severity of abuse among older persons by country: a European study. J Aggress Confl Peace Res. 2014;6:3–25. doi:10.1108/JACPR-06-2013-0015.
154. Strasser SM, Smith M, Weaver S, Zheng S, Cao Y. Screening for elder mistreatment among older adults seeking legal assistance services. West J Emerg Med. 2013;14:309–15. doi:10.5811/westjem.2013.2.15640.
155. Straus MA. Measuring intrafamily conflict and violence: The Conflict Tactics (CT) Scales. J Marriage Fam. 1979;41:75–88. doi:10.2307/351733.
156. Straus MA, Hamby SL, Boney-McCoy S, Sugarman DB. The revised conflict tactics scales (CTS2): development and preliminary psychometric data. J Fam Issues. 1996;17:283–316. doi:10.1177/019251396017003001.
157. Sumner SA, Mercy JA, Dahlberg LL, Hillis SD, Klevens J, Houry D. Violence in the United States: status, challenges, and opportunities. J Am Med Assoc. 2015;314:478–88. doi:10.1001/jama.2015.8371.
158. Teresi JA, Ocepek-Welikson K, Ramirez M, Eimicke JP, Silver S, Van Haitsma K, et al. Development of an instrument to measure staff-reported resident-to-resident elder mistreatment (R-REM) using item response theory and other latent variable models. Gerontologist. 2013;54:460–72. doi:10.1093/geront/gnt001.
159. Thornton M, Travis SS. Analysis of the reliability of the modified caregiver strain index. J Gerontol B Psychol Sci Soc Sci. 2003;58(2):S129. doi:10.1093/geronb/58.2.S127.
160. Tjaden P, Thoennes N, Prevalence, incidence, and consequences of violence against women: findings from the national violence against women survey. Research in Brief. Washington, DC: US Department of Justice, National Institute of Justice, and US Department of Health and Human Services, Centers for Disease Control and Prevention; 1998. Accessed 10 Nov 2015. https://www.ncjrs.gov/pdffiles/172837.pdf.
161. Touza C, Prado C, Segura MP. Detection scales for the risk of domestic abuse and self-negligent behavior in elderly persons

(EDMA). J Elder Abuse Negl. 2012;24:312–25. doi:10.1080/08946566.2012.661682.

162. UK Action on Elder Abuse, What is elder abuse?; 1995. Accessed 21 Dec 2015. http://elderabuse.org.uk/what-is-elder-abuse/.
163. US Preventive Services Task Force. Guide to clinical preventive services. 2nd ed. Baltimore: Williams & Wilkins; 1996.
164. Wang J-J. Psychological abuse and its characteristic correlates among elderly Taiwanese. Arch Gerontol Geriatr. 2006;42:307–18. doi:10.1016/j.archger.2005.08.006.
165. Wang J-J, Tseng H-F, Chen K-M. Development and testing of screening indicators for psychological abuse of older people. Arch Psychiatr Nurs. 2007;21:40–7. doi:10.1016/j.apnu.2006.09.004.
166. Wathen CN, MacMillan HL, Canadian Task Force on Preventive Health Care. Prevention of violence against women: recommendation statement from the Canadian Task Force on Preventive Health Care. Can Med Assoc J. 2003;169:582–4.
167. Winkworth G, McArthur M. A practice framework to guide screening and assessment in the Australian Family Relationship Centres and Advice Line. Child Fam Soc Work. 2009;14:410–9. doi:10.1111/j.1365-2206.2009.00612.x.
168. World Health Organization (WHO). World report on violence and health. Geneva: Author; 2002.
169. World Health Organization (WHO). A global response to elder abuse and neglect: building primary health care capacity to deal with the problem world-wide: main report. Geneva: Author; 2008.
170. Wu L, Chen H, Hu Y, Xiang H, Yu X, Zhang T, Cao Z, Wang Y. Prevalence and associated factors of elder mistreatment in a rural community in People's Republic of China: a cross-sectional study. PLoS One. 2012;7(3):e33857. doi:10.1371/journal.pone.0033857.
171. Yaffe MJ, Weiss D, Lithwick M. Seniors' self-administration of the elder abuse suspicion index (EASI): a feasibility study. J Elder Abuse Negl. 2012;24:277–92. doi:10.1080/08946566.2011.652930.
172. Yaffe MJ, Wolfson C, Lithwick M, Weiss D. Development and validation of a tool to improve physician identification of elder abuse: The Elder Abuse Suspicion Index (EASI). J Elder Abuse Negl. 2008;20:276–300. doi:10.1080/08946560801973168.
173. Yan E, Tang CS. Prevalence and psychological impact of Chinese elder abuse. J Interpers Violence. 2001;16:1158–74. doi:10.1177/088626001016011004.
174. Yan E, Tang C. Elder abuse by caregivers: a study of prevalence and risk factors in Hong Kong Chinese families. J Fam Violence. 2004;19:269–77. doi:10.1023/B:JOFV.0000042077.95692.71.

10 The Role of Technology in Elder Abuse Research

Scott R. Beach

10.1 Introduction

We are in the midst of a technological revolution that is changing the world in fundamental ways. The digital revolution has changed the way we learn, work, communicate, and how we spend our leisure time. Technology has also revolutionized the conduct of scientific research across disciplines. Computerized data collection, smartphone applications, video and sensor-based technologies, physiological monitoring, brain imaging techniques, and data mining algorithms for "big data" are just a few examples. This chapter focuses on the role of technology in elder abuse research. The primary goal of the chapter is to provide an overview of how technology has been used thus far in elder abuse research, and, more importantly, to stimulate thinking about how it might be used in the future.

The focus is on technology in three main areas: (1) technology for *direct data collection* from elder abuse victims, (2) technology for *indirect detection* of elder abuse and risk factors, and (3) the role of *information technology* (IT) in elder abuse research. The section on direct data collection describes work my own research group has done on using privacy-enhancing survey technologies to study elder abuse prevalence, including its potential for direct surveys of perpetrators. Use of technology in a community-based study of older Chinese adults living in the United States is also described. Then, use of survey technologies for elder abuse screening and detection in clinical settings is described. A brief discussion of the potential for computer-adaptive testing applications to elder abuse research is presented. The section concludes with a discussion of the intriguing potential for the use of video monitoring in long-term care (LTC) settings to study resident-to-resident aggression (RRA). Technologies for the indirect detection of elder abuse discussed include medical forensics technology, neuroscience/brain imaging, financial fraud detection data mining techniques, and individual physiological and home-based sensor monitoring. Technology for the indirect detection of elder neglect and self-neglect is also discussed. The discussion of IT and elder abuse research focuses on the need for a uniform national Adult Protective Services (APS) database, and describes two recent smaller scale projects that demonstrate the feasibility and effectiveness of IT applications in the APS context. The chapter incorporates illustrative examples of the use of technology in child abuse and intimate partner violence (IPV) research to inform work on elder abuse. The chapter concludes with a summary overview of use of technology to date for elder abuse research and potential future directions.

10.2 Technology for Direct Data Collection from Elder Abuse Victims

10.2.1 Survey Technologies for Elder Abuse Measurement

Among cognitively intact community-dwelling older adults, direct surveys have been used to measure the incidence and prevalence of elder abuse (e.g., [1, 34, 35]). These surveys have used interviewer-administered methods to obtain data on the occurrence of elder abuse, either telephone surveys [1, 35] or in-person interviews [34]. Prevalence estimates for various types of abuse have generally ranged from 5 to 10 %, although physical and sexual abuse prevalence is much lower (typically 1–2 %). However, questions remain as to whether prevalence has been underestimated, given the sensitive nature of elder mistreatment and the potential reluctance of victims to admit it to an interviewer using standard telephone or in-person methods [3].

The survey methodological literature on asking sensitive questions is relevant to any attempt to measure elder mistreatment directly from victims [57, 58]. Reports of sensitive behaviors are potentially subject to underreporting as a result of

S.R. Beach (✉)
University Center for Social and Urban Research, University of Pittsburgh, 3343 Forbes Avenue, Pittsburgh, PA, USA
e-mail: scottb@pitt.edu

X. Dong (ed.), *Elder Abuse*, DOI 10.1007/978-3-319-47504-2_10

social desirability concerns, perceived invasion of privacy, and fear of disclosure to third parties. Direct questions to older adults about mistreatment at the hands of family members or other trusted persons are likely subject to these concerns. These questions could potentially be seen as embarrassing or nobody's business (e.g., airing dirty laundry about intimate family matters). Potentially more important, questions about elder mistreatment may be seen as threatening, potentially resulting in family consequences (e.g., retaliation by the perpetrator if survey reports are revealed), or even legal consequences (removal or prosecution of the family perpetrator).

One of the most consistent findings in the survey literature on sensitive behaviors is that self-administered modes of data collection result in higher levels of reporting than interviewer-administered modes [57]. Although most studies do not involve a "gold standard," or "objective" record to verify individual reports of sensitive behaviors, researchers generally assume that, due to social desirability and other concerns, respondents tend to under-report behaviors that may reflect poorly on them or are less socially acceptable (e.g., drug use; illegal activity; abortions; same-sex relationships), and overreport behaviors that are more socially acceptable and make them look good (e.g., voting; church attendance; charitable donations). Thus, higher prevalence of "bad" things and lower prevalence of "good" things are generally seen as more valid or accurate. Self-administered methods of data collection are generally thought to increase validity in reporting sensitive behaviors by increasing perceived privacy through eliminating the need to disclose such information directly to an interviewer. In the case of elder mistreatment, self-administration may reduce at least some of the concerns mentioned above, including less embarrassment at having to report mistreatment to another person, as well as less threat of a potential perpetrator overhearing survey responses to an interviewer. Thus we would expect self-administration to result in increased reports of elder abuse relative to interviewer-administered modes.

Interviewer-administered surveys typically involve technology—computer-assisted telephone interviews (CATI) and computer-assisted personal interviews (CAPI)—which involve the interviewer reading questions from a computer screen and entering survey responses directly into the database. More recently, CATI and CAPI interviewing has been supplemented with new applications of technology that remove the interviewer in an attempt to enhance the perceived privacy of the interview (see [16] for an overview of technology trends in surveys). In the personal interview setting, *audio computer-assisted self-interviewing* (*A-CASI*) has been developed, in which the computer plays a recorded version of questions and answer choices over headphones while the respondent reads the questions/answer choices, and the respondent answers via keyboard, mouse, or touchscreen. One issue is whether or not the "audio" portion of A-CASI is actually adding anything over and above simpler computer-assisted self-interviews (CASI), where respondents read questions from the screen and respond using a laptop computer without hearing questions via headphones. However, among older adults with possible vision, hearing, literacy, or cognitive problems, giving respondents the option to simultaneously hear and see the questions may limit potential difficulties in responding. Traditional CATI telephone interviews have been supplemented with *Interactive Voice Response* (*IVR*), in which a recorded voice system administers questions and the respondent replies by using the keys on a touchtone telephone (see [38] for an overview). This has been applied in surveys by having a live interviewer initiate the call and administer nonsensitive items, then transferring the respondent to the IVR system for the sensitive questions, with the option of returning to the interviewer to complete the survey (e.g., [59]).

My research group conducted a study testing the feasibility, acceptability, and validity of technology-based survey methods for collecting self-reports about elder mistreatment among older adults in Allegheny County (Pittsburgh) Pennsylvania, USA [3]. We conducted a population-based survey of adults age 60 and over using random-digit dialing (RDD) telephone screening, with *random assignment* to one of four survey modes: (1) standard CAPI in-person interview; (2) "privacy enhanced" CAPI in-person interview with a switch to an A-CASI system for the elder mistreatment items; (3) standard CATI telephone interview; and (4) "privacy enhanced" CATI telephone interview with a switch to an IVR system for the elder mistreatment items. Interviews were conducted between May 2007 and January 2008 with 903 adults age 60 and older, with approximately equal numbers of interviews in each condition. The introductory recruitment script in the RDD phone call did not mention which condition the respondent had been assigned to until after the decision to participate was made to avoid potential confounding of experimental condition with nonresponse. In the telephone conditions, once a household was determined to be eligible and the respondent agreed to the interview, it was conducted at that time. For the in-person conditions, once eligibility was determined and the respondent agreed to the interview, an appointment was scheduled, and an address was obtained for those being conducted in the home. We focused on self-reports of elders regarding financial, psychological, and physical mistreatment by family members or other trusted persons using items developed from other surveys. The study addressed two major questions:

1. *Can older adults use newly developed A-CASI and IVR survey technologies to report data on elder mistreatment?* Will they accept the technology, or will they prefer simply responding to an interviewer?

2. If feasible and acceptable, *do these new methods actually produce more valid reporting of elder mistreatment?* Given the likelihood that older adults have a tendency to under-report mistreatment due to embarrassment, shame, or fear of reprisal, *do A-CASI and IVR increase elder mistreatment reporting relative to traditional CAPI and CATI approaches?*

We also asked follow-up questions for the A-CASI and IVR conditions about ease of use of the technology, privacy perceptions, and preference for the technology versus a human interviewer. Detailed methods and results are described in Beach et al. [3].

Looking first at feasibility and acceptance of A-CASI, among the 224 respondents initially assigned to this condition, about 83 % used the computer to answer the elder mistreatment items, although only about 55 % agreed to use the headphones to listen to the questions. Thus, about 28 % completed what is traditionally termed CASI (computer-assisted self-interviewing)—they read the questions silently and entered their own responses. Thirty-five respondents (16 %) in the A-CASI condition refused to use the computer for any responses and continued with a CAPI interview. Three respondents started with A-CASI, refused to finish, but answered the remaining questions via CAPI; and only one respondent refused to answer any elder mistreatment items. The majority of the problems or questions respondent's had were either general navigation issues—for example, not knowing to press "enter" to get to the next screen, or problems using the mouse. The majority refusing to use headphones simply said they "didn't need them," although a few mentioned issues with hearing aids.

Among the 227 respondents originally assigned to the IVR condition, about 83 % completed the elder mistreatment items using the system, the same figure as for A-CASI (see above). The main reason for non-completion of IVR was either lack of a touchtone phone ($n = 18$; 8 %) or difficulties using a cordless touchtone phone for response ($n = 7$; 3 %). Note that only one respondent refused to use the IVR system, which contrasts with the A-CASI findings, where about 16 % refused to use the system. Six respondents either began IVR but switched back to the interviewer to complete the elder mistreatment items either by choice ($n = 2$) or due to technical problems with the system ($n = 4$); while another five respondents quit IVR and refused to answer the remaining mistreatment items. Finally, only two respondents hung up or broke off during IVR, and both were recontacted by the interviewer immediately after the break-off and completed the mistreatment items in CATI. Both reported technical difficulties with the system. Turning to the impact of survey technology on elder abuse prevalence estimates, as shown in Fig. 10.1, 9.7 % reported experiencing some form of financial exploitation since turning 60 and 3.5 % reported experiencing this in the 6 months prior to the interview. Although the prevalence of financial mistreatment since turning 60 was highest in the A-CASI condition (15.6 %), neither Chi-Square test comparing A-CASI to CAPI nor IVR to CATI were statistically significant. When asked about financial mistreatment in the last 6 months, those in the A-CASI condition reported significantly ($p < 0.05$) more (7.3 %) than those in the interviewer-administered CAPI condition (2.5 %). IVR did not increase reporting of financial mistreatment in the last 6 months relative to CATI, which in fact produced a higher prevalence rate (3.2 vs. 1.8 %), though this difference was not significant.

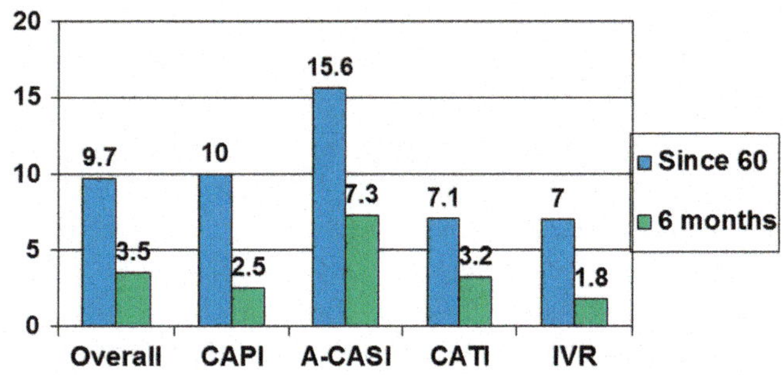

Fig. 10.1 Prevalence (%) of financial exploitation overall/by experimental condition [3]

The overall prevalence of psychological mistreatment since age 60 was 14.3 %, and the 6 month prevalence was 8.2 % (Fig. 10.2). The prevalence of psychological mistreatment since age 60 was highest in the A-CASI condition (22.5 vs. 13.6 % for CAPI; $p < 0.05$). The IVR condition also resulted in slightly higher prevalence of psychological mistreatment since 60 (14.0 vs. 9.1 % for CATI; n.s.). Results for psychological mistreatment in the last 6 months were clearer. In this case, once again, prevalence was highest in the A-CASI condition (16.4 vs. 5.0 % for CAPI; $p < 0.01$). The IVR condition also produced higher 6 month prevalence of psychological mistreatment (9.3 vs. 4.5 % for CATI), although the difference did not reach conventional levels of significance.

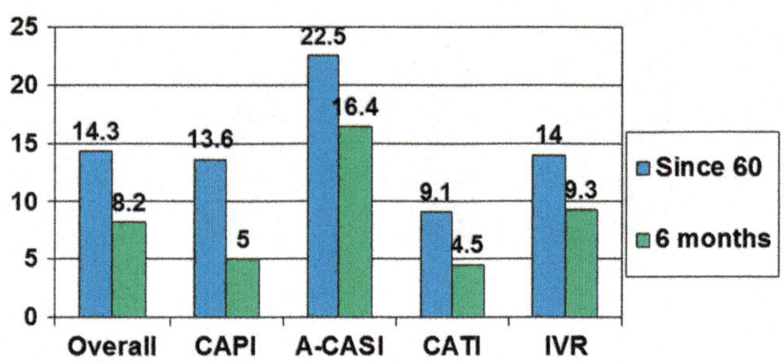

Fig. 10.2 Prevalence (%) of psychological mistreatment overall/by experimental condition [3]

The estimated prevalence of physical mistreatment since turning 60 was 4.4 and 1.8 % in the last 6 months. The experimental conditions had less effect on reports of physical mistreatment. The only significant finding was that IVR respondents were more likely to report physical mistreatment in the last 6 months (3.5 vs. 0.1 % for CATI; $p < 0.01$), but the results are highly unstable due to the fact that only one CATI respondent reported such an experience. One unexpected finding was that the interviewer-administered CAPI condition actually produced higher levels of reporting of physical mistreatment since turning 60 (6.1 %) than the A-CASI condition (2.8 %), although the difference was not statistically significant.

Figure 10.3 shows results for the follow-up questions on ease of use, perceived privacy, and preference for the technology versus a live interviewer for those in the A-CASI and IVR conditions. Approximately 70 % of older adults found both A-CASI and IVR "very easy to use," while A-CASI was seen as increasing privacy to a greater extent than IVR. When asked about preference for the technology versus a live interviewer in responding to "questions like these," slightly more than half in the A-CASI condition preferred the technology (vs. 20 % a live interviewer; 29 % expressed no preference). About 40 % preferred the IVR system (vs. 34 % live interviewer; 26 % no preference).

In summary, our study shows that new survey technologies like A-CASI and IVR can be used by older adults. A-CASI seems to be particularly effective in increasing reporting of financial and psychological mistreatment among older adults. The effectiveness of IVR technology is less clear in this context, although it did lead to generally higher prevalence estimates for psychological mistreatment. Neither technology appeared to affect reports of physical abuse. One way to interpret these findings is that while both A-CASI and IVR eliminate the need to report mistreatment to another person, thus reducing social desirability concerns, A-CASI can also reduce fear of disclosure to third parties who in fact may be perpetrators of the mistreatment. That is, in the home setting, A-CASI (or CASI for those not using headphones) eliminates the need for interviewers to read the abuse questions, and for verbal responding as in a CAPI survey, which may be overheard by third parties. In the CATI condition, this was less of an issue, as a family member could potentially only hear the respondent's half of the conversation, and the key elder mistreatment questions required only "yes" or "no" responses. Thus, IVR may have provided less relative benefit in terms of reduced disclosure compared to CATI, than A-CASI did to CAPI. Another explanation may be simply that older adults feel more comfortable in general in more personal face-to-face settings, where rapport can be established, and that A-CASI brings together increased rapport with increased privacy. We did find significantly higher prevalence of financial exploitation and psychological mistreatment in in-person versus telephone surveys (i.e., a significant mode effect). There may simply be more suspicion of telephone interviews among older adults (IVR included), given publicity about "phone scams" targeting older adults. Another possibility is that respondents in the IVR condition might have been suspicious as to whether the interviewer really got off the line, or was actually still listening in, as there was no way to objectively verify this. One caveat about A-CASI is that there was more reluctance to use the computer and headphones than to use the IVR system.

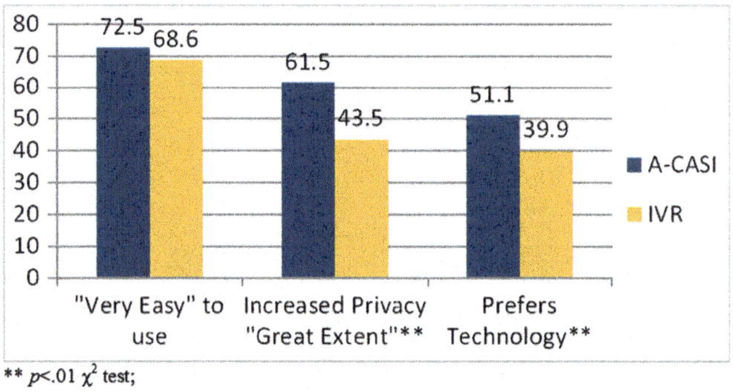

Fig. 10.3 Attitudes toward A-CASI and IVR technologies among older adults [3]

However, as the Pew Research Center has noted [43], Internet use among the population age 65 and older, although still low relative to younger age groups, has been steadily increasing over time (more than doubling from 28 % in 2005 to 58 % in 2015). This suggests that some of the A-CASI adoption issues may become less relevant as more technology-literate generations age. However, certain health-related factors such as vision, hearing, or cognitive deficits are less likely to disappear for subsequent cohorts, suggesting there may always be at least some difficulty in the use of technology for survey data collection among older populations. This suggests that new methods for assisting or "training" older adults in the use of technology like A-CASI, or new adaptations to the technology for the visually or hearing impaired, may be necessary. Similarly, while the IVR issue of not having a touchtone phone will certainly disappear over time for subsequent cohorts, problems in responding using a keypad on a cordless handset are more endemic to age-related factors like reduced manual dexterity. Assuming that voice recognition software continues to improve allowing spoken response to be the IVR standard, this may also become less problematic over time.

In conclusion, our work suggests that the current widely cited 5–10 % prevalence rates of elder abuse derived from interviewer-administered telephone and in-person surveys may be underestimates. This may be especially true for psychological abuse and financial exploitation, generally the most prevalent forms of abuse found in direct surveys. The most accurate reports may be obtained using A-CASI (or CASI) in the context of in-person surveys, which suggests the need for a national in-person prevalence study or the addition of elder abuse questions to existing aging-related national in-person surveys. The one other use of CASI in an elder abuse prevalence study that I could find was in Biggs and colleagues national prevalence survey conducted in the UK [7]. They note "As part of the [data collection] process, respondents were asked to complete a section themselves using a laptop computer (computer-assisted self-interviewing [CASI]) to cover particularly sensitive topic areas such as the experience of sexual abuse or mental health issues." Thus, Biggs et al. [7] did not use CASI to collect data psychological, physical, or financial abuse.

In another recent application of computer technology for the collection of elder abuse reports among older Chinese adults in Chicago, IL, Dong, Simon and colleagues used interviewer-administered IPAD technology as part of the *Population Study of Chinese Elderly in Chicago* (*PINE Study*; [19]). The IPADs used innovative web-based software to record simultaneously in English, Chinese traditional, and simplified characters, thus minimizing information that may have been "lost in translation" and providing deeper meaning to the data. It should be noted that these researchers trained the interviewers to hold the IPAD unobtrusively off to the side, so as not to interrupt rapport with the respondent. The study found that 24 % of Chinese elders had experienced some form of abuse, with psychological abuse (10 %) and financial exploitation (10 %) being the most common. Thus, use of IPAD technology in surveys of minority communities is feasible and appears to be effective in eliciting disclosures about elder abuse.

10.2.2 Potential for Use of Survey Technology in Abuser/Perpetrator Surveys

The findings on A-CASI and IVR are also relevant to the issue of obtaining elder abuse data directly from potential abusers/perpetrators/caregivers. In response to a 2011 Government Accountability Office (GAO) report on elder justice, the Department of Health and Human Services (HHS) noted that without understanding factors associated with elder abuse perpetration, prevention efforts are greatly hindered [25]. Direct surveys of potential perpetrators have proven to be very difficult in community-based surveys for various reasons, most obviously concerns about self-incrimination. One exception has been the literature on family caregivers of older adults with dementia-related disorders liked Alzheimer's Disease or physical health conditions like multiple sclerosis, who are willing to report resorting to potentially abusive behaviors in attempting to provide care, with some studies finding caregiver-reported prevalence rates approaching 50 % [15, 60]. I am not aware of the use of privacy-enhancing data collection methods like A-CASI/CASI or IVR in such studies, but one might imagine obtaining even higher prevalence rates by removing the need for caregivers to report potentially abusive behavior directly to an interviewer. More generally, community-dwelling perpetrators may also be more willing to report abusive behavior using privacy-enhancing methods. This should be explored in future research.

10.2.3 Technology and Screening for Elder Abuse in Clinical Settings

The potential utility of screening for elder abuse in clinical settings like physician offices, emergency departments, and dental clinics has been explored by researchers and practitioners as a cost-effective way to detect and potentially prevent abuse of older adults who may be unable or unwilling to respond to surveys [30, 41]. Recently, the Centers for Medicare and Medicaid Services (CMS; [9]) developed the *Elder Maltreatment Screen and Follow-up Plan* for inclusion in the Physician Quality Reporting System (PQRS). This measure tracks the percentage of patients age 65 or older with a documented elder maltreatment screen and follow-up plan on the date of the positive screen. However, in the first half of 2012, CMS reported that only *1438 of a possible 54 million* older adults eligible to receive screening for elder abuse were actually screened. Obviously, physicians have yet to incorporate elder abuse screening into routine practice. Although the U.S. Preventive Services Task Force [40] stated that "The evidence for screening elderly and vulnerable adults [for domestic violence abuse] remains insufficient [since 2004 guideline]; therefore the USPSTF was unable to make a recommendation in favor of or against screening," the American Medical Association, the American College of Emergency Physicians and other professional associations have recommended routine physician screening for elder abuse.

In addition to general lack of awareness about elder abuse and knowledge about how to screen for abuse, barriers to screening in clinical settings include time pressures and concerns about privacy and confidentiality. Technology like A-CASI could play a role in overcoming such barriers. Relatively few attempts have been made to screen for elder abuse in clinical settings. Fulmer and her colleagues have used brief screening instruments including the Elder Assessment Instrument (EAI; [23]) and the Hwalek–Sengstock Elder Abuse Screening Test (HS-EAST; [29]) in emergency departments (ED; [22, 23]); medical clinics [24]; and dental clinics [50]. Early studies in ED settings used traditional interviewer-administered data collection.

However, in more recent work in medical and dental clinics, Fulmer and colleagues have successfully used A-CASI technology to screen for elder abuse in waiting rooms [24, 50]. Older adults were willing to answer sensitive questions in these clinic settings using A-CASI technology, and did in fact report abuse at fairly high rates—35 % screened positive for abuse on the HS-EAST in the dental clinics; and over 30 % in the medical clinic reported verbal aggression with their caregivers in the past month. A new tool for physician screening for elder abuse—The *Elder Abuse Suspicion Index* (*EASI*)—has been developed by Yaffe and colleagues, including both physician-administered and self-administered (i.e., by the patient) versions [64, 65]. This six item scale could easily be administered using A-CASI, and a digitized version has been created.

In the area of interpersonal violence across the lifespan, Rhodes and colleagues have successfully used computer-assisted self- interviewing (CASI) for screening in the ED setting [46, 47]. In one study, they reported that 83 of 248 (33.5 %) ED patients screened positive for domestic violence using CASI methods, compared with only 1 of 222 cases receiving usual ED care/no formal screening [47]. In sum, A-CASI/CASI survey technologies have thus far been shown to be feasible, acceptable, and useful for elder abuse/domestic violence screening in clinic settings.

Another recent application of technology for screening and intervention in domestic abuse and neglect in clinical settings was described by Hawkins et al. [28]. In this study, *healthcare providers* (nurses and therapists) from Home Health VNA (HHVNA) in the Merrimack River Valley of New Hampshire and Massachusetts were trained to use *Personal Digital Assistants* (*PDA*) to screen for domestic abuse and neglect. An initial risk screening tool was administered, typically in the patient's home, on the PDA, and a positive screen resulted in a same-day follow-up risk assessment by a social worker, also collected via PDA. Mandated reporting of elder abuse was also done using PDA technology. All data went to a centralized, secure data repository. In general, screening for abuse and neglect was mainstreamed into routine care via streamlined communication and data sharing for resource mobilization, including same-day in-depth social work assessment and referrals to appropriate community agencies. Despite barriers and challenges involving software and collection, storage, and retrieval of sensitive and private health information, the authors concluded that wedding technology with healthcare professionals' skills and knowledge has great potential for both prevention and early intervention for domestic abuse and neglect. It should be noted that smartphones would likely be the current technology for implementation of healthcare provider screening tools as described by Hawkins et al. [28].

10.2.4 Computer-Adaptive Testing Applications to Elder Abuse

Another interesting and potentially valuable application of computerized data collection to the field of elder abuse is *computer-adaptive testing* (*CAT*). This technique involves use of item response theory (IRT) in development of unidimensional scales containing items of varying degree of severity or difficulty designed to measure a theoretical construct [18]. Once the items for the final scale are chosen, they can be placed on a "ruler" ordered from lowest to highest severity, or least to most "difficult." In a CAT application, the respondent is first presented with an item of medium severity/difficulty, and based on the response, *unique individualized* follow-up questions are then asked. For example, someone saying "yes" to an item of medium severity is then asked items measuring higher severity levels; while someone responding "no" to the initial medium severity item is funneled to less severe items. Based on each response, specific follow-up questions are asked to more precisely estimate individual severity scores, and the algorithm stops once a "best estimate" is achieved. The key feature that distinguishes CAT instruments from more traditional standardized surveys is that the respondent does not answer all of the questions. They only answer enough questions, contingent upon prior responses, to obtain a precise estimate. Thus, CAT applications reduce respondent burden without sacrificing precision of measurement. CAT methodology has been applied in many areas, including educational testing of abilities [36] and health-related quality of life (e.g., the Patient Reported Outcomes Measurement Information System [PROMIS] [45]).

In the elder abuse realm, Conrad and his colleagues have developed measures of financial exploitation (30 items; [10–13]) and psychological mistreatment (31 items; [10–13]) using state-of-the-art psychometric methods including concept mapping, expert panels, focus groups, and cognitive interviews. The measures were further developed using Rasch IRT rating scale modeling on data from Chicago area APS clients with confirmed cases of elder abuse. These analyses confirmed the unidimensionality of the measures and resulted in items ranked in severity, thus allowing more precise measurement "rulers" for potentially establishing cut-points and for CAT applications. Examples of financial exploitation items lower in severity include [Has trusted other] "borrowed money from you but not paid it back;" and "lied about how they were spending your money." Medium severity items include "have there been unauthorized withdrawals from your bank account;" and "Has trusted other persuaded you to sign any documents even though it was not in your best interest." High severity items include "has trusted other convinced you to turn the title of your home, property, car, etc. over to them;" and "changed the direct deposit destination so as to benefit him/herself." Although CAT algorithms have not yet been developed for the measures, they would work by starting with a medium severity item and, based on response to this question, following up with fewer higher or lower severity items to obtain a brief, precise measure the presence and severity of financial exploitation (or psychological mistreatment). Given the need for very brief screening instruments in the elder abuse field, CAT applications hold much promise. However, more psychometric work will be required to obtain reliable and valid items of ordered severity for the various subtypes of elder abuse before CAT could be usefully applied in practice. At a more basic level, elder abuse researchers will need to agree on common definitions and dimensional structures of the various subtypes of abuse in order to apply CAT methods.

10.2.5 Video Monitoring in Long-Term Care Facilities

Shifting focus from direct survey technologies, we now introduce other technology-based methods with potential to contribute to research on elder abuse. These methods could apply not only to cognitively intact older adults, but also to those with cognitive impairment or dementia-related disorders, such as those residing in long-term care (LTC) facilities. This section discusses the potential use of video monitoring in research on abuse occurring within LTC facilities. An emerging literature has noted that resident-to-resident elder mistreatment (RREM)/resident-to-resident aggression (RRA) is far more prevalent than staff-to-resident abuse [33, 49, 52]. A recent paper described the development of a research agenda on RRA based on a consensus conference of experts [37]. Among the top five research priorities identified was identification of environmental factors triggering RRA; incidence/prevalence of RRA; and identification of RRA perpetrator and victim characteristics (two others involved developing RRA interventions). Video monitoring of both public and private spaces in LTC facilities holds much promise in addressing this research agenda, despite obvious ethical barriers involving privacy concerns and logistical/cost concerns.

One example of an early attempt to implement video surveillance technology in public spaces (hallways, activity, and dining rooms) of LTC facilities is the *Care Media* project [5]. Digital cameras, microphones, and sensors captured raw, real-time video, with human coders specifying events of interest, such as pushing/shoving, punching, kicking, and other aggressive behaviors. Based on the human coding, computer algorithms were developed to automatically detect the event and its contextual characteristics. In this manner, the computer was "trained" to detect salient events, eventually reducing the need for human data coding to only those circumstances that are challenging even for human eyes. A feasibility study involving four ceiling-mounted video cameras and microphones in the public spaces of a locked dementia unit captured seven bouts of physical aggression (three un-witnessed by staff) among eight residents over 80 h of observation [5]. Following this, a more comprehensive study was conducted using 23 ceiling-mounted video cameras and microphones that recorded 15 consenting subjects with severe dementia 24 h a day for 25 consecutive days, amounting to 13,800 camera-hours of video data. Trained human coders identified 185 bouts of physical aggression in nearly 500 h of meal time (lunches and dinners) videos.

These researchers have written extensively on the ethical considerations around privacy and confidentiality, and on approaches to obtaining informed consent, enhancing privacy protection, and educational strategies for LTC residents, staff, administration, families, and visitors when implementing video monitoring for research [6, 53]. While admittedly challenging on many fronts, I would argue that use of video monitoring technologies in LTC settings is a "high risk/high reward" methodology. The rich, detailed, real-time objective data affords powerful opportunities to study RRA incidence/prevalence, triggers, and victim/perpetrator characteristics [37]. As monitoring technology evolves and machine learning algorithms become more sophisticated; and as more technology savvy baby boomer cohorts age, use of video monitoring in LTC care facilities to understand, and ultimately prevent, RRA will likely increase. Eventually, such technology should also be employed in private spaces (i.e., patient rooms), as studies have shown that a high proportion of RRA occurs in resident rooms [49, 52]. Finally, elder abuse researchers interested in video monitoring methods can also look to recent work in the area of *falls detection* in LTC using these methods [63].

10.3 Technology for Indirect Detection of Elder Abuse and Risk Factors

10.3.1 Medical Forensics Technology

Research in the area of medical forensics of elder abuse has examined potential physical markers of abuse and neglect [20]. Potential examples include bruises, fractures, burns, decubiti, malnutrition, pressure ulcers, dehydration, and hygiene, although there is little published research. The work of Mosqueda and colleagues on bruising as a forensic marker for elder abuse is a notable exception [39, 61, 62, 67]. In two studies funded by the National Institute of Justice (NIJ), Mosequeda and colleagues compared bruising patterns and characteristics between those caused by accidental falls ($n = 101$) versus physical abuse ($n = 67$; [39, 61, 62]). They found that abused elders had significantly larger bruises; were more likely to have bruising on the neck and head (face), the lateral aspect of the right arm, and the posterior torso (non-abuse bruises were more likely to be on the extremities); and abused elders were much more likely to know where the bruise came from. Using the same data, Ziminski et al. [67] reported that elders with head and neck bruises were more likely to report being choked, punched, or beaten up on the Revised Conflict Tactics Scales (CTS2) physical assault scale [56]. Lateral/anterior arm bruises were more likely for victims who reported being grabbed. The authors concluded that injuries resulting from physical abuse of elders were similar to those found in intimate partner violence among younger populations.

In more recent work, Rosen and his colleagues are comparing injury patterns, physical findings, forensic biomarkers, and photographic evidence from victims of confirmed physical elder abuse victims to those of geriatric patients presenting to the emergency department after an accidental fall [48]. The researchers are developing and evaluating a standardized protocol for photographing injuries in the acute care setting; and a comprehensive classification system/taxonomy to describe geriatric injuries. The goal of the study is to derive clinical decision rules to assist ED personnel in the detection of potential elder abuse for further screening and evaluation. The project also involves collaboration with radiologists to identify potential radiographic injury patterns suggestive of abuse. While this work offers much promise, it is also quite challenging, involving complex technical and ethical issues that must be confronted. For example, there are potential "false positives" and the resulting implications for families who may become reluctant to seek medical help. Use of data-based clinical decision rules will also likely lead to some situations where the older adult fitting criteria for abuse denies that abuse has occurred and refuses further screening/referrals. ED personnel will need to be sensitized to issues of the balance between objectively derived clinical observations versus the autonomy of the older adult. These situations are even more complicated when there are questions about older adults' cognitive capacity to refuse follow-up for suspected elder abuse.

While many potential physical markers of elder abuse rely on simple visual examinations by healthcare providers, some also involve use of standard medical technologies like X-rays, scans, etc. Another application is *postmortem evaluation* for suspected cases of elder abuse and neglect. For example, Knight and colleagues explored the utility of whole-body CT imaging in postmortem detection of elder abuse and neglect [32], although I could find no further published results of this work. Use of medical forensics technology to detect elder abuse (including postmortem) is clearly an area where additional research is warranted.

10.3.2 Neuroscience/Brain Imaging Technology

In a recent article related to the 2015 *White House Conference on Aging*, Pillemer et al. [44] argued that one of the key areas for action for the elder abuse field was "development of a knowledge base for addressing elder mistreatment." The authors included "connect brain science to elder mistreatment research" as a priority area. They argued for the study of how age-related declines in neurocognitive function, including memory and executive control, may operate as a risk factor for elder abuse. As executive control declines, individuals may be less able to flag self-detrimental or other disadvantageous behaviors, putting them at greater risk for elder abuse. Several studies in the area of child abuse have shown that mistreatment at an early age relates to brain changes and negative neurocognitive outcomes later in life [17, 26]. However, no work to date has directly linked structural and functional changes in the brain to elder abuse. *Functional magnetic resonance imaging (fMRI)* technology is one approach that could be applied. In an intriguing study, Griffith et al. [27] showed that reduced financial capacity/skill was associated with lower angular gyri volume (assessed via MRI) among individuals with mild cognitive impairment. Other work relating older age to less activation of the anterior insula region of the brain when making explicit judgments of trustworthiness of faces by Castle et al. [8] is also intriguing and may have implications for risk for financial exploitation. The use of fMRI and other neuroscience technologies will likely—and certainly should—play an increasing role in research on elder abuse.

10.3.3 Data Mining and Financial Fraud Detection

Another cutting edge technology with direct relevance to financial exploitation of older adults is the use of data mining to detect financial fraud [42]. Ngai et al. [42] presented a classification framework and review of the literature between 1997 and 2008. They describe four main types of financial fraud: (1) *bank fraud* (credit card fraud; money laundering); (2) *insurance fraud* (auto insurance fraud; crop insurance fraud; healthcare insurance fraud); (3) *securities and commodities fraud*; and (4) *other related financial fraud* (mass marketing fraud; corporate fraud). Further, they include six data mining techniques: classification; clustering; outlier detection; prediction; regression; and visualization, and describe specific statistical techniques within each class (e.g., neural networks; decision trees; regression models). The review of 49 published studies summarizes the data mining technique and the type of fraud for each study and finds that auto insurance fraud and corporate fraud are the most commonly studied. The most commonly used statistical techniques were logistic models (regression, classification and prediction) and neural networks (classification and clustering). The authors recommend more attention to mortgage fraud and mass marketing fraud (plus money laundering and securities and commodities fraud), and greater use of data visualization and outlier detection data mining techniques.

It should be noted that the vast majority of this work is focused on fraud in which an *institution is the victim* (i.e., a bank, insurance company, or corporation) rather than individuals, which is of most relevance for elder abuse. One study developed an algorithm to create a model of typical credit cardholder behavior and to analyze deviations in transactions to identify suspicious activity [66], which has become fairly common among major banks issuing credit cards. Financial fraud detection technology has obvious potential applications for research on elder financial exploitation. Automated systems alerting authorities to unusual financial transactions or activities in the accounts of older adults would enable more precise prevalence estimates, and more importantly, early detection and prevention.

10.3.4 Potential Technologies for Detecting Neglect by Caregivers and Self-Neglect

The next section discusses the potential for physiological monitoring and "smart home" technology to aid in detection of elder abuse and neglect. Neglect by caregivers/trusted others and self-neglect present special challenges for screening and detection, as they are often hidden and victims may not present clear clinical signs and symptoms. One approach has been development of *observational measures of neglect/self-neglect* (e.g., [31]), designed for use by APS workers, social workers, and case managers. These are checklists that are completed based on direct observation of older adults and the home environment. These measures could be unobtrusively administered with technology like IPADS, smartphones, etc. In addition, use of digital photography (e.g., of stairs condition; general clutter; cleanliness; contents of refrigerator and food pantry) and subsequent coding of the images has potential applications to the detection of neglect/self-neglect. Again, issues surrounding privacy and consent must be addressed to conduct such research ethically.

10.3.5 Physiological Monitoring and "Smart Home" Technology: Potential Applications to Elder Abuse Research

Earlier in the chapter, the potential for video monitoring in LTC facilities to detect resident-to-resident aggression (RRA) was discussed. Here I discuss technologies designed for *individual physiological monitoring* and *home-based monitoring* and their possible applications to elder abuse detection and prevention. Physiological and environmental sensor technologies with potential applications to dementia patients are being developed at a rapid pace (see [4] for an overview). Wearable devices have been developed that track physiological indicators like blood pressure, heart rate, EKG, respiration, temperature, blood glucose, and blood oxygen levels. Sensors for monitoring sleep quality have also been developed. Other devices are worn that enable activity and location monitoring, gait monitoring, and falls detection. Advanced integrated external sensor systems that use information from a variety of sensors (e.g., motion, temperature, pressure) to record day-to-day activity are also being developed. These systems are designed to monitor persons at risk for dementia, including whether he/she is in bed, using the toilet, operating appliances, opening a door, or moving around the home. Researchers have developed "smart homes," which are prototype apartments/homes with sensors embedded throughout to enable activity monitoring and provide early detection of health changes [54]. Despite these technology innovations, scholars have noted that there is very little evidence to date that they actually improve quality of life, health, and/or function in older adults in a cost-effective manner [51].

These technologies have potential applications for the detection and prevention of elder abuse in community-dwelling older adults. One application might be the early detection of signs of *self-neglect*, though this is not always included in discussions of elder abuse. These technologies could also be relevant for detection of *neglect by paid in-home caregivers* by family members not residing with the older adult. Most importantly, physiological and home-based monitoring may be useful for early detection of health declines, including declines in cognitive function that may put older adults at increased risk for abuse and neglect.

Of course, ethical issues around privacy noted above in the discussion of video monitoring in LTC settings are relevant here too, and may be an even larger barrier in the home setting. Aesthetics and unobtrusiveness of sensors will also be important to consider. In addition, as noted above, there is still much work to do to demonstrate that these technologies can be implemented in a cost-effective manner and shown to improve health and quality of life. Despite all this, these technologies are likely not going away and researchers should think creatively about how to design applications that may be useful in the detection and prevention of elder abuse.

10.4 Information Technology and Elder Abuse Research

10.4.1 The Need for Systematic Adult Protective Services (APS) Data Collection

In a 2011 report entitled, *Elder Justice: Stronger Federal Leadership Could Enhance National Response to Elder Abuse*, GAO recommended development and implementation of a uniform nationwide APS data collection system. The report notes that despite an increasing number of reported cases of elder abuse, and increased complexity of cases, APS lacks the financial resources to adequately respond. One of the basic issues is lack of adequate administrative data systems, which impedes APS ability to understand, track, and respond adequately to cases. Lack of systematic data also prevents studies of the outcomes of APS interventions. While nearly all states in the US have some type of automated APS data system, the value and quality of the systems varies widely. The specific type of information recorded during elder abuse investigations also varies by state. GAO [25] specifically recommended convening a group of state APS representatives to determine what types of data would be most useful to collect; which data elements should be uniformly collected in all states; and how the system should be technically designed. They also recommended a pilot study to determine feasibility and costs of collecting, compiling, and disseminating uniform APS data.

In a parallel effort, The Assistant Secretary for Planning and Evaluation (ASPE) of HHS released a *Congressional Report on the Feasibility of Establishing a Uniform National Database on Elder Abuse* [2]. The report provides an overview of current administrative data collection and reporting systems on elder abuse, including (1) APS; (2) law enforcement data, including FBI Uniform Crime Reports (UCR) and National Incident-Based Reporting System (NIBRS); and Bureau of Justice Statistics National Crime Victimization Survey (NCVS); (3) Center for Medicare and Medicaid Services (CMS) Online Survey Certification and Reporting System (OSCAR); and Minimum Data Set (MDS) Quality Indicators; (4) Medicaid Fraud Control Unit data; (5) long-term care ombudsman data; (6) guardianship and representative payee data; and (7) health indicator data. The report notes that all of the potential administrative data sources on elder abuse have weaknesses and limitations that would need to be addressed prior to the establishment of a uniform national database. These include variations across states in persons covered by elder abuse laws/reporting requirements; inconsistencies in definitional interpretations; inability of data systems to sort data by common data elements (e.g., age of victim); inconsistent staff training across states on identifying, coding, and reporting abuse; and inconsistent levels of technical sophistication and integration of paper and electronic records.

The report also describes efforts to establish national data collection systems in the areas of child abuse and intimate partner violence (IPV). The *National Child Abuse and Neglect Data System* (*NCANDS*) was established in 1990 as a way for state Child Protective Services (CPS) to voluntarily and systematically report child abuse. Currently, all states report at least some data and the majority report most data elements. The system has also evolved from collecting only aggregate data to case-level data. NCANDS is viewed as a potential model for developing a national elder abuse database. In contrast, there is no current comprehensive source of national data on IPV, although the Centers for Disease Control (CDC) published uniform definitions and recommended data elements for IPV surveillance in 2002.

The ASPE report concludes with a summary of considerations and recommendations in developing a uniform national elder abuse database. The authors mention the need for a national benchmark definition of elder abuse, noting the difficulties the field has had thus far in achieving a consensus definition, but stressing its importance in order to move forward. They also call for consistent definitions of important components of any elder abuse definition, such as “vulnerability” and “position of trust.” They discuss the need to carefully choose the correct *data elements for reporting* suggesting that *case-level* victim characteristics; type of incident; perpetrator characteristics; reporter of incident; victim–perpetrator relationship; setting and living arrangement; cognitive status/capacity of victim; general health of victim; substantiation decision; and APS system response disposition may be particularly useful. They note the importance of *ensuring confidentiality* for case-level data, including restricted access, de-identification/numeric identifiers, and encrypting names. Lastly, the report discusses cost and funding considerations, including (among other things) the need for a federal infrastructure; development and pilot testing; and collecting, validating, and analyzing data nationwide to produce profiles and reports. The report notes that the initial cost to design the NCANDS was approximately $1 million over 2 years; and that the current yearly cost to operate NCANDS is $1,385,000. The basic recommendation from the report was to use a multistep approach to the development of a national elder abuse database, including (1) addressing systemic weaknesses in existing elder abuse data collection systems; (2) compile a national database of state APS data; and (3) plan to build a comprehensive cross-disciplinary national database of administrative elder abuse data by combining sources incrementally. Related to the GAO and ASPE reports, the CDC is also working on uniform definitions and recommended data elements for elder abuse surveillance.

10.4.2 Smaller Scale Projects Demonstrating Applications of IT to APS Elder Abuse Data Collection and Management

As just noted, the APSE report recommended addressing systemic weaknesses in existing elder abuse data collection systems as a first step toward establishing a national database. Two recent smaller scale efforts along these lines illustrate the potential for information technology applications to improve APS assessment, service delivery, and outcomes tracking. The first is the *Elder Abuse Decision Support System* (*EADSS*) developed by Conrad et al. [14] (www.eadss.org) [21]. The EADSS is a web-based, multicomponent intake, assessment and reporting system designed for desktop computers, tablet PCs, or any other device that supports internet access. The EADSS includes real-time intake screener assessments for the various types of elder abuse; a more detailed suite of validated measures for each abuse type—the Older Adult Mistreatment Assessment (OAMA)—to support abuse investigations; a detailed client information form; an alleged abuser information form; an alleged abuser interview; and care plan recommendations for both victims and abusers. Statistical reports are generated on an "as needed" basis, by individual, agency, region, and statewide. Adoption of the EADSS includes training on its use which includes all steps in the APS intake, assessment, reporting, care planning, and follow-up procedures. The existence of an electronic record on a central server creates a living history of each case that is accessible by anyone who is authorized to access the system. Data encryption systems protect privacy and confidentiality. Field tests of the EADSS conducted in six Illinois Department of Aging (IDoA) APS provider agencies have shown that the system is generally acceptable to APS caseworkers and administrators, and that the system produced higher abuse substantiation rates (69.7 %) than all other IDoA agencies not using EADSS (44.3 %).

Another notable example is the development of the multidimensional *Tool for Risk, Interventions, and Outcomes* (*TRIO*) for use in APS settings by Sommerfeld et al. [55]. The goal of TRIO was "to develop an instrument that could be used to document and collect data related to multiple dimensions of a typical APS episode, including: (a) the investigation and assessment of allegations, (b) the identification of abuse and neglect risk factors, (c) the delivery of a range of potential interventions, (d) the achievement of specific outcomes, and (e) an assessment of the prognosis for future APS involvement at case closure. Ultimately, the TRIO was designed to allow for a comprehensive description of APS response to and involvement with clients and the resulting client outcomes" [55, pp. 497]. The TRIO was designed by APS administrators and social workers from Ventura County, California and is administered electronically. Initial tests of the TRIO indicated social worker "relevance and buy-in," and good inter-rater reliability (Kappa and ICC statistics ranging from 0.73 to 0.99). Concurrent validity was demonstrated via appropriate patterns of TRIO item differentiation based on the type of observed confirmed abuse or neglect. Predictive validity was demonstrated by prediction of the risk of actual APS recurrence by TRIO summary prognosis—25 % of those with a "poor" prognosis had a 180-day APS recurrence, versus 18 % with a "fair" prognosis, and only 1.3 % with a "very good" prognosis.

10.5 Conclusions

This chapter provides an overview of the use of technology in elder abuse research. The primary aim of the chapter was not necessarily to document what *has been done*, but to stimulate thinking about what *might be done* in the future to apply cutting edge technology to elder abuse research. First, I discussed technology for *direct data collection* from elder abuse victims, primarily *direct surveys/screening*. Here, the potential for technologies such as A-CASI/CASI, IVR, IPADS, and PDAs (smartphones) to enhance disclosure of elder abuse in both *home and clinical settings* with diverse populations was discussed. I note that CASI technology has also been effectively used to screen for IPV among younger populations in clinical settings. A brief discussion of the potential application of IRT-based CAT methods to develop brief but psychometrically sound measurement and screening tools for elder abuse was also included here. Finally, the potential for *direct behavioral observation in LTC settings* through video monitoring of public (and potentially private) spaces to detect RREM/RRA was discussed, with acknowledgement of the complex ethical challenges involved.

Next, technology for *indirect detection of elder abuse and risk factors* was discussed. Here, the use of *medical forensic methods* like bruising analysis and other physical signs and symptoms presenting in ED and clinical settings to form potential clinical decision rules were described. Then, the application of *neuroscience/brain imaging* technology like fMRI to the study brain function and risk for abuse was discussed, including work relating brain function and trust decisions with potential relevance to financial exploitation risk. *Data mining* techniques for *financial fraud detection* were discussed, highlighting the potential for "big data" analytics for the prevention of financial abuse. Potential technologies for detection of *neglect/self-neglect*, including computer-administered observation checklists and digital photography/coding of the older adult and the home environment were discussed. Then, a broader description of *physiological and "smart home" monitoring* technology for the potential detection of health declines, cognitive impairment and/or neglect by paid caregivers was provided, again acknowledging potential ethical barriers.

The chapter concludes with a discussion of the role of *information technology in elder abuse research*. The primary focus here was on the crucial need for a *systematic national APS data collection* system. I note several related efforts toward this goal by GAO, APSE, NIJ, and CDC including summaries of currently available sources of elder abuse data (e.g., state-level APS, CMS, MDS, OSCAR) and the corresponding weaknesses of each. These reports also note the NCANDS child abuse data system—which has been successfully implemented on a national level—as a potential model for a national elder abuse database. Then two recent smaller scale demonstrations of the application of IT to APS data collection—the EADDS and the TRIO tool—were described as potentially useful models for moving forward.

As anyone who has worked in the field knows, elder abuse research is fraught with methodological challenges, pitfalls, and barriers to implementation. Elder abuse is a generally hidden phenomenon—hidden by both victims and perpetrators—involving a range of behaviors that are rarely reported to authorities. There are numerous legal and ethical challenges confronting elder abuse researchers, including issues of mandatory reporting, elder autonomy, cognitive impairment, and IRB issues around privacy and confidentiality. Technology like that described in this chapter can be viewed as simultaneously helping to solve some of these challenges and pitfalls (e.g., A-CASI increases willingness to disclose abuse versus interviews; medical forensics or video monitoring can detect abuse in cognitively impaired elders who cannot report it) while at the same time potentially creating new problems to solve. For example, as electronic medical records systems become more sophisticated and integrated with technology-based data—computerized survey data; medical forensics data; physiological and home monitoring video data; brain scans; and other "big data"—new concerns about privacy, confidentiality, and HIPPA protections will also emerge.

The only confident prediction that can be made about the use of technology for research—including elder abuse research—is that it is here to stay. As society continues to rapidly adopt emerging technology, the still nascent field of elder abuse must embrace them and adopt creative applications that address fundamental problems that have impeded progress, while at the same time avoiding or minimizing new problems resulting from using technology. This will require working not only with our colleagues from IPV and child abuse research, but with the broader social, behavioral, and medical science communities engaged in research with frail elders. We need to develop protocols for the application of technology to elder abuse research that build a solid evidence base that will protect some of society's most vulnerable members from harm, and improve quality of life.

References

1. Acierno R, Hernandez MA, Amstadter AB, Resnick HS, Steve K, Muzzy W, Kilpatrick DG. Prevalence and correlates of emotional, physical, sexual, and financial abuse and potential neglect in the United States: the National Elder Mistreatment Study. Am J Public Health. 2010;100(2):292–7.
2. ASPE (Office of the Assistant Secretary for Planning and Evaluation). Congressional report on the feasibility of establishing a uniform national database on elder abuse. Washington, DC: U.S. Department of Health and Human Services, Office of the Assistant Secretary for Planning and Evaluation; 2010.
3. Beach SR, Schulz R, Degenholtz HB, Castle NG, Rosen J, Fox AR, Morycz RK. Using audio computer-assisted self-interviewing and interactive voice response to measure elder mistreatment in older adults: feasibility and effects on prevalence estimates. J Off Stat. 2010;26:507–33.
4. Bharucha AJ, Anand V, Forlizzi J, Dew MA, Reynolds CF, Stevens S, Wactlar H. Intelligent assistive technology applications to dementia care: current capabilities, limitations, and future challenges. Am J Geriatr Psychiatry. 2009;17(2):88–104.
5. Bharucha AJ, Atkeson C, Chen D. CareMedia: automated video and sensor analysis for geriatric care [abstract]. J Am Med Dir Assoc. 2006;7:B9.
6. Bharucha AJ, London AJ, Barnard D, Wactlar H, Dew MA, Reynolds CF. Ethical considerations in the conduct of electronic surveillance research. J Law Med Eth Fall. 2006;2006:611–9.
7. Biggs S, Manthorpe J, Tinker A, Doyle M, Erens B. Mistreatment of older people in the United Kingdom: findings from the first national prevalence study. J Elder Abuse Negl. 2009;21:1–14.
8. Castle E, Eisenberger NI, Seeman TE, Moons WG, Boggero IA, Grinblatt MS, Taylor SE. Neural and behavioral bases of age differences in perceptions of trust. Proc Natl Acad Sci. 2012;109:20848–52.
9. CMS. Physician quality reporting system. 2013. http://www.cms.gov/Medicare/Quality-Initiatives-Patient-Assessment-Instruments/PQRS/index.html?redirect=/PQRS. Accessed 01 Nov 2015.
10. Conrad KJ, Iris M, Ridings JW, Fairman KP, Rosen A, Wilber KH. Conceptual model and map of financial exploitation of older adults. J Elder Abuse Negl. 2011;23:304–25.
11. Conrad KJ, Iris M, Ridings JW, Langley K, Wilber KH. Self-report measure of financial exploitation of older adults. Gerontol. 2010;50(6):758–73.
12. Conrad KJ, Iris M, Ridings JW, Langley K, Anetzberger GJ. Self-report measure of psychological abuse of older adults. Gerontol. 2010;51(3):354–66.
13. Conrad KJ, Iris M, Ridings JW, Rosen A, Fairman KP, Anetzberger GJ. Conceptual model and map of psychological abuse of older adults. J Elder Abuse Negl. 2011;23:147–68.

14. Conrad KJ, Iris M, Riley BB, Mensah E, Mazza J. Developing end-user criteria and a prototype for an elder abuse assessment system. Research report submitted to the U.S. Department of Justice; 2013.
15. Cooper C, Selwood A, Blanchard M, Walker Z, Blizard R, Livingston G. The determinants of family carers' abusive behaviour to people with dementia: results of the CARD study. J Affect Disord. 2010;121:136–42.
16. Couper MP. Technology and the survey interview/questionnaire. In: Conrad FG, Schober MF, editors. Envisioning the survey interview of the future. Hoboken: Wiley; 2008. p. 56–76.
17. De Bellis MD, Woolley DP, Hooper SR. Neuropsychological findings in pediatric maltreatment: relationship of PTSD, dissociative symptoms, and abuse/neglect indices to neurocognitive outcomes. Child Maltreat. 2013;18:171–83.
18. DeMars C. Item response theory. New York: Oxford University Press; 2010.
19. Dong X, Chang E, Wong E, Simon MA. The perceptions, social determinants, and negative health outcomes associated with depressive symptoms among U.S. Chinese older adults. Gerontol. 2012;52(5):650–63.
20. Dyer CB, Connolly M, McFeeley P. The clinical and medical forensics of elder abuse and neglect. In: Bonnie RJ, Wallace RB, editors. Elder mistreatment: abuse, neglect, and exploitation in an aging America. Washington, DC: The National Academies Press; 2003. p. 339–81.
21. EADSS (Elder Abuse Decision Support System). http://eadss.org/. Accessed 01 Nov 2015.
22. Fulmer T, Guadagno L, Paveza G, VandeWeerd C, Baglioni A, Abraham I. Profiles of older adults who screen positive for neglect during an emergency department visit. J Elder Abuse Negl. 2002;14(1):49–60.
23. Fulmer T, Paveza G, Abraham I, Fairchild S. Elder neglect assessment in the emergency department. J Emerg Nurs. 2000;26 (5):436–43.
24. Fulmer T, Strauss S, Russell S, Singh G, Blankenship J, Vemula R, Caceres B, Valenti M, Sutin D. Screening for elder mistreatment in dental and medical clinics. Gerontology. 2012;29(2):96–105.
25. GAO. Elder justice: stronger federal leadership could enhance national response to elder abuse. Report to the Chairman, Special Committee on Aging, U.S. Senate. Washington, DC: United States Government Accountability Office; 2011.
26. Glaser D. Child abuse and neglect and the brain—a review. J Child Psychol Psychiatry. 2000;41:97–116.
27. Griffith HR, Stewart CC, Stoeckel LE, Okonkwo OC, den Hollander JA, Martin RC, Belue K, Copeland JN, Harrell LE, Brockington JC, Clark DG, Marson DC. Magnetic resonance imaging volume of the angular gyri predicts financial skill deficits in people with amnestic mild cognitive impairment. J Am Geriatr Soc. 2010;58:265–74.
28. Hawkins JW, Pearce CW, Skeith J, Dimitruk B, Roche R. Using technology to expedite screening and intervention for domestic abuse and neglect. Publ Health Nurs. 2009;26(1):58–69.
29. Hwalek MA, Sengstock MC. Hwalek–Sengstock elder abuse screening test-revised. J Appl Gerontol. 1986;5(2):153–73.
30. IOM (Institute of Medicine), NRC (National Research Council). Elder abuse and its prevention: workshop summary. Washington, DC: The National Academies Press; 2014.
31. Iris M, Conrad KJ, Ridings J. Observational measure of elder self-neglect. J Elder Abuse Negl. 2014;26:365–97.
32. Knight N. Whole-body CT imaging in post-mortem detection of elder abuse and neglect. Presented at the national institute of justice elder abuse workshop, Washington, DC, February 25–27, 2008.
33. Lachs M, Bachman R, Williams CS, O'Leary JR. Resident-to-resident elder mistreatment and police contact in nursing homes: findings from a population-based cohort. J Am Geriatr Soc. 2007;55(6):840–5.
34. Laumann EO, Leitsch SA, Waite LJ. Elder mistreatment in the United States: prevalence estimates from a nationally representative study. J Gerontol Soc Sci. 2008;63B:S248–54.
35. Lifespan of Greater Rochester, Inc., Weill Cornell Medical Center of Cornell University, and New York City Department for the Aging. Under the radar: New York State elder abuse prevalence study. In: Self-reported prevalence and documented case surveys. New York: New York State Office of Children and Family Services; 2011.
36. Lord FM. Applications of item response theory to practical testing problems. Hillsdale: Erlbaum; 1980.
37. McDonald L, Hitzig SL, Pillemer KA, Lachs MS, Beaulieu M, Brownell P, Burnes D, Caspi E. Developing a research agenda on resident-to-resident aggression: recommendations from a consensus conference. J Elder Abuse Negl. 2015;27:146–67.
38. Miller Steiger D, Conroy B. IVR: interactive voice response. In: De Leeuw E, Hox J, Dillman D, editors, International handbook of survey methodology. European Association of Methodology; 2008. p. 285–298.
39. Mosqueda L, Burnight K, Liao S. Bruising in the geriatric population. Research report submitted to the U.S. Department of Justice; 2006.
40. Moyer VA, on behalf of the U.S. Preventive Task Force. Screening for intimate partner violence and abuse of elderly and vulnerable adults: U.S. Preventive Services Task Force recommendation statement. Ann Intern Med. 2013;158(6):478–86.
41. National Research Council. Elder mistreatment: abuse, neglect and exploitation in an aging America. Washington, DC: The National Academies Press; 2003.
42. Ngai EWT, Hu Y, Wong YH, Chen Y, Sun X. The application of data mining techniques in financial fraud detection: a classification framework and an academic review of literature. Decis Support Syst. 2011;50:559–69.
43. Perrin A, Duggan M. Americans' Internet access: 2000–2015. Washington, DC: Pew Research Center; 2015.
44. Pillemer K, Connolly M, Breckman R, Spreng N, Lachs MS. Elder mistreatment: priorities for consideration by the White House Conference on Aging. Gerontol. 2015;55(2):320–7.
45. PROMIS—Dynamic tools to measure health outcomes from the patient perspective. http://www.nihpromis.org/. Accessed 01 Nov 2015.
46. Rhodes KV. The promise and problems with using information technology to achieve routine screening for intimate partner violence. Fam Violence Prev Health Pract. 2005;3:1–14.
47. Rhodes KV, Lauderdale DS, He T, Howes DS, Levinson W. "Between me and the computer": increased detection of intimate partner violence using a computer questionnaire. Ann Emerg Med. 2002;40(5):476–84.
48. Rosen T. Improving identification of and intervention for elder abuse in health care settings. Presented at NIH workshop on multiple approaches to understanding and preventing elder abuse, Bethesda, MD, October 30, 2015.
49. Rosen T, Pillemer K, Lachs M. Resident-to-resident aggression in long-term care facilities: an understudied problem. Aggress Violent Behav. 2008;13(2):77–87.
50. Russell SL, Fulmer T, Singh G, Valenti M, Vermula R, Strauss SM. Screening for elder mistreatment in a dental clinic population. J Elder Abuse Negl. 2012;24:326–39.
51. Schulz R, editor. Quality of life technology handbook. Boca Raton: CRC Press; 2013.

52. Shinoda-Tagawa T, Leonard R, Pontikas J, McDonough JE, Allen D, Dreyer PI. Resident-to-resident violent incidents in nursing homes. J Am Med Assoc. 2004;291(5):591–8.
53. Sifford KS, Bharucha A. Benefits and challenges of electronic surveillance in nursing home research. Res Gerontol Nurs. 2010;3 (1):5–10.
54. Skubic M, Rantz MJ, Miller SJ, Guevara RD, Koopman RJ, Alexander GL, Phillips LJ. Nonwearable in-home sensing for early detection of health changes. In: Schulz R, editor. Quality of life technology handbook. Boca Raton: CRC Press; 2013. p. 227–44.
55. Sommerfeld DH, Henderson LB, Snider MA, Aarons GA. Multidimensional measurement within adult protective services: design and initial testing of the tool for risk, interventions, and outcomes. J Elder Abuse Negl. 2014;26:495–522.
56. Straus MA, Hamby SL, Boney-McCoy S, Sugarman DB. The revised Conflict Tactics Scales (CTS2): development and preliminary psychometric data. J Fam Issues. 1996;17(3):283–316.
57. Tourangeau R, Yan T. Sensitive questions in surveys. Psychol Bull. 2007;133:859–83.
58. Tourangeau R, Rips LJ, Rasinski K. The psychology of survey response. Cambridge: Cambridge University Press; 2000.
59. Turner CF, Miller HG, Smith TK, Cooley PC, Rogers SM. Telephone audio computer-assisted self-interviewing (T-ACASI) and survey measurements of sensitive behaviors: preliminary results. In: Banks R, Fairgrieve J, Gerrard L, et al., editors. Survey and statistical computing. Chesham, Bucks, UK: Association for Survey Computing; 1996.
60. Wiglesworth A. Screening for abuse and neglect of people with dementia. J Am Geriatr Soc. 2010;58(3):493–500.
61. Wiglesworth A, Austin R, Corona M, Mosqueda L. Bruising as a forensic marker of physical elder abuse. Research report submitted to the U.S. Department of Justice; 2009.
62. Wiglesworth A, Austin R, Corona M, Schneider D, Liao S, Gibbs L, Mosqueda L. Bruising as a marker of physical elder abuse. J Am Geriatr Soc. 2009;57:1191–6.
63. Woolrych R, Zecevic A, Sixsmith A, Sims-Gould J, Feldman F, Chaudhury H, Symes B, Robinovitch SN. Using video capture to investigate the cause of falls in long-term care. Gerontol. 2015;55 (3):483–94.
64. Yaffe MJ, Weiss D, Lithwick M. Seniors' self-administration of the elder abuse suspicion index (EASI): a feasibility study. J Elder Abuse Negl. 2012;24(4):277–92.
65. Yaffe MJ, Wolfson C, Lithwick M, Weiss D. Development and validation of a tool to improve physician identification of elder abuse: the Elder Abuse Suspicion Index (EASI)©. J Elder Abuse Negl. 2008;20(3):276–300.
66. Zaslavsky V, Strizhak A. Credit card fraud detection using self-organizing maps. Inf Secur. 2006;18:48–63.
67. Ziminski CE, Wiglesworth A, Austin R, Phillips LR, Mosqueda L. Injury patterns and causal mechanisms of bruising in physical elder abuse. J Forensic Nurs. 2013;9(2):84–91.

A Multidisciplinary Approach to the Clinical Management of Elder Mistreatment

11

Nora OBrien-Suric, Avital Benson, XinQi Dong, and Terry Fulmer

11.1 Overview and Purpose of Chapter

Elder mistreatment is a serious and potentially fatal set of syndromes that affects nearly one in 10 older Americans [1]. The purpose of this chapter is to review the clinical management of elder mistreatment cases and to lay out the essential elements for detection, assessment, and intervention of these cases.

Mistreatment of any one of any age is not only a serious offense, but also presents a complex set of treatment modalities that requires sensitivity in addressing and treating the aftereffects for the victim as well as the perpetrator. However, there are special considerations when an older person is the victim of mistreatment because of the complex nature of the frailty of age and the issue of capacity. It is a compilation of many problems involving the older person, the caregivers, and the environment [3].

Elder mistreatment is associated with increased risk for morbidity and mortality especially among those with greater levels of vulnerability, cognitive impairment, physical disability, psychological distress, and social isolation [9, 26]. Elder mistreatment is associated with increased risk for mortality and for cardiovascular-related mortality, even after adjusting for an extensive list of potential confounders [9]. Moreover, elder mistreatment predicts increased rates of emergency department use, hospitalizations, readmissions, skilled nursing placement, and hospice utilization. Despite the frequency with which elder mistreatment victims interact with healthcare systems, most victims pass through these systems unrecognized. This represents a missed opportunity to improve quality of care and highlights the importance of integrating screening measures to detect elder mistreatment.

All states have some form of mandatory reporting of elder mistreatment and programming to address the report, policies, and procedures for addressing cases [12, 22] (Addressed in Chap. 10). It is clear that the legislative and regulatory mandates are important to have knowledge about, and also clear that every clinician who cares for older adults has a professional and ethical mandate to ensure that the possibility of elder mistreatment is ruled out during the clinical encounter. This means that regardless of setting, an elder mistreatment protocol, that includes a screening procedure, an assessment question or instrument, a set of care planning procedures that can guide a clinician in the event that elder mistreatment is suspected, and a follow-up procedure with the appropriate contact entities must be in place. Follow-up might include the utilization of adult protective services, law enforcement officials, the organization's administrators, primary care providers, and the family.

Important progress has been made related to these procedures and in particular, the National Center for Elder Abuse at University of Southern California [25, 36] and others have protocols to assist clinicians in this work. Further, the National Institute of Justice under the purview of the Elder Justice act has done an excellent job assembling protocols and procedures to the same end. Historically, there have been a number of protocols and programs that have been in place as the evidence base has been accruing. This includes the Beth Israel Elder Assessment Team [6] along with the University New Hampshire Family Violence Laboratory [31, 32]. Further, the Judge Baker laboratory, in Boston Massachusetts, which has focused on child abuse detection assessment and management, has lent a good deal of structure to the way that we use family violence protocols in the clinical setting. It is well appreciated that the earliest screening instruments were modeled after the child abuse assessment instruments, and while those in geriatrics are very clear about the dramatic differences between child abuse cases and elder abuse cases, there are structures and

N. OBrien-Suric · A. Benson · T. Fulmer (✉)
The John A. Hartford Foundation, 55 East 59th Street, 16th Floor, New York, NY 10022, USA
e-mail: terry.fulmer@johnahartford.org

N. OBrien-Suric
e-mail: nora.obsuric@johnahartford.org

X. Dong
Rush Institute for Healthy Aging, Rush University Medical Center, 1645 W. Jackson Blvd, Suite 675, Chicago, IL 60612, USA

X. Dong (ed.), *Elder Abuse*, DOI 10.1007/978-3-319-47504-2_11

protocols that have been extremely valuable in moving this field forward.

As a baseline, every clinical setting that provides care for older adults needs to have a protocol for elder mistreatment clinical management, and ensure it is being effectively monitored. This includes a screening mechanism, a clinical approach to care planning, and appropriate referrals to adult protective services and legal entities as needed.

As protocols are developed, it is extremely important to have the administrative support for these practice protocols for elder mistreatment. In the absence of such support, there is little chance that an effective protocol can be implemented and sustained. This means that clinicians should be afforded the time to develop protocols and procedures, and to process elder mistreatment cases similar to processing family violence cases. Each organization's agency will be different, but the fundamental question stands: is there any suspected elder mistreatment in the individual being assessed? There is evidence indicating that single-item screening can be equally as effective as longer protocols [35]. It is vitally important, whether one uses a single-item screen "are you safe at home?" or a longer battery of questions to get at the clinical nuances of the case, every older adult requires and deserves an elder mistreatment assessment. Finally, the Joint Commission on Accreditation of Healthcare Organizations does have a standard for victims of abuse or neglect rationale, for the standard explains the important role of healthcare workers in identifying victims [21].

As with any clinical protocol, the cultural context of the case as well as the structural situation of the living environment must be taken into account. Is the individual being cared for by a paid caregiver, such as a nurse, and therefore the question might be malpractice? Or is the individual being cared for by a frail elderly spouse? All of this should be considered as one addresses the clinical management of elder mistreatment. A solid understanding of family systems is extremely important, as well as establishing an interdisciplinary team to address these complex cases.

A 2015 article written by Dong in the Journal of the American Geriatric Society (JAGS) "Elder Abuse: Systematic Review and Implications for Practice" provides a curriculum's worth of references for more detailed information on prevalence, risk factors, and consequences [11]. In 2014 Lisa M. Gibbs and Laura Mosqueda edited a book on "The Medical Implications of Elder Abuse and Neglect" which provides explicit directions on treating the medical consequences of elder abuse [17]. Published in 2005 and still a valuable book edited by Georgia J Anetzberger "The Clinical Management of Elder Abuse" not only provides useful hands-on-information, but includes the perspective of various team members—physician, nurse, social worker, and attorney [2]. It is essential to consider the interdependence of team members' roles in providing clinical management of elder mistreatment.

According to Dr. Anetzberger, there are five steps in the clinical management of elder mistreatment: detection, assessment, planning, intervention, and follow-up [2]. The following will provide an overview of detection, assessment, intervention and management, and follow-up.

11.2 Detection: Screening Approaches in Clinical Settings

The first step is to detect the problem by screening for mistreatment. The American Medical Association (AMA) recommends that all geriatric patients receive elder mistreatment screening [5]. Also, the historic legislation of the Patient Protection and Affordable Care Act (ACA) of 2010 provides for the protections and expansion of services and resources for vulnerable people [18]. Although, as of 2015, Medicare does not specifically reimburse clinicians for their time in screening for mistreatment in their elderly patients. However, it is essential that screening is conducted, because elder mistreatment victims interact frequently with health systems, and therefore screening and treatment should be instituted at points of care [11].

In 2013, CMS held a national symposium on the role of elder mistreatment screening as a Physician Quality Reporting System (PQRS) measure among Medicare beneficiaries. Experts systematically examined the scope and impact of elder mistreatment, especially in healthcare settings. The VASS and H-S/EAST were recommended as suitable measures to detect elder mistreatment. CMS also recognized the limitations of existing knowledge and called for research and guidelines to support healthcare professionals. PQRS measure 181 is approved by CMS to screen for elder mistreatment and follow-up, but clinician utilization has been low. This PQRS measure could be an instrumental tool to improve reporting of elder mistreatment and quality measures in healthcare systems. This can further provide guidance for healthcare professionals to deal with the issues of elder mistreatment in clinical settings.

Each time older adults interface with the healthcare system, there are invaluable opportunities for healthcare providers to detect and intervene in abusive situations [29]. Since elder mistreatment victims often interact with health systems, increased screening and treatment could improve quality of care. Primary care outpatient practices, inpatient hospitalization episodes, as well as discharge planning and home health could play pivotal roles in identifying potentially unsafe situations that could jeopardize the safety and well-being of older adults [9]. Since elder mistreatment victims also disproportionally interact with the emergency department, hospital system, and nursing homes, brief screening measures should be incorporated as a part of the psychosocial and home safety assessment by physicians, nurses, therapists, and discharge planners. Increased screening and treatment should be instituted in the emergency departments and hospital settings, especially to those who frequently visit the healthcare setting despite adequate care and management plans. Discharge planning and home health services could play pivotal roles in identifying potential family conflict and dangerous environment and lifestyle choices that could jeopardize the safety and well-being of older adults in the community. Early detection and interventions, such as leveraging effective treatment of underlying issues, providing community-based and patient-centered services, and appropriately involving family, may help ameliorate or potentially stop elder mistreatment (Table 11.1).

By establishing screening protocols, clinicians will detect whether or not elder mistreatment is evident or suspected in a situation involving an older person who is currently under care or has been referred for evaluation or service [2]. Having policies and procedures in all clinical settings will help healthcare workers identify and assist victims as necessary [18]. Primary care outpatient practices, inpatient hospitalization episodes, discharge planning, home health, and community-based settings should be involved in screening protocols in order to also identify potentially unsafe situations that could jeopardize the safety and well-being of older adults [11].

The basic principle of screening programs is that they "do more good than harm" [28]. Among the criteria used to assess a screening program are: the condition should be an important health problem; the test should be simple, safe, and validated; the test should be acceptable to the population; there should be available effective interventions to follow up; there should be adequate staff available; and there should be evidence that the complete screening program is clinically, socially, and ethically acceptable to health professionals and the public [28].

Many screening tools exist to detect elder mistreatment through either potential victims and/or perpetrators in various settings (community, clinical, and institutional, etc.) and through various methods (telephone, in-person, computer assisted, self-administered, etc.). The two highlighted measures below are suggested by CMS based on available evidence. They provide a basis for heightening clinicians' suspicion for elder mistreatment, and asking additional questions to explore potential elder mistreatment (Table 11.2). The Hwalek-Sengstock Elder Abuse Screening Test (H-S/EAST) measures: violation of personal rights or direct abuse, characteristics of vulnerability, and potentially abusive situations. Vulnerability to Abuse Screening Scale (VASS) measures vulnerability, dependence, dejection, and coercion. These measures have been tested in diverse populations and racial/ethnic groups; VASS has demonstrated predictive validity.

The two measures noted above may not capture specific subtypes of elder mistreatment or the social, family, and cultural context of potential mistreatment. These measures have not been validated among those with cognitive impairment, who are particularly at high risk. False-positive results could cause psychological distress to patients and families, and potentially jeopardize the physician–patient relationship. False-negative results may negate the abusive situations and provide false assurance, which may further increase older adults' risk for adverse outcomes. In addition, there may be potential concern that screening and clinical management can put people at greater risk and actually result in harm from the potential perpetrator(s). Moreover, as there may be limited evidence on effective RTC intervention and prevention strategies to ameliorate elder mistreatment, there

Table 11.1 Brief screening measures for elder mistreatment

Hwalek-Sengstock Elder Abuse Screening Test (H-S/EAST)	Vulnerability to Abuse Screening Scale (VASS)
1. Has anyone close to you tried to hurt or harm you recently?	1. Are you afraid of anyone in your family?
2. Do you feel uncomfortable with anyone in your family?	**2.** Has anyone close to you tried to hurt or harm you recently?
3. Does anyone tell you that you give them too much trouble?	3. Has anyone close to you called you names or put you down or made you feel bad recently?
4. Has anyone forced you to do things that you didn't want to do?	4. Does someone in your family make you stay in bed or tell you you're sick when you know you aren't?
5. Do you feel that nobody wants you around?	5. Has anyone forced you to do things you didn't want to do?
6. Who makes decisions about your life… like how you should live or where you should live?	6. Has anyone taken things that belong to you without your OK?

Table 11.2 Clinical management strategies for elder mistreatment

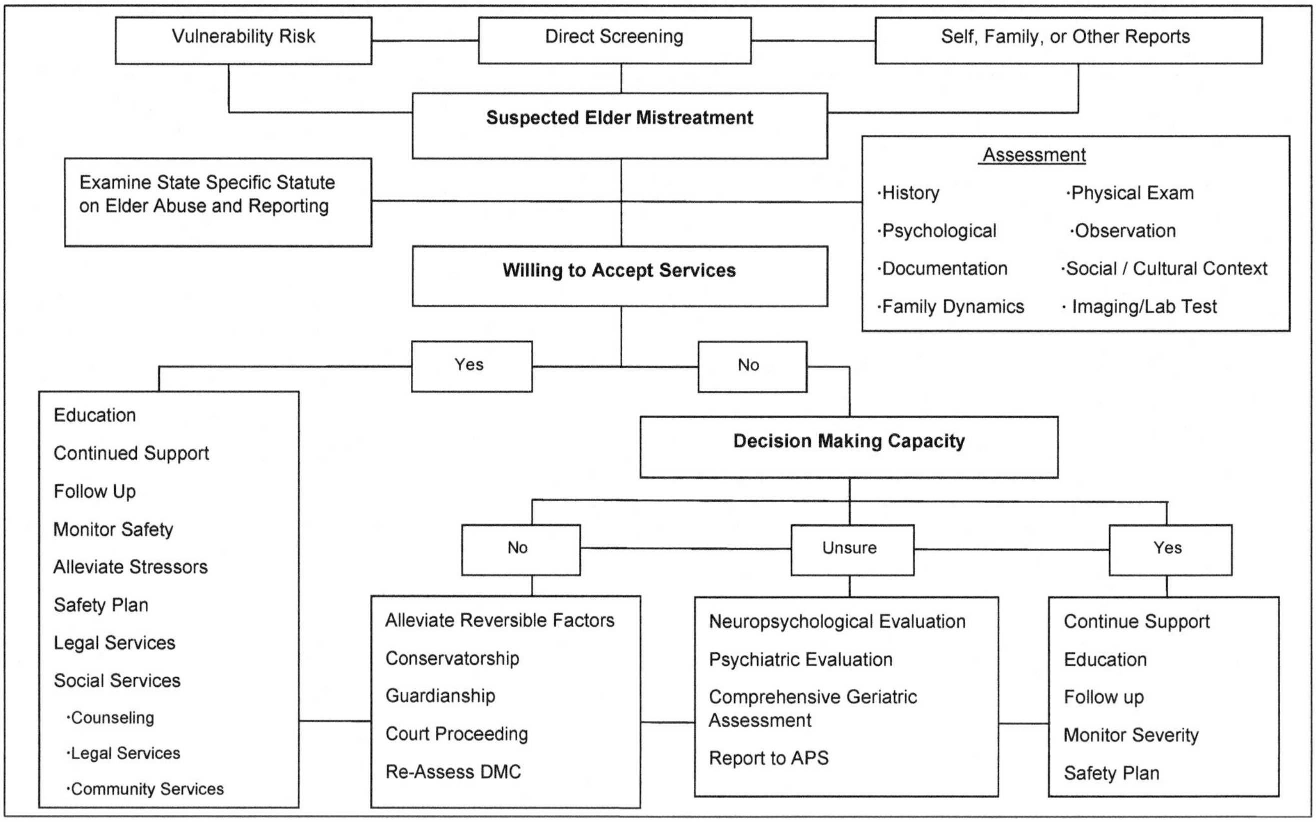

may be insufficient guidance within the healthcare systems to assist professionals, many of whom may not have the knowledge, time, or skills to deal with complex cases. Despite these potential limitations, many experts in the field concur that there is a great need for action. In 2013, the USPSTF report to US Congress suggested that elder mistreatment should be a priority research area, in order to better quantify these assumptions.

The physical examination is a foundation for detecting the many types of mistreatment [17]. There are six major categories of elder mistreatment: (1) physical abuse, (2) emotional or psychological abuse, (3) sexual abuse, (4) neglect by others, (5) self-neglect, and (6) financial exploitation [29]. Elder mistreatment is suspected through the identification of signs, which represent the consequence of mistreatment occurrence [2]. Physical abuse signs may include bruises, skin tears, fractures, burns, and other injuries [29]. Emotional abuse signs could be fear, silence, depression, and an inability to interview due to an ever-present or controlling caregiver [29]. Neglect may present as weight loss, dehydration, falls, fears, and poor hygiene [29]. Self-neglect can include depression or dementia with malnutrition, repeated falls, decubitus ulcers, contractures, medication non-adherence, missed appointments, and poor hygiene [29]. Additional warning signs of abuse and neglect include discrepancy in psychosocial and medical history between the elder and the possible abuser, vague, implausible explanation of illness or injuries; illnesses that do not appear to be responding to treatment; lab findings inconsistent with history provided; frequent visits to the emergency room; and unexplained injuries or illnesses [19]. Since older persons may present signs and symptoms of a multiplicity of factors due to aging, such as frail skin, a fall, or confusion, it is very important to always think more broadly in each circumstance and to be alert [28].

Providers who have suspicion for any type of elder mistreatment should first look for signs of physical injury. Healthcare providers who discover physical injuries during the course of an examination should be alert to the possibility of elder mistreatment. However, the physical finding is just one component of the assessment. It must be understood in the context of multiple factors including physiology, pathophysiology, medical history and function, and the mechanism of injury [17].

The main approach to detection of elder mistreatment is through identifying older individuals with high-risk profiles

[28]. Systematic screening for risk factors and indicators of mistreatment can make important differences in the frontlines of intervention, early detection, and prevention [5]. The main risk factors documented in the literature include: social isolation; frailty, functional disability, and/or cognitive impairment; pathology of the abuser (such as alcohol or other substance abuse), cognitive impairment, and/or mental-health problems; caregiver stress or anger; dependence of the older adult on the abuser or dependence of the abuser on the victim [28]. The characteristics of older adults associated with a greater likelihood of mistreatment include cognitive impairment, aggressive behaviors, psychological distress, lower levels of social network and social support, lower household income, need for activities of daily living assistance, and premorbid relationship to the abuser (Mosqueda and Dong [24]). The presence of chronic disease and chronic disability due to illness are both considered risk factors [2]. Abusers are typically effective at presenting themselves as overly concerned about the older victim and also at masking signs of mistreatment [19]. Careful attention to the psychosocial aspects of the older adult can assist in understanding the contextual factors that may be strong predictors of mistreatment [28].

Due to the many possible causes of mistreatment, it behooves all professionals to be knowledgeable about, and alert for, the different types of mistreatment. Using a team-based approach, there will be more opportunities to detect the varied signs of mistreatment.

11.3 The Assessment Team

Elder mistreatment by its very nature is a complex and multifaceted problem, for which assessment begins with a suspicion about its existence by any member of the healthcare team [2]. A team is helpful in confirming mistreatment, documenting impaired capacity, reviewing medications and medical conditions, and persuading the client or family to take action [24]. Group interviews enable the team to see victim/perpetrator interaction and separate interviews facilitate individual candor and enable comparison of accounts [2]. Effective actions pertaining to mistreatment rest on the collaboration and cooperation between practitioners [4].

The treatment of elder mistreatment requires clinicians to collaborate with other professionals by working in teams to provide an important strategy for elder mistreatment detection and intervention [2]. Working in teams will benefit the mistreatment detection and intervention process in three ways: (1) Offer a more holistic perspective to the situation of elder mistreatment than could be offered by a single discipline; (2) Assure that no single discipline has sole responsibility for handling complex and challenging situations; and (3) Forge relationships among professionals that transcend consideration of individual cases and promote a community-wide approach to elder mistreatment prevention and treatment [2].

All members of the team, physicians, nurses, and social workers, including others as needed, play a critical role in the treatment of elder mistreatment. Each clinical discipline brings a unique set of knowledge, skills, and perspectives to completing the steps in treating the medical condition [2].

11.3.1 Physicians

Physicians may see many of the sequelae of elder mistreatment. They have an ethical and, in most states, legal role in recognition and intervention where elder mistreatment is suspected [2]. The AMA recommends that physicians be able to institute measures needed to prevent further injury to the elder mistreatment victim, provide medical evaluation and treatment of injuries resulting from abuse and neglect while remaining objective and nonjudgmental, attempt to establish or maintain a therapeutic alliance with family, and report all suspected cases in accordance with local statutes [33]. Physicians are in a position to oversee screening and prevention of elder mistreatment because they often see their elderly patients five or more times per year [5]. They therefore have multiple opportunities to observe and discuss changes in cognition, function, mental health, social situation, living, and financial statuses [5]. The physician may notice a change in behavior over time that could be indicative of mistreatment [24]. During an office visit, the physician should ask direct questions of the patient and, if available, the caregiver. It is important to observe if the patient seems fearful of the caregiver and if so, to conduct a private interview and examination. Bruises, lacerations, burns, and other injuries, particularly if in unusual locations without adequate explanations as to cause, should raise a suspicion of mistreatment [24].

If there is suspicion of physical abuse, the physician has three responsibilities [2]. First, observations should be accurately and specifically documented. Second, an assessment should be made of whether the patient is in immediate danger and whether he or she should be hospitalized. Finally, suspicions of mistreatment should be reported to APS [2].

11.3.2 Nurses

Nurses play pivotal roles in all aspects of elder mistreatment [2]. They are the healthcare professionals who most often assume major responsibilities in assessing elder mistreatment situations. Nursing assessment of physical abuse and neglect focuses on the following aspects: nutrition, hydration, bruises and injuries, degree of frailty, and the presence of pathologic conditions. Assessment of bruises, swelling, injuries, lacerations, pressure ulcers, and other indications of physical harm is another important aspect of the detection of physical neglect or abuse. In situations of physical neglect, nurses may see any of the following indicators: leg ulcers, pressure ulcers, dependent edema, poor wound healing, burns from stoves, cigarettes, or hot water, and bruises and injuries from falls, especially repeated falls. Nurses may intervene in elder mistreatment situations as individual healthcare providers or as part of an interdisciplinary team [2].

11.3.3 Social Workers

Social workers, both in clinical settings and in community-based settings, bring a holistic perspective to elder mistreatment cases. Mistreatment often coexists with other social problems [28]. Social workers, by profession, apply a systems approach, taking into consideration all the factors that may be contributing to the abusive situation. An important approach in the social work profession is accepting individuals as they are, enhancing the dignity and worth of the person, assessing psychosocial functioning and the environment, identifying strengths, including the available support [2]. Studies have found that interventions that offer combinations of individual or family counseling, case management, skills training, and behavior management strategies can be quite effective [8]. Social workers can facilitate novel interventions addressing elder mistreatment, such as family care conferences to assist in identifying challenges and finding solutions to elder mistreatment [8]. Psychological interventions help to reduce the stress, anxiety, and depression of the victim as well as the perpetrators of mistreatment, which may assist in reducing the risk of elder mistreatment occurrence or reoccurrence [8]. Additionally, social workers are uniquely equipped to provide both the direct service and the advocacy needed to help victims become empowered, as well as to secure the resources needed to rebuild their lives [18].

11.3.3.1 Clinical Assessment and Interdisciplinary Approach

By conducting routine health and psychosocial assessments, it is more likely that, when a form of mistreatment becomes present, the clinician will be able to identify the change and investigate further to determine if mistreatment of the patient is taking place. The presence of elder mistreatment signs or risk factors will indicate the need for a more thorough assessment [24]. Without a comprehensive assessment of the bio/psychosocial context of elder mistreatment, any screening or assessment instrument will have significant limitations [28].

The Comprehensive Geriatric Assessments (CGA) are the gold standard for assessing the health and well-being of older adults [5]. These standardized tests are relatively quick and efficient and could be performed once or twice a year. It is important to follow up with vigilant monitoring of changes in status in subsequent visits [5]. Geriatric medical teams are trained in CGA and are accustomed to completing some combination of these assessments on a routine basis [5].

The Elder Assessment Instrument (EAI) is another instrument for the detection of elder mistreatment. This 46-item tool is clinically useful in the assessment and detection of elder mistreatment and is one of several available for this purpose. This screen, best used by clinicians, requires physical examination of the patient. Others do not have this requirement and may be more appropriate in community and home settings [6, 14–16, 34]. The other existing tools for detecting elder mistreatment include: the Brief Abuse Screen for the Elderly (BASE); the Caregiver Abuse Screen (CASE); and the Indicators of Abuse Screen (IOA). The Elder Assessment Instrument includes a general assessment of the older person as well as specific physical, social, and medical assessments and level of independence in lifestyle. The Elder Abuse Suspicion Index was developed with the goal of establishing a reasonable level of suspicion in order to justify referral to appropriate community services for in-depth assessment [28].

One of the first elements a practitioner should evaluate is the capacity for mistreated older adults to make their own decisions regarding their situation [4]. Assessing functional, cognitive, and psychological well-being is important for understanding the predisposing and precipitating risk factors associated with elder mistreatment [11]. It is necessary to assess the cognitive functioning in order to engage the older person in treatment and follow-up care. If there is no clear indicator of cognitive impairment, it must be presumed that an older adult has decision-making capacity and the clinician must accept the person's choices. If there are indications that the older person may have cognitive impairment, then the process of having the person declared incompetent must begin with the healthcare provider and the legal system determining that the person lacks capacity [24]. It is extremely difficult when a clinician feels the need to override a patient's personal wishes [24]. Capacity often fluctuates over time and clinicians must use their best judgment in determining if and what next steps need to be taken [24]. When necessary, a referral to assess decision-making capacity should be made to a neuropsychologist or psychiatrist [24]. When impaired capacity is identified, the clinician should look for reversible causes such as medications that impair cognition or illnesses that may manifest as impaired cognition [24].

The presence of lack of capacity is often the determining factor in deciding what healthcare professionals need to do next in pursuing treatment and intervention. However, capacity is not often completely present or completely absent. It is a gradient relationship between the issues in question and an older adult's ability to make these decisions. For complicated health issues, there is greater need to require higher levels of decisional capacity. At the same time, for simple issues, even a cognitively impaired adult could have decisional capacity. However, the healthcare providers are often forced to take a gray area and make it black or white for the purpose of guiding next steps such as guardianship or conservatorship. Commonly used brief screening testing, such as the MMSE, is inadequate for determining capacity except at the extremes of the score. Tests useful in assessing decision-making capacity are the Aid to Capacity Evaluation (ACE), the Hopkins Competency Assessment Test (HCAT), and Understanding Treatment Disclosure (UTD).

Overt physical abuse is generally easier to observe and assess than various forms of neglect where issues of caregiver responsibility, underlying patient condition, and the patient's wishes and capacity for self-determination may open matters to more interpretations [2]. People with dementia are particularly vulnerable to mistreatment because if there are impairments in memory, communication abilities, and judgment, it might make it difficult for them to avoid, prevent, or report mistreatment [17]. Therefore, if a person with cognitive impairment and/or dementia presents with suspicious physical signs of mistreatment it is easier for the clinician to decide to conduct an assessment.

Clinicians must presume an older adult has decision-making capacity (DMC) and accept the patient's choices until he or she is determined to lack capacity by a healthcare provider or the legal system. However, capacity is neither present nor absent; rather it is a gradient relationship between the issues in question and an older adult's ability to make these decisions. When a patient screens positive for cognitive impairment, health professionals, especially geriatricians, promote a patient's rights to autonomy and self-determination, maintain a family unit whenever possible, and provide recommendations for the least restrictive services and safety plan. Sometime, despite our best attempts, patients refuse services aimed to protect them.

While the screening and risk prediction for elder mistreatment are important steps, it is just as critical to assist healthcare professionals in taking appropriate steps if a patient screens positive. Elder mistreatment should be reported to APS whenever a reasonable suspicion of elder mistreatment arises. The goal is to make an informed referral to APS. While reporting is controversial and for many considered a barrier to inquiry and disclosure [28], clinicians should document with the knowledge that the medical record may be used in an elder mistreatment investigation, by social workers, law enforcement, or prosecutors [17]. Documentation is critical for supporting the interdisciplinary team and APS to ameliorate elder mistreatment and protect vulnerable older adults [11]. In some situations, immediate legal intervention may be critical, especially if there is a threat to life [2].

When health professionals suspect elder mistreatment, detailed histories should be gathered, including psychosocial, family, and cultural factors. In addition, specific findings from physical examinations that may further indicate elder mistreatment should be documented. Healthcare professionals should document observations of patient behavior, reactions to questions, as well as family dynamics and conflicts. Whenever indicated, healthcare professionals should order laboratory tests and imaging tests. These types of documentation are critical for supporting the interdisciplinary team and APS to ameliorate elder mistreatment and protect vulnerable older adults. Furthermore, healthcare professionals should devise patient-centered plans to provide support, education, and follow-up, as well as monitor ongoing mistreatment and institute safety plans.

11.3.4 Elder Mistreatment Reporting by Healthcare Professionals

All 50 states have procedures for reporting mistreatment and all but four states have made such reporting mandatory for healthcare providers to report a reasonable suspicion of elder mistreatment cases [19]. All states have established APS programs, which generally have the authority to investigate reported cases or to refer them to appropriate legal authorities [19]. APS is charged with taking a report and investigating alleged elder mistreatment if the older adults reside in the community. A long-term care ombudsman agency investigates alleged incidents that occur in licensed facilities such as skilled nursing facilities. According to the most recent data available, healthcare professionals were responsible for 11.1 % of elder mistreatment complaints or reports (citation, 2000 survey of state APS). Specifically, physicians made 1.0 % of the reports. A survey of APS workers in 43 states found that of 17 occupational groups, physicians were rated in the least helpful category for detecting elder mistreatment. The reasons physicians cite for not reporting include subtlety of signs, victim denial, and lack of knowledge about reporting procedures [26]. Other reasons described by primary care physicians include concern about losing physician–patient rapport, doubts about the impact of APS intervention on the patient's perceived quality of life, and perceived contradictions between mandatory reporting and healthcare provider's ability to act in the patient's best interests [30]. Despite these concerns, most healthcare providers in the U.S. are mandated to report suspected mistreatment. Failure to report may lead to legal consequences ranging from monetary penalties to jail sentences. To help overcome reluctance in reporting, a compassionate clinician could explain the need to make a report and the desire to help improve a dangerous situation. In doing so, such a report can help the APS worker have a more successful visit.

The scope and delivery of services provided by APS agencies vary due to differences in state laws, how enforcing laws are interpreted, and levels of funding and interest in different areas within the state. Irrespective of location, APS aims to provide the victimized older adults with coordinated, interdisciplinary care that encompasses social and health systems. This is done with an underlying philosophy that promotes a client's rights to autonomy and self-determination, maintains a family unit whenever possible, and provides recommendations for the least restrictive living situation. The APS worker must presume the client has decision-making capacity and must accept the client's choices until the client is determined to lack capacity by a healthcare provider or the legal system.

To make a referral to APS the clinician should contact either the local state number, ElderCare Locator (800-677-1116) or the National Center on Elder Abuse.

11.3.4.1 Psychosocial-Behavioral-Environmental Assessment

During the medical examination of the victim, the clinician will observe the injuries and the physical condition. When health professionals suspect elder mistreatment, detailed histories should be obtained, especially psychosocial and cultural aspects [11]. In addition, it is important for a member of the team, a nurse or a social worker, to conduct a psychosocial assessment of the victim and of the caregiver(s) if applicable. Older adults are often faced with multiple social complexities that can affect function and increase the risk for mistreatment, neglect, or self-neglect [17]. This psychosocial assessment will provide a summary of the issues that need to be addressed. A variety of factors need to be observed and assessed including the impact of the physical injuries on the psychological status of the patient, the results derived from psychological tests, legal status, descriptions of the problem(s), existing assets and resources, the prognosis or prediction of the outcome, and the plan designed to resolve the problem(s). The assessment is a communication tool to share pertinent information with other members of the team for case planning and referral purposes, as well as to establish in writing an account of the patient's physical and mental status. The psychosocial assessment account provides baseline information about the patient when he or she enters an agency for service.

Conducting a thorough assessment of all aspects of a person's situation will uncover issues that contribute to risk factors for elder abuse and neglect. The psychosocial-behavioral-environmental assessment will focus on areas that are risk factors and will obtain necessary information to assess the risk for mistreatment or continued mistreatment. The psychosocial assessment will determine the level of dependency and vulnerability of the victim. The behavioral part of the assessment will include a review of the relationship between the patient and the caregiver, including the dependence and deviance of the abuser. The environmental assessment will include housing, living arrangement, and the community which will flag the possibility of social isolation. Finally, the cultural assessment will provide a deeper understanding of the values of the patient and the caregiver as well as the potential resources of the community. The analysis of the completed assessment will provide a road map for the team in devising a plan for intervention and follow-up care.

The assessment should include information on the behavioral interaction between the victim and his/her abuser and others as pertinent to the situation. It will help uncover possible reasons for the cause of the mistreatment and can provide information on possible interventions, such as couples counseling to help prevent further mistreatment. It is important to be as specific as possible about the patient–caregiver relationship, including identification of specific sources of distress and the response to them [2]. The interview will begin to identify the caregiver who may be frustrated, angry, or exhausted and the interviewer should be alert for comments that would signal the possibility of abuse or neglect and thereby learn more about the relationship between caregiver and patient [2]. It will be helpful to watch for signs of general regard and empathy for the patient on the part of the caregiver [2]. Additionally, by inquiring about the relationship and the day-to-day activities of the victim and the caregiver, issues and causes of neglect can be uncovered. By understanding the behaviors and capabilities of all the people involved in caring for the older person, the team will be able to plan an intervention that will address the factors that lead to abuse or neglect.

Situations of frailty dependence of the older person, while a contributing factor to mistreatment, should be understood within the overall context of the relationship between the mistreated older person and the abuser along with the characteristics of the abuser [28]. The assessment should take into account the care recipient, the caregiver, housing, community factors as well as other environmental factors [19]. Loneliness and social isolation have been linked to elder mistreatment [7]. Therefore, it is important to assess support resources, such as caregivers and friends, who influence the older person's physical and psychosocial function, either positively or detrimentally [2]. If an older victim does not have an adequate social support network, it may be more difficult for them to recover from the psychological effects of the mistreatment [17].

The assessment requires speaking with the patient alone to get his or her perceptions on what is occurring and to understand their insight into the situation [2]. The caregiver should be interviewed separately as well. Health professionals should document observations of patient behavior, reactions to questions, and family dynamics and conflict.

There are three sections of the psychosocial assessment: Basic information, Background and Current Functioning; and Impressions, Assessment and Recommendations. The Basic Information should contain: Identifying Information, Referral, Presenting Problem, Sources of Data, and General Description of the patient. The Background and Current Functioning should include: Family Composition and Background, Educational Background, Employment and Vocational Skills, Religious/Spiritual Involvement, Physical Functioning, Health Conditions, and Medical Background, Psychological and Psychiatric Functioning and Background, Social, Community, and Recreational Activities, Basic Life Necessities, Legal Concerns, Other Environmental or Psychosocial Factors, and Client Strengths, Capacities, and Resources. The Impressions, Assessment, and Recommendations should provide a Clinical Summary, Impressions, and Assessment and the Goals and Recommendations for Work with the patient.

The major components of a psychosocial interview include: identifying the patient, the chief complaint, the history of presenting illness, psychiatric history, medical and surgical history, medication list, alcohol and drug use, violence risk assessment, family and social history, and the mental status examination. Other significant components to include are occupational history, educational history, legal history, developmental history, spiritual assessment, cultural assessment, financial assessment, coping skills, interests, and abilities.

Basic Patient Information and Presenting Medical Issue

The first step in any assessment is to adequately identify the patient. This should include the patient's name, gender, birth date/age, marital status, race/ethnicity, and languages spoken. The history of the present illness is the chronological account of what led up to the chief complaint. This section may include the problem's location, duration, severity, timing, context, modifying factors, and associated signs and symptoms.

Psychiatric and Psychological History

It is necessary to assess the strengths and limitations of the patient. Older people may have developed resiliency from past stresses or may have experienced trauma from which they have not fully resolved. Also, determining coping skills is an important part of the psychosocial assessment. The psychiatric/psychological assessment should include all mental-health issues in the past. The medical and surgical history is a listing of all medical illnesses and a listing of all surgeries including their date. All current and past medications should be listed including their dose and frequency. For medications currently taken, a listing of who prescribed them and why they are prescribed should be recorded. For past prescribed medications, a listing of why they were started and why they were stopped should be recorded. History of previous alcohol and drug use is an important part of the psychosocial assessment. The substances that are currently being used should be recorded, including the method of use (oral, inhalation, injection, intranasal), amount of use, frequency of use, and time period of use. Any substances used in the past should also be recorded. Common substances of mistreatment include: alcohol, heroin, opiates, marijuana, cocaine, crack, methamphetamines, inhalants, stimulants, hallucinogens, caffeine, and nicotine. The potential violence risk of the patient should also be assessed. Risk factors for violent behavior include: male gender, unemployment status, drug and alcohol use, active psychotic symptoms, and lower socioeconomic status.

Social and Educational History

The social history provides clues as to how one interacts with others. It is important to have an understanding of all social relationships in order to understand the social supports as well as the toxic relationships. The clinician should have the patient describe their social relationships including spouse/significant other, number of children, current living situation, military history (including type of discharge), and any other support or social networks should be reported. Any significant life event, such as a death or divorce should be reported. It is also important to determine the patient's abilities and interests in order to get a full picture of the patient. In addition, determining the patient's sexual orientation will help the team provide better care for the patient.

Determining the educational history will help the team understand the best way to interact with the patient.

Spiritual Beliefs

The spiritual assessment should note the patient's religious background. In addition, the degree of involvement within the religious community and any spiritual practices should be assessed. When spiritual concerns are identified, appropriate referrals (such as to the Chaplin) may help assure holistic wellness.

Cultural and Ethnic Background

The cultural assessment should list any important issues regarding the patient's ethnic and cultural background. It is impossible to have a full understanding of every culture, but a good cultural assessment will help the team understand the patient's cultural beliefs, values, and practices. These factors should be respected and considered when providing care.

Financial Status

The financial assessment should include a full inventory of income, assets, and debts. Understanding the patient's financial situation is important for multiple reasons. Clients with lower socioeconomic class are at higher risk for social isolation, which is a risk factor for mistreatment. In addition, clients who have limited financial resources may need help with money and would benefit from a consultation with a social worker. It is important to assess the financial situation of the caregiver as well. Awareness of financial resources is crucial in understanding caregiver needs, especially when the caregiver depends on the finances of the care recipient [29]. Should the financial resources be limited, a social worker can explore the possibility of eligibility for additional income, medical coverage, prescription costs, delivered or congregate meals, and assistance with housing and energy costs.

Environmental and Community Assessment

It is important to know about the patient's home, is it safe for the patient to return, is it habitable, are there dangerous steps, access to the bathroom, a working kitchen, etc. These factors are essential in planning the intervention and the best placement for the victim. When the team is not capable of doing a home assessment, it is imperative that the team include members from the community, such as a case manager or healthcare provider, who can do a home visit and conduct an environmental assessment. Understanding the type of community and gaining knowledge of available resources will help in planning appropriate interventions. Home-based and community-based resources must be accessed and individualized to address specific patient needs. Other factors involved in mistreatment include social and geographic isolation, which can produce loneliness and lack of oversight [29]. The home environment reveals clues to mistreatment that office or hospital visits may not [29]. Risk factors for abuse and neglect include shared living arrangements, which provide greater opportunity for tension and conflict. Residence in remote areas may include lack of readily available assistance and fewer support services [29]. This is also a risk factor for mistreatment which can go undetected. Low social support, or a lack of social connectedness and connectedness to the community is a risk factor for elder mistreatment. Elder mistreatment in the community setting is complicated by the sociocultural context; consideration of cultural issues needs to be included to effectively address the needs of the individuals within their communities [20]. The context of culture, community, and social support play a large role in the well-being of older adults. By knowing the ethnic and cultural dimensions of the victim and the caregiver, the practitioner can engage the appropriate community in providing supportive services that will be accepted by the pair.

11.4 Planning and Intervention

Training in interventions should target staff at all levels, encompassing both clinical and nonclinical aspects. Curricula for different health disciplines should incorporate gerontological approaches to case management and elder mistreatment training [20].

11.4.1 Clinical Team Management of Physical Sequelae of Elder Mistreatment

Clinical management for elder mistreatment is a complex matter; the intended benefits should be balanced against potential harms. Despite the incompleteness of the evidence, the benefits outweigh the harms of inaction. Because of the scope and impact of the issue, thoughtful assessment for elder mistreatment in healthcare settings should be a priority. Practical suggestions are provided to healthcare professionals to detect and treat cases of elder mistreatment. Health care professionals are well situated to screen for elder mistreatment and detect vulnerabilities [26, 27]. Assessing functional, cognitive, and psychosocial well-being are important factors to understand vulnerability associated with elder mistreatment. Dong et al. constructed a risk prediction index suggesting that older adults with three to four vulnerability factors have an almost-fold increased risk for elder mistreatment while those with ≥5 vulnerability factors have more than a 26-fold increased risk for elder mistreatment [10].

Interventions must first address the victim's acute medical problems, including any injuries and untreated illnesses, and acute emotional problems resulting from elder mistreatment, including fear and anxiety [2]. Second, clinicians should ensure the victim's safety [2]. Third, clinical procedures should help victims regain the sense of efficacy and control that the mistreatment eroded. Finally, clinicians should work with others to alleviate the underlying causes of elder mistreatment [2].

In clinical management, the intervention step will also involve the application of social services, laws, and clinical procedures to treat the consequences of elder mistreatment or to prevent occurrence or reoccurrence of the problem [2]. Effective intervention requires an understanding of the context of the situations and the relationships of the persons involved [2]. Intervention regarding older adult mistreatment raises many questions for clinicians [4]. They have to interact with the older person, the abuser and in many cases, with both at the same time [4]. The ideal goal is to help both the patient and the caregiver, though the prime duty is to the patient [2].

During a routine clinical physician office visit, answers to questions about how older adults manage their daily lives, potential family conflicts and struggles can suggest predisposing issues for elder mistreatment that will eventually impair the patient's ability to live independently. Difficulties in meeting the needs for the activities of daily living may be associated with current and future caregiver neglect, which may evolve and could progress in severity over time. Assessments of the patient's functional and cognitive status are important adjuncts to understanding the predisposing and precipitating risk factors associated with elder mistreatment.

11.4.2 Team Management of Psychosocial-Behavioral-Environmental-Cultural Issues

Psychosocial interventions are interpersonal or information activities, techniques, or strategies that target biological, behavioral, cognitive, emotional, interpersonal, social, and environmental factors with the aim of improving health functioning and well-being [24]. The two goals in planning elder interventions are preserving the victim's autonomy and promoting the victim's safety [2].

The first step for a successful intervention is to gain and build trust with the patient. A trusting relationship between the practitioner and the patient can make all the difference in breaking the cycle of mistreatment [28]. Improving trust and communication are central for dealing effectively with mistreatment [28]. There are five dimensions for building trust with patients: open communication, professional competency, a friendly practice style, a caring attitude, and emotional equality [28]. A victim of mistreatment can experience dramatic relief when a healthcare professional verbally recognizes an emotional state the patient is in or helps the patient express his or her emotions [28].

Interventions should maximize treatment of underlying conditions, provide community-based services, and appropriately involve family, which may help delay or prevent self-neglect and mistreatment by others [24]. Common forms of intervention programs include advocacy service, support groups care coordination, and public education [24]. Studies have found that interventions that offer combinations of individual or family counseling, case management, skills training, and behavior management strategies are more effective than interventions that only provide a support group [8]. In planning appropriate interventions, it is important to have knowledge of available health and community-based services and an understanding of the strengths and limitations of each service for any specific case [28].

Older adults who have been abused or neglected will be traumatized and should receive interventions to address the psychological distress. Psychiatrists, psychologists, or social workers trained in working with patients with psychological issues, posttraumatic stress disorders, and couples and family counseling should be involved in the treatment plan follow-up care. One other type of intervention is Trauma-Informed Approach. Trauma-Informed Care is an organizational structure and treatment framework that involves understanding, recognizing, and responding to the effects of all types of trauma. Trauma-Informed Care also emphasizes physical, psychological, and emotional safety and helps survivors rebuild a sense of control and empowerment.

According to the Substance Abuse Mental Health Services Association (SAMHSA) "A program, organization, or system that is trauma-informed: (1) *Realizes* the widespread impact of trauma and understands potential paths for recovery; (2) *Recognizes* the signs and symptoms of trauma in clients, families, staff, and others involved with the system; (3) *Responds* by fully integrating knowledge about trauma into policies, procedures, and practices; and (4) Seeks to actively resist *re-traumatization*" [13]. This approach can be adapted for elder mistreatment intervention and can be implemented in any type of service setting or organization.

The Trauma Affect Regulation: Guide for Education and Therapy (TARGET) is a model designed for use by organizations and professionals with a broad range of experience with trauma [13]. TARGET is an educational and therapeutic approach for the prevention and treatment of complex Post Traumatic Stress Disorder. This model provides practical skills that can be used by trauma survivors, such as mistreatment victims to de-escalate and regulate extreme emotions, manage intrusive trauma memories experienced in daily life, and restore the capacity for information processing and memory.

The Trauma Recovery and Empowerment Model (TREM) is intended for trauma survivors, particularly those with exposure to physical or sexual violence. This model is gender-specific: TREM for women and M-TREM for men. This model is appropriate for a full range of disciplines [13].

For victims of mistreatment, empowerment support groups discuss problems, strengths, solutions, and resources to safely maintain independence and protection from unwanted influence and mistreatment [29]. Support groups can be helpful in navigating the health, legal, and social systems and in addressing the victims' own needs and concerns [23].

It is important to understand that an older person with capacity may decline assistance and refuse interventions deemed appropriate by a mistreatment investigation, such as moving to alternative accommodations [7]. People with capacity have the right to make decisions that involve an element of risk. Should the victim refuse services and insist on returning to the situation that had resulted in mistreatment, it is imperative that the team plan to follow up with the patient and continue to establish trust and look for an opportunity to intervene with the patient's consent.

Caregivers who are being abusive or neglectful will also need assistance and ongoing support in order to best help vulnerable elders from being abused or neglected going forward [17]. Caregivers are subject to stress, illness, competing roles with other family concerns and loss of employment when caregiving results in work absences [23]. Often caregivers assume their roles with little preparation and no training for the skills required of them [23].

It is important that practitioners be aware of the extent to which caregivers are willing to collaborate whenever elder abuse or neglect occurs. Some caregivers will be willing to assume responsibility for neglectful or abusive behaviors. When the caregiver is willing to collaborate, he or she should be provided with the support and the resources available to ensure that the behavior will not continue. Resources for caregivers include web sites, support groups, individual counseling by social workers, and nursing personnel from hospital or home agencies [29]. Support groups for caregivers promote an opportunity to discuss circumstances that may lead to mistreatment, such as stress anger, feelings of entrapment, anxiety, sense of disruption in life, and role changes [23]. In addition to ensuring the termination of neglectful or abusive behaviors, practitioners should assist caregivers in addressing the specific issues that have led to elder abuse or neglect, such as financial burden or caregiver's burnout.

Because physical neglect can arise from the caregiver's lack of knowledge, it is essential to assess the caregiver's understanding of the dependent persons' needs and provide training and assistance as appropriate [2]. Opportunities for caregiver counseling and education, as well as changes in the care plan can be presented and explored [2].

The rationale for a collaborative approach with the caregivers relies on the fact that oftentimes caregivers are the only source of emotional, physical, and financial support for the victims.

For those caregivers who refuse to be held accountable for their behaviors, clinicians must recognize the important role that protective services plays in addressing situations of elder abuse and neglect.

11.5 Follow-up Interdisciplinary Care

Follow-up suggests the establishment of an ongoing relationship between victim (and perpetrator) and clinician [2]. A situation of elder mistreatment often requires long-term or intermittent intervention before resolution [2]. A survey of the APS workers who made referrals to the team indicated that the team was helpful in confirming mistreatment, documenting impaired capacity, reviewing medications and medical conditions, facilitating the conservatorship process, persuading the client or family to take action, and supporting the need for law enforcement involvement. Others that have used mixed quantitative and qualitative measures found that an elder mistreatment forensic center team consisting of APS and other community-based workers, medical professionals, and criminal justice professionals (police and district attorney) improved the efficiency and effectiveness of handling suspected elder mistreatment cases. Navarro et al. used a logic model to provide a framework for describing an elder mistreatment forensic center in which teams were rated as highly effective. While interdisciplinary teams may be an example of "action over evidence," the team members' belief that these meetings are highly effective implies the utility of this mechanism for handling elder mistreatment and deserves further study.

11.6 Exemplar of Case of Pressure Ulcers Caused by Drug Addicted Daughter

Mrs. Jones was brought into the emergency room by ambulance. Her neighbor found her on the floor of her apartment semi-conscious and bruised. Upon examination Mrs. Jones was dehydrated, she had bruises on her arms and left cheek, as well as pressure ulcers on her buttocks. She was admitted to the hospital. A social worker met with Mrs. Jones the next day.

During the psychosocial assessment it was discovered that Mrs. Jones was widowed and living on social security and supplemental security income. She barely had enough money to cover the rent for her one bedroom apartment. Mrs. Jones had two children, a son who lived in Atlanta and a daughter who moved in with her a few months ago. Mrs. Jones used to attend a Baptist church around the corner but had not been to a service in a couple months. She did not know how she obtained groceries. Her main source of food was toast with margarine and orange juice. She did not remember when she had her last meal before being admitted to the hospital. Mrs. Jones did not know how to contact her daughter or her son. She gave the social worker her home number. Mrs. Jones also did not know how to contact her neighbor other than going to the apartment down the hall and knocking on the door.

The social worker consulted the attending physician regarding Mrs. Jones injuries and conditions and possible discharge date so that she could develop the discharge plan. The physician stated that he suspected that bruises on Mrs. Jones were caused by punching her on her torso and head and twisting her arms. The physician felt that Mrs. Jones may not be safe in her home and wondered if she had been burglarized and beaten by an intruder. The social worker discussed the causes of the injuries with Mrs. Jones who refused to talk about it but did say that no one had broken into her home. The social worker called the home number several times during the day but did not receive an answer. One evening the social worker worked until 6 and called the home and the daughter answered. When questioning about Mrs. Jones, the daughter's speech was slurred and she became defensive saying that her mother was stingy and would not give the daughter any more money. The social worker called Adult Protective Services the following morning to report that she suspected physical and financial abuse by the daughter.

Mrs. Jones was kept in the hospital for 4 days and then discharged to a nursing home for follow-up care. The social worker started the procedure for applying for Medicaid for Mrs. Jones. It was hoped that Mrs. Jones would be able to return home when she was well and if her home situation was safe.

Adult Protective Services did investigate and found that the daughter was using drugs. The daughter was not cooperative. She refused drug treatment. She remained in the apartment while her mother was in the nursing home, never visiting her mother. The social worker in the nursing home had Mrs. Jones social security and SSI check sent directly into her checking account. Medicaid was obtained. Mrs. Jones remained in the nursing home. She said that she felt better and safer than she had while in her apartment. The social worker contacted the Baptist church where Mrs. Jones had previously attended and the pastor came to visit as did other members of the church including the neighbor that had first found Mrs. Jones on the floor in her apartment. The pastor was trying to locate Mrs. Jones son.

The daughter was evicted from the apartment as she was unable to pay the rent and her name was not on the lease. It was not known what happened to the daughter.

11.7 Summary and Conclusion

There were many opportunities for healthcare professionals to intervene with cases of elder mistreatment throughout the healthcare systems. While data are lacking, it is fair to surmise that maximizing function and linking older adults to rehabilitation, community programs, and/or social services may help prevent worsening self-neglect in the future. The complexities of elder mistreatment require the coordination of medical, social, and legal professionals as well as the broader community to balance the duty to protect and the duty to respect civil liberties. How different subtypes of elder abuse relate to each other is just beginning to be understood. Future longitudinal studies are critically needed to inform future practice and policy to protect this vulnerable population.

References

1. Acierno R, Hernandez MA, Amstadter AB, Resnick HS, Steve K, Muzzy W, Kilpatrick DG. Prevalence and correlates of emotional, physical, sexual, and financial abuse and potential neglect in the United States: The National Elder Mistreatment Study. Am J Public Health. 2010;100(2):292–7. doi:10.2105/AJPH.2009.163089.
2. Anetzberger GJ. Clinical management of elder abuse: General considerations. Clin Gerontol. 2005;28(1–2):27–41.
3. Anetzberger GJ. The clinical management of elder abuse. Abingdon: Routledge; 2012.
4. Beaulieu M, Leclerc N. Ethical and psychosocial issues raised by the practice in cases of mistreatment of older adults. J Gerontol Soc Work. 2006;46(3–4):161–86.
5. Burnett J, Achenbaum WA, Murphy KP. Prevention and Early Identification of Elder Abuse. Clin Geriatr Med. 2014;30(4):743–59.
6. Carr K, Dix G, Fulmer T, et al. An elder abuse assessment team in an acute hospital setting. The Beth Israel Hospital Elder Assessment Team. Gerontologist. 1986;26(2):115–8.
7. Cooper C, Livingston G. Mental Health/Psychiatric Issues in Elder Abuse and Neglect. Med Implic Elder Abuse Negl Issue Clin Geratric Med. 2014;30(4):839–850.
8. Dong X, Chen R, Chang E-S, Simon M. Elder abuse and psychological well-being: A systematic review and implications for research and policy-a mini review. Gerontology. 2013;59(2):132–42.
9. Dong X, Simon MA. Elder self-neglect: Implications for Health Care Professionals. CGS J CME. 2013;3(1):25–28. Retrieved June 16, 2016, from http://www.canadiangeriatrics.ca/default/index.cfm/linkservid/6D29E30B-98E7-31DA-625905BE874BE665/showMeta/0/.
10. Dong X, Simon MA. Vulnerability risk index profile for Elder abuse in a community-dwelling population. J Am Geriatr Soc. 2014;62(1):10–5. doi:10.1111/jgs.12621.
11. Dong XQ. Elder abuse: systematic review and implications for practice. J Am Geriatr Soc. 2015;63(6):1214–38.
12. Du Mont J, Macdonald S, Kosa D, Elliot S, Spencer C, Yaffe M. Development of a comprehensive hospital-based elder abuse intervention: an initial systematic scoping review. PLoS One. 2015;10(5):e0125105. doi:10.1371/journal.pone.0125105.
13. Elliott DE, Bjelajac P, Fallot RD, Markoff LS, Reed BG. Trauma-informed or trauma-denied: principles and implementation of trauma-informed services for women. J Commun Psychol. 2005;33(4):461–77.
14. Fulmer T. Elder abuse and neglect assessment. J Gerontol Nurs. 2003;29(6):4–5.
15. Fulmer T, Birkenhauer D. Elder mistreatment assessment as a part of everyday practice. J Gerontol Nurs. 1992;18(3):42–5.

16. Fulmer T, Guadagno L, Bitondo Dyer C, Connolly MT. Progress in elder abuse screening and assessment instruments. J Am Geriatr Soc. 2004;52(2):297–304.
17. Gibbs LM, Mosqueda L. Medical implications of elder abuse and neglect. Clin Geriatr Med. 2014;30(4):xv–xvi. doi:10.1016/j.cger.2014.08.015.
18. Hoffler EF, Clark EJ, Jackson E, Flynn M, Whitaker TR, Davis K, Zlotnik JL. Social work matters. Washington, DC: NASW Press; 2012.
19. Hooyman N, Kiyak HA. Social gerontology: a multidisciplinary perspective. Boston, MA: Pearson Education Inc; 2011.
20. IOM. Elder Abuse and Its Prevention. Washington: National Academies Press; 2014.
21. JCAHO. Accepted: standards revisions for deemed status hospices. Joint Comm Perspect. 2015;35(6).
22. Jogerst GJ, Daly JM, Brinig MF, Dawson JD, Schmuch GA, Ingram JG. Domestic elder abuse and the law. Am J Public Health. 2003;93(12):2131–2136. Retrieved from 14652346.
23. Medicine IO, Council NR. Elder abuse and its prevention: workshop summary. Washington, DC: The National Academies Press; 2014.
24. Mosqueda L, Dong XQ. Elder Asbuse and Self-neglect:"I Don't Care Anything About Going to the Doctor, to Be Honest…". JAMA. 2011;306(5):532–40.
25. Mosqueda L, Burnight K, Liao S, Kemp B. Advancing the field of elder mistreatment: a new model for integration of social and medical services. Gerontologist. 2004;44(5):703–8.
26. O'Brien JG. Elder abuse and the physician. Mich Med. 1986;85 (11):618–20.
27. O'Brien JG, Riain AN, Collins C, Long V, O'neill D. Elder abuse and neglect: a survey of irish general practitioners. J Elder Abuse Negl. 2014;26(3):291–9. doi:10.1080/08946566.2013.827955.
28. Perel-Levin S. Discussing screening for elder abuse at primary health care level by Silvia Perel-Levin. 2008.
29. Powers JS. Common presentations of elder abuse in health care settings. Clin Geriatr Med. 2014;30(4):729–41. doi:10.1016/j.cger.2014.08.004.
30. Rodriguez MA, Wallace SP, Woolf NH, Mangione CM. Mandatory reporting of elder abuse: between a rock and a hard place. Ann Fam Med. 2006;4(5):403.
31. Straus MA. Measuring intrafamily conflict and violence: The Conflict Tactics (CT) Scale—Form A. J Marriage Fam. 1979;41:75–88.
32. Straus MA, Brown B. Family measurement techniques: the conflict tactic scale. In: Touliatos J, Perlmutter B, editors. Handbook of family measurement techniques. Newbury Park, CA: Sage Publications Inc; 1978. p. 417.
33. Vognar L, Gibbs LM. Care of the victim. Clin Geriatr Med. 2014;30(4):869–80. doi:10.1016/j.cger.2014.08.012.
34. Wallace M, Fulmer T. Try this: best practices in nursing care to older adults. Fulmer SPICES: an overall assessment tool of older adults…reprinted with permission. The John A. Hartford Foundation Institute for Geriatric Nursing, 1(1), August 1998. J Gerontol Nurs. 1998;24(12):3.
35. Wasson JH, Jette AM, Anderson J, Johnson DJ, Nelson EC, Kilo CM. Routine, single-item screening to identify abusive relationships in women. J Fam Pract. 2000;49(11):1017–1022. Retrieved from 20543897.
36. Wiglesworth A, Mosqueda L, Burnight K, Younglove T, Jeske D. Findings from an elder abuse forensic center. Gerontologist. 2006;46(2):277–83.

12 Medical Decision-Making Capacity and Ethical Considerations

Elizabeth J. Santos and Corey Nichols-Hadeed

12.1 Introduction

Every day we bear witness to people making questionable decisions and for most people, these poor decisions result in minimal harm. However, when vulnerable older adults make poor decisions, we cannot help but wonder if we should intervene. We make recommendations, as treatment providers, as social service providers, and as advocates. When an older adult continues to reject our help or continues to make decisions that we believe will result in irreparable harm, we are compelled to intervene. But how can we intervene while still trying to keep an older adult's autonomy intact? To aid a vulnerable older adult who repeatedly makes poor decisions can be a very frustrating and arduous task that may lead one down the road of needing to assess capacity and then possibly pursue guardianship.

The most significant difference between working with abused children and adults is assessment of capacity. By default, children are presumed to lack capacity, whereas adults are presumed to have capacity. This is a very important distinction because the presumed ability of adults to make their own decision limits the interventions those who care for abused older adults can make. Adults with decision-making capacity are allowed to continue to choose to live with their abusers, can decide not to prosecute, and to make any number of bad decisions. This presents roadblocks, barriers, and frustrations for those of us trying to maintain the safety of older adults in our care.

This chapter will focus on medical decision-making capacity, but the assessment of capacity has generally the same guidelines as any other type of decision-making capacity evaluation. We will focus on medical decisions in order to give the reader concrete examples of the dilemmas faced when evaluating capacity, specifically with elderly patients that are victims of abuse. Any consideration of assessment of capacity necessitates that we also consider why we are assessing capacity and if this is an isolated incident regarding lack of capacity or if it will be an ongoing problem? The act of questioning another person's judgment and taking away the right to make decisions should never be made lightly and there are a number of concerns that we must always keep in mind to assure that we are acting in the most ethical manner possible. We will attempt to bring some of those concerns to light throughout this chapter while still focusing on a clinical case to illustrate the main points of discussion.

12.2 Paternalism Evolves to Shared Decision-Making and Patient-Centered Care

Before we can discuss the process of conducting a capacity assessment, we must first acknowledge the clinical, legal, and ethical landscape from which these assessments arise. For over a 100 years (1847 AMA Article II Ethical Code) physicians were trained to treat patients with a paternalistic attitude. The principle of paternalism has been present throughout our history and is still prevalent in many cultures. The practice of paternalism requires that there is someone in a position of authority over another and is embedded into many of our institutions and is antithetical to autonomy of persons [14]. This power and control relationship was the accepted by the medical community, but it is very easy to see how this can become a coercive relationship, especially when a patient has a mental illness or cognitive impairment [10, 23]. The physician ordered and the patient followed without question.

We must also be mindful that in many Asian cultures, paternalism also extends to interactions and decision-making within the family structure. The first-born son is often the main spokesperson and decision maker for the family. For example, 50 years ago, if a 70 year old Chinese-American

E.J. Santos (✉) · C. Nichols-Hadeed
Department of Psychiatry, University of Rochester Medical Center, 300 Crittenden Blvd. Box PSYCH, Rochester, NY 14642, USA
e-mail: Elizabeth_Santos@urmc.rochester.edu

X. Dong (ed.), *Elder Abuse*, DOI 10.1007/978-3-319-47504-2_12

female was diagnosed with cancer, the oncologist would most likely talk with the oldest son as head of the house, explaining diagnosis and treatment to him and expect that all the recommendations would be followed exactly. Today, if that 70 year old Chinese-American female was diagnosed with cancer, the oncologist would expect to have a discussion with the patient to talk about the diagnosis, treatment and her expectations, goals and wishes for treatment. However, the patient's son might intervene in the conversation, pull the oncologist out of the room and ask to speak with the physician alone before she talks with his mother. That son may even tell the physician that she should not tell his mother the diagnosis at all. This is not an uncommon scenario given the concept of filial piety that pits our model of working with the patients against a cultural norm that dictates otherwise [26, 42].

Over the past 20 years, the idea that there should be more of a discussion or dialogue between the patient and physician has gained a foothold in Western medicine and now models of Shared Decision-Making (SDM) and Patient-Centered Care (PCC) have emerged as the prevalent practice, or at least the model we strive to achieve [10, 33]. The premise that patients should be able to have a reasoned discussion to make decisions about their healthcare expands to the idea that all people should be able to make their decisions as a human right. The United Nations Convention on Persons with Disabilities achieved the highest number of signatories on the first day of any UN Convention on March 30, 2007 emphasizing the general acceptance of their guiding principles [43]. The first Guiding Principle of the Convention is "Respect for inherent dignity, individual autonomy including the freedom to make one's own choices, and independence of persons" speaks directly to this assumption. Thus, merely the idea that a clinical assessment or a ruling by a judge can eliminate a person's right to make his or her own decisions is in direct opposition to this presumed human right and is thought to be discrimination against vulnerable people.

In Europe, there is an outcry from many sectors to disengage from substituted or surrogate decision-making models and to change legislation to promote SDM and PCC [28, 34]. However, even with the support of the medical and legal community, there are numerous obstacles to overcome to achieve the goal of SDM and PCC [15, 33]. In the most basic doctor–patient relationship, both parties must desire to communicate and share their points of view and respect each others' experiences and wishes. We often focus on the doctor to facilitate this process, but the patient must also be willing to have a dialogue and express a choice. Even if the patient has the cognitive ability to participate in the process, he or she may be unwilling to disclose personal history. Should we force patients to disclose information that they would rather keep private?

For example, consider the case of a 21 year old female with a suspicious abdominal mass suspected to be ovarian cancer. Her male gynecologic oncologist presents a very conservative approach intended to try to preserve reproductive function because the patient is so young and has not started a family. The patient wants a more aggressive approach insisting that she does not intend to start a family and would like a total hysterectomy and bilateral oophorectomy if there is any possibility of cancer. He thinks that she is being rash and immature whereas she thinks that he is ignoring her wishes. She does not feel comfortable disclosing that she was repeatedly raped when she was young, had become pregnant several times resulting in miscarriages. She will not consider a male partner and does not wish to start a family. Additionally, her grandmother died from ovarian cancer and she recalls her grandmother's suffering. The rapes occurred after her grandmother's death and she always believed that if her grandmother had been alive she would have been protected. Should she be forced to disclose this history of abuse and trauma?

We must also consider that for many medical decisions, there is not one best choice, but rather a multitude of reasonable choices [10]. Consider the decisions about how to treat early stage breast cancer. It is not uncommon that patients and physicians have different opinions regarding preservation of their breasts. A lumpectomy may be the recommended course of action for some, radiation for others, and some may choose a mastectomy for any number of reasons. Many disagreements between physicians and patients necessitate an ongoing dialogue to work through them, but the current system is not equipped to allow the time for this process. Additionally, there will also be urgent decisions to be made that cannot allow for indecisiveness or discussion when only action must be taken to save someone's life where SDM does not have a place. For example, when a severe head injury is sustained after a car accident, there is no time for a dialogue about the decompressive craniectomy that must be performed to decrease the rising intracranial pressure.

Even when there is time to make decisions, people do not always want to make the choices themselves. Many older adults do not make advanced care decisions even when repeatedly presented with choices when they have the capacity to do so [15]. When an older adult no longer is able to communicate a wish, we will still need to act in his best interest. It is a fundamental tension that will likely always exist. This is the ongoing tension that exists between patient autonomy and physician beneficence. As physicians, care providers, and advocates for older adults, we automatically practice beneficence over maleficence. We strive to help the older adult by removing them from dangerous situations and preventing harm. For most of us, it is our duty to protect the older adult. Do we allow vulnerable people to participate in a

SDM model when they are not able or willing to understand the choices or communicate a wish or do we continue to enforce a paternalistic model of care that squashes patient autonomy?

Another important aspect to consider is what happens to the information that we gather in pursuit of the optimal case of SDM and PCC. Let us again ponder the case of the 21 year old female with suspected ovarian cancer. She has now disclosed her trauma history to the gynecologic oncologist who is able to have a more calm-reasoned discussion with her about the treatment options. He writes about their discussions in the medical record, including her history of trauma in an effort to have others be sensitive to her history. Does her ophthalmologist now get to see her entire record? Does he need to know about her history of trauma to do a routine eye examination? Who becomes privy to the information that our patients have disclosed in an effort to work collaboratively with us? We need to be aware of these ethical dilemmas as we push for patient autonomy in a patient-centered model of care.

12.3 Distinction Between Medical and Legal Determinations

Legal determinations concerning "competency" and "capacity" should be distinguished from clinical determinations of capacity. This is a distinction that is difficult to understand on the face of it because most legal statutes in the United States use the term "incapacity" and others use "incompetency" and neither are equivalent to "lacking capacity" as determined by a clinician [9, 16, 22]. A very simplified view is to say that legal "incapacity" or "incompetency" is a more permanent pronouncement whereas "lacking capacity" is usually intended only to encompass a specific decision at one point in time. Table 12.1 from Demakis [16] includes the relevant statutes from each states regarding incapacity or incompetence to make decisions. As one can see from the table, each state has different level of detail and guidance for the judiciary to determine whether or not a person should be deemed unable to make his or her own decisions.

Table 12.2 [16] outlines some relevant distinctions between the state statues regarding terminology. When one is deemed incapacitated by the court, then guardianship or conservatorship is granted and someone other than the older adult is charged with making decisions. These decisions may be limited only to health care decisions or financial, but most often they are both. The judges may take a clinical judgment of "lacking capacity" into consideration when making his or her ruling, but it is not required.

In this chapter, by "capacity," we mean a clinical judgment that can change over time and is specific to a certain decision [22]. One can have full capacity to make all decisions, or diminished capacity with limitations of ability to make certain decisions. In the case of someone who was previously assessed to have diminished capacity in some areas, the question becomes one of *sufficient* capacity to make certain decisions. "The gold standard for capacity assessment is the psychiatric interview" [11]. The medical decision-making capacity determination made by the physician is a cross sectional "snap shot" of the patient's decision-making capacity at that moment in time. Physicians may reevaluate a patient's capacity frequently throughout care.

Although the term "capacity" is used in certain legal contexts, we do not use "capacity" to refer to a legal determination for purposes of this chapter. In the legal sphere, for example, a judge or jury may be called upon to determine whether an individual lacks testamentary "capacity" to enter into a will or is "incapacitated" so as to require the appointment of a guardian or conservator. These legal "incapacity" determinations are made in a court of law, after a hearing or trial, based on evidence, and may be specific or global. By contrast, a physician makes "capacity" determinations in a clinical context, through an evaluation of a patient and determines medical decision-making capacity as to a specific decision at a given point in time. Depending on the physician's assessment, the patient is then deemed to have capacity to make the decision or to lack capacity to make the decision. Despite the different contexts, medical center versus legal setting, there are opportunities for interdisciplinary understanding. The American Bar Association (ABA) and American Psychological Association (APA) have recognized their dual roles and expertise in capacity assessments for older adults. In a collaborative effort they have provided informative handbooks aimed at Psychologists, Lawyer, and Judges. These handbooks and other pertinent information can be found on the APA website, http://www.apa.org/pi/aging/programs/assessment/ [5]. Given the numerous legal considerations involved in health care decision-making, the ABA's Commission on Law and Aging also provides comprehensive links to resources and state-specific guides, http://www.americanbar.org/groups/law_aging/resources/health_care_decision_making.html [3]. Interdisciplinary understanding of the nuances of capacity assessment in older adults has evolved into a distinct field [32]. In this chapter, we are focusing on "capacity" determinations in the clinical context.

Table 12.1 Definitions of incompetency/incapacity in state statutes as of May 24, 2012

State	Statute
Alabama	Incapacitated person. Any person who is impaired by reason of mental illness, mental deficiency, physical illness or disability, physical or mental infirmities accompanying advanced age, chronic use of drugs, chronic intoxication, or other cause (except minority) to the extent of lacking sufficient understanding to make or communicate responsible decisions (Ala. Code 1975 § 26-2A-20 (8))
Alaska	"Incapacitated person" means a person whose ability to receive and evaluate information or to communicate decisions is impaired for reasons other than minority to the extent that the person lacks the ability to provide the essential requirements for the person's physical health or safety without court-ordered assistance; "essential requirements for physical health or safety" means the health care, food, shelter, clothing, personal hygiene, and protection without such serious physical injury or illness is more likely than not to occur (Alaska Stat. § 13.26.005)
Arizona	"Incapacitated person" means an adult for whom a guardian has been appointed. A report filed pursuant to this section by a physician, psychologist or registered nurse acting within the person's scope of proactive shall include the following information: 1. A specific diagnosis of the person. 2. A comprehensive assessment listing any functional impairments of the alleged incapacitated person and an explanation of how and to what extent these functional impairments may prevent that person from receiving or evaluating information in making divisions or in communicating informed decisions regarding that person. 3. An analysis of the tasks of daily living the alleged incapacitate person is capable of performing with direction or with minimal direction (Ariz. Rev. Stat. Ann § 14-12102(7))
Arkansas	"Incapacitated person" means a person who is impaired by reason of a disability such as mental illness, mental deficiency, physical illness, chronic use of drugs, or chronic intoxication, to the extent of lacking sufficient understanding of capacity to make or communicate decisions to meet the essential requirements for his or her health or safety or to manage his or her estate (Ark. Code Ann § 28-65101 5(A))
California	(a) A conservator of the person may be appointed for a person who is unable to provide properly for his or her personal needs for physical health, food, clothing, or shelter, except as provided for the person as described in subdivision (b) or (c) of section 1828.5. (b) A conservator of the estate may be appointed for a person who is substantially unable to manage his or her own financial resources or resist fraud or undue influence, except as provided for that person as described in subdivision (b) or (c) of Section-1828.5. Substantial inability may not be proved solely by isolated incidents of negligence or improvidence (Cal. Prob. § 1801 (a-b))
Colorado	"Incapacitated person" means an individual other than a minor, who is unable to effectively receive or evaluate information or both or make or communicate decisions to such an extent that the individual lacks the ability to satisfy essential requirements for physical health, safety, or self-care, even with appropriate and reasonably available technological assistance (Colo. Rev. Stat. § 15-14-102 (5))
Connecticut	(c) "Incapable of caring for one's self or "incapable of caring for himself or herself means that a person has a mental, emotional or physical condition that results in such person being unable to receive and evaluate information or make or communicate decisions to such an extent that a person is unable, even with appropriate assistance, to meet essential requirements for personal needs. (d) "Incapable of managing his or her affairs" means that a person has a mental, emotional or physical condition that results in such person being unable to receive and evaluate information or make or communicate decisions to such an extent that the person is unable, even with appropriate assistance, to perform the functions inherent in managing his or her affairs, and the person has property that will be wasted or dissipated unless adequate property management is provided, or that funds are needed for the support, care or welfare of the person or those entitled to be supported by the person and that the person is unable to take the necessary steps to obtain or provide funds needed for support, care or welfare of the person or those entitled to be supported by the person (Conn. Gen. Stat. § 45a-644 (c-d))
Delaware	"Person with a disability" means any person who: (1) By reason of being under the age of 18 is legally unable to manage their own property or make decisions concerning the care of their own person; or (2) By reason of mental or physical incapacity is unable properly to manage or care for their own person or property, or both, and, in consequence thereof, is in danger of dissipating or losing such property or of becoming the victim of designing persons or, in the case where a guardian of the person is sought, such person is in danger of substantially endangering person's own health, or of becoming subject to abuse by other persons or of becoming the victim of designing persons; or (3) By reason of § 5703(1) or (2) of Title 16 is deemed legally incapable of giving informed consent to sterilization (Del. Code Annual § 3901)
Florida	"Incapacitated" means a judicial determination that a person lacks the capacity to manage at least some of the person's property or to meet at least some of the person's essential health and safety requirements. A minor shall be treated as being incapacitated (Fla. Stat. Ann. § 731.201 (21))
Georgia	The court may appoint a guardian for an adult only if the court finds that the adult lacks sufficient capacity to make or communicate significant responsible decisions concerning his or her health or safety. (Ga. Code. Ann. § 29-4-1 (a)) "Incapacitated person" means an individual who, for reasons other than being a minor, is unable to receive and evaluate information or make or communicate decisions to such an extent that the individual lacks the ability to meet essential requirements for physical health, safety, or self-care, even with appropriate and reasonably available technological assistance (Haw. Rev. Stat. Ann. § 560:5-102)

(continued)

Table 12.1 (continued)

State	Statute
Hawaii	"Incapacitated person" means an individual who, for reasons other than being a minor, is unable to receive and evaluate information or make or communicate decisions to such an extent that the individual lacks the ability to meet essential requirements for physical health, safety, or self-care, even with appropriate and reasonably available technological assistance (Haw. Rev. Stat. Ann. § 560:5-102)
Idaho	"Incapacitated person" means any person who is impaired, except by minority, to the extent that he lacks sufficient understanding or capacity to make or communicate responsible decisions concerning his person, provided, that the term shall not refer to a developmentally disabled person as defined in section 66-402 (5). (1) "Incapacity" means a legal, not a medical disability and shall be measured by function limitations and it shall be construed to mean or refer to any person who has suffered, is suffering, or is likely to suffer, substantial harm due to an inability to provide for his personal needs for food, clothing, shelter, health care, or safety, or an inability to manage his or her property or financial affairs; (2) Inability to provide for personal needs or to manage property shall be evidenced by acts or occurrences, or statements which strongly indicate imminent acts or occurrences; material evidence of inability must have occurred within twelve (12) months prior to the filing of the petition of guardianship or conservatorship; (3) Isolated instances of simple negligence or improvidence, lack of resources, or any act, occurrence, or statement, if that act, occurrence, or statement is the product of an informed judgment, shall not constitute evidence of inability to provide for personal needs or to manage property; (4) "Informed judgment" means a choice made by a person who has the ability to make such a choice, and who makes it voluntarily after all relevant information necessary to making the decision has been provided, and who understands that he is free to choose or refuse any alternative available and who clearly indicates or expresses the outcome of his choice; (Idaho Code § 15-5-101)
Illinois	At the hearing the court shall inquire regarding: (1) the nature and extent of respondent's general intellectual and physical functioning; (2) the extent of the impairment of his adaptive behavior if he is a person with a developmental disability, or the nature and severity of his mental illness if he is a person with mental illness; (3) the understanding and capacity of the respondent to make and communicate responsible decisions concerning his person; (4) the capacity of the respondent to manage his estate and his financial affairs; (5) the appropriateness of proposed and alternate living arrangements; (6) the impact of the disability upon the respondent's functioning in the basic activities of daily living and the important decisions faced by the respondent or normally faced by adult members of the respondent's community; and (7) any other area (Ill. Comp. Stat. Ann. § 755 11a-11)
Indiana	"Incapacitated person" means an individual who: (1) cannot be located upon reasonable inquiry; (2) is unable: (A) to manage in whole or in part the individual's property; (B) to provide self-care; or (C) both; because of insanity, mental illness, mental deficiency, physical illness, infirmity, habitual drunkenness, excessive use of drugs, incarceration, confinement, detention, duress, fraud, undue influence of others on the individual, or other incapacity; or (3) has a developmental disability (as defined in IC 12-7-2-61) (Ind. Code § 29-3-1-7.5)
Iowa	Incompetent means the condition of any person who has been adjudicated by a court to meet at least one of the following conditions: *a*. To have a decision-making capacity which is so impaired that the person is unable to care for the person's personal safety or to attend to or provide for necessities for the person such as food, shelter, clothing, or medical care, without which physical injury or illness may occur. *b*. To have a decision-making capacity which is so impaired that the person is unable to make, communicate, or carry out important decisions concerning the person's financial affairs. *c*. To have a decision-making capacity that is so impaired that both paragraphs "*a*" and "*b*" are applicable to the person (Iowa Code Ann. § 633.3 23)
Kansas	"Adult with an impairment in need of a guardian or a conservator, or both" means a person 18 years of age or older, or a minor who is considered to be of the age of majority pursuant to K.S.A. 38-101, and amendments thereto, or upon whom the rights of majority have been conferred pursuant to K.S.A. 38108, and amendments thereto, whose ability to receive and evaluate relevant information, or to effectively communicate decisions, or both, even with the use of assistive technologies or other supports, is impaired such that the person lacks the capacity to manage such person's estate, or to meet essential needs for physical health, safety or welfare, and who is in need of a guardian or a conservator, or both. No person who is being treated by prayer in the practice of the religion of any church which teaches reliance on spiritual means alone through prayer for healing shall be determined to be an adult with an impairment in need of a guardian under this act for that reason alone, nor considered to lack the capacity to meet essential needs for physical health, safety, or welfare because of such person's reliance upon such treatment (Kan. Stat. Ann. § 59-3051)
Kentucky	"Adult" means a person eighteen (18) years of age or older who, because of mental or physical dysfunctioning, is unable to manage his or her own resources, carry out the activity of daily living, or protect himself or herself from neglect, exploitation, or a hazardous or abusive situation (Ky. Rev. Stat. § 209.020)
Louisiana	"Adult" means any individual 18 years of age or older, or an emancipated minor who, due to a physical, mental, or developmental disability or the infirmities of aging, is unable to manage his own resources, carry out the activities of daily living, or protect himself from abuse, neglect, or exploitation (Louisiana Rev. Stat. §15: 1503)
Maine	"Incapacitated person" means any person who is impaired by reasons of mental illness, mental deficiency, physical illness or disability, chronic use of drugs, chronic intoxication, or other cause except minority to the extent that he lacks sufficient understanding or capacity to make or communicate responsible decisions concerning his person (Me. Rev. Stat. §5–101-1 (1))

(continued)

Table 12.1 (continued)

State	Statute
Maryland	Disabled persons–A guardian shall be appointed if the court determines that: (1) The person is unable to manage his property and affairs effectively because of physical or mental disability, disease, habitual drunkenness, addiction to drugs, imprisonment, compulsory hospitalization, confinement, detention by foreign power, or disappearance; and (2) The person has or may be entitled to property or benefits which require proper management (Md. Code Ann. § 13-201 (c))
Massachusetts	"Incapacitated person," an individual who for reasons other than advanced age or minority, has a clinically diagnosed condition that results in an inability to receive and evaluate information or make or communicate decisions to such an extent that the individual lacks the ability to meet essential requirements for physical health, safety, or self-care, even with appropriate technological assistance (Mass. Gen. Laws Ann. § 5-101 (9))
Michigan	"Incapacitated individual" means an individual who is impaired by reason of mental illness, mental deficiency, physical illness or disability, chronic use of drugs, chronic intoxication, or other cause, not including minority, to the extent of lacking sufficient understanding or capacity to make or communicate informed decisions (Mich. Stat. § 700.1105 (a))
Minnesota	"Incapacitated person" means an individuals who, for reasons other than being a minor, is impaired to the extent of lacking sufficient understanding or capacity to make or communicate responsible personal decisions, and who has demonstrated deficits in behavior which evidence an inability to meet personal needs for medical care, nutrition, clothing, shelter, or safety, even with appropriate technological assistance (Minn. Stat. Ann. § 524.5-102-Subd 6)
Mississippi	The chancery court of any county in which may be situated the property or any part thereof, or debt due to, or right of action of any citizens of this state who have not been adjudged to be of unsound mind, or may have been so adjudged in proceedings which did not fully comply with the law in effect at the time of such adjudication, may appoint guardians of the estates of such persons, provided such persons: (1) have been continuously confined in a mental hospital operated by the State of Mississippi or by the United States government within the State of Mississippi for a period of more than 1 year and are still so confined, (2) are of unsound mind, (3) are mentally incapable of taking care of their estates, and (4) are incapable of responding to process (Miss. Code SEC § 93-13-125)
Missouri	"Incapacitated person," one who is unable by reason of any physical or mental condition to receive and evaluate information or to communicate decisions to such an extent that he or she lacks capacity to meet essential requirements for food, clothing, shelter, safety or other care such that serous physical injury, illness, or disease is likely to occur. The term "incapacitated person" as used in this chapter includes the term partially incapacitated person unless otherwise specified or apparent from the context; 475.011. Nothing in this chapter shall be construed to constitute evidence of incapacity or partial incapacity of a person solely because such person refuses medical treatment upon the grounds that such person has consistently relied on prayer for healing in accordance with the religion of any church which teaches reliance on spiritual means for healing (Mo. Ann. Stat. § 475.010)
Montana	"Incapacitated person" means any person who is impaired by reason of mental illness, mental deficiency, physical illness or disability, chronic use of drugs, chronic intoxication, or other cause (except minority) to me extent that he lacks sufficient understanding or capacity to make or communicate responsible decisions concerning his person or which cause has so impaired the person's judgment that he is incapable of realizing and making a rational decision with respect to his need for treatment (Mont. Code Ann. § 72-5-101 (1))
Nebraska	Incapacitated person means any person who is impaired by reason of mental illness, mental deficiency, physical illness or disability, chronic use of drugs, chronic intoxication, or other cause (except minority) to the extent that the person lacks sufficient understanding or capacity to make or communicate responsible decisions concerning himself or herself; (Neb. Rev. Stat. § 30-2601 (1))
Nevada	"Incompetent" means an adult person who, by reason of mental illness, mental deficiency, disease, weakness of mind or any other cause, is unable, without assistance, properly to manage and take care of himself or herself or his or her property, or both. The term includes a person who is mentally incapacitated (Nev. Rev. Stat.§ 159.019)
New Hampshire	"Incapacity" means a legal, not a medical, disability and shall be measured by functional limitations. It shall be measured by functional limitations. It shall be construed to mean or refer to any person who has suffered, is suffering or is likely to suffer substantial harm due to an inability to provide for his personal needs for food, clothing, shelter, health care, or safety or inability to manage his or her property or financial affairs. Inability to provide for personal needs or to manage property shall be evidenced by acts or occurrences, or statements which strongly indicate imminent acts or occurrences. All evidence of inability must have occurred within 6 months prior to the filing of the petition and at least one incidence of such behavior must have occurred within 20 days of the filing of the petition for guardianship. Isolated instances of simple negligence or improvidence, lack of resources or any act, occurrence or statement if that act, occurrence or statement is the product of an informed judgment shall not constitute evidence of inability to provide for personal needs or to manage property (N.H. Rev. Stat. Ann. § 464-A: 2 XI)
New Jersey	"Incapacitated individual" means an individual who is impaired by reason of mental illness or mental deficiency to the extent that he lacks sufficient capacity to govern himself and manage his affairs. The term incapacitated individual is also used to designate an individual who is impaired by reason of physical illness or disability, chronic use of drugs, chronic alcoholism, or other cause (except minority) to the extent that he lacks sufficient capacity to govern himself and manage his affairs (N. J. Permanent Stat. § 3B: 1-2)

(continued)

Table 12.1 (continued)

State	Statute
New Mexico	F. "Incapacitated person" means any person who demonstrates over time either partial or complete functional impairment by reason of mental illness, mental deficiency, physical illness or disability, chronic use of drugs, chronic intoxication or other cause, except minority, to the extent that the person is unable to manage the person's personal affairs or the person is unable to manage the person's estate or financial affairs or both; G. "inability to manage the person's personal care" means the inability, as evidenced by recent behavior, to meet one's needs for medical care, nutrition, clothing, shelter, hygiene or safety so that physical injury, illness or disease has occurred or is likely to occur in the near future; H. "inability to manage the person's estate or financial affairs or both" means gross mismanagement, as evidenced by recent behavior, of one's income and resources or medical inability to manage one's income and resources that has led or is likely in the near future to lead to financial vulnerability; (N.M. Stat. ann. § 45-5-101 F-H)
New York	The determination of incapacity shall be based on clear and convincing evidence and shall consist of a determination that a person is likely to suffer harm because: 1. the person is unable to provide for personal needs and/or property management; and 2. the person cannot adequately understand and appreciate the nature and consequences of such inability. (c) In reaching its determination, the court shall give primary consideration to the functional level and functional limitations of the person. Such consideration shall include an assessment of that person's: 1. management of the activities of daily living, as defined in subdivision (h) of section 81.03 of this article; 2. Understanding and appreciation of the nature and consequences of any inability to manage the activities of daily living; 3. Preferences, wishes, and values with regard to managing the activities of daily living; and 4. The nature and extent of the person's property and financial affairs and his or her ability to manage them. It shall also include an assessment of (i) the extent of demands placed on the person by that person's personal needs and by the nature and extent of that person's property and financial affairs; (ii) any physical illness and the prognosis of such illness; (iii) any mental disability, as that term is defined in section 1.03 of this chapter, alcoholism or substance dependence as those terms are defined in section 19.03 of this chapter, and the prognosis of such disability, alcoholism, or substance dependence; and (iv) any medications with which the person is being treated and their effect on the person's behavior, cognition and judgment. (d) In addition, the court shall consider all other relevant facts and circumstances regarding the person's: 1. functional level; and 2. understanding and appreciation of the nature and consequences of his or her functional limitations (New York Code § 81.02 2b)
North Carolina	"Incompetent adult" means an adult or emancipated minor who lacks sufficient capacity to manage the adult's own affairs or to make or communicate important decisions concerning the adult's person, family, or property whether the lack of capacity is due to mental illness, mental retardation, epilepsy, cerebral palsy, autism, inebriety, senility, disease, injury, or similar cause or condition (N.C. Gen. Stat § 35A-1101 (7))
North Dakota	"Incapacitated person" means any adult person who is impaired by reason of mental illness, mental deficiency, physical illness or disability, or chemical dependency to the extent that the person lacks capacity to make or communicate responsibility decisions concerning that person's matters or residence, education, medical treatment, legal affairs, vocation, finance, or other matters, of which incapacity endangers the person's health or safety (N.D. Cent. Code § 30 1-26-01 (5-101))
Ohio	"Incompetent" means any person who is so mentally impaired as a result of mental or physical illness or disability, or mental retardation, or as a result of chronic substance abuse, that the person is incapable of taking proper care of the person's self or property or fails to provide for the person's family or other persons for whom the person is charged by law to provide, or any person confined to a correctional institution within this state (Ohio Rev. Code Ann. § 2111.01 (D))
Oklahoma	"Incapacitated person" means a person eighteen (18) years of age or older who is impaired by reason of: (1) mental illness as defined by section 1-103 of Title 43A of the Oklahoma Statues, (2) mental retardation or developmental disability as defined by section 1-818.2 of Title 63 of the Oklahoma Statutes, (3) physical illness or disability, (4) drug or alcohol dependency as defined by section 3-403 of Title 43A of the Oklahoma Statutes, or (5) such other similar cause, and b. whose ability to receive and evaluate information effectively or to make and to communicate responsible decisions is impaired to such an extent that said person: (1) lacks the capacity to meed essential requirements for his physical health or safety, or (2) is unable to manage his financial resources. Whenever in the Oklahoma Statues the term "incompetent person" appears and refers to a person who has been found by a district court to be an incompetent person because of an impairment or condition described in this paragraph it shall have the same meaning as "incapacitated person" but shall not include a person who is a partially incapacitated person; (Okla. Stat. Ann. § 30-1-111 12)
Oregon	"Incapacitated person" means a person eighteen (18) years of age or older who is impaired by reason of: (1) mental illness as defined by section 1-103 of Title 43A of the Oklahoma Statues, (2) mental retardation or developmental disability as defined by section 1-818.2 of Title 63 of the Oklahoma Statutes, (3) physical illness or disability, (4) drug or alcohol dependency as defined by section 3-403 of Title 43A of the Oklahoma Statutes, or (5) such other similar cause, and b. whose ability to receive and evaluate information effectively or to make and to communicate responsible decisions is impaired to such an extent that said person: (1) lacks the capacity to meed essential requirements for his physical health or safety, or (2) is unable to manage his financial resources. Whenever in the Oklahoma Statues the term "incompetent person" appears and refers to a person who has been found by a district court to be an incompetent person because of an impairment or condition described in this paragraph it shall have the same meaning as "incapacitated person" but shall not include a person who is a partially incapacitated person; (Okla. Stat. Ann. § 30-1-111 12)

(continued)

Table 12.1 (continued)

State	Statute
Pennsylvania	"Incapacitated person" means any adult whose ability to receive and evaluate information effectively and communicate decisions in any way is impaired to such a significant extent that he is partially or totally unable to manage his financial resources or to meet essential requirements for his physical health and safety (Pa. Cons. Stat. § 5512.1 (a))
Rhode Island	If, in any such action, the defendant is an infant, of unsound mind or otherwise incapacitated to take care of his or her right and estate, the court before which such action shall be pending shall appoint some discreet and disinterested person as guardian to defend the infant, person of unsound mind, or person otherwise incapacitated, against the action, and in case of judgment for partition, to attend to the partition to be made, and take charge of the interest of the person for whom he or she is appointed guardian (33-15-11). Elsewhere, the statute notes: The court shall authorize the guardian to make decisions for the individual in only those areas where the court finds, based on one or more decision-making assessment tools, that the individual lacks the capacity to make decisions (33-14-4) (R.I. Gen. Laws §§ 34-15-4 to 11)
South Carolina	"Incapacitated person" means any person who is impaired by reason of mental illness, mental deficiency, physical illness or disability, advanced age, chronic use of drugs, chronic intoxication, or other cause (except minority) to the extent that he lacks sufficient understanding or capacity to make or communicate responsible decisions concerning his person or property; (S.C. Code Ann. § 62-5-101 (1))
South Dakota	"Protected person," any individual for whom a guardian or conservator has been appointed other than for reasons of minority. Appointment of guardian where capacity lacking to meet requirements for health, care, safety, habilitation, or therapeutic needs. A guardian may be appointed for an individual whose ability to respond to people, events, and environments is impaired to such an extent that the individual lacks the capacity to meet the essential requirements for his health, care, safety, habilitation, or therapeutic needs without the assistance of protection of a guardian. A guardian for a minor may be appointed under this part if the minor meets the requirements of this section without regard to age and the minor's need for guardianship will likely continue into his adult years. 29A-5-303. Persons for whom conservator may be appointed. A conservator may be appointed for an individual whose ability to respond to people, events and environments is impaired to such an extent that the individual lacks the capacity to manage property or financial affairs or to provide for his support or the support of legal dependents without the assistance or protection of a conservator. A conservator may be appointed for an absentee whose estate or financial affairs require the attention, supervision and care of a conservator. A conservator for a minor may be appointed under this part if the minor meets the requirements of this section without regard to age and the minor's need for conservatorship will likely continue into his adult years (S.D. Codified Laws § 29A-5-102 (10))
Tennessee	"Disabled person" means any person eighteen (18) years of age or older determined by the court to be in need of partial or full supervision, protection and assistance by reason of mental illness, physical illness or injury, developmental disability or other mental or physical incapacity; (Tenn. Code Ann. § 34-1101(7))
Texas	"Incapacitated person" means: (A) a minor; (B) an adult individual who, because of a physical or mental condition, is substantially unable to provide food, clothing, or shelter for himself or herself, to care for the individual's own physical health, or to manage the individual's own financial affairs; or (C) a person who must have a guardian appointed to receive funds due to the person from any governmental source (Texas Stat. Ch. § XIII (14) Sec. 601)
Utah	"Incapacitated person" means any person who is impaired by reason of mental illness, mental deficiency, physical illness or disability, chronic use of drugs, chronic intoxication, or other cause, except minority, to the extent of lacking sufficient understanding or capacity to make or communicate responsible decisions (Utah Code Ann. § 75-1-201 (22))
Vermont	(1) "Person in need of guardianship" means a person who: (A) is at least 18 years of age; and (B) is unable to manage, without the supervision of a guardian, some or all aspects of his or her personal or financial affairs as a result of: (i) significantly subaverage intellectual functioning which exists concurrently with deficits in adaptive behavior; or (ii) a physical or mental condition that results in significantly impaired cognitive functioning which grossly impairs judgment, behavior, or the capacity to recognize reality. (2) "Unable to manage his or her personal care" means the inability, as evidenced by recent behavior, to meet one's needs for medical care, nutrition, clothing, shelter, hygiene, or safety so that physical injury, illness, or disease has occurred or is likely to occur in the near future. (3) "Unable to manage his or he financial affairs" means gross mismanagement, as evidenced by recent behavior, of one's income and resources which has led or is likely in the near future to lead to financial vulnerability (Vt. Stat. Ann. 14 § 3061 (1))
Virginia	"Incapacitated person" means an adult who has been found by a court to be incapable of receiving and evaluating information effectively or responding to people, events, or environments to such an extent that the individual lacks. Definitions. The capacity to (i) meet the essential requirements for his health, care, safety, or therapeutic needs without the assistance or protection of a guardian or (ii) manage property or financial affairs or provide for his support or for the support of his legal dependents without the assistance or protection of a conservator. A finding that the individual displays poor judgment alone shall not be considered sufficient evidence that the individual is an incapacitated person within the meaning of this definition. A finding that a person is incapacitated shall be construed as a finding that the person is "mentally incompetent" as that term is used in Article II, section 1 of the Constitution of Virginia and Title 24.2 unless the court order entered pursuant to this chapter specifically provides otherwise (Va. Code Ann. § 37.2-1000)

(continued)

Table 12.1 (continued)

State	Statute
Washington	(a) For purposes of this chapter, a person may be deemed incapacitated as to person when the superior court determines the individual has a significant risk of personal harm based upon a demonstrated inability to adequately provide for nutrition, health, housing, or physical safety, (b) For purposes of this chapter, a person may be deemed incapacitated as to the person's estate when the superior court determines the individual is at significant risk of financial harm based upon a demonstrated inability to adequately manage property or financial affairs. (c) A determination of incapacity is a legal not a medical decision, based upon a demonstration of management insufficiencies over time in the area of person or estate. Age, eccentricity, poverty, or medical diagnosis alone shall not be sufficient to justify a finding of incapacity. (d) a person may also determined incapacitated if he or she is under the age of majority as defined in RCW 26.28.010. (e) For purposes of giving informed consent for health care pursuant to RCW 7.70.050 and 7.70.065, an "incompetent" person is any person who is (i) incompetent by reason of mental illness, developmental disability, senility, habitual drunkenness, excessive use of drugs, or other mental incapacity, of either managing his or her property or caring for himself or herself, or both, or (ii) incapacitated as defined in (a), (b), or (d) of this subsection. (f) For purposes of the terms "incompetent," "disabled," or "not legally competent," as those terms are used in the Revised Code of Washington to apply to persons incapacitated under this chapter; those terms shall be interpreted to mean "incapacitated" persons for purposes of this chapter (Wash. Rev. Code Ann. § 11.88.010(a))
West Virginia	"Protected person" means any adult individual, eighteen years of age or older, who has been found by a court, because of mental impairment, to be unable to receive and evaluate information effectively or to respond to people, events, and environments to such an extent that the individual lacks the capacity: (A) To meet the essential requirements for his or her health, care, safety, habilitation, or therapeutic needs without the assistance or protection of a guardian; or (B) to manage property or financial affairs or to provide for his or her support or for the support of legal dependents without the assistance or protection of a conservator. A finding that the individual displays poor judgment, alone, is not sufficient evidence that the individual is a protected person within the meaning of this subsection (W. Va. Code § 44A-1-1 (13))
Wisconsin	(3)(a) A court may appoint a guardian of the person or a guardian of the estate, or both, for an individual based on a finding that the individual is in competent only if the court finds by clear and convincing evidence that all of the following are true: 1. The individual is aged at least 17 year and 9 months. 2. For purposes of appointment of a guardian of the person, because of impairment, the individual is unable effectively to receive and evaluate information or to make or communicate decisions to such an extent that the individual is unable to meet the essential requirements for his or her physical health and safety. 3. For purposes of appointment of a guardian of the estate, because of an impairment, the individual is unable effectively to receive and evaluate information or to make or communicate decisions relate to management of his or her property or financial affairs, to the extent that any of the following applies: The individual has property that will be dissipated in whole or in part. b. The individual is unable to provide for his or her support. c. The individual is unable to prevent financial exploitation (Wisc. Stat. Ann. § 54.10 3(a))
Wyoming	"Incompetent person" means an individual who, for reasons other than being a minor, is unable unassisted to properly manage and take care of himself or his property as a result of the medical conditions of advanced age, physical disability, disease, the use of alcohol or controlled substances, mental illness, mental deficiency or intellectual disability (Wy. Stat. § 3-1-101 (ix))

12.4 Physician Assessment of Capacity: Informed Consent and Ethical Considerations

As previously noted, adults are assumed to have capacity and one's capacity is not questioned until he/she makes an important decision that someone does not agree with. Every day, physicians determine patients' capacities to make decisions even when they do not think they are assessing capacity. When a physician asks a patient to agree to any treatment, the physician is making a judgment about the patient's capacity to make the decision—to agree to the treatment or refuse it. The understanding between the patient and physician is solidified through the informed consent process.

Informed consent is based on the ethical principals of autonomy and non-maleficence. The United States identified the following key ethical principals for informed consent of human research subjects in the Belmont report: respect for persons, beneficence, and justice [44]. When assessing decision-making capacity, the physician must be cognizant of the older adult patient's ability to make decisions for themselves but also recognize that certain characteristics of the older adult may make them vulnerable to harm. Does the older adult patient understand the risks and benefits and how they might impact overall health? Do they have the cognitive ability to analyze risk versus benefit? Does the patient appreciate that the concept of non-maleficence and the possibility of a double effect, weighing the risk of a good outcome versus a poor outcome? All these ethical considerations are paramount to obtaining informed consent for any patient or research subject and are particularly important to consider when capacity is in question.

There are a few common scenarios that call into question a patient's medical decision-making capacity

Table 12.2 Characteristics of state incompetency/incapacity statutes

Characteristic	n	States
Terminology		
Incapacitated	28	AL, AK, AZ, AR, CO, FL, HI, ID, ME, MA, MI, MN, MO
		MT, NE, NH, NJ, NM, NY, ND, OR, PA, RI, SC, TX, UT, VA
Incompetent	6	IA, NV, NC, OH, WI, WY
Other	16	CA, CT, DE, GA, IL,” KS, KY, LA, MD, MS, OK, [b] SD, TN, VT
		WA, WV
Characteristics of statute		
Estate [c] and other capacities together	20	AR, FL, ID, DE, KS, KY, LA, MD, NC, NV, NH, NJ, NY, ND, OH, PA, RI, SC, TX, WY
Estate and other capacities separated	14	CA, CT, IL, IN, IA, MS, [d] NM, OK, SD, VT, VA, WA, WV, WI
No explicit mention of estate	16	AL, AK, AZ, CO, GA, HI, ME, MA, MI, MN, MO, MT, NE, OR, TN, UT
Activities of daily living [e]	14	CA, FL, IN, KY, LA, MD, NV, NH, NK, NM, OH, TX, WA, WY
Communication/decision-making	7	AL, ME, MI, MT, NE, SC, UT
Both of the above	28	AZ, AK, AR, CO, CT, DE, GA, HI, ID, IL, IA, KS, MA, MN, MS, MO, NY, NC, ND, OK, OR, PA, RI, SD, VT, VA, WV, WI
Mention of undue influence or exploitation	7	CA, DE, IN, KY, LA, VT, [f] WI
Mention of technological assistance	6	CO, CT, HI, KS, MA, MN
Mention of isolated incidents or isolated negligence	3	CA, ID, NH
Mention of religious exemption	2	KS, MO

(1) When a patient refuses treatment, his/her capacity is not usually called into question unless the patient refuses and the physician thinks that the refusal of treatment is dangerous.
(2) When a patient seems to be confused, disoriented, and possibly is having fluctuations in consciousness.
(3) When the patient has known intellectual disability, the physician may not trust that the patient is able to understand the choices.
(4) When the patient has a mental illness that the physician thinks may be influencing the patient's refusal of treatment (e.g., a depressed patient refusing a life-saving procedure may be interpreted as a death wish/suicide).

The American Medical Association recognizes appropriate informed consent as both an ethical and legal issue [4]. Each state has specific informed consent requirements but there is a national expectation as well. The informed consent process is not adequate unless all pertinent medical information is disclosed and understood by the patient [4]. There are many challenges to effective informed consent, one of which is ensuring that steps were taken to deliver the information in a way best suited for the individual patient's comprehension [35]. The ultimate goal for informed consent is giving patients all the information needed to have autonomy over their health care [1].

There are certain situations where informed consent can be bypassed:

1. Emergency Treatment.
2. Therapeutic Privilege.
3. Patient waives the right to information (doesn't want to know).

There are several standard elements of a capacity assessment. Some institutions may utilize a standardized form for physician guidance, containing questions such as:

1. Does the patient express a preference/choice?
2. Is the patient able to attain a factual understanding of the relevant information provided?
3. Is the patient able to appreciate risks and benefits, and consequences of accepting or rejecting treatment?
4. Is the patient demonstrating rational thinking and logical decision-making?

Satisfying these elements of a capacity assessment is particularly relevant with patients that are critically ill and/or elderly. There is a large range of medical illnesses that impact capacity; it is not an issue limited to psychiatric illness [39]. Researchers have noted that over 50 % of patients admitted to general medical units had measureable indications of impairment [38]. Elderly patients referred to Adult Protective Services (APS) were found to be at an increased risk for diminished capacity when compared to a similar cohort of geriatric patients in an outpatient psychiatry clinic [40]. It is accepted that dementia and depression are independent risk factors for impaired executive function and are common among victims of abuse [24]. As noted by those who work with victims of abuse, "loss of executive function can prevent elders from seeking medical care or extracting themselves from an abusive or exploitive situation" [11].

12.5 A Case Study: Mrs. Smith

The case study of Mrs. Smith will be used throughout this chapter to illustrate the principles of medical decision-making capacity assessments in several common scenarios. This case is an amalgamation of many cases we have seen throughout the years and is not a description of one particular case. The case will evolve as a typical case would with discovery of information along the way.

Mrs. Smith is an 82 y/o female who lives with her 55 y/o son, Jake, and occasionally with her 25 y/o grandson, Billy. The patient has been to the hospital six times in the past 6 months with various fractures and syncopal episodes where she was hyperglycemic and/or hypertensive. During one of the emergency department (ED) presentations, adult protective services (APS) was called due to large bruises in various stages of healing on her upper right arm and lower back [45]. The Saturday night ED resident called APS recognizing that her injuries were suspicious. Unfortunately, when APS returned the call, it was several shifts later, the ED resident was not there, no one knew why APS was called and the patient was already discharged so no follow-up occurred. When the patient returned to the ED 5 days after the last visit, the patient was placed in observation as her condition had deteriorated. Her grandson showed up to the ED observation unit at 2 am. Staff heard him yelling at his grandmother, demanding to know where her purse was. When she was unable to answer him, he grabbed her arms. At this point, staff tried to intervene and he was very belligerent. Security was called and he was escorted out of the hospital. Staff members believe that he was intoxicated by drugs or alcohol.

Mrs. Peggy Smith went in and out of consciousness. She was admitted to the hospital for treatment of an infected right toe with osteomyelitis. The social worker on the unit was told about her grandson's visit to the observation unit. She called the number listed on the patient's record many times, but could not reach anyone. The patient became more ill and was very quiet until someone provided hands-on care and then she tried to swat him or her away. The surgeons determined that the osteomyelitis extended up her leg and she needed a below the knee amputation, but the patient refused. The treatment team called for a psychiatry consultant to determine her capacity to refuse treatment.

During the psychiatrist's capacity evaluation, the patient had trouble staying awake and maintaining attention. The psychiatrist had the surgery resident explain why she needed the amputation and the steps involved in the surgery and recovery process while she observed the interaction. The psychiatrist asked questions of the surgery resident in the patient's presence to simplify the language that the resident used. The patient had graduated from high school and had some experience in a business secretarial program, but had no medical training. The medical language was simplified to a 6th grade reading level, a reading level commonly recommended by institutional review boards. The psychiatrist also emphasized the need to slow down when explaining the procedure and give the patient time to process the information. Despite the simplification, the repetition of the information and the calm and unhurried manner in which they tried to discuss the reasoning for the surgery and necessary steps, the patient could not even repeat the information to them. She did make a choice in that she adamantly said, "No! Don't touch me!" However, she could not demonstrate a factual understanding of the relevant information. She also was not able to even repeat the basic steps of the amputation nor could she explain her refusal. She denied any problems with her mood. Initially, she was very pleasant speaking with them, but as they began to question her, she became very irritable. She denied any suicidal ideation or death wish and did not correlate her refusal of the surgery with a life threatening infection. Since the only positive element of capacity that she met was expressing a choice, she was determined to lack capacity to refuse the operation.

After the patient was determined to lack capacity, her son, Jake, showed up at the hospital in the late evening. He claimed to be her health care proxy (HCP) and that he did not want her to have surgery. He did not have any paperwork saying that he was her HCP. The staff observed Jake's interactions with Mrs. Smith—he was very rough with her and looked for her things in her room. He demanded his mother's personal belongings from the staff and was informed that her wallet and jewelry (wedding band) were sent to security. Staff was very suspicious of his intentions and called the resident on duty who came to speak with Jake about the need for the amputation. Jake refused to listen and stormed out of the hospital when the staff did not get his mother's things from security. The attending physician called the ethics committee because the patient's condition was rapidly deteriorating.

12.6 The Role of the Ethics Committee

Medical professionals, advocates, and others working with elderly victims of abuse may turn to ethics committees to give opinions on matters of capacity. In 1992, the Joint Commission for Accreditation of Healthcare Organizations (JCAHO) mandated that hospitals develop a process to address ethical issues arising from patient care. This sparked the formation of ethics committees, which continue to evolve and develop to date [12]. Despite a lack of standardization across hospitals, three "core competencies" of ethics committees have been identified: 1. Skills (ethical assessment, process, interpersonal), 2. Knowledge and 3. Good character [8]. A state by state and international review of Healthcare Ethics Committees explored the evolution of these committees and identified eight key areas: existence and availability, membership and composition, operating procedures, advisory roles, decision-making and gate keeping roles, confidentiality, immunity, and litigation and court cases [36]. Through historical exploration of these eight key areas, it becomes clear that ethics committees are an effective resource for those professional dealing with issues around capacity in elderly patients [36].

12.7 Return to Case Study: Ethics Committee Intervention

At the hospital, the attending physician contacted the ethics committee for an urgent consultation for guidance regarding treatment of the patient's osteomyelitis and sepsis. A member of the ethics committee discussed the case with the treatment team, reviewed the electronic medical record, and interviewed members of the staff and met with the patient. The committee member's interaction with the patient is similar to the psychiatrist's. The ethics committee member attempted several times to call the patient's family, calling all numbers listed in the chart, but could not reach anyone. The ethics committee convened with the patient's attending physician present and reviewed the information presented by the committee member.

The ethics committee determined that in the best interest of the patient, since she was determined to lack capacity and there is no evidence that the patient's son was her HCP and he cannot be reached, the surgery proceed. The patient underwent a right below the knee amputation. Jake and Billy came to the hospital as she is returned from surgery, caused a big commotion and security escorted them from the hospital. As the patient recovered and became more lucid, the social workers found out more about her life.

12.8 A History of Abuse

Peggy was married when she was 21 years old and was working as a secretary. Her husband, Ray was 35 years old and he was very possessive. She went to work for him. She had a series of miscarriages, probably due to being beaten by her husband when she was pregnant. During the first pregnancy, he punched her in the abdomen. During another pregnancy, he pushed her down the stairs. He was a prominent businessman in the community, but he was an abusive alcoholic. He kept her isolated from her family by either keeping her at work or home. He had convinced her that "he was the best she was ever going to get" and reminded her of that constantly. At 27 y/o, she finally had their son, Raymond Jacob Jr. (Jake) who was a difficult child. Jake and his father fought, but as the only son he was brought into the business. Eventually, the alcohol took its toll on Ray and he died 20 years ago. Jake inherited the business, but ran it into the ground. He spent more time getting high and drunk than he did at work. He lost his home, was in rehab five times and moved in with his mother after the last rehab stint 4 years ago. He was doing well with only short periods of relapse until he relapsed last year and had not yet gone into recovery. Jake's son, Billy, was also a troubled soul. Billy was the product of a one-night stand who looked like a younger and meaner version of Jake. He lived with his mother until she died when he was 15 years old of a heroin overdose. After that, he lived in a series of group homes, detention centers, and jails until he moved in with Jake when Jake was feeling generous during a period of sobriety and 12 step programs. As they each relapsed, their relationship became more chaotic and Billy intermittently moved in with Peggy. After Jake moved in with Peggy when he lost his house, Billy stayed with her more often. Jake and Billy were sometimes helpful to have around the house, shoveling the driveway in the winter and going to the grocery store, but they often helped themselves to her things, including her wallet. The police were called to the house on several occasions when arguments between Jake and Billy turned into brawls, with Peggy getting hurt a few times as she tried to intervene. But she was getting more physically frail and did not recover as well from each injury. This past year had been the worst yet. Both Jake and Billy had relapsed and had become more intimidating and demanding than ever before. Jake used the money reserved for her diabetes medication and Billy used the grocery money to party.

12.9 Return to Case Study: After the Surgery

Peggy became stronger and was able to start participating in rehabilitation at the hospital. Staff voiced some concerns about her memory because she repeatedly asked them the same questions. However, she was very pleasant and cooperative and since she did not have any odd or troublesome behaviors, no one pursued any formal cognitive testing. The physicians wanted her to be transferred to a skilled nursing facility for rehabilitation, but they were worried that because she was determined to lack capacity for the surgery, that she also lacked capacity to make any decisions. Additionally, the years of poor control of her diabetes led to chronic renal failure that now required dialysis which was being given in the hospital. The patient was agreeable to both transfer to a nursing home and continued dialysis, so the physicians did not ask for another capacity evaluation to determine if she had capacity to make those decisions.

Capacity evaluations are usually only requested if someone disagrees with the decision(s) that the older adult is making. When older adults are cooperative, we want to believe that they are making those decisions because they are being thoughtful rather than just compliant.

She was agreeable to transfer to a short-term rehabilitation center at a skilled nursing facility. At the rehabilitation center, her son visited her. He presented himself as very repentant. While she was in the hospital, he was admitted to a detoxification center and started outpatient chemical dependency treatment. Their interaction was strained and staff intervened when they saw Peggy crying and they asked Jake to leave. Peggy said that he had tried to get her to sign something, but she refused and he became angry. Over the next few weeks, the patient became more withdrawn, started staying in bed, refused to participate in physical therapy and intermittently refused to go to dialysis. Her physician asked for another medical capacity evaluation with consideration of pursuing guardianship through legal mechanisms.

12.10 Guardianship Law

Each state has its own specific guardianship or conservatorship laws (see Table 12.1). For example, under New York Mental Hygiene Law Article 81, a court may appoint a guardian for an individual if the court determines that the person is legally "incapacitated." For purposes of article 81, incapacitated means that the person is likely to suffer harm because he or she (1) is "unable to provide for personal needs and/or property management" and (2) is unable to "adequately understand and appreciate the nature and consequences of such inability" (MHL 81.02 [2] [b]; *see* N.Y. Pattern Jury Instr.-Civil 8:1, 2014). Although each state has its own guardianship laws, three Federally derived pieces of legislation influence the state-specific law: the Uniform Probate Code (UPC), the Uniform Guardianship and Protected Proceedings Act (UGPPA), and the Uniform Adult Guardianship and Protected Proceedings Jurisdiction Act (UAGPPJA). Center for Elders and the Court provides a comprehensive overview of these laws on their website at, http://www.eldersandcourts.org/Guardianship/Guardianship-Basics/State-Laws.aspx. The American Bar Association has complied specific state-by-state resources and compendiums for Adult Guardianship Law (American Bar Association, http://www.americanbar.org/groups/law_aging/resources/guardianship_law_practice.html) [2].

State-by-state adoption of federal guardianship legislation plays a key role in protecting abused elders [41]. For example in New York, legislation related to surrogate decision-making is codified in the Family Health Care Decisions Act (2010) by providing a prioritized list of those available to make decisions for an patient lacking medical capacity: (1) legal guardian under Mental Hygiene Law Article 81, (2) spouse or domestic partner, (3) adult child, (4) parent, (5) brother or sister, (6) close friend, and (7) outlines the procedure of the medical facility to make decisions on behalf of the patient.

12.11 Return to Case Study: Geriatric Psychiatrist Capacity Evaluation

A geriatric psychiatrist was asked to evaluate the patient's capacity to refuse treatment. The patient was surprised that anyone was concerned enough to ask her why she was refusing care. She answered the psychiatrist's questions very slowly with a very soft voice. Her speech was non-spontaneous and each answer was brief. In terms of the specific capacity evaluation criteria, she was able to communicate a choice, understood the relevant information, and demonstrated understanding of the situation and consequences of refusing physical therapy and dialysis regularly. However, she was not able to logically manipulate the information in a rational manner. Her primary reason for refusing treatment was that she deserved to die. When the psychiatrist explored the theme of death and suffering with the patient, she went on to describe her belief that she was a bad mother and had pushed her son to his addictions. She was quite hopeless that there was any quality left in her life. She also blamed herself for all of Jake and Billy's problems and denied any contribution from her abusive deceased husband who was also an alcoholic. The psychiatrist determined that Peggy did not have capacity at this time to refuse treatment due to her depression. She was making her decisions based on flawed and irrational reasoning due to depression.

12.12 The Impact of Mental Health on Capacity

The impact of depression on cognition is multifaceted. The symptoms of depression often include fatigue and decrease in concentration that can cause inattention and difficulty remembering or learning the facts important for decision-making. Decreased oral intake and sleep also contribute to fatigue. For medical decision-making, suicidal ideation and belief that he or she is worthless, a burden, or otherwise unworthy of the expense of treatment can greatly influence the older adult to refuse treatment. Depression can make older adults overgeneralize any setbacks in treatment. Any side effects can be distorted to reflect an older adult's negative self-image. Emotional reasoning causes the older adult to have a negatively skewed view of any facts presented and can lead to jumping to conclusions and fatalistic thinking. This type of thinking is not rational.

12.13 Return to Case Study: Lacking Capacity Due to Depression

The psychiatrist explained why she was not allowed to refuse treatment and deemed to lack capacity at this time. The patient agreed that depression was a significant factor in her refusal of treatment and she worked with the psychiatrist and a therapist to treat Major Depression. The psychiatrist said that the patient did not need to have a guardian appointed believing that her depression would go into remission and the patient would be able to regain capacity. The patient took an antidepressant and began psychotherapy. Unfortunately, her progression in physical therapy was very limited and she was transferred from the acute rehabilitation unit to long-term care. Her son and grandson both came to visit her during this time. Her mood was improving, but she had some setbacks every time they visited. The nursing home staff kept a watchful eye on her whenever Jake or Billy visited. Jake tried to get Peggy discharged home. He was unable to keep the house without her social security income. Peggy told the staff that she did not want to leave the nursing facility. She needed to have helped with toileting, bathing and other activities of daily living and she did not believe that Jake would be able to help her as he promised. She became more suspicious of his intentions as she started to care about herself more. She asked for a representative payee to be assigned to allow her social security income to be used for her care at the nursing home to protect it from Jake and Billy.

The nursing home staff became very attached to Peggy and for several years life was calm, but they noticed that her memory was starting to slip. Every 3 months, the nursing home social workers completed cognitive assessments that documented her worsening cognitive impairment. Her primary care physician started an acetylcholinesterase inhibitor (like donepezil) to try to slow the progression of her cognitive impairment. The next year, she had several complications related to her diabetes and dialysis. She needed revisions of her fistula, wounds that had trouble healing caused her to miss several dialysis sessions and lead to periods of fluid overload, congestive heart failure and subsequent hospitalizations. After the sixth hospitalization, Peggy decided that she no longer wanted to continue dialysis. Her nephrologist insisted on a capacity evaluation regarding her capacity to refuse dialysis treatment.

A geriatric psychiatrist was again called to complete a capacity evaluation since the patient has a history of depression that has rendered her without capacity in the past. Peggy's mood was noted to be down, but she was not clinically depressed. However, though she was not depressed, she did have notable cognitive impairment. She had some word finding difficulties and her immediate recall was impaired. She was oriented to herself and place and the situation. During the evaluation, Peggy and the psychiatrist had a frank discussion about why she is choosing to end dialysis. She clearly described what would likely happen as dialysis is stopped as she had recently experienced several occasions when dialysis could not be completed for several days. She denied any suicidal ideation or death wish, but she described understanding that dialysis cannot be continued indefinitely. She had many complications over the past year and described a realistic, rational, and logical appreciation of the risks and benefits of both continuing and discontinuing dialysis treatment. Despite her mood being down and having notable cognitive impairment, the psychiatrist determined that the patient did have the capacity to make the decision to stop dialysis treatment.

12.14 Research Challenges

It is clear that assessment of medical decision-making capacity is a complex task. Researchers have tried to mitigate the challenges that we face serving vulnerable older adults without compromising their autonomy. To do this, researchers all over the world have focused their efforts on creating tools that can be applied to every day situations. For decades, researchers have identified the difficulties in doing this complicated assessment and identified the need to be more specific in terms of type of decision-making and location. At the same time, there is also recognition now that an ongoing assessment of decision-making capacity is also invaluable for older adults that one is working with over time. Many studies still utilize the MacArthur Competence Assessment Tool for Treatment (MacCAT-T) [19] and build off of that foundation. However, each assessment tool still requires a semi-structured interview to evaluate the four areas required for a standard capacity assessment described above and takes over 15 min to complete.

Of course, when doing research, it is necessary to assess decision-making capacity in order to have the research subjects give informed consent [6]. Many researchers who require older adults with dementia as subjects are able to utilize the older adults' caregiver or identified guardian to give informed consent to participate in the research project. Unfortunately, victims of elder abuse are often victimized by a caregiver or trusted other who would not likely give consent for a study on elder abuse. This scenario is a common problem with institutional review board's approval of research in this area. The MacArthur Competence Assessment Tool for Clinical Research [7] and the University of California, San Diego Brief Assessment of Capacity to Consent (UBACC) are examples of capacity evaluation tools designed for specific use in research contexts [20].

Drs. Lai and Karlawish describe a model conceptualizing the assessment of capacity to solve functional problems that illustrates the interaction between a cognitive evaluation and a functional evaluation, shown in Fig. 12.1. The ability to answer questions testing cognition and the ability to perform activities of daily living are not equivalent. Many other variables that are not necessarily modifiable or easily identified such as psychological state can influence the ability of the older adult to make decisions to solve functional problems. This type of assessment goes beyond making singular medical treatment decisions and may be more relevant to the issue of guardianship or conservatorship as that involves appointing someone to make multiple decisions for the impaired older adult about almost all aspects of her life [21].

There are efforts to create and utilize capacity assessment tools around the world in order to take into account cultural variances. One example is use of the Chinese version of the Assessment of Capacity for Everyday Decision-Making

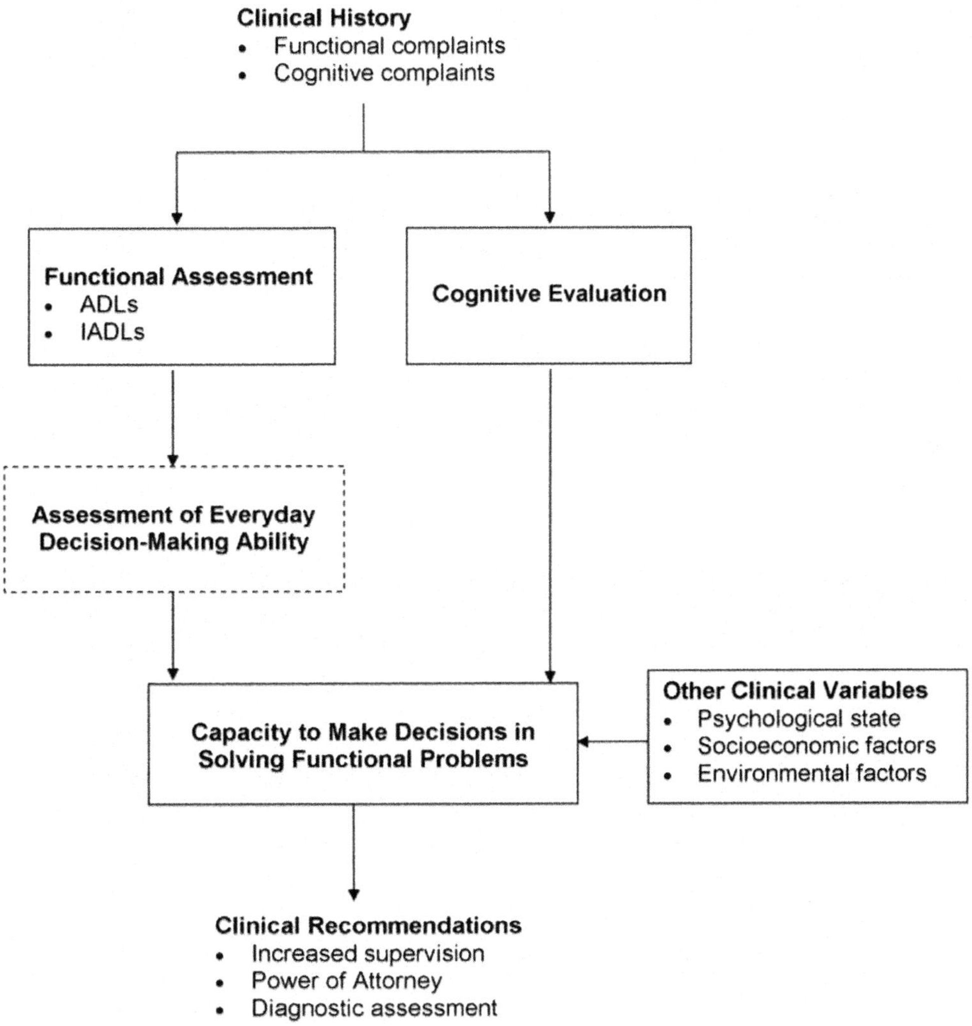

Fig. 12.1 Model for assessing the capacity to make decisions about how to solve functional problems

ADL: activities of daily living; IADL: instrumental activities of daily living.

(ACED) [27]. The MacCAT-T has been translated into Chinese, Greek, and Spanish and has been used in studies worldwide.

Efforts to create standardized and evidence-based tools for capacity assessment have improved screening methods for decision-making capacity. Making and Executing Decisions for Safe and Independent Living (MED-SAIL) is a screening tool created to identify those who may have impaired decision-making capacity [29, 30]. This may be a useful instrument, but it only screens and does not actually make the assessment that someone lacks capacity. Instead, the older adult is referred for a comprehensive assessment, but that is an important judgment for practitioners to make and can open the door to many other interventions. Increased interest in protecting a growing older adult population, the evolution of patient-centered care, and heightened awareness of ethical considerations all fuel the future of the field.

12.15 Future Directions

For practitioners dealing with older adults vulnerable to abuse and exploitation, the more pragmatic and salient developments are the methods being developed to evaluate decision-making capacity in specific situations. As the impact of elder abuse and financial exploitation is finally recognized as a significant and costly problem, research funding is focusing on ways to detect, mitigate and intervene. Multi-disciplinary teams are being created and studied around the country to evaluate their effectiveness and develop best practices. Tools to evaluate financial decision-making capacity are being created such as the Lichtenberg Financial Decision Rating Scale [25].

Many researchers are actively designing and validating capacity assessment tools. As they create these tools, it is important that we create a uniform vocabulary and framework in order to effectively utilize these tools no matter what realm we work in; whether it is medical, social services, or legal. The disparate legal definitions using both capacity and competency are confusing for practitioners, researchers, older adults and their families. Unfortunately, there does not seem to be much movement in this direction as we are overwhelmed with the everyday practicalities of working with vulnerable older adults. Hopefully, there will be more direction on a national scale to unify the legal definitions, but the current Elder Justice Roadmap has a focus on implementing existing laws rather than clarification or change of the laws. In the first wave of the Elder Justice Roadmap, the definitions to be clarified are related to research rather than policy.

In medicine, we often look to laboratory tests as more objective markers of a disease state. To translate that desire for an objective marker in terms of assessment of capacity or competency, some are looking at neuroimaging to fill that gap. Forensic psychiatrists have led the way with trying to associate neuroimaging findings with evaluations of competency to stand trial and to establish the mental state of an individual charged with a crime [17]. Dementia researchers are trying to link neuroimaging studies to specific areas of deficits and hope for the ability to detect changes in brain function before they develop into functional impairments but the results are not always consistent [31, 37].

In addition to these advances in science, practitioners across fields caring for older adults will look to patient-centered research to inform development of tools and policy to address decision-making capacity in older adults. Research from the patient and family perspective needs to be integrated into professional education and training. The process of informed consent carried out in professional practice still lags behind the more sophisticated understanding of the ethics found in the scientific literature despite best efforts to translate what is known into everyday practice [18]. To implement changes in practice, research must be coupled with effective dissemination and training opportunities for professionals.

12.16 Conclusion

It is clear that medical decision-making is a complex multifaceted process. Disagreements about treatment and lifestyle choices between older adults and their care providers do not necessarily indicate a lack of decision-making ability by the older adult. The determination that one is compelled to question an older adult's decision-making capacity must be carefully examined before pursuing that type of evaluation. There are multiple ethical quandaries that must be recognized before the inquiry proceeds. We must scrutinize our motivations to make sure that the intent and ultimate outcome of our questioning a person's autonomy is beneficial and justifiable. There must be recognition that each case is unique and that we are not discriminating based on an eccentric lifestyle choice or the person's perceived limitations.

The case above illustrated several examples of how medical decision-making capacity assessments can be utilized, even throughout one person's life. Recall that medical decision-making capacity is to be distinguished from legal determinations of incapacity in that the medical decision-making capacity we discussed is an evaluation of the older adult at one point in time, for one specific decision and is along a continuum of decision-making abilities. Medical decision-making capacity is based on the older adult meeting four required elements: expressing a choice, demonstration of understanding of the factual information, ability to appreciate the risks and benefits associated with each choice, and ability to rationally manipulate the information to make a logical decision. The older adult's decision may not necessarily be the one that the treatment team agrees with, but it may be logical nonetheless. When an older adult is determined to lack medical decision-making capacity that inability to make decision may be for only a short time and she may be able to regain medical decision-making capacity. If it is unlikely that the older adult will be able to regain medical decision-making capacity and is in danger of harming herself by making a number of illogical, irrational, and poor decisions, it may be necessary to pursue guardianship. We can hope that in the future, neuroimaging can identify vulnerable older adults early on and capacity assessment tools will be easy to utilize. Perhaps someday, no matter where in the world one lives and works, a vulnerable older adult will be treated with respect for her autonomy and even if she lacks decision-making capacity we will be able to come to her aid while maintaining her dignity.

References

1. Agency for Healthcare Research and Quality. Making Health Care Safer II; Rockville, MD; 2013. Retrieved from http://www.ahrq.gov/research/findings/evidence-based-reports/ptsafetyuptp.html. March 7, 2016.
2. American Bar Association. Guardianship Law and Practice. Retrieved from http://www.americanbar.org/groups/law_aging/resources/guardianship_law_practice.html. March 7, 2016.
3. American Bar Association. Health Care Decision Making. Retrieved from http://www.americanbar.org/groups/law_aging/resources/health_care_decision_making.html. March 7, 2016.
4. American Medical Association. Ethics Opinion 8.08, Informed Consent; 2006. http://www.ama-assn.org/ama/pub/physician-resources/medical-ethics/code-medical-ethics/opinion808.page?. March 7, 2016.
5. American Psychological Association. ABA/APA assessment of capacity in older adults. Retrieved from http://www.apa.org/pi/aging/programs/assessment/. March 7, 2016.
6. Appelbaum PS. Assessment of patients' competence to consent to treatment. N Engl J Med. 2007;357(18):1834–40.
7. Appelbaum PS, Grisso T. MacCAT-CR:MacArthur competence assessment tool for clinical research. Sarasota, FL: Professional Resource Press; 2001.
8. Aulisio MP, Arnold RM, Younger SJ. Health care ethics consultation: nature, goals, and competencies. Ann Intern Med. 2000;133:59–69.
9. Baker RR, Lichtenberg PA, Moye J. A practice guideline for assessment of competency and capacity of the older adult. Prof Psychol Res Pract. 1998;29(2):149.
10. Barry MJ, Edgman-Levitan S. Shared decision-making—the pinnacle of patient-centered care. N Engl J Med. 2012;366(9):780–1.
11. Brandl B, Dyer CB, Heisler CJ, Otto JM, Stiegel LA, Thomas RW. Elder abuse detection and intervention: a collaborative approach. New York, NY: Springer; 2007.
12. Caulfield SE. Health care facility ethics committees: new issues in the age of transparency. Am Bar Assoc Sect Civ Rights Soc Just. 2007;34(4). http://www.americanbar.org/publications/human_rights_magazine_home/human_rights_vol34_2007/fall2007/hr_fall07_caulfi.html. March 7, 2016.
13. Centers for Elders and the Court. Guardianship Basics. Retrieved from http://www.eldersandcourts.org/Guardianship/Guardianship-Basics/State-Laws.aspx. March 7, 2016.
14. Chin JJ. Doctor–patient relationship: from medical paternalism to enhanced autonomy. Singp Med J. 2002;43(3):152–5.
15. Daveson BA, Bausewein C, Murtagh FE, et al. To be involved or not to be involved: a survey of public preferences for self-involvement in decision-making involving mental capacity (competency) within Europe. Palliat Med. 2013;27(5):418–27.
16. Demakis GJ. State statutory definitions of civil incompetency/incapacity: issues for psychologists. Psychol Public Policy Law. 2013;19:331.
17. Edersheim JG, Brendel RW, Price BH. Neuroimaging, diminished capacity and mitigation. In: Simpson JR, editor. Neuroimaging in forensic psychiatry: from the clinic to the courtroom. Wiley; 2012.
18. Grady C. Enduring and emerging challenges of informed consent. N Engl J Med. 2015;372:855–62.
19. Grisso T, Appelbaum PS, Hill-Fotouhi C. The MacCAT-T: a clinical tool to assess patients' capacities to make treatment decisions. Psychiatr Serv. 1997;48(11):1415–9.
20. Jeste DV, Palmer BW, Appelbaum PS, Golshan S, Glorioso D, Dunn LB, et al. A new brief instrument for assessing decisional capacity for clinical research. Arch Gen Psychiatry. 2007;64(8):966–74.
21. Lai JM, Karlawish J. Assessing the capacity to make everyday decisions: a guide for clinicians and an agenda for future research. Am J Geriatr Psychiatry. 2007;15(2):101–11.
22. Leo RJ. Competency and the capacity to make treatment decisions: a primer for primary care physicians. Prim Care Companion J Clin Psychiatry. 1999;1(5):131–41.
23. Levin A. Coercion and autonomy sometimes collide in patient-care decisions. Psychiatric News; 2014;49(12).
24. Lichtenberg PA, Stickney L, Paulson D. Is psychological vulnerability related to the experience of fraud in older adults? Clin Gerontol. 2013;36(2):132–46.
25. Lichtenberg PA, Stoltman J, Ficker LJ, Iris M, Mast B. A person-centered approach to financial capacity assessment: preliminary development of a new rating scale. Clin Gerontol. 2015;38(1):49–67.
26. Liu YL. Autonomy, filial piety, and parental authority: a two-year longitudinal investigation. J Genet Psychol. 2013;174(5–6):557–81.
27. Lui VWC, Lam LCW, Chau RCM, Fung AWT, Wong BML, Leung GTY, et al. Structured assessment of mental capacity to make financial decisions in Chinese older persons with mild cognitive impairment and mild alzheimer disease. J Geriatr Psychiatry Neurol. 2013;26(2):69–77.
28. Mental Disability Advocacy Center. Legal capacity in Europe: a call to action to governments and to the EU. October 2013. Retrieved from http://mdac.info/en/resources/legal-capacity-europe-call-action-governments-and-eu. March 17, 2016.
29. Mills WL, Regev T, Kunik ME, Wilson NL, Moye J, McCullough LB, et al. Making and executing decisions for safe and independent living (MED-SAIL): development and validation of a brief screening tool. Am J Geriatr Psychiatry. 2014;22(3):285–93.
30. Mills WL, Snow AL, Wilson NL, Naik AD, Kunik ME. Conceptualization of a toolkit to evaluate everyday competence in planning transitions from nursing homes to the community. J Am Med Dir Assoc. 2013;14(8):626-e1.
31. Mortimer AM, Likeman M, Lewis TT. Neuroimaging in dementia: a practical guide. Pract Neurol. 2013;13:92–103.
32. Moye J, Marson D, Edelstein B. Assessment of capacity in an aging society. Am Psychol. 2013;68(3):158–71.

33. Munthe C, Sandman L, Cutas D. Person centered care and shared decision making: implications for ethics, public health and research. Health Care Anal. 2012;20(3):231–49. doi:10.1007/s10728-011-0183-y.
34. Nilsson A. Who gets to decide? Right to legal capacity for persons with intellectual and psychosocial disabilities. Council of Europe, Commissioner for Human Rights Issue Paper. February 20, 2012.
35. Pape T. Legal and ethical considerations of informed consent. AORN J. 1997;65(6):1122–7.
36. Pope TM. Legal briefing: healthcare ethics committees. J Clin Ethics. 2011;22(1):74–93.
37. Rudrauf D. Structure-function relationships behind the phenomenon of cognitive resilience in neurology: insights for neuroscience and medicine. Adv Neurosci. 2014;1–28.
38. Schillerstrom JE, Horton MS, Royall DR. The impact of medical illness on executive function. Psychosomatics. 2005;46(6):508–16.
39. Schillerstrom JE, Horton MS, Schillerstrom TL, Joshi KG, Earthman BS, Velez AM, et al. Prevalence, course, and risk factors for executive impairment in patients hospitalized on a general medicine service. Psychosomatics. 2005;46(5):411–7.
40. Schillerstrom JE, Salazar R, Regwan H, Bonugli RJ, Royall DR. Executive function in self-neglecting adult protective services referrals compared with elder psychiatric outpatients. Am J Geriatr Psychiatry. 2009;17(10):907–10.
41. Stiegel LA, Wood EF. Nine ways to reduce elder abuse through enactment of the uniform adult guardianship and protective proceedings jurisdiction act. Bifocal, e-journal of the ABA Commission on Law and Aging 2009;30(3):1–6.
42. Tai MC, Tsai T. Who makes the decision? Patient's autonomy vs paternalism in a confucian society. Croat Med J. 2003;44(5):558–61.
43. United Nations Convention on the Rights of Persons with Disabilities. Accessed online www.un.org/disabilities/default. March 7, 2016.
44. United States. The Belmont Report: ethical principals and guidelines for the protection of human subjects research. Bethesda, MD: The Commission; 1978.
45. Wigglesworth A, Austin R, Corona M, Schneider D, Liao S, Gibbs L, et al. Bruising as a marker of physical elder abuse. J Am Geriatr Soc. 2009;S57:1191–6.

13 Physician Quality Reporting System (PQRS) Quality Measure: The Elder Maltreatment Screen and Follow-Up Plan

Tara L. McMullen, Kimberly Schwartz, Sophia Autrey, Jane Lucas, Gary Rezek, Anita Somplasky, and Jeannette Shrift

13.1 Introduction

In 2013, the Centers for Medicare and Medicaid Services (CMS) convened a panel of experts in the field of elder abuse to explore the current state of elder maltreatment screening and elder care practices across CMS beneficiary populations and care settings. The *CMS Elder Maltreatment and Care Symposium* was comprised of researchers, healthcare providers, advocates, and government civil servants. Among discussion pertaining to elder maltreatment screening, participants of this symposium discussed the current Physician Quality Reporting System (PQRS) elder maltreatment screening quality measure, the *Elder Maltreatment Screen and Follow-Up Plan* (PQRS #181). Stakeholders discussed the usability of this measure, its value to PQRS program, and ultimately the measure's impact in protecting older adults who have been abused. Through expert input, elder abuse screening and intervention was determined to be of high value to PQRS reporting program as well as an important indicator of quality reporting.

13.2 Background

13.2.1 Elder Maltreatment

It has been estimated that each year, up to five million Americans experience some form of elder maltreatment [15]. Maltreatment may result in hospitalizations, increased rates of emergency room use, and mortality [11, 12]. However, many cases of elder abuse go unidentified and unreported [3]. The lack of efficient detection and reporting of elder abuse remains an issue, ultimately creating gaps in the reporting and tracking of maltreatment episode—limiting the evidence-base for this field. Elder abuse does not discriminate based on race, economic, or sexual identity. Of note, elder abuse does not limit itself to a specific living environment such as nursing homes or long-term care facilities.

In order to increase surveillance and collection of elder abuse data to fill these reporting gaps, the Centers for Medicare and Medicaid (CMS) developed a quality measure that provides an elder maltreatment screen, assessing for eight components of elder abuse including: (1) physical abuse, (2) emotional or psychological abuse, (3) neglect, (4) sexual abuse, (5) elder abandonment, (6) financial or material exploitation, (7) self-neglect and (8) unwarranted control [4]. The intent of this quality measure was to provide documentation around the event of detection of abuse, including recommended referrals, follow-up to include re-assessment, discussion with other providers, and/or direct intervention. Surveillance of elder abuse is necessary to ensure the safety of the victim, stopping the cycle of abuse, and ensuring collaboration between providers and agencies is occurring. However, this quality measure does have limitations including the breadth of providers who report the measure, which is limited due to a series of coding limitations, provider inclusion, or state regulations. In addition, the lack of a specific tool to measure and address elder abuse not only in the acute care but other care settings has created enormous roadblocks for the standardization of a measure and data across care providers and settings.

In addition to the development of this quality measure, CMS engaged with federal agencies to discuss whether a universal definition of elder maltreatment was achievable, how to better assess elder maltreatment through quality measures, and how to improve overall surveillance [13]. Additional findings from this federal engagement included discussion about screening tools and their varied use by providers, the impact of screenings and the education about screening for abusive events, and discussion pertaining to

T.L. McMullen (✉) · K. Schwartz · S. Autrey
Clinical Standards & Quality, Centers for Medicare and Medicaid Services, 7500 Security Boulevard, Baltimore, MD 21244, USA
e-mail: tara.mcmullen@cms.hhs.gov

J. Lucas · G. Rezek · A. Somplasky · J. Shrift
Quality Insights of Pennsylvania, King of Prussia, PA, USA

X. Dong (ed.), *Elder Abuse*, DOI 10.1007/978-3-319-47504-2_13

cultural diversity within the study and understanding of elder maltreatment [14].

Further, in order to address the increased need for surveillance due to either the underreporting of elder abuse or to increase education about what is abuse, a variety of strategic resources have been implemented to address the legal, social, health, and economic implications of elder abuse. One such example is the Elder Justice Roadmap Project, created to receive input from experts and stakeholders to "understand, prevent, identify, or respond to elder abuse, neglect, or exploitation" in order to prioritize action plans and identify key issues surrounding elder abuse [15]. The roadmap addresses four priority areas that provide further clarity for how each interrelates to elder abuse. Areas addressed in the roadmap are: (1) Direct Services related to the healthcare pathway which addresses the team, cultural sensitivity, care management, and geriatric expertise; (2) Education which entails public awareness, training, and cultural competency; (3) Policy encompassing adult protective services, infrastructure, funding, implementation of laws, and long-term care; and (4) Research which necessitates clarification of definitions, increasing the number of researchers, implementing national research centers, and furthering the cause [15].

Concurrent to efforts that aim to raise awareness and to enhance the response pertaining to events of abuse or neglect such as the roadmap, CMS continues to develop and improve upon quality measurement focused on elder abuse in order to fill the data gaps and to continue to address the needs for a more robust data collection pertaining to elder abuse/maltreatment. The assessment of elder abuse event requires ongoing engagement and prioritization. Below, you will find a description of the quality measure, *Elder Maltreatment Screen and Follow-Up Plan (PQRS #131)*, developed by CMS. This measure was developed to enhance the reporting of elder abuse to increase the response of abusive events.

13.2.2 The Centers for Medicare and Medicaid Services

The Centers for Medicare and Medicaid Services (CMS) is a federal agency that is a part of the United States Department of Health and Human Services (DHHS). Previously known as the Health Care Financing Administration (HCFA), CMS administers the Medicare and Medicaid programs. President Lyndon B. Johnson signed into law the bill that led to the development of the Medicare and Medicaid programs [5]. The Medicare program originally included Part A (Hospital Insurance) and Part B (Medical Insurance) [6]. Medicare has been expanded to include Part C (Medicare Advantage Plans) and Part D (prescription drug coverage) [6]. Medicaid is a federal and state program that aids individuals, those with limited income and resources, with their medical coverage [7].

In order to drive quality improvement for millions of beneficiaries, CMS has developed the CMS Quality Strategy, which guides that agency toward achieving the aims of better care, smarter spending, and healthier people and communities [8]. Built upon the foundation of the National Quality Strategy [1], the CMS Quality Strategies intent is to advance these three aims in coordination with the National Qualities Strategies priorities of:

> Making care safer by reducing harm caused in the delivery of care; Ensuring that each person and family is engaged as partners in their care; Promoting effective communication and coordination of care; Promoting the most effective prevention and treatment practices for the leading causes of mortality, starting with cardiovascular disease; Working with communities to promote wide use of best practices to enable healthy living; and making quality care more affordable for individuals, families, employers, governments, and communities by developing and spreading new health care delivery models (AHRQ [1]).

The CMS Quality Strategy was developed through a collaborative process of input from HHS and stakeholders (CMSd [8]). The CMS Quality Strategy is used to guide all program and quality objectives. Primarily, in order to address the principles of the National Quality Strategy, CMS leverages the aims and priorities in all measure development work in order to help promote better care and close quality gaps [8].

13.2.3 The Physician Quality Reporting System

The Centers for Medicare and Medicaid Services has various quality programs that report on the quality of care for many care settings in the United States. One of CMS's quality reporting programs is the Physician Quality Reporting System (PQRS), a program under the Medicare program. The PQRS is a quality reporting program that publicly reports on quality and performance of individual eligible professionals (EPs) and group practices in the United States [9]. The PQRS quality reporting is a voluntary CMS quality program that encourages health care professionals and group practices to report on health their care practices [15]. The information reported for this quality reporting program is located on the CMS Physician Compare website [10].

13.2.4 The Reporting of Screening for Elder Maltreatment: A Quality Measure for the Physician Quality Reporting System (PQRS)

In an effort to address the underreporting of elder abuse, CMS, in 2009, implemented a quality measure into the Physician Quality Reporting System (PQRS) that assisted eligible acute care providers in identifying suspected cases of elder maltreatment. This process-based quality measure, *Elder Maltreatment Screen and Follow-Up Plan (PQRS #181)*, is a claims-based measure that reports on the percentage of patients, 65 years and older, who have a documented elder maltreatment screen by way of an elder maltreatment screening tool. This quality measure reports on a documented elder maltreatment screen from the date of the medical encounter in addition to a documented follow-up plan on the date of the positive maltreatment screen.

The *Elder Maltreatment Screen and Follow-Up Plan (PQRS #181)* quality measure is to be reported once during the specified PQRS reporting period for which the patient was seen in the acute care setting. This measure is not collected in post-acute care settings. The reporting requirement for this quality measure is once per reporting period by means of the claim or registry. The denominator for this quality measure is comprised of all patients, ages 65 years and older who have had a patient encounter during the specified reporting period. The numerator for this quality measure is comprised of patients with a documented elder maltreatment screen using an Elder Maltreatment Screening Tool on the date of the encounter and follow-up plan documented on the date of the positive screen. Individuals that are not included in the data collection for this quality measure include: individuals who refused to participate and possess reasonable decisional capacity for self-protection, and/or individuals who have an urgent or emergent situation where time is of the essence and to delay treatment would jeopardize the patient's health status. In addition, screening for self-neglect is not included in this measure (please see Appendix A for public comment on this measure).

Conceptually, CMS has defined a screen for elder maltreatment to include an assessment and documentation of one or more of the following components: (1) physical abuse; (2) emotional or psychological abuse; (3) neglect (active or passive); (4) sexual abuse; (5) abandonment; (6) financial or material exploitation; and (7) unwarranted control. A follow-up plan for this quality measure includes documentation that abuse was reported to the individual's state or local Adult Protective Services Agency (APS). Additional quality measure definitions are listed below (Table 13.1).

Of note, this measure may be reported by eligible professionals who perform the quality actions described in the measure based on the services provided and the measure-specific denominator coding at the time of the qualifying visit. The documented follow-up plan must be related to a positive elder maltreatment screening. Cognitively impaired patients are included in the denominator of this measure and need to be screened using an elder maltreatment screening tool.

Table 13.1 Maltreatment screen components (2013): The Elder Maltreatment Screen and Follow-Up Plan (PQRS #181) quality measure

Physical abuse	Infliction of physical injury by punching, beating, kicking, biting, burning, shaking, or other actions that result in harm
Emotional or Psychological abuse	Involves psychological abuse, verbal abuse, or mental injury and includes acts or omissions by loved ones or caregivers that have caused or could cause serious behavioral, cognitive, emotional, or mental disorders
Neglect	Involves attitudes of others or actions caused by others—such as family members, friends, or institutional caregivers—that have an extremely detrimental effect upon well being Active—Behavior that is willful or when the caregiver intentionally withholds care or necessities. The neglect may be motivated by financial gain or reflect interpersonal conflicts Passive—Situations where the caregiver is unable to fulfill his or her care giving responsibilities as a result of illness, disability, stress, ignorance, lack of maturity, or lack of resources
Sexual abuse	Forcing of undesired sexual behavior by one person upon another against their will who are either competent or unable to fully comprehend and/or give consent. This may also be called molestation
Elder abandonment	Desertion of an elderly person by an individual who has assumed responsibility for providing care for an elder, or by a person with physical custody of an elder
Financial or material exploitation	Taking advantage of a person for monetary gain or profit
Unwarranted control	Controlling a person's ability to make choices about living situations, household finances, and medical care

Table 13.2 Eligible professional reporting: The Elder Maltreatment Screen and Follow-Up Plan (PQRS #181) quality measure

	2010	2011	2012	2013	2014
Eligible beneficiaries	Not available	Not available	Not available	22,699,320	Not available
Beneficiaries reported	Not available	Not available	Not available	103,277	Not available
Eligible EPs	66,877	69,780	589,553	550,715	Not available
# of EPs reporting	Not available	Not available	Not available	1955	4117*
% of EPs reporting	0.1 %	0.1 %	0.0 %	0.4 %	Not available
Performance rate	55.3 %	96.7 %	90.8 %	36.2 %	Not available

Source 2013 Physician Quality Reporting System Program Monitoring and Evaluation Report

In 2014, the National Quality Forum (NQF) reviewed the quality measure, the *Elder Maltreatment Screen and Follow-Up Plan (PQRS #181)* for consideration of initial endorsement. Data presented to the NQF for consideration of endorsement were based on testing conducted from January 1, 2010 through June 30, 2010. A total of 23 eligible professionals submitted data on the measure, *Elder Maltreatment Screen and Follow-Up Plan (PQRS #181)*. Due to the low number of eligible professionals submitting data on this quality measure, the NQF determined a performance gap could not be demonstrated and the measure was not endorsed (please see Appendices B–D for the NQF submission materials).

According to the 2013 Physician Quality Reporting System Program Monitoring and Evaluation Report, the quality measure, the *Elder Maltreatment Screen and Follow-Up Plan (PQRS #181)* was identified as one of the measures with large numbers of eligible professionals who could report but had "particularly low reporting rates." Data from 2010 illuminated there was a total of 558 valid claims submitted by 23 National Provider Identifiers (NPIs) during the first six months of the year. By 2012, eligible professionals reporting improved, resulting in 311 NPI and Taxpayer Identification Number (TIN) submitting data on this quality measure. While there has been an increase in the number of eligible professionals reporting the measure, the number is still at or below 0.4 % with performance rate varying from 36.2 to 96.7 % (Table 13.2). Although there was improvement, CMS has recognized that this measure has not been utilized as robustly as it was intended when developed. Reporting outcomes for this quality measure show low participation, stressing an important measurement gap and limitation [2, 14]. Typically, a varied group of professionals are included in the reporting of this measure including, Psychologists, Geriatricians, Occupational Therapists, Urologists, and Psychiatrists among various other health professionals.

13.2.5 The Elder Maltreatment Screen and Follow-up Plan (PQRS #181): Next Steps

The number of eligible professionals reporting this measure is low in comparison to other measures maintained for CMS. However, the number of eligible professionals reporting on the *Elder Maltreatment Screen and Follow-Up Plan (PQRS #181)* quality measure has increased significantly since the measure was tested in 2010. Overall, the number of eligible professionals reporting this measure more than doubled from 2013 (roughly 1955 eligible professionals reporting) to 2014 (roughly 4117 eligible professionals reporting). Due to this increase, CMS will continue to test this measure for reportability, usability, reliability, and validity purposes.

13.3 Conclusion

Elder maltreatment and events of abuse are a public health issue, and health professionals are faced with situations where they manage the care of a patient who may have been abuse. Improving the knowledge of what is abuse and what are abusive events will help make reporting of the abuse actionable, and will aid in the surveillance of maltreatment overall. This chapter has been a brief reflection of the efforts by CMS to improve this surveillance; however, the field has much room to grow in this type of data collection.

Final Public Comment Summary Report

Project Title:

2015 PQRS #181 Elder Maltreatment Screening and Follow-Up Plan

Dates:

- The Call for Public Comment was open from 8:00 A.M EDT on 9/11/14 to 5:00 P.M EDT on 10/22/14
- The Technical Expert Panel (TEP) met on 1/14/15, 1 P.M-2 P.M EDT
- The Public Comment Summary was made on January 15th 2015

Project Overview:

The Centers for Medicare & Medicaid Services (CMS) has contracted with Signature Consulting Group to maintain Measure 181 - Elder Maltreatment Screening and Follow-Up Plan. The contract name is Physician Quality Measures Maintenance. The contract number is HHSM-500-2013-00177C. As part of its measure maintenance process, CMS has requested interested parties to submit comments on this measure.

Project Historical Review:

CMS convened a national Elder Maltreatment & Care Symposium for all relevant stakeholders on March 8, 2013. The aim of this symposium was to assess the value of continuing the implementation and development of PQRS #181 Elder Maltreatment Screening and Follow-Up Plan.

Feedback from the Elder Maltreatment & Care Symposium was incorporated into the comprehensive review of the 2014 Elder Maltreatment Screening and Follow-Up Plan measure for use in PQRS. This comprehensive review also included a literature review, measure specifications review and an evaluation of the measure code sets.

Project Objectives:

- Assess relevance and value of elder maltreatment assessment within the clinical setting and patient behavioral response to support the continuation of development and implementation of PQRS #181: Elder Maltreatment Screening and Follow-Up Plan.
- Review public comments for consideration of potential revisions for implementation of the measure. This may include a comprehensive literature review, measure specifications review, and an evaluation of the measure code sets.

Information About the Comments Received:

- Technical Expert Panel members and other stakeholders were notified of the Public Comment Call via email
- The CMS Quality Measures Public Comment website was used to post the Public Comment Call: http://www.cms.gov/Medicare/Quality-Initiatives-Patient-Assessment-Instruments/MMS/CallforPublicComment.html
- 3 responses were received on this topic

Stakeholder Comments—General and Measure-Specific

Summary of comments:

- Agreement/support of measure
    - 3 comments supported the measure
- Recommendations to amend measure
    - 2 provider/organizations recommended changes related to:
        - Screening of the patient should be done privately with only the physician and elder in the room in order to encourage reporting of abuse by victims
    - 1 provider/organization recommended changes related to:
        - Removing the phrase "psychological abuse" from the definition of Psychological abuse" found in the Numerator section of the measure specification
        - Lowering the age criteria to 60 years as the threshold for defining elderly

- Utilizing this measure to gather data for use in research (i.e. support or refute the 2011 New York prevalence study)
- Screening with each visit rather than once per reporting period
- Addressing the "loop hole" created by the 'not eligible' definition "include patients who refuse to participate and have decisional capacity for self- protection"
- Using a single screening instrument to enhance data results

Overall Analysis of the Comments and Recommendations

The TEP met to address the public comments and make recommendations, as needed, based on the comments provided. Below is a summary of the TEP discussion and decisions.

Public Comments made by The Harry and Jeanette Weinberg Center for Elder Abuse Prevention at the Hebrew Home at Riverdale:

1. In support of the measure. Every client that enters is screened for elder abuse. The Weinberg Center team follows-up on every positive result and helps to create and implement a comprehensive care plan. They believe that integrating elder abuse screening into the healthcare services is critical.

Final Recommendations: The TEP acknowledges and thanks The Harry and Jeanette Weinberg Center for Elder Abuse Prevention at the Hebrew Home in Riverdale for the comment. The TEP feels passionately about this measure and the impact that it has on the elder population.

Public Comments made by NASOP:

1. The Definition of "Psychological abuse" within the measure specification currently uses the words "psychological abuse," NASOP suggests that the "psychological abuse" should not be defined with the terms "psychological abuse." Currently the measure states: Emotional or Psychological Abuse- involves psychological abuse, verbal abuse, or mental injury and includes acts or omissions by loved ones or caregivers that have caused or could cause serious behavioral, cognitive, emotional, or mental disorders.

Final Recommendation: The definition of Psychological abuse should be adapted from the definition listed on the NCPEA website. The TEP recommends deletion of the word "emotional" and amendment of the definition of Psychological abuse to, "infliction of mental or emotional anguish by threat, humiliation, or other verbal or nonverbal conduct."

2. NASOP suggests that when a physician administers a screen, it is to be done privately with only the physician and elder in the room. Oklahoma APS also states the screening needs to occur without the caretaker or family member present.

Final Recommendation: The TEP feels that this decision should be left to the discretion of the clinician, based on the situation at hand. Implementing this type of refinement within the Elder Maltreatment measure may constrict the measure and limit the clinician in his/her assessment. The TEP recommends retaining the current language.

Public comments made by Oklahoma APS:

1. Many states use 60 as the threshold for the elderly. Oklahoma APS suggests lowering the age to 60. If the age stands for this instrument, then a similar instrument needs to be developed for 18-64 who have conditions such as, intellectual, physical, or emotional disabilities.

Final Recommendation: The TEP recommends the age criteria for this measure remain at 65 in order to maintain consistency with the Medicare Beneficiary age criteria. This measure is primarily reported for Medicare Beneficiaries and most likely not reported for those 60-64, despite some states using 60 to define the elderly.

The TEP recommends the development of an abuse measure for those 18 to 64 years old who have conditions such as, intellectual, physical, or emotional disabilities.

2. Self-neglect was not included in this measure and is often reported to APS. A distinct screening instrument is needed for self-neglect.

Final recommendation: The TEP supports and reaffirms the 2013 TEP's recommendation of the development of a self-neglect measure.

3. Utilizing this measure to support or refute the 2011 New York Prevalence Study

Final Recommendation: The TEP agreed that the primary goal is to ensure the measure is valid and accurate and can be used for quality improvement and comparative purposes. In addition, the TEP recognizes the value of this data for observational studies contributing to the elder maltreatment literature and would encourage health services researchers to undertake such an analysis.

4. Currently the reporting instructions state that this measure is to be reported once per reporting period. Oklahoma APS suggests the screening should be administered with each contact.

Final Recommendation: The TEP does not want to dictate how often the eligible provider is to report, nor place an undue reporting burden on the provider by changing the reporting frequency to every visit, but would like to recommend changing the reporting frequency to "at a minimum of once per reporting period."

5. The "not eligible" definitions include patients who refuse to participate and have decisional capacity for self-protection; this is a loophole which could be used to avoid reporting.

Final Recommendation: Currently the 2015 "not eligible" definition states "patient refuses to participate and has reasonable decisional capacity for self-protection," based on direction received during the 2014 TEP meeting regarding this topic. The TEP recommends retaining the current language.

6. For consistency, Oklahoma APS recommends one instrument to be used instead of allowing multiple elder abuse screening instruments.

Final Recommendation: There is no single instrument that captures all the forms of abuse. The TEP agreed that they would not limit the provider to using one tool to assess abuse within the measure.

All comments and recommendations will be reviewed during the 2016 annual specifications update.

SIGNATURE
CONSULTING GROUP

Physician Quality Measures Management (PQMM)
Final Public Comment Summary Report

Public Comment Verbatim Report

Date Posted	Text of Comments
9/23/14	The Harry and Jeanette Weinberg Center for Elder Abuse Prevention at the Hebrew Home at Riverdale, the nation's first elder abuse shelter within a long-term care community, applauds Measure 181- Elder Maltreatment Screening and Follow-Up Plan. Every client who enters the Hebrew Home's healthcare system, which includes long-term care, short term rehabilitation, MLTC, ALP, CHAA, LIKSA, independent living and social and medical day programs, is screened for elder abuse. The Weinberg Center team follows up on every positive result and helps create and implement a comprehensive care plan that addresses the emergent abuse. We believe that integrating elder abuse screening into healthcare services is critical, both in servicing specific clients who disclose abuse via the screening process as well as in bringing elder abuse out of the shadows for both clients and professionals and acknowledging its prevention's central place in any older adult's health care plan. We view this measure as an important step towards promulgating that message nationwide.
9/24/14	The National Association of State Long-Term Care Ombudsman Programs (NASOP) thanks the Centers for Medicare and Medicaid Services for this opportunity to comment on the Draft PQRS #181 Elder Maltreatment Screening and Follow-Up Plan. NASOP is supportive of this screening and would like to make the following comments: In the document entitled, *"Measure Information Form"*, under Numerator Details 5.6., Definitions: Emotional or Psychological Abuse, the definition provided states, "involves psychological abuse, verbal abuse, or mental injury and includes acts or omissions by loved ones or caregivers that have caused or could cause serious behavioral, cognitive, emotional, or mental disorders." NASOP suggests the CMS should not define the term "psychological abuse" with the words psychological abuse. NASOP recommends that the phrase "psychological abuse" be deleted from definition. NASOP suggests that when a physician administers this screen, it should be done privately with only the physician and elder in the room. The presence of third party (potential abuser) could inhibit victims from disclosing whether or not abuse is occurring. We appreciate the opportunity to provide these comments. Please do not hesitate to contact me for additional information or clarification.

Date Posted	Text of Comments
10/01/14	Screening for adult maltreatment by health care professionals is desperately needed. Often, health care professionals are the gatekeepers for vulnerable adults. One of the dynamics of adult maltreatment includes isolation. The caregiver who mistreats a vulnerable adult will continue to seek medical care under their watchful eye. The screening needs to occur without the caretaker or family member present. If someone other than the health care professional is present, the chances for a false negative are very high. The stated age is 65. Many states use 60 as the threshold for elderly. Oklahoma APS does not consider 'elderly' as a condition. If the age stands for this instrument, then a similar instrument needs to be developed for adults 18 to 64 who have conditions such as, intellectual, physical, or emotional disabilities. Self -neglect was not included in this instrument. Self-neglect is often identified by medical professionals and reported to APS. A distinct screening instrument is needed for self- neglect. The results of this instrument can be the springboard needed for research for a validated prevalence and incidence study such as the one conducted by Cornell University in New York. This report was published in May 2011 and included New York residents. Research on results of this instrument could be used to support or refute the New York prevalence study. Often maltreatment does not occur as singular incidents. Maltreatment is insidious, and over time escalates in types and severity. Polyvictimization not only includes multiple types of maltreatment co-occurring but also a history of maltreatment 'events' which occur over time. It is not unusual to find financial exploitation co-existing with neglect and abuse. This screening also needs to be evaluated over time, and administered with each contact with a health care professional. The instructions state that the measure is to be reported once during the reporting period. The 'not eligible' definitions include patients who refuse to participate and have decisional capacity for self- protection. In many states, health care professionals are mandatory reporters and as such do not need the patient's permission or cooperation to report suspicions of maltreatment. This is a loophole which could be used to avoid reporting due to a litany of reasons why health care professionals shy away from reporting. The numerator note states that any elder maltreatment screening tool may be used. For consistency, one instrument needs to be used instead of allowing multiple elder abuse screening instruments chosen by the health care profession. Comparing results of multiple instruments dilutes the results. Thank you for asking for comments. I believe this is a good start on conducting and collecting information nationally. The results of this inquiry will inspire additional research into the role of health care professionals in preventing and reducing the incidence of maltreatment of vulnerable adults.

Print

NATIONAL QUALITY FORUM

Patient Safety
Measure #2426
Measure Title
Elder Maltreatment Screening and Follow-Up Plan
Last Edit Date

Introduction

Thank you for your interest in submitting a measure to NQF for possible endorsement.

What criteria are used to evaluate measures? Measures are evaluated on standardized criteria: importance to measure and report, scientific acceptability of measure properties, feasibility, usability and use, and related and competing measures. For your measure to be evaluated against these measure evaluation criteria (http://www.qualityforum.org/docs/Measure_Evaluation_Criteria.aspx), you must complete the measure submission form.

Why do I have to complete a form? Due to the volume and/or complexity of proposed measures, NQF provides measure information to committee reviewers in a standardized format to facilitate their evaluation of whether the measure meets NQF's measure evaluation criteria (http://www.qualityforum.org/docs/Measure_Evaluation_Criteria.aspx). This form allows the measure steward to present information demonstrating that the proposed measure meets NQF's criteria.

What is on the form? The information requested in this form is directly related to NQF's measure evaluation criteria (http://www.qualityforum.org/docs/Measure_Evaluation_Criteria.aspx).

Can't I just submit our files for consideration? No. Measures must be submitted through the online form to be considered. Requested information should be entered directly into this form and the required attachments for evidence and measure testing.

Can I submit additional details and materials? Additional materials will be considered only as supplemental. Do NOT rely on material provided in an appendix to provide measure specifications or to demonstrate meeting the criteria. The core information needed to evaluate the measure should be provided in the appropriate submission form fields and required attachments. Please contact **the designated project staff** regarding questions about submitting supplemental materials.

What do I do first? When you first start a new submission by selecting the type of measure form (e.g., quality or resource use measure), you will be directed to the "NQF Conditions" tab, which lists the conditions that must be met before your proposed measures may be considered and evaluated for suitability as NQF-endorsed voluntary consensus standards. You are asked to acknowledge reading and accepting the conditions.

Can I come back later to complete a submission once I have started? Yes. You can return to your submission at your convenience to complete the form until the designated deadline for the specific project. To save and return, simply click on the save-draft option anytime during the submission process. When you want to continue, please login to the National Quality Forum website, go to your Dashboard, and click on submission.

Can I make changes to a form once I have submitted it? No. Once you submit your measure, you will NOT be able to return to this submission form to make further revisions. You will need to contact project staff.

What if I need additional help? Please contact the project staff identified in the call for measures if you have questions regarding the information requested or submitting supplemental materials.

Please email us at web-help@qualityforum.org if you experience technical difficulties using the online submission form.

Thank you for your interest in submitting measures to NQF.

NQF Conditions

Conditions that must be met for consideration by NQF
Several conditions must be met before proposed measures may be considered and evaluated for suitability as voluntary consensus standards. If any of the conditions are not met, the measure will not be accepted for consideration.
A. The measure is in the public domain or a Measure Steward Agreement is signed. (All non-government organizations must sign a Measure Steward Agreement even if measures are made publicly and freely available.)
B. The measure owner/steward verifies there is an identified responsible entity and a process to maintain and update the measure on a schedule that is commensurate with the rate of clinical innovation, but at least every three years.
C. The intended use of the measure includes both accountability applications (including public reporting) and performance improvement to achieve high-quality, efficient healthcare.
D. The measure is fully specified and tested for reliability and validity.
E. The measure developer/steward attests that harmonization with related measures and issues with competing measures have been considered and addressed, as appropriate.
F. The requested measure submission information is complete and responsive to the questions so that all the information needed to evaluate all criteria is provided.
Do you agree to the condiitons?
☑ I have read and accept the conditions as specified above *

Specifications

Descriptive Information
De.1. Measure Type *(Patient-reported outcomes include HRQoL/functional status, symptom/burden, experience with care, health-related behavior.)**
Process
De.2. Measure Title*
Elder Maltreatment Screening and Follow-Up Plan
De.3. Brief description of measure (*including type of score, measure focus, target population, timeframe, e.g., Percentage of adult patients aged 18-75 years receiving one or more HbA1c tests per year*)
Percentage of patients aged 65 years and older with a documented elder maltreatment screen using an Elder Maltreatment Screening Tool on the date of encounter AND a documented follow-up plan on the date of the positive screen
De.4. IF PAIRED/GROUPED, what is the reason this measure must be reported with other measures to appropriately interpret results?
Not paired
De.5. Subject/Topic Areas Subject/Topic Areas(Check all the areas that apply):

☑ Behavioral Health : Behavioral Health
☐ Behavioral Health : Alcohol, Substance e/Abuse
☐ Behavioral Health : Attention Deficit 'peractivity Disorder (ADHD)
☐ Behavioral Health : Depression
☐ Behavioral Health : Post-Traumatic Stress ›order (PTSD)
☑ Behavioral Health : Screening
☐ Behavioral Health : Serious Mental Illness
☐ Infectious Diseases : Hepatitis
☐ Infectious Diseases : Human Immunodeficiency Virus/Acquired mune Deficiency Syndrome (HIV/AIDS)
☐ Infectious Diseases : Immunization
☐ Infectious Diseases : Respiratory
☐ Infectious Diseases : Sexually Transmitted
☐ Infectious Diseases : Tuberculosis
☐ Infectious Diseases : Screening
☐ Mental Health : Mental Health
☐ Mental Health : Alcohol, Substance Use/Abuse

☐Behavioral Health : Suicide
☐Behavioral Health : Tobacco Use
☐Cancer : Cancer
☐Cancer : Bladder
☐Cancer : Breast
☐Cancer : Colorectal
☐Cancer : Gynecologic
☐Cancer : Hematologic
☐Cancer : Liver
☐Cancer : Lung, Esophageal
☐Cancer : Pancreatic
☐Cancer : Prostate
☐Cancer : Screening
☐Cancer : Skin
☐Cardiovascular : Cardiovascular
☐Cardiovascular : Acute Myocardial Infarction
☐Cardiovascular : Atrial Fibrillation
☐Cardiovascular : Congestive Heart Failure
☐Cardiovascular : Hyperlipidemia
☐Cardiovascular : Hypertension
☐Cardiovascular : Ischemic Heart Disease, Coronary Artery Disease
☐Cardiovascular : Percutaneous Coronary Intervention (PCI)
☐Cardiovascular : Screening
☐Endocrine : Endocrine
☐Endocrine : Diabetes
☐Endocrine : Screening
☐Endocrine : Thyroid Disorders
☐Gastrointestinal (GI) : Gastrointestinal (GI)
☐Gastrointestinal (GI) : Appendicitis
☐Gastrointestinal (GI) : Cirrhosis
☐Gastrointestinal (GI) : GI Bleeding
☐Gastrointestinal (GI) : Gall Bladder Disease
☐Gastrointestinal (GI) : Gastroenteritis
☐Gastrointestinal (GI) : Gastro-Esophageal Reflux Disease (GERD)
☐Gastrointestinal (GI) : Polyps
☐Gastrointestinal (GI) : Screening
☐Gastrointestinal (GI) : Peptic Ulcer
☐GU/GYN : GU/GYN
☐GU/GYN : Incontinence
☐GU/GYN : Screening
☐Head, Eyes, Ears, Nose, Throat (HEENT) : Head, Eyes, Ears, Nose, Throat (HEENT)
☐Head, Eyes, Ears, Nose, Throat (HEENT) : Dental
☐Head, Eyes, Ears, Nose, Throat (HEENT) : Ear Infection
☐Head, Eyes, Ears, Nose, Throat (HEENT) : Hearing
☐Head, Eyes, Ears, Nose, Throat (HEENT) : Pharyngitis
☐Head, Eyes, Ears, Nose, Throat (HEENT) : Screening
☐Head, Eyes, Ears, Nose, Throat (HEENT) : Vision
☐Infectious Diseases : Infectious Diseases
☐Mental Health : Depression
☑Mental Health : Domestic Violence
☐Mental Health : Serious Mental Illness
☐Mental Health : Suicide
☐Musculoskeletal : Musculoskeletal
☐Musculoskeletal : Osteoarthritis
☐Musculoskeletal : Rheumatoid Arthritis
☐Musculoskeletal : Hip/Pelvic Fracture
☐Musculoskeletal : Joint Surgery
☐Musculoskeletal : Low Back Pain
☐Musculoskeletal : Osteoporosis
☐Neurology : Neurology
☐Neurology : Brain Injury
☐Neurology : Cognitive Impairment/Dementia
☐Neurology : Delirium
☐Neurology : Stroke/Transient Ischemic Attack (TIA)
☐Perinatal and Reproductive Health : Perinatal and Reproductive Health
☐Perinatal and Reproductive Health : Gynecology
☐Perinatal and Reproductive Health : Newborn
☐Perinatal and Reproductive Health : Perinatal
☐Perinatal and Reproductive Health : Screening
☐Prevention : Prevention
☐Prevention : Development/Wellness
☐Prevention : Immunization
☐Prevention : Malnutrition
☐Prevention : Obesity
☐Prevention : Physical Activity
☐Prevention : Screening
☐Prevention : Tobacco Use
☐Pulmonary/Critical Care : Pulmonary/Critical Care
☐Pulmonary/Critical Care : Asthma
☐Pulmonary/Critical Care : Chronic Obstructive Pulmonary Disease (COPD)
☐Pulmonary/Critical Care : Critical Care
☐Pulmonary/Critical Care : Dyspnea
☐Pulmonary/Critical Care : Pneumonia
☐Pulmonary/Critical Care : Sleep Apnea
☐Renal : Renal
☐Renal : Chronic Kidney Disease (CKD)
☐Renal : End Stage Renal Disease (ESRD)
☐Surgery : Surgery
☐Surgery : Cardiac Surgery
☐Surgery : General Surgery
☐Surgery : Perioperative
☐Surgery : Thoracic Surgery
☐Surgery : Vascular Surgery

De.6. Cross Cutting Areas Cross Cutting Areas(Check all the areas that apply):
☐Health and Functional Status : Health and Functional Status☐Disparities

- [ ] Health and Functional Status : Development/Wellness
- [ ] Health and Functional Status : Functional Status
- [ ] Prevention : Prevention
- [ ] Prevention : Immunization
- [ ] Prevention : Nutrition
- [ ] Prevention : Obesity
- [ ] Prevention : Physical Activity
- [x] Prevention : Screening
- [ ] Prevention : Social Determinants
- [ ] Access
- [ ] Care Coordination : Care Coordination
- [ ] Care Coordination : Readmissions
- [ ] Functional Status
- [ ] Overuse
- [ ] Palliative Care and End of Life Care
- [ ] Patient and Family Engagement
- [x] Safety : Safety
- [ ] Safety : Complications
- [ ] Safety : Healthcare Associated Infections
- [ ] Safety : Medication Safety
- [ ] Safety : Venous Thromboembolism
- [ ] Safety : Readmissions
- [ ] Safety : Workforce

Measure Specifications

S.1. Measure-specific Web Page *(Provide a URL link to a web page specific for this measure that contains current detailed specifications including code lists, risk model details, and supplemental materials. Do not enter a URL linking to a home page or to general information.)*

Under the subheading "Individual Measures" select the link entitled "2014 PQRS Individual Claims Registry Measure Specification Supporting Document; this link will open a zip file containing the 2014 PQRS measure specifications

S.2a. HQMF specificationsIf this is an eMeasure, HQMF specifications must be attached. Attach the output from the eMeasure authoring tool (MAT) - if the MAT was not used, contact staff. (Use the specification fields in this online form for the plain-language description of the specifications)

○ Available in attached file

○ No HQMF specs

S.2b. Data Dictionary, Code Table, or Value Sets *(and risk model codes and coefficients when applicable) must be attached. (Excel or csv file in the suggested format preferred - if not, contact staff. Provide descriptors for any codes. Use one file with multiple worksheets as needed.)*

◉ Available in attached Excel or csv file

Data_Dictionary-Code_Descriptions-635254597070481973.xlsx

○ No data dictionary/code table - all information provided in the submission form

S.3. For endorsement maintenance, please briefly describe any changes to the measure specifications since last endorsement date and explain the reasons.

S.4. Numerator Statement *(Brief, narrative description of the measure focus or what is being measured about the target population, i.e., cases from the target population with the target process, condition, event, or outcome)*

IF an OUTCOME MEASURE, state the outcome being measured. Calculation of the risk-adjusted outcome should be described in the calculation algorithm (S.18).

Patients with a documented elder maltreatment screen using an Elder Maltreatment Screening Tool on the date of the encounter and follow-up plan documented on the date of the positive screen

S.5. Time Period for Data *(What is the time period in which data will be aggregated for the measure, e.g., 12 mo, 3 years, look back to August for flu vaccination? Note if there are different time periods for the numerator and denominator.)*

This measure is to be reported once during the reporting period for patients seen during the reporting period. The reporting period is 12 months from January 1st to December 31st

S.6. Numerator Details *(All information required to identify and calculate the cases from the target population with the target process, condition, event, or outcome such as definitions, specific data collection items/responses, code/value sets - Note: lists of individual codes with descriptors that exceed 1 page should be provided in an Excel or csv file in required format at S.2b)*

IF an OUTCOME MEASURE, describe how the observed outcome is identified/counted. Calculation of the risk-adjusted outcome should be described in the calculation algorithm (S.18).

Definitions:

Screen for Elder Maltreatment - An elder maltreatment screen should include assessment and documentation of all of the following components: (1) physical abuse, (2) emotional or psychological abuse, (3) neglect (active or passive), (4) sexual abuse, (5) abandonment, (6) financial or material exploitation and (7) unwarranted control.

Physical Abuse - Infliction of physical injury by punching, beating, kicking, biting, burning, shaking, or other actions that result in harm.

Emotional or Psychological Abuse - Involves psychological abuse, verbal abuse, or mental injury and includes acts or omissions by loved ones or caregivers that have caused or could cause serious behavioral, cognitive, emotional, or mental disorders.

Neglect - Involves attitudes of others or actions caused by others-such as family members, friends, or institutional

caregivers-that have an extremely detrimental effect upon well-being.
Active - Behavior that is willful or when the caregiver intentionally withholds care or necessities. The neglect may be motivated by financial gain or reflect interpersonal conflicts.
Passive - Situations where the caregiver is unable to fulfill his or her care giving responsibilities as a result of illness, disability, stress, ignorance, lack of maturity, or lack of resources.
Sexual Abuse - The forcing of undesired sexual behavior by one person upon another against their will who are either competent or unable to fully comprehend and/or give consent. This may also be called molestation.
Elder Abandonment - Desertion of an elderly person by an individual who has assumed responsibility for providing care for an elder, or by a person with physical custody of an elder.
Financial or Material Exploitation - Taking advantage of a person for monetary gain or profit.
Unwarranted Control - Controlling a person's ability to make choices about living situations, household finances, and medical care.
Follow-Up Plan - Must include a documented report to state or local Adult Protective Services (APS) agency. Note: APS does not have jurisdiction in all states to investigate maltreatment of patients in long-term care facilities. In those states where APS does not have jurisdiction, APS may refer the provider to another state agency -- such as the state facility licensure agency - for appropriate reporting. Federal reporting: In addition to state requirements, some types of providers are required by federal law to report suspected maltreatment. For example, nursing facilities certified by Medicare and/or Medicaid are required to report suspected maltreatment to the applicable State Survey and Certification Agency.
For state-specific information to report suspected elder maltreatment, including self neglect, the following resources are available:
1. National Adult Protective Services Association- http://www.napsa-now.org/get-help/help-in-your-area/
2. Eldercare Locater: 1-800-677-1116 www.eldercare.gov
3. National Center on Elder Abuse
http://www.ncea.aoa.gov/NCEAroot/Main_Site/Find_Help/State_Resources.aspx

Not Eligible - A patient is not eligible if one or more of the following reasons is documented:
1. Patient refuses to participate
2. Patient is in an urgent or emergent situation where time is of the essence and to delay treatment would jeopardize the patient's health status

NUMERATOR NOTE: Documentation of an elder maltreatment screening must include identification of the tool used. Examples of screening tools for elder maltreatment include, but are not limited to: Elder Abuse Suspicion Index (EASI), Vulnerability to Abuse Screening Scale (VASS) and Hwalek-Sengstock Elder Abuse Screening Test (H-S/EAST).

G-codes are a defined as Quality Data Codes (QDCs), which are subset of HCPCs II codes. QDCs are non billable codes that providers will use to delineate their clinical quality actions, which are submitted with Medicare Part B Claims. There are 6 G-code options for this measure

Elder Maltreatment Screen Documented as Positive AND Follow-Up Plan Documented
G8733: Elder maltreatment screen documented as positive AND a follow-up is plan is documented
OR
Elder Maltreatment Screen Documented as Negative, Follow-Up Plan not Required
G8734: Elder maltreatment screen documented as negative, follow-up is not required
OR
Elder Maltreatment Screen not Documented, Patient not Eligible
G8535: Elder maltreatment screen not documented; documentation patient is not eligible for the elder maltreatment screen
OR
Elder Maltreatment Screen Documented as Positive, Follow-Up Plan not Documented, Patient not Eligible for Follow-Up Plan
G8941: Elder Maltreatment Screen Documented as positive, follow-up plan is not documented. Documentation that the patient is not eligible for follow-up plan
OR
Elder Maltreatment Screen not Documented, Reason not Given
G8536: No documentation of an elder maltreatment screen, reason not given
OR
Elder Maltreatment Screen Documented as Positive, Follow-Up Plan not Documented, Reason not Given
G8735: Elder maltreatment screen documented as positive, follow-up plan not documented, reason not given

S.7. Denominator Statement *(Brief, narrative description of the target population being measured)*
IF an OUTCOME MEASURE, state the target population for the outcome. Calculation of the risk-adjusted outcome should be described in the calculation algorithm (S.18).
All patients aged 65 years and older
S.8. Target Population Category *(Check all the populations for which the measure is specified and tested if any):*
☐Children's Health
☐Maternal Health
☐Populations at Risk : Populations at Risk
☐Populations at Risk : Dual eligible beneficiaries
☐Populations at Risk : Individuals with multiple chronic conditions
☐Populations at Risk : Veterans
☑Senior Care
S.9. Denominator Details *(All information required to identify and calculate the target population/denominator such as definitions, specific data collection items/responses , code/value sets - Note: lists of individual codes with descriptors that exceed 1 page should be provided in an Excel or csv file in required format at S.2b)*
IF an OUTCOME MEASURE, describe how the target population is identified. Calculation of the risk-adjusted outcome should be described in the calculation algorithm (S.18).
Patients aged = 65 years on date of encounter. Patient encounter during the reporting period (CPT or HCPCS): 90791, 90792,90832, 90834, 90837, 96116, 96150, 96151, 97003, 97802, 97803, 99201, 99202, 99203, 99204, 99205, 99212, 99213, 99214, 99215, 99304, 99305, 99306, 99307, 99308, 99309, 99310, 99318, 99324, 99325, 99326, 99327, 99328, 99334, 99335, 99336, 99337, 99341, 99342, 99343, 99344, 99345, 99347, 99348, 99349, 99350, G0101, G0270, G0402, G0438, G0439
S.10. Denominator Exclusions *(Brief narrative description of exclusions from the target population)*
A patient is not eligible if one or more of the following reasons is documented: Patient refuses to participate; Patient is in an urgent or emergent situation where time is of the essence and to delay treatment would jeopardize the patient's health status
S.11. Denominator Exclusion Details *(All information required to identify and calculate exclusions from the denominator such as definitions, specific data collection items/responses, code/value sets - Note: lists of individual codes with descriptors that exceed 1 page should be provided in an Excel or csv file in required format at S.2b)*
G8535: Elder maltreatment screen not documented; documentation the patient is not eligible for the elder maltreatment screen
S.12. Stratification Details/Variables *(All information required to stratify the measure results including the stratification variables, definitions, specific data collection items/responses, code/value sets - Note: lists of individual codes with descriptors that exceed 1 page should be provided in an Excel or csv file in required format with at S.2b)*
Not stratified
S.13. Risk Adjustment Type (Select type. Provide specifications for risk stratification in S.12 and for statistical model in S.14-15)
No risk adjustment or risk stratification
S.13a. If "Other", please describe:*
S.14. Identify the statistical risk model method and variables *(Name the statistical method - e.g., logistic regression and list all the risk factor variables. Note - risk model development and testing should be addressed with measure testing under Scientific Acceptability)*
No risk model
S.15. Detailed risk model specifications *(including coefficients, equations, codes with descriptors, and definitions. Note: if exceed 1 page, should be provided on a separate worksheet in the excel or csv file with data dictionary/code table at S.2b.)*

○ Available in attached Excel or csv file at S.2b

○ Provided in response box S.15a

S.15a. Detailed risk model specifications (if not provided in excel or csv file at S.2b) Detailed risk model specifications *(if not provided in excel or csv file at S.2b)*
S.16. Type of score:
Rate/proportion
S.16a. If "Other", please describe:
S.17. Interpretation of Score *(Classifies interpretation of score according to whether better quality is associated with a higher score, a lower score, a score falling within a defined interval, or a passing score)*
Better quality = Higher score
S.18. Calculation Algorithm/Measure Logic *(Describe the calculation of the measure score as an ordered sequence of steps including identifying the target population; exclusions; cases meeting the target process, condition, event, or outcome; aggregating data; risk adjustment; etc.)*
Performance Calculation: For performance purposes, this measure is calculated by creating a fraction with the following components: Numerator, Performance Denominator and Denominator Exclusions.

Numerator (A) Includes: Number of patients meeting numerator criteria
Performance Denominator (PD) Includes: Number of patients meeting criteria for denominator inclusion
Denominator Exclusions (B) Include: Number of patients with valid denominator exclusions
The method of performance calculation is determined by the following: 1) identify the patients who meet the eligibility criteria for the denominator (PD) which includes patients who are 65 years and older with an appropriate encounter, 2) identify which of those patients meet the numerator criteria (A); and 3) for those patients who do not meet the numerator criteria, determine whether an appropriate exclusion applies (B) and subtract those patients from the denominator.

Numerator (A) / (Performance Denominator (PD) - Denominator Exclusions (B))

Exclusion Calculation - The percentage of Denominator Valid (PD) patients with Denominator Exclusions (B).

Denominator Exclusions (B)/ Performance Denominator (PD)
S.19. Calculation Algorithm/Measure Logic Diagram URL or Attachment *(You also may provide a diagram of the Calculation Algorithm/Measure Logic described above at measure-specific Web page URL identified in S.1 OR in attached appendix)*

○ Available at measure-specific web page URL identified in S.1

○ Available in attached appendix at A.1

◉ No diagram provided
S.20. Sampling *(If measure is based on a sample, provide instructions for obtaining the sample and guidance on minimum sample size.)*
IF a PRO-based performance measure (PRO-PM), identify whether (and how) proxy responses are allowed.
Based on the entire population of providers reporting this measure with a total of 558 valid claims, it was decided that the entire population of providers would be sampled for the reliability testing. A maximum of 15 records were randomly selected from the population. This limitation was set so that the providers would not see this task as too burdensome and would be more likely to send in their records. A simple random sample of records for the 23 NPIs was drawn. From those 23 NPIs, a random sample of approximately 216 claims was identified.
S.21. Survey/Patient-reported data *(If measure is based on a survey, provide instructions for conducting the survey and guidance on minimum response rate.)*
IF a PRO-PM, specify calculation of response rates to be reported with performance measure results.
N/A
S.22. Missing data (specify how missing data are handled, e.g., imputation, delete case.)
Required for Composites, PRO-PMs, and eMeasures.
N/A
S.23. Data Source *(Check ONLY the sources for which the measure is SPECIFIED AND TESTED).*
If other, please describe in 2a1.26.

☑ Administrative claims
☐ Electronic Clinical Data : Electronic Clinical Data
☐ Electronic Clinical Data : Electronic Health Record
☐ Electronic Clinical Data : Imaging/Diagnostic Study
☐ Electronic Clinical Data : Laboratory
☐ Electronic Clinical Data : Pharmacy
☐ Electronic Clinical Data : Registry
☐ Healthcare Provider Survey
☐ Management Data
☑ Paper Medical Records
☐ Patient Reported Data/Survey
☐ Other

S.24. Data Source or Collection Instrument *(Identify the specific data source/data collection instrument e.g. name of database, clinical registry, collection instrument, etc.)*
IF a PRO-PM, identify the specific PROM(s); and standard methods, modes, and languages of administration.
Medicare Part B claims data
S.25. Data Source or Collection Instrument *(available at measure-specific Web page URL identified in S.1 OR in attached appendix)*

○ Available at measure-specific web page URL identified in S.1

○ Available in attached appendix at A.1

◉ No data collection instrument provided
S.26. Level of Analysis *(Check ONLY the levels of analysis for which the measure is SPECIFIED AND TESTED)*

☑ Clinician : Individual
☑ Clinician : Group/Practice
☐ Clinician : Team
☐ Facility
☐ Health Plan
☐ Population : Community
☐ Population : County or City
☐ Population : National
☐ Population : Regional

☐Integrated Delivery System☐Population : State

S.27. Care Setting *(Check ONLY the settings for which the measure is SPECIFIED AND TESTED)*

☐Ambulatory Care : Ambulatory Surgery Center (ASC)
☑Ambulatory Care : Clinician Office/Clinic
☐Ambulatory Care : Outpatient Rehabilitation
☐Ambulatory Care : Urgent Care
☐Behavioral Health/Psychiatric : Inpatient
☑Behavioral Health/Psychiatric : Outpatient
☐Dialysis Facility
☐Emergency Medical Services/Ambulance
☐Home Health
☐Hospice
☐Hospital/Acute Care Facility
☐Imaging Facility
☐Laboratory
☐Pharmacy
☐Post Acute/Long Term Care Facility : Nursing Home/Skilled Nursing Facility
☐Post Acute/Long Term Care Facility : Inpatient Rehabilitation Facility
☐Post Acute/Long Term Care Facility : Long Term Acute Care Hospital
☐Other

S.27a. If "Other", please describe*
undefined

S.28. COMPOSITE Performance Measure - Additional Specifications *(Use this section as needed for aggregation and weighting rules, or calculation of individual performance measures if not individually endorsed.)*

Importance

Importance to Measure and Report is a threshold criterion that must be met in order to recommend a measure for endorsement. All three subcriteria must be met to pass this criterion. See guidance on evidence.
Evidence (Measure evaluation criterion 1a)
1a. Attach evidence submission form (Click here to download Evidence Submission Form Template)
Elder_Maltreatment_MeasSubm_Evidence.docx

Performance Gap - Opportunity for Improvement (Measure evaluation criterion 1b)
1b.1. Briefly explain the rationale for this measure (e.g., the benefits or improvements in quality envisioned by use of this measure)
IF a COMPOSITE (e.g., combination of component measure scores, all-or-none, any-or-none), SKIP this question and answer the composite questions.
The aim of this quality measure is to assist eligible providers to identify suspected cases of elder maltreatment and refer these cases to the appropriate agency(s) for assessment and/or intervention for those who are being abused will receive services to stop the abuse. Elder maltreatment is prevalent and underreported. As a result of this, there is an increased rate of hospitalization and use of healthcare resources. As cited in Dong (2011), the Government Accounting Office reported spending $11.9 million dollars in 2009 for all activities related to elder abuse and this amount was not enough to provide basic protection for older adults from abuse, neglect and exploitation. Ultimately, halting abuse will improve the quality of life for these individuals and reduce the cost and use of healthcare resources.
1b.2. Provide performance scores on the measure as specified (**current and over time**) at the specified level of analysis. (This is required for endorsement maintenance. Include mean, std dev, min, max, interquartile range, scores by decile. Describe the data source including number of measured entities; number of patients; dates of data; if a sample, characteristics of the entities include). This information also will be used to address the subcriterion on improvement (4b.1) under Usability and Use.
N/A
1b.3. **If no or limited performance data on the measure as specified is reported in 1b2**, then provide a summary of data from the literature that indicates opportunity for improvement or overall less than optimal performance **on the specific focus of measurement.** Include citations.
N/A
1b.4. **Provide disparities data from the measure as specified (current and over time)** by population group, e.g., by race/ethnicity, gender, age, insurance status, socioeconomic status, and/or disability. (This is required for endorsement maintenance. Describe the data source including number of measured entities; number of patients; dates of data; if a sample, characteristics of the entities include.) This information also will be used to address the subcriterion on improvement (4b.1) under Usability and Use.

N/A
1b.5. **If no or limited data on disparities from the measure as specified is reported in 1b4**, then provide a summary of data from the literature that addresses disparities **in care on the specific focus of measurement.** Include citations.
N/A
High Priority (Measure evaluation criterion 1c)
1c.1. Demonstrated high priority aspect of healthcare

- [x] Affects large numbers
- [ ] Patient/societal consequences of poor quality
- [ ] A leading cause of morbidity/mortality
- [ ] Severity of illness
- [ ] Frequently performed procedure
- [ ] Other
- [x] High resource use

1c.2. If "Other", please describe:*
1c.3. Provide epidemiologic or resource use data that demonstrates the measure addresses a high priority aspect of healthcare). List citations in 1c.4.
"Most cases of elder abuse go unidentified and unreported" (Cohen, 2011, p.261). Elder maltreatment is prevalent and occurs predominantly in the community, not in nursing care facilities. One in ten seniors reported being abused, neglected or exploited in the past twelve months; 5.2% for financial abuse, 4.6% for emotional, 1.6% for physical abuse and 0.6% for sexual abuse. Financial exploitation by family members and by strangers was increased among the more physically disabled adults (Aceirno et al., 2010). Elder Abuse and Neglect: In Search of Solutions (2013), reports that every year an estimated 4 million older Americans are victims of physical, psychological, or other forms of abuse and neglect, and for every reported case there may be as many as 23 unreported. Although less prevalent, patients in nursing homes do experience maltreatment.
There are many complex reasons for underreporting; minimal screening, a lack of knowledge and skills for interventions (Cohen, 2011) on the part of health care providers and failure of the abused patient to report due to fear of retaliation by the abuser (APA, 2010), inability of the victim to report due to a cognitive deficit or initiating family discord. This lack of identifying victims of elder abuse leads to increased rates of hospitalization (Dong & Simon, 2013), morbidity (Cohen, 2011), mortality (Dong, et al., 2009) and admission into a nursing home (Lachs et al., 2011). These outcomes are costly. As cited in Dong (2011), the Government Accounting Office reported spending $11.9 million dollars in 2009 for all activities related to elder abuse and this amount was not enough to provide basic protection for older adults from abuse, neglect and exploitation. It is clear that additional screening, education of victims and health care providers and financial support is needed in order to unveil the depth of the problem and provide aid those who are being abused and neglected.
1c.4. Citations for data demonstrating high priority provided in 1c.3

Acierno, R., Hernandez, M.A., Amstadter, A.B., Resnick, H.S., Steve, K., Muzzy, W. & Kilpatrick, D.G. (2010). Prevalence and correlates of emotional, physical, sexual, and financial abuse and potential neglect in the United States: The national elder mistreatment study. American Journal of Public Health, 100, 292–297. doi:10.2105/AJPH.2009.163089

American Psychological Association (2013). Elder Abuse and Neglect: In Search of Solutions. Retrieved from http://www.apa.org/pi/aging/resources/guides/elder-abuse.aspx

American Psychological Association (2010). Elder Abuse and Neglect: In Search of Solutions. Retrieved from http://www.apa.org/pi/aging/resources/guides/elder-abuse.aspx

Cohen, M. (2011). Screening tools for the identification of elder abuse. Journal of Clinical Outcomes Management. 18(6), 261-270

Dong. X., & Simon, M. A. (2011). Enhancing national policy and programs to address elder abuse. JAMA: The Journal of the American Medical Association, 305(23), 2460-2461. doi: 10.1001/jama.2011.835.

Dong, X. & Simon, M.A. (2013). Elder abuse as a risk factor for hospitalization in older persons. JAMA: The Journal of the American Medical Association. doi:10.1001/jamainternmed.2013.238

Dong, X., Simon, M., Mendes de Leon, C., Fulmer, T., Beck, T., Hebert, L., . . . Evans, D. (2009). Elder self-neglect and abuse and mortality risk in a community-dwelling population. JAMA : The Journal of the American Medical Association, 302(5), 517-526. doi: 10.1001/jama.2009.1109.

1c.5. IF a PRO-PM (e.g. HRQoL/functional status, symptom/burden, experience with care, health-related behaviors), provide evidence that the target population values the measured PRO and finds it meaningful. (Describe how and from whom their input was obtained.)
N/A

Scientific Acceptability

Testing Attachment
2.1. Attach measure testing form (Click to here to download the Measure Testing Submission Form OR the Composite Measure Testing Form.)
Elder_maltreatment_MeasSubm_MeasTesting.docx

Feasibility

Extent to which the required data are readily available, retrievable without undue burden, and can be implemented for performance measurement.
Data Elements Generated as Byproduct of Care Processes (Measure evaluation criterion 3a)
3a.1. How are the data elements needed to compute measure scores generated? (Check all that apply)
Data used in the measure are:
☑ Generated "or collected" by and used by healthcare personnel during the provision of care (e.g., blood pressure, lab value, diagnosis, "depression score")
☑ Coded by someone other than person obtaining original information (e.g., DRG, ICD-9 codes on claims)
☑ Abstracted from a record by someone other than person obtaining original information (e.g., chart abstraction for quality measure or registry)
☐ Other
3a.2. If "Other", please describe:*
Electronic Sources (Measure evaluation criterion 3b)
3b.1. To what extent are the specified data elements available electronically in defined fields (**The specified data elements available electronically in defined fields***i.e., data elements that are needed to compute the performance measure score are in defined, computer-readable fields*)

○ ALL data elements are in defined fields in electronic health records (EHRs)

○ ALL data elements are in defined fields in electronic claims

○ ALL data elements are in defined fields in electronic clinical data (e.g., clinical registry, nursing home MDS, home health OASIS)

○ ALL data elements are in defined fields in a combination of electronic sources

○ Some data elements are in defined fields in electronic sources

◉ No data elements are in defined fields in electronic sources

3b.2. If ALL the data elements needed to compute the performance measure score are not from electronic sources, specify a credible, near-term path to electronic capture, OR provide a rationale for using other than electronic sources.
Some data elements are in electronic sources... For this test in 2010, the majority of providers were still documenting on a paper based product.
3b.3. If this is an eMeasure, provide a summary of the feasibility assessment in an attached file or make available at a measure-specific URL. If this is an eMeasure, provide a summary of the feasibility assessment in an attached file or make available at a measure-specific URL.

○ Available at measure-specific web page URL identified in S.1

○ Available in attached file

○ No feasibility assessment

Data Collection Strategy (Measure evaluation criterion 3c)
3c.1. Describe what you have learned/modified as a result of testing and/or operational use of the measure regarding data collection, availability of data, missing data, timing and frequency of data collection, sampling, patient confidentiality, time and cost of data collection, other feasibility/implementation issues.
IF a PRO-PM, consider implications for both individuals providing PRO data (patients, service recipients, respondents) and those whose performance is being measured.
Quality Insights of Pennsylvania (Quality Insights obtained data 202 randomly generated Medicare Part B claims records for all 23 unique NPIs/eligible professionals who reported one of the G-codes for the measure during the 1/1/2010 - 6/30/2010 time period. As stated in 2a2.4 reliability testing demonstrated disparate agreement rates observed between IRR vs. Claims. This disparity suggests that providers are using a broad interpretation of what

needs to be included in the medical record to document the eight components that comprise the screening. Modifications have been made to the specifications which are intended to improve claims reliability. These changes are being applied to the 2014 version of the specifications.

Lessons Learned from operational use Underutilization of this measure was thought to be the result of a poorly defined 'follow-up plan' and the requirement that the patient screening included all 8 components of abuse. In addition, no single tool exists no screening tool exists which addresses all 8 types of abuse which adds burden to the implementation of the measure. Also, there was no requirement for the use of an Elder Maltreatment screening tool. As a result of these findings, the following modifications were made to the measure: (1)('self-neglect' was removed as a screening component due to the discordant nature of this form of abuse as compared to the other 7 types of abuse (self-abuse vs. abuse by another individual), (2) removed the requirement that all types of abuse must be part of the screening process allowing the practitioner to select from a number of available screening tools (examples of elder abuse screening tools which were vetted by subject matter experts in the Elder Maltreatment Technical Expert Panel (TEP)) and (3) the follow-up plan was modified to include a report to a state or local Adult Protective Services or another appropriate state or federal agency as guided by law for positive screens. In addition, state specific contact information (organization names, websites, phone numbers) were included to facilitate the reporting process.
3c.2. Describe any fees, licensing, or other requirements to use any aspect of the measure as specified (e.g., value/code set, risk model, programming code, algorithm)?
N/A

Usability and Use

Extent to which intended audiences (e.g., consumers, purchasers, providers, policy makers) can understand the results of the measure and are likely to find them useful for decision making.
NQF-endorsed measures are expected to be used in at least one accountability application within 3 years and publicly reported within 6 years of initial endorsement in addition to performance improvement.
4.1. Current and Planned Use *(check all the current and planned uses; for any current uses that are checked, provide a program name and URL for the specific program)*
Current and Planned Use

Use	Planned	Current	For current use, provide Program Name and URL
a. Public Reporting	○	◉	Program Name:* Physician Quality Reporting System URL:* http://www.cms.gov/PQRS
b. Public Health/Disease Surveillance	○	○	Program Name:* URL:*
c. Payment Program	○	◉	Program Name:* Physician Quality Reporting System URL:* http://www.cms.gov/PQRS
d. Regulatory and Accreditation Programs	○	○	Program Name:* URL:*
e. Professional Certification or Recognition Program	○	○	Program Name:* URL:*
f. Quality Improvement with Benchmarking (external benchmarking to multiple organizations)	○	○	Program Name:* URL:*
g. Quality Improvement (Internal to the specific organization)	○	○	Program Name:* URL:*

h. Not in use	○
i. Use Unknown	○

Accountability/Transparency (measure evaluation criterion 4a)
4a.1. For each CURRENT use, checked above, provide:

- Name of program and sponsor
- Purpose
- Geographic area and number and percentage of accountable entities and patients included

Name of program and sponsor
Public Use: Physician Quality Reporting System is sponsored by Centers for Medicare and Medicaid Services; PQRS is a national reporting program that uses a combination of incentive payments and payment adjustments to promote reporting of quality information by eligible professionals (EPs). The program provides an incentive payment to practices with EPs. EPs satisfactorily report data on quality measures for covered Physician Fee Schedule (PFS) services furnished to Medicare Part B Fee-for-Service (FFS) beneficiaries.
Refer to the following link for additional information: http://www.cms.gov/PQRS
4a.2. If not currently publicly reported OR used in at least one other accountability application (e.g., payment program, certification, licensing) what are the reasons? (*e.g., Do policies or actions of the developer/steward or accountable entities restrict access to performance results or impede implementation?*)
Accountability application
N/A
4a.3. If not currently publicly reported OR used in at least one other accountability application, provide a credible plan for implementation within the expected timeframes -- any accountability application within 3 years and publicly reported within 6 years of initial endorsement. (*Credible plan includes the specific program, purpose, intended audience, and timeline for implementing the measure within the specified timeframes. A plan for accountability applications addresses mechanisms for data aggregation and reporting.*)
Credible plan
N/A
Improvement (measure evaluation criterion 4b)
4b.1. Progress on Improvement. (Not required for initial endorsement unless available.)
Performance results on this measure (current and over time) should be provided in 1b.2 and 1b.4. Discuss:

- Progress (trends in performance results, number and percentage of people receiving high-quality healthcare)
- Geographic area and number and percentage of accountable entities and patients included

Progress on Improvement
N/A
4b.2. If no improvement was demonstrated, what are the reasons? If not in use for performance improvement at the time of initial endorsement, provide a credible rationale that describes how the performance results could be used to further the goal of high-quality, efficient healthcare for individuals or populations.
Credible rationale
N/A
Unintended Consequences (measure evaluation criterion 4c)
4c.1. Were any unintended negative consequences to individuals or populations identified during testing; OR has evidence of unintended negative consequences to individuals or populations been reported since implementation? If so, identify the negative unintended consequences and describe how benefits outweigh them or actions taken to mitigate them.
Any unintended negative consequences
No

Related and Competing Measures

If a measure meets the above criteria and there are endorsed or new related measures (either the same measure focus or the same target population) or competing measures (both the same measure focus and the same target population), the measures are compared to address harmonization and/or selection of the best measure.
Relation to Other NQF-endorsed® Measures (Measure evaluation criterion 5)
Are there related measures (conceptually, either same measure focus or target population) or competing measures (conceptually both the same measure focus and same target population)? If yes, list the NQF # and title of all related and/or competing measures. (Can search and select measures.)Related Measure

○ Yes

◉ No

5.1a.

Related Measure(s):
5.1b. If related or competing measures are not NQF endorsed please indicate measure title and steward.Non endorsed measures
Harmonization (Measure evaluation criterion 5a)
5a.1. If this measure conceptually addresses EITHER the same measure focus OR the same target population as NQF-endorsed measure(s):
Are the measure specifications completely harmonized?

○ Yes

○ No

5a.2. If the measure specifications are not completely harmonized, identify the differences, rationale, and impact on interpretability and data collection burden.
Competing Measure(s) (Measure evaluation criterion 5b)
5b.1. If this measure conceptually addresses both the same measure focus and the same target population as NQF-endorsed measure(s):
Describe why this measure is superior to competing measures (e.g., a more valid or efficient way to measure quality); OR provide a rationale for the additive value of endorsing an additional measure. (Provide analyses when possible.)

Additional

Authorized Users
Developer Steward

Steward	Developer	Username	First Name	Last Name	Organization
○	◉	JSHRIFT	Jeannette	Shrift	Quality Insights of Pennsylvania

View / Edit My Account
Appendix
A.1. Supplemental materials may be provided in an appendix. Supplemental Materials
All supplemental materials (such as data collection instrument or methodology reports) should be organized in one file with a table of contents or bookmarks. If material pertains to a specific submission form number that should be indicated. Requested information should be provided in the submission form and measure testing attachment. There is no guarantee that supplemental materials will be reviewed.

○ Available at measure-specific web page URL identified in S.1

◉ Available in attached file
Elder_Maltreatment_Summary_Materials-635255523288135916.docx

○ No appendix
Contact Information
Co.1. Steward Point of Contact
Co.1.1. Organization
Centers for Medicare & Medicaid

Co.1.2. First Name
Sophia
Co.1.3. Last Name
Autrey
Co.1.4. Email Address
sophia.autrey@cms.hhs.gov
Co.1.5. Phone Number
(
410
)
786
-
2004
ext.
Co.2. Developer Point of Contact
☑*Uncheck to Edit*
Co.2.1. Organization
Centers for Medicare & Medicaid
Co.2.2. First Name
Sophia
Co.2.3. Last Name
Autrey
Co.2.4. Email Address
sophia.autrey@cms.hhs.gov
Co.2.5. Phone Number
(
410
)
786
-
2004
ext.
Additional Information
Ad.1. Workgroup/Expert Panel Involved in Measure Development
List the workgroup/panel members' names and organizations.
Describe the members' role in measure development.
Through a collaborative process, the Technical Expert Panel (TEP) reviewed the current 2013 measure specifications (description, numerator, denominator, definitions, clinical recommendation, and environmental scan); reviewed and considered the Beta Testing results, analysis, finding and recommendations based on testing.
Jean Carter, PhD, TEP Member, Washington Psychological Center, P.C., Washington, DC

Mirean Coleman, MSW, LICSW, CT, TEP Member, National Association for Social Workers, Washington, DC

Susan M. Levy, MD, TEP Member, Levindale Hebrew Geriatric Center and Hospital, Baltimore, MD

Katherine C. Nordal, PhD, TEP Chair, American Psychological Association, Washington, DC

Kevin M. Schuer, PA-C, MSPAS, MPH, TEP Member, Kentucky College of Health Sciences & Center for Enterprise Quality and Safety Leadership, Lexington, KY

Jan Towers, PhD, NP-C, CRNP, FAANP, TEP Member, American Academy of Nurse Practitioners, Washington, DC

Donna M. Ulteig, LCSW, TEP Member, Psychiatric Services, SC, Madison, WI

Kathleen M. Quinn, MA, TEP Member, National Adult Protective Services Association, Fredericksburg, VA
Measure Developer/Steward Updates and Ongoing Maintenance
Ad.2. Year the Measure Was First Released
2009
Ad.3. Month and Year of Most Recent Revision
092013
Ad.4. What is your frequency for review/update of this measure?

Annually
Ad.5. When is your next scheduled review/update for this measure?
082014
Ad.6. Copyright Statement
Current Procedural Terminology (CPT®) copyright 2013 American Medical Association. All Rights Reserved. CPT is a registered trademark of the American Medical Association.
Fee schedules, relative value units, conversion factors and/or related components are not assigned by the AMA, are not part of CPT, and the AMA is not recommending their use. The AMA does not directly or indirectly practice medicine or dispense medical services. The responsibility for the data contained in this file is with the Centers for Medicare and Medicaid Services and no endorsement by the AMA is intended or implied. The AMA disclaims responsibility for any consequences or liability attributable to or related to any use, non-use, or interpretation of information contained or not contained in this file.
Any use of CPT beyond the terms of the license Agreement that you agreed to for personal non-commercial use, including by way of illustration and not by way of limitation, making copies of CPT for resale and/or license, transferring copies of CPT, creating any modified or derivative work of CPT, or making any commercial use of CPT, requires a separate license from the AMA. Applications for license are available at the AMA Web site, www.ama-assn.org/go/cpt.
Ad.7. Disclaimers
This measure and specifications are provided "as is" without warranty of any kind. This measure does not represent a practice guideline.
Ad.8. Additional Information/Comments

NATIONAL QUALITY FORUM—Evidence (subcriterion 1a)

Measure Title: Elder Maltreatment Screening and Follow-Up Plan
IF the measure is a component in a composite performance measure, provide the title of the Composite Measure here: Click here to enter composite measure title

Date of Submission: 1/17/2014

Instructions

- *For composite performance measures:*
    - *A separate evidence form is required for each component measure unless several components were studied together.*
    - *If a component measure is submitted as an individual performance measure, attach the evidence form to the individual measure submission.*
- Respond to all questions as instructed with answers immediately following the question. All information needed to demonstrate meeting the evidence subcriterion (1a) must be in this form. An appendix of *supplemental* materials may be submitted, but there is no guarantee it will be reviewed.
- If you are unable to check a box, please highlight or shade the box for your response.
- Maximum of 10 pages (*incudes questions/instructions*; minimum font size 11 pt.; do not change margins). ***Contact NQF staff if more pages are needed.***
- Contact NQF staff regarding questions. Check for resources at Submitting Standards webpage.

Note: The information provided in this form is intended to aid the Steering Committee and other stakeholders in understanding to what degree the evidence for this measure meets NQF's evaluation criteria.

Subcriterion 1a. Evidence to Support the Measure Focus
The measure focus is a health outcome or is evidence-based, demonstrated as follows:

- Health outcome:[3] a rationale supports the relationship of the health outcome to processes or structures of care.
- Intermediate clinical outcome, Process,[4] or Structure: a systematic assessment and grading of the quantity, quality, and consistency of the body of evidence[5] that the measure focus leads to a desired health outcome.
- Patient experience with care: evidence that the measured aspects of care are those valued by patients and for which the patient is the best and/or only source of information OR that patient experience with care is correlated with desired outcomes.
- Efficiency:[6] evidence for the quality component as noted above.

Notes

3. Generally, rare event outcomes do not provide adequate information for improvement or discrimination; however, serious reportable events that are compared to zero are appropriate outcomes for public reporting and quality improvement.
4. Clinical care processes typically include multiple steps: assess → identify problem/potential problem → choose/plan intervention (with patient input) → provide intervention → evaluate impact on health status. If the measure focus is one step in such a multistep process, the step with the strongest evidence for the link to the desired outcome should be selected as the focus of measurement.
5. The preferred systems for grading the evidence are the U.S. Preventive Services Task Force (USPSTF) grading definitions and methods, or Grading of Recommendations, Assessment, Development and Evaluation (GRADE) guidelines.
6. Measures of efficiency combine the concepts of resource use and quality (NQF's Measurement Framework: Evaluating Efficiency Across Episodes of Care; AQA Principles of Efficiency Measures).

1a.1. This is a measure of:

Outcome

- ☐ Health outcome: Click here to name the health outcome

  Health outcome includes patient-reported outcomes (PRO, i.e., HRQoL/functional status, symptom/burden, experience with care, health-related behaviors)
- ☐ Intermediate clinical outcome: Click here to name the intermediate outcome

☒ Process: Screening for elder maltreatment and documenting a follow up plan

☐ Structure: Click here to name the structure

☐ Other: Click here to name what is being measured

HEALTH OUTCOME PERFORMANCE MEASURE *If not a health outcome, skip to 1a.3*

1a.2. Briefly state or diagram the linkage between the health outcome (or PRO) and the healthcare structures, processes, interventions, or services that influence it

1a.2.1. State the rationale supporting the relationship between the health outcome (or PRO) and at least one healthcare structure, process, intervention, or service.

Note: For health outcome performance measures, no further information is required; however, you may provide evidence for any of the structures, processes, interventions, or service identified above.

INTERMEDIATE OUTCOME, PROCESS, OR STRUCTURE PERFORMANCE MEASURE

1a.3. Briefly state or diagram the linkages between structure, process, intermediate outcome, and health outcomes. Include all the steps between the measure focus and the health outcome.

1. Identified suspected risk of current elder maltreatment
2. Report to appropriate local or state Adult Protective Services (or federal agency as appropriate for nursing home residents)for assessment and possible intervention
3. Assessment/Potential intervention to improve the health and well-being of the patient and less use of healthcare resources.

1a.3.1. What is the source of the systematic review of the body of evidence that supports the performance measure?

☐ Clinical Practice Guideline recommendation – ***complete sections 1a.4, and 1a.7***

☒ US Preventive Services Task Force Recommendation – ***complete sections 1a.5 and 1a.7***

☐ Other systematic review and grading of the body of evidence (*e.g., Cochrane Collaboration, AHRQ Evidence Practice Center*) – ***complete sections 1a.6 and 1a.7***

☒ Other – ***complete section 1a.8***

Please complete the sections indicated above for the source of evidence. You may skip the sections that do not apply.

1a.4. CLINICAL PRACTICE GUIDELINE RECOMMENDATION

1a.4.1. Guideline citation (*including date*) and **URL for guideline** (*if available online*):

1a.4.2. Identify guideline recommendation number and/or page number and **quote verbatim, the specific guideline recommendation.**

1a.4.3. Grade assigned to the quoted recommendation with definition of the grade:

1a.4.4. Provide all other grades and associated definitions for recommendations in the grading system. (*Note: If separate grades for the strength of the evidence, report them in section 1a.7.*)

1a.4.5. Citation and URL for methodology for grading recommendations (*if different from 1a.4.1*):

1a.4.6. If guideline is evidence-based (rather than expert opinion), are the details of the quantity, quality, and consistency of the body of evidence available (e.g., evidence tables)?

☐ Yes → ***complete section 1a.7***

☐ No → ***report on another systematic review of the evidence in sections 1a.6 and 1a.7; if another review does not exist, provide what is known from the guideline review of evidence in 1a.7***

1a.5. UNITED STATES PREVENTIVE SERVICES TASK FORCE RECOMMENDATION

1a.5.1. Recommendation citation (*including date*) and **URL for recommendation** (*if available online*):

Screening for Intimate Partner Violence and Abuse of Elderly and Vulnerable Adults, Topic Page. U.S. Preventive Services Task Force. Recommendation Statement U.S. Preventive Services Task Force Annals of Internal Medicine, 158(6), 478-487.

URL: http://www.uspreventiveservicestaskforce.org/uspstf12/ipvelder/ipvelderfinalrs.htm

1a.5.2. Identify recommendation number and/or page number and **quote verbatim, the specific recommendation.** No numbering provided; date is January 2013

The United States Preventive Services Task Force (USPSTF) concludes that the current evidence is insufficient to assess the balance of benefits and harms of screening all elderly or vulnerable adults (physically or mentally dysfunctional) for abuse and neglect

1a.5.3. Grade assigned to the quoted recommendation with definition of the grade:

I statement - The USPSTF concludes that the current evidence is insufficient to assess the balance of benefits and harms of the service. Evidence is lacking, of poor quality, or conflicting, and the balance of benefits and harms cannot be determined.

1a.5.4. Provide all other grades and associated definitions for recommendations in the grading system. (*Note: the grading system for the evidence should be reported in section 1a.7.*)

A.— The USPSTF strongly recommends that clinicians provide [the service] to eligible patients. *The USPSTF found good evidence that [the service] improves important health outcomes and concludes that benefits substantially outweigh harms.*

B.— The USPSTF recommends that clinicians provide [this service] to eligible patients. *The USPSTF found at least fair evidence that [the service] improves important health outcomes and concludes that benefits outweigh harms.*

C.— The USPSTF makes no recommendation for or against routine provision of [the service]. *The USPSTF found at least fair evidence that [the service] can improve health outcomes but concludes that the balance of benefits and harms is too close to justify a general recommendation.*

D.— The USPSTF recommends against routinely providing [the service] to asymptomatic patients. *The USPSTF found at least fair evidence that [the service] is ineffective or that harms outweigh benefits.*

1a.5.5. Citation and URL for methodology for grading recommendations (*if different from 1a.5.1*):
URL: http://www.uspreventiveservicestaskforce.org/uspstf/grades.htm

Complete section 1a.7

1a.6. OTHER SYSTEMATIC REVIEW OF THE BODY OF EVIDENCE
1a.6.1. Citation (*including date*) and **URL** (*if available online*):

1a.6.2. Citation and URL for methodology for evidence review and grading (*if different from 1a.6.1*):

Complete section 1a.7

1a.7. FINDINGS FROM SYSTEMATIC REVIEW OF BODY OF THE EVIDENCE SUPPORTING THE MEASURE
1a.7.1. What was the specific structure, treatment, intervention, service, or intermediate outcome addressed in the evidence review?
The information in the following questions is based on the USPSTF review cited in sections 1a.5 unless otherwise specified.

Screening women of childbearing age and elderly and vulnerable adults for intimate partner violence (IPV) and elderly and vulnerable adults for abuse and neglect was studied for its benefits of detection and early intervention. It also examined the accuracy of screening tools for identifying IPV and elder abuse.

1a.7.2. Grade assigned for the quality of the quoted evidence with definition of the grade:
The USPSTF concludes that the benefits and harms of screening elderly or vulnerable adults for abuse are uncertain, and that the balance of benefits and harms cannot be determined.

1a.7.3. Provide all other grades and associated definitions for strength of the evidence in the grading system.
Levels of Certainty Regarding Net Benefit
High: The available evidence usually includes consistent results from well-designed, well-conducted studies in representative primary care populations. These studies assess the effects of the preventive service on health outcomes. This conclusion is therefore unlikely to be strongly affected by the results of future studies.
Moderate: The available evidence is sufficient to determine the effects of the preventive service on health outcomes, but confidence in the estimate is constrained by such factors as:
• The number, size, or quality of individual studies.
• Inconsistency of findings across individual studies.
• Limited generalizability of findings to routine primary care practice.
• Lack of coherence in the chain of evidence.
As more information becomes available, the magnitude or direction of the observed effect could change, and this change may be large enough to alter the conclusion Low: The available evidence is insufficient to assess effects on health outcomes. Evidence is insufficient because of:
• The limited number or size of studies.
• Important flaws in study design or methods.
• Inconsistency of findings across individual studies.
• Gaps in the chain of evidence.
• Findings not generalizable to routine primary care practice.

• Lack of information on important health outcomes.
More information may allow estimation of effects on health outcomes.

1a.7.4. **What is the time period covered by the body of evidence? (*provide the date range, e.g., 1990-2010*). Date range**: 2002- 2012. This includes studies of both childbearing women and vulnerable adults. The date range for evidence related only to abused and vulnerable adults is 2006-2008.

QUANTITY AND QUALITY OF BODY OF EVIDENCE

1a.7.5. **How many and what type of study designs are included in the body of evidence?** (*e.g., 3 randomized controlled trials and 1 observational study*)

The vast majority of the studies in the body of evidence were conducted on women of childbearing age. The USPSTF found no valid, reliable screening tools to identify abuse of elderly or vulnerable adults in the primary care setting. The following studies were conducted on abused and vulnerable adults: (1) descriptive study and (1) screening instrument

1a.7.6. **What is the overall quality of evidence across studies in the body of evidence?** (*discuss the certainty or confidence in the estimates of effect particularly in relation to study factors such as design flaws, imprecision due to small numbers, indirectness of studies to the measure focus or target population*).

The information in the following questions is based on Evidence Synthesis Number 92, Screening Women for Intimate Partner Violence and Elderly and Vulnerable Adults for Abuse: Systematic Review to Update the 2004 U.S. Preventive Services Task Force Recommendation (Nelson, Bougatsos, & Blazina, 2012). URL: *http://www.ncbi.nlm.nih.gov/books/NBK97297/pdf/TOC.pdf*

Grades for quality of evidence were developed by the USPSTF. The USPSTF grades the quality of the overall evidence for a service on a 3-point scale (good, fair, poor).

No overall grade was provided by the USPSTF or Evidence Synthesis Number 92. The quality of evidence was associated with each of 5 key questions and no RCTs or controlled observational studies were identified or met inclusion criteria for any of the key questions. The articles in the body of evidence addressing screening of the elderly for abuse and neglect were limited to two studies. See below

One diagnostic accuracy study with cross-sectional data: The screening tool Elder Abuse Suspicion Index - rated poor quality. There is conflicting information on the quality of evidence of this study. USPSTF source 1a.5 rates the quality as fair, and Nelson, Bougatsos & Blazina (2012) rate the overall quality as poor due to its low applicability and small sample size of a single study.

One descriptive retrospective study: rated poor quality.

Definitions of Grades

Fair: Evidence is sufficient to determine effects on health outcomes, but the strength of the evidence is limited by the number, quality, or consistency of the individual studies, generalizability to routine practice, or indirect nature of the evidence on health outcomes

Poor: Evidence is insufficient to assess the effects on health outcomes because of limited number or power of studies, important flaws in their design or conduct, gaps in the chain of evidence, or lack of information on important health outcomes

.

ESTIMATES OF BENEFIT AND CONSISTENCY ACROSS STUDIES IN BODY OF EVIDENCE

1a.7.7. What are the estimates of benefit—magnitude and direction of effect on outcome(s) across studies in the body of evidence? *(e.g., ranges of percentages or odds ratios for improvement/ decline across studies, results of meta-analysis, and statistical significance)*
The USPSTF was not able to estimate the magnitude of net benefit for screening all elderly or vulnerable adults (physically or mentally dysfunctional) for abuse and neglect because there were no studies on the accuracy, effectiveness, or harms of screening.

The following information is based on the review of Evidence Synthesis Number 92, Screening Women for Intimate Partner Violence and Elderly and Vulnerable Adults for Abuse: Systematic Review to Update the 2004 U.S. Preventive Services Task Force Recommendation (Nelson, Bougatsos, & Blazina, 2012). URL: http://www.ncbi.nlm.nih.gov/books/NBK97297/pdf/TOC.pdf

No quantitative analysis, such as meta-analysis, was conducted. Summary of studies included below:

Outcome: Identified Abuse: A descriptive study of elderly abused veterans who were identified in primary care clinics and referred to case management found that 5.4 percent were reported to Adult Protective Services over a 3-year period. Case Management outcomes were varied, including conservatorship arrangements, nursing home placement, board or assisted living, remaining in the home, refusal of services as well as unknown outcomes. This study is consistent with the direction in favor of increased identification and reporting of abuse.

Outcome: Analysis of Screening Tools: A single instrument, the Elder Abuse Suspicion Index, was evaluated for diagnostic accuracy and had sensitivity and specificity of 9 to 47 percent and 75 to 97 percent, respectively, depending on the number of positive responses to specific questions. This analysis also supports the use of an elder maltreatment screening tool to identify suspected abuse.

1a.7.8. What harms were studied and how do they affect the net benefit (benefits over harms)?
There were no studies on the accuracy, effectiveness, or harms of screening.

"Although there is no direct evidence, the existing evidence about the lack of harms resulting from IPV screening suggests that the harms of screening elderly and vulnerable adults might also be small. Some potential harms of screening include shame, guilt, self-blame, fear of retaliation or abandonment by perpetrators, and the repercussions of false-positive results" (Moyer, 2013 p. 481).

.

UPDATE TO THE SYSTEMATIC REVIEW(S) OF THE BODY OF EVIDENCE

1a.7.9. If new studies have been conducted since the systematic review of the body of evidence, provide for each new study: 1) citation, 2) description, 3) results, 4) impact on conclusions of systematic review.

1a.8 OTHER SOURCE OF EVIDENCE

If source of evidence is NOT from a clinical practice guideline, USPSTF, or systematic review, please describe the evidence on which you are basing the performance measure.

1a.8.1 What process was used to identify the evidence?

1. AHRQ Guideline summary NGC-9711: *Mistreatment detection*.

Locating the best evidence in the published research is dependent on framing a focused, searchable clinical question. The PICO format—an acronym for population, intervention (or occurrence or risk factor), comparison (or control), and outcome—can frame an effective literature search. The editors enlisted the assistance of the New York University Health Sciences librarian to ensure a standardized and efficient approach to collecting evidence on clinical topics. A literature search was conducted to find the best available evidence for each clinical question addressed. The results were rated for level of evidence and sent to the respective chapter author(s) to provide possible substantiation for the nursing practice protocol being developed.

In addition to rating each literature citation as to its level of evidence, each citation was given a general classification, coded as "Risks," "Assessment," "Prevention," "Management," "Evaluation/Follow-up," or "Comprehensive." The citations were organized in a searchable database for later retrieval and output to chapter authors. All authors had to review the evidence and decide on its quality and relevance for inclusion in their chapter or protocol. They had the option, of course, to reject or not use the evidence provided as a result of the search or to dispute the applied level of evidence.

2. Elder Maltreatment and Care Symposium sponsored by Centers for Medicare and Medicaid

The Centers for Medicare and Medicaid Services (CMS) developed the Elder Maltreatment Screening Quality Measure in Physician Quality Reporting System as a vehicle to help protect CMS beneficiaries' well-being and safety as well as demonstrate their deep commitment to their patients. Over the tenure of this measure, the Elder Maltreatment Technical Expert Panel provided Subject Matter Expert (SME) support to continue the use of the screening for Elder Maltreatment quality measure despite the lack of strong clinical evidence to align this quality measure with the NQF National Priority, healthy living and well-being.

In response to the lack of strong evidence in the literature to support screening for elder maltreatment in this NQF National Priority/ Patient Safety Project, the Centers for Medicare and Medicaid Services (CMS) began making plans to convene a national Elder Maltreatment and Care symposium for all relevant stakeholders, held on March 8, 2013. The aim of this symposium was to assess the value of continuing the implementation and development of PQRS #181 Elder Maltreatment Screening and Follow-up Plan (Beach et al., 2013). The symposium was preceded by months of review of the literature by subject matter experts, stakeholders, researchers and policy makers. The symposium agenda included the review of prevalence statistics, recommendations and evidence related to screening tools, discussion of controversies surrounding the benefits and harms of screening and the determination of appropriate follow-up steps for suspected elder maltreatment. At the conclusion of this symposium, it was determined there was sufficient expert consensus to support the value of screening this vulnerable population. Although there are gaps in the science, CMS will move forward to support the further development of the standing PQRS #181 Elder Maltreatment Screening and Follow-Up Plan measure (T. McMullen & K. Schwartz, personal communication, January 17, 2014).

In support of this conclusion, there have been many qualitative reports on the benefits of screening and recommendations by stakeholder organizations for screening for IPV in all patients. Some groups have specific, targeted opinion statements/recommendations on screening for all forms of abuse, including screening all elderly patients for abusive or violent treatment by family, caretakers, or others. The American Medical Association and the American Academy of Neurology both have specific position statements on screening elderly patients for abuse (Moyer, 2012). As a subset to screening all elderly patients for abuse, the Agency for Healthcare Research and Quality (AHRQ), NGC-008596 Elder Abuse Prevention (Daly, 2010), supports screening of potential victims with screening tools, and identifies specific elder maltreatment screening tools. In addition, there are studies reporting elder maltreatment is prevalent and rate of prevalence is underreported.

"It is important to remember that incompleteness of gold standard criteria, does not suggest there is no evidence at all supporting the screening of elder abuse" (X. Dong, personal communication, December 20, 2013).

3. Institute of Medicine: Elder Abuse and Its Prevention Workshop Summary, Forum on Global Violence Prevention
The 2-day workshop was dedicated to elder abuse and its prevention to shed light on an underappreciated and frequently overlooked form of violence. The aim was to move beyond what is known and foster discussions on ways to improve prevention, intervention and mitigation of the victims' needs through collaborative efforts.

4. AHRQ Guideline summary NGC-8569: Elder abuse prevention.
Description of Methods Used to Collect/Select the Evidence
To determine the current status and quality of elder abuse research, a comprehensive review of the health sciences literature was performed. An expert reference librarian conducted the electronic search with input from study investigators. Sixteen databases were searched: AgeLine Database; American Theological Library Association (ATLA) Religion Database with AtlaSerials; Cochrane Database of Systematic Reviews; Cumulative Index to Nursing and Allied Health Literature (CINAHL) Plus; Education Resources Information Center (ERIC); Index to Legal Periodicals; LegalTrac; LexisNexis Academic; LexisNexis Government Periodicals Index; National Criminal Justice Reference Service (N CJRS) Abstracts Database; PsycINFO; PubMed, which included MEDLINE; Social Work Abstracts; and the Web of Science three indexes: Social Sciences Citation Index (SSCI), Science Citation Index Expanded (SCI-EXPANDED), and the Arts & Humanities Citation Index (A & HCI). In addition, two other mechanisms were used to retrieve the elder abuse research: a manual search of the reference list of publications dated prior to 1990 and a reference search of elder abuse reviews or annotations.
All literature searches were conducted from inception of each index through December 31, 2008. Elder abuse research publication inclusion criteria were: English-language articles reporting completed research on abuse of people aged 55 years and older, from any country.
The databases were searched using combinations of the following keywords: abuse, aged, elder, elder abuse, neglect, and exploitation

1a.8.2. Provide the citation and summary for each piece of evidence.
1. Caceres, B. & Fulmer, T. (2012). *Mistreatment detection*. In: Evidence-based geriatric nursing protocols for best practice. 4th ed. Boltz, M., Capezuti, E., Fulmer, T., Zwicker, D. (Eds.). New York (NY): Springer Publishing Company. AHRQ Guideline summary NGC-9711. National Guideline Clearinghouse. Rockville (MD): Agency for Healthcare Research and Quality (AHRQ); [cited 2014 Jan 06]. Available: http://www.guideline.gov/content.aspx?id=43923&search=elder+mistreatment#Section405

The following is summary of the guideline: Definitions of levels of evidence will appear at the end of the Major Recommendations

Guideline Objective: To provide a standard of practice protocol to identify best practices in identifying and responding to cases of elder mistreatment
Major Recommendations:

a. Nursing Care Strategies

•Detailed screening to assess for risk factors for elder mistreatment (EM) using a combination of physical assessment, subjective information, and data gathered from screening instruments (Perel-Levin, 2008 [Level I]).
•Strive to develop a trusting relationship with the older adult as well as the caregiver. Set aside time to meet with each individually (Perel-Levin, 2008 [Level I]).
•The use of interdisciplinary teams with a diversity of experience, knowledge, and skills can lead to improvements in the detection and management of cases of EM. Early intervention by interdisciplinary teams can help lower risk for worsening abuse and further deficits in health status (Jayawardena & Liao, 2006 [Level V]; Wiglesworth et al., 2010 [Level IV]).
•Institutions should develop guidelines for responding to cases of EM (Perel-Levin, 2008 [Level I]; Wiglesworth et al., 2010 [Level IV]).
•Educate victims about patterns of EM such that EM tends to worsen in severity over time (Cowen & Cowen, 2002 [Level VI]; Phillips, 2008 [Level II]).
•Provide older adults with emergency contact numbers and community resources (Cowen & Cowen, 2002 [Level VI]).
•Referral to appropriate regulatory agencies

b. Follow-up Monitoring of Condition: Follow-up monitoring in the acute care setting is limited compared to the follow-up that may be performed in the community or long-term care settings

Levels of Evidence

Level I: Systematic reviews (integrative/meta-analyses/clinical practice guidelines based on systematic reviews)
Level II: Single experimental study (randomized controlled trials [RCTs])
Level III: Quasi-experimental studies
Level IV: Non-experimental studies
Level V: Care report/program evaluation/narrative literature reviews
Level VI: Opinions of respected authorities/consensus panels

2. Elder Maltreatment and Care Symposium sponsored by Centers for Medicare and Medicaid

Beach, S., McMullen, T., Schwartz, K., & Yaffe, M. (2013*)*. II.6 Elder abuse and its prevention: Screening and detection. In *Elder abuse and its prevention: Workshop summary*. Washington, DC: The National Academies Press. Manuscript submitted for publication.

The Centers for Medicare and Medicaid (CMS) explored the current state of elder maltreatment screening and elder care practices across Medicare and Medicaid beneficiary populations and care settings. The aim of this symposium was to develop a framework to build more robust measure specifications for the quality measure PQRS# 181 Elder Maltreatment Screening and Follow-Up Plan. Preliminary findings from the symposium suggest:

- There is consensus for the need to develop a definition of elder maltreatment that can be utilized across Health and Human Services (HHS) agencies
- Crosscutting tools were identified which could be implemented in a variety of care settings and by multiple providers. Among these tools, the EASI, HS-EAST and the VASS scale were identified for increased use in practice, consistency with PQRS #181 measure specification, their ability to assess multiple types of abuse.
- The impact of screening on the provider-patient relationship should be considered

- Cultural diversity should always be taken into account during elder maltreatment measurement; including screening and measurement
- Awareness of feasibility and provider burden should be considered

3. Institute of Medicine and the National Research Council of the National Academies. Elder abuse and its prevention: Workshop summary (2013). Washington, DC: The National Academies Press. Manuscript submitted for publication.

The Institute of Medicine and the National Research Council of the National Academies sponsored a 2-day workshop dedicated to elder abuse and its prevention in order to shed light on an underappreciated and frequently overlooked form of violence. The aim was to move beyond what is known and foster discussions on ways to improve prevention, intervention and mitigation of the victims' needs through collaborative efforts. Workshop topics included measuring and conceptualizing elder abuse, risk factors and health outcomes, ethical considerations, screening and prevention and how to move the field of elder abuse research and prevention forward.

4. Daly, J. M. (2010). Elder abuse prevention. AHRQ Guideline summary NGC-8569. National Guideline Clearinghouse. Rockville (MD): Agency for Healthcare Research and Quality (AHRQ); [cited 2014 Jan 06]. Available: http://www.guideline.gov/content.aspx?id=34018&search=elder+abuse+prevention

The objective of this guideline is to facilitate health care professionals to assess older persons in domestic and institutional settings who are at risk for elder abuse, excluding self-neglect, and to recommend interventions to reduce the incidence of mistreatment. It is intended for use by advanced practice nurses, healthcare providers, nurses and social workers within the clinical specialties of Family Practice, geriatrics, Nursing, Preventive Medicine and Psychology. A systematic review and synthesis of current evidence followed by critique and analysis yielded the following recommendations (evidence grades are defined at the end of this summary):

1. Assessment Criteria were defined for patients most likely to benefit the most from utilizing this practice guideline (*Evidence Grade = C1*): Persons with physical, functional, or cognitive impairment, persons who have mental illness, alcoholism, or drug abuse problems, persons who are socially isolated or have a poor social network. persons who are dependent on others, persons with a past history of abusive relationships, persons with financial or other family problems, persons who reside in inadequate housing or unsafe conditions, persons who are depressed, persons who have delusions, persons who are in poor health, persons whose caregiver is stressed/frustrated with the difficult task of caring for an older person, persons whose caregiver has mental illness, alcoholism, or drug abuse problems, persons whose caregiver has inadequate financial resources, persons whose caregiver has health problems
2. Assessment tools are identified to assess potential victims. The following having an evidence grade = C1: Elder Abuse Suspicion Index©, Elder Assessment Instruments (EAI), Hwalek-Sengstock Elder Abuse Screening Test (H-S/EAST), Index of Spouse Abuse, Indicators of Abuse Screen (IOA), Mini-Mental Status Examination (MMSE), Partner Violence Screen (PVS) and Vulnerability to Abuse Screening Scale (VASS)
3. Description of Practice: a definition, defining characteristic, related factors, nursing interventions, nursing outcomes and risk factors are provided for each form of abuse

4. Implementation of the Practice: a step-by-step guideline including assessment and referral protocol is suggested for the health care provider

Potential benefits identified included reduced incidence of elder abuse and mistreatment. No potential harms were stated.

Rating Scheme for the Strength of the Evidence
Evidence Grading
A1 = Evidence from well-designed meta-analysis or well-done systematic review with results that consistently support a specific action (e.g., assessment, intervention, or treatment)
A2 = Evidence from one or more randomized controlled trials with consistent results
B1 = Evidence from high quality evidence-based practice guideline
B2 = Evidence from one or more quasi experimental studies with consistent results
C1 = Evidence from observational studies with consistent results (e.g., correlational, descriptive studies)
C2 = Inconsistent evidence from observational studies or controlled trials
D = Evidence from expert opinion, multiple case reports, or national consensus reports

5. Moyer, V.A. (2013). *Screening for intimate partner violence and abuse of elderly and vulnerable adults: A U.S. preventive services task force recommendation statement*. Annals of Internal Medicine, 158(6), 478-487. doi:10.7326/0003-4819-158-6-201303190-00588.
Available: http://annals.org/article.aspx?articleid=1558517
This guideline has been summarized within this submission document.

National Quality Forum—Measure Testing (subcriteria 2a2, 2b2-2b6)

Measure Title: Elder Maltreatment Screening and Follow-Up Plan
Date of Submission: 1/17/2014
Type of Measure:

☐ Composite – ***STOP – use composite testing form***	☐ Outcome (*including PRO-PM*)
☐ Cost/resource	☒ Process
☐ Efficiency	☐ Structure

Instructions

- Measures must be tested for all the data sources and levels of analyses that are specified. ***If there is more than one set of data specifications or more than one level of analysis, contact NQF staff*** about how to present all the testing information in one form.
- **For all measures, sections 1, 2a2, 2b2, 2b3, and 2b5 must be completed.**
- **For outcome and resource use measures**, section **2b4** also must be completed.
- If specified for **multiple data sources/sets of specificaitons** (e.g., claims and EHRs), section **2b6** also must be completed.
- Respond to all questions as instructed with answers immediately following the question. All information on testing to demonstrate meeting the subcriteria for reliability (2a2) and validity (2b2-2b6) must be in this form. An appendix for *supplemental* materials may be submitted, but there is no guarantee it will be reviewed.
- If you are unable to check a box, please highlight or shade the box for your response.
- Maximum of 20 pages (*incuding questions/instructions;* minimum font size 11 pt; do not change margins). ***Contact NQF staff if more pages are needed.***
- Contact NQF staff regarding questions. Check for resources at Submitting Standards webpage.

Note: The information provided in this form is intended to aid the Steering Committee and other stakeholders in understanding to what degree the testing results for this measure meet NQF's evaluation criteria for testing.

2a2. Reliability testing [10] demonstrates the measure data elements are repeatable, producing the same results a high proportion of the time when assessed in the same population in the same time period and/or that the measure score is precise.

2b2. Validity testing [11] demonstrates that the measure data elements are correct and/or the measure score correctly reflects the quality of care provided, adequately identifying differences in quality.

2b3. Exclusions are supported by the clinical evidence; otherwise, they are supported by evidence of sufficient frequency of occurrence so that results are distorted without the exclusion; [12]
AND
If patient preference (e.g., informed decisionmaking) is a basis for exclusion, there must be evidence that the exclusion impacts performance on the measure; in such cases, the measure must be specified so that the information about patient preference and the effect on the measure is transparent (e.g., numerator category computed separately, denominator exclusion category computed separately). [13]

2b4. For outcome measures and other measures when indicated (e.g., resource use):
• **an evidence-based risk-adjustment strategy** (e.g., risk models, risk stratification) is specified; is based on patient factors that influence the measured outcome (but not factors related to disparities in care or the quality of care)

and are present at start of care; [14,15] and has demonstrated adequate discrimination and calibration
OR
- rationale/data support no risk adjustment/ stratification.

2b5. Data analysis of computed measure scores demonstrates that methods for scoring and analysis of the specified measure allow for **identification of statistically significant and practically/clinically meaningful** [16] **differences in performance**;
OR
there is evidence of overall less-than-optimal performance.

2b6. If multiple data sources/methods are specified, there is demonstration they produce comparable results.

Notes
10. Reliability testing applies to both the data elements and computed measure score. Examples of reliability testing for data elements include, but are not limited to: inter-rater/abstractor or intra-rater/abstractor studies; internal consistency for multi-item scales; test-retest for survey items. Reliability testing of the measure score addresses precision of measurement (e.g., signal-to-noise).
11. Validity testing applies to both the data elements and computed measure score. Validity testing of data elements typically analyzes agreement with another authoritative source of the same information. Examples of validity testing of the measure score include, but are not limited to: testing hypotheses that the measures scores indicate quality of care, e.g., measure scores are different for groups known to have differences in quality assessed by another valid quality measure or method; correlation of measure scores with another valid indicator of quality for the specific topic; or relationship to conceptually related measures (e.g., scores on process measures to scores on outcome measures). Face validity of the measure score as a quality indicator may be adequate if accomplished through a systematic and transparent process, by identified experts, and explicitly addresses whether performance scores resulting from the measure as specified can be used to distinguish good from poor quality.
12. Examples of evidence that an exclusion distorts measure results include, but are not limited to: frequency of occurrence, variability of exclusions across providers, and sensitivity analyses with and without the exclusion.
13. Patient preference is not a clinical exception to eligibility and can be influenced by provider interventions.
14. Risk factors that influence outcomes should not be specified as exclusions.
15. Risk models should not obscure disparities in care for populations by including factors that are associated with differences/inequalities in care, such as race, socioeconomic status, or gender (e.g., poorer treatment outcomes of African American men with prostate cancer or inequalities in treatment for CVD risk factors between men and women). It is preferable to stratify measures by race and socioeconomic status rather than to adjust out the differences.
16. With large enough sample sizes, small differences that are statistically significant may or may not be practically or clinically meaningful. The substantive question may be, for example, whether a statistically significant difference of one percentage point in the percentage of patients who received smoking cessation counseling (e.g., 74 percent v. 75 percent) is clinically meaningful; or whether a statistically significant difference of $25 in cost for an episode of care (e.g., $5,000 v. $5,025) is practically meaningful. Measures with overall less-than-optimal performance may not demonstrate much variability across providers.

1. DATA/SAMPLE USED FOR ALL TESTING OF THIS MEASURE

Often the same data are used for all aspects of measure testing. In an effort to eliminate duplication, the first five questions apply to all measure testing. If there are differences by aspect of testing,(e.g., reliability vs. validity) be sure to indicate the specific differences in question 1.7.

1.1. What type of data was used for testing? (*Check all the sources of data identified in the measure specifications and data used for testing the measure. Testing must be provided for all the sources of data specified and intended for measure implementation.* ***If different data sources are used for the numerator and denominator, indicate N [numerator] or D [denominator] after the checkbox.***)

Measure Specified to Use Data From: (*must be consistent with data sources entered in S.23*)	**Measure Tested with Data From:**
☒ abstracted from paper record	☒ abstracted from paper record
☒ administrative claims	☒ administrative claims
☒ clinical database/registry	☐ clinical database/registry
☒ abstracted from electronic health record	☐ abstracted from electronic health record
☐ eMeasure (HQMF) implemented in EHRs	☐ eMeasure (HQMF) implemented in EHRs
☐ other: Click here to describe	☐ other: Click here to describe

1.2. If an existing dataset was used, identify the specific dataset (*the dataset used for testing must be consistent with the measure specifications for target population and healthcare entities being measured; e.g., Medicare Part A claims, Medicaid claims, other commercial insurance, nursing home MDS, home health OASIS, clinical registry*).

Medicare Part B claims

1.3. What are the dates of the data used in testing? 1/1/2010 – 6/30/2010

1.4. What levels of analysis were tested? (*testing must be provided for all the levels specified and intended for measure implementation, e.g., individual clinician, hospital, health plan*)

Measure Specified to Measure Performance of: (*must be consistent with levels entered in item S.26*)	**Measure Tested at Level of:**
☒ individual clinician	☒ individual clinician
☒ group/practice	☒ group/practice
☐ hospital/facility/agency	☐ hospital/facility/agency
☐ health plan	☐ health plan
☐ other: Click here to describe	☐ other: Click here to describe

1.5. How many and which measured entities were included in the testing and analysis (by level of analysis and data source)? (*identify the number and descriptive characteristics of measured entities included in the analysis (e.g., size, location, type); if a sample was used, describe how entities were selected for inclusion in the sample*)

Eligible professionals (EPs) who reported the measure for PQRS were identified through claims data. Twenty-three (23) EPs were identified, reporting a total of 558 claims.

The entire population of 23 EPs was used for reliability testing. A maximum of 15 records from each EP were randomly selected. This limitation was set so that the providers would not see this task as too burdensome and would be more likely to send in their records. The resulting sample was comprised of 216 claims.

Providers were mailed a letter requesting that they provide the documentation to support the assignment of the numerator code that they had submitted on the claim.

Documentation for 202 claims was received and reviewed.

1.6. How many and which <u>patients</u> were included in the testing and analysis (by level of analysis and data source)? (*Identify the number and descriptive characteristics of patients included in the analysis (e.g., age, sex, race, diagnosis); if a sample was used, describe how patients were selected for inclusion in the sample*)

Description of the total population (558) reporting the measure via claims:

3.4% were reported as performance exclusions with a total reported performance rate of 96.5%.

99.3% Urban
0.7% Rural

66.2% Female
33.8% Male

91.5% Non-underserved
8.5% Underserved (racial/ethnic minority)

9.1% Aged 65 – 69
13.5% Aged 70 – 74
77.4% Aged 75+

The entire population of 23 EPs was used for reliability testing. A maximum of 15 records from each EP were randomly selected. This limitation was set so that the providers would not see this task as too burdensome and would be more likely to send in their records. The resulting sample was comprised of 216 claims. Documentation from 202 claims was returned and reviewed.

1.7. If there are differences in the data or sample used for different aspects of testing (e.g., reliability, validity, exclusions, risk adjustment), identify how the data or sample are different for each aspect of testing reported below.

The random sample of 202 claims of the total of 558 claims submitted for this measure during the 6 month time period. They include records from all 23 providers who reported the measure.

2a2. RELIABILITY TESTING

***<u>Note</u>**: If accuracy/correctness (validity) of data elements was empirically tested, separate reliability testing of data elements is not required – in 2a2.1 check critical data elements; in 2a2.2 enter "see section 2b2 for validity testing of data elements"; and skip 2a2.3 and 2a2.4.*

2a2.1. What level of reliability testing was conducted? (*may be one or both levels*)
☒ **Critical data elements used in the measure** (*e.g., inter-abstractor reliability; data element reliability must address ALL critical data elements*)
☐ **Performance measure score** (e.g., *signal-to-noise analysis*)

2a2.2. For each level checked above, describe the method of reliability testing and what it tests (*describe the steps—do not just name a method; what type of error does it test; what statistical analysis was used*)

Quality Insights of Pennsylvania (Quality Insights) oversees the abstraction of 202 randomly generated Medicare Part B claims records for all 23 unique NPIs/eligible professionals who reported one of the G-codes for the measure during the 1/1/2010 – 6/30/2010 time period. Quality Insights requests the medical record documentation from the NPI/eligible professional for the randomly selected encounter date. The documentation is abstracted and a G-code is assigned by two registered nurse (RN) abstractors, one from Quality Insights and one from ALPS Services, Inc. (ALPS), an independent reviewer contracted with Quality Insights, according to the measure specifications.

Crude agreement rates, Prevalence Adjusted Kappa (PAK) and Kappa scores are calculated to assess the reliability of the measure.

2a2.3. For each level checked above, what were the statistical results from reliability testing? (e.*g., percent agreement and kappa for the critical data elements; distribution of reliability statistics from a signal-to-noise analysis*)

Results of IRR between 2 independent reviewers were as follows:
Crude agreement 94.3%
Kappa .77 (95% CI .53 – 1.00)
Prevalence adjusted kappa .92 (95% CI .82 – 1.00)

Agreement rates suggest very good reliability based on 2 independent reviews of the submitted documentation.

However, agreement rates between an independent reviewer and the claims submission were poor.

Crude agreement 22.8%
Kappa .05 (95% CI .03 - .08)
Prevalence adjusted kappa .14 (.09 - .19)

2a2.4 What is your interpretation of the results in terms of demonstrating reliability? (i.*e., what do the results mean and what are the norms for the test conducted?*)

Agreement rates suggest very good reliability based on 2 independent reviews of the submitted documentation.
The disparate agreement rates observed between IRR vs. Claims suggest that providers are using a broad interpretation of what needs to be included in the medical record to document the eight components that comprise the screening.

Modifications have been made to the specifications which are intended to improve claims reliability. These changes are being applied to the 2014 version of the specifications. Refer to section 3c.1

2b2. VALIDITY TESTING

2b2.1. What level of validity testing was conducted? (*may be one or both levels*)

☐ **Critical data elements** (*data element validity must address ALL critical data elements*)

☒ **Performance measure score**

☐ **Empirical validity testing**

☒ **Systematic assessment of face validity of performance measure score as an indicator** of quality or resource use (*i.e., is an accurate reflection of performance on quality or resource use and can distinguish good from poor performance*)

2b2.2. For each level checked above, describe the method of validity testing and what it tests (*describe the steps—do not just name a method; what was tested, e.g., accuracy of data elements compared to authoritative source, relationship to another measure as expected; what statistical analysis was used)*

Quality Insights of Pennsylvania conducts an Environmental Scan to evaluate the most current research and evidence-based guidelines. The TEP, composed of subject matter experts with technical measure expertise, evaluates the results of the review and provides recommendations related to quality measure improvement. The TEP also reviews and evaluates the measure's ability to capture what it is designed to capture using a consensus process.

The initial measure development process included alpha-testing in the field with select providers and a public comment period. During the Reliability Testing, Quality Insights again convened a TEP for an Environmental Scan review as well as, a detailed analysis of the beta testing results. Based on the process of multiple stakeholder input, expert panel discussion and public comment, face and content validity of CMS/Quality Insights measures can be assumed to be established.

2b2.3. What were the statistical results from validity testing? (*e.g., correlation; t-test*)
Face validity is established by subject matter specialists and experts who determine that the measure represents the process of interest.

2b2.4. What is your interpretation of the results in terms of demonstrating validity? (i.*e., what do the results mean and what are the norms for the test conducted?*)

Based on the process of multiple stakeholder input, expert panel discussion and public comment, face and content validity of CMS/Quality Insights measures can be assumed to be established.

2b3. EXCLUSIONS ANALYSIS

NA ☐ no exclusions — ***skip to section 2b4***

2b3.1. Describe the method of testing exclusions and what it tests (*describe the steps—do not just name a method; what was tested, e.g., whether exclusions affect overall performance scores; what statistical analysis was used*)

Based on review of the medical documentation crude agreement rates, Prevalence Adjusted Kappa (PAK) and Kappa scores are calculated to assess the reliability of the assignment of exclusion criteria.

2b3.2. What were the statistical results from testing exclusions? (*include overall number and percentage of individuals excluded, frequency distribution of exclusions across measured entities, and impact on performance measure scores*)

Results of IRR for exclusion criteria between 2 independent reviewers were as follows:
Crude agreement 100.0%
Kappa n/a
Prevalence adjusted kappa n/a

Agreement with exclusion criteria from claims was as follows:
Crude agreement 95.0%
Kappa 0.0 (95% CI -0.0 - 0.0)
Prevalence adjusted kappa .90 (.84 - .96)

2b3.3. What is your interpretation of the results in terms of demonstrating that exclusions are needed to prevent unfair distortion of performance results? (*i.e., the value outweighs the burden of increased data collection and analysis. Note: **If patient preference is an exclusion**, the measure must be specified so that the effect on the performance score is transparent, e.g., scores with and without exclusion*)

Instances of reported exclusions were relatively small (3.4% of the entire reported population) and include patient refusal and urgent or emergent situations where delay of treatment would jeopardize the patient's health status.

2b4. RISK ADJUSTMENT/STRATIFICATION FOR OUTCOME OR RESOURCE USE MEASURES
If not an intermediate or health outcome, or PRO-PM, or resource use measure, skip to section 2b5.

2b4.1. What method of controlling for differences in case mix is used?
☒ **No risk adjustment or stratification**
☐ **Statistical risk model with** Click here to enter number of factors **risk factors**
☐ **Stratification by** Click here to enter number of categories **risk categories**
☐ **Other,** Click here to enter description

2b4.2. If an outcome or resource use measure is not risk adjusted or stratified, provide rationale and analyses to demonstrate that controlling for differences in patient characteristics (case mix) is not needed to achieve fair comparisons across measured entities.

n/a

2b4.3. Describe the conceptual/clinical and statistical methods and criteria used to select patient factors used in the statistical risk model or for stratification by risk (*e.g., potential factors identified in* *the literature and/or expert panel; regression analysis; statistical significance of p<0.10; correlation of x or higher; patient factors should be present at the start of care and not related to disparities*)

n/a

2b4.4. What were the statistical results of the analyses used to select risk factors?

n/a

2b4.5. Describe the method of testing/analysis used to develop and validate the adequacy of the statistical model or stratification approach (*describe the steps—do not just name a method; what statistical analysis was used*)

n/a

Provide the statistical results from testing the approach to controlling for differences in patient characteristics (case mix) below.

if stratified, skip to 2b4.9

2b4.6. Statistical Risk Model Discrimination Statistics (*e.g., c-statistic, R-squared*)**: **

n/a

2b4.7. Statistical Risk Model Calibration Statistics (*e.g., Hosmer-Lemeshow statistic*):

n/a

2b4.8. Statistical Risk Model Calibration – Risk decile plots or calibration curves:

n/a

2b4.9. Results of Risk Stratification Analysis:

n/a

2b4.10. What is your interpretation of the results in terms of demonstrating adequacy of controlling for differences in patient characteristics (case mix)? (*i.e., what do the results mean and what are the norms for the test conducted*)

n/a

***2b4.11. Optional Additional Testing for Risk Adjustment** (*not required, but would provide additional support of adequacy of risk model, e.g., testing of risk model in another data set; sensitivity analysis for missing data; other methods*)

2b5. IDENTIFICATION OF STATISTICALLY SIGNIFICANT & MEANINGFUL DIFFERENCES IN PERFORMANCE

2b5.1. Describe the method for determining if statistically significant and clinically/practically meaningful differences in performance measure scores among the measured entities can be identified

(describe the steps—do not just name a method; what statistical analysis was used? Do not just repeat the information provided related to performance gap in 1b)

While *reported* performance was high (mean provider performance 91.2%) with little variation (10th percentile 100.0%, 5th percentile 14.3%) the documentation review revealed opportunity for improvement.

Based on QIP review of documentation from 23 providers, mean performance was only 16.8%.
Min – 0.0%, Max – 100.0% Std Deviation .375
99th percentile – 100.0%
95th percentile – 100.0%
90th percentile – 100.0%
75% percentile – 0.0%

2b5.2. What were the statistical results from testing the ability to identify statistically significant and/or clinically/practically meaningful differences in performance measure scores across measured entities? (e.g., *number and percentage of entities with scores that were statistically significantly different from mean or some benchmark, different from expected; how was meaningful difference defined*)

Based on review of documentation review from the 23 providers who reported the measure, the majority show a 0.0% performance rate.

2b5.3. What is your interpretation of the results in terms of demonstrating the ability to identify statistically significant and/or clinically/practically meaningful differences in performance across measured entities? (*i.e., what do the results mean in terms of statistical and meaningful differences?*)

Only 23 providers reported the measure via Medicare claims during the 1/1/2010 through 6/30/2010 time period. While the reported performance rate was high, a review of the documentation provided to support these rates demonstrated a large opportunity for improvement.

2b6. COMPARABILITY OF PERFORMANCE SCORES WHEN MORE THAN ONE SET OF SPECIFICATIONS
If only one set of specifications, this section can be skipped.

Note: *This criterion is directed to measures with more than one set of specifications/instructions (e.g., one set of specifications for how to identify and compute the measure from medical record abstraction and a different set of specifications for claims or eMeasures). It does not apply to measures that use more than one source of data in one set of specifications/instructions (e.g., claims data to identify the denominator and medical record abstraction for the numerator).* ***If comparability is not demonstrated, the different specifications should be submitted as separate measures.***

2b6.1. Describe the method of testing conducted to demonstrate comparability of performance scores for the same entities across the different datasources/specifications (*describe the steps—do not just name a method; what statistical analysis was used*)

n/a

2b6.2. What were the statistical results from testing comparability of performance scores for the same entities when using different data sources/specifications? (*e.g., correlation, rank order*)

n/a

2b6.3. What is your interpretation of the results in terms of demonstrating comparability of performance measure scores for the same entities across the different data sources/specifications? (*i.e., what do the results mean and what are the norms for the test conducted*)

n/a

References

1. (The) Agency for Healthcare Research and Quality. The National Quality Strategy (NQS). 2016. http://www.ahrq.gov/workingforquality/.
2. (The) American Medical Association. Measure #181: elder maltreatment screen and follow-up plan—national quality strategy domain: patient safety. 2015. http://www.nethealth.com/wp-content/uploads/2016/09/2016_PQRS_Measure_181_11_17_2015-2.pdf
3. (The) Center for Excellence on Elder Abuse and Neglect. Fact sheet. 2011. http://www.centeronelderabuse.org/docs/ea_stats_fact_sheet_2011.pdf. Accessed 4 March 2016.
4. (The) Centers for Medicare and Medicaid Services. Technical Expert Panel (TEP) summary report elder maltreatment screening and follow-up plan. 2013. https://www.cms.gov/Medicare/Quality-Initiatives-Patient-Assessment-Instruments/MMS/Downloads/Elder-Maltreatment-Screening-and-Follow-Up-Plan.pdf
5. (The) Centers for Medicare and Medicaid Services. CMS's program history. 2016a. https://www.cms.gov/About-CMS/Agency-Information/History/index.html?redirect=/History/.
6. (The) Centers for Medicare and Medicaid Services. What is medicare? 2016b. https://www.medicare.gov/sign-up-change-plans/decide-how-to-get-medicare/whats-medicare/what-is-medicare.html.
7. (The) Centers for Medicare and Medicaid Services. What is medicaid? 2016c. https://www.medicare.gov/your-medicare-costs/help-paying-costs/medicaid/medicaid.html.
8. (The) Centers for Medicare and Medicaid Services. CMS quality strategy 2016. 2016d. https://www.cms.gov/Medicare/Quality-Initiatives-Patient-Assessment-Instruments/QualityInitiativesGenInfo/Downloads/CMS-Quality-Strategy.pdf.
9. (The) Centers for Medicare and Medicaid Services. Physician quality reporting system. 2016e. https://www.cms.gov/Medicare/Quality-Initiatives-Patient-Assessment-Instruments/PQRS/index.html?redirect=/pqri/.
10. (The) Centers for Medicare and Medicaid Services. Physician compare. 2016f. https://www.medicare.gov/physiciancompare/search.html.
11. Dong X, Simon MA. Elder abuse as a risk factor for hospitalization in older persons. JAMA. 2013;173(10):911–7.
12. Dong X, Simon MA. Association between elder abuse and use of ED: findings from the Chicago Health and Aging Project. Am J Emerg Med. 2013;31:693–8.
13. McMullen T, Schwartz K. The Centers for Medicare and Medicaid Services (CMS) Elder Maltreatment and Care Symposium. Not published; 2012.
14. McMullen T, Schwartz K, Yaffe M, Beach S. Elder abuse and its prevention: Screening and detection. In: IOM (Institute of Medicine) and NRC (National Research Council). 2014. Elder abuse and its prevention: workshop summary. Washington, DC: The National Academies Press; 2014.
15. (The) National Center on Elder Abuse. The Elder Justice Roadmap: a stakeholder initiative to respond to an emerging health, justice financial and social crisis. http://ncea.acl.gov/library/gov_report/docs/ejrp_roadmap.pdf (n.d.). Accessed 4 March 2016.

Part IV

Practices and Services

14 The Aging Network

Jeanine Yonashiro-Cho, Kylie Meyer, and Kathleen H. Wilber

14.1 Introduction

Mr. B, a retired builder, has always prided himself on being independent. Over the years, Mr. B's sight began to decline as a result of worsening glaucoma, and for the past few years he has had difficulty with household chores. Even more troubling, he had to give up his driver's license after he went off the road and hit a tree, causing significant damage to his car. He was subsequently unable to pass the vision test required to reinstate his license. The inability to drive has been a significant inconvenience for him, as he lives in a rural area outside of the city and is now otherwise unable to get to his medical appointments or visit his friends in the city. Mr. B must rely on his 42-year old son for help driving into the city and completing household tasks. At first, this seemed to be a timely arrangement, as his son had recently moved back in with Mr. B after being served by his wife with a restraining order and eviction notice barring him from their home on the grounds of ongoing physical and emotional abuse. Over time, however, Mr. B's son has become increasingly hostile and aggressive toward his father. When Mr. B asked his son to wash the dishes, his son threw a dirty plate at Mr. B, resulting in lacerations to his arm. In another instance, his son came home intoxicated and proceeded to shove and threaten Mr. B, who fled into his room. Concerned about his safety, Mr. B would like to obtain a Restraining order and evict his son, but he is afraid of living by himself with his diminishing vision and is reliant on his son for help with household chores and transportation to medical appointments and social visits in the city. And, he reasons, his son needs his help and is trying to get his life back on track.

Like Mr. B, Mrs. D is an older adult who wants to live independently in the community. Mrs. D was once a buyer for a major department store and lives in an upscale apartment in an affluent area of town. Over the past year, family and friends have noticed some changes and have become increasingly concerned about Mrs. D's well-being. Although throughout her life, she was known for her glamorous appearance and designer clothes, she recently lost weight and is increasingly unkempt, disheveled, and malodorous. Her apartment manager has expressed concerned that she is behind on her rent, even though her family reports that she has sufficient funds in her account. The homeowner's association in her building is complaining about the smell coming from her apartment and her violation of by-laws, including subletting a room in her apartment to someone she met while eating at a fast food restaurant. Mrs. D has severe arthritis affecting her hands and her ability to cook, clean, and care for her personal needs. A few years ago, her husband died after sustaining a hip fracture from a fall. Since then, Mrs. D has become increasingly fearful of falls and avoids taking baths out of concern that she will fall in the tub and die alone. Her loneliness and fear of being socially isolated prompted her to solicit short-term renters who can keep her company. Mrs. D's husband also managed the family's finances; since his death she struggles to pay her bills and, increasingly postpones financial tasks and decisions. She assumes that her renter is a good and honest person who will pay her the correct amount. Several months ago, one of the renters, with Mrs. D's consent, stayed on and appears to have become well entrenched in her home.

The case examples of Mr. B and Mrs. D illustrate the diverse and complex needs of abuse victims and the intricate ecologies and relationships from which these needs emerge. Intervening in cases of maltreatment and self-neglect and preventing further victimization requires interpersonal and professional skills of client assessment and treatment, coupled with an extensive knowledge about available resources and services, including the ability to identify which resources offer the best potential to provide ongoing support to victims.

Most countries have developed unique service delivery structures, public service institutions, and methods of

J. Yonashiro-Cho · K. Meyer · K. H. Wilber (✉)
Leonard Davis School of Gerontology, University of Southern California, 3715 McClintock Avenue, Los Angeles, CA 90089, USA
e-mail: wilber@usc.edu

X. Dong (ed.), *Elder Abuse*, DOI 10.1007/978-3-319-47504-2_14

accessing supportive resources. In some countries, informal long-term care support systems have traditionally been comprised of family members and neighbors, though such care disproportionately burdens women and is unsustainable [107]. Because addressing each country's individual approach is beyond what can be done in a chapter, we focus primarily on lessons learned by examining the United States' Aging Network, an approach that seeks to balance national standards, a consistent structure, and core services with opportunities for local innovation based on the needs of individual communities.

The Aging Network is an extensive and diverse nationwide network of government-funded providers serving older adults in their local communities. Despite the important role that the Aging Network can play in supporting victims and potentially helping older adults avoid victimization, collaboration between protective services and aging services does not seem to routinely occur in many communities. To examine the role of the Aging Network and the ways in which its diverse services can address the needs of abused, neglected, and at-risk older adults, we begin with a discussion of the background and history of both the Aging Network and protective service programs. We compare and contrast the approaches and services offered by each and discuss ways in which they can effectively work together to prevent abuse, address it when it occurs, and reduce the likelihood that victims will suffer from recurring maltreatment.

14.1.1 Legislative Efforts to Support Older Adults

Both the Aging Network and Adult Protective Services (APS) have been in existence since the 1960s, in one form or another. Although they have a long history and there are potentially promising outcomes through collaborations, in many communities they remain distinct and siloed. Examining their evolution over the years, it appears that their histories do not intersect as much as one would expect. Perhaps this is because they have distinctly different missions, philosophies, approaches, origins, structure, and to some extent different clients, all of which make joint efforts challenging. Both programs grew out of embryonic efforts in the 1960s and both saw infusions of interest and monies in the 1970s. Since their inception both programs have focused primarily on elders living in the community. And importantly, services supplied by the Aging Network and APS are both universal—serving all who require support—rather than need-based—as well as targeted to older adults (most often considered to be people aged 60 and older) as well as adults with disability in the "greatest social and economic need." In other ways, however, the Aging Network and APS are distinctly different.

The foundation for the Aging Network was laid with the passage of the Older Americans Act in 1965 as part of President Lyndon Johnson's Great Society [38, 100]. What came to be known as the Aging Network—the backbone of an intricate web of services shown in Fig. 14.1, began to develop with the passage of amendments in 1973 that created a structure of state and local entities designed to deliver core services to older adults. Under the auspices of the Administration on Aging, the revised act called for designation of a State Unit on Aging in each state. Moreover, based on a formal planning process, service areas were designated within states and Area Agencies on Aging (AAAs) were developed within each locality. This process created a uniform structure to distribute resources, information, and program ideas both up and down organizational hierarchies. Each level (federal, state, and local) is expected to coordinate with other parallel departments and units; thus this network impacts local, state, and national programs and services. However, the structure also funnels monies down to the local level, including funding for meals, senior centers, in-home services, and other programmatic areas, which we discuss below. In this way, structure of the Aging

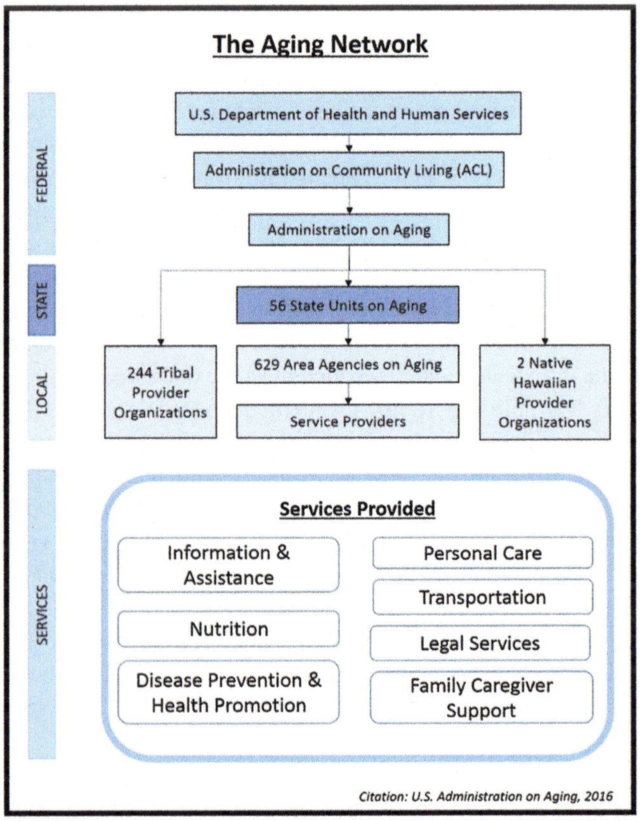

Fig. 14.1 The Aging Network. Citation: U.S. Administration of Aging (2016)

Network allows for local input and innovation based on the specific needs of each community, as well as direction and support from the state and federal level.

At its core, the Aging Network is a system of government agencies and service providers engaging in advocacy, planning, policy and program development, and service provision in order to promote the well-being of older Americans [87]. Under the authority of the U.S. Administration on Aging (AOA), the federal Older Americans Act establishes the Aging Network's infrastructure, identifies basic types of services to be provided through the Network, and provides funding for these services. As of 2012, the AOA and OAA programs were brought together with the Administration on Intellectual and Developmental Disabilities and the Health and Human Services Office on Disability to become the Administration on Community Living, part of the U.S. Department of Health and Human Services. Although there are somewhat disparate goals of the aging and disability communities, the intent of this transition was to meet the needs of people with disability from early to late life.

While the Department of Health and Human Services, the Administration on Community Living, and the Administration on Aging provide key leadership and guidance on aging services, the Aging Network is a federalist program and is, thus, significantly shaped by state and local governments. On the state and local levels, programs are defined and implemented to meet the needs of older adults within specified Service Planning Areas, resulting in a nationwide network of community-centric programs and services that fulfill local needs in a variety of different ways.

In addition, recognizing of the autonomy and needs of indigenous populations, the Administration on Aging provides funding for agencies which serve American Indian, Alaskan Natives, and Native Hawaiian populations. Currently, 244 tribal organizations and 2 Native Hawaiian organizations receive funding to implement Older Americans Act services among their respective communities [95]. This chapter describes services that are generally available in most areas while highlighting notable unique model programs which may be of interest to elder abuse practitioners. Contact information for agencies providing information and assistance with obtaining local services is available through the U.S. Administration on Aging's Eldercare Locator (http://www.eldercare.gov/eldercare.NET/Public/index.aspx; 1-800-677-1116).

A closer look at the OAA shows that the topic of elder abuse has been an increasing focus starting with amendments in 1984 [38]. Title VII of the Older Americans Act authorizes funds for long-term care Ombudsman program, which is described in detail elsewhere in this volume, and the Prevention of Elder Abuse, Neglect, and Exploitation Program, which allocates funds to State Units on Aging to support strategic planning, research, and programs intended to prevent and address elder abuse [61, 98]. Funds can be spent at the state level or distributed to local Area Agencies on Aging for their use or distribution to local service providers. Title VII also authorizes the institution of the National Center on Elder Abuse (NCEA; http://www.ncea.aoa.gov). The NCEA seeks to prevent elder abuse by providing training, technical assistance and support to elder abuse professionals and the general public, serving as a reliable and highly visible clearinghouse of resources and information [61, 97]. While Title VII specifically addresses elder abuse, other provisions offer more general services that nonetheless can be employed to support victims and help reduce the risk of abuse.

The Aging Network has been able to rely on a consistent (although constricting) funding stream over the years. This federal source of authorization is one reason why OAA programs have a comprehensive and standardized structure depicted in Fig. 14.1.

Although the OAA remained in limbo after 2011, past due for reauthorization but unable to pass in a contentious political climate, it was reauthorized in 2016. With the most recent iteration of the OAA, several new program requirements address elder abuse more specifically [20]. Although this chapter does not endeavor to assess these in detail given their very recent implementation, they are worth nothing. First, the recent legislation requires the Office for the Long-Term Ombudsman to collect best practices to respond to elder abuse. Again at the federal level, the AOA must ensure that OAA-supported programs include training to prevent elder abuse, as well as services capable of addressing elder justice. In addition, the AOA is required to ensure grants to State Units on Aging to support health screenings also assess for elder abuse, neglect, and exploitation. State Units should also find ways to promote data submission on reported elder abuse to designated databases, and support communities in developing partnerships addressing elder justice to prevent, investigate, and prosecute in cases of abuse. Finally, the reauthorized OAA requires local AAA plans to include plans to increase awareness about elder abuse, neglect, and exploitation. Each of these measures supports promising ways to prevent and address elder mistreatment at all levels of OAA infrastructure.

In contrast to the Aging Network, Adult Protective Services (APS) appear to have been much more organic and locally driven. APS, described as "the backbone of community-based efforts to respond to elder mistreatment" [8, p. 124], has relied on a variety of funding streams that are not earmarked specifically for protective services. A major catalyst for the development of APS was the Social Service Block Grant program funding through Title XX of the Social Security Act, 1975 [62, 71]. As a block grant, this funding was not designated for specific programs, but was directed toward a vulnerable target population that included older and disabled adults who were abused, neglected, exploited, or living in dangerous conditions [71]. Thus, for many communities, the Social Security Block Grants (SSBGs) provided a much needed resource for local government, some of which could be directed at what was then called "granny bashing," a term used at congressional hearings to cast light on disturbing cases of abused elders. Because APS had been established in many communities before the SSBGs became available, these grants breathed new life into addressing a long-standing yet newly discovered problem. However, unlike the OAA-funded Aging Network, funds were not designated specifically for older adults, and thus programs had to compete for these monies with other social service entities.

Currently, all states have policies on reporting abuse and the vast majority requires mandatory reporting by most professionals in fields such as health care, social services, and long-term services, and support provision. An ongoing challenge, however, is to make sure that the role of APS is understood by professionals and others who might report abuse.

Bonnie and Wallace [8] note that APS has several core tasks which include:

(1) intake, screen, and determine priorities for future action for reported victims of abuse, neglect, and exploitation
(2) investigate abuse allegations; and
(3) engage in case planning to address and mitigate the abuse.

Given limited funding, much of APS' resources are directed toward meeting the first two functions—taking in and investigating allegations of abuse. However, using information garnered from this task to intervene and stop abuse is challenging for several reasons. Unlike those affected by child abuse, victims of elder abuse can exercise their rights as adults and decline to participate in an investigation or refuse APS services. And like victims of intimate partner violence, elder abuse victims may deny that abuse has occurred because they are conflicted about the situation and/or wish to protect their abuser. In many jurisdictions, APS may also be limited by legislative or procedural constraints which restrict agency activities to largely a crisis management approach. Thus, collaboration with Aging Network agencies may offer APS both a challenge and an opportunity.

A recent study sheds light on the challenges APS faces as it seeks to address abuse and collaborate with other services in the community. Focus groups comprised of APS workers and others with healthcare professionals both identified similar constraints and barriers to abuse reporting and subsequent interagency collaborations to address it [23]. From their perspective, APS workers reported difficulties in transitioning clients to the larger service delivery system, especially given the limited time for care planning and the need to respect the autonomy of victims who do not always want to pursue cases. In turn, health service providers felt frustrated because they did not fully understand the role of APS and the boundaries that APS worked within, especially with regard to maintaining client confidentiality and autonomy. Indeed, in cases involving clients who are unwilling to permit a referral to an outside agency, APS confidentiality mandates make a handoff to an Aging Network organization nearly impossible. It is important to recognize these constraints and at the same time examine how agencies can work together to address elder abuse. We begin this discussion by briefly exploring what APS and other community providers need to know to identify abuse risk.

14.1.2 Risk Factors for Abuse

What makes one older person more at risk of experiencing abuse than another older adult? Researchers have identified risk factors or characteristics that increase the likelihood that an older person will experience elder abuse. Each additional risk factor contributes to increased vulnerability to mistreatment in unique ways, tilting the scales such that an outcome of abuse or mistreatment is more likely. Mosqueda et al. [60] integrated this concept into the Abuse Intervention Model (AIM) framework which categorizes risk factors for abuse into three major categories: characteristics of the potential victim, characteristics of the possible perpetrator, and the contextual environment in which possible victims and alleged abusers interact. While a more extensive review of abuse risk factors is available elsewhere in this volume, we will discuss a few key risk factors that may be addressed by Aging Network services.

14.1.2.1 Social Isolation

Older adults who are socially isolated from formal (e.g., service providers) and informal (e.g., family members, friends, neighbors, etc.) social networks appear to be at greater risk for experiencing abuse and neglect [1, 8]. Social isolation may emerge organically, due to an individual's decline in health, functional ability, or cognition, or even from a death within the victim's existing social network. In other cases, isolation may be intentionally orchestrated and maliciously perpetrated in order to increase the victim's vulnerability to maltreatment by creating a dependency on the perpetrator and preventing would-be interveners from learning about inappropriate activities [102]. Having higher levels of social support has been found to be protective against abuse [48, 55]. Acierno et al. [1] found an association between not using social services and financial abuse, implying, perhaps, that engagement in formal supportive service networks might reduce isolation and prevent financial abuse.

14.1.2.2 Cognitive Impairment

Cognitive impairment increases an individual's vulnerability by raising their need for support and assistance while simultaneously diminishing their ability to protect themselves from abuse. A review of the literature found that individuals with cognitive impairment are at significantly higher risk of being abused [48]. In their longitudinal analysis, Lachs et al. [52] found that cognitively impaired older adults had two times greater odds of experiencing abuse compared to non-impaired older adults. The odds of abuse increased more than fourfold among those who had recently experienced a decline in cognitive function, compared to those with no cognitive impairment and those who were impaired but had not experienced a change in their cognitive status, suggesting that older adults may be especially vulnerable during and immediately following this period of transition in cognitive status. Possible reasons for this increased risk of abuse among cognitively impaired older adults may include being targeted by perpetrators who assume victim accounts of abuse will be disregarded, but also the need to rely on others who might misuse this trust. More recently, Dong et al. [27] identified declines in Mini-Mental State Examination score, global cognitive functioning, perceptual speed, and episodic memory, specifically, as being associated with having a higher risk of experiencing elder abuse.

14.1.2.3 Functional Limitations

Functional limitations are often defined by an individual's ability to independently perform Activities of Daily Living (ADLs) which include eating, walking, bathing, dressing, grooming, and toileting, and Instrumental Activities of Daily Living (IADLs), such as meal preparation, managing money and medications, completing housework, shopping, use of a telephone, and accessing transportation. Older adults with greater functional limitations have greater risk of experiencing financial, physical, or emotional abuse [1, 13]. There is also evidence to suggest that the level of risk increases with each additional ADL impairment reported [31, 52]. Although it is important to remember that most caregivers are not abusers, functional impairment can cause individuals to seek care from those who may eventually exploit, abuse, or neglect them. Victims of abuse may be reluctant to seek help or leave the situation because their abuser proves instrumental assistance with daily tasks.

14.1.2.4 Abuser Characteristics

Characteristics of the abuser and the relationship between the abuser and victim may also increase the risk of abuse occurrence and are important factors to consider and address [48, 60]. Contrary to what might be expected, studies have found that abusers are often more dependent on their victims than their victims are upon them [8]. Thus, it is not surprising that risk factors for being an abuser include mental health issues, substance or alcohol abuse, and poor abuser–victim relationship quality [48].

Some have proposed multiple abuser typologies to describe the characteristics and modus operandi of abusers [43, 47, 79, 93]. Characteristics which may contribute to risk of abuse vary by the particular abuser typology. For instance, in situations involving extensive caregiver burden, a caregiver's inability to cope with the stressful caregiving situation may increase the likelihood of abuse [48].

14.2 Effects of Abuse

Elder abuse and mistreatment have multiple detrimental effects on victims, who not only endure the direct impacts of abuse (e.g., physical injury and lost assets), but also its reverberating consequences. Victims may face anger, disappointment, or grief following abuse [18]. Abuse can also render a severe blow to independence in later life: victims face an increased likelihood of functional impairments [25] as well as a higher risk of institutionalization than non-victims [28]. Longitudinal work also demonstrates an increased risk of death following abuse [3, 26, 29, 30, 53, 81]. It is important to understand, however, that the effects of abuse will vary by victim [76].

Recognizing the protective and contextual factors surrounding abuse leads one to suspect that elder abuse prevention is enhanced by environmental factors, such as the availability of services and supports provided by the Aging Network. Although the U.S. Administration on Aging is currently funding studies related to the prevention of abuse [99], we were unable to find any studies addressing the role of the Aging Network in directly reducing risk and incidence of abuse. Still, there is some evidence to suggest different mechanisms through which services may prevent elder abuse. For example, in their focus group study, Enguidanos et al. [34] found that participants feared reporting abuse due to fear of nursing home placement. The availability of supportive services within the home, such as those offered through the Aging Network, could potentially mitigate nursing home placement and thereby increase older adults' willingness to report abuse.

In this chapter, we suggest that the services and supports provided to older Americans via the Aging Network have the potential to counterbalance risk factors for abuse and help to prevent vulnerability in old age. These services also offer support for victims that may help them overcome risk factors once the abuse occurs. The case studies at the beginning of this chapter illustrate needs that Aging Network intervention and support could help address to reduce the risk of abuse. Another consideration in the list of harms caused by elder abuse is the effects abuse can have on others, impacting families, neighbors, and communities who are left to respond to the consequences of elder abuse [74].

Finally, while some survivors of abuse may be able to cope well and recover, others may be less equipped to do so. Providing adequate supports to improve recovery may help to mitigate negative consequences of abuse. For example, older victims of domestic violence reported significant improvements in well-being after attending support groups, including reduced isolation, peace of mind, and even self-reported improvements in health [9]. Earlier research reiterates these findings, suggesting that victims who have higher levels of social support experience less psychological distress than victims with lower levels of social support [18]. Thus, the effects of abuse may, in part, be mediated by the support that follows.

14.3 Long-Term Services and Supports for Secure Community Living

Given the choice, most older adults would prefer to "age-in-place," remaining in their homes and communities. A recent AARP survey found that 87 % of people ages 65 and older indicated they preferred to remain in their current home [44]. While reasons for this preference are vast and vary by individual, there is some indication that such reluctance may stem from strong place attachment [56] and resulting identity formation [84], as well as proximity to existing social networks and familiarity with the existing community.

Home- and community-based long-term services and supports, such as those provided by the Aging Network, are programs intended to provide older adults with instrumental assistance to enable them to continue living in the community. While long-term care can be effectively provided within an institutional setting like a nursing home, and may be appropriate for some, for many, services that support older adults to remain in the community are most suitable. Moreover, depending on the needs of the older adult, home care may also be more cost-effective. For example, whereas 4 h of in-home assistance cost $84 in 2010 on average, 1 day of nursing home care averaged $205 per day for a shared room [57].

Provision of long-term services and supports may enable victims of abuse, neglect, or self-neglect to receive sufficient support to enable them to continue living safely in the community. As in the case studies presented in the introduction, Mr. D may have been reluctant to report the abuse or obtain a restraining order because of his reliance on the abuser for transportation to medical appointments. With the receipt of transportation services through an Aging Network provider, the abused victim may no longer feel dependent on the abuser and be empowered to seek assistance with obtaining a protective order to halt the abuse or agree to report the abuse to law enforcement to facilitate the arrest his abuser. Similarly, Mrs. B may have initially been unwilling to bathe regularly because she is fearful of slipping and falling in the bathtub. However, with the receipt of personal care assistance from an Aging Network provider or through the Aging Network Information and Assistance service, she may be able to bathe safely and manage other personal care, enabling her to remain in the community rather than moving to an Assisted Living Facility.

14.4 The Aging Network: A Key Resource to Address Elder Mistreatment

Aging Network providers offer a wide array of programs and services intended to support community-dwelling older adults. While government agencies sometimes provide direct services, they often contract with local agencies and organizations to provide these services. Providers may be organizations serving older adults at large or may serve specific cultural, social, or religious subpopulations. As described more fully below, these service programs are important resources available to practitioners seeking to assist older victims of mistreatment or self-neglect and those at-risk for these conditions. Programs provide integral support to alleviate the detrimental effects of maltreatment, and can also provide support to reduce dependency and vulnerability, thus preventing/reducing future abuse and self-neglect. The services described below are presented in order of applicability to victims.

14.4.1 Aging and Disability Resource Centers

Aging and Disability Resource Centers were created to assist consumers to access services. In general, social services "networks" are comprised of a variety of service providers who may have different program goals, funding streams, eligibility requirements, and protocols [49, 108]. As a result, it can be difficult for older adults and those helping them to identify programs and services that help them continue living in the community. In the 1980s, Aging Network and Medicaid programs in some areas began to create interagency Resource Centers to improve consumer access to services, adopting consumer-friendly approaches which would increase the likelihood that consumers would be able to obtain necessary information and services [72]. In Centers adopting the "single point of entry" approach, consumer inquiries and requests for information or services were directed to a central entity designed to connect consumers with appropriate and available service providers [58, 72, 94]. Other Centers adopted a "no wrong door" approach in which workers at participating agencies were trained in the types of services available from other member agencies, and were thus equipped to refer clients to providers who might be better able to meet their needs [72, 94]. In this way, consumers could access services from the appropriate providers despite contacting an agency that would otherwise be unsuited to fulfill their service needs.

In 2003, the Administration on Aging and Centers for Medicare and Medicaid Services provided funding to replicate the interagency Resource Center model by establishing Aging and Disability Resource Centers (ADRCs) in twelve states under the Real Choice Systems Change Grants for Community Living [72]. The Centers were designed to bring together and streamline access to providers offering services for elder and disabled adults. In 2006, the Older Americans Act was amended such that each state was required to have an ADRC, and as a result, this model program has been replicated in all 50 states and several U.S. territories [72]. To date, at least 535 ADRCs have been established nationwide with at least 41 states establishing an ADRC presence online to promote greater accessibility [94].

While the individual protocols and participating agencies may differ between ADRC programs, ADRCs are intended to provide an array of services designed to aid consumers of all ages and levels of need. These services may include, but are not limited to, (1) information and referral services, (2) long-term services and supports options counseling, (3) eligibility determination for programs and services, (4) person-centered transition support, and (5) quality assurance and continuous improvement services [94]. Some ADRCs include or are colocated with local Adult Protective Services agencies, thus promoting APS's integration with other aging and disability service providers [63].

The integration of aging and disability resources is a logical step that offers support for agencies serving elder and dependent abuse victims and those at risk for abuse. Traditionally these systems have been operated independently, requiring older adults to identify and access services from each of these systems and personally coordinate eligible services. With the growth of ADRCs, there is increasing potential that practitioners can support at-risk elders or victims as they seek assistance through ADRCs.

14.4.2 Senior Centers

Senior Centers often serve as "one-stop shops," providing services to older adults as well as opportunities for social engagement and interpersonal interaction for community-dwelling elders. In general, Senior Centers have dedicated staff members who plan social, educational, and health-related activities for older adults at little or no cost to participants. Aging Network services typically are available to older adults through their local Senior Centers. For instance, many centers operate congregate nutrition programs. Some offer evidence-based health promotion and disease prevention programs and/or house case managers who can assist older adults with accessing additional services. Many of these programs are targeted to low-income older adults who may have limited ability to pay. Often, programs are supported in whole or in part by federal, state, and local government funds including Older Americans Act funds, although participants are given the opportunity to make a suggested donation if they are able and willing to do so.

By providing services in a centralized location where older adults come together, Senior Centers offer a means to combat social isolation, a noted risk factor for abuse. Older adults who frequent their local Senior Center may develop friendship with other community members, as well as staff. Such opportunities may be particularly important, as positive social engagement and strong social support is associated with lower mortality [82], greater survival after serious health events [5, 39], higher self-rated health [22], and better cognitive functioning [83].

Continued participation in senior center activities may also foster opportunities for informal monitoring of participant well-being and their physical and cognitive functioning. In some cases, program staff may be among the first to suspect that a participant is in an abusive, exploitive, or neglectful situation. When a client has suspicious injuries or begins to arrive disheveled and malodorous, senior center staff may be the ones who contact APS and/or law enforcement to notify them about their concerns and request that they investigate the situation. In some states this report may be required under mandatory reporting laws [70]. Such referrals can help to ensure that the older adult is safe and able to adequately care for his or her personal needs.

Moreover, Senior Center programs' emphasis on social engagement and encouragement of positive social interactions may be especially beneficial for victims of abuse and neglect who may have experienced social isolation and/or negative and detrimental social interaction. Regular interaction with program staff and participants offers an alternate support system to fill the social and emotional void left by the removal or desertion of the abuser. Such social engagement may also provide sufficient support to empower individuals experiencing abuse to remove their abusers from their life. Additionally, given that abuse has been estimated to recur in 4–33 % of cases [19, 32, 35, 89], senior center staff may be well positioned to act as vigilant observers and to make a report and seek assistance from elder abuse professionals if concerns occur after an investigation is closed [16, 60].

14.4.3 Nutrition

The Older Americans Act funded Title IIIC nutrition program to promote the health and well-being—physical, emotional, and social—of older adults through the provision of nutrition services [17]. To ensure that older adults have access to at least one nutritious meal a day, the Administration on Aging provides funding for Area Agencies on Aging to contract with nutrition providers who prepare and distribute meals to older adults either in the community or at home. In general, programs are required to provide these meals at least five times a week, though there are allowances for programs in rural areas that may be unable to meet this requirement. Program staff is also required to provide participants with nutrition counseling and other nutrition services as needed. Older adults aged 60 and older and their spouses of any age are eligible to participate in the program.

Congregate nutrition programs (IIIC-1) provide older adults with hot meals that meet federal nutrition standards. Meals are offered in a specified physical location, such as a senior center or other program provider. Participants have the opportunity to share a meal, often over friendly conversation and social interaction. Like other Senior Center programs, older adult nutrition programs were developed with a joint goal of providing nutritious food and facilitating social interaction among program participants.

Older adults who are frailer or chronically ill, and therefore unable to attend congregate meals, can receive meals delivered to their homes (III C-2). The Aging Network addresses the unmet need of such individuals through programs providing "Meals on Wheels," which may offer social interaction at the time of the meal delivery or at the very least someone who checks on the older adult's welfare on a regular basis. Volunteers delivering the meal may interact with home-bound older adults and may also be trained to look for signs that the older individual may be in need of added services or supports. For example, volunteers might recognize signs of disarray in the home, or an empty refrigerator. Some pilot programs have sought to partner elder abuse protection with home-delivered meal providers to provide education and training to meal delivery persons about suspicious signs of abuse [66].

14.4.4 Personal Care

Personal care services include providing assistance with a range of ADLs, such as bathing and dressing. These can also include "chore" services addressing IADL needs, including meal preparation and light housekeeping. Personal care may be provided on a temporary basis, as when an older person is returning from the hospital and needs extra assistance while recovering, or long-term, where recovery or return to an independent level of functioning is unlikely.

Although many states have their own state-specific personal care service programs, Area Agencies on Aging oversee the distribution of personal care services in a number of ways. This happens most directly though the Older Americans Act Title IIIB funding meant to support independent living. Often these services are provided to clients who meet certain target criteria (e.g., low income) and are provided via contracted agencies. Under Title III-E, AAAs can also provide respite care services, which frequently entail personal care assistance. Finally, at the most basic level, AAAs may provide information and advice on local business and organizations providing these services. Older adults, including those accessing personal care through Medicaid, out-of-pocket, or with long-term care insurance, may benefit from such information and assistance services.

Personal care services provided by the Aging Network may prevent elder abuse by addressing unmet needs and reducing neglect and self-neglect. In addition these services may also prevent additional loss of functioning, declines in physical health, dependency, and social isolation. For example, assistance with dressing may prevent dangerous falls and other injuries that leave older adults more vulnerable and in need of additional assistance. Interactions with personal care service providers may also buffer against possible social isolation, as these relationships may develop into what is recognized as friendship [73]. Although there are cases implicating the role of home care aides in elder abuse, this is likely the exception; state plans are required to address quality assurance in home care, a possible safeguard against mistreatment.

14.4.5 Transportation

Data from the 2012 Health and Retirement Survey revealed that one in five older Americans likely needs transportation services [40]. American's heavy reliance on cars shapes communities in ways that pose a challenge to older people who can no longer drive, face constraints when driving (e.g., cannot drive after dark), or cannot afford a car. For example, in some communities, public transport options are disjointed and unpredictable, making these less suitable to meet the needs of older people who do not drive.

Since 1974, the Older Americans Act has addressed these challenges by providing Title III transportation services via state and local agencies [38, 95]. Although these agencies are required to plan for the transportation needs of older adults, they have great flexibility in doing so. Area agencies might meet transportation needs through voucher programs that provide transport at a reduced cost or by providing information on curb-to-curb, escort, volunteer, public transport and taxi services, for example. In fiscal year 2012, states spent $68.8 million on transportation services (e.g., public transport) and $3.3 million on assisted transportation (e.g., escorting to front door), money that was used to serve 31,950 older adults [40]. State and local agencies also are encouraged to advocate and work with communities to systemically address transportation systems to better fit the needs of older adults. Since 2006, Title IV of the Older Americans Act includes a section supporting the creation of more innovative and cost-effective transportation services.

Transportation services can be used to offset potential risk factors for elder abuse by connecting older people to services and supports outside the home and decreasing dependency on less trustworthy others as illustrated in Mr. B's case. Transportation services can enhance access to social activities, such as senior centers. Transportation to certain services may also result in opportunities to screen for abuse, as when older people receive transportation to attend doctors appoints where physical signs of abuse may become evident. Neglect, too, may be offset through the availability of transportation services. Older people who do not drive may need assistance to get to the grocery store or pharmacy, thereby allowing older adults to address nutrition and medication needs independently rather than rely upon less dependable and potentially neglectful caregivers.

It should be noted that transportation services will likely change over time. The advent of the shared economy, including ride-sharing options, will likely transform how transportation needs are met in later life. In addition, the increased availability of delivery options for certain goods, including groceries, will likely lessen some of the need for transportation services among some older people. Still, there is little information on what the future may hold. Continued concerns with rideshare programs is their ability to serve people with disabilities, access in rural communities, as well as their safety for more vulnerable older people—these and related issues will need to be addressed.

14.4.6 Legal Services

The Older Americans Act includes provisions to fund civil legal services for older adults through the Aging Network. Legal providers can offer a range of services, including education, outreach, advice, and support. While elder abuse is often addressed in a criminal context through the arrest and prosecution of the suspected abuser, there are also a number of different civil actions that can be undertaken to address the abuse, protect the victim, and prevent future mistreatment. Aging Network-funded legal services may be able to provide older adults with information about civil legal recourses and, in some cases, even practical legal counsel.

The specific legal services needed to assist victims of elder mistreatment or self-neglect or those at-risk for these conditions may vary by the type of abuse involved and the level of vulnerability of the victim. For example, protective orders, also known as restraining orders, can be instituted to prevent suspected abusers from interacting with the person they are suspected of abusing. Often thought of as an intervention to prevent future physical abuse and promote client safety, protective orders may also be beneficial in cases of undue influence, financial abuse, or emotional abuse as well. In such situations, legally removing the suspected abuser from accessing the older adult disrupts their ability to manipulate, coerce, or otherwise exert control over the client's decision-making and emotional well-being. Moreover, physically removing the suspected abuser from the client's immediate physical environment may restrict access to private financial information and banking documents, preventing future financial loss.

Advance Directives include several different kinds of documents that clients can complete. These can be used to designate a surrogate decision maker, also known as an agent, to make financial or medical decisions on the older adult's behalf if the individual lacks the capacity to make his or her own decisions. Adults with capacity can also designate a surrogate if they need assistance managing a specific issue such as selling property [103]. In situations where clients do not already have an Advance Directive, providers can assist them with information and resources to help them complete the necessary forms and establish a trustworthy agent who can make decisions or act on their behalf. In some cases of financial exploitation, designated surrogates abuse their influence or Power of Attorney designation for personal gain at the expense of the client's well-being. In such situations, legal service providers may be able to provide information and assistance to modify existing Advance Directives and negate the authority of suspected abusers while helping to see that more trustworthy agents are legally appointed.

14.4.7 Disease Prevention and Health Promotion Services

Many older adults, including victims of abuse and neglect, experience negative health events or health decline over time. Poor health status and/or chronic conditions may not only result from abuse and neglect [3, 26, 29, 30, 53, 81] but also are risk factors that increase the likelihood of such events occurring [1, 48]. Through the Older Americans Act, the Administration on Aging provides funding for disease prevention and health promotion programs and activities (OAA Title IIID). Many such programs are offered through Senior Centers or congregate meal sites. By October 1, 2016, all programs offered through federal Older Americans Act funding will be required to be evidence-based, such they will have to demonstrate effectiveness through scientific, peer-reviewed evaluation and successfully translate this into a community site [96]. This mandate was designed to promote the dissemination and implementation of more effective programs.

As with the other Aging Network services, the availability of specific programs vary across the country. Nevertheless, there are several notable programs that may be useful to victims of abuse or neglect, their friends, family members, and caregivers. These programs are varied and address medication management, chronic disease self-management, fall risks, muscle strengthening, and depression [2, 4, 15, 46, 59, 85, 92]. By helping elderly victims of abuse or neglect and those at-risk better manage their health, elder abuse practitioners may reduce future abuse or neglect. Moreover, use of these strategies may be an effective intervention to help medically self-neglecting older adults better manage their health and care for themselves.

14.4.8 National Family Caregiver Support Program

Family caregivers play an integral role in providing support and services to family members who need care. Recognizing the immense contributions of these informal caregivers, the Administration on Aging provides the Aging Network with funding for programs to provide caregivers with information and assistance, counseling, training, respite, and other services (OAA Title IIIE). Supportive services such as those listed above may help to address caregiver burden and stress, factors that have been associated with abuse by some caregivers [54, 75]. However, the availability of programs and services and their local administration varies greatly between states [36]. Caregiver service providers may include adult day care providers, healthcare organizations, disease-specific service organizations, and general social services providers [101].

In addition to providing services for family members caring for older or developmentally disabled adults, the National Family Caregiver Support Program also strives to provide support for older adult caregivers providing care for minors (OAA Title IIIE). There is an increasing number of grandparents providing care for their grandchildren [45]. Unfortunately, research among grandparent caregivers notes greater stress and difficulty within the caregiving population [45]. Caregiver program services are intended to support such caregivers and provide training and resources to aid them in this role. Victims of abuse or exploitation who are in this role may benefit from services provided by programs supporting grandparent caregivers.

14.4.9 Tribal Organizations

Native populations face social and health-related challenges which stem from their displacement from their lands, ensuing discriminatory attitudes and practices, and exposure to lower socioeconomic conditions throughout their life course [11, 12, 51]. Additionally, studies have noted that some cultural values and approaches to care as well as service provision within indigenous cultures differ from mainstream Western cultures, resulting in the potential provision of services offered in culturally inappropriate or offensive ways [12].

In recognition of the autonomy of indigenous populations and the unique barriers these communities encounter, the Older Americans Act establishes special funding to support the provision of long-term services and supports to Native American, Alaskan Natives, and Native Hawaiians [87]. Funding is available to tribal governments and organizations serving native elders, enabling them to provide Aging Network long-term services and support programs within their communities. These Title VI services, referring to the section of the Act which governs these programs, vary by provider and area but may include information and referral assistance, congregate and home-delivered nutrition services, senior center programs and activities, telephone reassurance or friendly visitors, health and wellness programs, nonmedical transportation, shopping or commodity distribution, and respite care services [14, 65].

Title VI programs serving indigenous populations have been successful in developing culturally appropriate interventions to support older adults within their communities. The Family Support Center of Jamestown S'klallam is one example of an elder justice program developed with funding from the Administration on Aging's Native American Caregiver Support Program [70]. This restorative justice intervention brings together "talking circles" of individuals supportive of the elder from the older adult's family, friends, and community to educate families about caregiving issues and develop care plans using the culturally significant "medicine wheel" approach to address the physical, emotional, spiritual, and social needs of the elder [70]. The development and implementation of such culturally appropriate interventions may help indigenous communities better identify and address abuse. There is a growing emphasis among indigenous Aging Network providers to prevent and address elder abuse within their communities. The National Indigenous Elder Justice Initiative (NIEJI; www.NIEJI.org) was formed in 2011 to focus on the development and dissemination information, tools, and resources to indigenous communities and their service providers [11, 65]. In addition to these resources, the initiative also provides a compilation of tribal codes regarding elder abuse and a listing of elder abuse reporting hotlines serving tribal populations. Since its establishment in 2011, many Title VI providers have sought to provide elders with elder abuse prevention and intervention services including abuse investigation services, case management for victims and those at-risk for experiencing abuse, neglect or self-neglect, adult guardianship services, community education and training, victim or witness services, and short-term emergency victim services [65]. Providers report partnering with law enforcement, APS, domestic violence advocates, and legal, medical, and social services professionals to identify and respond to abuse, and about 20 % participate in on an elder abuse Multidisciplinary Team (MDT) [65]. Elder abuse MDTs are discussed in greater detail in Dr. Georgia Anetzberger's chapter within this volume.

14.4.10 Cultural Considerations

Building and expanding work with tribal organization and indigenous peoples, it is important to recognize that a client's cultural identity and community may affect their help-seeking behavior and willingness to accept formal services and supports. Seeking to connect clients with service providers who have a specific mission, expertise, history or competency in working with individuals of that cultural group is often key. Such providers may be a part of the Aging Network in the client's local area and can be identified by contacting the local Area Agency on Aging (AAA) or Aging and Disability Resource Center (ADRC). Readers are encouraged to review the textbook chapters on culture in this volume.

14.5 Coordination Between the Aging Network and Service Providers

14.5.1 Collaboration with APS

The work of Title VI Aging Network providers to prevent, identify, and address abuse and neglect (discussed above) is exemplary and demonstrates multiple ways the Aging Network can seek to promote elder justice and safety independently, and in partnership with APS and other service providers. Despite their unique developmental histories, authorizations, and funding sources, the Aging Network and APS have a shared goal and responsibility to promote the physical, emotional, and social well-being and safety of America's older adults. While in the majority of cases, these programs operate in separate silos, interacting primarily when practitioners take the initiative to refer cases between agencies, in some areas, programs have sought ways to better collaborate and establish formal or informal partnerships.

The state of New Mexico has sought to better integrate aging service provision through its Aging and Disability Resource Center (ADRC). New Mexico's APS program is a member agency of the ADRC (a program described earlier in this chapter), and APS Intake staff are co-located in the ADRC facility [63]. ADRC staff is cross-trained in APS intake, enabling them to provide backup support for APS as needed. Once the report is received, it is transmitted to the APS field offices where field supervisors and staff evaluate, investigate, and intervene in cases of abuse according to established program protocols. In cases where the referred individual is deemed ineligible for services or APS is unable to definitively confirm the abuse, APS clients are referred back to the ADRC where a Resource Options Coordinator works with the consumer to provide information, referrals, and resources that may provide some support [63]. In this promising practice, efforts to streamline client intake and establish clear referral protocols help consumers better access APS services and ensure that vulnerable elders continue to receive supportive services after their APS case is closed.

In another promising practice, the Region One Area Agency on Aging and local APS in Maricopa, Arizona have established the Service Coordination Program (SCP) to actively collaborate on serious cases of abuse and

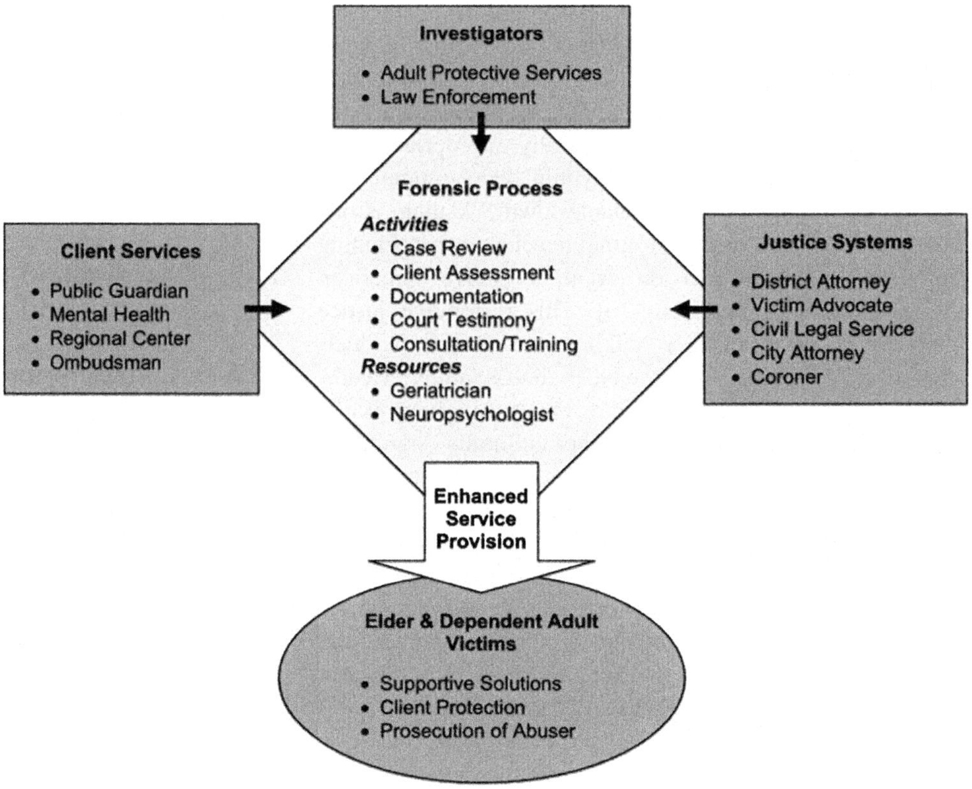
Investigators
• Adult Protective Services
• Law Enforcement
Forensic Process
Activities
• Case Review
• Client Assessment
• Documentation
• Court Testimony
• Consultation/Training
Resources
• Geriatrician
• Neuropsychologist
Client Services
• Public Guardian
• Mental Health
• Regional Center
• Ombudsman
Justice Systems
• District Attorney
• Victim Advocate
• Civil Legal Service
• City Attorney
• Coroner
Enhanced
Service
Provision
Elder & Dependent Adult
Victims
• Supportive Solutions
• Client Protection
• Prosecution of Abuser

Fig. 14.2 Elder Abuse Forensic Center Conceptual model. *Note* This model builds on an initial model laid out in Navarro et al. [68]. *Source*: Gassoumis et al. [37] Aging and Mental Health, 19, 790–798. doi:10.1080/13607863.2014.962011. Copyright © 2014 Taylor & Francis

neglect [64]. Specifically, community-dwelling APS clients in need of immediate services are enrolled in the 90-day program and are eligible for immediate home- and community-based services through the Area Agency on Aging (AAA). Within 48 hours of a client's referral to the SCP, an AAA case manager visits with the client to assess their needs and develop a service plan. The benefit of this approach is that highly vulnerable older adults are able to meet with program staff who is knowledgeable about the range of services available and access services quickly rather than being placed on waiting lists, resulting in improved service coordination, faster APS investigation, and a lower rate of APS case recurrence [50, 64].

14.5.2 Collaboration with Other Elder Abuse Professionals

Collaboration through elder abuse Multidisciplinary Teams (MDTs) is one way that Aging Network providers work with elder abuse professionals to improve communication and service delivery to victims of abuse and neglect. MDTs are dedicated to preventing, investigating, and addressing cases of abuse and neglect within the community [70, 88]. Teams are comprised of interested professionals who gather together to perform specific tasks related to elder abuse, such as providing consultation to professionals providing direct services to abuse victims, identifying structural or systemic barriers to service delivery, advocacy, member training, or sponsoring educational forums and events [88]. A nationwide survey of AAAs found that in communities with an elder abuse MDT present, 79.3 % of local AAAs participated on the team [86]. And Teaster et al. [88] found that Aging Network providers participate on more than half of MDTs surveyed as part of a nationwide survey. In addition, State Units on Aging and Area Agencies on Aging played key roles in convening and coordinating MDTs, provided key leadership and support through direct funding, in-kind support, technical assistance, and meeting coordination [88]. However, it is important to note that as with Aging Network services, there is no singular MDT model and the availability and functions of local MDTs vary significantly.

While there has not been much standardization of the MDT approach, Congress has sought to support the nationwide development of the Elder Abuse Forensic Center model, a type of MDT, by authorizing their replication under the Elder Justice Act [33]. First developed and introduced at University of California, Irvine [106], the Forensic Center brings together legal (e.g., prosecutors, law enforcement, civil attorneys), medical (e.g., geriatricians, registered nurses, psychologists, mental health professionals), and social services (e.g., APS, Long-Term Care Ombudsman, public guardian) professionals to review complex cases of abuse or neglect and provide services and supports to investigators and direct service providers already involved in abuse investigation and intervention [37, 68, 80, 106]. The accompanying figures present a conceptual model of the intervention (Fig. 14.2) and a case processing map (Fig. 14.3) outlining the process used by the MDT to assess, investigate, and intervene in cases of suspected financial abuse. The model has demonstrated effectiveness in increasing safety through expanding the use of appropriate conservatorships for vulnerable older adults [37] and decreasing rates of APS case recurrence [104]. Use of the Forensic Center increases abuser prosecution rates [67], which prosecutors attributed to the immediate availability of key decision-makers, provision of forensic medical and psychological assessment and case review, and cross-discipline learning [24]. As with other MDTs, Forensic Centers may integrate Aging Network providers into their multidisciplinary team or may rely on them for coordination and support [80].

14.6 Future Directions

Future directions in applied research may help the Aging Network strengthen their service delivery approach and identify community-based interventions to effectively support efforts to prevent, identify, investigate, and intervene in cases of abuse and neglect.

14.6.1 Research and Practice

As communities seek ways to effectively resolve abuse, scientific evidence evaluating intervention approaches is largely lacking [77, 78].

As previously discussed, the use of the Elder Abuse Forensic Center multidisciplinary team intervention has demonstrated effectiveness in promoting client safety, reducing short-term recurrence, and achieving criminal justice [37, 67, 104]. In addition, in their systematic review of the literature for elder abuse interventions, Ploeg and colleagues [78] identified eight abuse interventions which demonstrated effectiveness in improving victim outcomes. These include providing abuse victims with discussion and support groups, enhanced provision of social or legal services and supports, community education in public housing developments, enhanced police and social services home response following abuse report, caregiver interventions, and provider training and education, many of which can be or are already provided by the Aging Network [78].

In 2013, the Administration on Aging instituted the Elder Abuse Prevention Interventions Program, a three-year demonstration project providing five states with funding to enact and evaluate elder abuse prevention interventions [99]. Although the demonstration has not concluded, the Administration's investment in the establishment and research of these pilot interventions provide an important starting point to inform future abuse prevention research and service provision. Similar investments in translational and evaluation research are needed in order to continue moving the field forward.

Future work may also seek to implement successful interventions with diverse ethnic, religious, or social minority groups. The translation of promising practices into different cultures, countries, and communities may help to address abuse round the world. The creation of novel, culturally tailored, interventions can draw on the unique perspectives, preferences, and practices of these groups. Alternatively, the existing evidence-based interventions can be adapted to be culturally relevant and appropriate for use with diverse populations. Replicating evidence-based programs with fidelity to the evaluated program model has been used within the Aging Network in areas such as health promotion and disease prevention programs with minority populations [90, 91]. This approach may be most efficient and cost-effective for smaller organizations as they have already been rigorously evaluated and demonstrated successful among the general population. Adoption of adapted interventions may be strengthened and encouraged if program planners partner with existing community leaders. We encourage interested parties to consider using Community-Based Participatory Research methods to facilitate this process [6, 10].

14.6.2 Technological Interventions

Technological interventions may also play a role in bridging relationships between Aging Network service providers and elder abuse professionals. The development of mobile phone applications can assist providers in determining whether abuse may have occurred and knowing what to do after these suspicions arise. The Guide for Elder Abuse Response (GEAR) mobile application and website (http://guideforelderabuse.org) equips direct service providers and law enforcement personnel with information on the signs and symptoms of abuse and links them to APS' online abuse reporting system. The app also includes a searchable map with local resources for victims of abuse, including senior centers and other Aging Network resources. Developed through a collaboration between the University of Southern California, Davis School of Gerontology and the Los Angeles County Elder Abuse Forensic Center, the app is designed with providers in mind and even includes an age calculator to quickly determine whether a particular individual meets reporting or program age requirements. Although the app is specifically designed for use in Los

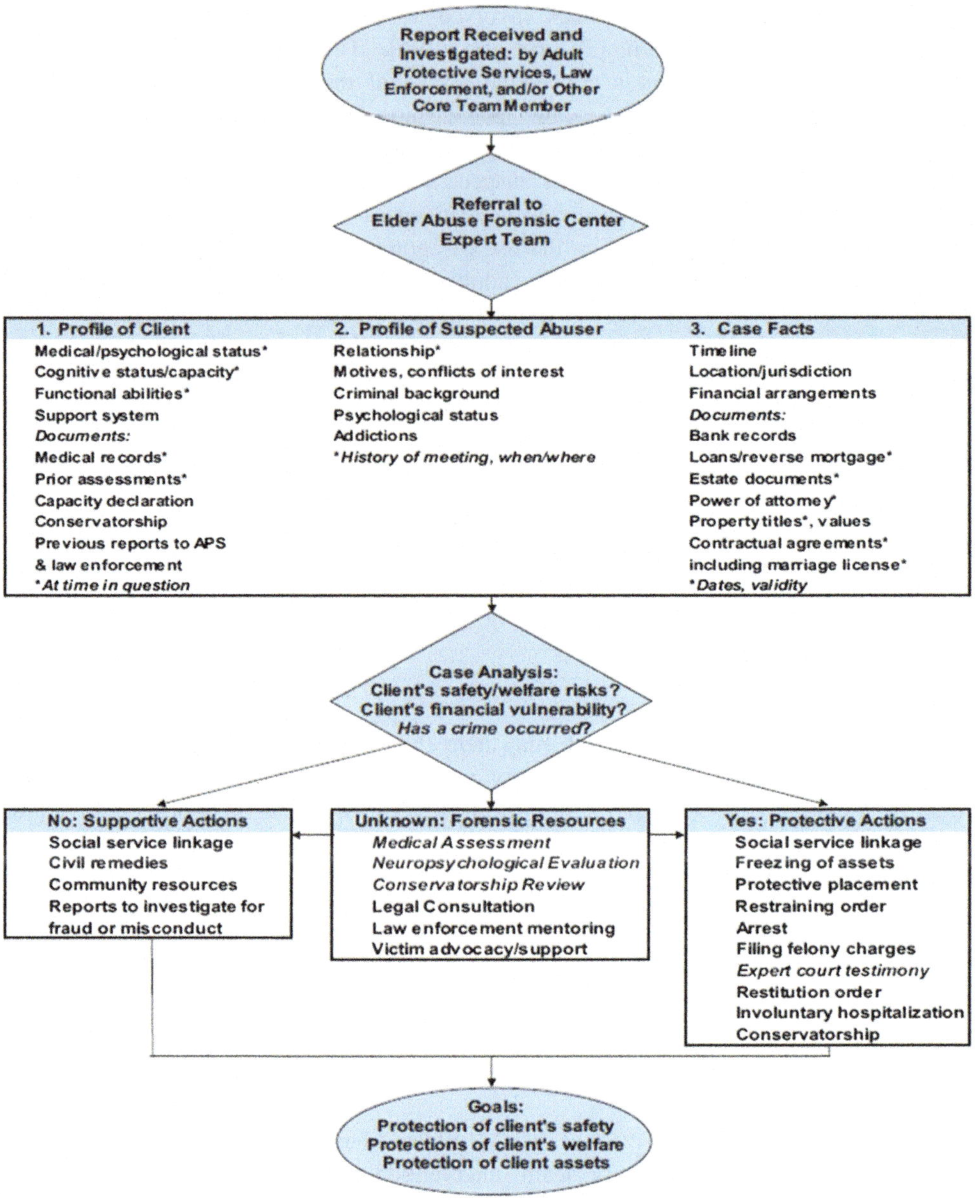

Fig. 14.3 Elder Abuse Forensic Center Case Processing Map. *Source*: Navarro et al. [69], The Gerontologist

Angeles, it is a model intervention that can be replicated in other geographic areas.

The use of telecommunication technologies may also seek to improve interagency collaboration and resource-sharing. In a study of Elder Abuse Forensic Centers in California, Centers reported using teleconferencing technologies to enable practitioners who would otherwise be unable to participate in the multidisciplinary team's meetings [105]. This has been especially important in Los Angeles which serves a large geographic area larger than some states and houses rural providers who need to drive over an hour to reach resources located in the City of Los Angeles.

14.6.3 Data Collection and Analysis

The lack of available data on elder abuse has been cited as a major impediment to work in the field [8]. To date, much of the research on abuse and abuse interventions have been cross-sectional, and the development and use of longitudinal datasets is important to inform the field and evaluate interventions [8].

On the federal level, the Aging Network has taken significant steps to move the field forward in data collection. The U.S. Department of Health and Human Services is in the process of developing a national APS reporting system with standardized data definitions and services [109]. The National Adult Maltreatment Reporting System (NAMRs) collects data on (1) reporting agency policies and practices and (2) report-level case data on nonidentifiable client and perpetrator characteristics and services or, if report-level data are unavailable, key indicator data on aggregate investigation and victim statistics.

Although participation in the NAMRS will be voluntary, the information collected will provide researchers and policy makers with critical data to inform policies and practices regarding elder abuse. Researchers will be able to identify abuse across states and geographic locations over time. Moreover, data collected through the database may also help practitioners identify promising practices across geographic regions.

14.6.4 Strengthening Systems

Despite efforts by Aging Network agencies and providers, a recent Government Accountability Office [41] report cites a substantial unmet need for services among older Americans. The Aging Network requires sustained funding to support the infrastructure required to serve and support community-dwelling older adults and work with elder abuse professionals to prevent and address abuse. Aging Network funding flows through appropriations made to the Administration on Aging as authorized by the Older Americans Act. Given that the most recent authorization of the Older Americans Act was five years overdue at the time of its passage, it is unsurprising that funding for Aging Network programs has been relatively stagnant during this time despite the increasing size of the older adult population [41, 61]. To support the essential work of these federal, state, and local agencies and their innumerable and integral local service providers, efforts must be made to increase federal Aging Network funding.

In addition to these efforts, the Aging Network may need to identify ways to align with other potential funding streams. The former Assistant Secretary for Aging Kathy Greenlee, once head of the U.S. Administration on Aging, has suggested that the Aging Network should adapt to better collaborate and align with health care, including Medicaid, Medicare, Accountable Care organizations, the Veterans Administration and private insurers [42]. Under the Affordable Care Act of 2010, healthcare providers are required to meet quality standards in order to maintain their current funding levels [7]. Strategic planning, self-assessment, and creativity can enable Aging Network programs and providers to identify means for partnering with healthcare providers to enable them to better serve their patients and provide them with quality health and social service supports and interventions [42].

The Aging Network should also continue to expand its efforts to integrate supports and services across sectors. With the aging of the Baby Boomer population, the Aging Network is more important than ever in its efforts to support older adults and share their lessons learned over decades of service to this population. Through partnerships with legal services providers, housing programs, transportation, mental health services, and elder abuse professionals, the Aging Network can seek to find more efficient and effective ways of serving our nation's older adults. Moreover, through partnership with these groups, providers can gain knowledge and experience to better inform their support and service delivery systems.

14.6.5 Moving Forward

In 2014, the U.S. Department of Justice and U.S. Department of Health and Human Services sponsored an initiative to identify the resources, knowledge, and skills needed to understand, prevent, identify, and respond to elder abuse [21]. The massive, national initiative sought input from over 750 public and private stakeholders representing direct service providers, educators, policy makers, and researchers [21]. The resulting Elder Justice Road map is a strategic plan outlining key priorities needed to move the field forward in the future. These include:

(1) increased public awareness of abuse
(2) research to better understand and assess capacity and mental health issues among victims and perpetrators
(3) caregiving support and training
(4) quantification of elder abuse costs to victims, families and society; and
(5) investment in resources for services, education, and research.

Readers are encouraged to consult the Elder Justice Roadmap for greater insight into the future directions needed to strengthen and expand efforts to prevent, identify, investigate, intervene, and resolve cases of elder abuse and neglect. The Elder Justice Roadmap is available online at: https://www.justice.gov/elderjustice/research/roadmap.html.

14.7 Conclusion

First implemented to deliver in-home supports and services to community-dwelling older American across the country, the Aging Network was not specifically designed to prevent, identify, investigate, or address cases of elder abuse or neglect. Nevertheless, this nationwide system spanning all levels of government and thousands of service providers is well positioned to support those at-risk for maltreatment and victims of abuse—both while the abuse is occurring and after its cessation. The provision of timely and appropriate resources and services can reduce the risk of abuse by addressing client vulnerabilities (e.g., social isolation, functional limitations, poor physical, or mental health), lowering abuser opportunity (e.g., fostering client dependency and isolation), and instilling protective contextual factors, such as vigilant providers and social support. In situations where abuse or neglect has already occurred, engagement in Aging Network programs and services may provide victims with the support and encouragement needed to report the abuse or seek assistance from those outside the situation. Moreover, the social, emotional, and instrumental support available through the Aging Network may help victims as they recover from the incident and seek to establish a new "normal."

In Mr. B's case, relief came when his doctor contracted with an agency to provide a part-time case manager. The case manager listened to Mr. B's concerns about his inability to drive and difficulty with household tasks. She was able to enroll him in a transportation program that would send a shared-bus driver to his home to transport him to his appointments or social gatherings. The case manager also got him in touch with an Aging Network agency, which agreed to pay for a home attendant to visit his home and help him with household tasks for two hours, twice a week. Mr. B was relieved that he would no longer need to ask his son for help with these tasks. A few months later, during one of his son's drunken outbursts, Mr. B realized that he was no longer dependent on his son for care and called the police for help. When the police arrived, he reported the abuse and agreed to press charges against his son. With his son in jail, Mr. B went down to the courthouse to file for a protective order against his son and begin eviction proceedings. Although he was troubled by this outcome, he believed that he had done the right thing in taking these steps to regain his independence.

For Mrs. D, this adjustment came after receiving supportive services from a host of Aging Network providers after her building manager called Adult Protective Services for help. The APS worker connected Mrs. D with the area's Aging and Disability Resource Center (ADRC). The ADRC was able to enroll Mrs. D in a personal care program, which assessed her needs and sent a personal care assistant to her home three times a week to help her with bathing and personal hygiene. She also received support through a housekeeping program that provided a few hours a week of light housekeeping. In order to determine what other services Mrs. D might need, ADRC staff interviewed Mrs. D and conducted brief cognitive, social, and emotional assessments. The assessments indicated that Mrs. D did not appear to be cognitively impaired but was experiencing severe depression and anxiety. Staff at the ADRC referred Mrs. D to a senior center near her home which offered case management services coupled with an Aging Network-funded evidence-based health promotion and disease prevention program to provide counseling and support for older adults with depression and anxiety. The case manager helped Mrs. D sign up for a Life Alert program and provided her with information about equipment that might help reduce risk of falls in the bathroom. The case manager was also able to refer Mrs. D to a money management program to help her pay her back rent, establish a reasonable budget, and pay her future bills on time. After a several sessions with the case manager, Mrs. D began to feel less depressed and anxious. She began to attend the senior center's congregate meal program and made friends with two other widows in her neighborhood. As she became more social, she also began to pay more attention to her appearance, once again taking the time to style her hair and put on makeup—things she had not done since her husband died. With social support from new friends and formal service providers, Mrs. D no longer felt it necessary to have anyone live with her. The money management company found that the boarder living with Mrs. D had given her less than half of what was actually owed her and she no longer wanted the renter in her home. Mrs. D contacted an Aging Network legal provider to assist with evicting her unwanted tenant. A year after the original APS report was made and she became connected to the Aging Network, Mrs. D is happier and more socially engaged.

References

1. Acierno R, Melba A, Hernandez AB, Amstadter HS, Resnick KS, Muzzy W, Kilpatrick DG. Prevalence and correlates of emotional, physical, sexual, and financial abuse and potential neglect in the United States: The National Elder Mistreatment Study. Am J Public Health. 2010;100(2):292–7.
2. Alkema G, Enguidanos S, Wilber K, Trufasiu M, Simmons J, Frey D. The role of consultant pharmacists in reducing medication problems among older adults receiving Medicaid waiver services. Consult Pharm. 2009;24(2):121–33.
3. Baker MW, LaCroix AZ, Wu C, Cochrane BB, Wallace R, Woods NF. Mortality risk associated with physical and verbal abuse in women aged 50 to 79. J Am Geriatr Soc. 2009;57 (10):1799–809.
4. Belza B, Snyder S, Thompson M, LoGerfo J. From research to practice: EnhanceFitness, an innovative community-based senior exercise program. Top Geriatr Rehabil. 2010;26(4):299–309.
5. Berkman LF, Leo-Summers L, Horwitz R. Emotional support and survival after myocardial infarction: a prospective, population-based study of the elderly. Ann Intern Med. 1992;117(2):1003–9.
6. Blair T, Minkler M. Participatory action research with older adults: key principles in practice. Gerontologist. 2009;49(5): 651–62.

7. Blumenthal D, Abrams M, Nuzum R. The affordable care act at 5 years. N Engl J Med. 2015;372(25):2451–8.
8. Bonnie RJ, Wallace RB (eds). Elder mistreatment: abuse, neglect, and exploitation in an aging America. Washington: National Academies Press; 2003.
9. Brandl B, Hebert M, Rozwadowski J, Spangler D. Feeling safe, feeling strong support groups for older abused women. Violence Against Women. 2003;9(12):1490–503.
10. Braun KL, Nguyen TT, Tanjasiri SP, Campbell J, Heiney SP, Brandt HM, Ma GX. Operationalization of community-based participatory research principles: assessment of the National Cancer Institute's Community Network Programs. Am J Public Health. 2012;102(6):1195–203.
11. Browne CV, Carter P, Gray JS. National resource centers focus on indigenous communities. Generations. 2014;38(4):70.
12. Browne CV, Mokuau N, Lana S, Kim BJ, Higuchi P, Braun KL. Listening to the voices of Native Hawaiian Elders and 'Ohana Caregivers: discussions on aging, health, and care preferences. J Cross Cult Gerontol. 2014;29(2):131–51.
13. Burnes D, Pillemer K, Caccamise PL, Mason A, Henderson CR, Berman J, Cook AM, Shukoff D, Brownell P, Powell M, Salamone A, Lachs MS. Prevalence of and risk factors for elder abuse and neglect in the community: a population-based study. J Am Geriatr Soc. 2015;63(9):1906–12.
14. Carpio E, Kunkel SR, Straker JK, McGrew KB. 2011 Title VI Survey Results. Scripps Gerontology Center: Ohio; 2012.
15. Ciechanowski P, Wagner E, Schmaling K, Schwartz S, Williams B, Diehr P, LoGerfo J. Community-integrated home-based depression treatment in older adults: a randomized controlled trial. JAMA. 2004;291(13):1569–77.
16. Cohen LE, Felson M. Social change and crime rate trends: a routine activity approach. Am Sociol Rev. 1979;44(4):588–608.
17. Colello KJ. Older Americans act: Title III nutrition services program (RS21202). Washington: Congressional Research Service; 2011.
18. Comijs HC, Penninx BW, Knipscheer KP, van Tilburg W. Psychological distress in victims of elder mistreatment: the effects of social support and coping. J Gerontol B Psychol Sci Soc Sci. 1999;54(4):P240–5.
19. Comijs HC, Pot AM, Smit JH, Bouter LM, Jonker C. Elder abuse in the community: prevalence and consequences. J Am Geriatr Soc. 1998;46(7):885–8.
20. Congress.gov. S.192—Older Americans Act Reauthorization Act of 2016 (Summary). 2016, April. Retrieved online from 9th May 2016. https://www.congress.gov/bill/114th-congress/senate-bill/192.
21. Connolly M, Brandl B, Breckman R. The elder Justice roadmap: a stakeholder initiative to respond to an emerging health, Justice, financial and social crisis. Washington: Department of Justice; 2014.
22. Cornwell EY, Waite LJ. Social disconnectedness, perceived isolation, and health among older adults. J Health Soc Behav. 2009;50(1):31–48.
23. DeLiema M, Navarro AE, Enguidanos S, Wilber KH. Voices from the frontlines: examining elder abuse from multiple professional perspectives. Health Soc Work. 2015;40(2):e15–24.
24. DeLiema M, Navarro AE, Moss M, Wilber KH. Prosecutors' perspectives on elder justice using an Elder Abuse Forensic Center. Am J Crim Justice. In Press.
25. Dong XQ. Elder abuse: systematic review and implications for practice. J Am Geriatr Soc. 2015;63(6):1214–38.
26. Dong X. Medical implications of elder abuse and neglect. Clin Geriatr Med. 2005;21(2):293–313.
27. Dong X, Simon M, Beck T, Evans D. Decline in cognitive function and elder mistreatment: findings from the Chicago Health and Aging Project. Am J Geriatr Psychiatry. 2014;22 (6):598–605.
28. Dong X, Simon MA. Association between reported elder abuse and rates of admission to skilled nursing facilities: findings from a longitudinal population-based cohort study. Gerontology. 2013;59(5):464–72.
29. Dong XQ, Simon MA, Beck TT, Farran C, McCann JJ, Mendes de Leon CF, et al. Elder abuse and mortality: the role of psychological and social wellbeing. Gerontology. 2011;57 (6):549–58.
30. Dong X, Simon M, de Leon CM, Fulmer T, Beck T, Hebert L, et al. Elder self-neglect and abuse and mortality risk in a community-dwelling population. JAMA. 2009;302(5):517–26.
31. Dong X, Simon M, Evans D. Decline in physical function and risk of elder abuse reported to social services in a community-dwelling population of older adults. J Am Geriatr Soc. 2012;60(10):1922–8.
32. Dunlop BD, Rothman MB, Condon KM, Hebert KS, Martinez IL. Elder abuse: risk factors and use of case data to improve policy and practice. J Elder Abuse Negl. 2001;12(3–4): 95–122.
33. Elder Justice Coalition. Elder justice act summary (fact sheet). 2016. Retrieved online from April 11, 2016. http://elderjusticecoalition.com/sites/default/files/documents/Elder%20Justice%20Act%20Facts%20Funding%20Resources.pdf.
34. Enguidanos SM, DeLiema M, Aguilar I, Lambrinos J, Wilber KH. Multicultural voices: attitudes of older adults in the United States of America about elder mistreatment. Ageing Soc. 2014;34 (5):877–903.
35. Ernst JS, Smith CA. Assessment in adult protective services: do multidisciplinary teams make a difference? J Gerontol Soc Work. 2012;55(1):21–38.
36. Feinberg LF, Newman SL. A study of 10 states since passage of the national family caregiver support program: policies, perceptions, and program development. Gerontologist. 2004;44(6): 760–9.
37. Gassoumis ZD, Navarro AE, Wilber KH. Protecting victims of elder financial exploitation: the role of an Elder Abuse Forensic Center in referring victims for conservatorship. Aging Ment Health. 2015;19(9):790–8.
38. Gelfand D. The Aging Network: programs and services. 5th ed. Springer Publishing Company: New York; 1999.
39. Glass TA, Maddox GL. The quality and quantity of social support: stroke recovery as psycho-social transition. Soc Sci Med. 1992;34(11):1249–61.
40. Government Accountability Office. Transportation for Older adults: measuring results could help determine if coordination efforts improve mobility. (Publication no. GAO-15-158). 2014, December. Retrieved online from April 1, 2016. http://www.gao.gov/assets/670/667375.pdf.
41. Government Accountability Office. Older Americans Act: Updated Information on Unmet Need for Services. (Publication no. GAO-15-601R). 2015, June. Retrieved online from on April 1, 2016. http://www.gao.gov/assets/680/670738.pdf.
42. Greenlee K. Assistant secretary for aging sees network at a crossroads—and a place of new opportunities. Aging Today. 2016;37(2):1.
43. Hafemeister TL. Financial abuse of the elderly in domestic settings. In: Bonnie RJ, Wallace RB, editors. Elder mistreatment: abuse, neglect, and exploitation in an aging America. Washington, DC: The National Academies Press; 2003. p. 382–445.

44. Harrell R, Lynott J, Guzman S, Lampkin C. What is livable? Community preferences of older adults. 2014. Retrieved online from April 1, 2016. http://www.aarp.org/content/dam/aarp/research/public_policy_institute/liv_com/2014/what-is-livable-report-AARP-ppi-liv-com.pdf.
45. Hayslip B, Kaminski PL. Grandparents raising their grandchildren: a review of the literature and suggestions for practice. Gerontologist. 2005;45(2):262–9.
46. Hunkeler EM, Katon W, Tang L, Williams JW, Kroenke K, Lin EH, Hargreaves WA. Long term outcomes from the IMPACT randomised trial for depressed elderly patients in primary care. BMJ. 2006;332(7536):259–63.
47. Jackson SL. all elder abuse perpetrators are not alike: the heterogeneity of elder abuse perpetrators and implications for intervention. Int J Offender Ther Comp Criminol. 2014;60 (3):265–85.
48. Johannesen M, LoGiudice D. Elder abuse: a systematic review of risk factors in community-dwelling elders. Age Ageing. 2013;42 (3):292–8.
49. Kane RL, Kane RA. A guide through the maze of long-term care. West J Med. 1981;135(6):503.
50. Kasunic ML. Tool for addressing elder abuse: multi-disciplinary coalitions. Presented at international network for the prevention of elder abuse (INPEA) 8th world conference in Seoul, South Korea on June 23, 2013.
51. Ka'opua LS, Braun KL, Browne CV, Mokuau N, Park CB. Why are native Hawaiians underrepresented in Hawai 'i's older adult population? Exploring social and behavioral factors of longevity. J Aging Res. 2011.
52. Lachs MS, Williams C, O'Brien S, Hurst L, Horwitz R. Risk factors for reported elder abuse and neglect: a nine-year observational cohort study. Gerontologist. 1997;37(4):469–74.
53. Lachs MS, Williams CS, O'Brien S, Pillemer KA, Charlson ME. The mortality of elder mistreatment. JAMA. 1998;280(5): 428–32.
54. Lee M. Caregiver stress and elder abuse among Korean family caregivers of older adults with disabilities. J Fam Violence. 2008;23(8):707–12.
55. Litwin H, Zoabi S. A multivariate examination of explanations for the occurrence of elder abuse. Soc Work Res. 2004;28 (3):133–42.
56. Low SM, Altman I. Place attachment. Berlin: Springer; 1992.
57. LTC.gov. Costs of care. 2016. Retrieved online from February 5, 2016. http://longtermcare.gov/costs-how-to-pay/costs-of-care/.
58. Mollica R, Gillespie J. Single entry point systems: state survey results. New Jersey: CSHP, Rutgers Center for State Health Policy; 2003.
59. Moore-Harrison TL, Johnson MA, Quinn ME, Cress ME. An evidence-based exercise program implemented in congregate-meal sites. J Phys Act Health. 2009;6(2):247.
60. Mosqueda LC, Gironda MW, Olsen BJ, Burnight K. An elder abuse prevention intervention: sample characteristics of persons with dementia and caregivers. Gerontologist. 2015;55(S2):177.
61. Napili A, Colello KJ. Funding for the older Americans act and other aging services programs. Washington, DC: Congressional Research Service; 2013. p. 196.
62. National Association of Protective Services Agencies. History of adult protective services. 2016. Retrieve online from Feb 4, 2016. http://www.napsa-now.org/about-napsa/history/history-of-adult-protective-services.
63. National Adult Protective Services Resource Center. Integrated information, training and access to services at an ADRC: New Mexico's experience. National Adult Protective Services Resource Center; 2012.
64. National Adult Protective Services Resource Center. The APS/AAA service coordination program, Maricopa County. Arizona: National Adult Protective Services Resource Center; 2016.
65. National Association of Area Agencies on Aging and Miami University. 2014 Title VI survey results. National Association of Area Agencies on Aging; 2014.
66. National Center on Elder Abuse. Sentinels: reaching hidden victims. Washington, DC: National Center on Elder Abuse; 2002.
67. Navarro AE, Gassoumis ZD, Wilber KH. Holding abusers accountable: an Elder Abuse Forensic Center increases criminal prosecution of financial exploitation. Gerontologist. 2013;53 (2):303–12.
68. Navarro AE, Wilber KH, Yonashiro J, Homeier DC. Do we really need another meeting? Lessons from the Los Angeles County Elder Abuse Forensic Center. Gerontologist. 2010;50(5):702–11.
69. Navarro AE, Wysong J, DeLiema M, Schwartz EL, Nichol MB, Wilber KH. Inside the black box: the case review process of an Elder Abuse Forensic Center. Gerontologist. 2016;56(4):772–81.
70. Nerenberg L. Communities respond to elder abuse. J Gerontol Soc Work. 2006;46(3–4):5–33.
71. Nerenberg L. Elder abuse prevention: emerging trends and promising strategies. New York: Springer Publishing Company; 2008.
72. O'Shaughnessy C. Aging and Disability Resource Centers can help consumers navigate the maze of long-term services and supports. Generations. 2011;35(1):64–8.
73. Piercy KW. When it is more than a job close relationships between home health aides and older clients. J Aging Health. 2000;12(3):362–87.
74. Pillemer K, Connolly MT, Breckman R, Spreng RN, Lachs MS. Elder mistreatment: priorities for consideration by the White House conference on aging. Gerontologist. 2015;55(2):320–7.
75. Pillemer K, Finkelhor D. Causes of elder abuse: caregiver stress versus problem relatives. Am J Orthopsychiatry. 1989;59(2): 179–87.
76. Pillemer K, Finkelhor D. The prevalence of elder abuse: a random sample survey. Gerontologist. 1988;28(1):51–7.
77. Pillemer KA, Mueller-Johnson KU, Mock SE, Suitor JJ, Lachs MS. Interventions to prevent elder mistreatment. In: Doll LS, Bonzo SE, Sleet DA, Mercy JA, editors. Handbook of injury and violence prevention. New York: Springer; 2007. p. 241–54.
78. Ploeg J, Fear J, Hutchison B, MacMillan H, Bolan G. A systematic review of interventions for elder abuse. J Elder Abuse Negl. 2009;21(3):187–210.
79. Ramsey-Klawsnik H. Elder-abuse perpetrators: a typology. Generations. 2000;24(2):7–22.
80. Schneider DC, Mosqueda L, Falk E, Huba GJ. Elder Abuse Forensic Centers. J Elder Abuse Negl. 2010;22(3–4):255–74.
81. Schofield MJ, Powers JR, Loxton D. Mortality and disability outcomes of self-reported elder abuse: a 12-year prospective investigation. J Am Geriatr Soc. 2013;61(5):679–85.
82. Seeman TE. Health promoting effects of friends and family on health outcomes in older adults. Am J Health Promot. 2000;14 (6):362–70.
83. Seeman TE, Lusignolo TM, Albert M, Berkman L. Social relationships, social support, and patterns of cognitive aging in healthy, high-functioning older adults: MacArthur studies of successful aging. Health Psychol. 2001;20(4):243.
84. Shenk D, Kuwahara K, Zablotsky D. Older women's attachments to their home and possessions. J Aging Stud. 2004;18(2):157–69.
85. Smith ML, Ory MG, Ahn S, Kulinski KP, Jiang L, Horel S, Lorig K. National dissemination of chronic disease

self-management education programs: an incremental examination of delivery characteristics. Front Public Health. 2014;2:227.
86. Straker JK, Lackmeyer AL, Kunkel S. Elder abuse and legal assistance AAA results (research brief). Oxford, OH: Scripps Gerontology Center; 2008.
87. Takamura JC. Getting ready for the 21st century: the aging of America and the older Americans Act. Health Soc Work. 1999;24 (3):232.
88. Teaster PB, Nerenberg L, Stansbury KL. A national look at elder abuse multidisciplinary teams. J Elder Abuse Negl. 2003;15(3–4): 91–107.
89. Terracina KA, Aamodt WW, Schillerstrom JE. Executive function impairment and recidivism in adult protective services clients referred for a decision making capacity assessment. J Elder Abuse Negl. 2015;27(2):91–9.
90. Tomioka M, Braun KL. Implementing evidence-based programs a four-step protocol for assuring replication with fidelity. Health Promot Pract. 2012;14(6):850–8.
91. Tomioka M, Braun KL, Compton M, Tanoue L. Adapting Stanford's chronic disease self-management program to Hawaii's multicultural population. Gerontologist. 2012;52(1):121–32.
92. Towne SD Jr, Smith ML, Ahn S, Altpeter M, Belza B, Kulinski KP, Ory MG. National dissemination of multiple evidence-based disease prevention programs: reach to vulnerable older adults. Front Public Health. 2014;2:156.
93. Tueth MJ. Exposing financial exploitation of impaired elderly persons. Am J Geriatr Psychiatry. 2000;8(2):104–11.
94. U.S. Administration on Community Living. Aging and disability resource centers in a no wrong door system [fact sheet]. Washington, DC: U.S. Administration on Community Living; 2016.
95. U.S. Administration on Aging. Administration on Aging (AoA): Historical evolution of programs for older Americans. 2015. Retrieved online from April 1, 2016. http://www.aoa.gov/AoA_Programs/OAA/resources/History.aspx.
96. U.S. Administration on Aging. Disease prevention and health promotion services (OAA Title IIID). 2016a. Retrieved online from Feb 1, 2016. http://www.aoa.acl.gov/AoA_Programs/HPW/Title_IIID/index.aspx.
97. U.S. Administration on Aging. National Center on Elder Abuse (Title II). 2016b. Retrieved f from Feb 4, 2016. http://www.aoa.acl.gov/AoA_Programs/Elder_Rights/NCEA/index.aspx.
98. U.S. Administration on Aging. Prevention of elder abuse, neglect, and exploitation (Title VII-A3). 2016c. Retrieved online from April 1, 2016. http://www.aoa.acl.gov/AoA_Programs/Elder_Rights/EA_Prevention/Index.aspx.
99. U.S. Administration on Aging. The elder abuse prevention interventions program. 2016d. Retrieved online from April 1, 2016. http://www.aoa.acl.gov/AoA_Programs/Elder_Rights/EA_Prevention/Demonstration/Index.aspx.
100. Wacker RR, Roberto KA. Chapter 2: Legislative foundations for programs, services, and benefits supporting older adults. In: Community resources for older adults: programs and services in an era of change. 4th edn. Thousand Oaks, CA: Sage Publications; 2014.
101. Whittier S, Scharlach A, Dal Santo TS. Availability of caregiver support services: implications for implementation of the National Family Caregiver Support Program. J Aging Soc Policy. 2005;17 (1):45–62.
102. Wilber KH, Reynolds SL. Introducing a framework for defining financial abuse of the elderly. J Elder Abuse Negl. 1997;8(2):61–80.
103. Wilber KH, Yonashiro-Cho J, Navarro AE, Alkema GE. Policies related to competency and proxy issues. In: Kaplan D, Berkman B, editors. The Oxford handbook of social work in health and aging. 2nd ed. New York: Oxford University Press; 2016. p. 661–70.
104. Wilber KH, Navarro AE, Gassoumis ZD. Evaluating the Elder Abuse Forensic Center model. Submitted to the National Institute of Justice; 2014.
105. Wilber K, Gironda M, Yonashiro-Cho J, DeLiema M, Gassoumis Z, Torres-Gil M, Wysong J. Cross site evaluation of four Elder Abuse Forensic Centers: final report to the Archstone Foundation. California: University of Southern California; 2013.
106. Wiglesworth A, Mosqueda L, Burnight K, Younglove T, Jeske D. Findings from an Elder Abuse Forensic Center. Gerontologist. 2006;46(2):277–83.
107. World Health Organization. World report on ageing and health. Geneva: World Health Organization; 2015.
108. Yip JY, Myrtle RC, Wilber KH, Grazman DN. The networks and resource exchanges in community-based systems of care. J Health Hum Serv Adm. 2002;25(2):219–59.
109. Yuan Y, Leelaram S, Dahbour S, Greene M, Acker A, Swartz E. Development of a National Adult Protective Services Data System: final report. Submitted to the office of the assistant secretary for planning and evaluation, U.S. Department of Health and Human Services; 2015.

15 Adult Protective Services and the Long-Term Care Ombudsman Program

Joseph Snyder and William F. Benson

Adult Protective Services (APS) and the Long-term Care Ombudsman Program (LTCOP) are critical components of states' protection and advocacy services for the nation's elderly and other vulnerable adults, including those in long-term care facilities. These services are critical and indispensable for elders and vulnerable adults in communities across the nation. Yet, the two programs have very different and distinct purposes, roles, and structures. For the most part they can collaborate and complement each other. But in some circumstances they can be at odds with each other. The distinctions are significant enough that it is a conflict for an Ombudsman to also serve as an adult protective service worker or for one to be answerable to the other.

Adult Protective Services is the single, dedicated, authorized victim service system for elder and vulnerable adult abuse victims who live in community settings (in about half the states, APS also investigates abuse in various facility settings). APS, which exists in every community in the United States, operates under state law. APS receives and investigates reports of abuse, neglect, and financial exploitation of older adults, and in most states, of younger adults with severe disabilities as well.

The Long-term Care Ombudsman Program (LTCOP) was created to provide long-term care residents with an independent advocate who would help them resolve complaints and help protect their rights, and who also would work on a systemic level to change policies and practices on statewide, corporatewide, or facilitywide bases in order to promote quality care and quality of life for all long-term care facility residents.

This chapter will explore how APS and LTCOP originated and how they work today, their similarities and differences across the states, and the key issues, recent developments and future directions in both programs.

As noted earlier, APS exists in every community in every state to investigate complaints of abuse, neglect and financial exploitation against elders and vulnerable adults. APS is often compared to child protective services, but there is a critical difference: APS works with adults, who unless adjudicated as lacking capacity by a court of law, get to live their lives as they see fit. This includes making "bad" decisions, or at least decisions that do not follow the norm. A central function of APS is to determine whether a person is capable of making informed decisions about critical issues affecting their lives, or whether to take action to protect the individual against their will.

15.1 Day in the Life of APS and Ombudsman

15.1.1 A Day in the Life of an APS Investigator

An APS investigator starts each day with a list of challenges starting with how to balance their caseload activity when each case is potentially someone who is in crisis and needs protective services. Each case must be monitored and

Several Long-Term Care Leaders were consulted for this chapter. Among those who must be singled out with gratitude for their contributions are Louise Ryan, Ombudsman Program Specialist, U.S. Administration for Community Living; Lori Smetenka, former Director of the National Ombudsman Resource Center (NORC) and now Executive Director, Consumer Voice (host organization for NORC); Deanna Clingan-Fischer, J.D., State Long-Term Care Ombudsman, Iowa Department of Aging; and Cindy Englert, Regional Ombudsman Director, Centralina Area Agency on Aging, NC and President, National Association of Local Long-Term Care Ombudsmen.The authors express their gratitude to Kelli White of Philadelphia APS and Kendra Kuehn of Health Benefits ABCs for their technical know-how and assistance in preparing this chapter.

J. Snyder (✉)
Older Adult Protective Services, Philadelphia Corporation for Aging, 642 N. Broad St., Philadelphia, PA 19130, USA
e-mail: Jsnyder@pcaphl.org

W.F. Benson
National Adult Protective Services Association, Health Benefits ABCs, 11101 Georgia Avenue, #320, Silver Spring, MD 20902, USA

X. Dong (ed.), *Elder Abuse*, DOI 10.1007/978-3-319-47504-2_15

prioritized and when combined with agency and administrative challenges makes every day an adventure.

An investigator must close cases that need to be closed and help clients navigate the various systems engaged in their care. This includes working with other systems while upholding the confidentiality requirements written in the particular statute. This often causes conflict between professionals working together and must be overcome for the welfare of the mutual client. An investigator must also be ready for the new case that may take precedence over his/her best laid plans.

Depending on the funding, size of the workforce and frequency of reports, this challenge can happen on a daily basis. The investigator may have to change plans and drop everything to investigate a new report. States have different time frames on when they have to begin the investigation and indeed what even constitutes the beginning of an investigation. The investigator will analyze the report, see if is a repeat case and go out to see the client. The investigator will hope the client is in the location reported and if not will try to find the client. Once engaged, the investigator will use observation and conversation to determine if there is an actual real emergency that requires immediate attention and act accordingly. If not, the investigator will begin the process of gaining rapport with the client and support system to set the stage for future action. The APS investigator is always walking the fine line between protecting the individual client's civil and constitutional rights and advocating and arranging for his/her safety.

15.1.2 Case Example

The 24 h hotline receives a report of need that states there is a 73-year-old female living alone, slightly confused, house is dirty and cluttered, the bills are not being paid, and the bank account is depleted. Reporter is the neighbor.

Neighbor observes that the niece comes every first of the month and the older person's check is direct deposited to the client's account. Reporter alleges that niece is exploiting her aunt. Based on the information provided, the report is given a non-priority response status and is assigned to an investigator the following day.

Investigator who is assigned the case looks into the system to see if case was previously open to the agency and finds that it is new to everyone so there are no records to review. Investigator contacted the reporter before going out because the information needed to open a case is not the information needed to investigate a case. The purpose of the contact is to determine if there is additional information that will help the investigation, and to discover if the neighbor is a first-hand reporter, i.e., actually witnessed maltreatment. Reporter states that consumer is constantly asking for food for herself and her cats and appears to have lost weight. Reporter says that she recently visited the alleged victim to deliver food and observed a pile of bills, most of which were unopened.

Investigator drives to the home, arrives at the door and meets the client, who is reluctant to let her in. The consumer speaks to the investigator through the screen door, eventually shutting the door without letting the investigator into the home. Investigator goes back to the car and calls the neighbor on the cell phone to explain the reason why she is there. Some helpful hints for gaining access: if the program had known that the consumer had cats, the Investigator could have arrived with a couple cans of cat food that might have gotten her in the door. Intake could have asked the neighbor at the time of the report if she thought that there was going to be a problem with access, and if so, can she be of help? Investigator would then call the neighbor on the phone from the car. We would also explore if anyone else might help us get in the house, such as a neighbor, friend, family, church member etc. *After talking with the neighbor, the client agrees to let the Investigator in the home.*

Investigator meets with client and documents the initial face-to-face visit, observing empty cat food containers in the living room and dining room, heavy drapes on the windows, dust on the table, bills mostly unopened on the table, and very little food in the house except for spoiled food in the refrigerator (Investigator had asked for permission to look around in the refrigerator and other parts of the house). Client appears unkempt and disheveled, and cannot answer questions about medications or her doctor. Investigator asks if there were any medication bottles and there were a bunch of old medication bottles that the consumer brought to the investigator. When asked about the finances, our client replies "I don't have time for that anymore." Client score on a cognitive capacity screening tool indicates severe impairment.

Client reports that her niece comes to visit every now and then to help her, but she was not able to supply the niece's phone number and name. Investigator makes the decision that the client does not understand or comprehend what investigator was saying, so she does not ask the client to sign the various forms. Investigator drives back to the office and starts to analyze the case.

Investigator decides from the initial face-to-face visit that she will substantiate for self-neglect, and put in meals and heavy cleaning to address those issues as she continues with the financial exploitation investigation. Investigator checks the utilities, deed and taxes to make sure there were no impending shut off notices or other issues. Investigator pulls the information from the old med bottles and calls pharmacy and physician to see if they can provide any information. The doctor's office manager states client had been a patient but has not been seen in many years, and because of that she could not comment on their capacity or whether or not abuse or neglect was occurring. Investigator decides a comprehensive capacity evaluation will be ordered, due to the obvious confusion on the part of the client and the allegation of financial exploitation.

Investigator now has to decide whether she should ask the client for permission to open her mail and look at the bank statements since she doubts her capacity? Investigator decides against asking permission and returns to the office. Her first call is to the bank and explains the situation. Bank contact asks for a release of information but investigator cannot form a good faith belief that client has capacity to understand what she is signing. Bank states they will consider giving copies if we have legal authority to act on behalf of the client. Investigator meets with supervisor and decision is made to file for guardianship and then send copy of petition to the bank and request the records.

Investigator contacts the niece to set up an appointment to talk about consumer's finances and the management of money in this case. Niece agrees to a meeting at the agency. Niece claims to be the Power of Attorney (POA) and was asked to bring the documents and any bills or other expenses that she has been paying for the consumer. Niece comes to the interview with some hand written receipts, and when asked to explain the numerous ATM withdrawals and provide receipts, she is unable to do so. Niece doesn't bring official POA documents with her but still insists that she is the POA.

Capacity evaluation is completed and it was determined that the client lacks capacity as to person and estate. The decision is made to file the guardianship petition and a copy is sent to the bank. After analyzing 6 months of statements, the opening balance was $60,000 and the current balance was $8500. Bank makes the independent decision to limit the withdrawals pending the outcome of the APS case.

Investigator calls the niece to ask her again to provide documentation as to why the money was spent and if she could not, to notify her that we will be going to court and asking that a guardian be appointed for her aunt. Niece does not respond to any more inquiries from us. Petition is filed asking for a neutral person to serve as to both and a hearing date is set. Case is taken to court and a neutral attorney is appointed as guardian of both person and estate. Case is transferred to the aging services' care management program. Investigator and Supervisor meet to decide whether there is enough here to make a referral to criminal justice. It was decided there is, and we turn over all the case records to the court-appointed guardian as well as to law enforcement. This is made easier as the APS agency is part of a Task Force which includes both the District Attorney and the police.

There are many and varied issues in the case example, and different points of intersection that could change the nature of the case. What is clear is how complex and intensive these investigations have become and how different they are from child protective services due to the issues of capacity and informed consent.

15.1.3 A Day in the Life of a Long-Term Care Ombudsman

Under the Older Americans Act and many state-specific statutes, the Office of the State Long-Term Care Ombudsman does not exist without an individual identified and empowered as the State Long-Term Care Ombudsman. The title of "State Long-Term Care Ombudsman" (SLTCO) is at the heart of the Office of the State Long-Term Care Ombudsman (LTCOP) and virtually all of the "Office's" authority and responsibility emanates from the SLTCO including heading up the LTCOP. No other individual may carry out the duties of the SLTCO without the blessing of the SLTCO, including provision of Ombudsman services at the local or community levels, even if such individual is located in, hired by and directly supervised by another organization. Such organization may not perform Ombudsman services without being designated to do so by the SLTCO and no individual within such designated organization may carry out SLTCOP responsibilities without being recognized as a "representative" of the Office of the State Long-Term Care Ombudsman.

As a result, the daily work of the State Long-Term Care Ombudsman can differ significantly from those who serve as representatives of the SLTCO including those who serve as Ombudsmen on a voluntary rather than paid basis. The SLTCO is at the center of the Office of the State Long-Term Care Ombudsman; his or her daily responsibilities include a great deal of activity to ensure the program operates with all the proper designations, certifications and associated activities to carry out its statutory duties and to serve its client population as fully as possible.

The daily work of the SLTCO and those who work within the direct Office of the State Long-Term Care Ombudsman at the state level (typically in a state unit on aging or other state agency), can encompass a broad array of activities. Examples include:

- Providing technical assistance to and problem solving with local LTC Ombudsman programs about individual complaints, volunteer management, program operations, working with regulatory and provider organizations and many other matters.
- Providing quality assurance over the program statewide including doing quality assurance (QA) and management reviews of local Ombudsman programs, as well as QA reviews of individual cases handled by local Ombudsman programs.
- Representing the program in dealings with a complex and wide array of organizations and agencies at the state and

national levels (e.g., U.S. Administration for Community Living (ACL), Centers for Medicare and Medicaid Services; Attorney General; State Licensing and Certification agencies for nursing homes and board and care homes; State Medicaid Agency; Medicaid Fraud Control Unit; Quality Improvement Organization; long-term care provider organizations; state organizations of area agencies on aging).

- Designating "representatives" of the Office of the SLTCO and ensuring that certification training of representatives takes place.
- Responding to complaints about local or "substate" Long-Term Care Ombudsman programs.
- Engaging in systems advocacy by representing the program and long-term care facility residents before legislative bodies (federal, state, and local), including drafting and providing testimony; educating legislators and their staff and in general working the legislative process. Systems advocacy also includes representing the program and residents in the rulemaking and other regulatory processes.
- Drafting and updating state program policies (the new federal LTCOP regulation promulgated by the ACL effective July 1, 2016 will require many states to examine and amend state policies and procedures if not state laws and regulations to ensure compliance with the new rule).
- Staying on top of legislative, regulatory, and other policy changes and trends that may affect long-term care facility residents (e.g., facility requirements, Medicaid policy, consumer rights), and communicating and interpreting such changes to the representatives of the Office.
- Ensuring fiscal support for the program by engaging in the state's budget formulation and oversight process.
- Ensuring recognition of volunteers serving as representatives and in other program roles.
- Representing the program with the media.
- Overseeing the state's reporting of data through the National Ombudsman Reporting System (NORS).

On occasion, the State LTCO may have to initiate a process for finding a new organization to serve as a local designated Ombudsman program, whether the former entity was "de-designated" or voluntarily withdrew from the program. There may be an interregnum between one local Ombudsman program closing its door and a new one opening. During such time the State LTCO may have to serve as the Ombudsman receiving and resolving individual complaints in jurisdictions without an operating local Ombudsman program. As a former SLTCO noted, when this happened she or her deputy then responded to individual facility residents' complaints and worked to resolve their complaints including representing residents at administrative or fair hearings (e.g., regarding involuntary discharges from a facility). On any given day her anticipated plan for the day could be entirely up-ended by an unexpected urgent matter or a crisis. For example, the sudden decision of a large long-term care facility to shutter its doors may require the SLTCO and her representatives to spring into action to protect the rights of affected residents and to assist in finding suitable alternatives for them. Similarly, a demand from a legislator for information or input on a legislative matter could consume the SLTCO's time on any given day. The SLTCO also noted the importance of calling upon accessible and capable legal counsel to assist with programmatic issues, advice on complaint resolution, and legislative other systems advocacy work.

Most states carry out the day-to-day complaint response and casework operation of their program through designated local or substate long-term care ombudsman programs. These local programs are largely responsible for a variety of activities especially responding to complaints made by or on behalf of facility residents and the direct visitation to long-term care facilities and their residents and staff. In most communities this work is carried out by both paid and volunteer ombudsmen. Many local LTCOPs operate with very limited funding thus paid staffing is very thin and may often consist of one paid person on a part-time basis.

A "typical day" of a local ombudsman is elusive to describe because it depends to a great extent upon the number of paid staff and whether or not the program relies upon volunteers, and what the volunteer ombudsmen actually do. In theory, however, a certified local ombudsman, paid or volunteer, does the same kind of work centered around the receiving and resolution of residents' complaints. The focus here is on a typical day for a local LTCOP director.

As described by a long-tenured local ombudsman director, her day typical begins going through phone messages received from the previous day while she was out visiting facility residents and facilities in responses to complaints received and prioritizing which to respond to first. She first tries to handle those that can be dealt with simply by providing information or technical assistance to someone. Examples include a person who is looking for a placement in a long-term care facility or someone in a hospital who has been handed a list of facilities and needs some guidance on how to proceed. In particular, she wants to quickly provide information to help residents or those calling on their behalf to do self-advocacy to resolve their problem. This might involve helping someone figure out what questions they should ask about a prospective facility placement. Once done she then moves to the matters that will require more time including go to meet with the resident or family. She attempts to figure out which are most pressing or urgent and give them priority. A complaint about a pending transfer or discharge from a facility, or that a facility will not readmit a resident who was sent to a hospital, will take precedence over a complaint that the food is cold or that a call-bell has not been answered. Yet, with time, all will be responded to.

Around mid-morning she visits facilities mostly to actively investigate cases that the ombudsman has opened. After talking with the resident who has made a complaint or upon whose behalf one was made, and talking with others who may be pertinent to the matter, she tries to talk with other residents, facility staff, any visiting family members and others, to communicate who she is and what her role is. Even if she does not have an active complaint or case in a particular facility she works hard to build relationships with the facility administrator and others in hopes that it will help to stave off or mitigate other complaints. Visits to facilities also provide the opportunity to determine if a matter was resolved, where the changes agreed to by the facility (and others) put into place, was the matter resolved to the satisfaction of the affected resident(s), can the case be closed?

She notes that "all-too-often" the planned 1-h facility visit turns into 3 h. She said when she first started she was mortified by this but over time has learned that it is essential to not only helping residents fully appreciate the role of the Ombudsman but also to develop and sustain relationships with family members, facility staff, and others who may have reason to be in the facility. In a typical day she is able to visit one or two facilities. Facilities can of course be many miles from the Ombudsman's office. If she can make it back to her office by day's end then it is time for "paperwork," to input data into the Ombudsman reporting system, to do appropriate document in case files.

In addition to these responsibilities there are many others for the local ombudsman program director. Noting "There are days when it feels like I'm doing everything but seeing residents" because of meetings, and follow-up interactions with others who may have a stake in a resident's case or problem, such as APS, guardians, Department of Social Services or Medicaid staff, hospital discharge planners, and of course regulatory personnel to determine if they have jurisdiction or a role to play in a particular complaint or problem. And of course some days are just paperwork days.

Because volunteers are so crucial to the Ombudsman program there is also time spent on managing the program's volunteers. Volunteers need to be recruited, trained, deployed, supported, and sustained. Their work (as with all employees) must be supervised and quality assurance activities undertaken. Sometimes, volunteers are the subject of complaints made by facilities or others (including family members) who do not understand or support the ombudsman's role as an independent voice for the resident. In these situations, the local coordinator must address such complaints. Depending upon the numbers of volunteers and the roles they play this can be a full-time pursuit, although rarely at the local level is there full-time time staff assigned to handle volunteers.

Local Ombudsmen are also expected to engage in "systems advocacy," to improve conditions and circumstances for facility residents on a broader basis, by pursuing policy and practice changes within facilities, among facility corporate sponsors, by local and state government entities and others.

As the local coordinator noted, "There isn't really a typical day; it's more like a typical week. I do all this in a typical week. All of it has to be done in order to solve problems, satisfy residents, and close their cases".

15.1.4 Major Issues Confronting APS and Ombudsman

APS is often dealing with a client who has "slipped through the cracks" and has not come to the notice of the many systems that serve a person throughout the life span. Isolation is a major issue for APS clients and a primary tool of the perpetrators of abuse, neglect and exploitation. Working with clients who have diminished capacity, especially financial capacity, is another major issue for APS. Medication misuse complicated by the increased frequency of major illness, and the fact that a person may have multiple physicians who do not know what the others are prescribing, presents another major challenge. Noncompliance with medical care plans can lead to serious self-neglect, and intervention can be difficult and time-consuming. The fact that we are living longer, and frequently living alone with no family or support system nearby, is a major challenge for all of us. Working through family dysfunction and getting reluctant clients to accept services is a major obstacle for all APS investigators and a skilled clinician is often able to overcome insurmountable odds to make this happen. It is a remarkable thing to see and is often not appreciated by the community at large.

The availability of services and the willingness to prioritize services for APS clients is uneven at best across the country. The cooperation of the financial industry in providing victims' financial records and in a timely fashion so the damage to the client is not permanent and all-encompassing, is something that is problematic for many APS programs across the country. The expectation that an APS worker becomes adept at reading all manners of financial documents or at least has access to this expertise has changed the nature of how we do our social services work. Conducting victim and perpetrator interviews in a manner that facilitates the end of the victimization is a skill that requires the presence and availability of this highly specialized training. Educating and cooperating with the criminal justice system, including referring cases that reach the level necessary for criminal prosecution, is a challenge that is met with variable success across the country. There has been much written about the problems with guardianship in this country, and APS professionals have hope they live in jurisdictions where the hearings are scheduled in a timely manner, deference is given to the client's wishes, and there are professionals or agencies available to serve as guardians in the absence of available and reliable family or others close to the client and those individuals serving are monitored closely by the court.

Lack of adequate and reliable funding for APS leads to a plethora of issues, including unmanageable caseloads, lack of training, and no standardization among the states, leading to the inability to move the field forward. There is also an appalling lack of public awareness both about elder abuse and APS, despite the sheer number of cases and the rapid aging of the population. Experts have been trying to figure out for years why this is so with little success. The reason most often cited is ageism, and the fact that people tend to deny they are aging and are certain that this would never happen to them.

It is good to see that research in this area is accelerating and becoming more broadly accepted. This has not always been the case and research has lagged behind despite how long the issue of elder abuse, neglect, and exploitation has been discussed by policymakers. Attracting more researchers to this problem as the demographic explosion continues is a major challenge that must be met.

A report is received by the local APS agency concerning an 80-year-old female living with her granddaughter. Client is bed-bound and the allegations are caregiver neglect and physical abuse. The reporter is the home health agency serving the consumer. Reporter states consumer told her that the granddaughter is sometimes mean to her and have hit her in the past. There also the beginnings of skin breakdown, pink areas are starting to appear on the hip. Client is clear and can express her wishes. The aide has noticed on several occasions that the client is sitting in urine and needs to be cleaned up. The Intake Supervisor reviews the case and makes it an Emergency, based on the fact that the reporter alleged physical abuse, has access to the client and the client is bed-bound.

Investigator receives the case while in the field. Investigator, because it is an Emergency, calls the care manager to get more details including the dynamics in the household. Investigator then calls the reporter at the Home Health Agency to get the pertinent information and asks the reporter to expand on what she reported to the hotline. Investigator finds out that it is a second-hand report as the reporter, the Nurse from the Home Health Agency, got the information from the aide working the case.

The Investigator asks for the schedule for the aide and a good time to talk to her. The Nurse says that the aide comes in the morning and often finds the client sitting in urine as if she had not been changed or cleaned during the night. The aide reported to the Nurse that the granddaughter is not always there so there can be a problem with access, and that the client appears afraid of the granddaughter and covers up for her. She also reports that there are beginnings of skin break down in the hip area. Aide reported to the Nurse that the client reported to the aide that her granddaughter handles consumer roughly at times and grabbed her the last time they were together, and there were bruises visible on the arms and shoulders. Nurse tells investigator that client lives in area with heavy drug traffic and in fact, drugs are sold openly on the corner of the block where consumer lives.

Investigator arrives at the home and granddaughter is present and answers the door. Investigator comes in and asks to speak with the client and the granddaughter to do an assessment.

After conducting the original assessment to determine if there is a real emergency that has to be dealt with right away, and starting the process of gaining rapport, Investigator asks if she could have a few minutes of privacy with the client to finish the assessment because that is part of our process. Investigator asks to check the alleged skin break down on the hip and the client refuses. Investigator then asks permission to look at medication bottles and the name of client's doctor. Investigator asks how the client is paying her bills, who pays them, and where she banks. Investigator asks if there are other family members or friends or neighbors involved in her care. Investigator then asks client to sign a release of information so that we can get more information. The client requests more explanation about the release of information and investigator explains it further and she agrees to sign.

Investigator calls the care manager and leaves a message as she gets voicemail and also reaches out to the Doctor's office. Doctor is not sure that the patient is always getting her meds appropriately and says the caregiver appears to be trying but sometimes can be abrasive and hard to work with as far as the doctor's office is concerned. Investigator asks if the skin breakdown occurs regularly or is something new, and doctor says that occasionally there is some breakdown and it could be because patient is not getting turned frequently enough. Doctor has seen the bruises but is not sure where or when the bruises occurred and the consumer has denied physical abuse to the doctor.

Investigator reaches out to the aide who is the first-hand reporter to discuss the allegations on the report and what she has observed personally. Aide stated she often arrives and the client is sitting in urine and has not been changed, and the aide also confirmed that the client made an admission to her that the she was being handled roughly by the caregiver. She has not witnessed abuse directly however.

Investigator discusses initial finding with Supervisor and a meeting is set up with the care management staff. Investigator questions the care management team, who tells us that this not an ideal situation and that the caregiver sometimes can be difficult. There are no reports of physical abuse from the care manger, and the care management team offers to increase services if the need arises.

There are no other collaterals in this case to interview. Investigator checks utilities, deed and bills and everything comes up ok on that side of the case. We now are ready to conduct an in depth interview with the consumer.

We want to do this interview alone with the client so we ask the aide if there a time when the granddaughter is not home. The aide provides us with a time and we make a visit to the client then. The client admits that the granddaughter is rough at times but she does not want to get her in trouble because she does a lot for her and she still loves her. We now have an admission and substantiation. Investigator asks the client if she thinks her granddaughter needs more help because she is being overwhelmed with the care. The client says that she definitely can benefit from more help, and that her goal is to stay at home for the rest of her life. Investigator asks the client about the wound and if she is turned frequently, changed frequently enough, etc. Client says that she does not want to bother granddaughter during the night because after all she has to care for her the rest of the time, so client chooses to wait until the morning.

Investigator comes back and reviews findings in supervision, and the supervisor sets up another meeting with the care management team to discuss our concerns and findings. We meet with the care management team and we conclude that there are some care issues, but it looks like an overwhelmed caregiver and we recommend increasing services. Care management team agrees to the increase. The substantiation decision occurs before the meeting so we can share certain things with care management as part of our care plan. This is allowable under Pennsylvania Law. Investigator and supervisor agree that they do not think we have a malicious abuser, but an overwhelmed caregiver, who can benefit from services and the client agrees. We have no other witnesses but we do have an admission from the client. So we are now ready for the perpetrator interview to hear her side of the story.

The granddaughter states that things are really tough, sometimes she does not do everything great and sometimes that there may be rough handling. Eventually we ask specifically about the bruises that the client has and how they got there. The granddaughter said clearly that she does not physically abuse her grandmother, and that she loves her but it is getting harder to care for her. She states that her grandmother is not the person that she used to be, and she cannot be getting up every night to change her because she is the only one doing the care. Investigator talks a little bit about how to prevent abuse by keeping the care manager in the loop when things are getting too tough for her. We asked the granddaughter if she still thinks she is up to doing this task and if she can continue to do this task with the additional help to be provided. She says yes, she is going to do it as long as she can and she wants to do it for her grandmother.

Care management has agreed to the increase in services and Investigator goes out for one more visit and does a reassessment to make sure the plan is working and closes the case to APS.

Issues that emerge in this case are: will the physician cooperate and give the investigator useful information? The APS investigator has to make a decision and decide even though the care is not perfect, can the risk be relieved or eliminated by offering services. What does the client want? Will removing the perpetrator undermine the support system that does exist and will that removal actually make the situation worse? There are also issues around worker safety since ideally, investigators would travel in pairs, but limited resources and heavy caseloads often make that impractical. Will not removing the perpetrator make the surrounding community unhappy? One major complaint that APS professionals hear constantly is that, "we called you and you did nothing". What the complainant often means is that APS did not do what I wanted done. Sometimes folks think APS has more power than they actually do and do not realize that adults get to make decisions that do not conform to the norm.

It is clear from the case examples the skills set that a good investigator must possess. It is also clear that the commitment and passion has to be there when you consider that only thirteen states reported having 25 cases or less on the caseload of an individual investigator (see Table 15.1).

15.1.5 Major Issues Confronting the Long-Term Care Ombudsman Program

As with Adult Protective Services, many Long-Term Care Ombudsman Programs are confronting a number of significant challenges and issues. Several are structural and others are substantive issues affecting long-term care facility residents.

A major immediate challenge for many states' Long-Term Care Ombudsman Programs is making the policy and program changes necessary to ensure compliance

Table 15.1 National Adult Protective Services Association (or APS) Code of Ethics

NAPSA (or APS) Code of Ethics [1]
APS workers are guided by a code of ethics and guiding principles that permeate all aspects of the practice. The code of ethics was developed by NAPSA members representing a wide cross section of states highlighting some of the significant differences between APS practitioners and those practicing in other fields of family violence
Adult Protective Services programs and staff promote safety, independence, and quality of life for older persons and persons with disabilities who are being mistreated or in danger of being mistreated, and who are unable to protect themselves
Guiding value
Every action taken by Adult Protective Services must balance the duty to protect the safety of the vulnerable adult with the adult's right to self-determination
Secondary value
Older persons and persons with disabilities who are victims of mistreatment should be treated with honesty, caring, and respect
Principles
• Adults have the right to be safe
• Adults retain all their civil and constitutional rights, i.e., the right to live their lives as they wish, manage their own finances, enter into contracts, marry, etc. unless a court adjudicates otherwise
• Adults have the right to make decisions that do not conform with societal norms as long as these decisions do not harm others
• Adults have the right to accept or refuse services
NAPSA (or APS) practice guidelines
APS worker practice responsibilities include:
• Recognize that the interests of the adult are the first concern of any intervention
• Avoid imposing personal values on others
• Seek informed consent from the adult before providing services
• Respect the adult's right to keep personal information confidential
• Recognize individual differences such as cultural, historical and personal values
• Honor the right of adults to receive information about their choices and options in a form or manner that they can understand
• To the best of one's ability, involve the adult as much as possible in developing the service plan
• Focus on case planning that maximizes the vulnerable adult's independence and choice to the extent possible based on the adult's capacity
• Use the least restrictive services first whenever possible—community-based services rather than institutionally based services
• Use family and informal support systems first as long as this is in the best interest of the adult
• Maintain clear and appropriate professional boundaries
• In the absence of an adult's expressed wishes, support casework actions that are in the adult's best interest
• Use substituted judgment in case planning when historical knowledge of the adult's values is available
• Do no harm. Inadequate or inappropriate intervention may be worse than no intervention

with the new federal regulations governing the LTCOP promulgated by the U.S. Administration for Community Living that took effect July 1, 2016 (see discussion under the LTCOP portion of this chapter). These include states in which the LTCOP has been a mandatory reporter of abuse, which is specifically not permitted under federal law, and states in which the LTCOP has had jurisdiction under state law for receiving and investigating reports of abuse in long-term care facilities. The new rules clarify in considerable detail the role of the LTCOP in responding to residents' complaints about abuse and how it differs significantly from that of entities authorized as finders of fact with respect to abuse reports, such as APS. The new regulations will require other challenges for some state LTCOPs including those related to addressing potential conflicts of interest within the program, the roles of volunteer ombudsmen, and in some cases reassessing the entity in which the LTCOP is housed. They also require LTCOPs to develop policies concerning promptness of complaint response, as well providing narrow circumstances in which a LTCO can disclose information provided by a resident.

An ongoing challenge for many ombudsman programs, dating to the origins of the program, are the common circumstance is which local ombudsmen directors/coordinators "serve two masters." A state's Office of the State Long-Term Care Ombudsman is headed by the State Long-Term Care Ombudsman. All who carry out Ombudsman responsibilities in a state, particularly related to responding to and resolving resident complaints do so only with the direct approval of the SLTCO; they are "representatives" of the SLTCO. They have no authority to act (and to receive the protections provided in law for ombudsmen for the "good faith performance" of their responsibilities) without being formally recognized and approved by the SLTCO. Yet, at the local level, many local Long-Term Care Ombudsman Programs are administratively housed in agencies and organizations that are not part of the state agency/organization in which the State Ombudsman is housed. Very often, these local Ombudsman Programs are located within area agencies on aging (AAAs) These local Ombudsman Programs often receive funding from the host AAA, as well as from the Office of the State Long-Term Care Ombudsman and other sources. And the local Ombudsman Program Directors/ Coordinators are hired and fired by the local host AAA or other entity. Ombudsman work of necessity involves conflict and requires the Ombudsman to frequently take a stance on behalf of facility residents that may be at odds with other interests and decisions, including those of facility management, but also of other entities within the community (or state). For example, if in response to a resident's complaint, the Ombudsman questions or challenges the actions of a case management entity for its placement decisions related to long-term care facilities, or for failing to adequately monitor the resident's circumstances, the Ombudsman may be challenging a case management program funded or even directly operated by the Ombudsman Program's local host organization. As many Ombudsmen have noted this can lead to conflicts for the Ombudsman with respect to their employment status and raises the "serving two masters:" the State Long-Term Care Ombudsman and the local entity funding or operating the local Ombudsman Program. The new federal LTCOP regulations should help to further mitigate such challenges.

Another long-running challenge for the LTCOP has been ensuring that all representatives of the Office of the State Long-Term Care Ombudsman have adequate access to legal counsel. Under federal law all LTCOPs must have access to legal counsel but major challenges exist in some programs as to the source and the payment for such counsel. As a local Ombudsman Director commented that while we serve at the pleasure of the State LTC Ombudsman, who is a state employee, as her representatives, "Our state's Attorney General says ombudsmen located in area agencies on aging are not state employees and therefore not entitled to representation by the AG. So who is responsible for us legally? Who has our backs for 'good faith performance?" Again, the new federal rules may help to lessen this challenge but it is likely to not resolve it for all programs.

Adequate funding of the LTCOP is an ongoing major challenge. Without question the program is inadequately funded and is likely to become even more so—certainly in the near term—with the demographic growth of the older adult population, particularly among those of very advanced age who are the likeliest candidates for becoming residents of long-term care facilities. A look at the program's recent federal appropriations history—from Federal Fiscal Year (FY) 2006 to FY 2016 is illuminating. With an appropriation of $15 million in Fiscal Year FY 2006 the program's funding increased in incremental steps to its high-water mark during this period of $16.825 in FY 10. Annual appropriations then dropped somewhat over the next several fiscal years reaching $15.885 million in FY 13, a level at which it has remained constant until FY 16.[1] The $15.885 million amount is $885,000 more than the FY 2006 appropriation. If that amount were to be equally divided among the 50 states (not taking into account the District of Columbia, Puerto Rico and the territories for their programs), it represents a $17,700 increase for each state from 2006. The absurdity of this amount is obvious.

The LTCOP also faces significant issues because of the challenges facing long-term care facility residents. A key one that has vexed the LTCOP for many years as well as other consumer advocates is the absence of federal regulation or oversight of the assisted living industry and similar levels of care. Unlike residents of nursing homes, there is no federal "Bill of Rights" to ensure the protection of the basic rights of assisted living residents. There is no federal system for ensuring quality in such facilities or responding to major quality problems. Oversight of assisted living is left to states. To be sure some states have regulatory schemes governing assisted living but not all do, some stronger than others. And there is not consistency from state-to-state. Moreover, if assisted living or similar types of facilities (e.g., board and care homes) are not licensed by the state, the LTCOP may have difficulties identifying such facilities or guaranteeing residents' access and rights to a Long-Term Care Ombudsman, much less to a regulatory or other formal oversight body.

Long-Term Care Ombudsmen are also challenged to provide consistent access to residents in board and care settings, currently reaching 29 % of all board and care residents through quarterly visits to such facilities. This is in contrast to the 69 % of all nursing homes reached by LTCOs on a quarterly basis. The needs of board and care residents for the services of a LTCO are no less than those of nursing home residents. Some argue their needs may even be greater.

Residents with limited capacity to manage their finances or affairs are often under the control (of finances, estate, of the person) of fiduciaries or third parties who have been given this authority by the resident or others (e.g., courts, Social Security Administration). This often poses significant

[1]As of this writing FY 17 appropriations have not yet been finalized.

challenges for facility residents and for the LTCOP. Residents under the control of others may have limited ability (if any at all) for reaching out to an Ombudsman to voice their concerns. Ombudsmen may have difficulty getting access to such residents or to the resident's fiduciary. Fiduciaries are to act in the best interest of the resident but many don't have the education or knowledge about their roles as decision-makers for another. They often do not know or understand the requirements for performing as a fiduciary. And, sadly, they often do not make decisions that are in the best interest of a resident, inadvertently or intentionally. A State Long-Term Care Ombudsman cited financial exploitation of residents as the source of many involuntary discharges of residents from long-term care facilities. She noted that the "number one reason" for involuntary discharges is lack of payment. It is her program's belief that financial exploitation of residents' funds by the person with responsibility for paying the bills for the care is the chief reason they are no longer to pay for their care. Gaining access to residents with third-party decision-makers or helping such residents with their complaints poses many challenges for LTCOs. It requires them to work with guardians, conservators, representative payees, trustees, attorneys-in-fact, as well as the courts of jurisdiction, the Social Security Administration (for representative payees) and other authorities. The new federal LTCOP regulations provide new guidance to help Ombudsmen navigate their way through the very sticky thicket of third-party decision-makers but major challenges will continue and new ones will emerge.

The ever-transforming world of health care and long-term services and supports (LTSS) poses challenges for LTCOPs and will continue to do so. In particular, as the trend continues to attempt to move facility residents to non-facility-based forms of care or to prevent people from entering facilities in the first place, Ombudsmen have their hands full trying to ensure that the rights of residents are ensured through any change or upheaval and to ensure that former residents continue to have their rights protected and opportunities for expressing their grievances. While the jurisdiction of some States' LTCOPs has expanded to include various forms of nonresidential home and community-based services (HCBS) for LTSS thus allowing them to serve HCBS clients including following residents who've left facility care, many other state LTCOPs do not have this authority. As a result, older adult and other disabled adults utilizing nonresidential forms of HCBS may not have access to a LTCOP for responding to their complaints and problems. Moreover, they may not have access to other forms of consumer advocacy in lieu of no access to an Ombudsman. As one State Ombudsman noted, "In the rush to move people from facility-based care to HCBS, sometimes not appropriate or safe".

And of course any effort to expand the LTCOPs jurisdiction to cover HBCS clients raises important issues related to the adequacy of funding. If such expansion is not accompanied by an appropriate increase in funding and other resources (e.g., for staffing, training with regard to HCBS) then it is adding to the current demands upon LTCOPs. In fact, LTCOP funding provided by the Older Americans Act may only be used for Ombudsmen services to long-term care facility residents. In discussing this, an Ombudsman commented, "We can only reach as many people today as yesterday with the same resources. It is not like people stop going into nursing homes and all are shifting to HBCS. Do not pile onto the existing workforce with the current level of support." The outcome may well be diluted capacity to serve residents of long-term care facilities and inadequate ability to reach out to and be responsive to ever-growing numbers of HCBS clients.

15.1.6 History of Adult Protective Services

According to recent testimony, there are more elder abuse victims in the United States as there are domestic violence and child abuse victims combined; an estimated 5 million victims of elder abuse versus 1.25 million child abuse victims and 2.3 million battered women [2]. Federal investment in the child protective services and domestic violence systems has led to significantly reduced rates of both child abuse and domestic violence [3]. It is hard to believe that elder abuse as a national policy issue has been around for over a half-century without any federal investment in the system (see Table 15.2).

The history of APS and elder abuse as a national policy issue can be traced back to 1950, when the Department of Health, Education and Welfare awarded demonstration projects for protective service units. A long gap of inaction followed, until in 1974, APS was authorized under Title XX of the Social Security Act. States then started creating their own APS programs. Congress conducted various hearings on elder abuse, with the first hearing being held in 1978 in the House of Representatives. The second, in 1979, was entitled *Elder Abuse: A Hidden Problem*. In 1981 a report from Congress stated that the problem of elder abuse existed in epidemic proportions, that the incidence of such abuse appeared to be growing, and that few states had allocated the resources needed to meet the problem [12]. A 1985 hearing, *Elder Abuse: A National Disgrace* found that states spent $22.14 per child for child protective services compared to $2.91 per person for adult protective services. In 1987, nursing home reforms through the Omnibus Budget and Reconciliation Act (OBRA) and elder abuse prevention sections were added to the Older Americans Act. Another congressional report was issued in 1990, *Elder Abuse: A*

Table 15.2 Federal funding for victims of crime and abuse

Estimates	Child abuse	%	Domestic violence	%	Elder abuse	%	Total	General crime victims
No. of victims	1.25 M [4]	13.5	2.3 M [5]	25	5.7 M [6]	61	9.25 M	21.2 M [7]
Federal funding for *All* victims services	$7.4B [8]	93	$551.8 M [9]	5	$10.9 M [10]	2	$7.97B	635 M [11]
Federal funds specifically for *Elder Abuse* (but not for services)					$9.1 M[a]	100	$9.1 M	9.5 M[b]
Per victim spending	$5920		$240		$1.91[c]		$862	

[a]$5.1 M in elder abuse prevention funding under the Older Americans Act and $4 M new appropriation under the Elder Justice Act. None of the funds go to direct victims' services
[b]Based on 1.5 % of VOCA victims served being older [7]
[c]Based on victims' **services'** funds only ($10.9 M)

Decade of Shame and Inaction [13]. None of this spurred any action on the part of the federal government except on small fronts; for example, the National Center on Elder Abuse (NCEA) was created and funded in 1990 and in 1992, amendments to the Older Americans Act included the creation of Title VII, the Elder Abuse Prevention Chapter. The early 2000s saw hearings by the Senate Special Committee on Aging. In 2002, advocates and public policy officials were excited by the introduction of the Elder Justice Act (EJA).

APS professionals across the country were very excited about the introduction of the Elder Justice Act and the promise that it held to finally begin to address the long-term funding inequities that had existed for over 50 years. The EJA hit some roadblocks along the way and was reintroduced four times, finally passing in 2010 as part of the Affordable Health Care Act. The EJA in its original form had many robust provisions including the creation of the Elder Justice Coordinating Council (EJCC), an Advisory Board on Elder Abuse, Neglect and Exploitation, Forensic Center grants, grants for state ombudsman programs, a National Nursing Home Surveyors Institute, incentives for long-term care staffing and a national nurse aide registry study and report.

The EJA was and is at its heart, however, an APS bill in that it authorizes the first dedicated federal funding for APS. The original proposed funding of $300 million to fund APS programs was passed by the Senate Finance Committee at $100 million. There was also $25 million for APS demonstration grants and $3–$4 million to the Department of Health and Human Services to provide a federal "home" for APS.

There was great jubilation among APS professionals when the EJA was enacted in March 2010 but this joy was tempered when not a single penny was appropriated in FY 11, 12, 13, or 14. In FY 2015, the President's budget requested $25 million, and for the first time, the words "adult protective services" appeared in a federal budget document. In FY 2015, $4 million was appropriated; $3 million for grants to states (10 grants for $300,000 each to implement a new national APS data collection system and to improve practice), and $1 million for administration, data collection and technical assistance to programs. In FY 2016, $25 million was requested again by the President.

The results of this federal negligence for over a half-century is that states were forced to develop programs on their own without thought of cross-state standardization necessary to establish minimum standards and consistent practices. Some of the issues resulting from the lack of standardization that have emerged are: lack of consistency in APS programs, a lack of research on adult abuse, its causes, prevention and effective interventions, and even more telling, a lack of awareness, in fact the invisibility, of elder and vulnerable adult abuse and APS. These all pale in comparison to the untold suffering, impoverishment and death of older and vulnerable adults.

15.1.7 What We Know

Although lack of information and data has been cited as a problem, there is much that we have come to know especially around elder abuse. We know that seniors who are abused, neglected and exploited are three times more likely to die prematurely [14]. We also know that elder abuse victims are four times more likely to go into a nursing home [15]. Elder abuse victims use healthcare services at higher rates, in fact 2.5 times as often as non-abused elders [16]. We also know that 90 % of reported abusers are family members [17]. According to the 2006 census data, 90 % of seniors live in the community. This information would seem to be sufficient to satisfy those who think that we do not have enough evidence-based data to address this horrific epidemic both from a human perspective and from a cost perspective.

Incidence studies continue to establish the enormity of this problem. Acierno reports that 1 in 9 seniors report being abused, neglected or exploited in the past 12 months [18]. Another study points to the vast problem of underreporting of the abuse. Only 1 in 23.5 cases is reported to any agencies; for financial abuse 1 in 44 cases are reported and for neglect only 1 in 57 cases are reported [19]. A study in Utah showed that almost 1 in 10 financial abuse victims will turn to Medicaid as the direct result of their own money being stolen from them [20]. The Met Life Mature Market Institute study estimates that at a minimum $2.9 billion dollars is lost annually to financial exploitation [21]. A 2015 study estimates losses at $36.48 billion dollars a year [22].

The General Accountability Office (GAO) conducted three studies on the subject of elder abuse, neglect and exploitation. The studies consistently recommended a coordinated federal response to the needs of APS, including funding, public awareness, prevention, intervention, coordination, and research. The GAO studies further illustrate the years of federal neglect of this vulnerable population and the system and staff that serves them. Resulting challenges include the increased number of cases reported; shrinking state and local revenues to use to fund APS programs; inadequate staffing levels; limited information on how to resolve complex cases and difficult to use or inadequate data systems across the country [23].

15.1.8 Differences and Similarities Across States

These differences were encapsulated and put into focus by a 2012 survey of states conducted by the National Adult Protective Services Association (NAPSA) and the National Association of States United for Aging and Disabilities (NASUAD) through a federal grant for the National APS Resource Center. One hundred percent of the states responded to the survey. This report was conducted with the cooperation of state APS agency staff from around the country and produced startling results except for those in the field who knew of the differences if not their extent. For look at some of the differences, see Table 15.3.

There are a number of conclusions that can be drawn from this report, but it is obvious that the strain put on APS systems in many remarkably understaffed and underfunded states cries out for more funding and standardization.

15.1.9 Recent Developments Affecting APS

NAPSA has emerged as a force in the field for many years. NAPSA is the only national organization that represents the professionals in APS and the victims they serve. NAPSA is a membership organization with representation in every state, hosts the only national conference on elder abuse, abuse of adults with disabilities and APS, provides technical assistance to states, produces technical assistance and research-to-practice briefs, and, perhaps most importantly, offers critical networking opportunities for APS professionals and those in related fields. NAPSA was funded by the Administration on Aging/ Administration of Community Living to establish the first National APS Resource Center; to provide training, technical assistance and to provide access to research to APS practitioners.

Elder and vulnerable adult abuse has become recognized as a public health and human rights issue, complicated by the underlying principles that APS practice is based on: self-determination and the least restrictive alternative. There are countless practical and ethical dilemmas faced everyday by the professionals who have been fighting this hidden scourge for many years with limited resources and no federal support and leadership. There is increased hope as recent developments have shined some light at the end of the tunnels for those dedicated professionals and the victims that they serve.

Under the leadership of Assistant Secretary of the Administration for Community Living/Administration on Aging, Kathy Greenlee, elder abuse has received long overdue recognition in the federal government. Some of the highlights include:

- The previously mentioned first-ever funding for a national APS resource center which was awarded to NAPSA in 2012.
- Leadership of the Elder Justice Coordinating Council (EJCC) created by the Elder Justice Act. This marks the first time that major federal agencies, including include the Social Security Administration, Securities and Exchange Commission, Department of Justice, Federal Trade Commission, Department of Labor, United States Postal Inspection Service and the Administration on Community Living/Administration on Aging, must report on what they are doing to address elder abuse. The creation of the EJCC marks the first time that all federal departments with a stake in elder justice have come together to identify gaps, make recommendations and coordinate activities. The EJCC has concluded that there is a great need for strengthening support of APS as well as a need for greater public awareness of both elder justice and APS. One of the major recommendations out of the EJCC is to develop a national adult protective service system to include a federal home for APS and recommended program guidelines.
- Another major federal initiative, the Elder Justice Roadmap Project, which took place in 2013–2014, was a stakeholder engagement process to bring to light the most

Table 15.3 APS differences and similarities across states

• About half of APS programs work within the State Unit on Aging, while the others are in the states' departments of social or human services. Two programs are independent state agencies
• In two-thirds of the states, APS is state-administered (i.e., all APS employs are state employees). In seven states, APS is county-administered
• In about a third of the estates, APS investigators and supervisors work in other programs in addition to APS (child protective, aging or disability services)
• Almost 9 in ten (87 %) of the programs saw the number of reports and caseloads increase between 2007 and 2012, with the increases ranging up to 100 %
• Almost half of the reporting states had reductions in APS staff during that same time period
• Thirty-eight APS programs serve all vulnerable adults 18 and older; five serve persons with disabilities ages 18–59 and all older persons; one serves only persons with disabilities, ages 18–59; and seven serve older victims only
• All APS programs investigate abuse, neglect, and exploitation in community settings. Almost half (45 %) investigate in nursing homes; 59 % in assisted living facilities; 69 % in board and care homes; 41 % in developmental disability facilities; and 39 % in mental health facilities
• Fifteen states require all citizens to report to report suspected elder abuse to APS. All but one of the remaining states (New York) mandates a range of professionals to so report
• Three-quarters of states receive intake reports 24 h a day; nineteen respond to reports 24 h a day
• A significant majority of states:
○ triage reports at intake;
○ maintain regular contact with the client during the case; and
○ are required to report at least some cases to law enforcement
• Two states provide no preservice training for new workers. Forty-three provide annual in-service training to APS investigators and caseworkers
• Forty APS programs train APS supervisors; of those, twenty states provide APS-specific training, and twenty do not. Nine provide no training to APS supervisors
• Forty-six states now have automated APS data systems. In 28 states, the system is integrated with another system, such as child protective services or elder case management
• At least 32 states report that APS participates in multidisciplinary teams, 80 % of which operate without funding. The majority of teams include representatives from civil, legal and criminal justice agencies as well as domestic violence, healthcare, mental health, and developmental disabilities organizations. Eighty-eight percent focus on handling specific cases
• Twenty states operate abuser registries. In 11 states, the registry is limited to APS; in nine, it is operated by another program [24]

important issues for the elder justice field and to identify priority actions that the federal government as well as others should and could focus on. Once again, APS figured prominently in the discussion. Specific discussion and recommendations focused on developing national APS definitions, training requirements, data collection, technical assistance, creating a national office for APS and standards for realistic caseloads. For practitioners of APS, realistic caseloads have been on the top of the list for many, many years.

- An Office of Elder Justice and APS was established at ACL in 2014. This expanded upon the current operations and administration of the elder abuse prevention programs by officially designating this Office as the "home" for APS in the federal government. This office will lead and support the development and implementation of a comprehensive national infrastructure for preventing, detecting and responding to adult maltreatment.
- Another very important step was the development of a national APS data collection system. In 2013, in partnership with the HHS Office of the Assistant Secretary for Planning and Evaluation, ACL began a two-year effort to design and pilot test a national reporting system based on data from current APS information systems. The goal of the system is to provide consistent accurate, national data on adult maltreatment as reported to APS in all of the jurisdictions in the United States. The system, currently designated as the National Adult Maltreatment Reporting System (NAMRS), is designed to collect quantitative and qualitative data on victim and perpetrator characteristics, types of abuse, the practices and policies of adult protective service systems and the outcome of investigations into adult maltreatment. The testing was completed in September of 2015 and it is anticipated that the NAMRS system will be deployed by 2016, with the first states submitting data between

October and December 2016. The first annual report on NAMRS is targeted to be completed in early 2017. Submission of data by states will be voluntary but supported and encouraged by ACL. The child protective system has had success with the submission of voluntary data.

- Developing national guidelines for APS is another project tackled by ACL. Based on guidelines already produced by NAPSA, the proposed federal guidelines aim to insure consistency in all programmatic areas in order to afford similar protections and services regardless of the state. It will also allow researchers and funders to be able to compare and contrast similar data across the states.

15.1.10 Financial Exploitation Emerges as a Catalyst to Move the Field Forward

The issue of financial exploitation has emerged as an issue of great interest and is moving the field forward. There are many reasons for this including the fact that it is about money, which resonates across the spectrum. The increased awareness has presented opportunities for collaboration with other fields, including the field of medicine and the financial services industry, which is aware of the primary role that APS plays to combat this epidemic.

The issue of financial exploitation has been prominent in the world of APS for some time. There have been many successful partnerships between APS and the financial industry and many of the Multidisciplinary Teams or Task Forces have coalesced around the issue of financial exploitation. Financial industry leaders and regulators are starting to recognize that more is needed if we are going to protect the life and health of our mutual customers. The Financial Services Roundtable has produced two papers, working with APS, to encourage and guide financial institutions in establishing fraud prevention programs for elderly and vulnerable adults [25]. The Financial Industry Regulatory Authority (FINRA) recently put out a proposed rule that would allow institutions to delay a transaction where financial abuse is suspected while they make a report to APS and law enforcement [26]. The North American Security Administrators Association (NASAA) has proposed a change that would require a report to APS when exploitation is suspected and the subsequent sharing of records [27]. The issue of financial exploitation has figured prominently in federal activity including the EJCC and the Elder Justice Roadmap Project.

There have been many studies addressing the role of the aging brain and the issue of financial capacity and the connection to the vulnerability to financial exploitation as we age. The concept of mild cognitive impairment (MCI) has been researched and discussed as leading to increased vulnerability to financial exploitation. A 2006 study found that MCI patients are four times more likely to make errors than patients without MCI [28]. Researchers have also found that damage to the prefrontal cortex makes affected elders less risk adverse and thus more willing to gamble more with their finances [29]. The Institute of Medicine (IOM) published a 2015 report on cognitive aging that made recommendations to the banking and financial services industry and federal banking and financial regulators to develop and disseminate banking and financial policies, services and information material that help older adults and their families make decisions that meet their means and objectives and protect against and mitigate harms of such decisions. The report further recommended strengthening systems that take action against potential fraud, exploitation and abuse [30]. These changes would greatly benefit APS programs throughout the country.

Collaboration between Baylor College of Medicine, Investor Protection Trust, Investor Protection Institute, National Adult Protective Services Association, North American Securities Administrators Association and State Securities Regulators resulted in a program to educate medical professionals, who routinely see older Americans as part of their practice, about elder investment fraud. The Elder Investment Fraud and Financial Exploitation (EIFFE) Prevention Program is currently running in 28 U.S. states and jurisdictions [31].

NAPSA has been in front of this issue for many years now, forming a Financial Exploitation Advisory Board (FEAB) with representatives from many different and related professions, including the financial services industry and APS. One of FEAB's major accomplishments has been holding annual Financial Exploitation Summits, in concert with NAPSA's annual conference, since 2010. NAPSA has also participated or held national events on World Elder Abuse Awareness Day (WEAAD) on June 15. The WEAAD event in 2015, which was sponsored by NAPSA and two partnering organizations, focused on financial abuse. It was held at the Securities and Exchange Commission and featured prominent government officials as well as professionals from related fields who are interested in this issue. A major announcement at the 2015 WEAAD event was the formation of the National Institute on Elder Financial Exploitation (NIEFE), a partnership between NAPSA, the Brookdale Center for Healthy Aging of Hunter College, and the University of Texas Medical School at Houston. NIEFE was created to serve as the first national think tank on the complex issues of elder financial abuse.

The adult protective services system has emerged without federal support and leadership, necessitating states to build their own systems. Research and funding has lagged significantly behind the other forms of family violence, such as child abuse and domestic violence, while the number of cases has eclipsed the combined total of those fields. The call for evidence-based research resonates throughout the field without consideration to those that say that evidence-based research does not work in the social welfare field. While this debate goes on and the search for evidence-based research continues, millions of victims suffer and APS staff faces overwhelming caseloads and an indifferent response to their calls for help. While we certainly need the research and the documentation of the problem, it is time to put it in line behind the action that is sorely needed. APS staff everywhere looks forward to that day.

15.2 Long-Term Care Ombudsman Program

As noted at this chapter's outset, Adult Protective Services and the Long-Term Care Ombudsman Program are critical components of states' protection and advocacy services for the nation's elders and other vulnerable adults, including those in long-term care facilities.

To complement the discussion of APS, the rest of this chapter addresses the Long-Term Care Ombudsman Program, established under the Older Americans Act [32]. While an overview of the history, purpose and roles of the LTCOP is provided, the discussion emphasizes the LTCOP's role in responding to complaints involving elder abuse and in dealings with APS and other entities charged with investigating abuse, neglect and exploitation.

Long-Term Care Ombudsmen are advocates for residents of long-term care facilities. As noted in the federal government's final rule governing the LTCOP, effective July 1, 2016, "State Long-Term Care Ombudsman programs (Ombudsman programs) serve as advocates for residents of nursing homes, board and care homes, assisted living and similar adult care facilities. They work to resolve problems of individual residents and to bring about improvements to residents' care and quality of life at the local, state and national levels". [33]. This role has been central to the LTCOP since its creation in the 1970s.

Each state, the District of Columbia, as well as Puerto Rico and Guam, have a State Long-Term Care Ombudsman Program. States' Long-Term Care Ombudsman Programs are typically located within state's State Unit on Aging (e.g., Department of Aging) but in several states are administratively located in other settings including other state entities and not-for-profit organizations. Most States' Long-Term Care Ombudsman Programs empower local entities to perform many of the LTCOP's duties—including complaint investigation and resolution—through a formal process of "designation" [34].

In federal fiscal year 2014 state LTCOPs received to 188,599 complaints. Of these, the LTCOPs opened 126,336 cases. In FY 2014 LTCOPs closed 124,484 cases [35].

15.2.1 Background

The Long-Term Care Ombudsman Program has its origins in the Nixon Administration when President Nixon proposed in 1971 as part of his "8-point plan" for improving conditions in nursing homes, the creation of "state investigative ombudsman units" that "focus exclusively on the resident, thereby compensating for the limitations of regulations and other quality assurance strategies" [36]. As a result, in 1972 the Health Services and Mental Health Administration at the U.S. Department of Health, Education and Welfare (HEW) funded "Nursing Home Ombudsman" demonstration programs in five states. Administrative responsibility for the demonstration projects was moved to the U.S. Administration on Aging (AoA) at HEW in 1973. As a result of the demonstration projects, AoA offered the State Units on Aging a small grant to hire a "Nursing Home Ombudsman Developmental Specialist," to begin the development of a state's long-term care ombudsman program. All but two states accepted the money and the development of today's nationwide system of states' long-term care ombudsman programs was underway [36].

In 1978 the Nursing Home Ombudsman Program was given a statutory foundation when it was incorporated into the Older Americans Act amendments of 1978. The 1978 amendments required every state to have an ombudsman program. Other key provisions included: mandates for ombudsman programs to investigate complaints; involve volunteers in ombudsman programs; and engage in systems advocacy by providing information to public agencies about issues facing long-term care facility residents and monitoring the development of federal, state and local laws, regulations and policies affecting facility residents [36].

Significant amendments were made to the LTCOP provisions in 1981 when the program was required to include residents of board and care homes within its purview. Correspondingly, the program's name was changed to the Long-Term Care Ombudsman Program dropping the label "Nursing Home". This was a significant change in the program's scope and was part of the federal government's efforts to find a "hook" for addressing the growing concerns about the quality of many board and care homes and about protecting the rights of the residents of those facilities. As there was no federal oversight or funding provided for board and care homes (for the most part this remains true today) efforts to create federal "reach" into these facilities had been limited and unsuccessful.

The 1987 and 1992 OAA reauthorizations added significant new amendments to the LTCOP provisions strengthening its authority, independence, structure, and organization, and clout. For example, the 1987 amendments required states to provide ombudsmen with access to facility residents and to their records, and provided ombudsmen with immunity for good faith performance of their responsibilities [37]. States were also required to ensure that the ombudsman program is able to "pursue administrative, legal and other appropriate remedies on behalf of residents," and that the program has adequate legal counsel. The 1992 amendments incorporated the LTC Ombudsman provisions into a new title of the OAA, Title VII, the "Vulnerable Elder Rights Protection" title. Among the numerous 1992 amendments to the LTCOP provisions of the OAA, the roles of local ombudsmen were clarified and strengthened under the auspices of the State LTC Ombudsman, as was the authority of the State LTC Ombudsman. An Elder Abuse, Neglect and Exploitation Prevention Program were also incorporated into the new OAA title [38].

In addition to the federal OAA many states have also adopted state LTCOP enabling laws further strengthening or expanding the roles and responsibilities of ombudsman under state law. For example, some states have expanded the scope of the ombudsman's role to include non-facility-based consumers of long-term services and supports. The 2006 amendments to the OAA explicitly clarified that "assisted living facility" is included in the definition of long-term care facilities, reflecting many states' interpretation of the OAA and states' enabling laws and practice [37].

From the outset of the LTCOP under the OAA, it has been a resident-centered advocacy program driven by the wishes and instructions of facility residents who have brought complaints to the attention of an ombudsman or upon whose behalf complaints have been made. There is no ambiguity about this role. The person-centered role of the ombudsman has consistently been clarified, strengthened and reinforced through successive OAA reauthorizations and other means, including federal regulations governing the program recently promulgated by the Administration for Community Living/Administration on Aging at the U.S. Department of Health and Human Services [33].

Long-Term Care Ombudsmen (LTCOs) have two overarching duties: to work to resolve complaints of individual long-term care facility residents in ways satisfactory to those individual residents (individual advocacy); and to work to bring about systemic changes on behalf of long-term care facility residents (systems advocacy). LTCOs are to "identify, investigate and resolve complaints that are made by, or on behalf, of residents (of LTC facilities)" [39]. The scope of residents' complaints to be investigated and resolved is very broad, encompassing complaints that "relate to action, inaction, or decisions, that may adversely affect the health, safety, welfare, or rights of the residents (including the welfare and rights of the residents with respect to the appointment and activities of guardians and representative payees)". Moreover, the ombudsman's purview explicitly includes responding to complaints relating to "action, inaction, or decisions" of [40]:

- Providers, or representatives of providers, of long-term care services
- Public agencies
- Health and social services agencies

A common misperception about the LTCOP is that it responds only to residents' complaints (or those made on behalf of residents) that involve behavior by or conditions in nursing homes and other long-term care facilities. While the majority of complaints handled by LTCOPs do relate to such matters, residents' complaints may equally be related to "action, inaction, or decisions" of public agencies, as well as health and social services agencies. In other words, a resident's (or group of residents) complaint(s) may relate to an adverse (in the eyes' of the resident) action, inaction or decision of a state's Medicaid agency, a state or federal regulatory agency, an area agency on aging, or state or local APS, and many others.

Put another way, the LTCO is empowered, indeed required, to pursue resolution of complaints about matters adversely affecting the health, safety, welfare, or rights of residents regardless of the source of the adverse action, inaction or decision. For example, a resident's complaint that her welfare has been adversely affected by denial of Medicaid coverage for her nursing home stay could involve an ombudsman pursuing resolution from the state's Medicaid agency. Another example would be a resident's complaint to an ombudsman that their welfare or rights are adversely affected by an action or decision of an APS agency.

The responsibilities of the State LTCOP, carried out by the State LTC Ombudsman or her or his representatives,[2] are many and broad. A "primer" on the State LTCOP issued by two national organizations detailed the "unique role of an ombudsman within the aging network" in the following way [37]:

According to the Older Americans Act, the State LTC Ombudsman shall:

[2]LTCOP Representatives are individuals who work on behalf of the State Long-Term Care Ombudsman and have been recognized by the State Ombudsman to serve as her or his representative. Representatives can be employees of the State Ombudsman or be employed by other organizations that are designated to serve as local or "substate" ombudsman programs, or may be volunteers in such programs. Representatives have no authority to act as ombudsman representatives without the express recognition of the State LTC Ombudsman.

1. Identify, investigate, and resolve complaints that are made by or on behalf of residents and relate to action, inaction or decisions that may adversely affect the health, safety and welfare of the residents of long-term care facilities;
2. Provide services to assist residents in protecting the health, safety, welfare, and rights of residents;
3. Inform residents on ways of obtaining services for which they are entitled;
4. Ensure that residents have regular and timely access to the services provided through the Office and that the residents and complainants receive timely responses from the Office to complaints;
5. Represent the interests of the residents before governmental agencies and seek administrative, legal, and other remedies to protect the health, safety, welfare, and rights of the residents;
6. Analyze, comment on, and monitor the development and implementation of federal, state, and local laws, regulations and other governmental policies and actions, that pertain to the health, safety, welfare, and rights of long-term care residents with respect to the adequacy of long-term care facilities and services in the State. They will recommend changes in such laws, regulations, policies and actions as appropriate and facilitate public comment;
7. Promote the development of and provide assistance to citizen advocacy groups that want to protect the well-being and rights of residents;
8. Provide for training representatives of the Office;
9. Provide technical support for the development of resident and family councils to protect the wellbeing and rights of residents; and
10. Carry out other activities as the Assistant Secretary[3] determines to be appropriate.

While the LTCOP is one of many programs and services authorized by the Older Americans Act (OAA) it is indeed unique among OAA programs, differing in several remarkable ways. As the preamble to the proposed federal rule governing the State LTCOP (now final rule, effective July 1, 2016) noted,

> Long-Term Care Ombudsman programs were designed by Congress to have several features which are uncharacteristic of other programs created by and funded under the Act. Among those features are independence (a characteristic of any type of ombudsman program), unusually stringent disclosure requirements, a public policy advocacy function, and the Ombudsman responsibility to designate local staff and volunteers to serve as representatives of the Office even if they do not report to the Ombudsman for personnel management purposes [41].

The overarching unique feature of the LTCOP is its unwavering resident-centered mission. The preamble to the Administration on Aging's proposed (now final) rule describes the steps involved in the ombudsman person-centered focus in their complaint processing role: "…regardless of the source of the complaint, the Ombudsman or representative of the Office shall discuss the complaint with the resident in order to determine the perception of the resident, request consent in order to investigate the complaint, **determine the wishes of the resident**, advise the resident of his or her rights, work with the resident to develop a plan of action, investigate the complaint, and **determine whether the complaint is resolved to the satisfaction of the resident**" (emphasis added) [41].

Undergirding the resident-centered role is the program's independence. While federal law—and often state law, too—provides numerous authorities and protections for ombudsmen to enable them to do their job freely,[4] they do not have authority or power to compel changes in behavior or action on the part of others in response to complaints they investigate. While states are obligated to provide sanctions for those who willfully interfere with an ombudsman in the performance of her or his duties (e.g., deny ombudsman access to a facility or resident), ombudsmen do not have authority to sanction others for behavior or actions that adversely impact facility residents. To the extent there may be any exceptions to this they are anomalous at best.

Rather, the ombudsman's authority or "power" rests in his or her ability to give "voice" to the preferences and rights of facility residents who lack the ability or power to effectively communicate their complaints or problems, much less convince others to do right by them. Frequently ombudsmen do this through persuasion, cajoling or otherwise convincing others to address and remedy residents' grievances or circumstances adversely affecting their health, safety, welfare, and rights. The key to doing this effectively is to "function as a program with an independent voice" [37].

Moreover, the majority of cases handled by State LTCOPs are generated by complaints made by facility residents themselves. In FY 2014, 39.78 % of cases were generated by complaints from residents followed by relatives or friends of relatives (18.94 %) and facility staff (18.56 %) [35]. The Ombudsman's independence is essential to establishing herself or himself as a trusted person to whom a resident or someone on the resident's behalf can confide and

[3]Assistant Secretary for Aging at the Administration for Community Living, USDHHS.

[4]Immunity for good faith performance of duties, unlawful to willfully interfere with the duties of an ombudsman, strict confidentiality requirements, access to facilities, residents and resident's records, engage in legislative and regulatory advocacy, to name some.

expect to pursue the matter with the resident's interests foremost. Moreover, the resident (or their representative) can trust that the Ombudsman's actions in response to the complaint will be guided by the resident's wishes including seeking an outcome that the resident believes to be satisfactory. The OAA's strict confidentiality and disclosure provisions help to ensure the Ombudsman can be entirely trusted with knowledge of the resident's concern or problem. Furthermore, under the OAA it is unlawful to retaliate or commit reprisals against persons filing complaints with, providing information to, or cooperating with States' LTCOPs [42]. These and other OAA provisions reinforce the importance of the independence of the State LTCOP so that it may most fully serve as advocates for residents.

While the State LTCOP is administratively located within state government agencies (and in a few cases delegated to non-state government entities), the OAA structures the LTCOP to operate with a remarkable degree of independence in its ability to investigate and work to resolve residents' complaints on a person-centered basis; to determine who may act as a representative on behalf of the State Ombudsman; and, perhaps most notably, to engage in policy and other forms of advocacy to bring about changes in law, policy and practice to alleviate adverse impacts on facility residents. Nowhere is the ombudsman's independence most empowering and important than in freely giving voice to residents' problems, concerns and wishes in the legislative, regulatory and other policy arenas, sometimes pursuing remedies that may be at odds even antithetical to the desires, values and policies of others including the Ombudsman's superiors. To be sure, this mandate of the LTCOP is easier to articulate in law than to execute in practice but it has steadily gained attention and adherence in acknowledging and respecting the Ombudsman's duties and rights in this regard. As the National Association of States United for Aging and Disabilities (the organization representing SUAs) and the National Ombudsman Resource Center note, "Challenges occur when an Ombudsman's resident-centered view of laws, regulations, policies and practices differ from those of their own agency or any state agency...education to other state agencies and/or the governor's office needs to occur so that there is a full understanding of the unique role the Ombudsman has in making recommendations which may differ from others in state government" [37].

15.2.2 Complaints Made to Ombudsman Programs by or on Behalf of Facility Residents

The states' Long-Term Care Ombudsman Programs deal with a very broad array of complaints brought to them by or on behalf of facility residents.[5] According to AoA's FY 2014 NORS data, the five most frequent complaints pertaining to nursing facilities and for board and care facilities received by States' LTCOPs were [43]:

Most Frequent Nursing Facility Complaints

- Improper eviction or inadequate discharge/planning
- Unanswered requests for assistance
- Lack of respect for residents, poor staff attitudes
- Quality of life, specifically resident/roommate conflict
- Administration and organization of medications

Most Frequent Board and Care Complaints

- Improper eviction or inadequate discharge/planning
- Quality, quantity, variation and choice of food
- Administration and organization of medications
- Lack of respect for residents, poor staff attitudes
- Quality of life, specifically resident/roommate conflict

Although elder abuse-related complaints are not among the five most frequent complaints they are a significant volume of complaints handled by states' LTCOs. In FY 2014 ombudsman reported responding to 10,453 complaints from (or on behalf of) nursing facility residents and 3805 complaints from board and care facility residents in the "Abuse, Gross Neglect and Exploitation" complaint category, for a total of 14,285 complaints concerning abuse, gross neglect and exploitation, or 7.72 % of all complaints reported by State LTCOPs against facilities [35]. The number of elder abuse-related complaints brought to LTCOs may be affected by the fact that in most states the primary responder to abuse, neglect and exploitation allegations are APS programs, facility regulatory bodies and even law enforcement, rather than the LTCO, Furthermore, as noted later, the new LTCOP regulation promulgated by the Administration for Community Living prohibits the LTCOs from being the primary official finder of fact with respect to abuse reports.

The following chart shows the total numbers of all complaints by category against nursing and board and care facilities made to State LTCOPs by or on behalf of facility residents in FY 2014 [35]. The referenced website defines in

[5]Ombudsmen may also initiate complaints on behalf of facility residents when they identify a problem that affects multiple residents or is systemic, or when they witness or have independent knowledge of a matter that falls within their purview. The program's strict confidentiality and disclosure requirements limit the capacity of ombudsmen to share information that would reveal the identity of individual residents except under certain circumstances when a resident is unable (not unwilling) to provide consent. The AoA's final rule (effective July 1, 2016) goes into considerable detail about exception circumstances and requirements.

Table 15.4 Complaints against the facility by category (50 states and DC) [35]

Category	Nursing facilities	Board and care and similar facilities	Total	Percentage (%)
Total	126,077	43,625	169,702	100.00
Resident rights: abuse, gross neglect, exploitation	10,453	3805	14,258	8.40
Resident rights: access to information by resident or resident's representative	3814	1284	5098	3.00
Resident rights: admission, transfer, discharge, eviction	10,942	3508	14,450	8.51
Resident rights: autonomy, choice, preference, exercise of rights, privacy	16,592	5805	22,397	13.20
Resident rights: financial, property (except financial exploitation)	6831	3197	10,028	5.91
Resident care: care	35,590	8730	44,320	26.12
Resident care: rehabilitation or maintenance of function	6090	759	6849	4.04
Resident care: restraints—chemical and physical	511	298	809	0.48
Quality of life: activities and social services	8492	3102	11,594	6.83
Quality of life: dietary	8708	3644	12,352	7.28
Quality of life: environment	11,546	5684	17,230	10.15
Administrations: policies, procedures, attitudes, resources	1643	1546	3189	1.88
Administration: staffing	4865	2263	7128	4.20

great detail what each of the categories below includes. As defined by the Administration on Aging, "A complaint is about a problem of commission or omission" [44] (see Table 15.4).

As noted, the State LTCOPs' scope includes complaints related to "action, inaction, or decisions that may adversely affect the health, safety, welfare or rights of the residents" and that such action, inaction or decisions can be those of public agencies, health and social services agencies, or others, in addition to those of providers, or representatives of providers, of long-term care services. The following chart shows the number of complaints made in FY 2014 to State LTCOPs that come under the "Problems with Outside Agency, System or People (Not Against Facility)" categories. These include agencies that survey, certify and license LTC facilities, states' Medicaid agencies and numerous others [45]. As with the complaint categories above, the Administration on Aging provides considerable detail about the types of complaints that fall within the categories below. As an example, a complaint about a state's "Certification/Licensing Agency" that falls within the "Decertification/closure" subcategory is used when an individual's complaint is "about decertification/closure (of a facility) and if agency fails to decertify/close a facility when within residents' best interests or with disregard to residents' rights [44].

Other subcategories that fall within the "System/Other" category in the chart below include, among many others [44]:

- Abuse/neglect/abandonment by family member/friend/ guardian, or while on a visit outside of facility, any other person" (No. 117, p. 17).
- Financial exploitation or neglect by family or other not affiliated with facility (No. 121, p. 18)
- Legal—guardianship, conservatorship, power of attorney, wills (No. 122, p. 18)
- Protective Services agency (No. 126, p. 18)

This last category, Protective Services agency, is "for complaints **involving the agency in the State charged with investigating reports of adult abuse or exploitation and providing protective services for victims of abuse and exploitation**" (emphasis added) (see Table 15.5).

Table 15.5 Complaints not against the facility by category (50 states and DC) [35]

Category	Nursing facilities	Board and Care and similar facilities	Total	Percentage (%)
Total	10,686	4605	15,291	100.00
Certification/licensing agency	382	131	513	3.35
State medicaid agency	1189	424	1613	10.55
System/other	9115	4050	13,165	86.10

15.2.3 Ombudsman Program and Elder Abuse

Perhaps the most dramatic and powerful example of the person-centered duty of the Ombudsman as an advocate for the resident is to be found in their response to complaints related to elder abuse, neglect and exploitation. In many ways abuse cases can represent a genuine conundrum for Ombudsmen and have in fact been a source of debate, contention and confusion among some states' LTCOPs, yet the statutory and regulatory guidance is clear. A case example from a State LTCOP will illustrate this.

A local representative of the State LTCOP is told by a nursing home resident that she has been raped by a facility employee. The resident names the employee. The resident is cognitively alert and tells the ombudsman that she wants the matter to be brought only to the attention of the facility administrator and to have the employee fired. She specifically instructs the ombudsman that she does not want it brought to the attention of law enforcement or other authorities. The ombudsman knows that the law governing the LTCOP prohibits the ombudsman from divulging information that would or may identify the resident who made the complaint without his or her express consent to do so. This resident is unwilling to do so. The local ombudsman is deeply troubled by this and goes to the state's nursing home regulatory agency (the survey and certification authority) and tells them that she is aware of a resident who has been raped but that she cannot reveal the identity of the victim or the alleged perpetrator given to her because of Ombudsman confidentiality requirements. The survey and certification agency official is understandably deeply distressed by this as he now knows there is an allegation of a rape in one of the homes within his jurisdiction. He demands the identifying information (e.g., name of victim, alleged perpetrator, the facility). The ombudsman refuses to provide. The Survey and Certification official contacts the State LTC Ombudsman and angrily complains about the "noncooperative" and "obstructionist" Ombudsman representative in his county. The State Ombudsman who had been unaware of this matter speaks with the local ombudsman and after hearing the details from her informs the survey and certification official that he has no choice under federal and state law than to uphold his representative. The frustrated, indeed incensed, official then goes to his state-level superiors and protests the response. The senior state survey and certification officials protest to the state's Department of Aging, where the State LTCOP is located but the State Ombudsman and the county representative do not change their position. Eventually the state's Attorney General's office is brought into the dispute and ultimately rules that the federal OAA's LTCOP confidentiality requirements are clear and as a result neither the State LTCO nor the program's local representative may violate the OAA confidentiality requirements.[6]

To be sure, this was not all the Ombudsman did or could do in response to this case. The representative tried to persuade the resident to relent and allow her to bring it to the attention of the proper authorities explaining such considerations as the perpetrator could do it again to others and that his behavior was a major crime. Moreover, she explained that by bringing it to the facility administrator's attention, the administrator was then under a duty to report the rape to law enforcement under the state's mandatory reporting law, and failure to do so would violate state law.

This is an unfortunate case but it underscores the unambiguous nature of the Ombudsman's duty to the resident complainant. The Ombudsman not only offers confidential handling of information brought to his or her attention but guarantees it to the extent the resident wants the matter kept confidential or the sharing of information pertaining to it disclosed only to those for whom the resident grants consent.

The LTCOP is but one resource for making complaints about or reporting abuse, neglect or exploitation involving residents of LTC facilities. Other key resources include law enforcement, states' facility survey and certification or licensing agencies, and Adult Protective Services. Depending upon the jurisdiction and circumstances there may be others such as the state's Medicaid Fraud Control Unit, licensing or credentialing bodies for various professionals (e.g., nursing home administrators, nurses), or civil attorneys.

It is important to note that while the LTCOP is but one resource for making complaints or reports about abuse, neglect or exploitation, the LTCOP's response differs significantly from that of other key entities such as APS or regulatory bodies. Ombudsman investigations are not done to meet the same standards as other agencies (e.g., compliance with

[6]This case occurred during the tenure as a State LTC Ombudsman of one of this chapter's coauthors.

regulatory requirements, a particular evidentiary standard). Rather, the Ombudsman gathers facts to determine what happened then turns to the affected resident as to what course of action to next take, including possibly bringing the matter to the attention of other authorities.

When the Ombudsman receives the complaint the ombudsman responds to the resident who either made the complaint or on whose behalf the complaint was made with a process, as discussed in the Administration on Aging's Proposed Rule governing the State LTCOP (now final) [41]. Key steps in this process include:

- Discussing the complaint with the resident in order to determine the perception of the resident
- Requesting consent in order to investigate the complaint
- Determining the wishes of the resident
- Advising the resident of his or her rights
- Working with the resident to develop a plan of action
- Investigating the complaint, and
- Determining whether the complaint is resolved to the satisfaction of the resident

In many cases the Ombudsman as the resident's advocate becomes in effect their "navigator" for the handling of the case that results from their complaint, helping to guide the resident through the information they may need to understand their rights, their options for resolution of their complaint, assisting them as necessary through the process of any investigation, and ensuring their rights are protected. When the resident consents to the complaint being investigated or otherwise responded to by other authorities or officials, whether LTC facility management, regulatory agencies, law enforcement or others, the Ombudsman will do what they can to ensure proper, full and timely response from those authorities and officials. The Ombudsman's role is to hold others accountable for performing their responsibilities, and to stick with the matter until the complaint is resolved to the satisfaction of the resident to the greatest extent possible or appropriate.

In an abuse complaint, an Ombudsman can typically be expected to describe for the resident the options available for reporting an abuse case and seeking remedies for the abuse that occurred, what each option would entail and the consequences associated with each. In the case example described above, the resident's wish that the matter only be divulged to the nursing home administrator likely means the administrator would then have the duty to report the matter to appropriate authorities. Assuming the administrator in fact does report it, his report will likely trigger investigations on the part of such authorities and may result in various consequences. Helping a resident understand options and possible scenarios, coupled with the knowledge that the Ombudsman is there to help them achieve resolution to their satisfaction, may overcome a resident's reluctance to refer the matter elsewhere. A resident may be fearful of retaliation or reprisal, or their family members may have such fear and persuade the resident to not pursue the matter. Understanding that federal and state law prohibits retaliation or reprisal may also help overcome any such reluctance.

Assuming the resident consents to her or his abuse complaint being divulged to other parties, such as APS, the state survey and licensing agency or law enforcement, the expectation is that the complaint will be treated seriously and in a timely manner. If it is not, or if the effort seems to be less than thorough or eventually dropped, or if sanctions are not imposed if the complaint is deemed substantiated, the Ombudsman, as the resident's advocate, may then do what they can to ensure the matter is pursued more vigorously or outcomes reconsidered. The Ombudsman's primary objective is to see the complaint resolved to the satisfaction of the resident. In some cases, particularly if there appear to be similar unsatisfactory outcomes for other residents, the Ombudsman may engage in their systems advocacy responsibility by seeking more favorable outcomes or redress through the legislative or regulatory processes, the courts (e.g., through referral to civil attorneys), or the "court of public opinion". Two key OAA provisions that underscore this role of State LTCOPs are:

- It is the duty of the State LTC Ombudsman (or her/his designee) to "represent the interests of residents before government agencies and seek administrative, legal and other remedies to protect the health, safety, welfare and rights of the residents" [46].
- As part of a required annual report, States' LTCOPs will provide, "policy, regulatory, and legislative recommendations to solve identified problems, to resolve the complaints, to improve the quality of care and life of residents, to protect the health, safety, welfare, and rights of residents, and to remove the barriers" [47].

Despite the OAA's statutory language requiring strict limits on Ombudsman disclosure of residents' identities or other confidential information, and the role of the Ombudsman as the residents' advocate, adhering to these restrictions and limits has been difficult for some State LTCOPs. In some states Ombudsmen were made mandatory reporters under their state's law. In some other jurisdictions Ombudsmen found it difficult to not report abuse so reported it to law enforcement without obtaining a resident's consent, or perhaps reported it despite a resident's wishes to the contrary. A 2009 report from the California Legislature noted, "Many (local ombudsman programs) fail to get consent at all, even from the long-term care resident. Some intentionally ignore consent requirements when they consider the case too serious" [48].

In proposing its new regulations governing the State LTCOP, the Administration on Aging sought to address inconsistencies among states in ways in which the State LTCOPs were administered or operated. In its Notice of Proposed Rulemaking AoA noted, "There has been significant variation in the interpretation and implementation of the provisions of the Act among States. This has resulted in residents of long-term care facilities receiving inconsistent services from Ombudsman programs in some states compared to other states. **An example of this inconsistency in approach is the way that various States respond to complaints to the Ombudsman program that a facility has abused a resident**" (emphasis added) [41]. It is important to note, however, that most State LTCOPs have handled abuse cases consistent with what Congress intended in the Older Americans Act. In fact, as AoA noted in their Preamble to the Proposed Rule, "In most States, the Ombudsman program is available to assist and resolve the complaint to the satisfaction of the resident, working with the resident to assure his or her well-being. **In those States, the Ombudsman program explains to the complainant that another agency represents the State as the official finder of fact, but that the Ombudsman serves as a victim advocate to support the resident through the official investigation process and to assist the resident in voicing and realizing his or her goals**" (emphasis added) [41].

As part of the preamble, AoA described in considerable detail the different ways some State LTCOPs were handling abuse complaints, as follows [41]:

- However, in some States, the same abuse complaint gets the same response that the Ombudsman program is not the official finder of fact for abuse complaints, and the complainant is immediately referred to another State or local agency. However, in some cases, the resident receives no additional assistance from the Ombudsman program related to the abuse allegation.
- In still other States, the Ombudsman program is designated by the State as the official finder of fact to determine whether the abuse is substantiated. It refers substantiated cases to law enforcement, at times without (or even in violation of) the wishes of the resident.
- In still other States, the Ombudsman is designated by the State as the official finder of fact, but in order to not violate the wishes of the resident or the disclosure provisions of the Act, it does not refer substantiated cases to law enforcement without resident consent.

In completing the discussion about State LTCOPs' inconsistencies in the handling of abuse complaints AoA states, "The Act requires that Ombudsman programs both assist residents in protecting their health, safety, welfare and rights as well as to provide the resident with the option to consent to disclosure of information about his or her complaint. This proposed rule is intended to provide the clarity and consistency needed to ensure that residents receive needed protections, and, at the same time, that resident choice is honored, regardless of the State in which a resident lives" [41].

The few states that have made the State LTCOP responsible for the official formal investigation of abuse cases in LTC facilities or have made Ombudsmen mandatory reporters of abuse will likely have to change state law or policy to ensure they operate fully consistent with federal law. In responding in the Final Rule for States LTCOPs to comments received during the NPRM phase of the rule, AoA offered important commentary to not only fully clarify the Ombudsman's role in abuse-related complaints but also to differentiate it from that of other entities with responsibility for investigating abuse especially Adult Protective Services. Several paragraphs from the Final Rule are particularly noteworthy [49].

> The services of the Ombudsman program are distinct from, and as indicated in §1327.21(c), may even conflict with the responsibilities of protective services. An individual resident, may, for example, have a complaint about protective services or may seek support from the Ombudsman program to realize a goal that is inconsistent with his or her protective services plan.
>
> While the complaint resolution function of the Ombudsman program requires 'investigation," an Ombudsman investigation is not for the same purposes as an investigation by protective services, licensing and regulatory agencies, law enforcement or other entities. This may result in confusion regarding the appropriate investigatory role of such entities. When an Ombudsman program receives any complaint (including, but not limited to, an abuse-related complaint), the goal is to resolve the complaint to the resident's satisfaction, rather than to substantiate whether the abuse or other allegation occurred. The Ombudsman program does not have a duty to collect sufficient evidence to meet the higher legal standards of proof that protective services, licensing or regulatory agencies, or law enforcement may need to meet their respective purposes. The Ombudsman program investigates solely for the purpose of gathering necessary information to resolve the complaint to the resident's satisfaction, not to determine whether any law or regulation has been violated for purposes of a potential civil or criminal enforcement action.
>
> With the Ombudsman program fulfilling its duties, the priorities and interests of the individual resident can be supported and advocated for. If the protective services and other government systems charged with taking protective or enforcement actions are not providing the outcomes that serve the health, safety,

welfare or rights of residents, the Ombudsman program is available to address the larger systemic problems. Therefore, it is critically important that each of these agencies is able to fully and distinctly fulfill their duties.

With respect to the conflict imposed upon State LTCOPs in states making Ombudsmen mandatory reporters of abuse under state law, AoA's Final Rule makes clear that Ombudsmen are prohibited from being mandatory reporters. In response to an inquiry to the Administration on Aging specifically asking, "Does the final rule prohibit us from being mandated reporters?" AoA responded, "Yes. The Rule (and the OAA) prohibit reporting of resident-identifying information without resident's permission and, by logical extension, mandated reporting of suspected abuse which discloses such information". In explaining their response AoA provides a very thoughtful and useful explanation for the rationale: [50]

Through the strict disclosure limitations within the OAA, Congress has indicated its intent for the Ombudsman program to be a safe, person-centered place for residents to bring their concerns. Residents can be assured that their information will not be disclosed without their consent, the consent of the resident representative, or court order. OAA Sect. 712(d)(2)(B). Despite numerous Congressional reauthorizations of the Act, Congress has never provided an exception for abuse reporting in the Act. While the Rule provides limited exceptions for reporting resident-identifying information where residents are unable to communicate informed consent, we do not believe that the Act provides ACL with the authority to promulgate a rule that would permit Ombudsman program reporting of resident identifying information if a resident or his/her representative, who is unable to communicate informed consent, has not provided consent. Nor does ACL support such reporting over the resident's objections, as a matter of policy.

The Ombudsman Program is designed to represent the interest of the resident (and not necessarily the interest of the State) in order to support the resident to make informed decisions about the disclosure of his or her own information. Residents may be concerned about retaliation if their concern is known or have other reasons why they do not want the Ombudsman program to disclose their information. While Congress intends for the Ombudsman program to resolve complaints related to the health, safety, welfare and rights of residents, and while that intent logically includes response to and protection from abuse, Congress provided the resident – and not the Ombudsman program – with the authority to make the decision about when and where resident-identifying information can be disclosed by the Ombudsman program. That is as it should be.

AoA promulgated its final rule on February 11, 2015 making it effective July 1, 2016, thus giving any State needing to make statutory or regulatory changes necessary to comply with federal law, the time to adopt such changes in their law or other policy.

For those wishing to understand in greater detail the role of the State LTCOP in abuse-related complaints, AoA's Final Rule provides considerable detail and insight including the Ombudsman's role vis-à-vis other entities charged with investigating abuse especially APS. It also provides detailed guidance for circumstances when a resident is unable to give consent, when a resident's representative (when the resident is unable to do so) does not give consent and may not be acting in the resident's best interest, and when an ombudsman personally witnesses incidents of abuse.

The restrictions on disclosure of information and the strict confidentiality requirements notwithstanding, the Ombudsman has an exceptionally important role to play in bringing to light and remedying the effects of abuse of facility residents. In fact, no one has a more significant role to play. Other than facility personnel, no other party of authority is in LTC facilities and sees residents more frequently than do Ombudsmen. A key hallmark of the LTCOP is the notion of "presence" in the facility—simply being in the facility on a regular basis. Regular presence is a critical goal of State LTCOPs and most State LTCOPs do their best to ensure facilities are visited by Ombudsmen on a regular basis.

Regular "presence"[7] in facilities provides the opportunity for Ombudsmen to get to better know the residents, the facility staff and even family members, and over time to establish that they are an independent voice for the resident whom the resident can trust with their complaints and fears, including those related to abuse, neglect and exploitation. Presence is best achieved by in-person visits to facilities and residents but can also be enhanced through other means such as speaking to residents or family councils, visible posters in strategic locations in facilities, and interaction with others who may have reason to visit facilities and interact with residents, family members and staff, and other means.

The fact that the preponderance of cases handled by State LTCOPs originate with complaints from residents themselves (38 %) followed by relatives or friends of residents (19 %) and facility staff (17 %) says it all with respect to the importance of being seen and known in facilities. Residents especially are highly unlikely to bring complaints to an Ombudsman if they do not interact personally with an Ombudsman. They are unlikely to pick up the phone and make a cold call much less go to an Ombudsman's office. As a California legislative report noted,

"Research has shown that the presence of ombudsmen increases abuse reporting. A 1995 evaluation of the national long-term care ombudsman program by the Institute of Medicine called the phenomenon "a sentinel" effect. Local (Ombudsman) coordinators in California say they've seen it firsthand. The posters that facilities are required to put up telling residents how to contact an ombudsman aren't enough

[7]The landmark 1995 Institute of Medicine report on the LTCOP (*Real People Real Problems*) noted, "The regular presence of persons from outside of facilities has been identified as an important factor in improving quality of care and quality of life in facilities," cited numerous studies supporting this.

to reach those who are bedridden or suffer from dementia. Only repeated visits from an ombudsman can" [48].

The ability of State LTCOPs to have regular presence in facilities is largely a function of adequate resources including personnel. Most State LTCOPs cannot accomplish this without a substantial corps of volunteer ombudsmen. As a result, most State LTCOPs and their local designees expend considerable effort in recruiting, training and managing volunteers. Visiting all of a state's LTC facilities especially board and care and assisted living facilities is an enormous undertaking, much less visiting them on a regular basis. Given this, nationally State LTCOPs visit a remarkable number of facilities. In FY 2013 a combined total of 1283.64 full-time equivalent staff and 8155 volunteers visited 69 %of all nursing homes and 29 % of all board and care, assisted living and similar homes at least quarterly. They also conducted 5260 trainings sessions for facility staff on such topics as residents' rights, and participated in 22,205 resident council and 2230 family council meetings [35].

More frequent Ombudsman visits to and therefore presence in the nation's long-term care facilities logically suggests that more complaints about abuse, neglect and exploitation of facility residents (and other matters) would emerge. Without an Ombudsman available it is likely that many incidents of abuse will never come to light to other authorities including APS and law enforcement.

15.2.4 LTCOP Systems Advocacy and Elder Abuse

When the LTC facility resident complains to a State LTCOP that he or she is a victim of abuse, neglect or exploitation the resident is entitled, if they so wish, to have their abuse investigated, remedies put in place and appropriate sanctions imposed. In addition to the Ombudsman, other entities clearly have major roles to play in responding to allegations and complaints including Adult Protective Services, certification and licensing agencies, law enforcement and others.

In addition to the unique and unambiguous resident advocacy role of the State LTCOP the other unique overarching feature of State LTCOPs is its responsibility, indeed mandate, to engage in "systems advocacy;" to independently and freely pursue legislative, regulatory and other policy changes to redress circumstances and conditions adverse to the health, safety, welfare, or rights of residents in the nation's LTC facilities. The policy advocacy purview of State LTCOPs is huge. It can be brought to bear to improve standards of care in LTC facilities, payment policy to ensure better staffing and care, changes in guardianship and conservatorship requirements and so forth. It can also be brought to bear to improve policy to prevent abuse, neglect and exploitation of residents, to better identify abuse when it occurs, to create more effective sanctions against those who commit, enable or ignore abuse, and to improve services and supports for those that have been abused.

Each of these objectives of policy advocacy are of great importance to all who are dedicated to addressing elder abuse, whether they are Ombudsmen, APS, law enforcement, prosecutors, regulators (e.g., certification and licensing), mental health professionals, long-term care providers, aging services professionals, and others. And each of them should have a keen interest in collaborating with States LTCOPs to help shape and support the LTCOPs' systems advocacy agendas and strategies. Adult Protective Services, for example, could look to the State LTCOP's systems advocacy to support increased funding, improved staffing and training, stronger investigative and forensics tools, improved support services for victims (e.g., emergency funds, shelters, transportation), to name a few, with the ultimate goal of protecting LTC facility residents from abuse or redressing its effects. There is common cause among State LTCOP, APS and the other key players in addressing elder abuse. The LTCOP's systems advocacy role can be a powerful tool in combatting elder abuse.

To locate the State LTCOP in individual states, contact the National Long-Term Care Ombudsman Resource Center, operated by the National Consumer Voice for Quality Long-Term Care (or Consumer Voice) [51].

15.3 Future Directions

So what are the big questions for Adult Protective Service system and the Long-Term Care Ombudsman as the baby boomer generation begins to flood both systems? For APS, funding is and has long been a major issue. The promise of the Elder Justice Act still remains unfilled and we await movement from a Congress that has not shown any indication that we will see any action. The regulatory and membership arms of the financial services industry have shown an increasing awareness of an adequately funded APS system to be absolutely critical to combatting this problem which is robbing their customers of their wealth and health. This looks like a promising place for an alternative source of funding and another partner to work with on this critical policy issue.

Public awareness remains low despite our efforts over the last half-century but is increasing daily. This has been cited by both The National Policy Summit on Elder Abuse in 2001 and the Elder Justice Roadmap as the top or near the top recommendation in combating elder abuse. We need to engage the services of a top tier marketing agency to help us promote the message that any of us can be victims or any of us can be a perpetrator of abuse, neglect or exploitation.

What we have lacked that other movements had was the voices of the victims themselves. This has been problematic as many of the victims by definition are vulnerable and cannot speak for themselves. The APS community has not been an effective political voice in this process despite the efforts of the National Adult Protective Services Association and unlocking the key to make this happen is one of the great challenges facing the next generation of protective service professionals.

We in the field are all waiting to see if the National Adult Maltreatment Reporting System mentioned earlier in the chapter will take hold and begin to let us have increased standardization in the field. As reported, this is a voluntary system and will allow us to measure and discuss things in a similar manner and will help move the field forward. I think this is a very important step and will hopefully attract more research and funding to the field.

As Elder Mistreatment is finally being recognized as a public health and human rights issue around the world, it is time for all of us to join forces and recognize and support the work of adult protective service investigators and the long-term care ombudsman. They are the front line workers and the first line of defense for all of us as we meet the needs of the largest and oldest cohort in the history of mankind.

As previously discussed, the Long-Term Care Ombudsman Program faces many challenges. Looking ahead to future directions several major themes are clear. After a hiatus of almost a quarter-century since the 1992 amendments to the Older Americans Act, the Administration for Community Living has promulgated a set of regulations for the LTCOP to complement and provide further guidance to statutory law governing the program. These new regulations, effective July 1, 2016, should help to provide greater consistency across and among states' LTCOPs, addressing and hopefully mitigating if not resolving long-standing challenges within LTCOPs. Key examples are the role of LTCOPs in dealing with abuse complaints as well as such matters as conflicts of interest, roles of volunteers, program independence and other matters discussed in this chapter.

There are several certainties in long-term care. First, the numbers of people needing some form of long-term services and supports, including facility-based care, will continue to grow. The demographics of aging society guarantee that. Second, there will be continuing pressure to reduce expenditures for LTSS especially for nursing home and other facility-based forms of care, as well as in-patient hospital costs. As a result, our health care and LTSS systems will continue to transform. And, third, all-too-often residents of LTC facilities and other consumers of nonresidential LTSS will have their rights violated, be provided less than optimal care and sometimes horrid care, and will need independent trusted outlets for expressing their fears and complaints. Each of these certainties undergirds the importance of having a strong consumer advocacy system in place for LTSS residents and clients. The LTCOP is an essential component of consumer advocacy for facility residents and increasingly nonresidential HBCS clients. Yet, to perform its role adequately, funding will have to increase for the LTCOP to carry out its current roles much less to expand to other forms of LTSS. This author believes neither the Older Americans Act nor other sources of state and local funding will be available to meet the need, and that ultimately Medicare and Medicaid should contribute to support the LTCOP. The recently established Medicaid Managed Care Ombudsman services in some states (and in some states associated with the state's LTCOP) is an important precedent.

References

1. National Adult Protective Services Association. Adult protective services code of ethics. http://www.napsa-now.org/about-napsa/code-of-ethics. Accessed 10 Nov 2015.
2. United States. Cong. Senate. Special Committee on Aging. Broken trust: combating financial exploitation of vulnerable seniors. Feb. 4, 2015. 114th Cong. 1st sess. Washington. (statement of Kathleen Quinn, Executive Director, National Adult Protective Services Association).
3. United States., Mrena C, Weisberg E, United States. Elder justice: stronger federal leadership could enhance national response to elder abuse: report to the Chairman, Special Committee on Aging, U.S. Senate. Washington, D.C.: U.S. Govt. Accountability Office; 2011.
4. Sedlak AJ, Mettenburg J, Basena M, Petta I, McPherson K, Greene A, Li S. Fourth national incidence study of child abuse and neglect (NIS–4): report to congress. Washington, DC: U.S. Department of Health and Human Services, Administration for Children and Families; 2010. http://www.acf.hhs.gov/programs/opre/abuse_neglect/natl_incid/index.html.
5. Department of Health and Human Services: Office of Women's Health. One department: overview of activities on violence against women 2008–2009. Department of Health and Human Services. 2009. http://www.womenshealth.gov/owh/pub/violence-against-women.cfm.
6. Acierno R, Hernandez-Tejada M, Muzzy W, Steve K. National elder mistreatment study. Report. National Institute of Justice. 2009. https://www.ncjrs.gov/pdffiles1/nij/grants/226456.pdf.
7. United States. Bureau of Justice Statistics. Violent crime rate remained unchanged while theft rate declined in 2008. Press Release. Bureau of Justice Statistics. 2009. http://bjs.ojp.usdoj.gov/content/pub/press/cv08pr.cfm.
8. Administration for Children and Families. FY 2010 Congressional justification. 2010. http://archive.acf.hhs.gov/programs/olab/budget/2010/cj2010.html.
9. Women's Policy Inc. FY 2010 appropriations summary. 2009. http://www.womenspolicy.org/wp-content/uploads/2013/10/FY2010_Appropriations_Summary.pdf.
10. National Network to End Domestic Violence. Funding and appropriations. 2016. http://nnedv.org/policy/issues/funding.html.
11. National Association of VOCA Assistance Administrators. VOCA funding. 2016. http://www.navaa.org/budget/index.html.
12. United States. Elder abuse: a national disgrace: a report by the Chairman of the Subcommittee on Health and Long-Term Care of the Select Committee of the Subcommittee on Aging, House of Representatives, Ninety-ninth Congress, first session. Washington, DC: U.S. Government Printing Office; 1985.

13. United States. Elder abuse: a decade of shame and inaction: a report. Washington: U.S. Government Printing Office; 1990.
14. Lachs M, Williams C, O'Brien S, Pillemer K, Charlson M. The mortality of elder mistreatment. J Am Med Assoc. 1998;280 (5):428–32.
15. United States. Cong. Senate. Special Committee on Aging. Justice for all: ending elder abuse, neglect and financial exploitation. March 2, 2011. 112th Cong. 1st sess. Washington. (statement of Mark Lachs, Director of Geriatrics, New York Presbyterian Health System, Co-Chief, Division of Geriatric Medicine and Gerontology, Weill Medical College of Cornell University).
16. Koss MP, Heslet L. Somatic consequences of violence against women. Arch Fam Med. 1992;1:53–9.
17. National Center on Elder Abuse. The national elder abuse incidence study: final report. Report. Administration for Children and Families and Administration on Aging. 1994. http://aoa.gov/AoA_Programs/Elder_Rights/Elder_Abuse/docs/ABuseReport_Full.pdf.
18. Acierno R, Hernandez M, Amstadter A, Resnick H, Steve K, Muzzy W, Kilpatrick D. Prevalence and correlates of emotional, physical, sexual, and financial abuse and potential neglect in the United States: the national elder mistreatment study. Am J Public Health. 2010;100(2):292–7.
19. Lifespan of Greater Rochester, Inc., Weill Cornell Medical Center of Cornell University, New York City Department for Aging. Under the radar: New York state elder abuse prevalence study: Self-reported prevalence and documented case surveys. Report. William B, Hoyt Memorial New York State Children and Family Trust Fund, and the New York State office of Children and Family Services. 2011. http://www.ocfs.state.ny.us/main/reports/Under%20the%20Radar%2005%2012%2011%20final%20report.pdf.
20. Gunther J. The Utah cost of financial exploitation. Report. Utah Division of Aging and Adult Services. 2011. http://victimsofcrime.org/docs/default-source/financial-fraud/2011-economic-cost-of-financial-exploitation.pdf?sfvrsn=2.
21. MetLife Mature Market Institute, Virginia Tech, National Committee for the Prevention of Elder Abuse. The MetLife study of elder financial abuse: Crimes of occasion, desperation, and predation against America's elders. Report. MetLife Mature Market Institute, Virginia Tech, National Committee for the Prevention of Elder Abuse. 2011. https://www.metlife.com/assets/cao/mmi/publications/studies/2011/mmi-elder-financial-abuse.pdf.
22. True Link Financial. The true link report on elder financial abuse 2015. Report. True Link Financial. 2015. https://www.truelinkfinancial.com/research.
23. U.S. Government Accountability Office. Elder justice: stronger federal leadership could enhance national response to elder abuse. Report. Government Accountability Office. 2011. http://www.gao.gov/assets/320/316224.pdf.
24. Quinn K, Benson B. The states elder abuse victim services: a system still in search of support. Generations. 2012;36(3):66–71.
25. BITS, Financial Services Roundtable. Protecting the elderly and vulnerable from financial fraud and exploitation. Report. BITS, Financial Services Roundtable. 2010. http://www.bits.org/publications/fraud/BitsProtectingVulnerableAdults0410.pdf.
26. Financial Industry Regulatory Authority. Financial exploitation of seniors and other vulnerable adults. Regulatory Notice. FINRA. 2015. http://www.finra.org/industry/notices/15-37.
27. North American Securities Administrators Association. Proposed model legislation or regulation to protect vulnerable adults from financial exploitation. Model Legislation. NASAA. 2015. www.nasaa.org.
28. Okonkwo O, Wadley V, Griffith H, Ball K, Marson D. Cognitive correlates of financial abilities in mild cognitive impairment. J Am Geriatr Soc. 2006;54(11):1745–50.
29. Denburg N. The orbitofrontal cortex, real-world decision-making, and normal aging. Ann N Y Acad Sci. 2007;1121:480 98.
30. Institute of Medicine. Cognitive aging: progress in understanding and opportunities for action. Washington: Institute of Medicine; 2015.
31. Investor Protection Trust. Elder investment fraud and financial exploitation prevention program. Resource. Investor Protection Trust. 2016. http://www.investorprotection.org/IPT-activities/?FA=EIFFE-pp.
32. Sec. 712 and following, Older Americans of 1965, as amended.
33. Final Rule, 45 CFR Parts 1321 and 1327, State Long-Term Care Ombudsman Programs, Administration on Aging, Administration for Community Living, HHS, Federal Register, February 11, 2015.
34. Older Americans Act, Sec. 712 (a)(5).
35. National Ombudsman Reporting System. Administration on Aging, Administration for Community Living, USDHHS. 2014. http://www.agid.acl.gov/DataGlance/NORS/.
36. Institute of Medicine. Real people real problems: an evaluation of the long-term care ombudsman programs of the Older Americans Act. Washington: Institute of Medicine; 1995.
37. National Association of States United for Aging and Disabilities and the National Ombudsman Resource Center at the National Consumer Voice for Quality Long-Term Care. State long-term care ombudsman programs: a primer for state aging directors and executive staff. Report. NASUAD and Consumer Voice. 2013. http://www.nasuad.org/documentation/nasuad_materials/NASUAD%20Ombudsman%20Report%20final.pdf.
38. Public Law 102-375.
39. OAA, Sec. 712(a)(3)(A).
40. OAA, Sec. 712 (a)(3)(ii)(I)-(III).
41. Proposed Rule, 45 CFR Parts 1321 and 1327, RIN 0985-AA08, State Long-Term Care Program, Administration on Aging, Administration for Community Living, HHS, June 18, 2013.
42. OAA, Sec. 712 (j)(2).
43. Administration on Aging. Long-term care ombudsman program. http://www.aoa.acl.gov/AoA_Programs/Elder_Rights/Ombudsman/index.aspx#data.
44. Administration on Aging. Long-term care ombudsman complaint codes. http://www.aoa.acl.gov/AoA_Programs/Elder_Rights/Ombudsman/docs/Complaint-Code-2019.pdf.
45. Administration on Aging. 2013 national ombudsman reporting system data tables. http://www.aoa.acl.gov/AoA_Programs/Elder_Rights/Ombudsman/National_State_Data/2013/Index.aspx.
46. OAA Sec. 712 (a)(5)(B)(iv).
47. OAA Sec. 712 (h)(1)(F).
48. Hill J. California's elder abuse investigators: Ombudsman shackled by conflicting laws and duties. Report. California Senate Office of Oversight and Outcomes. 2009. http://sooo.senate.ca.gov/sites/sooo.senate.ca.gov/files/ombudsmanreport10_29.pdf.
49. Final Rule, 45 CFR Parts 1321 and 1327, State Long-Term Care Ombudsman Programs, Administration on Aging, Administration for Community Living, HHS, Federal Register, February 11, 2015, pp. 102–103.
50. Correspondence from Becky A. Kurtz, Director, Office of Long-Term Care Ombudsman Programs, AoA/ACL, to Joseph Rodrigues, State LTC Ombudsman, California Department of Aging, October 15, 2015.
51. Consumer Voice. Locate an ombudsman. Consumer Voice. 2016. http://theconsumervoice.org/get_help.

16 Elder Abuse Victims' Access to Justice: Roles of the Civil, Criminal, and Judicial Systems in Preventing, Detecting, and Remedying Elder Abuse

Lori A. Stiegel

16.1 Introduction

Recent high-profile cases of elder abuse—including those involving New York City philanthropist Brooke Astor and entertainer Mickey Rooney—have drawn attention to the fact that the three components of the US justice system—civil, criminal, and judicial—have crucial roles in preventing, detecting, and remedying elder abuse, neglect, and exploitation (referred to generally as "elder abuse" unless otherwise indicated). Following this overview and comparison of the goals of the civil justice and criminal justice systems, the chapter focuses on impediments that victims may face in accessing the three system components and the ways in which lawyers, judges, and allied professionals can protect older persons from elder abuse, make victims whole, and hold perpetrators accountable. This chapter also addresses ideas and promising practices for improving the justice system's response to elder abuse, and the potential benefits of involving justice system professionals in efforts to enhance the response of other systems that are relevant to elder abuse victims.

Elder abuse can occur in many forms. Categories, terminology, and definitions vary among State and Federal laws, but the National Center on Elder Abuse has developed seven general classifications: physical abuse, sexual abuse, psychological/emotional abuse, neglect, abandonment, self-neglect, and financial exploitation [1]. Elder abuse can occur in different settings, which are commonly grouped as domestic and institutional (the latter term generally referring to long-term care and residential care facilities) [1]. No matter the form or the setting of elder abuse, there is some purpose that one or more components of the justice system can serve.

All three systems have a role in preventing, detecting, and remedying elder abuse, but each has a different purpose and distinct goals. The civil justice system is both proactive and reactive, focused on individual victims and with the ability to prevent elder abuse and to remedy it when it does occur. The criminal justice system is reactive, focused on protecting society by punishing criminal conduct and preventing its reoccurrence. The judicial system also is reactive, focused on the parties in cases brought before the courts, with judges and juries making decisions primarily related to remedies or punishment for elder abuse.

Table 16.1 highlights key distinctions between the civil justice and criminal justice systems. The remainder of this chapter elaborates on these characteristics.

16.2 Elder Abuse Victims' Attitudes About the Justice System

In 1993, the State Justice Institute funded the American Bar Association Commission on Law and Aging (ABA Commission) to conduct a groundbreaking study of barriers to consideration of cases involving elder abuse by the state courts and develop recommended guidelines for overcoming those barriers. Nearly 300 professionals were involved in the project. They included judges, court administrators, private and publicly funded lawyers, prosecutors, staff of state Attorneys General Offices, Medicaid Fraud Control Unit staff, state legal services developers, Adult Protective Services (APS) administrators and staff, and other non-legal professionals [2].

Study participants identified practices and barriers that inhibited entry of cases involving elder abuse into the state courts. These fell into two categories: abuse victims' attitudes about the courts and about the pursuit of legal remedies, and systemic practices in or related to the courts. The

The author is not writing on behalf of her employer and the views expressed are her own and do not necessarily represent an official position of her employer unless otherwise indicated.

L.A. Stiegel (✉)
American Bar Association Commission on Law and Aging, 1050 Connecticut Avenue, NW, Suite 400, Washington, DC 20036, USA
e-mail: lori.stiegel@americanbar.org

X. Dong (ed.), *Elder Abuse*, DOI 10.1007/978-3-319-47504-2_16

Table 16.1 Key distinctions between the civil justice and criminal justice systems

Issue	Civil justice system	Criminal justice system
Key goals	• Protect the victim • Determine whether actions were lawful and undo those that were not, or order that certain actions be taken • Resolve disputes • Compensate the victim for harm caused	• Protect society • Determine whether criminal laws were violated • Punish/hold accountable the perpetrator • Protect the victim • Order the perpetrator to provide restitution to the victim
Types of cases	• Civil rights • Contract disputes • Family matters such as divorce and adoption • Guardianship/conservatorship • Health care and insurance • Mental health commitments • Personal injury/medical malpractice • Protective orders • Real estate matters such as foreclosures, landlord/tenant disputes, and property disputes • Wills and estates	• Criminal matters
Burden of proof	"Preponderance of the evidence" "Clear and convincing evidence"	• "Beyond a reasonable doubt"
Victim's role	• Subject of the legal proceeding • Usually has some control over the case • Has constitutional or statutory rights	• Witness to the events that are the subject of the legal proceeding • Has no control over the case • Has constitutional or statutory rights

victims' attitudinal barriers are listed below; the courts' systemic barriers are discussed in Sect. 5.

- Older abused persons are commonly reluctant to press charges against abusive family members or caregivers because "they do not want to get that person in trouble."
- Often, the abused person is dependent on the abuser for care or companionship, and, therefore, believes that he or she has "no choice" but to continue in the abusive relationship.
- Older persons also fear that involving APS or law enforcement in their problems will lead to their removal from their home and placement in a nursing home. They also fear that APS or court intervention will not prevent further abuse or retaliation.
- Older abused persons are sometimes so afraid of testifying in court or so ashamed to have their abusive situation aired in public that they are willing to forego pursuit of their legal rights.
- Older persons' lack of knowledge about their rights and about the judicial system also inhibits their pursuit of appropriate legal remedies.
- Older abused persons may have no means of traveling to the courthouse for hearings or may have no one to assist their care-dependent spouse, partner, or child while they are meeting with lawyers or testifying at trial.
- Older abused persons often are ignorant of the availability of APS and other services that may be able to help them correct an abusive situation. Additionally, even if they are aware of these services they may not think of themselves as abused and recognize that such services may benefit them [2].

16.3 Civil Justice System

Civil lawyers who advise and represent older persons or organizations that serve them have significant opportunity to prevent, detect, and remedy elder abuse. Civil lawyers also have valuable knowledge to share in system-improvement activities such as multidisciplinary initiatives, professional and public education, and legislative and policy development.

This section covers the roles of civil lawyers regarding elder abuse, the systemic barriers that may impede victims' access to the civil justice system, and promising practices and other potential improvements to reduce those barriers.

16.3.1 Roles of Civil Lawyers

Civil lawyers, often assisted by paralegals under their supervision, work in a variety of settings. They may provide free legal services under the auspices of legal aid agencies or other programs to people who are over age 60 or who have low incomes, work in private law firms and charge for their services, work in the private sector, or work for Federal, State, or local government agencies. Regardless of their employment setting, civil lawyers can have myriad vital proactive and reactive roles in elder abuse.

To assist older persons directly in preventing or remedying elder abuse, civil lawyers can:

- Screen and assess whether an older person might already may be experiencing elder abuse in some form;
- Counsel an older person about the forms and risks of elder abuse and about taking steps to prevent it, for example by including provisions in a power of attorney that limit the agent's opportunity to misuse his or her authority and commit financial exploitation;
- Advise a victim how to obtain a civil protection order against an abuser;
- Help an older client obtain appropriate housing and government benefits, which may enable the older person to avoid or escape from an abusive situation;
- Help an older client obtain Medicaid eligibility through a hardship exemption by demonstrating that the client did not make a "gift" to another person that would render the client ineligible, but rather was financially exploited; and
- Bring lawsuits in civil court on behalf of an elder abuse victim to terminate an abuser's control over the victim, evict an abuser from a shared home, seek financial compensation for physical harm caused by a caregiver intentionally or through neglect, terminate the legal authority of an agent or guardian who is exploiting the victim, or recover misappropriated assets.

Additionally, civil lawyers can indirectly prevent or remedy elder abuse by:

- Advising and representing public sector organizations (APS, long-term care ombudsman programs, law enforcement, or other government agencies) in fulfilling their legal responsibilities to elder abuse victims;
- Litigating civil lawsuits on behalf of government agencies against individuals or businesses to stop abusive or exploitative practices;
- Helping the private sector to interpret laws and regulations and to develop policies and protocols to facilitate prevention, detection, and reporting of elder abuse; and
- Participating in multidisciplinary teams, task forces, legislative study committees, and other collaborative efforts to develop and advocate for improved laws, regulations, and policies.

The discussion of barriers, promising practices, and potential improvements that follows is focused on the needs of victims and the role of civil lawyers in meeting those needs. It will not address further the role of civil lawyers in advising and representing public or private sector organizations regarding elder abuse.

16.3.2 Barriers of the Civil Justice System

The ability of the civil justice system to prevent, detect, and remedy elder abuse offers considerable benefits to older persons. Recent research on the impact of providing civil legal services to victims of domestic violence demonstrates that legal aid facilitates the independence of victims and also may indirectly benefit the government agencies and businesses that serve them [3, 4]. It seems likely that civil legal services for elder abuse victims would result in similar outcomes.

There are substantial barriers to using the civil justice system, however. Many older persons face significant challenges in obtaining civil legal help because they:

- Lack information about what elder abuse is, that it raises legal issues, and that civil lawyers can help to prevent or rectify it;
- Lack information about how to find legal help;
- Have difficulty finding civil lawyers who are knowledgeable about elder abuse; or
- Are unable to obtain free legal services or pay for a private lawyer.

Additionally, even if legal problems are recognized and capable civil legal help can be obtained, existing civil laws may be inadequate to prevent or stop elder abuse.

Inadequate data collection about the civil justice system also poses an impediment, by making it difficult to obtain needed funding and other resources to overcome the barriers that directly affect victims.

These obstacles, promising practices that address them, and other potential improvements are discussed next.

16.3.2.1 Lack of Public Awareness

The public lacks awareness of elder abuse *and what to do about it* (emphasis added) [5]. Compounding this problem, anecdotal data about elder abuse victims indicates that even when they do recognize they are being victimized, they often fail to realize that their problems may have legal solutions.

Efforts to enhance public awareness about elder abuse and what to do about it must furnish information about the role of civil legal services and how to access them, including the possibility that free or reduced-cost legal assistance may be available to elder abuse victims.

16.3.2.2 Professionals' Lack of Awareness of the Role of the Civil Justice System

Professionals and other service providers, agencies, and businesses interacting with older persons also often lack awareness that elder abuse raises civil legal issues and that civil lawyers can help prevent or remedy the problem. Referring victims or their caring family members and friends to a legal aid program or to a lawyer referral service is equally important as a referral or report to APS, aging and disability services, the long-term care ombudsman program, law enforcement, prosecutors, regulators, and other services that may prove useful. Each system has different resources and goals, and no one system can holistically meet all of a victim's needs [6].

Raising the awareness of non-legal professionals about the availability and importance of civil legal services is necessary. Accomplishing that requires regular cross-training with civil lawyers, as well as the development and dissemination of routinely updated materials to help allied professionals understand the role of civil legal services and to identify situations in which a referral to civil legal services is appropriate. Many professionals who interact with older persons are mandated by state law to report suspected elder abuse to APS, law enforcement, another government agency, or some combination thereof, so there are excellent opportunities to include information about the role of civil legal services in broader trainings about recognizing and reporting elder abuse [6, 7].

16.3.2.3 Civil Lawyers' Lack of Knowledge About Elder Abuse

Efforts to raise awareness among the public and non-legal professionals about the civil justice system's role in preventing, detecting, and remedying elder abuse have limited impact if older persons are unable to find civil lawyers who are knowledgeable about the complex and multi-faceted problem. A civil lawyer's ability to provide competent advice and representation regarding elder abuse may require knowledge of an array of substantive legal topics including banking and securities law; contract law; decision-making capacity; domestic violence; family law; guardianship and conservatorship, as well as their alternatives such as financial and health care powers of attorney; laws governing health care, long-term care, and residential care facilities; public benefits eligibility; real property, trust and estate law; and undue influence [8 10].

Awareness of the law is necessary but not sufficient. To effectively advise clients about options and remedies, assess the merits of cases, and determine what evidence is available or needed, civil lawyers also must have knowledge about:

- the indicators and consequences of all forms of elder abuse [11];
- the availability and effectiveness of an array of elder abuse interventions, which might include APS; alternative dispute resolution; appointment and monitoring of substitute decision makers such as guardians, conservators, agents under a power of attorney, or representative payees; housing options including emergency options such as elder abuse or domestic violence shelters as well as longer-term options; and long-term care ombudsman programs [8, 11]; and
- the growing body of scientific research about decision-making capacity and susceptibility to exploitation and undue influence [10].

Currently, lawyers are rarely exposed to the problem of elder abuse in law school. Aging issues are generally not incorporated into traditional doctrinal law school courses, such as contracts, criminal law, evidence, real property, torts, trusts and estates [12]. Nearly half of all law schools do not offer a doctrinal class on elder law [12], and elder law classes survey an array of issues and do not place much emphasis on elder abuse. Yet Kohn and Spurgeon's survey of elder law practitioners and professors indicated that respondents most often listed elder abuse and ethics as the subjects necessitating additional legal education.

Clinical elder law courses are even less common than doctrinal elder law classes. Clinical students may assist older clients on an array of matters including elder abuse, but the only known clinical program devoted to elder abuse is the University of Illinois College of Law Elder Financial Justice Clinic [13].

Continuing legal education (CLE) on elder abuse shares the same limitations as law school education. Aging issues in general and elder abuse in particular are not usually incorporated into relevant topics such as planning for incapacity, estate planning, torts (with the exception of long-term care facility abuse and neglect cases), family law, domestic violence, and other substantive issues. Elder law CLE programs usually either survey several issues or focus on Medicaid planning, planning for incapacity, and guardianship and conservatorship; no matter which approach is used, relatively little time is spent on the topic of elder abuse.

Improving legal education and continuing legal education about elder abuse would increase lawyers' awareness of elder abuse and how to prevent or remedy it. Content on elder abuse in CLE and other on-the-job training programs is becoming more common. Additionally, there are two recent national training efforts that deserve mention.

- The Legal Services Corporation (LSC), which funds free legal services to low-income individuals, collaborated with the US Department of Justice through its Elder Justice Initiative, Office for Access to Justice, and Office for Victims of Crime to develop free, online training for LSC grantees' staff. Four hours of free online training are available at https://www.ovcttac.gov/views/dspLegalAssistance.cfm?tab=1#onlinetraining. The four modules are titled: What Every Legal Services Lawyer Needs to Know About Elder Abuse, Practical and Ethical Strategies, Domestic Violence and Sexual Assault, and Financial Exploitation.
- Another initiative to educate civil lawyers is the Elder Investment Fraud and Financial Exploitation Prevention Program—Legal, a collaboration of the ABA Commission on Law and Aging and the Investor Protection Trust (IPT) and Investor Protection Institute (IPI). Working with state securities regulators and state or local bar associations, the ABA Commission, IPT, and IPI are developing, testing, and then implementing a national model curriculum for civil lawyers on detecting elder investment fraud and financial exploitation and what to do about it [14].

These two education initiatives are promising, but much more needs to be done to reach other civil lawyers, to expand the range of topics covered, and to provide more advanced training.

In addition to law school education and CLE programs on elder abuse, civil lawyers could benefit greatly from other resources to help them provide high-quality, cost-effective civil legal services. These resources could include case analyses, brief banks, case consultations and mentoring, more opportunities for communication and networking, information about finding qualified expert witnesses, and statutory analyses [10]. Congress appropriates millions of dollars for providing similar training and resources to civil lawyers who represent victims of child abuse and of domestic violence, but only a small amount of funding to inform civil lawyers representing older persons–and those funds are not earmarked for education about elder abuse.

16.3.2.4 Lack of Access to Civil Legal Assistance

Enhancing awareness that elder abuse raises civil legal issues and expanding lawyer education about elder abuse will be hollow victories if older persons or their caring family members or friends who are trying to prevent or remedy victimization cannot afford a private lawyer or obtain free legal services.

The challenges that low- or middle-income individuals face in access to the civil justice system are not unique to elder abuse. National studies of unmet legal needs of low-income persons and state-specific studies of unmet legal needs of older persons have demonstrated clearly that Legal Services Corporation- and Older Americans Act-funded free civil legal aid programs are unable to serve a substantial majority of persons who need help [15–17].

So serious is the problem that almost every state, plus the District of Columbia and Puerto Rico, has established an access to justice commission or initiative [18]. The Conference of Chief Judges and Conference of State Court Administrators have reported that the growing numbers of litigants who are not represented by civil lawyers have negative consequences on the courts as well as the parties involved in a case [19]. President Obama also has recognized the critical importance of civil legal services in American society, first by establishing the Office for Access to Justice within the Department of Justice and then by creating the White House Legal Aid Interagency Roundtable to bring together relevant Federal agencies to address the problem of access to justice and how it impacts programs administered by those agencies [20].

Older persons with limited incomes who need preventive or remedial assistance related to elder abuse do face additional challenges in obtaining civil legal services from providers of free legal aid and from private lawyers, however.

The LSC is an independent, non-profit agency that funds and regulates free civil legal aid programs across the country. It is the largest source of funding for free civil legal services; the amount of financial support provided to LSC grantees is set by Congressional appropriations. LSC-funded programs provide services to clients who have incomes below 125 % of the poverty level and have limited resources [21]. LSC collects case data on "juvenile neglected/abused/dependent" and "domestic abuse," but does not have a case data code specifically for elder abuse [22]. The fact that elder abuse is not a case category for which grantees are required to report service data indicates that it is not a priority issue for the LSC. Nonetheless, LSC-funded programs do represent lower-income older persons in case categories related to elder abuse, including consumer fraud, domestic violence, evictions, home foreclosure, other housing matters, and public benefits.

Title III-B of the federal Older Americans Act (OAA) authorizes funding for programs providing free legal aid for persons over age 60 regardless of income and assets. While OAA legal assistance programs do not apply an income and assets test to determine eligibility for services as LSC grantees do, OAA programs must be targeted towards individuals in greatest social and economic need. Title VII of the OAA funds other elder rights activities relevant to elder abuse prevention and redress, including some state Senior Legal Helplines whose staff telephonically provides advice, some brief services, referrals to aging services or other government agencies, and referrals to legal aid programs for more intensive services including representation in court.

The OAA is administered by the Administration for Community Living (ACL), part of the US Department of Health and Human Services. Federal OAA monies flow to state units on aging, and then (in most states) to area agencies on aging (AAAs), which select and fund local providers of free legal assistance. The OAA states that the AAAs are supposed to give priority to legal assistance on an array of fundamental problems including abuse, neglect, and income (which would include financial exploitation).

Some of the OAA-supported legal assistance providers also receive LSC funding, some are non-profit agencies but are not LSC grantees, and some are attorneys in private practice who receive small contracts to provide a limited array of free services. Funding of these programs varies widely, from six figures to a few thousand dollars. Accordingly, the array and nature of services offered, including efforts related to elder abuse, also vary widely. Some service providers prioritize elder abuse and make concerted efforts to raise public awareness, provide preventive legal advice and brief services, and seek remedies in court [23]. Other grantees have such limited funding that they simply provide advice and assistance with planning for incapacity.

Many lawyers volunteer to provide free legal services (known as *pro bono*) to individuals with low incomes, but their efforts are usually administered by LSC-funded programs and subject to the same eligibility criteria for income and assets. Lawyers also may charge a reduced fee (now being called "low bono") to certain categories of clients, including older persons, but even a reduced fee may be too expensive for a victim of elder abuse, especially one who has suffered financial exploitation. Lawyers providing pro bono and low bono services may lack expertise in elder abuse, and the challenging elder abuse cases that most legal aid programs lack resources to take may prove too burdensome for volunteers or lawyers accepting reduced fees.

Some law schools have elder law or other types of clinics (for example, on consumer issues) that educate students by providing free services to older persons, including advice and counseling, preparation of legal documents, and representation in court. All clinical programs face challenges in providing services due to lack of expertise, student vacation and examination schedules, and turnover when the courses end. For these reasons, clinical programs are unlikely to be able to represent elder abuse victims in complex cases requiring litigation.

In elder abuse lawsuits brought against defendants with financial resources or insurance—particularly health care providers, hospitals, long-term and residential care facilities, financial institutions, and other businesses—private lawyers are often willing to accept payment on a contingency fee basis. This means the lawyers take a percentage of damages awarded by the judge or jury to the victim, and bear the financial risk if those lawsuits are not successful.

In contrast, older persons or their concerned family members and friends carry the financial burden if they need legal advice about ways of preventing elder abuse. They also shoulder the burden of paying for legal representation if they wish to sue individuals or businesses without extensive resources or insurance, such as family members, caregivers, "sweetheart scammers" and "new best friends," or substitute decision-makers named by the victim, a government agency, or a court (e.g., agents under a power of attorney, representative payees, guardians, or conservators). Lawyers generally will not take cases on a contingency fee basis if there is a low chance of winning the case or of collecting financial assets from the abuser after winning the case. Obviously elder abuse victims who are not wealthy will face significant challenges in paying for the services of a private civil lawyer, as will wealthier individuals who have lost control over their assets due to decision-making incapacity or financial exploitation [24].

The unmet need for free legal assistance and the challenges of paying for a civil lawyer in private practice demonstrate that increased funding for LSC and OAA grantees is imperative.

Having recognized the importance of civil legal services in preventing and remedying elder abuse, the ACL is striving to improve the ability of OAA-funded legal assistance programs to recognize and address legal issues related to elder abuse. It is doing this by supporting the development or enhancement of state systems that provide training and technical assistance, as well as facilitate multidisciplinary coordination, about the problem. Increased funding would allow the ACL to expand these efforts—known as Model Approaches Phase II—more rapidly, and to continue to support these important initiatives after the initial funding period ends.

Multidisciplinary collaboration between legal aid programs and APS programs may be a promising practice that can help overcome the fact that both systems are woefully underfunded. A recent evaluation of the Jewish Association Serving the Aging Legal/Social Work Elder Abuse Prevention Program in New York City demonstrated that its legal and social work services resulted in reduced elder abuse risk at the time cases were closed [25].

16.3.2.5 Inadequate Civil Laws

Inadequate civil laws add to the challenges that victims and concerned family members or friends face in accessing civil legal representation and in obtaining civil remedies that protect older persons, recover assets, or provide financial remuneration for physical or financial harm. To avoid repetition, specific examples of impediments and of statutory provisions that might address them are discussed below.

Private practitioners could be encouraged to provide representation in civil elder abuse cases if laws provided clear civil remedies for physical or sexual abuse, neglect, or financial exploitation; allowed lawsuits to continue if the victim died prior to verdict; required judges to award punitive or treble damages to victims if statutory conditions were met; and required judges to order defendants who lose elder abuse cases to pay the victim's attorney's fees and costs [9, 13, 24]. Some states have enacted one or more of these useful statutory provisions; they include Arizona, California, Florida, Illinois, Minnesota, Oregon, Utah, and Washington [9, 13, 24].

Laws governing civil protection orders could be expanded to include more situations commonly experienced by victims of elder abuse. Examples include adding financial exploitation, physical abuse by a caregiver, or physical abuse by a family member who is not an intimate partner to the reasons why a person could obtain a protection order [26].

Enacting statutory presumptions of fraud or undue influence when real estate or other assets are transferred in certain circumstances (e.g., without the older person having independent legal advice, to caregivers or fiduciaries) commonly seen in elder financial exploitation cases could facilitate civil lawsuits. These presumptions would either render the transaction void or transfer the burden of proving the transfer's legitimacy from the victim to the defendant. States with statutory presumptions like these include California, Illinois, Maine, and Nevada [27, 28].

Expanding "slayer statutes"—civil laws that prohibit a murderer from inheriting from his or her victim—to include perpetrators of elder abuse could reduce motivation to harm an older person. As of 2013, seven states had amended their laws to include such provisions: California, Illinois, Kentucky, Maryland, Michigan, Oregon, and Washington [29].

Strengthening guardianship and conservatorship laws, as well as practices, to enhance court monitoring of guardians and conservators could help prevent, detect, and redress abuse, neglect, and exploitation. The handful of states and territories that have not yet enacted the Uniform Adult Guardianship and Protective Proceedings Jurisdiction Act (UAGGPJA) should do so because the UAGPPJA reduces the jurisdictional barriers that can impede attempts to redress elder abuse cases that cross state lines [9, 30]. Excellent information about the intersection of elder abuse with the guardianship system is provided in Chap. 17.

The states and territories that have not yet adopted the Uniform Power of Attorney Act (UPOAA) should do so. The UPOAA clarifies the responsibilities and duties of an agent under a power of attorney and contains numerous other provisions that protect against or redress power of attorney abuse, which is a common form of financial exploitation [31].

16.3.2.6 Insufficient Data Collection

The lack of data about civil legal services for elder abuse victims stymies efforts to obtain additional funding for legal aid programs and pro bono services, to enhance training of allied professionals about the importance of the civil justice system to elder abuse victims, to expand law school education and CLE programming, and to advocate for better laws. As discussed earlier, the LSC does not include elder abuse in its case categories for data collection [22]. OAA-funded legal assistance programs are required to report basic, combined output, but those data do not even indicate the legal issues addressed [32]. Law school clinic programs appear to collect some data for internal decision-making and fundraising purposes, or if they receive funding from government agencies or private foundations. Civil lawyers in private practice generally do not share data about the cases they handle.

There are opportunities to collect valuable output and outcome data from legal aid programs supported by the LSC and the OAA. In a 2006 white paper prepared for the National Center on Elder Abuse, Wood opined that LSC grantees and OAA-funded legal assistance programs and senior legal hotlines (now known as helplines) could become sources of data on incidence and prevalence of elder abuse [22]. Additionally, requiring LSC and OAA legal assistance grantees to capture and report data about outcomes in addition to outputs could provide extremely useful data about the effectiveness of civil legal interventions and about the financial costs of elder abuse to victims, their families, businesses, and governments. Examples of such outcome data might be the value of financial accounts or homes that are recovered from an exploiter and the resulting savings to banks that do not have to absorb the losses or to a state's Medicaid program, for which a victim impoverished due to exploitation would become eligible. Recent studies conducted by Utah's and Wyoming's APS programs of the costs of financial exploitation demonstrate that this can be done [33, 34]. A recent study demonstrated that the provision of civil legal assistance to victims of domestic violence reduces the incidence of that problem and results in costs savings to the criminal justice, medical, and mental health systems [4]. Effective in 2016, the LSC started requiring its programs to provide outcome data [35]. Some states require their OAA-funded legal assistance providers to report more data than is required by the Administration for Community Living, but of those states fewer than half require outcome data and generally those states do not require specific data about elder abuse cases [32].

16.3.3 Involving Civil Lawyers in Efforts to Strengthen Laws, Policies, and Practices

Civil lawyers who represent older persons and the government agencies and private sector businesses that serve older persons can and should be involved in local, State, and Federal initiatives to strengthen laws, policies, and practices related to elder abuse. Their knowledge is crucial to efforts to study the problems and implement the solutions described earlier. Civil lawyers also need to be involved in identifying new challenges and developing new ideas as our understanding of elder abuse and of civil legal remedies for it evolve.

Civil lawyers have ethical limitations in their ability to share information about their cases and clients, so their ability to participate in multidisciplinary teams that focus on finding solutions for difficult cases may pose issues that need to be addressed. They are not, however, precluded from participating in multidisciplinary or other initiatives concerned with legislative reform and policy development, and can bring their knowledge of civil law and its impact on elder abuse victims to the table. They also can educate other lawyers and non-legal professionals about preventing and remedying elder abuse through civil law.

16.4 Criminal Justice System

The many actors of the criminal justice system play critical roles in detecting and stopping elder abuse that constitutes criminal conduct, and by punishing perpetrators to protect society, as well as individual victims, from further harm. The system's involvement also serves to communicate to society that elder abuse will not be tolerated [8].

After briefly describing the criminal justice agencies and professionals most involved in cases involving elder abuse, this section covers the systemic barriers that limit the system's response to elder abuse victims, as well as promising practices and other improvements that might lessen those obstacles.

16.4.1 Roles of Criminal Justice Professionals

The criminal justice system involves an array of participants who work to protect society and individual victims in a variety of government agencies. Brief descriptions of the agencies' and participants' roles in relation to victims are provided. The roles of two types of agencies that are focused on defendants (those who have been charged with crimes) or offenders (those who have been found guilty of or pled guilty to crimes) are also reviewed. Coroners and medical examiners, who have a different relationship to victims, are not discussed in this chapter; their role is addressed in Chap. 18.

- Law enforcement agencies, which may be local or regional police departments and sheriffs' offices, or state or federal law enforcement agencies. These agencies receive reports of and otherwise detect alleged criminal behavior, conduct investigations, and, if warranted, take steps to protect the victim and to hold the alleged perpetrator accountable [6]. Some local law enforcement agencies also conduct "welfare" or "wellness" checks on an older or vulnerable person about whose safety someone (for example, a relative, neighbor, or a postal worker) has expressed concern [6]. Often there are multiple local law enforcement agencies within a jurisdiction; more than one agency may have authority to become involved in a case [6]. If violations of both state and federal laws are suspected, state and federal agencies may investigate the alleged perpetrator(s).
- Prosecutors' offices, which employ investigators and prosecutors and which may be local or state agencies (where they may be known as district attorneys, state's attorneys, commonwealth attorneys, or county attorneys) or federal agencies (known as the US Attorney's Office, there is one or more in each state). Every state except North Dakota also has a Medicaid Fraud Control Unit (MFCU), which is responsible for prosecuting fraud and abuse by providers, including long-term care facilities and home health care agencies [36]. Most MFCUs are housed in the state attorney general's office [37]. Additionally, state attorneys general sometimes have authority to bring criminal proceedings or to assist local prosecutors with prosecutions. If both state and federal laws are violated, multiple state and federal agencies may have authority to prosecute the alleged perpetrator.
- Community corrections agencies, which provide pre-trial, probation, parole, and community-based corrections services. Community corrections officials have the potential to detect and prevent elder abuse in several ways. They can discourage criminal defendants and offenders from finding employment in settings that are

frequented by or home to vulnerable elders, or supervise more carefully defendants and offenders who work in such settings. Also, they may supervise offenders who live with older family members or in close proximity to older individuals who are not family [38].

- Corrections agencies, which administer jails and prisons. Professionals who are concerned about elder abuse victims should be aware of policy initiatives to reduce the prison population by eliminating or shortening sentences for non-violent offenders, as well as more specific initiatives supporting early release of older offenders who require extensive, expensive health care.
- Victim services agencies, which may be system-based (meaning that they are part of law enforcement agencies or prosecutors' offices) or community-based (meaning that they are or are a part of a private community organization) [6]. Providers of victim services may be known as victim advocates, victim services professionals, victim-witness coordinators, or victim assistance (or services) providers. No matter their title, these professionals help crime victims navigate the criminal justice process by providing services including information, emotional support, notification of hearings or other key events such as the release of the offender from jail or prison, transportation to and/or accompaniment at court hearings, referrals to other services (including civil legal services), help preparing applications for protective orders, guidance in writing victim impact statements, and assistance in claiming victims' compensation funds. In all states, victims' compensation may be used to help eligible crime victims pay for costs associated with experiencing physical crimes (e.g., recouping money paid for medical care, mental health treatment, funeral costs; recouping lost wages; paying the costs of changing door locks or even relocating) [6]. Some states have chosen, as they are allowed to do by federal regulation, to allow victims of financial crimes to receive victims' compensation for financial losses.

16.4.2 Barriers of the Criminal Justice System

Some states and communities have made substantial progress during the past 10–15 years in strengthening the criminal justice system's response to elder abuse. Improvements are scattered and often fleeting, however. Victims and non-criminal justice professionals face challenges in seeking help from criminal justice professionals, and those professionals face systemic obstacles in their work on elder abuse cases.

- Victims lack information about what elder abuse is, that it raises legal issues, and that criminal justice professionals can help protect them and punish offenders.
- Non-criminal justice professionals lack information about the criminal justice system.
- Criminal justice system professionals lack knowledge about elder abuse and how it often violates criminal laws.
- Lack of resources and other systemic barriers impede the ability of criminal justice professionals to handle elder abuse cases.
- Existing criminal laws may be inadequate.

As with the civil justice system, inadequate data collection raises hurdles to funding and other system improvements.

These obstacles, promising practices that address them, and other potential improvements are discussed next.

16.4.2.1 Lack of Public Awareness

The public's lack of awareness [5] about elder abuse extends to the fact that it is usually also criminal conduct and that abusers should be held accountable by the criminal justice system to protect society as well as individual victims.

Public education campaigns need to inform the public on that issue, and also should recognize and address the concerns and misconceptions that older people have about seeking help from the criminal justice system.

Criminal justice professionals, civil lawyers, and allied professionals including APS continue to report that elder abuse victims are reluctant to contact law enforcement agencies. The attitudinal barriers discussed earlier, derived from the results of the early-1990s ABA Commission study about whether elder abuse cases were being heard in the judicial system [2], remain relevant. Professionals' anecdotes indicate that victims commonly explain their reticence by saying that although they want the abuse to stop, they do not want their abuser to get in trouble or go to jail. Professionals also indicate that many older persons, especially those from cultural, ethnic, or racial minority groups, distrust the criminal justice system [6]. Others want to keep their personal problems private. Some may fear that the process will endanger their health and independence, or that of a loved one for whom they provide care.

An older victim's concerns may be perfectly valid. Nevertheless, it is important to educate older victims about the criminal justice system so they can make informed decisions about the consequences, both good and bad, of contacting law enforcement. Older persons should be made aware of the assistance that may be available from victim services professionals and of the possibility of obtaining victim compensation for physical or, in some states, financial harm. They should be educated that imprisonment is not the only outcome for an abuser. Judges usually have discretion to order that offenders receive needed treatment for substance abuse or mental health problems in lieu of incarceration, and community corrections officials can supervise offenders and take further action against offenders who do not comply with judicial orders.

16.4.2.2 Professionals' Lack of Awareness of the Role of the Criminal Justice System

Non-criminal justice professionals who engage with older persons also lack awareness that elder abuse often violates criminal laws. They also lack an understanding of the duties of criminal justice system professionals, how those professionals do their jobs, and how to communicate with those professionals. This limits the ability of allied professionals to know when referrals or reports to law enforcement are appropriate or, in some instances depending on the type of professional or the type of harm that has occurred, required by state law. Lack of awareness hinders counseling an older person about the protections and services that may be available through the criminal justice system to either the victim or the offender. Moreover, failure to recognize that a crime has occurred may result in the loss of evidence needed to build a criminal case and further harm to a victim [39].

It also is very important for these allied professionals to learn how to communicate effectively with criminal justice professionals [39]. Once professionals acquire that skill they should counsel older victims or victims' concerned family members and friends on how to do the same. Using civil legal or social work lingo such as "the victim experienced financial exploitation through power of attorney abuse" or "the victim lacked cognitive capacity to engage in sexual behavior" when reporting suspected elder abuse will have less impact than using criminal justice terminology such as "the victim's adult child stole her money and her house through fraud" or "the victim could not consent to sex and was raped."

Additionally, allied professionals, victims, and victims' concerned family members and friends need to understand that victims do not have to "press charges" against an alleged perpetrator for law enforcement or prosecutors to act. In the United States, crimes are committed against society, as embodied by the State or Federal government, and the victim is regarded as a witness to the crime. (This explains why prosecutors are known as district attorneys or state's attorneys or US attorneys.) A victim's refusal or inability to provide physical evidence or verbal information and testimony may prevent law enforcement officers from investigating a case and prosecutors from proving beyond a reasonable doubt that a crime occurred. But elder abuse prosecutors say that if victims had to press charges and testify, homicides could never be investigated and prosecuted. If an elder abuse victim will not or cannot participate, law enforcement officers and prosecutors need to try to build a case through other sources of evidence just as they have been taught to do in cases of child abuse and domestic violence [39, 40].

Training by law enforcement professionals about their duties and responsibilities is the first step to raising the awareness of allied professionals. Resource materials that help allied professionals understand the terminology used by law enforcement officers and prosecutors can be very useful. Building rapport, as well as knowledge, through multidisciplinary initiatives—whether general case review teams, financial (or fiduciary) abuse specialist teams (FAST), elder abuse fatality or death review teams, forensic centers—are widely believed to be of enormous benefit to all professionals directly involved, and indirectly to their colleagues as well (Chaps. 18 and 19).

16.4.2.3 Criminal Justice System Professionals' Lack of Knowledge About Elder Abuse

Lack of knowledge about elder abuse greatly impedes the ability of criminal justice system professionals to protect victims and society, and to hold perpetrators accountable [39]. As discussed previously regarding civil lawyers, prosecutors are unlikely to learn about elder abuse in law school or in CLE programs about criminal law [41]. Law enforcement officers also are unlikely to get much, if any, education about this problem in the law enforcement academy curriculum [39, 41, 42].

To competently detect, investigate, analyze, and pursue elder abuse cases, law enforcement officers, other investigators, and prosecutors require information about the different types of elder abuse; how elder abuse relates to criminal conduct; risk factors and indicators; the role of APS in assisting victims as well as in being a potential source of evidence; whether they are mandated to report to or receive reports from APS; whether mandatory reporters commit a crime if they fail to fulfill their reporting duty; how to work with older victims and witnesses who may have physical or cognitive impairments or other challenges; and special skills for investigating and prosecuting elder abuse cases. Additionally, they will need some familiarity with an array of substantive civil law concepts, documents, and tools including banking and securities law; consent, capacity, and undue influence; contract law; deeds and life estates; domestic/family violence; the duties of guardians, conservators, agents under financial or health care powers of attorney, representative payees, trustees, and Veterans' Administration fiduciaries; long-term care and residential care facilities; public benefits eligibility and Medicaid planning; reverse mortgages; and wills [6, 41, 42].

Due to their different roles and responsibilities, community corrections officials also need to know whether offenders under their supervision are allowed by state law to work with or live near older persons, and they need to consider whether offenders' living and employment situations necessitate enhanced or otherwise different supervision [38].

Through a variety of means and with funding from an array of sources, states and localities have implemented training programs and developed training materials. Agencies that are part of the US Department of Justice have supported some of those efforts, as well as national initiatives to train criminal justice system professionals about domestic violence in later life and elder abuse; to train community corrections officials about elder abuse; and to develop and disseminate a pocket guide and a desk guide for law enforcement about legal issues related to elder abuse. The Department's Elder Justice Initiative has developed a website that, among other things, provides extensive information of use to CJS professionals; that website is found at https://www.justice.gov/elderjustice/.

16.4.2.4 Systemic Impediments to Elder Abuse Cases

Resources are needed to support the work of law enforcement, prosecutors, and community corrections officials in these cases. Absent public and professional awareness resulting in reports and cases, however, it can be difficult to obtain resources when there are so many competing priorities.

Nonetheless, some communities across the nation have devoted substantial resources to training, detection, investigation, and prosecution of elder abuse despite the lack of Federal resources that have made a significant difference in the criminal justice response to other problems such as child abuse and domestic violence [39]. Often these efforts have been led by an individual who was inspired by a terrible case outcome or a situation in his or her own family. Experience has demonstrated that these important efforts are often not institutionalized, however, and they evaporate if the leader is moved into another position in the agency or leaves the agency.

Professionals who handle elder abuse cases say that they are often very difficult to investigate and prosecute, requiring more time and resources to pursue than many other crimes. Investigators and prosecutors will need to develop proficiency and at times will also need to retain consultants and expert witnesses to analyze complex financial transactions, provide medical expertise, or assess whether a victim had decision-making capacity when an event occurred [41]. This is not simply a funding issue. Supervisors and policymakers need to recognize that professionals working on elder abuse cases may need smaller caseloads or longer timeframes for case-handling than their colleagues who are handling less complex and time-consuming matters. Supervisors also may need to adopt different standards of determining success in these cases for purposes of personnel evaluation and promotions, so that professionals who handle elder abuse matters do not experience—or perceive that they will experience—limitations in their career advancement as a result [39].

In addition to training, resources, and agency support for work on elder abuse, criminal justice system professionals, particularly prosecutors who have litigated elder abuse cases, have indicated that several practices are meritorious. The ABA has policy calling for implementation of these practices.

- Specialization in elder abuse by individual law enforcement officers, prosecutors, and victim assistance professionals, or the establishment of specialized units on elder abuse within a law enforcement agency or prosecutor's office [6, 39, 41, 43].
- Use of "vertical prosecution" in the absence of a specialized prosecutor or unit, so the victim works with only one prosecutor through all phases of the prosecution to minimize trauma to the victim and to maximize evidence-development by the prosecutor [6, 39, 43].
- Multidisciplinary, collaborative investigations in either domestic or institutional settings can benefit both victims and professionals. Examples include joint investigations by law enforcement and APS, or collaborative unannounced visits to long-term care facilities by law enforcement, regulatory, and victim advocacy agencies (Operation Spot Check in Florida and Operation Guardian in California are examples of the latter); and the US Department of Justice's ten new, regional Elder Justice Task Forces that will take collaborative action against providers of substandard nursing home care. Combining different professional perspectives at an investigation can enhance evidence detection and preservation; eliminate the need for cross-referrals and multiple investigations; minimize trauma to victims; and facilitate immediate efforts to meet victims' needs [6, 39, 43, 44].
- Meaningful support for professionals' active participation in multidisciplinary teams and other initiatives is crucial. Although team meetings are time-consuming, participants indicate that benefits outweigh costs because they learn more about the responsibilities of other professionals, educate those professionals how to make more timely, appropriate, and information-filled referrals; and learn who to call when they need the assistance of another professional [6, 39, 43, 45]. A recent evaluation of the Los Angeles County Elder Abuse Forensic Center demonstrated that cases examined by the Forensic Center

were more likely to be sent to the prosecutor's office for review than cases handled only by APS [46, 47].

16.4.2.5 Inadequate Criminal Laws

Acts of elder abuse that constitute criminal conduct can be charged and prosecuted as violations of numerous criminal laws. For example, physical abuse might be charged as assault, battery, manslaughter, or murder; psychological abuse might be charged as stalking; sexual abuse might be charged as rape or sexual assault; and financial exploitation might be charged as embezzlement, forgery, fraud, larceny, or theft [6, 9, 48]. Although some states have statutes that explicitly criminalize elder abuse [2], such laws are generally unnecessary for prosecutions to occur; the exception is criminal elder neglect, for which prosecutors indicate a specific statute is often needed.

It may be valuable to enact tougher penalties for elder abuse by classifying crimes as felonies rather than as misdemeanors or by enhancing penalties for physical or financial crimes of older persons because their age or vulnerability is deemed to be an aggravating factor [39]. Measures of productivity and success within criminal justice agencies often motivate professionals to place priority on cases that can generate tougher penalties. Thus, tougher penalties may result in more elder abuse prosecutions, which in turn may generate more public and professional awareness, more funding, and more messages to perpetrators that they may not get away with their actions.

Another benefit of prosecutions is that information about convictions may become available when criminal background checks are conducted, thus potentially preventing elder abuse by caregivers in domestic or institutional settings, by non-caregiving staff in institutional settings, and even by other residents in institutional settings [7].

Criminal justice system professionals also have expressed support for criminal laws that encourage or require their involvement in multidisciplinary teams and other collaborative efforts; that allow financial institutions to temporarily freeze and protect the assets of an alleged victim of financial exploitation while an investigation is conducted; and that authorize or require judges to allow prosecutors special latitude in questioning or preserving the testimony of an older victim [2, 6, 39, 41, 43].

16.4.2.6 Insufficient Data Collection

Although the ability to prosecute most acts of elder abuse using traditional criminal laws means that specific laws creating the crime of elder abuse or exploitation are not necessary, there are negative consequences for state data collection about criminal cases involving elder abuse [39].

Collecting elder abuse crime data across states also is hampered by differences in definitions and categories. Moreover, the federal government's three methods for collecting and combining state crime data—the FBI's Uniform Crime Reports, the FBI's National Incident-Based Reporting System, and the National Crime Victim Survey—largely or completely fail to capture elder abuse data [22, 49].

The lack of data impedes criminal justice professionals from demonstrating to policymakers the need for funding, training, and resources to pursue elder abuse cases and provide assistance to victims. It also limits the ability of researchers to evaluate the efficacy of interventions, which is especially problematic given the increased focus in the criminal justice field on supporting evidence-based practices. State laws criminalizing elder abuse, neglect, or exploitation might alleviate the data problem but would not eliminate the issues of comparability and collection. Policymakers, practitioners, and researchers should consider whether existing data can be analyzed in new ways or whether relatively minor revisions to the categories of data collected might facilitate new information about elder abuse.

16.4.3 Involving Criminal Justice Professionals in Efforts to Strengthen Laws, Policies, and Practices

Criminal justice professionals, like civil lawyers, have ethical and legal restrictions that affect their ability to disclose case information, and these challenges must be considered and addressed thoughtfully. But the growing number of multidisciplinary teams with members from criminal justice agencies indicates that the challenges are not insurmountable, and the study of the Los Angeles County Elder Abuse Forensic Center demonstrates that their participation is beneficial [46, 47]. Criminal justice professionals bring critical knowledge to efforts intended to protect individual victims, to enhance the safety of other service providers, and to improve laws, policies, practices, and procedures [6, 39, 41, 42].

16.5 Judicial System

Elder abuse may involve civil laws, criminal laws, or both. It may be appropriate for an elder abuse case to be heard by a judge in a civil court, a criminal court, or in both types of courts. As discussed previously and illustrated in Table 16.1, the civil and criminal justice systems have distinct goals and purposes. They hear different types of cases (lawyers refer to this as "jurisdiction"), the burdens of proof are dissimilar, and the victim's role in each type of court varies significantly.

This delineation between civil and criminal courts is fundamental yet simplistic. State court systems are structured in divergent ways and a wide array of names or descriptors are used for their courts. Many communities—particularly those in less populated or rural areas—have courts of general jurisdiction that hear both civil and criminal cases. Other communities have separate civil courts and criminal courts. Moreover, there exist specialty courts that fall under the rubric of either the civil or criminal court systems. Many communities have probate courts that commonly handle civil matters such as guardianship/conservatorship, mental health commitments, protective proceedings, and wills and estates cases. Some communities have family courts that hear civil matters including divorce, custody, visitation, paternity, adoption, and domestic and family violence. Sometimes specialty courts handle both civil and criminal cases. For example, a growing number of communities have one or more problem-solving courts that hear both criminal and civil matters related to a certain problem or population group; these may be domestic violence, drug, elder, housing, or veterans courts. The goal of problem-solving courts, as the name suggests, is to bring together legal services, social services, and other resources to address the underlying problem that is causing or contributing to an individual's legal problem(s).

Federal courts also hear cases involving elder abuse. The US District Courts, which are the frontline trial courts in the Federal judicial system, handle both civil and criminal matters. The similarities and differences outlined in Table 16.1 also apply to the federal courts. Bankruptcy proceedings, which may be a consequence of elder financial exploitation, are governed by a distinct law and heard by bankruptcy divisions within the US District Courts.

16.5.1 Roles of Judges

Growth of the older population, increasing detection and/or incidence of elder abuse, training of lawyers and allied professionals about civil remedies and criminal prosecution, and state legislative action have expanded emphasis on the use of the legal system to redress elder abuse and thus also the role of the judicial system in addressing the problem [24, 39].

As highlighted in the Introduction, judges handle elder abuse cases—whether they occur in domestic or institutional settings—in both civil and criminal courts, including specialty courts that hear matters including guardianship and conservatorship, family issues, domestic violence, and elder protection. Elder abuse cases may arise in numerous contexts:

- criminal cases such as assault, battery, elder abuse/neglect/exploitation, forgery, fraud, manslaughter, murder, rape, sexual assault, or theft (some of which may carry enhanced penalties when committed against an older person);
- civil fraud or conversion matters to regain misappropriated property;
- personal injury actions;
- guardianship or conservatorship;
- mental health commitment;
- special protective proceedings initiated through APS agencies;
- cases involving health care decisions for an incapacitated patient; and
- criminal or civil cases regarding institutional care in nursing homes or other long-term care facilities [2].

Increasingly, judges are hearing petitions for civil orders of protection from victims of elder abuse as victims learn that such protection is available and as states expand their statutory criteria to include more situations of elder abuse (e.g., physical violence committed by a family member other than a spouse or intimate partner).

16.5.2 Barriers of the Judicial System

As previously discussed, the ABA Commission's early-1990s study of cases involving elder abuse in the state courts indicated that there were two categories of practices and barriers that inhibited entry of cases: the abused person's attitudes about the courts and about the pursuit of legal remedies, and systemic practices in or related to the courts. As the attitudinal barriers related to the civil justice, criminal justice, and judicial systems, they were provided earlier in this chapter. Study participants identified systemic practices connected with the judicial system.

- The lack of knowledge about and sensitivity to elder abuse by judges was seen as inhibiting prosecutors, civil lawyers, and abused persons from bringing cases into the courts.
- The failure of court staff to explain the judicial process to older abused persons, particularly to those who have a mental or cognitive disability or who may be intimidated or confused, was considered to be a barrier to the pursuit of legal remedies by abused persons.
- The courts' failure to recognize that older persons who are homebound or bedbound may be incapable of traveling to the courthouse even though they are capable of testifying was also considered to be a barrier to elder abuse cases.
- Court delays—typical or otherwise—were thought to be particularly onerous to older abused persons who are nearing the end of their life span, and who may be losing their capacity to remember the abuse and testify about it.

- Lack of knowledge about elder abuse among prosecutors, law enforcement officers, and civil lawyers was also viewed as a barrier by the participants [2].

To address both categories of barriers, the ABA Commission promulgated 29 recommended guidelines for state courts. The recommended guidelines were subsequently adopted as ABA policy by its House of Delegates in August 1996 [50]. As the guidelines remain timely and relevant 20 years later, they are provided in their entirety.

1. Judges should receive training about elder abuse. Topics should include: dynamics of elder abuse and family violence; types of cases involving elder abuse; capacity issues; State laws concerning elder abuse; the APS system and aging services; case management issues and procedural innovations; and crafting effective orders in elder abuse cases. Training should be designed and presented with the input and involvement of advocates, APS, prosecutors, law enforcement, and aging services providers and should include coverage of their roles and resources.
2. Court staff should receive training about elder abuse. Topics should include: dynamics of elder abuse and family violence; types of cases involving elder abuse; capacity issues; APS system; aging network and other social services; case management issues and procedural innovations; and data collection about elder abuse cases. Training should be designed and presented with the input and involvement of advocates, APS, prosecutors, law enforcement, and aging services providers and should include coverage of their roles and resources.
3. Courts should ensure that prosecutors, investigators, lawyers, law enforcement officers, APS workers, social workers, bank and financial institution officials, health care providers, and any other professionals appearing before them in cases involving elder abuse are familiar with the dynamics and issues of elder abuse and with the role of the courts in addressing elder abuse. To achieve that objective, courts should encourage and support the development and implementation of cross-training for victim/witness programs, APS staff, aging services providers, lawyers, prosecutors, law enforcement, banking officials, health care providers, and any other relevant professionals about the resources and assistance offered by each of them to older abused persons and about the ways in which they need to coordinate those efforts.
4. Courts should provide accommodations for persons with physical and mental deficiencies and, if necessary, hold hearings in cases involving elder abuse in the setting that best accommodates the needs of the abused older person.
5. Courts should recognize that the capacity of older persons may fluctuate with time of day, medications, etc. and should be flexible in scheduling hearings to accommodate those individual variations.
6. Courts should expedite cases involving elder abuse on the calendar.
7. Courts should use expert witnesses, evaluators, guardians *ad litem*, court investigators, court visitors, or interdisciplinary teams who are trained and knowledgeable about the problems of older persons to assess the older person's capacity.
8. Courts should understand gradations of diminished capacity in order to more effectively manage and adjudicate cases involving elder abuse.
9. Courts should consider that incapacity could increase the likelihood of abuse and, if necessary, order a qualified evaluator to conduct an unbiased assessment of the older person's capacity.
10. Courts should understand and use limited guardianship and other alternatives to guardianship appropriately.
11. When counsel for the older person is required to be appointed, or is otherwise appointed, the appointment should be at the earliest possible stage of the proceedings.
12. Courts should allow prosecutors special latitude in questioning older abused persons and in offering additional witnesses and corroborating evidence.
13. Courts should ensure that plea agreements meet the needs of the older abused person, including protection from further abuse, and be willing to be creative in negotiations and sentencing, exploring the alternatives available to the older abused person.
14. Further analysis and study should be undertaken of the ramifications of courts more readily allowing an older abused person's testimony to be videotaped before capacity is lost or the individual dies.
15. Further analysis and study should be undertaken of the ramifications of courts taking steps when necessary to reduce the level of fear experienced by an older person who is testifying against his or her abuser such as allowing the hearing to be held in a less confrontational setting, allowing testimony and cross-examination of the older abused person by videotape or closed-circuit television, and closing the courtroom to the public.
16. Further analysis and study should be undertaken of the ramifications of courts more readily allowing admission of evidence from collateral sources if the older abused person's capacity is at issue, as has been done by the

Department of Justice regarding child witnesses and child abuse cases.

17. Courts must develop ways of ensuring that judges become aware of cases involving older abused persons that might be underway simultaneously in different divisions or that might previously have been heard and have some influence on a current case.
18. Further study should be given to the concept of consolidation of the courts handling cases involving elder abuse, for example into a "family court."
19. The use of alternative dispute resolution (ADR) in cases involving elder abuse is not recommended at this time. The possible use of ADR should be studied further.
20. Newly appointed guardians should receive training about their role and responsibilities as guardians, and about preventing, recognizing and reporting elder abuse.
21. Victim/witness advocates should be available and involved in assisting older abused persons throughout the judicial process in both non-criminal and criminal court proceedings.
22. All victim/witness advocates should be trained about the dynamics of elder abuse and about the APS system and other aging network services available to assist older abused persons. Additionally, there should be an elder abuse specialist at every victim/witness program.
23. Especially if there are no victim/witness advocates available to help an older abused person, court staff should help explain and de-mystify the court process for older abused persons who may be intimidated or confused, or who may have some type of mental or cognitive disability.
24. Courts should: encourage and support the development and continuing operation of a state or local task force or coordinating council on elder abuse issues; lend their support to existing task forces or coordinating councils on elder abuse; or encourage evolving or existing task forces or coordinating councils on family violence or domestic violence to incorporate elder abuse advocates into their membership and elder abuse issues into their agenda. Task force or coordinating council members should include judges and court personnel, representatives of the Attorney General, representatives of the Medicaid Fraud Control Unit, public and private lawyers, law enforcement officers, APS administrators or workers, social services providers, health care providers, banking and financial institution officials, victim/witness advocates, representatives of the long term care ombudsman program, and other relevant professionals. In addition to addressing systemic problems faced by the courts and the council members in preventing and responding to elder abuse, these task forces or coordinating councils should develop materials that explain their roles and their relationships to each other and the court system, and disseminate those materials to each other, the courts, and the public.
25. Courts should include APS and aging services on court advisory councils or develop other mechanisms for establishing linkages with those organizations and others that address elder abuse.
26. Courts should encourage and support the development and continued operation of multidisciplinary teams on elder abuse.
27. Courts should encourage and support the development of protocols or memoranda of understanding between various entities involved in elder abuse cases as to their roles and relationships.
28. Judges and court personnel should have familiarity with APS, aging, and social services providers in their community or brochures or other materials from those agencies so that they can direct an older abused person to appropriate service providers.
29. Courts should encourage and support the development of a "court social worker" or "court ombudsman" program using trained volunteers to help older, disabled, incapacitated or other individuals by giving them information about social services and other community organizations; linking, rather than just referring, them to social services and other community organizations; assisting them with the completion of *pro se* documents; and helping them to understand the nature of the court process [2].

In March 2006 the Center on Aging at Florida International University (FIU) produced recommendations for adapting the US Department of Justice Bureau of Justice Assistance's *Trial Court Performance Standards with Commentary* [51] to an aging society in three contexts: guardianship, self-service, and criminal cases involving elder abuse and domestic violence [52].

The FIU recommendations were organized into the five categories used in the Trial Court Performance Standards. A synopsis by category of the FIU recommendations most pertinent to elder abuse cases follows; the FIU recommendation numbers are provided.

1. Access to justice: older court users receive escort assistance (1.2.A); older criminal defendants receive a standardized medical and mental health assessment (including dementia and cognitive impairment) unless they have had one in the past 30 days (1.3.F); judges, court-appointed counsel, and all other court staff receive standardized, current training on physical and psychosocial issues related to aging (1.4.A).
2. Expedition and timeliness: multiple cases involving the same older person should be heard by a single court if

possible, and if impossible then court staff should ensure that the judges involved are aware of all related cases (2.1.A).

3. Equality, fairness, and integrity: determinations of diminished capacity of an older litigant are made in accord with professional standards and with input from appropriate professionals (3.1.C); capacity assessments are performed in the alleged incapacitated person's home or other familiar environment (3.1.C); courts are cautious about recommending or requiring mediation in cases involving elder abuse or domestic violence (3.1.F); the court balances the goal of minimizing delays in cases involving older persons with the need to provide accommodations to litigants whose ability to participate necessitates that proceedings move at a slower pace than normal (e.g., more breaks, later start or earlier end to a court day) (3.1.H); guardianship and conservatorship cases are monitored by court staff, the judge is notified if reporting requirements are not met, and the judge initiates an investigation or appropriate legal proceedings for non-compliance or reports that evidence malfeasance (3.5.A and 3.5.C); all newly-appointed guardians and conservators are provided with jurisdiction-specific information about their roles and duties, including preventing, detecting, and reporting elder abuse, and subsequently updated about any legal changes in their duties (3.5.D); and the court maintains an electronic information system and staff capable of monitoring and compiling case data including litigant demographics (3.6.B).
4. Independence and accountability: the court cultivates and continues relationships with aging, health, and mental health service providers in its jurisdiction, including APS (4.1.A); and in partnership with those service providers, the court conducts and updates education programs for older persons and for those service providers about court services and relevant substantive topics (4.4.A and 4.4.B)
5. Public trust and confidence: courts create and then comply with standards about data collection and maintenance, including case-outcome data and demographic data about older court users, and issue annual reports summarizing that data (5.2.A) [51, 52].

16.5.2.1 Lack of Knowledge of Elder Abuse Among Judges and Court Personnel

Judges need training and technical assistance on addressing systemic barriers and on substantive legal issues and scientific knowledge about decision-making capacity, physical abuse, exploitation, and neglect. Judges and court administrators do not have access to or time to read lengthy journal articles about research and therefore could benefit from simple, practical tools about research findings. They need to learn about developments in scientific research about decision-making capacity, physical abuse, and neglect to inform their judgments in many civil and criminal cases, and about any research on the effectiveness of interventions that may occur in the future [53].

The State Justice Institute funded the ABA Commission to develop curricula on elder abuse for judges and courts personnel in the late 1990s [2]. The US Department of Justice Office on Violence Against Women has provided judicial training through its Enhanced Training and Services to End Abuse in Later Life Program. The National Center for State Courts has, with a combination of Federal and foundation funding, established the Center for Elders and the Courts, developed new resources and made training available online. Other judicial organizations, such as the National College of Probate Judges and the National Council of Juvenile and Family Court Judges, have offered training to their members about elder abuse. State judicial education programs have addressed the problem as well. Ongoing technical assistance and the development and dissemination of additional practical materials for judges and court staff are necessary, however.

16.5.2.2 Data Collection and Evaluation by the Judicial System

Understanding the extent, nature, and outcomes of the judicial system's role in elder abuse cases is critical. It is also quite challenging. The failure to place a high priority on evaluation, lack of resources, varying practices among local jurisdictions and states, and engagement with multiple definitions and relevant laws make it difficult to consistently categorize cases and allow meaningful comparison statewide or nationally.

In 2006, ABA Commission research demonstrated that only three state courts systems (Kansas, Vermont, and Wisconsin) had elder abuse as a distinct case type reported by trial courts to the state courts' administrative office [22]. Three years later the Conference of Chief Justices and the Conference of State Court Administrators supported a policy resolution urging state court systems to collect data on elder abuse [54].

Stiegel and Teaster's assessment [45] of the five court-focused elder abuse initiatives discussed in the following section indicated that each was doing very little to collect data on their impact and outcomes. Only two of the initiatives had developed a client satisfaction survey, and they had received very few responses. None of the initiatives were making any formal attempt to obtain feedback from their professional stakeholders. Moreover, court case files in all five study sites contained very little information about the victims and perpetrators beyond the most basic demographic-type data. There was very little information about the circumstances and outcomes of the case that would be needed for an evaluation. Indeed, in four of the five study sites it was usually impossible to tell from the court's data cover sheet that a case involved elder abuse, and that is the data reported to and by the state court administrative offices. In other words, these cases are not "counted" as elder abuse cases. Clearly these limitations have significant policy and practice implications.

16.5.3 Involving Judges and Court Personnel in Efforts to Strengthen Policies and Practices

Fueled by the ABA Commission's recommended guidelines or the same problems that those guidelines addressed, between 1999 and 2006 five jurisdictions established court-focused elder abuse initiatives, defined as "an initiative that serves victims or potential victims of elder abuse through either a court or a court-based program, or a program conducted in partnership with a court" [45].

With funding from the National Institute of Justice, which is the research agency of the US Department of Justice, researchers from the ABA Commission and the University of Kentucky College of Public Health/Department of Gerontology assessed those five initiatives. Descriptions of their activities at the time of the research project follow, organized alphabetically by county of location.

- The "Elder Protection Court" (EPC) in Alameda County, California, offered a special civil and criminal docket for elder abuse cases, including elder abuse protection order cases, in the Superior Court of Alameda County. It was the first specialized elder court.
- The "Elder Justice Center" (EJC) in Hillsborough County, Florida, a program of the 13th Judicial Circuit Court, provided residents aged 60 and older with assistance—but not legal advice—in completing court documents, such as applications for protective orders, referrals to legal and social services programs, and case management services in guardianship matters. The EJC staff monitored guardianship cases. Additionally, staff advocated for older crime victims and, if the victim desired, could help older criminal defendants by providing referrals to diversionary programs such as mental health or substance abuse treatment programs.
- The "In-Home Emergency Protective Order Initiative" (IEPOI) in Jefferson County, Kentucky, helped medically fragile/homebound victims of abuse aged 60 and older to obtain emergency protective orders and longer-term domestic violence orders by telephone. Initiative partners included: ElderServe, Inc., an aging services nonprofit that managed the IEPOI, the Circuit Court Clerk's office, the Family Court, APS, and the sheriff's office.
- The "Elder Temporary Order of Protection" Initiative (ETOP) in Kings County, New York, was sponsored by the New York City Family Justice Center in Brooklyn. The ETOP assisted eligible victims of domestic violence (aged 60 or older and unable to appear in court because infirmity or disability made it impossible or a great hardship to travel) obtain temporary orders of protection. Social workers and lawyers from the New York City Department for the Aging and the Jewish Association for Services for the Aged Legal/Social Work Elder Abuse Program were available to provide emergency counseling, direct services, and other information regarding services for the elderly. The Family Court and its Clerk's Office also had significant roles in the initiative.
- The "Elder Justice Center" (EJC) in Palm Beach County, Florida, a program of the Board of County Commissioners in collaboration with the 15th Judicial Circuit Court. The EJC helped residents aged 60 and older who were arrested for certain crimes, involved in guardianship proceedings, or in need of other court-related help. The program provided assistance—but not legal advice—to older persons in completing court documents such as applications for protective orders, referrals to legal and social services programs, and accompaniment to civil and criminal hearings. Staff also monitored and investigated guardians at the probate judge's request. In certain cases the EJC identified older criminal defendants who might have dementia or other cognitive problems, and arranged assessments that helped judges decide whether to divert the defendants from jail into mental health or substance abuse treatment programs [45].

Interviews with initiative participants, other professionals in the community, and three older persons who had been helped demonstrated that the initiatives improved handling of elder abuse cases and enhanced the criminal justice response to elder abuse by:

- Facilitating greater access to justice and better court outcomes for victims through court accommodations, increasing judges' and other professionals' knowledge about elder abuse, and providing emotional support throughout the court process;
- Providing services to courts or to victims that enhance victim safety and prevent further abuse;
- Connecting victims with services that may help address underlying problems and prevent future court cases;
- Providing services to courts or to victims that may facilitate prosecution of elder abuse cases; and
- Handling elder abuse cases more efficiently and with fewer delays [45].

Other elder protection courts were established in Contra Costa and Ventura counties in California. One is under development in Charleston, South Carolina. Other communities have expressed interest in the concept. The Elder and Miscellaneous Remedies Division (ELMRD) of the Circuit Court of Cook County in Chicago, Illinois, combined the elder protection court concept with the elder justice center concept; it also hosts a law school clinical program. The ELMRD is the largest and most ambitious CFEAI to date, implemented after several years of multidisciplinary input into its planning. It hears both civil and criminal cases, involves law students in its activities, enhances public and professional awareness of elder abuse and legal problems affecting older persons, continues to be advised by a multidisciplinary task force, and is collaborating with researchers to ensure that data about the effectiveness of the ELMRD's services are collected and analyzed [55, 56].

Aware of the impending impact on the courts of the burgeoning population of older persons, the Supreme Courts of three states—Alaska, Pennsylvania, and South Carolina—have established task forces to examine the judicial system's response to elder abuse and other elder law issues. Judges also participate in and often serve as leaders of state and local task forces or multidisciplinary collaborations that have not been established by a state's highest court.

The Conference of Chief Justices and the Conference of State Court Administrators have adopted resolutions supporting development of problem-solving courts, widespread implementation of the principles driving those courts, and development and promotion of state judicial leadership on efforts to improve courts' recognition of and response to elder abuse [57–59]. The ABA also has policy urging state, territorial, tribal, and local courts to address the problems referenced earlier by applying principles based on the practices implemented by the five CFEAI assessed by Stiegel and Teaster [45] and by subsequent initiatives [60].

16.6 Conclusion/Overarching Policy and Research Issues/Recommendations

This chapter has discussed numerous promising practices and suggestions that should be developed and institutionalized throughout the country. Therefore, this conclusion will focus on five overarching recommendations that would benefit all three components of the justice system and the elder abuse victims who interact with them.

1. While some states and communities are doing important and exciting work with very few resources, substantial funding for Federal, State, and local agencies, for training and education, for resource development and technical assistance, and to support data collection is essential to enhance access to justice for elder abuse victims.
2. Assessment and elimination of barriers other than lack of funding—such as laws, regulations, policies, and practices—that inhibit victims' access to justice and the ability of justice system professionals to meet victims' needs.
3. Implementation of existing recommendations about data collection to obtain prevalence or incidence data or data about the financial costs of elder abuse and to establish a stronger foundation for research and evaluation of the justice system's role in preventing, detecting, and remedying elder abuse.
4. Research on the outcomes of justice system interventions, including whether they are what victims want, making victims safer, preventing further victimization, reducing costs to businesses and government agencies, etc. Assess whether different cultural groups have greater difficulties accessing the justice system and whether they are disparately impacted by it. Consider justice system interventions or approaches that are used in other countries or cultures and whether they might have merit in the United States.
5. Research about decision-making capacity—particularly financial capacity—and susceptibility to undue influence, and about markers and consequences of neglect. The results of this research must be made accessible and understandable to civil lawyers, criminal justice professionals, and judges, as well as adult protective services, financial institutions, health care providers, and myriad other professionals and providers of services to older persons.

References

1. National Center on Elder Abuse. 2016. FAQs. www.ncea.aoa.gov/faq/index.aspx. Accessed 25 Feb 2016.
2. Stiegel L. Recommended guidelines for state courts handling cases involving elder abuse. 1995. Available via ABA. http://www.americanbar.org/groups/law_aging/resources/elder_abuse.html. Accessed 9 Mar 2016.
3. Farmer A, Tiefenthaler J. Explaining the recent decline in domestic violence. Contemp Econ Pol. 2003;21(2):158–72. doi:10.1093/cep/byg002.
4. Rosenberg JS, Grab DA. Supporting survivors: the economic benefits of providing civil legal assistance to survivors of domestic violence. 2015. Available via Institute for Policy Integrity. http://policyintegrity.org/publications/detail/supporting-survivors. Accessed 9 Mar 2016.
5. Connolly MT, Brandl B, Breckman R. The elder justice roadmap: a stakeholder initiative to respond to an emerging health, justice, financial and social crisis. 2014. Available via National Center on Elder Abuse. http://ncea.acl.gov/Library/Gov_Report/docs/EJRP_Roadmap.pdf. Accessed 1 Mar 2016.

6. Brandl B, Dyer CB, Heisler CJ, Otto JM, Stiegel LA, Thomas RW. Elder abuse detection and intervention: a collaborative approach. New York: Springer; 2007.
7. Connolly MT. Where elder abuse and the justice system collide: police power, parens patriae, and 12 recommendations. J Elder Abuse Neglect. 2010;22(37–93):2010. doi:10.1080/08946560903436338.
8. Quinn MJ, Heisler CJ. The legal response to elder abuse and neglect. J Elder Abuse Neglect. 2002;14(1):61–77. doi:10.1300/J084v14n01_04.
9. Stiegel LA. An overview of elder financial exploitation. Generations. 2012;36(2):73–80.
10. Stiegel LA. White paper on civil legal services for the elder justice coordinating council. Prepared for the Elder Justice Coordinating Council meeting, Washington DC, 11 Oct 2012. Available via Administration for Community Living. http://www.aoa.gov/AoA_programs/Elder_Rights/EJCC/docs/Stiegel_White_Paper-Civil_Legal_Services.pdf. Accessed 9 Mar 2016.
11. Stiegel LA. Financial abuse of the elderly: risk factors, screening techniques, and remedies. Bifocal 2002;23(4):1–11. Available via ABA. http://www.americanbar.org/content/dam/aba/migrated/aging/publications/bifocal/summer02.authcheckdam.pdf. Accessed 11 Mar 2016.
12. Kohn NA, Spurgeon ED. A call to action on elder law: an assessment and recommendations based on a national survey. Elder Law J. 2014;21(2):345–74.
13. Andres MN. Making elder financial exploitation cases part of a sustainable practice: tips from the experiences of the University of Illinois College of Law's elder financial justice clinic. Elder Law J. 2015;23(3):101–44.
14. Stiegel LA. Elder investment fraud and financial exploitation prevention program—legal. Bifocal. 2014;35(6):175–7. Available via ABA. http://www.americanbar.org/publications/bifocal/vol_35/issue_6_august2014/eiffe_legal_ipt_ipi_grant.html. Accessed 13 Mar 2016.
15. Godfrey D. In search of adequate funding for legal assistance for low-income seniors. Bifocal. 2010;32(1):8–12.
16. Legal Services Corporation. Documenting the justice gap in America. 2009. Available via Legal Services Corporation. http://www.lsc.gov/sites/default/files/LSC/pdfs/documenting_the_justice_gap_in_america_2009.pdf. Accessed 9 Mar 2016.
17. Legal Services Corporation. FY 2017 budget request. 2016. Available via Legal Services Corporation. http://www.lsc.gov/media-center/publications/fy-2017-budget-request. Accessed 13 Apr 2016.
18. Directory and Structure. American Bar Association, Access to Justice Commissions, Chicago. 2016. Available via ABA. http://www.americanbar.org/groups/legal_aid_indigent_defendants/initiatives/resource_center_for_access_to_justice/atj-commissions/commission-directory.html. Accessed 27 Mar 2016.
19. Conference of Chief Justices and Conference of State Court Administrators. The importance of funding for the Legal Services Corporation from the perspective of the Conference of Chief Justices and the Conference of State Court Administrators. 2013. Available via Conference of Chief Justices. http://ccj.ncsc.org/Policy-Resolutions.aspx. Accessed 13 Apr 2016.
20. U.S. Department of Justice. White House legal aid interagency roundtable: civil legal aid research workshop report. U.S. DOJ National Institute of Justice and Office for Access to Justice with NSF. 2016. Available via U.S. DOJ. https://www.justice.gov/lair/select-publications-and-research. Accessed 13 Mar 2016.
21. Legal Services Corporation. What is legal aid. Washington, DC. 2016. Available via Legal Services Corporation. http://www.lsc.gov/what-legal-aid. Accessed 28 Mar 2016.
22. Wood E. The availability and utility of interdisciplinary data on elder abuse: a white paper for the National Center on Elder Abuse. 2006. Available via National Center on Elder Abuse. http://www.ncea.aoa.gov/Resources/Publication/docs/WhitePaper060404.pdf. Accessed 13 Mar 2016.
23. Martin J, Culley D. No higher calling—representing victims of financial exploitation. Bifocal. 2013;34(5):89–92. Available via ABA. http://www.americanbar.org/publications/bifocal/vol_34/issue_5_june2013/no_higher_calling.html. Accessed 13 Apr 2016.
24. Stiegel L. The changing role of the courts in elder-abuse cases. 2000. Available via ABA. http://www.americanbar.org/content/dam/aba/administrative/law_aging/2011_aging_arta2260_chgrolecrts_tb.authcheckdam.pdf. Accessed 13 Mar 2016.
25. Rizzo VM, Burns D, Chalfy A. A systematic evaluation of a multidisciplinary social work-lawyer mistreatment intervention model. J Elder Abuse Neglect. 2015;27(1):1–18. doi:10.1080/08946566.792104.
26. Brandl B, Meuer T. Domestic abuse in later life. Elder LJ. 2000;8:297–335.
27. Wagley S. Maine's improvident transfers act: a unique approach to protecting exploited elders. Bifocal. 2014;36(1):18–20. Available via ABA. http://www.americanbar.org/publications/bifocal/vol_36/issue_1_october2014/maines_improvident_transfers_act.html. Accessed 13 Apr 2016.
28. Barton R, Lukaszewski LM, Lau ST. Gifts to caretakers: acts of gratitude or disguised malfeasance? New statutes may decide for us. Prob Prop May/June 2015;22–27.
29. Kisabeth LK. Slayer statutes and elder abuse: good intentions, right results? Does Michigan's amended slayer statute do enough to protect the elderly? Quinnipiac Prob L J. 2013;26:373–402.
30. Stiegel LA, Wood EF. Nine ways to prevent elder abuse through enactment of the uniform adult guardianship and protective proceedings jurisdiction act. Bifocal. 2009;30(3):35, 37–40. Available via ABA. http://www.americanbar.org/content/dam/aba/migrated/aging/publications/docs/Feb_09_0ABA_Bifocal_J.authcheckdam.pdf. Accessed 13 Mar 2016.
31. Stiegel LA, Klem EV. Power of attorney abuse: what states can do about it. AARP Public Policy Institute. 2008. Available via AARP. http://www.aarp.org/money/scams-fraud/info-11-2008/2008_17_poa_1.html. Accessed 13 Mar 2016.
32. Hommel P, Lisi LB. Report on the national survey of statewide reporting practices for Older Americans Act Title III-B legal services. 2015. Available via The Center for Social Gerontology. http://www.tcsg.org/law/surveyreport2015.pdf. Accessed 9 Mar 2016.
33. Gunther J. The 2010 cost of Utah financial exploitation. Available via Utah Division of Aging and Adult Services. 2011. http://www.nlrc.aoa.gov/NLRC/Docs/2010_Cost_of_FE_5_24_LE.pdf. Accessed 14 Mar 2016.
34. Thomas DE. The Wyoming cost of financial exploitation, 2011, 2012 and 2013. Wyoming Department of Family Services. 2014. Available via National Association of States United for Aging and Disabilities. http://www.nasuad.org/sites/nasuad/files/Wyoming%20Cost%20of%20Financial%20Exploitation%20FINAL%202011-13.pdf. Accessed 13 Apr 2016.
35. Legal Services Corporation. Civil legal outcomes. (n.d.). Available via Legal Services Corporation. http://clo.lsc.gov/. Accessed 13 Apr 2016.
36. National Association of Medicaid Fraud Control Units (NAMFCU). What is Medicaid fraud. (n.d.) Available via NAMFCU. http://www.namfcu.net/what-is-medicaid-fraud1.php. Accessed 13 Mar 2016.
37. Medicaid Fraud Control Unit. National Association of Medicaid Fraud Control Units (NAMFCU). (n.d.). Available via NAMFCU.

http://www.namfcu.net/medicaid-fraud-control-unit1.php. Accessed 13 Mar 2016.
38. DeMichele MT, Crowe A, Stiegel LA. Elder abuse: identifying and responding to probation and parole practices. Perspectives. American Probation and Parole Association. 2007. Available via ABA. http://www.americanbar.org/content/dam/aba/administrative/law_aging/2011_aging_arta2254_prbtaprleprac_tb.authcheckdam.pdf.
39. Heisler CJ, Stiegel LA. Enhancing the justice system's response to elder abuse: discussions and recommendations of the 'improving prosecution' working group of the national policy summit on elder abuse. J Elder Abuse Neglect. 2002;14(4):31–54.
40. Heisler CJ. Elder abuse and the criminal justice system: new awareness, new responses. Generations. 2000;24(2):52–8.
41. Ulrey P. Confusion on the front lines: the response of law enforcement and prosecutors to cases of elder abuse. Prepared for the Elder Justice Coordinating Council meeting, Washington, DC, 11 Oct 2012. Available via Administration for Community Living. http://www.aoa.gov/AoA_programs/Elder_Rights/EJCC/docs/Ulrey_White_Paper.pdf. Accessed 13 Mar 2016.
42. Thomas RW. Law enforcement and the elder justice act. J Elder Abuse Neglect. 2002;12(2/3):205–8.
43. American Bar Association. 105A: resolution supporting vigorous prosecution of elder abuse. Adopted by the ABA House of Delegates, 11 Feb 2008. Available via ABA. http://www.americanbar.org/content/dam/aba/directories/policy/2008_my_105a.authcheckdam.pdf. Accessed 13 Mar 2016.
44. U.S. Department of Justice. Department of Justice launches 10 regional elder justice task forces 30 Mar 2016. Available via U.S. DOJ. https://www.justice.gov/opa/pr/department-justice-launches-10-regional-elder-justice-task-forces. Accessed 30 Mar 2016.
45. Stiegel LA, Teaster PB. Final technical report to the National Institute of Justice on "A multi-site assessment of five court-focused elder abuse initiatives." 2011. Available via ABA. http://www.americanbar.org/content/dam/aba/administrative/law_aging/2011/2011_aging_ea_multi_assess.authcheckdam.pdf. Accessed 13 Mar 2016.
46. Navarro AE, Gassoumis ZD, Wilber KH. Holding abusers accountable: an elder abuse forensic center increases criminal prosecution of financial exploitation. Gerontologist. 2013;53(2):302–12.
47. Taylor T, Mulford C. Evaluating the Los Angeles County Elder Abuse Forensic Center. Nat'l Inst Just J. 2015;276:32–7. Available via National Institute of Justice. http://www.nij.gov/journals/276/Pages/elder-abuse-forensic-center.aspx. Accessed 9 Mar 2016.
48. Heisler C, Tewksbury J. Fiduciary abuse of the elderly: a prosecutor's perspective. J Elder Abuse Neglect. 1991;3(4):23–40.
49. Acierno R. Elder mistreatment: epidemiological assessment methodology. In: Bonnie RJ, Wallace RB, editors. Elder mistreatment: abuse, neglect, and exploitation in an aging America. Washington DC: National Academies Press; 2003. p. 261–302.
50. American Bar Association. 102: resolution supporting efforts to improve the response of the state courts to elder abuse. Adopted by the House of Delegates, Aug 1996. Available via ABA. http://www.americanbar.org/content/dam/aba/directories/policy/1996_am_102.authcheckdam.pdf. Accessed 13 Mar 2016.
51. Bureau of Justice Assistance. Trial court performance standards with commentary. The U.S. Department of Justice, Bureau of Justice Assistance. 1997. Available via National Criminal Justice Reference Service. https://www.ncjrs.gov/pdffiles1/161570.pdf. Accessed 13 Mar 2016.
52. Rothman MB, Dunlop BD, Seff LR. Adapting trial court performance standards to an aging society: guardianship, self-service, and criminal cases involving elder mistreatment and domestic violence. 2006. Available via The Center of Aging, Robert Stempel School of Public Health, College of Health and Urban Affairs, and Florida International University. http://www2.fiu.edu/~coa/downloads/elder%20justice/SJI4-03-06.pdf. Accessed 13 Mar 2016.
53. Stiegel LA. White paper on the judicial system for the elder justice coordinating council. Prepared for the Elder Justice Coordinating Council meeting, Washington DC, 11 Oct 2012. Available via Administration for Community Living. http://www.aoa.gov/AoA_programs/Elder_Rights/EJCC/docs/Stiegel_White_Paper-Judicial_System.pdf. Accessed 9 Mar 2016.
54. Conference of Chief Justices and Conference of State Court Administrators. Encouraging collection of data on adult guardianship, adult conservatorship, and elder abuse cases by all states. 2009. Available via Conference of Chief Justices. http://ccj.ncsc.org/Policy-Resolutions.aspx. Accessed 13 Apr 2016.
55. Banks P. A new age and a new court for older litigants. Experience. 2012;22(2):12–6.
56. Banks P. Bridging the access gap for older litigants: an elder court model. Prepared for the Elder Justice Coordinating Council meeting, Washington, DC, 11 Oct 2012. Available via Administration for Community Living. http://www.aoa.gov/AoA_programs/Elder_Rights/EJCC/docs/Banks_White_Paper.pdf. Accessed 13 Mar 2016.
57. Conference of Chief Justices and Conference of State Court Administrators. In support of the NCSC concept paper, state courts and elder abuse: ensuring justice for older Americans. 2008. Available via Conference of Chief Justices. http://ccj.ncsc.org/Policy-Resolutions.aspx. Accessed 13 Apr 2016.
58. Conference of Chief Justices and Conference of State Court Administrators. In support of problem-solving courts. 2000. Available via Conference of Chief Justices. http://ccj.ncsc.org/Policy-Resolutions.aspx. Accessed 13 Apr 2016.
59. Conference of Chief Justices and Conference of State Court Administrators. In support of problem-solving courts. 2004. Available via Conference of Chief Justices. http://ccj.ncsc.org/Policy-Resolutions.aspx. Accessed 13 Apr 2016.
60. American Bar Association. 106C: resolution urging state, territorial, tribal, and local courts and community organizations to collaborate in establishing court-focused elder abuse initiatives. Adopted by the ABA House of Delegates, 6–7 Aug 2012. Available via ABA. http://www.americanbar.org/content/dam/aba/directories/policy/2012_hod_annual_meeting_106c.doc. Accessed 13 Mar 2016.

Guardianship Systems

17

Erica Wood and Mary Joy Quinn

17.1 Introduction

In the United States, all adults are considered capable of handling their own personal and financial affairs unless a court determines that they cannot do so [51, 58]. In those situations, an individual or an agency may petition the court for the appointment of a guardian of person or estate or both to handle the person's personal and financial affairs under court supervision. Guardianships can also be seen as a way to remove an alleged abuser from having decision-making power over a vulnerable adult, and it can be useful when an adult is unable to manage personal care or financial assets or real estate. On the other hand, guardianship can remove significant rights from the individual, such as the right to contract to purchase goods and services, the right to marry, the right to control assets, and the right to make medical decisions or to choose a place to live. State law and the scope of the court order determine which rights will be removed from the person in guardianship. In addition, most courts do not have the resources or staff to closely monitor existing guardianships. Guardians—much like anyone handling someone else's affairs—may need assistance, and can become neglectful or abusive especially where money is concerned.

The National Center on Elder Abuse lists the following types of elder abuse:

- Physical Abuse—Inflicting, or threatening to inflict, physical pain or injury on a vulnerable elder, or depriving them of a basic need.
- Emotional Abuse—Inflicting mental pain, anguish, or distress on an elder person through verbal or nonverbal acts.
- Sexual Abuse—Nonconsensual sexual contact of any kind, coercing an elder to witness sexual behaviors.
- Exploitation—Illegal taking, misuse, or concealment of funds, property, or assets of a vulnerable elder.
- Neglect—Refusal or failure by those responsible to provide food, shelter, health care or protection for a vulnerable elder.
- Abandonment—The desertion of a vulnerable elder by anyone who has assumed the responsibility for care or custody of that person [52].

Petitions for guardianship may allege one or more of the above types of elder abuse or neglect. In addition, a petition may allege self-neglect—perhaps the person is not providing food, clothing, shelter, medical care, or basic grooming for him or herself, or is not able to handle financial matters. Finally, petitions may state that an individual has become a victim of predatory telemarketers or lottery scammers, and that the victim keeps sending money even when told this is impoverishing the estate. In such cases a guardianship can protect their money——from themselves and the predators.

In theory, any of the types of abuse and neglect also can take place after a guardianship order is in place, and can be perpetrated or exacerbated by the guardian. In reality, the most common abuse by guardians is financial. The guardian may take advantage of the person's finances or manipulate the funds for his or her own benefit. In rare instances, guardians have also been known to desert the person they are charged with protecting.

17.1.1 The Guardianship System

The guardianship system in each state is unique because it is determined by that state's guardianship laws. There is no federal nationwide system of guardianship. While state laws

Erica Wood is not writing on behalf of the American Bar Association, and the views expressed are her own and do not necessarily represent an official position of the ABA, unless otherwise indicated.

E. Wood (✉)
American Bar Association Commission on Law and Aging, 1050 Connecticut Ave NW, #400, Washington, 20036, DC, USA
e-mail: erica.wood@americanbar.org

M.J. Quinn
San Francisco Superior Court San Francisco, California, USA

X. Dong (ed.), *Elder Abuse*, DOI 10.1007/978-3-319-47504-2_17

may have some similarity, they are not identical. For instance, in many states guardianship proceedings take place in the probate court while in other states, the family court or the civil court may be involved. The criteria for guardianship differ in each state, as do the powers that are granted to the guardian. Even the terminology is different from state to state. Many states use the terms "guardianship of the person" and "guardianship of the estate (or property)" but some states (and the Uniform Guardianship and Protective Proceedings Act [76] use the term "guardianship" to refer to guardianship of the person and "conservatorship" to refer to financial matters. Three states (California, Connecticut, and Tennessee) do not use the term "guardianship" at all for adults, but use the term "conservatorship" exclusively for person and for estate of adults.

The manner in which judges are assigned to appoint guardians and to oversee existing guardianships also differs from state to state. For instance, 14 states have specialized probate courts. Judges in those states are elected or appointed to serve in probate court although they may have to stand for reelection [51]. Four states have specialized probate courts in urban areas and general jurisdiction judges in rural areas. The remaining states and the District of Columbia have judges who are assigned to serve in the probate court for a period of time but may have had assignments in other parts of the court, such as criminal, and may rotate out of probate court to other assignments.

17.1.2 Data on Guardianships

Researchers at the National Center for State Courts have noted that quality data on petitions for adult guardianships, as well as existing guardianships, currently is generally unavailable. Most states do not collect statistics on adult guardianships although they may collect statistics on probate civil matters in general. The lack of data on existing guardianships makes it challenging to track guardianship cases, which are frequently open for years [26].

Taking data from four jurisdictions (Arkansas, District of Columbia, Ohio, and Vermont) that do have reasonably reliable data, researchers found that there were 664 existing guardianships of the person per 100,000 adults. When applied to the U.S. adult population, this would mean there were 1.5 million existing adult guardianship of person cases in 2008. However, the variance between states is high, and the number of active pending adult guardianship cases could range from fewer than 1 million to more than 3 million. Moreover, these figures do not include guardianships of estate. The ongoing challenges in documenting the number of adult guardianship and conservatorship petitions and existing guardianship and conservatorship cases have been the subject of numerous reports and calls for action over recent years [74, 75, 71].

While we do not know the exact number of adults under guardianship, we do know that the need for guardianships or other decision-making options is increasing across the country due to the following:

- The population growth of people 65 and older. The population 65 and over has increased from 35.9 million in 2003 to 44.7 million in 2013 (a 24.7 % increase) and is projected to more than double to 98 million in 2060 [1]. The 85+ population is projected to triple from 6 million in 2013 to 14.6 million in 2040. This is the group of older adults most subject to physical and mental disabilities due to chronic diseases and conditions commonly associated with aging [1].
- Alzheimer's disease, a devastating chronic, terminal disease, affects approximately 5.1 people over 65 in 2015. By 2025, that number is estimated to increase to 7.1 million people, a 40 % increase, barring medical breakthroughs to prevent or cure the disease [5].
- Growth in the numbers of adults with developmental disabilities due to medical advances and better health practices.
- Rising numbers of reported cases of elder abuse and neglect.

17.1.3 The Guardians

A wide variety of agencies and individuals serve as guardians [50, 58]. Most guardians are family members and indeed, laws of most states reflect a clear preference for family members to be appointed as guardians. However, family members may not be available or willing to serve. Or the family member may have been abusive or neglectful or unsuitable to serve for other reasons.

Individuals or agencies also serve as guardians—including neighbors, friends, or professional associates such as lawyers or accountants. Agencies may be nonprofit, for-profit, or state or local public guardianship programs. Some states permit trained volunteers to serve and in a few states, adult protective services (APS) professionals also serve as guardians, at least on a temporary basis (although this may be a conflict of roles).

In the early 1980s, people designating themselves as private professional guardians began petitioning courts to be appointed to serve as guardians. These individuals had experience handling finances, perhaps as trust officers in banks or they were social workers looking to have a private practice. They petitioned to serve as a guardian because there were no family members to serve, or the family members were in conflict, or they were not appropriate to serve because they were abusive or neglectful, or perhaps they could not be bonded (insured) to handle assets. They also petitioned when public guardianship programs were unable to add cases to an already burdened caseload, or where there were no public guardianship programs. Such professionals continue to serve in many localities.

Only a few states have licensing or certification requirements for private professional guardians—such as, for example, Florida, Arizona, California, Texas, and Washington [7, 50]. In general, courts may hold professional guardians to a higher standard of practice than family members, although there is little or no differentiation in state law. Their fees come from the estate of the person in guardianship and must be approved by the court.[1]

At the same time, state and local public guardianship programs that serve as a last resort, when there is no one else willing and qualified to serve, have been increasing over the past 25 years—at least in some areas of many states. In 2007, a national study found that 27 states had explicit, generally statutory, public guardianship programs with at least some degree of state funding, and since that time, two additional states (Oregon and Nebraska) have added statewide public guardianship programs. In addition, most of the remaining states generally assign the role of guardianship of last resort to a designated state agency such as human services [66].

17.1.4 Elders in Guardianship

People come into guardianship for a variety of reasons. The causes include dementia, a catastrophic illness or accident, a substance abuse problem, mental illness, or significant developmental disabilities [51]. A large proportion of people in guardianship are elders. Some states allow people to nominate a specific guardian in advance should they become incapacitated. Certainly, not everyone who has a disability has or needs a guardian. First, the state law criteria must be met. Once that is clear, concrete reasons dictate whether a petition for guardianship may be filed, and whether guardianship is necessary:

1. The elder has lost or partially lost ability due to growing dementia and did not make any plans for care or the handling of finances.
2. There is a pending lawsuit, or divorce, or annulment, and the person is not able to participate in discussions with an attorney.
3. The person experiences a sudden and catastrophic loss of cognitive functioning due to a cerebral vascular accident (stroke) or head injury from an automobile accident—and no advance directives or surrogate decision-makers are in already in place.
4. The person does not grasp the severity of a situation and does not understand that assistance is needed, or refuses desperately needed support. For instance, a home may be in foreclosure but the elder is sure all mortgage payments have been made and cannot be convinced otherwise.
5. Other decision-making options cannot be implemented because the person may not cooperate, even after explanations of the need, and there is a risk of substantial harm.
6. A family is quarreling over custody or assets of the elder. Sibling rivalry can persist even among people in their 70s and 80s. The court may appoint a neutral guardian in these situations to make certain the elder is taken care of and assets are protected.
7. The elder has nominated a person to a serve as guardian as part of estate planning. The elder loses capacity due to a medical condition, and the nominee files a petition with the court for guardianship as the elder wished.
8. An elder has been financially exploited by a telemarketer or other scam artist who uses undue influence. A guardianship is the only way to stop the person from continuing to send money, often to another country, and thus impoverishing him or herself.
9. A less restrictive option, such as a power of attorney or a trust, has been abused; the person who is the principal is not able to serve; or the agent or trustee will not cooperate in correcting the abuses [59].

17.2 Options for Decision-Making Without Guardianship

Not everyone who needs help with decision-making requires a guardian. Since guardianship can remove fundamental rights, it is critical to explore other options first. Such options include "various legal arrangements, social services, and governmental programs that may delay or prevent the appointment of a guardian …" [63]. None of the options has the court oversight of a guardianship but none of them partially or fully remove civil rights in the same way a guardianship does. In addition, guardianships involve expense, time, and the courts. For all those reasons, less restrictive options need to be considered before a petition for guardianship is filed. Many state laws require that courts consider such options before appointing a guardian, and the National Probate Court Standards advise judges to consider them [51].

[1]See "Guardian Fees" at Sect. 17.4.6 in this chapter.

Each of the options has pluses and minuses just as guardianships do. They may be more easily abused because there is minimum or no oversight. The person whose assets and perhaps health care decisions are to be managed must be cognitively capable of agreeing to the arrangement and there must be a trustworthy person willing to assume the decision-making role. Selection of an option short of guardianship needs to be tailored to the elder's situation. Ideally such an option can delay or negate the need to file for a guardianship.

There is an array of legal and practical solutions for both financial and health care decision-making, including financial powers of attorney, representative payees, trusts, joint ownership, single court actions, health care powers of attorney, advance directives, and state default surrogate consent laws—as well as other options that do not require legal steps, such as provision of services and supports to meet the person's needs.

17.2.1 Options for Health Care Decision-Making

17.2.1.1 Durable Power of Attorney for Health Care

The health care power of attorney is a very common option in which a document is signed between two people authorizing one person (the agent) to act for or represent another (the principal). It can take effect at the time it is signed or later with a "springing" clause. For it to "spring" or take effect later, one or more physicians must determine that the elder has lost decisional capacity. It is a private relationship and if a guardianship is needed at a later date, the court may consult the document and depending on state law, recognize it even if a guardianship is established, making the guardian look to the agent's decisions in the areas of authority set out in the power of attorney. An advantage of the health care power of attorney is that it can be as broad or narrow as the elder wishes. It can also include end of life wishes and directions. Disadvantages include the lack of supervision of the person (agent) making the decisions, and the realities that the authority may not be fully recognized from one state to another—although the document will provide key evidence of the person's wishes. Also, people and medical treatments change over time. For instance, an agent may be unable to serve or may move to another state. But for some people, those are not major considerations, especially if there is an alternate agent available.

17.2.1.2 Health Care Advance Directives

Advance directives are comprehensive planning documents in case of decisional inability in the future. They appoint an agent as decision-maker, and also may give direction to others in case of inability to make medical decisions. In most states there is one document that is called a health care advance directive and it can include both instructions and appointment of an agent under a power of attorney for health care. In other states, the same information is separated into two documents: a power of attorney for health care and a living will. A living will often applies only to the very end of life and contains directions for physicians regarding procedures wanted or not wanted, as well as comfort care. The power of attorney for health care is the more useful and versatile advance directive, because it applies to all health care decisions and empowers the agent to make decisions in the way the person would like, and according to the person's values. Two-thirds of all adults have no living will or other advance directive [60].

17.2.1.3 Physician Orders for Life-Sustaining Treatment (POLST)

These are doctor orders for the treatments a person wants at the very end of life [57]. They are used when there is already a serious, progressive, chronic illness. The patient decides what kinds of care he or she wants and the doctor makes an order. This means that all health care providers are legally bound to follow the directions on the order. The order covers treatments such as resuscitation, ventilators, feeding tubes, and other end of life procedures as well as pain control. A guardian or an agent under a health care power of attorney can make the decisions if the patient is unable to do so. The original order is kept with the patient and copies are put in medical records. A POLST order moves with the patient from one care setting to another [69].

17.2.1.4 Default Health Care Consent Laws

By law, medical practitioners can provide emergency care and routine care to adults who cannot give informed consent. No decision-maker is needed. But major nonemergency medical care requires a decision-maker to consent to the treatment, such as surgery, medication, placement of feeding tubes, use of antibiotics, and breathing tubes. If there is no guardian and no advance directive, over 40 states provide that designated family members or others can make at least some health care decisions. The laws have a priority list of people who can make medical decisions. If there is no guardian, family members come in order of relationship to the elder. A "close friend familiar with the person's values" may be at the end of the list in some states [78]. State laws differ as to what decisions family and friends can make. Usually these situations come up when someone is in a nursing home or a hospital. Sometimes, when there is no one to make the decisions, doctors are left to decide what to do and they have to act according to the ethics of their profession [42].

17.2.1.5 Care Managers

Care managers are public or private professionals who come and go to the elder's home and help elders and families determine which supports and services are needed to help the person stay at home. Care managers are familiar with the services available in the community. Such services include arranging for medical, dental and podiatry care, retaining in-home help for grocery shopping and meal preparation, and if needed, personal care such as bathing and dressing. Other services include home-delivered meals, congregate meals, chore services, homemaker assistance, transportation, counseling services, and the various services at senior centers. Care managers may make referrals to adult day care programs, or arrange for assistive equipment to be installed in the home. They can also help to make medical or therapy appointments. Private fee geriatric care managers are available in some areas and can help for longer periods of time. The Aging Life Care Association is a voluntary member organization for private care managers [3].

The largest no-fee care manager service in the country is adult protective services (APS) which exists in every state and is funded by the federal government. APS sees elders in their homes but elders can refuse the service. APS staff can perform all the functions of a care manager but time involvement is usually limited. APS staff also receives and investigates complaints about mistreatment of elders or adults with disabilities [49]. In most states, the law requires them to investigate such complaints (NGN).

17.2.2 Options for Managing Finances

17.2.2.1 Durable Power of Attorney for Finances

A financial durable power of attorney is the most common option for handling financial affairs without a guardianship. As with a durable power of attorney for health care, a financial power of attorney is a written, witnessed document between two people that authorizes one person to act for or represent the other. The person who is designated to handle the elder's affairs is called an "agent." The durable power of attorney may take effect at the time it is signed or later, with a "springing" clause, which means it takes effect only when the elder is declared by one or more physicians to have lost decisional capacity. Powers of attorney are private arrangements, and if a guardianship is needed at a later date, the court may consult them. Depending on state law and on the situation at hand the court may recognize them even if the guardianship is established, directing the guardian to look to the agent for decisions within the scope of the power of attorney.

The main advantages of the financial power of attorney are privacy, ability to tailor wishes and directions, less expense than guardianship, and empowerment of an individual in assuming control of his or her future. Some banks require that their bank power of attorney forms be used for bank transactions; they will not honor any other form. Sometimes title companies may fail to honor powers of attorney. Major disadvantages are that there is no supervision or accountability for the agent, with the added issue that this power of attorney cannot address a living situation or personal care needs. The largest disadvantage is that there is no bonding, which means that the agent can easily use the money for him or herself and there is no insurance to reclaim the assets if the misuse is detected. Guardianship petitions often stem from an agent's financial abuse, and thus powers of attorney have sometimes been called a "license to steal." A guardian can attempt to reclaim assets and possibly file a lawsuit if needed [55].

17.2.2.2 Representative Payees

Several federal governmental agencies offer programs whereby a designated person can receive and use monthly payments on behalf of an agency beneficiary, for the individual's basic needs. The agencies include

- Social Security Administration
- Veteran's Administration
- Department of Defense
- Railroad Retirement Board
- Office of Personnel Management (retirement pensions for former employees or their survivors).

The person or institution who receives the check is termed a representative payee, or federal fiduciary. This arrangement is meant to assist adults who are unable to handle their own benefits. The agency accepts physician statements as well as those by relatives and friends as evidence that a representative payee may be needed. Each program has its own rules as to who can serve as a representative payee, and what accounting is required. There is no cost to set up a representative payee arrangement. If the benefits are the only income source, representative payment can be a very helpful arrangement. If there is other income or assets, additional arrangements will need to be made. The disadvantages include minimal oversight and enforcement of the requirement for accountings, and the lack of investigation of a proposed representative payee (NGN).

17.2.2.3 Trusts

Trusts are also private arrangements for handling decision-making if an elder becomes unable to do so. Typically, an attorney is involved in preparing the trust documents. Trusts can be expensive to create, and generally are most useful for substantial estates. There are three types of trusts: testamentary, special needs, and revocable living trusts. Testamentary trusts take effect on the death of the elder. Special needs trusts are established for the sole benefit of a person with a disability, usually a person under the age of 65. The unique provisions of these special needs trusts enable people to continue to receive public benefits while at the same time trust assets are dispersed under strict federal law definitions.

Revocable living trusts are the most common type of trust. They take effect during the person's lifetime and thus can help avoid guardianship of the estate. They do not address the personal needs or living situation of an elder. Most people name themselves as the initial trustee and name another person or institution to serve as successor trustee should one be needed. The trustor (the elder) can modify the trust at any time and must be careful to include in the trust all assets acquired after the trust has been created—otherwise the court may need to be involved, even though the trust was established to avoid a court process.

While having a trust means that there is no probate process including attorney fees, there is no tax benefit to this type of trust. However, there are attorney fees as there are many legal issues to be settled before and after an elder dies. As with a power of attorney for finances, there is no oversight and no bonding. Thus, if a successor trustee mismanages or takes the elder's money, there may be no way to recover the money. On the other hand, a trustee can usually act more quickly than an executor to distribute the assets of a deceased elder, providing there is no controversy or outstanding claims and taxes.

In recent years, so-called "trust mills" have sprung up. Employees of these organizations telephone people promising they can avoid taxes, costly attorney services, and the probate court process if only they have a revocable living trust. The elder may never see an attorney because a "trust advisor" is the representative who makes personal contact and prepares the "one-size-fits all" document. Typically the trust is of poor quality and is not tailored to the elder's circumstances, which makes it a target for litigation in the probate department.

17.2.2.4 Joint Ownership

Another decision-making option is joint ownership of cash assets and real property, established either at the initiation of a bank account or purchase of the real property or at a later date. Once a second person is officially on the account or property, half belongs to her or him. There are tax and other consequences for both people. The original owner loses exclusive control of assets. State law and local bank practices determine which type of joint accounts is available. Most states allow the type that gives the joint asset to the surviving person after the elder dies. Joint ownership has distinct advantages in that it allows one person to help another who is unable to get to the bank or pay bills or manage property. Banks have the forms. Putting real property into joint ownership may require the assistance of an attorney or a real estate agent [62]. Of course, a downside is that a joint owner may exploit the situation, withdrawing funds for his or her own use rather than using the funds for the benefit of the elder. Thus, joint ownership can be a doorway to abuse.

17.2.2.5 Money Management Assistance

Daily money management programs offer assistance to people who have problems managing their personal financial affairs. The elder continues to make the decisions, but receives practical help. Money management programs provide a wide variety of services for people with various disabilities. They can assist with bill paying, prepare checks for signature, make deposits to the bank, and dispense cash to their clients. They may manage more complex tasks such as maintaining payroll records for home attendants and preparing documents for accountants for annual federal and state tax preparation. Some programs are nonprofit but there are an increasing number of for-profit money management programs.

Money management programs are valuable for people who have disabling arthritis or visual disabilities, those who are widowed and have little experience managing money, those who have limited ability to read and write or are unfamiliar with bank practices. They are also helpful for people with mild to moderate cognitive impairment. Some programs ask their clients to sign a power of attorney for finances that allows them to continue providing services in case of disability. The programs are flexible and there is no court process. The qualifications of people who act as money managers vary considerably and the field is unregulated. There is a professional organization that has standards of practice and a code of ethics, the American Association of Daily Money Managers (AADMM) [12].

17.2.2.6 Single Court Actions

Many state laws have provisions that provide for single transactions that involve court action. In addition to medical decisions, depending on state law, courts can make orders that freeze assets if there is evidence that someone is draining a bank account. An attorney may be appointed to represent an elder who is alleged to be unable to speak for him or herself and make necessary decisions [58].

17.2.3 Other Options for Decision-Making Without Guardianship

17.2.3.1 Options for Supporting Decision-Making

Most of the above options name a surrogate to act on behalf of an individual with a disability. However, sometimes an individual may be able to make decisions on his or her own with needed support. Under "supported decision-making" arrangements, individuals with a disability use trusted others to help in understanding choices so they can make their own decisions when possible—moving away from surrogacy toward self-determination [20]. In addition to supporters, there is an array of practical solutions that may enhance an individual's ability to make his or own decisions. Supported decision-making is a growing movement that is incorporated in the United Nations Convention on the Rights of Persons with Disabilities and is being recognized as a viable approach less restrictive than guardianship.[2]

17.2.3.2 Mediation and Guardianship

Mediation can be very helpful in resolving family conflicts that have led to a petition for guardianship or even after a guardianship has been established when issues of visitation and the amount of money being spent on the elder arise [85]. Using mediation standards and communication techniques geared toward problem-solving and settlement of the dispute, the mediator helps the parties understand their issues, become sensitive to each other's point of view, and work toward mutually acceptable solutions. Often when people state their positions in a mediation session, a skilled mediator can assist the parties in finding their own solutions. If a petition for guardianship already has been filed, the presence of the elder's attorney at the mediation session can help to safeguard rights—but it is the parties themselves who do the talking, with the facilitation of the mediator. Mediation can be empowering for all involved, and can give the elder a voice. It also has the advantage of being more flexible than court procedures. One disadvantage is that it can be difficult to locate a mediator who is familiar with elders and the issues they face. The Association for Conflict Resolution has developed "Mediation Training Objectives for Adult Guardianship Cases" as part of its guidelines on elder mediation training [18].

Some egregious guardianship conflicts have gone beyond the ability of mediation to address. There may be allegations of abuse or exploitation, and some family members may be isolating an elder from others [85]. For such high conflict cases, the Association for Conflict Resolution in 2014 approved a new court-based dispute resolution process called "eldercaring coordination" [19, 21]. The process "assists elders, legally authorized decision-makers, and others who participate by court order or invitation, to resolve high conflict disputes impacting the elder's autonomy and safety" [18]. Eldercaring coordination uses problem-solving skills, education and resources, development of an eldercare plan, mediation—and in some cases the trained eldercaring coordinator may be authorized to make certain decisions within the scope of a court order or with the parties' prior agreement.

[2]See Sect. 17.4.3 in this chapter for more on supported decision-making.

17.3 Court Process of Establishing a Guardianship

The guardianship process begins when someone becomes concerned about the cognitive functioning and decision-making capacities of another person, and less restrictive options hopefully have been explored and will not work. The concerned person may be a physician, a hospital or long-term care facility, a family member, a banker, a real estate broker, an attorney, adult protective services professional, or a friend or neighbor. The elder may not be making decisions that are in keeping with previous values or is making decisions that are not in his or her own best interests such as giving money to lottery scammers. Or the elder is failing to take care of basic personal needs such as food, clothing, shelter, and medical care and managing bill paying. Perhaps a family member appears from another state and "takes over" the elder and threatens to move the elder. The concerned person thinks "something needs to be done" and may contact others who are also concerned. The subject of guardianship and other decision-making options get raised as a way for decision-making to be placed in the hands of someone other than the person who seemingly has diminished decision-making ability.

The process of establishing of guardianship and appointing a guardian unfolds in a predictable fashion: petition, court hearing, ongoing guardianship, and (possible) termination of the guardianship. Each step of the guardianship process is or should be accompanied by due process protections which mean

1. The person who is the subject of a proposed guardianship receives a personal visit from someone with written notice of the pending guardianship in a way that maximizes the chance that the person can understand it.
2. There is sufficient time for the person to respond to the petition and prepare a defense if desired.
3. The person is furnished with the information that supports the petition.
4. The notice, and in some cases court officers, inform the person of the right to attend the hearing, object to the

proposed guardianship or the proposed guardian. In addition, the person receives information about the right to have a jury trial to determine the need for the guardianship, and the right to an attorney.

In reality, not all court jurisdictions have the resources and personnel to ensure that due process rights are observed evenly.

17.3.1 Petition

The first formal step in establishing a guardianship is to file a formal request with the court, which is termed a petition. The contents of the petition are determined by state law but in general include basic information about the person and the facts that support the appointment of a guardian. Some states have standard petition forms. Courts typically do not search for a guardian; one must be named in the petition. The petitioner also may file medical reports and psychological reports, either in conjunction with the petition or following the petition. Once the petition is filed, the court sets a date and time that it will be considered by the court.

17.3.2 Notice

Just after the petition is filed, the petitioner or the court or a neutral party must personally take the petition to the person who is alleged to need a guardianship. A copy of the petition is sent to the spouse if there is one and to relatives within a stated degree of relationship. Depending on state law requirements, others may receive notice: governmental agencies, agents with powers of attorney, trustees, nieces or nephews or even cousins who live in other countries. The goal is for the fact of the proposed guardianship to be transparent to those parties or agencies that are concerned with the incapacitated person [14]. Ideally the notice should state the rights of the person in the hearing, as well as the rights that may be lost as a result of court appointment, and should be in plain language and readable type, but in practice the notice is not always clear or understandable.

17.3.3 Counsel

The person is who is alleged to need a guardian has the due process right to be represented by an attorney and can hire one, but only approximately 22 states require the court to appoint an attorney. Other states note that the individual has a right to be represented or state the circumstances under which the court may appoint an attorney—such as if the court investigator recommends it, the judge determines it is necessary, or the individual requests it [6]. Most state laws are silent as to the role an attorney for the individual should take. Some state laws specify the attorney should advocate for the wishes and preferences of the person, but others provide the attorney should act as a "guardian ad litem" representing the person's best interests A national guardianship consensus conference in 2001 outlined the tasks of an attorney representing the person alleged to need a guardian: (a) advise the client of all options and the probability of success in pursuing any one of those options; (b) give the advice in language, mode of communication, and terms that the client is most likely to understand; and (c) zealously advocate the course of actions chosen by the client [40, 81]. Court-appointed attorney fees must be approved by the court and are drawn from the guardianship estate.

17.3.4 Emergency Appointment

In some situations, a guardianship may be urgently needed before the hearing for the formal appointment of a guardian. In most states, the court can act within a few days to give limited powers to the proposed guardian to deal with the situation. For instance, the family home may be in foreclosure because the mortgage has not been paid, or there is evidence that a bank account is being actively drained or that the person is accompanied to the bank by someone who urges that the person to take out money in a way that is inconsistent with past habits. Perhaps the person needs immediate surgery or has a medical condition and is unable to consent to treatment. In some cases, someone may be trying to quickly move the person to an isolated and undisclosed location.

In such cases, a court may appoint an "emergency" or "temporary" guardian if it is alleged there is risk of substantial harm to the person's health, safety, or welfare and there is no other person with authority to act. Almost every state has provisions for emergency guardianship setting out a streamlined process with less rigorous notice requirements [9]. There may be a time limit on the duration of the order, or the temporary authority may last until a permanent guardian is in place or there is a determination that none is needed. Emergency orders are generally narrower in scope, limited to the specific powers needed to address the problem. Emergency guardianships can be a welcome relief from abusive situations—but on the other hand they can be misused is there is no real emergency and the petitioner simply wants to get a guardianship in place quickly.

17.3.5 Review and Investigation

The time between the filing of the petition and the court hearing is the time for the court to review the petition and to take various actions depending on state law and the particular court. For instance the court may do a criminal background check on the proposed guardian. Perhaps a neuropsychological examination is warranted and the court may require that it take place before the hearing.

Some courts have employees or trained volunteers who will visit the person alleged to need a guardianship and inform them of the proposed guardianship and their rights. These court visitors also investigate the circumstances of the petition in more detail. Sometimes the court appoints attorneys as "guardian ad litem" to inform individuals of their rights and conduct investigations—ideally a function very different from the advocacy undertaken by an attorney representing the individual. These court appointees then report back to the judge as to the situation of the person and may recommend appointment of a guardian—yet could in fact identify less restrictive options.

Court personnel will also make certain that all the documents submitted are in order and comply with state law. Finally, when all the information has been assembled and put in order, the judge will review the pleadings and documents looking for consistency with state law examining the situation at hand. This is the time that a judge should consider whether a less intrusive decision-making option is appropriate. The judge does not make a final determination as to need for guardianship until after listening to the testimony at the formal court hearing.

17.3.6 Court Hearing

The conduct of a hearing can vary substantially from court to court depending on the judge, the number of cases to be considered, and the complexity of the cases. The hearing is usually in a court room and there may be a court reporter. Generally, it is the judge who makes the decision, not a jury. Many courts schedule all guardianship matters for a single morning. The main purpose of the hearing is for the judge to literally hear first-hand what people have to add to the documents that have already been submitted. The second purpose is to appoint a guardian, whether it is the person who petitioned to be the guardian or another entity or person. The third purpose is to determine which powers the guardian should have in order to manage the needs and limitations of the person in guardianship.

Ideally, all persons concerned about the person with diminished capacity will be present at the time of the hearing, including the person who is alleged to need a guardian—who has a right to be present. This is another part of due process. In reality, most people who are alleged to need a guardian do not attend the hearing out of embarrassment, physical weakness, disability, or because they implicitly trust the person who is willing to be their guardian [58]. However, it is critical that the person who is alleged to need a guardian attend if possible, both to promote his or her participation, and to give the judge an opportunity to observe the person. Under the Americans with Disabilities Act, courts must make accommodations to allow for attendance at the hearing—for example by holding the hearing at a more accessible place. Most likely the proposed guardian, often the person who petitioned for the appointment, will be appointed as long as the person seems suitable and there are no objections from any of the parties, the person who is alleged to need a guardian.

At the time of hearing or directly following the hearing, the judge will issue a court order that both establishes a guardianship and appoints the guardian. The order should be limited to the powers that are needed to administer the estate (guardianship of estate) or to manage the person's needs (guardianship of person). The myth is that a guardianship removes all the civil rights of a person. In truth, many rights are retained depending on individual state law and the court order.[3]

At the time of the hearing, the judge may order that the guardian of the estate post a bond. The bond is a form of insurance for the person in guardianship, and amount of the bond may well increase when all the assets have been located and identified by the newly appointed guardian. Conversely the bond may be lowered as liquid assets are spent for the person in guardianship. Bonding companies do background checks of proposed guardians of the estate to determine if they are "bondable," which means the guardian has good credit.

17.3.7 Termination of Guardianship

In most cases, a guardianship terminates upon the death of the person. However, in some instances, the person in guardianship may recover and be able to handle his or her own affairs again. Or, the guardianship may have been established for a distinct purpose such as a divorce action or a real estate transfer. Once that action is completed, there is no need for the guardianship and it can be terminated upon court order. Or, a plan may be put into place that will assist the incapacitated person with all activities of daily living and with financial matters. For instance, a trust may be established that handles the finances; the person may move to a group home, and there is a health care agent in place. In

[3]For a discussion of limited guardianship orders, see Sect. 17.4.1 in this chapter.

these instances, where supports and services are involved and are likely to continue, the court may terminate the guardianship—but someone has to petition the court for termination and restoration of rights.

Termination of the guardianship restores the rights of the individual and increases self-determination. However, it can be difficult for the person who has a guardian to hire an attorney to assist in filing a petition for termination since the person likely has no access to her or his finances and may not legally have the ability to contract due to the provisions of the guardianship. In jurisdictions where there is court review, people who have a guardian can voice their wish to the court visitor or investigator. An attorney can then be appointed to represent the individual and can file for termination of the guardianship. At times, a guardian may petition the court for termination—or may actively oppose a termination requested by the individual. The guardian has access to the person's assets and thus, with court approval, can pay an attorney.

The process for terminating a guardianship is not well articulated in state law, national standards, or in practice. Key issues policy and legislative issues include: court appointment of counsel; the required evidentiary standard; the role of the guardian when a person files for termination and restoration; and the need for ongoing court review concerning changes that might warrant termination [22].

17.4 Duties and Roles of the Guardian

17.4.1 Guardian Authority

Serving as guardian is one of society's most challenging roles. A guardian of the person must make decisions about medical treatment including end-of-life care, where the person will live, what long-term services and supports are needed, and in some cases who will visit the person. A guardian of property must manage the person's estate, paying bills, making investments, securing public benefits, and maintaining or buying and selling property. To make these decisions, guardians should be knowledgeable and up-to-date about community aging and disability resources, accounting and financial management, real estate, public benefits, health care and health insurance, housing, accessibility, long-term care, mental health, and abuse, neglect and exploitation. Yet often family members, the most common guardians, come to the job unprepared—having never done it before and unlikely to do it again. They may not know what is expected of them and have little or no training. Even professional guardians may not have all the guidance they need [83].

In each state, the duties of guardians of person and property are set out in statute. The state statute the first place to look to understand a guardian's role and responsibilities. But state statutes may be very broad. The statute may provide, for instance, that the guardian is to make decisions about the person's "support, care, education, health, and welfare" but offer no specific instruction as to how this should be done [83]. The statute also may set out certain rights that are automatically retained by the individual unless specifically removed in the court order—for example the right to vote or to marry. Some state and local courts have rules to clarify guardian duties and powers. That is the second place to check.

Courts use the statute and any relevant rules in writing specific orders in each case. That is the third place to look to determine guardian powers and duties. The court order may be very inclusive and general—it may be a "plenary" order transferring all of the person's rights to the guardian; or it may be a more specific "limited" order including powers and duties only in areas in which the judge determines the person cannot make decisions for him or herself. For example, the order may specify that the guardian is to manage property, but that the person retains the authority for day–to-day expenditures—or that the person retains the authority to decide where to live or who may visit. When interacting with a guardian, it is important to get a copy of the court order, to understand the breadth of the guardian's authority. Some areas of guardianship readily suitable for tailoring in the court order (depending on state law) are

- Handling a small bank account
- Consenting to medical treatment
- Paying usual monthly bills
- Making usual birthday and holiday gifts to family members.

The main obstacle to limiting guardianships may be that judges do not always receive the detailed, objective, neutral information that would enable them to tailor the order. In one research study where court visitors recommended that guardians be given limited powers, the court more often than not followed the recommendation or denied the petition for guardianship [45]. Other obstacles may include the additional time and attention required by the court, the possible expense for the person's estate in returning to court if conditions change, and lack of clarity for third parties. Such challenges can be overcome, and the Uniform Guardianship and Protective Proceedings Act and the National Probate Court Standards, as well as most state statutes, promote the use of limited orders.

17.4.2 Guardian Standards of Practice

Because statutes and court rules often give little practical guidance, there is a need for standards to flesh out the specifics and instruct the guardian, especially when problems or competing priorities arise. The National Guardianship Association has an extensive set of *Standards of Practice* that offers ready tools for guardians, and some measure of expectation for those working with guardians [53]. The NGA Standards are intended to be applicable to both professional and family or other lay guardians. The Preamble for the Standards states that the aim is "to strike a consistent balance between standards that represent an ideal and those that recognize practical limitations, whether for a family guardian or for a professional guardian."[4]

The Center for Guardian Certification uses the NGA *Standards* as the basis for certifying guardians nationally. Additionally, some states have adapted the NGA *Standards* or developed their own guardian standards, and a growing number have instituted their own certification or licensing programs [23, 24, 37]. A few states, such as Florida, New York, and Ohio have required training for professional and family or other lay guardians by statute or court rule.

Guardians are accountable both to the court and to the individual. The guardian is an agent of the court and must report to court. At the same time, the guardian must put the needs and wishes of the person foremost. At least as to financial matters, the guardian is a "fiduciary"—a person "invested with rights and powers to be exercised for the benefit of another person," and who relates to the person with the utmost trust and confidence [68]. Thus, even if the court has not specifically directed the guardian in a certain action or it is not specifically provided in statute or rule, the guardian should be acting as a fiduciary in the person's interests. As a fiduciary, the guardian must avoid all conflicts of interest—and even the appearance of a conflict; and may not make decisions that benefit someone else—including the guardian him or herself—at the person's expense [70]. A guardian must take actions to prevent or address any abuse, neglect or exploitation; and must ensure that he or she does not commit such abuse, neglect or exploitation, or give the appearance of doing so [84].

Statutes, court rules, court orders, and standards all offer important direction for guardians. However, in practice, the conduct of guardians does not always follow these dictates, and has remained uneven. Press stories have profiled grave problems with the guardianship system.[5] The Government Accounting Office identified a substantial number of allegations of abuse by guardians—but "could not determine whether allegations of abuse by guardians are widespread" [73]. Because guardianship data and empirical research is scant [75], we do not know the extent of the problems highlighted by the press. "Anecdotal evidence says guardianship practice ranges widely from quietly heroic to satisfactory to unknowingly deficient to malfeasant, but the proportions are not clear" [83]. It is important to be alert to guardians who may be abusing or exploiting individuals in their care, and report to the court and to adult protective services. Some courts have complaint processes and will investigate and take action, possibly removing the guardian. However, it is also important not to assume that because the guardian is subject to court oversight, abusive actions are recognized and dealt with. Notifying APS—and law enforcement if fraud or criminal action is suspected—are critical steps in protecting the individual who has a guardian.

17.4.3 Guardian Standards of Decision-Making

Guardians are surrogates. They make decisions on behalf of someone else. There are basically four paths of surrogate decision-making that in practice tend to merge and overlap: (1) using explicit instructions; (2) offering support so the individual can take a lead in or participate in making the decisions on his or her own or jointly with the surrogate; (3) making decisions according to the "substituted judgment" model in which the surrogate aims to make the decisions the person would have made, using the person's values and preferences; and (4) making decisions using the

[4]NGA Standards of Practice, Preamble, p. 1 (2013), www.guardianship.org.

[5]Leonnig, C., Hun, L. & Cohen, S. "Under court, Vulnerable Become Victims: Attorneys Who Ignored Clients or Misspent Funds Rarely Sanctioned," *The Washington Post,* A01, June 15, 2003; Cohen, S., Leoning, & Witt, A., "Rights and Funds Can Evaporate Quickly, Attorneys' Powers Thwarted D.C. Residents Trying to Remain Independent," *The Washington Post,* A01, June 16, 2003; Leonard, J., Fields, R. & Larrubia, E., "Guardians for Profit: Judges' Inaction, Inattention Leave Many Senior at Risk," *The Los Angeles Times,* A1, November 14, 2005; Glaberson, W., "Grand Jury Urges Overhaul of Legal Guardianship System, *The New York Times,* B1, March 3, 2004; Jarman, J., Riepenhoff, J., Sullivan, L. & Wagner, M., "Unguarded," *Columbus Times Dispatch,* May 18–22, 2014, http://dispatch.com/unguarded.html; Smith, B. P., "The Kindness of Strangers," *Sarasota Herald Tribune,* December 7–9, 2014, http://guardianship.heraldtribune.com; Bauman, K., "Family Speaks Out About Guardianship System, *Contact 13,* February 2, 2015, http://www.scrippsmedia.com/ktnv/news/contact-13/contact-13-investigates/Family-speaks-out-about-guardianship-system-290598431.html; Jones, A. & Campo-Flores, A., "Abuse Plagues System of Legal Guardians for Adults," *The Wall Street Journal,* October 30, 2015, http://www.wsj.com/articles/abuse-plagues-system-of-legal-guardians-for-adults-1446225524.

"best interests" model in which the surrogate makes choices that the surrogates determines are beneficial and enhance the person's welfare [80].

A guardian may have explicit instructions about health care in an individual's advance directive, particularly an advance directive designed to elucidate values and preferences such as the Aging with Dignity "Five Wishes" form [4]. There are also a growing number of tools encouraging people to record their health care values and wishes and discuss these with trusted others (The Conversations Project). Or the individual may have written a letter or discussed choices with his or her doctor, which are recorded in the doctor's files.

Without explicit instructions, or combined with explicit instructions, the guardian may provide the person with the support he or she needs to make, or participate in making, his or her own decisions when possible—moving from "surrogate decision-making" toward "supported decision-making" [20]. Through communication strategies, a circle of trusted supporters, assistive technology and practical community supports, guardians may give individuals a voice in decisions that affect them and enhance their self-determination.

Such a right to support in decision-making is recognized in the United Nations Convention on the Rights of Persons with Disabilities [77]. The National Guardianship Association "supports policies that help maximize the participation of the person and provide the person under guardianship with every opportunity to exercise those individual rights that the person might be capable of exercising" [54]. Numerous findings that show that being able to make choices about one's life can benefit overall health and well-being [20]. Moreover, with sufficient support, an individual may not need a guardian and may be able to have the guardianship terminated and have his or her rights restored. For example, in a New York case, a woman with intellectual disabilities had developed a system of supports through relative, friends, and provider staff, and thus the court found "guardianship is no longer warranted because there is now a system of supported decision-making in place that constitutes a less restrictive alternative …"[6]

In supporting the person in making choices, guardians must guard against undue influence or outright conflicts of interest. A guardian's position of authority and full knowledge of the person's affairs makes it easy to improperly influence the individual in a choice that directly or indirectly benefits the guardian or third parties. Indeed, a guardian could attempt to hide exploitation under the cover of supporting a person in making a choice that wrongly benefits others. The need for safeguards in supported decision-making is well-recognized [46, 54, 77].

If there are no explicit instructions and the person is not able, even with supports, to make or participate in making choices, the guardian must use a "substituted judgment" standard, being guided by the individual's values and preferences—"stepping into the shoes" or "living the life" of the individual [65, 80]. The Uniform Guardianship and Protective Proceedings Act provides that a guardian "shall consider the expressed desires and personal values of the ward to the extent known to the guardian" (although it references best interest as well).[7] The National Guardianship Association *Standards of Practice* define "substituted judgment" as "the principle of decision-making that substitutes the decision the person would have made when the person had capacity as the guiding force in any surrogate decision the guardian makes." The Standards point out that substituted judgment "promotes the underlying values of self-determination and well-being of the person."[8]

According to the *Standards of Practice*, the guardian may not use substituted judgment only when either the result would cause substantial harm to the person or when there is insufficient evidence of what the person would have wanted.[9] In such a case, a guardian is left with the "best interest" principle, determining what the guardian believes to be best for the individual's welfare. But the *Standards* note that in using the best interest principle, the guardian should still "consider the least intrusive, most normalizing, and least restrictive course of action possible."[10]

Whitton and Frolik examined guardianship statutes in 52 U.S. jurisdictions (all 50 states, the District of Columbia and the Virgin Islands), and found that 28 have no general decision-making standard for guardians; 18 have provisions with substituted judgment language, sometimes in combination with a best interest component; and six reference a best interest standard [80]. They also surveyed guardians about factors that influenced them in making surrogate decisions. The survey showed that generally guardians do not use either a strict substituted judgment or best interest standard, but rather consider both the person's best interest and what the person would want. They also found that statutory decision-making standards do tend to have some influence on the way in which guardians make decisions.

[6]*In Re the Guardianship of Dameris L.*, 2012 NY Slip Op 22386 Decided on December 28, 2012 Sur Ct, New York County.

[7]Sec 314 UGPPA 1997.

[8]NGA Standard #7.

[9]NGA Standard #7, 2013.

[10]NGA Standard. #7, 2013.

17.4.4 Duties of Guardian of the Person

Consistent with the scope of the court order and with the person's preferences if possible, a guardian of the person must ensure and coordinate needed care, support, services, education and training, and social opportunities. The guardian begins by meeting with the person, and making a plan for identifying needs and carrying out responsibilities. The plan should document the person's known values, lifestyle, history, and wishes. In some states, the guardian must submit a forward-looking plan to court, but in other states, it is simply a tool of good practice, and recommended by the NGA *Standards of Practice*.

The guardianship plan ideally is based on any functional assessment showing strengths, weaknesses, and needs for support. If there was not a thorough assessment during the appointment process, the guardian may need to secure an assessment from a social worker, psychologist, gerontologist, psychologist, or multidisciplinary evaluation team. A functional evaluation may be couched in terms of the person's abilities concerning "activities of daily living" such as eating, dressing, toileting, walking, transferring, bathing, and grooming; and "instrumental activities of daily living" such as shopping, taking medications, using transportation, using the telephone, and maintaining the home. If the person is in a nursing home or in assisted living, the staff's care plan may offer a useful basis for preparing a guardianship plan.

Along with the personal interviews with the person and the assessment, the guardian must find and collect relevant legal documents such as an advance directive. If another person or agency is serving as a guardian of the estate, the guardian of the person must consistently coordinate—for instance, the guardian of the estate must authorize funds for an apartment or assisted living care, or for medical treatment outside of health plan coverage. The guardian may or may not be serving as a Social Security representative payee or VA fiduciary to receive benefits and use them for the individual's needs. If a different person is serving in these roles, coordination is critical [71, 72].

The guardian must communicate with and manage service providers such as care managers, physicians, nurses or nurse aides, home care workers, housecleaning, and repair workers. The guardian must arrange for meals, clothing, travel, social and religious events, physical or occupational therapy—essentially "living the life of another." The guardian should be knowledgeable about community resources such as agencies on aging, centers for independent living, local departments of human services, protection and advocacy agencies, housing agencies and long-term services and supports.

To fully understand and react to the person's changing needs and preferences, the guardian must visit regularly. The NGA *Standards* require a visit "no less than monthly,"[11] but some states allow less frequent visits or do not specify. If the guardian is an agency or attorney, the guardian sometimes sends staff such as a social worker to visit and report back—and this arrangement may or may not be acceptable or adequate to meet the needs.

Guardians must "encourage and support the person in maintaining contact with family and friends, as defined by the person, unless it will substantially harm the person."[12] It may be difficult to determine whether visitation by relatives is desired by the person, or possibly harmful to the person—but the guardian must avoid interfering with family and established relationships unless abusive, and should ask the person what he or she wants. Guardians must be alert to any abuse, neglect, or exploitation by others and report to adult protective services—and may in some cases need to remove the abuser or remove the individual from access by the abuser, which may require court approval. The guardian may have been appointed for this very reason—because the adult son or daughter is living off the person's Social Security, isolating the person from other family members, and draining bank accounts.

17.4.4.1 Making Health Care Decisions

Among the most challenging of guardian responsibilities is making health care choices, which may range from everyday care decisions to determinations about health plans and choice of physicians, treatment for chronic conditions, surgery, medications, alternative medicine remedies, psychiatric care, hospital admission and discharge, and end-of-life care including tube feeding, do-not-resuscitate orders, hospice and palliative care. Some health care decisions, especially end of life decisions, require court approval in some states (ABA Commission "Guardianship Law and Practice").

The NGA *Standards of Practice* set out clear steps specifically for making health care decisions or seeking court approval for such a decision, based on the overall decision-making standards noted above: "maximize the participation of the person; acquire a clear understanding of the medical facts; acquire a clear understanding of the health care options and the risks and benefits of each option; and encourage and support the individual in understanding the facts and directing a decision." If the patient cannot participate in the decision, the guardian must make a choice based on what the patient would want or otherwise what would be best for the person. The guardian must exercise due diligence in asking questions, getting second opinions when needed, and seeking out resources (ABA Commission, "Making Health Care Decisions," 2009) [67]. The guardian

[11]NGA Standard #13.

[12]NGA Standard #4.

is the person's advocate in the hospital or other medical setting, and with the patient's health plan, and must stay informed about the person's condition and options, ask questions, and be assertive with the often-changing medical team.

17.4.4.2 Making Residential Decisions

Few things are as important as where you live, where you call home. One of the toughest tasks of a guardian often is determining where the person will live, and seeking the least restrictive setting while considering risks. A guardian may be faced with a situation in which a person is living at home alone in an uncleanly or unsafe environment, but does not want to move to other housing, assisted living or to a nursing home—or such options are not affordable or available in the area.

The NGA *Standards* direct the guardian to "have a strong priority for home or other community-based settings, when not inconsistent with the person's goals and preferences."[13] This could mean bringing in home care, housecleaning, and arranging for transportation and home-delivered meals, as well as making accessibility modifications to the home if the person wants to stay there. The guardian needs to assess the person's support system in the area, and whether living at home will maintain longstanding contacts—or isolate the person, possibly inviting abuse and exploitation. Selected guardianship programs, such as the Vera Institute Guardianship Project in New York City, have prioritized home and community-based care options, and developed strategies to keep people at home if that is where they want to be, even saving Medicaid funds by avoiding costly institutional care [79].

Often, an individual goes to the hospital in an emergency, and the guardian quickly must be ready to participate in and consent to a discharge plan to a nursing home, assisted living or other residential setting. This may be a squeeze. In a 2010 survey of guardians on making residential decisions, many expressed frustrations with the limits of money, time, and quality resources. "Usually there is no choice, it's just advocate for what you can get" and "It's less a decision than the only course available," they explained [41]. In particular, affordable, accessible housing is at a premium in many communities.

If the person ends up in a nursing home or assisted living, even if temporarily for rehabilitation, the guardian must "monitor the quality of care on an ongoing basis and take any necessary action when the setting does not meet the individual's current goals, needs and preferences."[14] This means attending regular care conferences, getting to know the staff, becoming familiar with the facility's care plan, voicing any complaints, and perhaps working with the long-term care ombudsman to ensure quality care, settle disputes, and target any abusive actions. Guardians may need to explain their role to facility staff, which may not differentiate their court-appointed role from that of a health care of financial agent or a family caregiver. In some states, a guardian must get court approval to move an individual to a higher, more restrictive level of care such as from home to assisted living or a nursing home [41].

[13]NGA Standard #12.

[14]NGA Standard #13.

17.4.5 Duties of Guardian of the Estate

A "guardian of the estate" also may be called a "guardian of property" or, as in the Uniform Guardianship and Protective Proceedings Act and a growing number of states, a "conservator." Unless limited by court order, a guardian of the estate has broad powers over the person's money and property.

17.4.5.1 Financial Management

Following appointment, the guardian must submit an inventory to court, and in many states buy a bond. The inventory may involve an extensive search for assets.[15] The NGA *Standards of Practice* require the guardian to "develop and implement a financial plan and budget,"[16] the National Probate Court Standards reference "an asset management plan,"[17] and many states require that a financial plan be submitted to the court. The guardian must provide for the person's support, receive the income and manage the expenses, pay the bills and debts, review bank accounts, pay taxes, make investments if there are sufficient funds, and secure any insurance needed.

The guardian of the estate may also serve as the guardian of person but if not, must coordinate with the guardian of person and with any representative payee or VA fiduciary. If the guardian of the estate and of the person disagree, the court may need to decide. If the guardian of the estate is also the beneficiary of the estate, as is often true for family members, the guardian may have a natural conflict. The guardian must put the interest and welfare of the person first [70]; and must give priority to the goals, needs and preferences of the person [53].

The NGA Standards on duties of the guardian of the estate set out broad mandates including transparency, competent management, sound record-keeping, prosecuting a case if it is in the person's best interest, defending the estate, managing according to the person's estate plan, and using

[15]For a discussion of asset protection, see Sect. 17.5.2 in this chapter.

[16]NGA Standard #18.

[17]National College of Probate Judges, National Probate Court Standards, 3.3.16 (2013).

the prudent person or investor rule [32]. The Standards also require the guardian to secure the property, apply for public benefits, "value the well-being of the person over the preservation of the estate," ensure that the financial plan emphasizes "a person-centered philosophy," and consider the previously expressed or current desires of the person in considering whether to dispose of property.[18]

17.4.5.2 Fiduciary Duty of Guardian of the Estate

A guardian of the estate is a fiduciary, with a high duty of accountability to the person and to court. The NGA *Standards* require that the guardian "as a fiduciary, shall manage the financial affairs of the person under guardianship in a way that maximizes the dignity, autonomy, and self-determination of the person."[19] With full access to the individual's assets, some guardians may fail to seek the person's involvement, may exert undue influence on how the money should be spent, or may even engage in exploitation —which is theft by the very person the court has appointed to guard against such theft. The Consumer Financial Protection Bureau has set out four basic duties of a guardian of the estate as a fiduciary [70]:

(1) Act only in the person's best interest, rather than in the guardian's interest or the interest of others. The guardian must follow the court order, involve the person as much as possible, avoid conflicts of interest or even the appearance of a conflict of interest, and refrain from borrowing or loaning estate funds to him or herself or to others.
(2) Use care in managing the assets. This means ensuring that the inventory is complete and timely filed with the court. The guardian also must safeguard the assets by taking charge of the income and bills, locking away valuables, reviewing financial statements regularly, ensuring upkeep of property, investigating eligibility for public benefits, and consulting with accountants and financial advisors if necessary. A guardian may be needed to apply for Medicaid for health care or long-term care coverage. A guardian must be alert to any scams or any exploitation by third parties.
(3) Keep the estate assets separate. Guardians must never commingle the person's money and property with their own, and must maintain an "arm's length" in financial transactions. The guardian must maintain separate accounts for the estate funds, titled as a fiduciary account.
(4) Maintain good records and report to court. A guardian must consistently keep detailed records of income and expenses, supported by receipts, and must use this record to complete the annual accounting for the court. The guardian also must submit a final accounting after the death of the individual.

17.4.6 Guardian Fees

Guardians are generally entitled to reasonable compensation for their services. The fee usually is taken from the estate of the individual served, and the guardian must seek approval of the court for the fees. The fee may be a percentage of the value of the assets, an hourly rate, or in some cases for nonprofit entities a flat sum per case [34, 50].

The court must determine that the fees are "reasonable," based on factors such as what services the guardian provided, whether the services were necessary, the guardian's expertise and experience level, the difficulty of the work and the skill required, the degree of risk, and the fees customarily paid in the community.[20] Family members serving as guardian often are not paid—although they may be entitled to compensation. Their compensation may not necessarily be at the same level as a professional, and they may not be entitled to payment for services that family members generally provide [61].

Guardian fees can be substantial, and fee disputes have been frequent. In some cases, press stories have highlighted excessive guardian fees that drain the estates of those served. If the guardian is an attorney, it is important to determine whether the fees sought are at the rate for legal services or for guardianship services, which may be different, with the attorney rate substantially higher [61]. If the guardian is a professional, it is important to determine if the fees sought are for services that could only be performed by the skilled professional, or whether a staff member could have performed the services at a lower rate—for example, shopping for clothes or groceries.

Another key question is what the guardian should do if the person's money runs out—should the guardian continue to perform services without fees? The NGA Standards require that the guardian report to the court on "any likelihood that funds will be exhausted and advise the court whether the guardian intends to seek removal when there are no longer funds to pay fees. A guardian may not abandon the person when estate funds are exhausted and shall make appropriate succession plans."[21] Some courts require that the

[18] NGA Standards #17, 18, 19.
[19] NGA Standard #17.
[20] NGA Standard #22.
[21] NGA Standard #22.

guardian designate a successor before leaving the case. Other questions are how courts should best resolve fee disputes, and what information about anticipated fees the guardian should provide up front at appointment. Court practices vary significantly on all of these issues.

The NGA *Standards of Practice* state that the guardian must "bear in mind at all times the responsibility to conserve the person's estate" when charging a fee for services. The *Standards* further state that the guardian should "disclose in writing the basis for the fee" at the guardian's first appearance in the case; report to the court "any likelihood that funds will be exhausted;" may "not abandon the person when estate funds are exhausted;" and must "make appropriate plans."[22]

Some states provide for guardianship of last resort mechanisms or public guardianship programs if the estate is insufficient to pay a private guardian [66]. For example some state laws require that if there is no one willing and able to serve as guardian, a state agency such as the department of human services will serve, or a panel of paid professionals will serve, paid from state funds. Other states have an explicit office of public guardianship staffed to handle a range of indigent cases—supported by state appropriations, but often insufficiently funded to meet the full need. While some public guardianship programs have staffing ratios beyond which they may not accept cases, and some may have discretion in accepting cases, others must accept "unbefriended" individuals in need, making for caseloads that are detrimental to good care [66].

17.4.7 Guardian Training and Assistance

Although serving as guardian is clearly a challenging role with a high duty of accountability, many guardians have little or no training. Professional guardians may be certified at the state or national level [23, 24], but family guardians come to the role unprepared and without knowing what is expected. A few states have a minimum training requirement for guardians. Some courts have developed pamphlets, instructions and training videos for prospective guardians (ABA Commission, "Guardianship Law and Practice;" Karp and Wood [43]—and a few courts designate staff to provide guardians with orientation and technical assistance. In some states, guardianship handbooks provide forms, information on decision-making, reporting requirements and links to community resources (ABA Commission, "Guardianship Law and Practice"). Recently the U.S. Consumer Financial Protection Bureau has developed a series of guides called *Managing Someone Else's Money* for family financial caregivers including guardians of property [70]. These plain language guides set out basic fiduciary duties and alert guardians to possible financial exploitation and consumer scams. But generally, training for guardians is clearly needed, and "lack of guardianship training is especially apparent in cases where family or friends are assigned as guardian with little guidance on the boundaries of their authority or knowledge of appropriate actions" [74].

17.5 Guardian Accountability and Court Oversight

Adult guardianship can be seen as having a "front end" (encompassing all the steps in the appointment process) and a "back end" consisting of court oversight procedures. Sometimes judges and judicial staff may view a case as "closed" once a guardian is appointed, but in fact the job of the court is just beginning. Under the ancient concept of *parens patriae,* the king, and later the state, is responsible for those who cannot take care of themselves or their property. The court, on behalf of the state, appoints a guardian as an agent to carry out this responsibility, and must provide supervision.

Over the past 25 years advocates have called for stronger monitoring procedures [11, 74; Stetson Law Review 2002], and many states have enacted statutory provisions bolstering oversight (ABA Commission, "Guardianship Law and Practice"). The 1997 Uniform Guardianship and Protective Proceedings Act states that courts must "establish a system for monitoring guardianships, including the filing and review of annual reports."[23] The National Probate Court Standards commentary observes that "Although probate courts cannot be expected to provide daily supervision of the guardians' or conservator's role, they should not assume a passive role, responding only upon the filing of a complaint.

The safety and well-being of the respondent and the respondent's estate "remain the responsibility of the court following appointment."[24] In practice, however, monitoring is uneven—and sometimes, as press stories highlight, next to nonexistent. Courts are strapped by budget limitations and competing priorities, and often cannot invest staff as needed, or in some cases simply may not devote the attention required.

[22]NGA Standard #22.

[23]Uniform Guardianship and Protective Proceedings Act, Sec. 317.

[24]National Probate Court Standards, National College of Probate Judges, Sec. 3.3.19 (2013).

17.5.1 Signs of Problem Guardianship Cases

Courts must be alert to guardians who are having difficulties, or who may be malfeasant or abusive. Adult protective services, long-term care ombudsmen, and aging/disability agency staff also should be knowledgeable about "red flags" indicating problems that need court investigation.

The National Association for Court Management has a list of such flags that should trigger more rigorous court review.[25] For example, under "financial/accounting irregularities" the list includes that the guardian: does not pay the bills or pays irregularly; does not pay for needed clothing or services; does not apply for Medicaid when needed; does not renew a bond when required, or the bond is revoked; and has questionable accounting entries such as utility charges when the person is not living at home, checks written for case, numerous ATM withdrawals, or missing entries. Under "compliance/quality of care issues" the list includes that the guardian does not cooperate with service providers or "is reluctant to spend money on the respondent;" says the person cannot afford needed services when this may not be the case; does not file reports on time; is not visiting regularly; or there are repeated complaints from family or friends about the guardian's care [50, 59].

Other factors that might indicate high risk and call for extra scrutiny are that the person has no relatives or friends, the estate is large, the guardian has used multiple attorneys or attorneys withdraw from the case, the guardian has health or personal problems, the guardian has little experience; or there are signs of financial problems such as tax liens, judgments, or bankruptcy [43].

17.5.2 Asset Protection

Courts use various methods to prevent or target exploitation of assets. If the court assesses high risk of exploitation, it can freeze assets pending review and possible sanctioning or removal of the guardian.

Courts, and many state statutes, generally require a guardian of property to submit an inventory of the estate following appointment. The National Probate Court Standards recommend that courts require an inventory and appraisal of the assets within 60 days of the guardian's appointment.[26] The guardian must find and list for the court all of the income, assets, debts and any legal claims. This might include bank accounts, cash, annuities, public benefits, real estate, cars, insurance policies, trusts for which the person is a beneficiary, stocks and bonds, jewelry, furniture, collections, and household items [59, 70].

Preparing an inventory and appraisal can be an arduous task. It may involve sorting through the person's home and through accumulated mail, locating financial records, and speaking with friends and professionals. It may be especially difficult where there has been hoarding, and cash and financial records may be found among stacks of papers or in unlikely places [59].

Some courts require the guardian of property to post a bond, which is the most effective way to protect the person's assets [59].[27] As reflected in state law, the requirement for a bond for all liquid assets plus annual income has not been standard over the years in many states. It has been considered discretionary. The presumption has been that no guardian would ever co-mingle assets or take assets from the person in guardianship. That perspective has changed with the negative media publicity courts and guardianships have received in recent years. This change is reflected in the revised National Probate Court Standards, which states that "except in unusual circumstances, probate courts should require all conservators to post a surety bond in an amount equal to the liquid assets and annual income of the estate.[28] The National Guardianship Association Standards state that "the conservator shall take all steps necessary to obtain a bond to protect the estate, including obtaining a court order."[29] Approximately 20 state statutes require a guardian of property to post bond, and the remainder allow courts some or complete discretion. These statutes vary in the specifying exceptions as well as the amount of the bond [36].

By bonding, courts can remove a major cause of financial abuse of people in guardianship. If guardians mismanage the assets or take money from the guardianship, the bonding insurance can restore the lost money. The cost of bonding is typically low for the protection it provides and it is paid for by the guardianship estate, not the guardian or the court. In addition, bonding companies may alert the court if the guardian is not paying the annual bond premiums—a serious event may indicate that financial abuse is taking place.

Courts must check to see that any required bond actually is in place, and some require filing of a "proof of bond." Another important court practice is to periodically review the sufficiency of the bond to see whether the amount needs to be adjusted. Having ensured the bond is in place and

[25]National Association for Court Management, Adult Guardianship Guide, 2014, based on a list of red flags from Quinn and Krooks [59, pp. 1663–1665]. Also see National Probate Court Standards, 3.3.17.

[26]National College of Probate Judges, National Probate Court Standards, 3.3.16 (2013), http://ncsc.contentdm.oclc.org/cdm/ref/collection/spcts/id/240.

[27]For a discussion of bonds, see Sect. 17.3.6 in this chapter.

[28]Standard 3.3.15, National Probate Court Standards.

[29]Standard #18(IV), National Guardianship Association Standards of Practice.

sufficient to cover needs, courts must call in the bond when financial exploitation has occurred [43, 59].

An alternative—or additional—approach to protecting assets is to restrict accounts. The court may require approval for expenditures above a certain amount or for expenses that are out of the ordinary and beyond routine needs—such as home modification or purchase of medical equipment. Sometimes the court may require that accounts above a specified amount be restricted or "blocked" by the bank, and that the guardian must file a "proof of restricted account" [43]. However, this technique may not be effective if there are bank mergers or reorganizations that could make it difficult to maintain and trace records on the account restrictions. Some banks no longer accept restricted accounts [59]. Yet another strategy is to require court approval for specific transactions such as sale of a residence, gifts or loans above a designated amount, building repairs or renovations, or reverse mortgages.

17.5.3 Reports and Accounts

All states require guardians of property to submit regular—generally annual—accountings to court, and some also require forward-looking financial plans. The guardian must report income, expenses, and assets. Many courts require the guardian to submit supporting bank statement, brokerage statements, and receipts [43, 50].

Virtually all states require guardians of the person to submit personal status reports on the well-being of the individual, significant changes in the person's condition, the actions taken by the guardian, and whether the guardian thinks the guardianship should be modified or terminated. Some states also require the submission of forward-looking guardianship care plans [43].

For both accountings and reports, some states have uniform accounting forms, but in others the forms differ from court to court. Some courts have posted the forms on their websites. An increasing number of courts allow or require guardians to file electronically. Ideally, courts should have a tracking system to enter accountings and reports received in a database, and identify cases in which accountings and reports are not timely received. Through such a database, courts may be able to generate reminders of accountings and reports coming due or overdue, and flag late filings for investigation. The Minnesota Judicial Branch operates a pioneering conservator tracking software system called MyMNConservator—an online conservator account reporting application through which conservators file their inventory and annual accountings electronically (Minnesota Judicial Branch). However, generally court technology, case management systems, court staff dedicated to tracking of filings, and court financial resources vary—and thus the consistency of filings is uneven [2, 44, 71].

What happens if a guardian fails to timely file an accounting or report? Some courts are overloaded with cases and unable to respond. In other courts, staff may contact the guardian to inquire, and if the filings are still not made, may schedule a compliance conference or hearing, send out an investigator, and eventually may remove the guardian (Karp and Wood [43].

In addition to regular filing of accountings and reports, many courts require guardians to notify them of significant events such as a change in residential setting, move outside the state or death of the individual. Often the court sends a notice of the filing of reports or accountings, or of significant changes, to interested parties listed in the petition or to certain designated parties. This allows third parties to maintain current information about the case and alert the court about problems.

17.5.4 Court Review, Investigation, and Sanctions

While requirements to file accountings and reports may spur guardians to comply with their duties, the filings themselves serve little purpose if the court does not review them. The judge may personally review the filings, but more frequently designates court staff, contracted accountants, attorneys or other qualified examiners, including trained volunteers, to conduct the review. Judges and court staff surveyed about court oversight agreed that "specialized court staff are essential to raise guardianship monitoring standards" [74]. It is easier to audit a financial accounting than to assess the adequacy of a status report on the person's well-being, given changing needs and conditions.

Some courts, overwhelmed with cases, conduct random audits of accounts rather than reviewing every filing. A few leading courts are piloting the use of risk assessment strategies in reviewing the filings. They list specific factors that might be signs of possible abuse, neglect or exploitation, and place a priority on intensive review of those cases. Cases may be assigned to different review categories depending on the risk involved (National Association for Court Management 2014).

Another approach to identifying problems is through complaints. The National Probate Court Standards recommend that courts "establish a clear and easy-to-use process for communicating concerns about guardianships and conservatorships and the performance of guardians/conservators."[30] Courts should make the complaint procedure known to

[30]National Probate Court Standards 3.3.18.

individuals under guardianship, family members, interested parties and the public; and should develop a protocol for timely court review [59; National Association for Court Management 2014].

In some instances, courts have ordered in depth accountings by certified public accountants which focus on all the financial assets of the person, including bank accounts and investments from the beginning of the account until the current time. This type of accounting, termed a "forensic accounting," focuses on where the assets came from, how they were dispersed, to whom, and when. It is different than a court accounting in that it is a complete investigation of the assets conducted by a neutral party. Courts may order a forensic accounting when it is alleged that someone has been taking the person's money.

If the court review uncovers a problem—such as a guardian needing assistance with his or her fiduciary duties or a guardian whose own condition may be declining—or instances of abuse, the court may call the guardian in for a hearing or send out an investigator or appoint an attorney for the person. Some courts have supplemented court staff with a trained cadre of volunteer visitors to serve as the "eyes and ears of the court." These programs train community volunteers or students to review records, gather data, make visits and report to the court [9].

If the court finds guardian fraud, malfeasance, or abuse, it must act quickly to protect the individual. The *National Probate Court Standards* provide that "When probate courts learn of a missing, neglected, or abused respondent or that a respondent's assets are endangered, they should take timely action to ensure the safety and welfare of that respondent and/or the respondent's estate."[31] The court may fine or remove the guardian, appoint a co-guardian or a successor guardian, and call in a bond when necessary. In some instances, the court may use mediation to address disputes and problems with high conflict families. The court also may report the matter to a state professional licensing or certification agency, such as a guardianship certification board or a bar association disciplinary committee. In addition, in many states judges and court personnel are mandatory reporters of abuse, neglect, and exploitation, but in any case should report to adult protective services (NACM 2014), and if they suspect a crime has been committed, to law enforcement.

17.6 Guardianship Around the Globe

In the United States, by state law, history, and long tradition, guardianship is lodged in the courts [43, 51, 82]. However, in other countries around the world, the guardianship system is structured differently, and non-court entities may play a substantial role. In Dayton, *Comparative Perspectives on Adult Guardianship* [27], guardianship experts from all over the world have described their country's practices. The following profiles for a sample of nations show the diversity of structures and processes.

In Tribal Nations in the U.S., there is a great deal of diversity in guardianship law and practice. There are 566 federally recognized tribal government in the country. State courts do not have jurisdiction over guardianship proceedings involving a tribal member domiciled in Indian lands. Instead, with some exceptions, the tribal court has jurisdiction over guardianship of person and estate. One example is the Navajo Nation, which governs the largest Indian reservation in the U.S. The Navajo Nation Code includes guardianship provisions enacted in 1945. Any person can file a petition for the appointment of a guardian, and a social worker conducts an investigation for a court decision. There is little guidance in statutory standards on procedural due process and use of less restrictive options, and thus the courts look to Navajo traditions that respect individual liberty [28].

In Canada, responsibility for guardianship lies with the superior courts of the provinces and territories. As with the U.S., there is no federal jurisdiction. Recent legislative changes reflect a greater emphasis on less restrictive options, including supported decision-making, which is recognized by a number of Canadian jurisdictions. For instance, British Columbia has enacted a Representation Agreement Act that allows adults to enter into a legally recognized supported decision-making agreement (Canadian Center for Elder Law). In addition, some jurisdictions are exploring the use of mediation in contested guardianship situations.

Canadian provincial and territorial public guardian and trustee services monitor private guardians appointed by the courts. These services receive and review guardian accountings; report annually to government agencies; and are subject to independent audits [35].

In England, adult guardianship law is rooted in the Mental Capacity Act of 2005, which is based on: (1) functional, decision-specific and time-specific determinations of capacity; and (2) a requirement for surrogate decisions to be in the best interests of the individual. The Court of Protection may appoint a "deputy" to make decisions on behalf of another. The court may require the deputy to give security to and submit reports and account to the Public Guardian. The Public Guardian supervises deputies appointed by the court. In addition, bonds are required of both lay and professional deputies, and "General Visitors" regularly contact deputies as part of the Public Guardian supervision [47].

In Sweden, the "chief guardian" of a local jurisdiction receives applications for appointment of a custodian ("god man") or trustee ("administrator"), and collects medical and

[31]National Probate Court Standards 3.3.19.

other documentation before sending the application to a district court with a request for appointment. Sometimes a relative is appointed, but often the court names an outside party. In most custodianship cases, the person consents. The custodian and trustee must assert the individual's rights, administer the property and care for the person. Custodians and trustees must submit annual reports including accountings to the chief guardian or the chief guardian board in the municipality. County administrative boards supervise the local chief guardian or board. [31, 82].

In France, according to a 1968 law and reforms added in 2007, there are a range of legal mechanisms for individuals needing help in decision-making. A "judicial safeguard" is a temporary protection through which a fraudulent transaction can be declared null and void. In a "curatelle" the court appoints legal counsel to advise and check when an individual engages in legal transactions that can affect his or her estate. The person retains rights and can disagree with the counselor, and then a judge must make a determination. With a stronger "tutelle," there is a court-appointed surrogate decision-maker akin to a guardian. A guardian must submit an inventory to the head clerk of the court, and must submit annual accountings. There is no requirement for a report on the welfare of the person. The clerk may ask for assistance from various state agencies such as the French Treasury or other financial bodies. In certain cases, the judge can name a surrogate guardian or form a family council to monitor the guardian. If a problem is identified, the judge or district attorney can order injunctions and fines or remove the guardian [48].

In Israel, guardianship is guided by the 1962 Legal Capacity and Guardianship Act, and the Legal Capacity and Guardianship Regulations of 1970, which allow a court to appoint a guardian for a person deemed unable to manage his or her affairs. A family member or local welfare officers may initiate a proceeding. Since 1996, family courts have had jurisdiction over guardianship, and aim to use less formal, more family-oriented procedures. Israel's Public Guardian has responsibility for monitoring guardians. Guardians must submit an annual report. A 2013 critique of Israel's guardianship system addressed the lack of data, need for additional procedural protections, lack of guidelines for capacity assessment, and need for limited orders [29].

In China, there is no formal judicial declaration of incapacity and appointment of a guardian. Instead, the *General Principles of Civil Law* provide that family members are guardian for an individual in a listed order of priority—spouse, parent, adult child, other near relative—or other willing relative or friend having approval from the unit to which the person belongs or from the neighborhood or village committee where he or she lives. According to Confucian teachings, it is the family and not the individual that is most important, and the emphasis is on family and community obligations rather than individual rights. However, there is no oversight of family guardians nor guidance in their role, leaving the door open to possible exploitation or neglect despite the cultural priority on family. There have been calls for reform of guardianship in China to provide for the protection, welfare, and autonomy of adults [25].

In Japan, with its rapidly growing aging population and marked decline in birth rate, guardianship is gaining greater visibility, and is guided by a 2000 Adult Guardianship Law that sought to introduce a more rights-based approach. There are two types of adult guardianship. The first is statutory guardianship—consisting of gradations of "guardianship," "curatorship," and "advisorship." In addition to the individual, a family member or mayor of the village or city where the person lives may petition for guardianship. The second type of guardianship is a "continuing power of attorney" in which a person may select a guardian and provide instructions while able to do so. Once created, the power of attorney is registered, and a family court appoints a supervisor to oversee it [17].

Two important international documents address adult guardianship reform. In many countries, the 2006 U.N. *Convention on the Rights of Persons with Disabilities* has triggered changes in guardianship law and practice by stating that "persons with disabilities enjoy legal capacity on an equal basis with others in all aspects of life;" and that governments must provide necessary supports to enable individuals to exercise their rights to make their own decisions. This represents a dramatic shift in the perception of guardianship, and drives changes to enhance self-determination. In 2010, the First World Congress on Adult Guardianship Law in Yokohama, Japan offered an international exchange of ideas and practices, and resulted in a *Yokohama Declaration* setting out key principles, while recognizing and affirming the principles of the U.N. Convention [86].

17.7 Future Directions

Three landmark adult guardianship reform conferences in the United States, bolstered by the two guiding international documents described above, have set out a distinct and challenging set of future directions for improving guardianship and other options for decision-making. In 1988, the First National Guardianship Symposium sponsored by two American Bar Association Commissions gathered an interdisciplinary group at the "Wingspread" conference facility in Wisconsin and came out with sweeping recommendations to better safeguard the rights while providing for the needs of individuals. Thirteen years later, the Second National Guardianship Conference (known as "Wingspan"), at the Stetson University School of Law, identified clear steps in education, training, practice, data collection, funding, and research. Some of these recommendations found their way into state law, court rules, and uniform acts [38]. In 2011, a Third National Guardianship Summit sponsored by the National Guardianship Network set out standards for guardian performance and decision-making. Taken together, these key recommendations urge action on a number of fronts:

- Data Collection. Tackling guardianship reform without data remains problematic. A major hope lies in improving court databases and tracking technology such as the online system used by the Minnesota Judicial Branch, currently being adapted by other states [30].
- A Range of Decision-Making Options, including Supported Decision-Making. Boosted by the U.N. Convention on the Rights of Persons with Disabilities, reform is beginning to acknowledge that there are a range of decision-making abilities and needs, and these must be addressed by a range of options and supports that strengthen self-determination where possible.
- Procedural Safeguards. While most state statutes require procedural due process rights in guardianship proceedings, practice varies greatly on the quality of the notice provided, the efforts to ensure the individual can be present at the hearing, the provision of hearing rights, and perhaps most important of all, the appointment of effective counsel to give the individual a voice in the system and ensure that all evidence and possibilities are examined.
- Determination of Need for a Guardian. Years ago, the court's determination triggering appointment of a guardian was based primarily on medical conditions such as dementia, mental illness, or intellectual disability. Statutes now envision a more robust determination based on functional abilities and needs for support [13, 16, 8, 15]. Attorneys and judges must not only examine abilities, but must ensure attention to less restrictive options before looking to guardianship. The American Bar Association is developing a tool for attorney to operationalize the "least restrictive alternative" principle and find ways to provide supports short of guardianship where possible [10].
- Limited Orders; Restoration of Rights. While most state statutes clearly provide for or prefer limited guardianship orders, in practice such orders appear rarely sought, since tailoring orders requires additional effort; returning to court if conditions change is expensive; and third parties may find it more difficult to recognize and enforce limited orders. Nonetheless, if rights are to be lost in guardianship, they should be limited to those areas in which help or protection is actually needed [33]. Moreover, a person's condition may improve over time, or the person may gain necessary supports. A periodic reexamination of the need for guardianship, as well as a readily usable process for termination of the order and restoration of rights, is critical to self-determination [22].
- Guardian Standards and Qualifications. As detailed above, lay and professional guardians need standards to give guidance in decision-making and conduct. The National Guardianship Association 2013 *Standards of Practice* offer detailed instructions, and may be used or adapted by states.
- Court Monitoring. Courts must strengthen guardian accountability and deter abusive practices through measures to protect assets, ensure the timely filing of reports and accounts, identify and address "red flag" problems; review reports and investigate problems, and train, sanction or remove guardians. Additionally, programs for courts to assist family guardians could catalyze better performance.

Court-Community Partnerships. While courts are responsible for oversight of guardianship in the United States, executive branch and community agencies can play an important role. For example, frequently, guardianship cases come to the attention of the courts through adult protective services; and once a guardian is appointed, APS may receive reports if a guardian is suspected of abuse, neglect, or exploitation. Long-term care ombudsman programs regularly interact with individuals under guardianship, and can contact the court if they spot problems. Local Social Security field offices appoint representative payees to manage benefits for a beneficiary unable to manage his or her own benefits, and coordination between the court and the Social Security office is essential, as they are serving largely the same population [71, 72]. Mental health agencies and developmental disabilities councils serve individuals who may be under guardianship and need to ensure strong relationships with the court. Local or regional area agencies on aging provide or support many services an individual under guardianship needs. Moreover, community agencies can provide training for guardians and court staff, and can help supply volunteers for monitoring.

For all of these reasons, the 2011 Third National Guardianship Summit recommended that states create "working interdisciplinary networks of guardianship stakeholders" (WINGS) to improve adult guardianship and offer a continuing forum for evaluation of strengths and weaknesses of the guardianship system. By combining the efforts of all public and private stakeholders (such as adult protective services, the state protection and advocacy agency, agencies on aging, bar associations and mental health agencies) under court initiatives, states can strengthen judicial processes, enhance services, better protect individual rights and promote fiduciary standards and guardian accountability (Symposium, Third National Guardianship Summit [55, 56, 64]. As of 2015, the National Guardianship Network—including 11 national organizations dedicated to effective adult guardianship law and practice—has sponsored court-initiated WINGS groups in 10 states, and 4 additional states independently have developed similar groups [55, 56]. These ongoing court-community partnerships use "collective action" strategies to make important changes benefiting the lives of at-risk individuals [56, 39].

17.8 Conclusion

Guardianship is a substantial intervention that should be a last resort—after careful examination shows that other decision-making options are not feasible. With effective court supervision, adult guardianship can be a bulwark against elder abuse, neglect, and exploitation. To provide needed care and protection, and to maximize the person's self-determination as much as possible, family and other lay guardians—as well as professional guardians—need support, training, clear standards of practice, and consistent oversight. While data is not available on the frequency, some guardianships do "go bad." Courts require systems and funding for screening potential guardians, methodically receiving and reviewing guardian reports, identifying red flags in problematic cases, and removing or sanctioning guardians that fail to abide by their fiduciary duties. Courts and community stakeholders, including adult protective services, must partner to improve guardian accountability and the guardianship system.

References

1. Administration on Community Living. http://www.aoa.gov/Aging_Statistics/Profile/2014/2.aspx (2014). Retrieved 20 Nov 2015.
2. Administrative Conference of the United States. SSA Representative Payee: survey of state guardianship laws and court practices. https://www.acus.gov/documents/report (2015). Retrieved 29 Nov 2015.
3. Aging Life Care Association. http://www.aginglifecare.org/ALCA/About_Aging_Life_Care/ALCA/Features/The_Transition.aspx. Retrieved 2 Jan 2016.
4. Aging with Dignity. Five wishes: changing the way we talk about and plan for care at the end of life. https://agingwithdignity.org/five-wishes/about-five-wishes. Retrieved 22 Nov 2015.
5. Alzheimer's Association. 2015 Alzheimer's facts and figures. http://www.alz.org/facts/overview.asp (2015). Retrieved 30 Nov 2015.
6. American Bar Association Commission on Law and Aging, Hurme S. Representation and investigation in guardianship proceedings. http://www.americanbar.org/groups/law_aging/resources/guardianship_law_practice.html (2014). Retrieved 2 Jan 2016.
7. American Bar Association Commission on Law and Aging, Hurme S. http://www.americanbar.org/content/dam/aba/administrative/law_aging/CHARTStateGuardianCertification.authcheckdam.pdf (2015).
8. American Bar Association Commission on Law and Aging. Making health care decisions for someone else: a how-to guide. http://www.americanbar.org/groups/law_aging/resources/health_care_decision_making.html. Retrieved 24 Nov 2015.
9. American Bar Association Commission on Law and Aging. Volunteer guardianship monitoring and assistance: serving the court and the community. http://www.americanbar.org/groups/law_aging/resources/guardianship_law_practice/court_volunteer_guardianshipmonitoring.html (2011). Retrieved 29 Nov 2015.
10. American Bar Association Commission on Law and Aging, with Commission on Disability Rights, Section on Civil Rights and Social Justice, and Section on Real Property, Trust and Estate Law. PRACTICAL checklist for attorneys for supporting decision-making (2016).
11. American Bar Association Commission on the Mentally Disabled & Commission on Legal Problems of the Elderly. Guardianship: an agenda for reform: recommendations of the national guardianship symposium (1989).
12. American Association of Daily Money Managers. http://aadmm.com. Retrieved 2 Jan 2016.
13. American Bar Association Commission on Law and Aging. Guardianship law and practice. http://www.americanbar.org/groups/law_aging/resources/guardianship_law_practice.html. Retrieved 25 Nov 2015.
14. American Bar Association Commission on Law and Aging, Hurme S. Notice in guardianship proceedings. http://www.americanbar.org/groups/law_aging/resources/guardianship_law_practice.html (2014). Retrieved 2 Jan 2016.
15. American Bar Association Commission on law and Aging, American Psychological Association & National College of Probate Judges. Judicial Determination of Capacity of Older Adults in Guardianship Proceedings: A Handbook for Judges. 2006.
16. American Bar Association Commission on Law and Aging. http://www.americanbar.org/content/dam/aba/administrative/law_aging/Emergency_Guardianship_Chart.authcheckdam.pdf (2014). Retrieved 2 Jan 2016.
17. Arai M. Guardianship in Japan under the adult guardianship law of 2000. In: Dayton AK, editor. Comparative perspectives on adult guardianship. Carolina: Carolina Academic Press; 2014. p. 167–79.
18. Association for Conflict Resolution. Elder care and elder family decision-making mediation: training objectives and commentary. http://acreldersection.weebly.com/ (2012). Retrieved 11/30/15.
19. Association for Conflict Resolution. Guidelines for eldercaring coordination. http://acreldersection.weebly.com/ (2014). Retrieved 11/30/15
20. Blanck P, Martinis J. The right to make choices the national resource center for supported decision-making. Inclusion. 2015;3 (1):24–33.
21. Bronson S, Fieldstone L. From friction to fireworks to focus: eldercaring coordination sheds light in high conflict cases, experience. ABA Senior Lawyers Division, Fall/Winter; 2015.
22. Cassidy J. Restoration of rights in the termination of adult guardianship. Elder Law J. 2015;23:83–122.
23. Center for Guardianship Certification. http://www.guardianshipcert.org/. Retrieved 25 Nov 2015.
24. Center for Guardianship Certification. http://guardianshipcert.org/become_certified_states.cfm. Retrieved 24 Nov 2015.

25. Chan C, Lee R. Adult guardianship law in China: traditional values and modern international developments. In: Dayton AK, editor. Comparative Perspectives on Adult Guardianship. Durham: Carolina Academic Press; 2014. p. 123–36.
26. Conference of State Court Administrators. The demographic imperative: guardianships and conservatorships. National Center for State Courts. http://www.eldersandcourts.org/Guardianship/Guardianship-Basics/Guardianship-Data.aspx (2010). Retrieved 29 Nov 2015.
27. Dayton AK, editor. Comparative perspectives on adult guardianship. Durham: Carolina Academic Press; 2014.
28. Deer S, Routel C. Adult Guardianship and Tribal Nations in the U.S. In: Dayton AK, editor. Comparative perspectives on adult guardianship. Durham: Carolina Academic Press; 2014. p. 71–81.
29. Doron I, Waksman Y. Elder guardianship in Israel. In: Dayton AK, editor. Comparative perspectives on adult guardianship. Durham: Carolina Academic Press; 2014. p. 153–65.
30. Elders and the Courts, National Center for State Courts. Conservator Accountability Project. http://www.eldersandcourts.org/Guardianship/Conservatorship-Accountability-Project.aspx. Retrieved 1 Mar 2016.
31. Fjordevik C. Adult guardianship in Sweden: a chief guardian's perspective. In: Dayton AK, editor. Comparative perspectives on adult guardianship. Durham: Carolina Academic Press; 2014. p. 207–14.
32. Fleming RB, Morgan RC. Standards of financial decision-making: legal, ethical, and practical issues. Utah Law Rev. 2012;3:1275–328.
33. Frolik L. Promoting judicial acceptance and use of limited guardianship. Wingspan—the second national guardianship conference. Stetson Law Rev. 2002;XXXI(3):735–55.
34. Frolik L, Kaplan R. Elder law in a Nutshell 2014. 6th ed. St Paul: West Academic Publishing; 2014.
35. Gordon RM, Soden A. The guardianship of incapable adults and their property in Canada. In: Dayton AK, editor. Comparative perspectives on adult guardianship. Durham: Carolina Academic Press; 2014. p. 109–22.
36. Gorski K. Conservatorship and Guardianship Bonds: State Statutory Requirements. Bifocal. ABA Commission on Law and Aging. 2014;35(5).
37. Hurme S. State guardian certification chart. http://www.americanbar.org/groups/law_aging/resources/guardianship_law_practice.html (2015). Retrieved 30 Nov 2015.
38. Hurme S, Wood E. Introduction. Symposium—third national guardianship summit: standards of excellence. Utah Law Rev. 2012;3.
39. Kania J. & Kramer M. Collective Impact. Stanford Social Innovation Review. Winter 2011.
40. Kapp MB. Reforming guardianship reform: reflections on disagreements, deficits, and responsibilities. Stetson Law Rev. 2002; XXXI(3):1047–55.
41. Karp N, Wood E. Choosing home for someone else: guardian residential decision-making. Utah Law Rev. 2012;2012(3):1445–90.
42. Karp N, Wood E. Incapacitated and alone: health care decision-making for the unbefriended elderly. ABA Commission on Law and Aging; 2003.
43. Karp N, Wood E. Guarding the guardians: promising practices for court monitoring. AARP Public Policy Institute, #2007-21; 2007.
44. Karp N, Wood E. Guardianship monitoring: a national survey of court practices. AARP Public Policy Institute, #2006-14. http://www.aarp.org/money/estate-planning/info-2006/2006_14_guardianship.html (2006). Retrieved 29 Nov 2015.
45. Keith PM, Wacker RR. Older wards and their guardians. Westport, CT: Praeger; 1994.
46. Kohn N, Blumenthal J, Campbell A. Supported decision-making: a viable alternative to guardianship? Penn State Law Rev. 2013;117:1111–57.
47. Lush D. Guardianship in England and Wales. In: Dayton AK, editor. Comparative perspectives on adult guardianship. Durham: Carolina Academic Press; 2014. p. 137–52.
48. Mercat A. Guardianship and surrogate decision-making in France: additional flexibility and protections. ABA Commission on Law and Aging. Bifocal. 2008;30(1).
49. National Adult Protective Services Resource Center. State of adult protective services: 2012: survey of adult protective services. Springfield: National Adult Protective Services Association. www.napsa-now.org/resource-center/main/ (2012). Retrieved 29 Nov 2015.
50. National Association for Court Management. Adult guardianship guide: a guide to plan, develop and sustain a comprehensive court guardianship and conservatorship program. https://www.nacmnet.org/sites/default/files/publications/AdultGuardianshipGuide_withCover.pdf (2013–2014). Retrieved 24 Nov 2015.
51. National College of Probate Judges. National probate court standards. National Center for State Courts. http://ncsc.contentdm.oclc.org/cdm/ref/collection/spcts/id/240 (2013). Retrieved 29 Nov 2015.
52. National Center on Elder Abuse. FAQs. www.ncea.aoa.gov/faq/index.aspx (2016). Retrieved 2/25/16.
53. National Guardianship Association. Standards of practice. http://www.guardianship.org/documents/Standards_of_Practice.pdf (2013). Retrieved 21 Nov 2015.
54. National Guardianship Association. Position statement on guardianship, surrogate decision-making, and supported decision-making. http://www.guardianship.org/ (2015). Retrieved 22 Nov 2015.
55. National Guardianship Network. www.nationalguardianshipnetwork.org. Retrieved 24 Nov 2015.
56. National Guardianship Network. Decision making without guardianship. http://www.naela.org/NGN/About_Guardianship/Decision_Making_Without_Guardianship (2014). Retrieved 24 July 2015.
57. National POLST Paradigm. http://www.polst.org/about-the-nationa-polst-paradigm/. Retrieved 29 Nov 2015.
58. Quinn MJ. Guardianship of adults: achieving justice, autonomy, and safety. New York: Springer; 2005.
59. Quinn MJ, Krooks HS. The relationship between the guardian and the court. Utah Law Rev. 2012;2012(3):1611–66.
60. Sabatino C. Top ten myths and facts about health care advance directives. Bifocal. 2015;37(1):6–9.
61. Seal C, Crona S. Standards for guardian fees. Utah Law Rev. 2012;3:1575–610.
62. Sickler S. Use joint tenancy only with extreme caution. Elder's Advis. 1999;1(2):35–7.
63. Stiegel L. Alternatives to guardianship: substantive training materials and module for professionals working with the elderly and persons with disabilities. Washington: American Bar Association, Commission on Law and Aging; 1992.
64. Symposium—Third National Guardianship Summit: Standards of Excellence. Utah Law Rev. 2012;2012(3).
65. Teaster P. When the state takes over a life: the public guardian as public administrator. Public Adm Rev. 2003;63:396.
66. Teaster P, Wood E, Schmidt W, Lawrence S. Public guardianship after 25 years: in the best interest of incapacitated people? Kentucky: University of Kentucky & ABA Commission on Law and Aging; 2007.
67. The Conversation Project. http://theconversationproject.org/. Retrieved 22 Nov 2015.

68. The Law Dictionary. Black's law dictionary online legal dictionary, 2nd ed. http://thelawdictionary.org/fiduciary. Retrieved 21 Nov 2015.
69. The National POLST Paradigm. http://www.polst.org. Retrieved 2 Jan 2016.
70. U.S. Consumer Financial Protection Bureau. Managing someone Else's money guides. http://www.consumerfinance.gov/managing-someone-elses-money (2013). Retrieved 21 Nov 2015.
71. U.S. Government Accountability Office. Guardianships: collaboration needed to protect incapacitated elderly people, GAO-04-655; 2004.
72. U.S. Government Accountability Office. Incapacitated adults: oversight of federal fiduciaries and court appointed guardians needs improvement. GAO-11-678; 2011.
73. U.S. Government Accountability Office, Guardianships: Cases of Financial Exploitation, Neglect and Abuse of Seniors, GAO-10-1046; 2010.
74. Uekert B. Center for elders and the courts. In: National Center for State Courts, editor. Adult guardianship court data and issues: results from an online survey, Conference of chief justice and conference of state court administrators; 2010.
75. Uekert B, Van Duizend R. A 'best guess' national estimate and the momentum for reform. In: National Center for State Courts, editor. Future trends in state courts, pp. 107–112. http://www.eldersandcourts.org/Guardianship/Guardianship-Basics/Guardianship-Data.aspx (2011). Retrieved 21 Nov 2015.
76. Uniform Law Commission. Uniform guardianship and protective proceedings act. http://uniformlaws.org/Act.aspx?title=Guardianship (1997). Retrieved 25 Nov 2015.
77. United Nations. Convention on the rights of persons with disabilities. http://www.un.org/disabilities/convention/conventionfull.shtml (2006). Retrieved 2 Jan 2016.
78. Valanejad D. Health care decision-making authority of guardians and agents: an update. Bifocal. 2015;36(6).
79. Vera Guardianship Project, The Vera Institute of Justice. Guardianship practice: a six-year perspective. http://www.vera.org/pubs/guardianship-practice-six-year-perspective-0 (2011). Retrieved 24 Nov 2015.
80. Whitton L, Frolik L. Surrogate decision-making standards for guardians: theory and reality. Utah Law Rev. 2012;3:1491–539.
81. Wingspan—The Second National Guardianship Conference. Stetson Law Rev. 2002;31(3).
82. Wood E. Guardian accountability: key questions and promising practices. In: Dayton AK, editor. Comparative perspectives on adult guardianship. Durham: Carolina Academic Press; 2013.
83. Wood E. Recharging adult guardianship reform: six current paths forward. Touro Law Rev. 2016.
84. Wood E. The paradox of adult guardianship: a solution to—and a source for—elder abuse. Generations. 2012; 36:79–82.
85. Wood E. ADR and aging: what is the nexus and where do we stand? Experience. 2015;24(3):4–7, 38 (American Bar Association Senior Lawyers Section).
86. World Congress on Adult Guardianship Law 2010. Yokohama declaration. http://www.international-guardianship.com/yokohama-declaration.htm. Retrieved 1 Mar 2016.

18 Elder Abuse Forensics: The Intersection of Law and Science

Candace J. Heisler

18.1 Introduction[1]

Historically knowledge of elder abuse has been hampered by limited and inadequate funding to support research and development of evidence-based practices [12, 118]. At the same time the approach to elder abuse has changed from a social services problem to a complex issue that often involves many systems in addition to protective services and social services including medicine, mental health, and civil, and criminal justice. Who can or must intervene, the extent to which an older person can be forced to accept involuntary services, and the kinds of remedies that may be available all begin with the identification of elder abuse, neglect, and exploitation.

In the absence of a body of scientific knowledge specific to older adults and elder abuse, recognition of abuse often mimicked what had been learned from child abuse, and domestic violence research [172] without an assessment if it was the same or different when dealing with older adults. In other situations, protective services and others relied on field experience which was not validated and was based on family-systems' approaches and a belief that elder abuse occurred because of the stress of caregiving for an older adult [171].

The effects of elder abuse are devastating, so identifying elder abuse in all its forms—physical, sexual, financial, psychological/emotional, abandonment, and neglect—is critical. As Dong [53] has written:

> The medical implications of elder abuse and neglect can be devastating. The quality of life can be jeopardized in the forms of declining functional abilities, progressive dependency, a sense of helplessness, social isolation, and a cycle of worsening stress and psychologic decline. The health implications of abuse and neglect include its associations with premature mortality and morbidity. It can induce fractures, depression, dementia, malnutrition, and death. It was found that the risk of death for elder abuse and neglect victims are three times higher than for non-victims. The direct medical costs associated with these violent injuries are estimated to add over $5.3 billion to the nation's annual health expenditures (Dong [53, at p. 293], cites omitted).

As recognition of the extent and complexity of elder abuse has grown, particularly since the late 1980s, legal approaches have expanded to include criminalization of acts of elder abuse, neglect, and exploitation; creation of elder abuse protective and restraining orders; identification of new elder abuse phenomenon, including undue influence and strangulation and suffocation; mandatory reporting in nearly every state and territory and possession of the United States; creation of civil causes of action and enhanced penalties for elder abuse; and expansion of protective proceedings, including guardianships, to protect victims of abuse, neglect, and exploitation and their assets.

All of these changes are predicated on a finding that abuse, neglect, or exploitation has occurred. And it is at this intersection of law and science that this chapter focuses. How are findings of abuse and neglect assessed? Are there other possible explanations and if so, how is abuse or neglect differentiated? In cases of exploitation, the older person's capacity to understand, make a gift, enter into a contract, and/or manage his or her assets may determine if an act is lawful or actionable. What is capacity? How is it assessed? Can a person appear able to manage his or her affairs and have significant brain impairment? What do screening test scores mean? Is brain research changing our understanding of capacity? Is capacity inevitably linked to aging?

As scientific knowledge about injuries and capacity grow, how is new information conveyed to professionals so identification of abuse, neglect, and exploitation improves? And finally what promising practices are developing to improve interventions in elder abuse cases?

[1]Throughout this chapter the term elder abuse refers to older adults as defined by statute. There is no distinction made between older persons with cognitive, mental, or physical disabilities and those older adults without them.

C.J. Heisler (✉)
Heisler and Associates, San Bruno, CA, USA
e-mail: cjheisler@aol.com

X. Dong (ed.), *Elder Abuse*, DOI 10.1007/978-3-319-47504-2_18

This chapter will discuss each of these topics: Part I focuses on the "Context" in which elder abuse cases are heard. Part II will address "Causation", that is the identification of abuse and neglect; Part III will discuss "Capacity" and its assessment; Part IV will focus on Competency and Availability of Critical Experts to recognize and assess abuse; and Part V "Collaboration" concludes with a review of multidisciplinary approaches to improve case assessment and management.

This chapter will focus on "Forensics"; that is "relating to or dealing with the application of scientific methods to legal problems" [102]. Forensic science is "the application of science to questions in a legal system…It involves utilizing experts from differing disciplines to investigate and resolve cases of abuse and neglect" [136, at p. 256].

18.2 Part I Context in Which Forensic Issues Arise

Forensic issues arise in the context of legal actions. Generally, legal actions in elder abuse matters most often arise in criminal, civil, and probate proceedings. Criminal actions focus on whether particular acts are crimes for which an abuser (called a defendant) should be held accountable. Civil actions are brought by a victim or a victim's representative to seek redress for abuse and may take the form of civil lawsuits for damages or recovery of money and other assets and issuance of restraining and protective orders to limit or direct certain conduct between the parties (typically the older adult and the abuser). Probate courts may be part of or separate from the Civil Justice System but hear matters related to Probate, including will contests and protective proceedings, typically leading to creation of guardianships and/or conservatorships. Other chapters in this book describe court systems and guardianships/conservatorships in much greater detail.

Each of these proceedings require that the moving party, e.g., The State, People, or Government in criminal cases; the plaintiff in civil actions, produces a certain amount of evidence to prevail, called the burden of proof.

There are two common burdens of proof: preponderance of the evidence and beyond a reasonable doubt. "Preponderance of the evidence" applies in most civil actions and means "a superiority in weight, force, importance, etc. In legal terms, a preponderance of evidence means that a party has shown that its version of facts, causes, damages, or fault is *more likely than not*…"[163], or that the evidence on one side "outweighs, preponderates over, is more than, the evidence on the other side, not necessarily in number of witnesses or quantity, but in its effect on those to whom it is addressed" (Glage v. Hawes Firearms Co [180] 226 Cal. App.3d 314, 325, 276 Cal.Rptr. 430, quoting People v. Miller [183] 171 Cal. 649, 652, 154 P. 468; In re Angelia P [181] 28 Cal.3d 908, 918, 171 Cal.Rptr. 637, 623 P.2d 198).

"Beyond a reasonable doubt" is a far higher burden of proof, and indeed is the highest burden of proof in law. It applies in a criminal case and means "proof that leaves you (the jury) with an abiding conviction that the charge is true. The evidence need not eliminate all possible doubt because everything in life is open to some possible or imaginary doubt" [184–186].

An attorney considering the filing of a legal action must evaluate what can be proven, who can be shown to be culpable, and if what can be proven meets the legal definition of a crime or civil cause of action. Legal and ethical rules and codes often establish guidelines for such decisions, and especially when the action is brought by state and federal prosecutors.[2] Case evidence is particularly compelling when there is forensic evidence which was collected in a timely fashion and properly analyzed and documented by knowledgeable experts who are well-informed on research and accepted science in their field.

Evidence form experts is commonly received and accepted in the legal system. Generally, the expert must be shown: (1) to have experience, skill, training, education, or knowledge beyond that of an average juror (or fact finder such as the judge or judicial officer hearing a case without a jury); and (2) the expert's information will assist the trier of fact. Of course the information must be relevant, that is, goes to a matter in dispute. Scientific evidence is subject to certain foundational challenges. The evidence (theory, method, or practice) must be shown to be reliable, which historically meant it met the "Frye Test", a showing that there is general consensus in the scientific community about the reliability of the information, theory, or test [179] Frye, a federal case, was widely adopted by states in their case law or statutes [66, 93].

Frye was replaced at the federal level by Daubert v. MerrellDow Pharmaceuticals [182] creating a standard for admissibility that the evidence must be shown to be based on reliable scientific methodology, defined as based on hypotheses that could be replicated or falsified; whether the research was peer-reviewed and published, whether the technique had a known error rate, and whether the findings were generally accepted in the scientific community [66].

[2]See e.g., American Bar Association Model Rules of Professional Conduct [5, 177] 295 U.S. 78, "The [prosecutor] is the representative … of a sovereignty whose obligation to govern impartially is as compelling as its obligation to govern at all; and whose interest, therefore, in a criminal prosecution is not that it shall win a case, but that justice shall be done…." "The [prosecutor] may prosecute with earnestness and vigor—indeed, he should do so…. It is as much his duty to refrain from improper methods calculated to produce a wrongful conviction as it is to use every legitimate means to bring about a just one" (page 88).

States are free to develop their own rules of admissibility. Some have adopted Daubert while many others have adopted the Frye rule. As new markers are identified and tests developed they may face challenge to their admissibility on Frye, Daubert, or another state-standard grounds.

18.3 Part II Causation[3]

It is hard to imagine a more fundamental forensic question than "Is this abuse or neglect"? Distinguishing abuse and neglect from non-abusive causes can be difficult. Older adults may have underlying or chronic medical conditions that leave marks similar to abuse, leading to false positives (skin conditions that mimic bruising attributed to physical abuse). Conversely, "false negatives" may result from misidentifying abuse as age-related or chronic medical conditions (fracture caused by abuse misidentified as a pathologic fracture related to osteoporosis) [95].

In cases resulting in death causation requires more than identification of forensic markers. While there may be proof of elder abuse or neglect, unless the abuse or neglect caused the death the expert will be unable to say that the abuse was the cause of death. "Regarding cause of death determination, it is important to note that, just because elder maltreatment is present, this does not mean that it necessarily caused death. Likewise, just because an individual has severe underlying natural disease that may be sufficient to explain death, this does not mean that the natural disease necessarily caused death. In order to implicate the maltreatment as contributory, it must be linked to a physiological explanation/mechanism of death" [129, at p. 272].

There is no gold standard test for abuse or neglect [57]. To date, and unlike the field of child abuse, researchers have been unable to identity injuries clearly diagnostic of abuse [168]. Elder abuse may be present in many different ways including falls, fractures, dehydration and malnutrition, bruises, pressure ulcers, burns, etc. Physicians and others dealing with possible elder abuse victims rely on forensic markers. Unfortunately, there is often a great overlap among the markers of disease and abuse and neglect [57].

An elder abuse forensic marker indicates if elder abuse, neglect, or exploitation should be suspected or has occurred [43]. "Medical forensic markers of elder abuse and neglect are factors that are relevant to medical and legal determinations of whether elder abuse and neglect has occurred" [57, at p. 341]. They should be evaluated in light of other available information and evidence [95].

Forensic markers [57] may include physical findings, injury patterns, and medical or laboratory signs. Existing literature primarily has focused on suspicious physical injury patterns including bruising, lacerations, fractures, and burns [99]. But there is a growing body of research evaluating medical and laboratory markers that support increased suspicion of elder abuse or neglect including indicators of malnutrition, dehydration, alterations in status of chronic illness, rhabdomyolysis, toxicological findings, hypothermia/hyperthermia, and postmortem biochemical values [79, 99]. Laboratory markers will corroborate a medical finding of abuse or neglect.

In addition, older adults may have conditions associated with physical frailty and psychological and cognitive problems [70, 118]. As a result, they may be unable to describe what happened and how an injury occurred. "The consideration of these underlying conditions must be balanced with the realization that these patients are vulnerable to abuse and neglect. History obtained from several sources, review of records, and careful examination of patterns of injuries can be useful in evaluating these cases" [78, at p. 683].

The remainder of this section will describe forensic markers of abuse and possible alternative explanations that may be offered to counter the conclusion that abuse or neglect has occurred. These alternative explanations should be considered by the health care provider or investigator when assessing information and conclusions. In a court setting, these alternative explanations are likely to be offered by the other side to counter expert opinion that an older person is the victim of abuse.

Table 18.1 describes forensic markers for physical and sexual abuse and neglect, non-abusive explanations for medical findings, and distinguishing characteristics of abuse and neglect. It summarizes the remainder of the content of this section.

18.4 Identification of Physical Abuse

The most common injuries of physical abuse are unexplained bruises, skeletal fractures, abrasions, and head injury [96, 174]. Physical abuse signs may include bruises, skin tears, fractures, burns, and other injuries. Clues to physical abuse may be found after inspection of the injuries, which commonly involve skin, the head, and bone [128]. Bite marks are established evidence of abuse [9, 57].

Most often, the physical injury must be evaluated in the context of the history for a determination of abuse to be made… [128, at p. 735].

[3]Throughout this chapter the term "elder abuse" is used to refer to abuse and neglect. At times the forms are differentiated, most often when the information is specific to a specific f form.

Table 18.1 Distinguishing injuries from other causes: a summary of the chapter content on causation

Injury	Other possible explanations	Indicators of abuse
Falls and fractures	• Medications, illness, environmental factors • Poor bone health (osteoporosis, pathologic fractures)	• Location (head, spine, trunk) • Fracture with rotational component • Multiple injuries in different healing stages • Context of fall or fracture • Patterned injuries
Burns	• Accidental due to reduced pain sensation	• Splash marks in mobile elder • Lack of splash marks in immobile elder • Uniformity of injury depth throughout the injury • Bilateral, stocking, or glove injuries • Patterned injuries
Bruising and other skin injuries	• Age-related skin changes • Senile purpura • Medication	• Size of injury • Location (lateral right arm, head, neck, abdomen, genitalia, buttocks, palms, soles, and ears) • Patterned injuries • Multiple bruises in varying stages of healing (not color)
Blunt force head injuries	• Advanced age, • Accidental falls, • underlying dementia • Anticoagualant medications	• Location of injury • Bleeding patterns
Strangulation and suffocation	• Not detected due to lack of external injuries • Heavy coughing, forceful defecation, skydiving • Age • Underlying medical conditions	• Hoarseness (aphonia) • Difficulty swallowing • Sore throat (odynophagia), dyspnea • Shortness of breath (stridor) • sniffing position to assist with breathing • Patterned injuries • Defensive injuries to anterior neck • Petechiae on neck, head, face, forehead, eyes, ears, conjunctive, and buccal mucosa; at autopsy, undersurface of the scalp and internal organs
Sexual assault	• Attempt to catheterize a patient • Rough perineal care • Age-related skin breakdown • Consensual sexual contact	• Oral venereal lesions • Bruising of the uvula, bleeding • Bruising of the anogenital area • Difficulty sitting and walking • Abdominal bruising • Bruising of the soft palate at the junction of the hard palate • Behavior changes • STDs in nursing home patients • Multiple bladder or urinary tract infections at same time in nursing home setting
Neglect	• Poor quality care • Elder refused care or medical treatment • Underlying medical condition • Cachexia • Medications	• Pressure ulcers • Malnutrition • Dehydration • Poor hygiene • Inadequate or inappropriate clothing • Missing, needed assistive devices • An unexpected deterioration in a person's health • Laboratory findings

18.4.1 Falls and Fractures

Falls can lead to fractures, subdural hematomas, chronic pain, and death [88]. They can be caused by abuse, e.g., being pushed or thrown to the floor or against a hard surface. They may also be an outcome of medications, illness, environmental factors such as a slippery floor, uneven surface, or loose rug, and changes in position or movement [21].

Falls are common. For example, one-third of community-dwelling older persons fall at least once annually. Half of nursing home residents and adults over 80 years fall annually [78]. However, data from 2009, found that falls were both the most common type of unintentional injury in older adults as well as the seventh leading cause of violence-related injury in older adults [31, 176].

The bones of older persons are thinner and less dense, increasing susceptibility to fractures resulting from bone disease or injury. Pathologic fractures[4] can occur to older women with osteoporosis and hip fractures. Prolonged bed rest, chronic limb paralysis, and non-weight bearing status increase the risk of pathologic fractures [86].

Underlying medical conditions can increase the risk for fractures. Osteoporosis, characterized by low bone mass, deterioration of bone tissue, disruption of bone architecture, and compromised bone strength afflicts more than 9.9 million Americans. An additional 43.1 million have low bone density. Half of Caucasian women and 20 % of men will experience an osteoporosis-related fracture during their lifetime. Although osteoporosis is less frequent in African Americans, those with osteoporosis have the same elevated fracture risk as Caucasians [47].

Other conditions associated with older adults that increase the risk of falls without abuse include arthritis, heart conditions, and neurological conditions such as Parkinson's Disease and stroke [78, at p. 682]. Additionally, frailty, a clinical state of increased vulnerability resulting from age-related declines in reserve and function across multiple physiologic systems [173], is associated with falls, hospitalization, comorbidity, functional limitations, disability, and death [62], and is a risk factor for elder abuse [82]. These conditions can be present where abuse is present and where it is not. Therefore, while their presence can increase the risk of falls and fractures, that alone will not distinguish if abuse has occurred. Nor will it eliminate the possibility that abuse has occurred.

Location of the fracture is significant. Fractures in the elderly resulting from bone disease, e.g., osteoporosis, or injury, such as an accidental fall, commonly occur in the vertebrae and hips for women over age 75 and wrists for women under age 75. Fractures to the head, spine and trunk are more likely to be assault injuries than limb fractures, sprains or strains, or musculoskeletal injuries in adults. A spiral fracture of a large bone without a history of gross injury and fractures with a rotational component are diagnostic of abuse [57]. Suspicion of abuse should be raised when persons who are not alcoholics present with fractures at locations other than hip, wrist or vertebrae [57].

Distinguishing falls resulting from abuse from other causation requires an understanding of the context in which they occurred. Patterns of injury and multiple injuries in varying stages of healing should raise a suspicion of abuse [174]. In addition, implausible explanations for the injury, an elder's report of being pushed, and a person accompanying the elder who refuses to let the elder speak, speaks for or over an elder, or refuses to allow the health care provider or investigator to see the older person alone should raise a suspicion of abuse [26].

18.4.2 Burns

Burns often are indicative of elder abuse. It is estimated that 40–70 % of burns in older adults are linked to elder abuse [25]. Clinical and forensic investigations of burn patterns in older adults resemble those found in child abuse [68] and where present should increase a suspicion of abuse [31] and work in child abuse has informed the evaluation of burns in older adults.

Such findings include scalds from hot water with or without the presence of splash marks. If a victim is able to struggle, burns are likely to include splash marks [69]. Splash marks may not be present when victims are immobile and unable to struggle because of movement disorders or contractures suffer burns or have impaired pain sensation. Uniformity of depth throughout the injury is thought to indicate that the victim was held still in the water. Bilateral, or stocking and glove injuries, imply that the person was forcibly immersed. Skin sparing with a surrounding burn area may be evident in flexed surfaces, palms, soles of the feet, or buttocks when in contact with a surface, such as a bath or sink. Patterned injuries may be present when an older person is burned with cigarettes, heated metal objects such as irons, and electrical shocks [65].

18.4.3 Bruising and Other Injuries to Skin

Blunt force traumatic skin injuries caused by elder abuse include bruises, contusions, skin tears, lacerations, and abrasions. Many are overlooked or considered non-abusive because of assumptions about aging and changes in skin. However, skin findings from abuse can often be distinguished from accidental causes by applying forensic knowledge to an awareness of the possibility of abuse [65].

Skin thickness and elasticity decrease with age and chronic sun exposure. Tensile strength also declines increasing susceptibility to various injuries associated with shearing force trauma. Abrasions are superficial scraping injuries to the outer layer of the skin. Lacerations are full thickness splitting of the skin. Abrasions are caused by movement of the skin over rough surfaces; lacerations are caused by direct blunt impact [48, 57]. Skin tears, a common type of laceration commonly seen in older adults, are a splitting of the epidermis layer of skin from the underlying

[4]A pathologic fracture is one that occurs in diseased bone (e.g., due to osteoporosis or metastatic cancer), where the amount of force would not break a healthy bone, but because of the underlying bone disease, a small force will break a weakened bone.

connective tissue resulting in a flap of skin. Skin tears typically appear on the forearms and less often the legs. They usually result from bumping into objects, falls, and wheelchairs but can also be caused by rough handling and abuse of an older person [57].

Bruises result from blunt force trauma causing rupture of small blood vessels under the skin. Bruises can appear on the skin surface hours to days after the trauma was inflicted, depending on the depth of the wound. Blood can track through fascial planes causing visible bruising away from the injury site. Common areas include the face, where injury on the scalp or above the eye may result in bruises forming below the eye; a subgalael hematoma, i.e., bleeding leading to swelling between the skull and scalp typically caused by head trauma such as from a fall, in which blood travels to the forehead can indicate traumatic hair pulling,[5] and tracking in the perineum after genital trauma. Basilar skull fractures are also associated with blood tracking, producing "raccoon eyes" [65]. Eyelids, neck, and scrotum are very susceptible to bruising [57, 65].

Historically child abuse studies were used to age and stage bruises in the elderly. Important research on accidental versus intentional bruising and the aging of bruises by color changes has been conducted and has shown that reliance was misplaced. Mosqueda et al. [112] studied the occurrence, progression, and resolution of accidental bruises compared to non-accidental traumatic bruising. This observational study revealed that 90 % of accidental bruises occurred on the extremities. No accidental bruises were found on the neck, ears, genitalia, buttocks, or soles. In addition, 15 % of the bruises were yellow within the first 24 h of onset. Many bruises did not follow standard and then-widely accepted notions of color progression, in which, as the hemoglobin is broken down, the color of the bruising changes from red to blue and purple and then yellow and green.

This 2005 study was followed by another observational study, [168] which chronicled the appearance of bruises known to result from physical elder abuse. Locations of bruises from abuse differed significantly from those from accidental bruising. In addition, the inflicted bruises were larger than 5 cm in size. Almost 90 % of victims recalled the cause of at least one bruise compared with only 25 % of their peers with accidental bruises. Bruises associated with abuse occurred on the lateral right arm, and to the head and neck. Other research has shown that the most severe injuries in elder abuse occur on the head (61 %) and torso (31.7 %) [63, 65].

Suspicious or traumatic bruises may also occur in atypical locations, such as the head, neck, chest, abdomen, genitalia, buttocks, palms, soles, and ears [29, 48, 57]. In addition, bruises in varying stages of healing are suggestive of abuse [57, 65].

Bruises may show the pattern of the striking object if the bruise is superficial. When the bruise is in the deeper dermis, or subcutaneous tissues, borders are poorly circumscribed or hazy. Examples of pattern bruises are fingertip or pad bruises, shoe stamps, belt buckles, and tramline bruises, i.e., formed by cylindrical objects and appear as a pale linear central area bordered on both sides by linear bruises, bite marks, and abrasions from identifiable material [65]. Bruises may also retain the shape of knuckles or fingers; parallel marks suggest a stick [48, 57] or a cane.

Because bruises may retain the shape of the object that caused them, careful documentation of the injury is critical, especially if it can be matched to items left at a crime scene or linked to an alleged perpetrator. Skin tears in locations other than the arms or legs or multiple tears and abrasions should raise suspicion. Lacerations heal with scarring; skin tears heal without scarring. "Abrasions or lacerations are most commonly seen in cases involving physical abuse though they can occur in cases of caregiver neglect" [57, at p. 345].

There are causes for bruises, skin tears, and abrasions other than abuse. For example, older adults may have what appear to be bruises on the dorsal (exterior) surfaces of hands and arms. These "bruises" may be blunt force trauma from very minor contact but are not due to abuse. These so-called "senile purpura" results from increased blood vessel fragility, thinning skin, skin atrophy, and lack of elasticity associated with sun exposure [65, 94]. Chronic sun exposure contributes to wrinkling and loss of tone in the skin [78]. Unlike bruises, purpura is flat, without swelling, and painless and requires no treatment to clear.

Some medications and conditions can increase an older adult's risk for bruising. For example, aspirin, clopidogrel, and warfarin may increase bleeding time and propensity for bruising. Diseases such as cirrhosis or myelodysplasia could cause disruptions in the clotting mechanism, predisposing the older adult to bruising or bleeding [78, at p. 673, 94].

18.4.4 Blunt Force Head Injuries

Head trauma may cause injuries to the head, face, and neck; including skull fractures, traumatic brain injury (TBI), and facial fractures. These injuries are the most common types in intimate partner violence (IPV) and elder abuse and can cause asphyxia and TBI [65]. TBI is craniocerebral trauma associated with decreased consciousness, cognitive or neurologic abnormalities, skull fracture, or intracranial injuries [83]. In older adults, trauma to the face and head is more likely to result in serious injury and death than in younger

[5] Subgaleal hematoma is not specific to a single causation but may result from hair pulling as well as head blunt impact trauma.

persons. Use of anticoagulant medications increases the risk of intracranial bleeding, even in the absence of symptoms [98].

Sadly, such injuries may be overlooked such as when signs of cognitive impairment are assumed to be caused by advanced age, accidental falls, or underlying dementia. Additionally, brain injury may be missed if facial bruising that indicates deeper injury is not recognized. When such injuries are caused by elder abuse, these assumptions will result in overlooked injuries and misattribution to non-abuse causes.

Basilar skull fractures, while common, are missed because bruising near the eyes and ears is mistaken for facial trauma. Bruising from direct trauma to the eye region must be distinguished from anterior basilar skull fractures ("raccoon eyes"). Trauma to the eye causes a black eye at the injury site. Trauma to the periorbital area causes blood vessels to rupture sending blood through connective tissue and downward with gravity around the affected eye(s). Cerebrospinal fluid discharge from the ear with bruising over the mastoids causes "battle sign" injuries which may be mistaken for direct trauma behind the ear [65]. Such a mistaken conclusion may not be supported by physical evidence and witness accounts and may raise a doubt that abuse caused the injury.

A scalp injury may signal intracranial injury. Coup and contrecoup injuries may occur. A brain contusion, the coup injury, may occur inside the head under the site of impact from the blow to the head. If the blow to the head is followed by a fall or striking a wall, the victim may sustain the contrecoup injury opposite to the point of contact as the brain rebounds from the initial impact against the skull [83].

Subdural hematomas are more common in older adults, because the veins that connect the brain to sinuses are susceptible to tears. Some subdural hematomas may result from relatively minor trauma. Brain atrophy in older persons may allow bleeding to continue without symptoms, causing a delay in seeking medical care and diagnosis. Symptoms, if they develop, include headaches, light-headedness, slowness in thinking, apathy and drowsiness, unsteady gait, and occasionally, seizures [65]. Anticoagulant medication exacerbates these injuries.

18.4.5 Strangulation and Suffocation

Strangulation is a form of asphyxia in which blood vessels and air passages are closed as a result of *external* pressure on the neck [147]. It can produce unconsciousness in seconds and death within minutes. Death often occurs without any external injuries or marks [75, 108, 147].

Suffocation is impeding the flow of oxygen through such means as covering the face with a hand or pillow, covering he victim's mouth and pinching nostrils to prevent breathing; forcing the victim's face down into floor or bed to prevent breathing; sitting or straddling a victim's chest or abdomen preventing the chest wall from expanding to breathe, or placing a plastic bag over the victim's head or duct tape across the victim's face.

Strangulation has long been recognized as a form of physical abuse in intimate partner violence (IPV), and the severity of episodes increases over time [170]. Smith et al. [142] found that 34 % of strangulation victims had been strangled multiples times, increasing the risk of recurrent hypoxia. Most studies of strangulation have focused on younger persons though there are many case reports of strangulation of older adults [87, 126, 148]. The study of nonfatal strangulation began with intimate partner violence research; more recently IPV findings have been evaluated in older adults.

The victim's initial presentation is not a reliable predictor of seriousness or case outcome. Findings are often subtle and underappreciated by responders [74]. External markings do not necessarily reflect the severity of the strangulation [76]. Victims may have no visible injuries even if the strangulation or suffocation causes death [67, 76]. Hoarseness (aphonia) occurs in roughly half of strangulation cases [144] and some victims may have difficulty in swallowing and sore throat (odynophagia), dyspnea, and shortness of breath (stridor) [60] as well as assuming a sniffing position to assist with breathing. Some signs of injury, such as swelling to the neck, may be absent in the initial assessment [144].

Table 18.2 describes injury sites and clinical signs and symptoms associated with strangulation assaults.

When victims do have visible injuries from strangulation or suffocation, common physical signs include patterned abrasions or contusions of the anterior neck caused by fingernails, finger pads, ligatures, or clothing. Hand marks may be found on the perpetrator and/or the victim and in the case of the victim, were self-inflicted by a victim while trying to break free. The hyoid bone and thyroid cartilage are more susceptible to fracture in older adults compared with younger victims [144].

Petechiae, small red or purple spots caused by rupture of capillaries with resultant bleeding into skin, may be found on the neck, head, face, forehead, eyes, ears, conjunctive, and buccal mucosa [60]. On autopsy, petechiae may be found on the undersurface of the scalp and internal organs. Petechiae are a sign of asphyxia from multiple causes, including strangulation [76], and are also noted to occur with increased vascular congestion [60]. In strangulation cases petechiae are found above the location where the pressure was applied. In suffocation petechiae are non-localized.

Neurologic consequences of strangulation may include cerebral cortical infarct, anoxic encephalopathy, and mental status changes caused by cerebral hypoxia and intracranial injury [60]. Although uncommon, damage to the intimal

Table 18.2 Strangulation injuries: location, signs, and symptoms

Location	Clinical signs	Clinical symptoms
Skin	Fingernail abrasions, ligature abrasion, patterned abrasion or contusion, finger contusions, blunt impact contusions	Local pain, specific point tenderness (mastoid process)
Muscles and ligaments	Local tenderness to palpation, swelling on soft tissue radiographs, diminished mobility of the larynx upon manual external examination due to pre-vertebral hematoma	Deep pain, tenderness, swelling, odynophagia
Recurrent laryngeal nerve	No external signs, fiberoptic laryngoscopy for vocal cord paralysis	Hoarsness, aphonia
Jugular veins	Geographic petechiae, darkly pigmented skin may not reveal petechiae	Asymptomatic
Carotid arteries	Absence of petechiae, can be fatal in a few seconds, arteriography	Confusion, loss of consciousness
Laryngeal skeleton: thyroid, aretynoid, cricoid and tracheal cartilage, hyoid bone	Respiratory stridor, subcutaneous emphysema, DROOLING	Shortness of breath, palpable crepitus
Cervical spinal bone	Pain on movement, paralysis, radiographic findings	Pain
Central nervous system	unconsciousness; cerebral infarcts, hyperventilation, disorientation, memory loss, agitation, nausea, vomiting: (as a complication from getting air in stomach when hyperventilating)	Fainting, incontinence of urine or feces, seizure, headache
Miscarriage	Intrauterine fetal demise	Loss of fetal movement, spotting, labor

Source Dr. Dean Hawley, Indiana University School of Medicine

layer of the carotid artery may induce thrombosis of the artery or an embolus to distal cerebrovascular circulation. [144]. Progressive, irreversible encephalopathy and neurologic sequelae caused by cerebral cortical infarcts may present after strangulation [60].

Although death from the carotid sinus reflex is uncommon, older persons may be more susceptible to cardiac arrest from sustained pressure on the carotid body caused by atherosclerosis [81].

Strangulation is more difficult to detect in elder death investigations [39, 133] in part due to the victim's advanced age and underlying medical condition [133], and the low priority elder death investigations historically have received from coroners and medical examiners [17]. Nonetheless, strangulation as the cause of death increases with victim's age [133, 148]. Consistent with other age groups, women over the age of 65 are more likely to die from strangulation than men of the same age [65, 148], and because of aging physiology, comorbid conditions, history of cognitive impairment, dementia, or stroke, the elderly are especially susceptible to cerebral injury [65].

18.5 Identifying Sexual Abuse

Women experience age-related changes to the genital tract. Estrogen and progesterone levels decline, causing changes to the shape of the vagina and increased dryness and thinning of the vaginal walls. Altered acidity of vaginal secretions makes older women more susceptible to vaginal and bladder infections [57].

Clinical findings suggestive of elder sexual abuse include presence of oral venereal lesions; bruising of the uvula, bleeding and bruising of the anogenital area as well as difficulty sitting and walking, and abdominal bruising [57]. Lacerations and abrasions in the genital area should raise suspicions of sexual abuse [65]. Explanations for such injuries may be an attempt to catheterize a patient or rough perineal care [27].

Burgess et al. [29] conducted a retrospective study of 125 cases of elder sexual abuse using the Comprehensive Sexual Assault Assessment Test (CSAAT), an instrument specifically designed to be used with elderly sexual assault victims. They found that

(1) Bruising injuries from sexual abuse are often located on the labia majora, labia minora, or posterior fourchette;
(2) Victims of elder sexual assault sustain significant injury to nongenital parts of their bodies, most often the head, legs, chest, and abdomen;
(3) Nearly half of elderly victims sustained vaginal trauma; and
(4) The majority did not have forensic findings of presence of sperm.

Bruising of the soft palate at the junction of the hard palate may indicate forcible oral copulation. In long-term care facilities, urinary tract infections in nursing home patients are suggestive of sexual abuse if several cases occur in a cluster. Any diagnosis of STDs in a nursing home resident is a strong indicator of sexual abuse [57].

In addition to clinical signs, studies have shown that victims of sexual assault change their behavior after an attack. Victims, including those with dementia, experienced psychosocial trauma whether or not they could verbally discuss what had occurred. There was **no** significant difference in trauma reactions between elders with and without dementia. Symptoms included sleep disturbances, incontinence, increased anxiety, crying spells, withdrawal, depressive symptoms, heightened startle reflex, agitation, restlessness, decreased enjoyment in activities, intrusive memories, and attempts to leave facilities in which they were assaulted [30]. At a minimum, careful documentation of a victim's behaviors and behavior changes after an alleged sexual assault may provide convincing corroborating evidence of the attack.

18.6 Role of Medications

Older adults comprise about 13 % of the population but are prescribed more than 40 % of all prescribed drugs [80]. On average, individuals aged 65–69 years are prescribed 14 different drugs per year [14]. The high rate of prescription drug use is associated with substantial rates of serious adverse drug events [18, 61]. Additionally, some medications with the potential for negative effects on cognition are available over the counter.

In the hands of an abuser, medications may be given to an older adult in an attempt to "chemically restrain" the elder or with the intention of killing the elder [129]. Obtaining many kinds of medications that can be tools of abuse and neglect, whether prescribed or over the counter is relatively simple. Health care providers may not know the adverse consequences of common drugs and may be unaware of the full extent of what an elder is prescribed and receiving. "The role of health care professionals who are interested in preventing adverse effects from medication is made more difficult by a steady influx of new knowledge about the effects and interactions of these medications, by the complex medication regimens that are required to treat many diseases, and by the multiple health care providers that are involved in the care of many older people" [80, at p. 150].

Certain classes of medicines can cause cognitive decline and impairment; these potentially preventable adverse events have risks that are a function of dose, duration, and individual susceptibility including preexisting cognitive impairment, dementia, or genetic makeup [80].

The usage of anticholinergic and benzodiazepine drugs is especially common and is especially risky for use by older individuals. Anticholinergic Drugs, including antihistamines, are widely prescribed for the elderly [35]. While helpful in the treatment of allergies, nausea, depression, muscle spasm, etc., these medications are overprescribed when less toxic alternatives exist. Anticholinergic drugs are associated with both short-term and long-term adverse cognitive effects in older adults, including delirium, cognitive impairment, and dementia [35, 36, 85, 150] and increase the risk of hospitalization for confusion and dementia [85]. A 10-year longitudinal study of older women, especially those who developed dementia in later life, found a high prevalence of inappropriate medication use and high anticholinergic load [80].

Benzodiazepines are often used to treat anxiety, sleeplessness, and agitation in older persons. They are associated with a markedly increased risk for delirium, cognitive impairment, falls, fractures, and motor vehicle accidents [22, 51, 150].

As discussed previously, conditions such as arthritis, osteoporosis, heart conditions, and neurologic conditions such as Parkinson's Disease and stroke are treated with multiple medications which can increase the risk of falls and other injuries [78]. Some medical conditions are treated with anticoagulant medications, aspirin, or antiplatelet agents which can affect bleeding, clotting rates, and bruising [78].

Medications can cause delirium, an acute decline in cognitive functioning, which is marked by rapid onset, inattention, impaired consciousness, and cognitive disturbance including disorientation, memory impairment, and language changes. Behaviors include restlessness, agitation, and hallucinations while delirious [78]. Delirium can be an outcome of abuse or neglect due to improper administration of medications, or failure of a caregiver to provide proper care causing development of an infection or other illness.

A list of medications commonly prescribed for older adults is located in Elder Abuse Pocket reference: A Medical/Legal Resource for California Judicial Officers, Appendix C, available at http://www.courts.ca.gov/documents/ElderAbusePDoc.pdf.

18.7 Identifying Neglect

There are two kinds of neglect—self-neglect and caregiver neglect. The primary distinction is whether or not there is a caregiver, that is, someone with a legal duty of care, who is responsible for causing or preventing neglect of an older adult. Identification of neglect may be made more difficult by personal values based in cultural or religious beliefs [37, 72].

18.7.1 The Role of Cultural Beliefs and Values

Beliefs and values may play out in whether a person will seek or permit others to seek Western-type medical care, or will seek help from a healer or practitioner of other forms of care. In some traditions it is considered inappropriate to place an older family member in a nursing home or other skilled care setting, and in others cultural expectations are that certain family members, often daughters, will care for an aging and frail elder irrespective of their caregiving abilities, economic situation, or capacity or the needs of the elder [149, at p. 11]. In others, sharing resources, including food and medicine, even when needed by the older adult may not be considered abuse or neglect [33]. Conversely, other conduct, not defined as abuse or neglect in the dominant community, may be considered neglect by a particular cultural community but may not qualify for certain legal interventions or remedies. For example, some traditions may define elder abuse in terms of the elder adult being disrespected, or being denied access to cultural, spiritual, or religious practices [26, 52 at p. 54].

Immigrants and refugees may tolerate abuse and neglect rather than face deportation of themselves or their family member abuser if they report. They may accept abuse and neglect as a better alternative than what they left in their country of origin [34].

Cultural beliefs and values may also guide what remedies or interventions may be acceptable [28, 141]. For example, it may be acceptable to seek help from the tribe or community elder but not from the criminal justice system. Or a person may be willing to seek help from, for example, a tribal court or healing circle but not from a state court.

Even how a provider may ask about abuse or neglect may have cultural implications. There may not be language for abuse, neglect, or self-neglect and if questions are framed in such terms, will be unlikely to lead to disclosure; instead, providers must learn to communicate in culturally acceptable terminology.

The role of resources must also be considered. The cultural or religious community may not have social services or nursing facilities available even if an elder wanted to use them. Supportive housing where dietary restrictions, medical needs, and religious or spiritual observance are supported may not exist. An understanding of these and other cultural perceptions must be incorporated in collaborative responses, professional training and education, and legal and other interventions.

18.7.2 Self-Neglect

The Elder Justice Act defines self-neglect as an adult's inability, due to physical or mental impairment or diminished capacity, to perform essential self-care tasks including: (A) obtaining essential food, clothing, shelter, and medical care; (B) obtaining goods and services necessary to maintain physical health, mental health, or general safety; or (C) managing one's own financial affairs [187]. Self-neglect "results from an individual's difficulty in obtaining, maintaining, and/or managing the necessities of life independently [130]

Self-neglect includes such categories as hoarding, obsessive–compulsive disorder (OCD) [10], living in squalor [1], and Diogenes Syndrome. It is the most common form of elder abuse reported to Adult Protective Services programs throughout the United States and while not a crime, is litigated in legal actions in civil and probate courts as, for example, lawsuits to abate a public nuisance, code enforcement actions, and guardianships and conservatorships. Identification of self-neglect raises serious legal and moral questions such as:

- Does the person have the capacity to manage his or her life? People with decision-making capacity are allowed to make their own decisions, even if those choices appear unwise (self-determination). Society places enormous value and importance on letting people live their own lives.
- How can safety be balanced with autonomy?
- To what extent can the person be offered assistance and services either voluntarily or involuntarily?
- If services can be imposed on the person, how can services be provided in the most humane manner so as to avoid or minimize greater emotional or psychological harm?
- Is the apparent self-neglect causing harm to someone else?
- Is the apparent self-neglect an outcome of elder abuse or a prior crime victimization?

18.7.3 Caregiver Neglect

Unlike all other forms of elder abuse, caregiver neglect requires a failure to act, an omission, by someone with a duty to act on behalf of an older person who requires care or other assistance. Restated, that someone (a caregiver) failed to act, to do something that he or she should have done resulting in harm to the older person. The omission is something that a reasonable person would have done in similar circumstances.

The older adult is a person with a significant disability which is why the person requires a caregiver. The disability may be medical, cognitive, or both, but it is so significant that the person cannot live safely without assistance. The care can be for basic needs including food, clothing, shelter, health care needs, or management of assets and finances.

A person may become a caregiver in a variety of ways, including

- Through a contract to provide care
- Through a legal relationship which carries with it a duty to provide care, such as a spouse. Some states impose a duty of care on adult children with the ability to provide care; many do not [110]. Examples of other legal relationships include a court appointed guardian or conservator, agent or attorney—in fact under a power of attorney, or trustee.
- By assuming the duty of care of a person who requires care, whether paid or not (e.g., People v. Heitzman [182]). A duty may be created when someone assumes care for a person who requires it even in the absence of a legal obligation: "However, it is a long-standing theory of the law that a person who voluntarily provides care to someone in need of care has a duty to continue providing care or seek help from others in providing that care rather than abandon the care recipient" [145, p. 3].

There are many legal and moral questions in establishing that caregiver neglect has occurred

- Does someone have a duty to provide care for an older adult, i.e., is there a legally recognized caregiver?
- What is the caregiver's legal responsibility? Is it to provide personal care, to pay for the care of another through a contractual duty, or to arrange for care? Is the duty limited to financial responsibility?
- What are the available resources for the elder's care from the care recipient and from community services? A caregiver is not required to expend personal resources for an elder's care absent an agreement or special duty.
- What is the caregiver's capacity to provide care? What are their physical, cognitive, educational, intellectual, and other abilities to provide care?
- What is the relationship between the caregiver and care recipient? Is the caregiver dominated by the care recipient?
- What are the long standing personal preferences of the care recipient?
- What is the care recipient's capacity to make their own decisions?

The elements of neglect typically are those for negligence and include a duty of care, an awareness or appreciation of the general consequences of failing to carry out the legal duty, failure to exercise that degree of care that a reasonable person in a like position would exercise (breach of duty), and resulting harm. While neglect criminal laws vary across the US, the level of negligence is far greater than that of simple negligence required in a civil case such as a traffic accident. Criminal statutes describe the requisite intent as criminal negligence, reckless disregard, or malicious negligence [160], all of which are considerably higher levels of intent.

Identification of neglect is difficult for health care providers and Adult Protective Services and law enforcement investigators. "Clinicians are frequently challenged to make a definitive diagnosis of neglect. Unlike other forms of elder mistreatment where injuries are more obvious (fractures, burns, contusions, and lacerations), neglect may present with subtler findings. Awareness of red herrings and maintaining a high index of clinical suspicion are necessary to detect and assess neglect" [49, at p. 769]. It may be difficult to distinguish between neglect and poor care quality, especially when pressure ulcers, malnutrition, and/or dehydration are present [129]. Neglect may also be explained as cachexia [154], a wasting disease associated most often with end-stage cancer.

Among those subtler clues are

- Missing and needed assistive devices, such as walkers, hearing aids, eyeglasses, and dentures which help the older person aware of what is around them. Their absence increases the risk of falls, fractures, and decreased function.
- An unexpected deterioration in a person's health which may signal lack of medical care or withholding of medications and treatments needed to manage health conditions [49].

Medical markers of both neglect and self-neglect are the same and include malnutrition, dehydration, poor hygiene, and inadequate or inappropriate clothing. Malnutrition, nutritional deficits, and poor hygiene are all risk factors for pressure ulcers [38].

Dehydration is a common finding in neglect cases [41] and must be severe to be outwardly noticed. Medical signs include dry mucous membranes, sunken eyes, decreased skin turgor, and fecal impaction. Additional findings (often seen at autopsy) include skin tenting and "sticky," dry serosal surfaces. Vitreous electrolyte evaluation (especially elevated sodium, chloride, creatinine, and urea nitrogen) is useful in making a postmortem diagnosis of hypernatremic dehydration [129] where hypernatremia, a serum sodium level greater than 145 mmol/L, is the most commonly noted laboratory finding [99].

High sodium levels are associated with elder mortality. One study found a 33 % mortality rate for patients admitted to a geriatrics ward with serum sodium levels in the range of 151–153 mEq/L. Another investigation found that nearly 50 % of patients hospitalized with dehydration died within a year, and among those with a sodium level higher than 154 mEq/L, mortality was 71.4 % [165]. Collins and colleagues reported the results of forensic evaluations of eight elder neglect cases; in three cases in which dehydration was the cause of death, vitreous chemistries revealed sodium levels ranging from 164 to 180 mmol/L and urea nitrogen 76–310 mg/dL [99].[6]

Malnutrition is a state in which a deficiency, excess, or imbalance adversely affects the body's form, function, and clinical outcome. Malnutrition is the outcome of the body not receiving proper calories/energy, water, fiber, and nutrients such as vitamins, minerals, protein, carbohydrates, and fats needed [79]. Signs of malnutrition include decreased body mass, loss of muscle mass, recurrent infection, decreased total protein, decreased albumin, and decreased total iron binding capacity (TIBC) [129].

Malnutrition has been identified by medical examiners as particularly important in identifying abuse or neglect [91]. A retrospective 10-year review of elder abuse cases of a State Medical Examiner's Office serving a large metropolitan area revealed that 36.4 % of postmortem elder neglect cases were severely malnourished [Body Mass Index (BMI) < 17.5 kg/m^2], 40.9 % were underweight (BMI 17.5–20.0 kg/m^2), and only 22.7 % had a BMI of greater than 20.0 kg/m^2 [99, 140]

Laboratory markers suggestive of malnutrition and nutritional status include serum proteins synthesized by the liver, especially albumin. Low serum albumin (<3.5 g/dL) has been shown to predict mortality and morbidity [99, at p. 717]. Thus the presence of high levels of albumin and/or sodium with other indications of neglect will provide significant scientific support for a civil or criminal action for caregiver neglect.

When conducting an autopsy in an alleged death case "investigative information is vital in determining the specific situation involved in the death. Pertinent medical historical information, including noting the physical and mental abilities and limitations of the decedent, must be ascertained. Medication history, care provider capabilities/expectations, and other factors/issues may also be important. Findings in elder neglect cases should be documented grossly, histologically, and via a variety of ancillary studies (i.e., radiographs, toxicology, microbiology, and chemistry tests" [129, at p. 268, 40].

18.8 Pressure Ulcers

A pressure ulcer, also called a decubitus ulcer or bedsore, is caused by the breakdown of skin integrity resulting in an ulcer. Pressure ulcers result from circulatory failure due to pressure; pressure on the skin causes vein obstruction or thrombosis of the microcirculation, i.e., blockage of blood in small blood vessels. The affected skin is thus devitalized of oxygen and nutrients causing hypoxia and ischemia to the skin and its ultimate death [79]. Pressure ulcers can be caused by a failing to properly reposition an immobile person or placing a person on bed restraints for prolonged periods of time [49, at p. 770].

The most common areas for development of pressure ulcers are the sacrum, hip and heels. Their presence could result from severe end-stage diseases affecting mobility and malnutrition or they may also indicate caregiver neglect [31, 32]. Pressure ulcers should alert the health care professional of the possibility of neglect. A sixfold increase in mortality has been linked to pressure ulcers that have failed to heal [53].

The duration of time for ulcer development depends on many factors, including the habitus of the individual, area of pressure, extent of pressure (e.g., prolonged), and underlying medical conditions. Ulcers can take hours [101] to days to develop and there is no standard formula for determining this period [65]. However, the size and depth of each ulcer is related to its duration, as they increase in size with time.

Deep pressure ulcers in multiple sites may indicate neglect. Failure to provide proper care to high risk persons to prevent the development of ulcers may indicate neglect. Failure to seek medical care for or to provide proper care for an infected or necrotic pressure ulcer is an indicator of neglect [57].

Older adults are more susceptible to pressure ulcers due to disease states, not age alone. Risk factors such as acute illness, neurological and peripheral vascular disease, incontinence, and poor nutritional status, are not predictive of their development when appropriate care is provided; but are predictive when the standard of care is not provided [20, 57]. Failure to provide appropriate standard of care can be due to medical, institutional, or caregiver neglect. Medical conditions that can lead to poor wound healing and increased risk for pressure ulcers, include diabetes mellitus, vascular diseases, and wounds that occur at the end of life, also known as Kennedy Terminal Ulcers [49, at p. 770]. Because pressure

[6]Vitreous sodium is only loosely correlated with blood sodium so these vitreous levels do not mean the same as blood levels (Personal communication with Dr. Dean Hawley, December 31, 2015).

ulcers often develop in older adults with serious underlying medical conditions, and the multiple risk factors present in the development of ulcers, many experts believe that pressure ulcers can develop, even with the best care [65].

When considering an action for neglect, the presence of pressure ulcers alone is most likely insufficient to prove the legal case, instead it may be more helpful to explore if ulcers were treated and treated promptly and professionally. In addition, the case will be stronger if there is evidence that

- The caregiver was instructed in the care needs of the older adult
- The caregiver was offered assistance and if so, did not accept such help
- The victim had financial resources to pay for needed care
- The caregiver benefitted financially or otherwise by not providing proper care
- Other victim health issues were not attended to such as filling medications or failing to provide needed nutrition or liquids
- The victim was left alone for long periods of time

In short, because criminal neglect cases are some of the most challenging and difficult cases to prove, proper identification and development of such cases require the combined efforts and expertise of many disciplines and professionals. Not only are medical and laboratory findings critical in identifying neglect and differentiating it from other causation but the surrounding circumstances, any refusal of offered services, complexity of the elder's medical needs, capacity of the caregiver to meet caregiving responsibilities, financial benefit to the caregiver of denying care, and other information will be essential in distinguishing situations of carelessness or poor care from criminal cases where the caregiver acted recklessly, maliciously, or with disregard for the likely and foreseeable consequences.

18.9 Part III Capacity and its Assessment

The intersection of law and science is not limited to identifying forensic markers of abuse and neglect and differentiating them from other possible causation. Attorneys, investigators, and courts frequently rely on the expertise of the mental health and medical fields to determine if an older person is responsible for their decisions and the consequences of those decisions. An assessment of capacity will be used to determine case theory and in some cases, if there is a basis for a case at all.

A person must have the ability to make decisions and carry out decisions with respect to his or her needs [116] Adults are presumed to have capacity to live independently, make their own decisions, and "suffer" the consequences of those decisions. "A finding that a person is incapacitated in some or all areas is a joint medical and judicial decision, based on expert clinical opinion" [131, at p. 817]. "In the past 2 decades, capacity assessments have shifted from being a fairly minor part of legal and clinical practice to a distinct field of legal, clinical, and behavioral practice and research" [58, at p. 853].

The legal setting in which capacity issues may arise may vary: some arise in criminal and civil proceedings (e.g., ability to testify; give consent; engage in various kinds of transactions), while others are specific to criminal cases (ability to understand the proceedings; sanity) or probate matters (should case be heard in a protective proceeding such as a guardianship or conservatorship, where should a person reside).

If that person is an alleged perpetrator the kinds of issues that arise include

- Is that person legally able to form the requisite intent (mental state such as intent to kill, premeditate and plan, permanently deprive) to commit certain crimes?
- Is that person able to understand the legal proceedings and assist counsel?
- Is a person legally sane?
- Should a case proceed in the criminal courts or should it be handled in the mental health system
- Can that person refuse medical treatment?

If that person is the alleged victim, examples of the kinds of issues that may arise include:

- Could that person give "legal" consent?
- Could that person appreciate the nature of the act to which they allegedly agreed
- Could that person engage in the act at issue, e.g., enter into a contract, change a will, make a gift, consent to sexual contact, consent to a medical procedure, create a power of attorney
- Can the person testify as a witness?
- Is the person susceptible to undue influence and/or can the person resist undue influence?
- Is the person able to plan and execute a course of action, or are there deficits in executive function?
- Can the person live independently?

Capacity assessments can guide law enforcement and protective services in determining the extent to which a victim may be able to participate in an investigation or legal process. In many types of neurocognitive disorders, particularly Alzheimer dementia, verbal and social skills may remain intact when memory and other cognitive domains are compromised. The presence of a dementing illness may make it difficult to assess the accuracy of a person's report of abuse, and a capacity evaluation may improve understanding of the nature and extent of the person's cognitive deficits. A capacity evaluation explains why an adult with a neurodevelopmental disorder (formerly called intellectual disability/mental retardation) was unable to understand the implications of signing over the deed to a home left to him by his mother can assist prosecutors in charging the case, developing their case theory, and evaluating the witness' strengths, weaknesses, and need for accommodations [58].

These determinations require an understanding of how the brain functions, how deficits in various parts of the brain affect function, what is executive function and its role, what is capacity and cognition, and how capacity is related to function. Each of these requires the assessment of an expert. This chapter is not a discussion of dementia and other cognitive conditions; that information is available in other chapters of this book. Instead, this section focuses on forensic issues related to capacity.

Capacity refers to "a cluster of mental skills, such as memory and logic, as well as physical and behavioral functioning that people use in everyday life." (Mosqueda and CA Judicial Council 2012, at p. 19). In the legal arena, the terms "competency" and "legal capacity" are typically used and refer to a judicial determination of capacity to do something in issue, e.g., execute a contract, make a gift, understand the nature of the proceedings and assist counsel, testify as a witness. Determinations of legal capacity are based in significant part, on assessments of capacity by experts.

Critical mental skills are those involved in attention, thinking, understanding, learning, remembering, solving problems, and making decisions. They are directly related to a person's ability to engage in activities, accomplish goals, and successfully negotiate the world. Although cognition is sometimes equated with memory, cognition is multidimensional involving various interrelated abilities that depend on brain anatomy and physiology. Distinguishing among these abilities is important as each plays a different role in processing information and behavior. Each is affected by aging, but in different ways [80].

Once seen as a global, all or nothing determination, capacity is now understood to involve many different abilities or capacities [114]. The law recognizes there are numerous kinds of capacity. Some examples are included in Table 18.3.

It is now understood that a person may have some capacities but have deficits in others. In general, the greater the consequences of the decision, the higher the level of capacity, that is required. Therefore, an older adult can have the capacity to engage in one activity (e.g., make a decision about a minor medical procedure), but not another (e.g., make a decision about high-risk surgery). Each type of decision requires different cognitive abilities; a proficient evaluation will link a person's strengths and weaknesses to the specific decision for which his or her capacity is being assessed. A cognitive assessment alone will not necessarily reveal information about a person's ability to function in everyday life, but it does reveal information that may be important in understanding abuse, neglect, or undue influence in the determination of capacity [58, 115].

Table 18.3 Determinations of legal capacity

Type of capacity	Definition
Testamentary	Execute or change a will
Donative	Make a gift
Decisional	Execute a power of attorney or advanced directive
Contractual	Enter into agreements, contracts, and other financial transactions
Medical	Consent to legal treatment
Testimonial	Provide testimony in a legal proceeding
Present ability of a defendant to participate in criminal proceedings	Understand the nature of the proceedings and assist counsel in the defense

Capacity is neither static nor global. Instead it may vary according to time of day, illness, mental condition, medications, setting, grief, loneliness, etc. Older persons may have deficits but these do not usually affect every aspect of their lives. Because capacity is no longer understood to be global, all or nothing, the first question that should be addressed by anyone conducting an assessment is "capacity to do what?"

Capacity requires more than a medical diagnosis, such as dementia. A diagnosis may serve as a framework for understanding a person's limitations with declining cognitive skills, a diagnosis alone is insufficient for a determination of capacity [58]. A finding of a specific incapacity can be made even without a medical diagnosis. The process of capacity assessment involves more than a diagnosis, especially with the move away from merely making a diagnosis to describing cognitive and functional abilities [6]. "Some persons, especially those with high intelligent quotients who are highly educated, maintain excellent verbal skills while lacking insight, good judgment, or the physical ability to care for themselves in a safe manner. In such "gray" cases the determination can be difficult for highly trained and skilled physicians. Such determinations are fraught with difficulties for APS workers who are differently skilled and trained" [55, at p. 435].

Any medical diagnosis must be linked to functional decline, such as inability to manage finances or resist undue influence, for a court to make a legal determination of a particular incapacity.

Legal determinations are based on local laws and statutes defining incapacity. In civil and probate proceedings, most standards are based on the functional abilities of the person to meet, or arrange to meet, the essential requirements for physical health, safety, or self-care [8].

Courts evaluating evidence relating to capacity typically consider the "Six Pillars of Judicial Determination" which include:

- Medical condition
- Cognition
- Everyday Functioning
- Values and Preferences
- Risk and Level of Supervision
- Means to Enhance Capacity [8].

An aspect of capacity is executive function, a person's ability to plan, organize, sequence, monitor and inhibit complex goal-driven behaviors. Executive function allows the person to engage in purposeful, self-directed activities including taking initiative and respond to novel events and conditions [97, 153]. Generally, executive function declines with age [175]. Deficits in executive functioning are linked to risk for financial exploitation.

Specific regions of the brain are involved in executive function. The prefrontal controls the planning and multi-tasking required for complex actions, such as cooking a meal. In contrast, the hippocampus controls memory that is required to remember the food items that must be obtained to cook that meal. Other brain areas play key roles in other functions [80].

A person with intact executive functions may have significant cognitive deficits but can remain independent, self-supporting, and productive [97]. However, deficits in executive functions due to changes in the brain structures that manage planning, initiation, and sequencing, may leave the older adult unable to manage successfully and independently [56, 80]. Interpersonal relationships may be negatively affected. A person may begin to neglect personal hygiene, act impulsively, or lack self-control. They may be unable to initiate activities, manage time, and may lack motivation, be noncompliant with medical treatment, and have difficulty with completing tasks [58]. Their ability to make decisions, inhibit responses, and simultaneously process relevant and irrelevant information are all affected. These declines have been linked to the ability to perform instrumental activities of daily living (IADLs), such as medication management [19, 80].

Executive function is particularly important in executional capacity, the ability to implement a decision which must evaluated separately from decisional capacity, the ability to make a decision.

Decisional capacity is determined by:

- the ability to understand the basic facts about a decision
- the ability to appreciate how the decision relates to one's situation, including strengths and limitations and requires adequate memory.
- the ability to reason, rationally evaluate, and compare options and evaluate the consequences of alternative choices
- the ability to make an informed decision [13, 58, 116].

Executional capacity requires that a person is able to:

- formulate a plan
- adapt the plan in response to novel or changing conditions
- delegate tasks to appropriate others when physically unable to carry out the plan [44, 58, 116, 132, 135].

18.9.1 Financial Capacity

Understanding financial capacity is critical in many civil and criminal legal contexts in assessing the older person's ability to give legal consent. The determination whether a person had the capacity to consent to a transaction, gift, transfer of assets, or designation of a surrogate decision maker all begin with an assessment of capacity.

Financial capacity is defined as 'the capacity to manage money and financial assets in ways that meet a person's needs and which are consistent with his or her values and self-interest" [104, 105]. No single capacity underlies it [58]. Instead, financial capacity comprises a broad range of conceptual, pragmatic, and judgment abilities, ranging from basic skills, such as counting coins, to more complex skills, such as paying bills and managing a checkbook [106, 107].

Financial capacity includes several domains of activity each with its specific clinical relevance, including:

- Basic monetary skills (recognize and count money, understand debts and loans,)
- Carrying out cash transactions (identify correct amount of money needed, count change)
- Managing a checkbook and bank statement (pay bills)
- Exercising financial judgment (maintain ability to act prudently and avoid scams, exploitation) [89]
- Financial literacy (knowledge of basic financial investment concepts) declines in later life and is reflected in increasingly rash and irrational financial decision-making [100].

Financial capacity is one of the first abilities to decline as cognitive impairment and early dementia occur [155] and may be identified as mild cognitive impairment. Decline in an older adult's financial skills may signal impending Alzheimer's type dementia [105] and may be detectable before a diagnosis of Alzheimer's Disease. Financial capacity shows relatively rapid decline over one year in patients with mild Alzheimer's Disease. Studies have found that written arithmetic abilities are the primary predictor of financial capacity performance in groups across the dementia spectrum: normal elderly, patients with amnestic MCI, and patients with mild Alzheimer's Disease [139]. Declines in financial capacity increase the risk that older adults will become victims of financial fraud and abuse [2, 50, 134].

Warning signs include *memory lapses* (forgets to pay bills, pay the same bill more than once); *disorganization* (disorganization and unable to find financial and other documents, miss deadlines); *decline in checkbook management skills* (changes in ability to handle check register and checkbook); *arithmetic errors* (noticeable decline in everyday math skills, errors in making change or computing a tip); *conceptual confusion* (loss of knowledge of basic financial concepts and such as mortgage, will, annuity); and *impaired judgment* (loss of judgment about investments and money, unfounded anxiety about extent of wealth, new and abiding interest in financial get rich schemes) [156]. Recognition of early warning signs requires knowledge of the person's prior level in functioning.

Financial capacity questions typically arise in the context of older adults with neurodegenerative diseases such as Alzheimer's disease (AD), Parkinson's disease (PD), and frontotemporal dementia (FTD). Recent studies have demonstrated that financial skills are highly vulnerable to the early cognitive changes found in mild cognitive impairment (MCI) and early Alzheimer's disease [73, 103, 155]. Declines in financial skills are often the first functional change to be identified in declining cognitive ability and incipient dementia. A recent study showed that declines over 1 year in checkbook management and overall financial skills predicted conversion to Alzheimer's disease in patients with amnestic mild cognitive impairment (MCI)[7] MCI has been retitled in DSM-5 as "Mild Neurocognitive Disorder". Declining skills are detectable long before a diagnosis of Alzheimer's Disease [155].

Changes to specific regions of the brain appear to increase susceptibility to financial frauds. Persons with behavioral variant frontotemporal dementia (bvFTD) are less able to understand another person's perspective, and their use of sarcasm or deceit. This inability to discern appears to increase their susceptibility to fraudulent schemes and scams, and exploitation [138]. Persons with damage to the ventromedial prefrontal cortex region of the brain (vmPFC) are less able to doubt incoming information (skepticism) referred to as the "doubt deficit." Those with damage to their vmPFC have difficulty assessing incoming information and determining whether to doubt it [15]. As a result, they make poor decisions and may fall victim to scams and deception [100].

18.9.2 Assessing Capacity

Assessment of capacity in a court or other legal setting is intended to identify an older person's strengths and weaknesses, and integrating them into an evaluation of their effect on function. There are two different categories of evaluation: screening and assessment. Screening gives a "snapshot" of how a person is at a moment in time. Its value is in giving information about general level of overall cognitive impairment and can suggest when a more comprehensive assessment should be obtained. They can be helpful when an individual has such severe impairment that the person cannot complete any other tests [8, 11]. Assessment is a more comprehensive evaluation using testing, clinical interview, functional assessment, information gathered from collaterals (witnesses), medical history, and in some cases, a home visit.

Assessments should be conducted by clinicians with specific expertise in administering, scoring, and interpreting the results. For example, neuropsychologists and neuropsychologists are able to use standardized tests to assess the full range of cognitive functioning. Standardized tests are helpful in avoiding vague and subjective findings and use normed findings to inform the conclusion [58].

Both screening tests and assessments have limitations. Not all assessments include many or each of the components just highlighted. Historically, assessments were based on a clinical interview or general mental status evaluation. These were subject to variability based on the clinician's expertise, theoretical orientation, and experience, personal values, and attitudes [7, at p 12].

"…(A)lthough many instruments and protocols exist, they are a disparate group, and do not, taken together, achieve the uniformity necessary to support an effective and coherent response from the medical, social service, public safety, and legal communities" [57, at p. 368]. There is disagreement as to which tools are best for each cognitive domain and population group. While some capacity areas, including capacity to give medical consent, have well developed tools, others, such as capacity to consent to sexual

[7]Mild cognitive impairment (MCI) is "subjective and objective impairment in memory or other cognitive domains that represents a decline and is greater than expected for age, but is of insufficient severity to significantly affect activities of daily living" [157, at p. 828]. Although persons with MCI may well be able to function in a home setting, they may have memory difficulties, compromised executive skills, and other cognitive impairments that interfere with their ability to understand complex financial decisions, placing them at risk for financial exploitation [167, 84]. Mild dementia is characterized by short-term memory loss and subtle but noticeable impairment in judgment, difficulty with complex tasks such as managing finances or medication regimens (bill and pills), are unable to work, and may have difficulty driving (Tronetti at p. 829).

contact and testamentary capacity, do not. Some tools have been developed for research purposes; others for clinical use.

In American Indian/Alaska Native (AI/AN) communities "physical complaints are normalized as part of life, and memory loss and dementia are minimized by family members and the tribal community. The diagnostic criteria of the Diagnostic and Statistical Manual of Mental Disorders (DSM) may not be applicable to members of the community due to differences in tribal beliefs about mental illness, cultural labeling of different emotions, and conceptual language differences [77]. These differences carry over to medical and mental health screenings and assessments. Unless the testing includes culturally applicable elements, the person may appear less capable than he or she actually is" [34, at p. 19].

Tools must be culturally validated. For example, using usual scales of ADLs and IADLs may test for tasks never undertaken by the person. These tests typically evaluate tasks such as the older adult's ability to manage a checkbook and use a telephone. If the elderly person grew up in a tribal community or less developed rural community in another country these tasks may well be irrelevant to the person's life experiences which may have involved chopping wood, carrying water, weaving, or simple farming [77].

Western measures of depression may not be valid either because the term "depression" is not used or because Western scales are not culturally appropriate. For example, the Indian Depression Scale (IDS) was developed to incorporate the American Indian cultural context [77].

Screening tools are often used by persons who may be unaware of their limitations. "A wide variety of tools and measures are available to test for cognitive change; however, not all may be relevant to real-world activities. Studies use different methods, measures, and definitions that make comparison difficult, and the cognitive aging literature has some significant gaps." [80]. "There is a paucity of evidence-based data and a lack of uniformity among existing practices [57]. Absent validation, uniform standards, and implementation such tools will not gain general use, provide an accurate picture of the phenomenon, or supply a useful base of data for research" [57, at p. 363]. In addition, most "lack adequate reliability, validity, and normative properties for older adults" [7, at pp. 12–13].

Tools have also been criticized for failing to evaluate the impact of living with abuse and neglect on decision-making capacity. Persons living with abuse and/or neglect and their willingness and ability to take action against an abuser and/or accept services, leave, etc., are evaluated the same way as a person who is not living with abuse and neglect [124].

Examples of commonly used screening tools include: the Mini Mental State Examination (MMSE), a 30-point screening test that measures orientation, attention and calculation, short-term memory, and visual construction. It does not measure executive function; the CLOCK test which can detect MCI and dementia; the Montreal Cognitive Assessment (MoCA) which has been validated for identifying Mild Cognitive Impairment and Mild Alzheimer's disease [117]; and the Saint Louis University Mental Status Examination (SLUMS) which can detect MCI and early stage dementia.[8] None of these tests, by itself, should be used to diagnose a cognitive disease. New screening and assessment testing instruments continue to be developed and validated. The US Department of Justice released a research report "Building Consensus on Research Priorities in Elder Mistreatment" which addresses recommendations for enhancing the assessment of capacity [143].

18.9.3 Retrospective Assessment of Capacity

It is not uncommon for there to be late discovery of a transaction or execution of a document which is believed related to elder abuse, neglect, or exploitation. While the older person is clearly cognitively impaired today, critical events happened 18 months ago. The older person's financial or decisional capacity in the past becomes critical to a criminal or civil lawsuit. Was the person cognitively impaired then? Could s/he understand the nature of the transaction or act? Could s/he appreciate the ramifications of that act? Was the impairment evident to the alleged perpetrator at that time?

It is sometimes possible to conduct a retrospective determination of capacity. Such evaluations are document-intensive, requiring the expert to carefully review historical information including medical records, psychological test results, if they exist, collateral sources of information, including witness statements, depositions, and affidavits, law enforcement investigative reports, notes, diaries, and other writings, APS reports, and electronic communications [24]. The clinician should conduct a complete cognitive assessment to establish current cognitive abilities, assuming the older adult is alive. In reviewing the historical information, the clinician is seeking information about the elder's cognitive abilities at an earlier time when questioned events occurred. "The success of these evaluations depends upon the quality of the records, the available collateral information collected during the relevant time frame, and the degree of cognitive impairment that the victim demonstrates when the assessment is conducted" [59, at p. 287].

Investigators should attempt to identify people who were part of the older adult's life at times when questioned events

[8]For other common tests see American Bar Association et al. [7, at p. 48].

occurred and interview them. These include friends, neighbors, and family members as well as professionals such as doctors, pharmacists, veterinarians, bank tellers and other personnel, long standing financial advisors and attorneys, and service providers who frequently may have seen the older adult, like hair dressers and postal carriers. If the older adult was active in a faith, social, professional, or cultural organization, leaders and other participants should be sought out. All relevant records and documents should also be collected. A comprehensive investigative effort to locate supporting information is required for a credible retrospective assessment of capacity to be made. If such an investigation is absent, the expert may be unable to offer an opinion or may offer an opinion which is subject to attack as based on an incomplete knowledge of the evidence. Either can undermine the strength of an elder abuse case or make it impossible to bring a case at all.

Whether the forensic issue is identification of injuries through forensic markers or assessment of capacity, well-trained and highly qualified experts must be located. In the next section barriers to obtaining competent experts will be discussed.

18.10 Part IV Competency of and Availability of Critical Experts

Prior sections of this chapter have identified some of the forensic complexities of identifying and responding to elder abuse. In short, the law cannot operate fairly and objectively without qualified, competent experts able to distinguish abuse, and neglect from other causation and able to assess capacity to testify participate in proceedings, engage in a variety of transactions, understand and give consent, and control their own lives. Successful prosecution, in particular, requires both collaboration **and** expertise across disciplines [26, 43]. Qualified experts are often difficult to locate [146]. The expertise of some may be little understood by public and private attorneys who handle elder abuse civil and criminal cases. Ultimately, most important is the expert's qualifications rather than the professional's discipline [103].

Barriers to locating competent experts include lack of professional training opportunities resulting in under detection and reporting. This part of the chapter will highlight these points.

Table 18.4 describes some of those experts, the types of cases in which they may be needed, and the nature of their forensic opinions.

Adding to the difficulty locating such experts is the historical lack of training and education for a variety of professionals, including:

- **First responders** [123, 125, 127] who are critical in initially identifying abuse, collecting evidence, and sometimes, contacting experts
- **Front line clinicians** Most front line clinicians, however, are not experienced or knowledgeable in capacity assessment, and are not qualified to offer such a judgment, which can carry inordinate weight with families, financial institutions, and legal professionals [103].
- **Health care professionals** "Because many health care professionals may not be able to detect the signs of elder abuse, or know how to screen for it, enhanced training in geriatric medicine is needed to improve prevention and early detection of elder abuse" [31 at p. 747]. In one study, 98 % of physicians stated that there should be more education on elder mistreatment, 96 % thought education should be included in medical training, and 80 % believed they had not been trained to diagnose elder mistreatment [90].
- **Geriatric trained medical professionals** (Bardash and Rowles 2012) Currently, there are only 1.7 geriatricians for every 10,000 adults aged 65 years and older, with this ratio expected to *decline* in the future [16, 3]. Connolly [43] argues there is a need for a medical subspecialty in forensic geriatrics, akin to that in child abuse where forensic pediatricians are cross trained in both forensic pathology and pediatrics. The absence of such experts "hinders both the identification and reporting of elder abuse and neglect" [43, at p. 61]. Forensically trained geriatricians would be more capable of identifying possible signs of abuse and neglect, know when and where to report, and be more confident with involvement in legal matters [43].
- Nurse Investigators who understand how facilities are supposed to operate and can understand and analyze medical and other health care records, particularly in cases filed against facilities [43].
- Wound care specialists who understand the proper treatment and care of pressure ulcers [43].
- Medical Examiners and Coroners. A majority of deaths occurring in elderly individuals represent natural deaths. Because of this fact, and the fact that many deaths in the elderly are considered expected deaths, the identification of a nonnatural death in this population may require a high index of suspicion [129, at p. 269]. While such professionals are critical to identifying, reporting, and handling elder abuse cases, historically they have been offered little elder abuse training. These include medical examiners and coroners who decide if elder deaths are autopsied [71].
- Forensic accountants who can review and analyze financial records and transactions in financial exploitation cases [43].

Table 18.4 Forensic experts in elder abuse cases

Expert	Nature of information	Type/form of elder abuse case
Mental health professionals, including geropsychologists, geropsychiatrists, neuropsychologists, psychologists, psychiatrists	Capacity assessments, functional abilities, susceptibility to undue influence, mental health conditions, witness legal capacity to testify; Capacity to consent, capacity to consent in past	All types of elder abuse cases in civil, criminal and probate matters
Mental health professionals, including geropsychologists, geropsychiatrists, neuropsychologists, psychologists, psychiatrists	Ability of defendant to stand trial, defendant's sanity	Criminal elder abuse cases
Geriatrician and other doctors with geriatric training, including family medicine, cardiology, gerontologist	Identification of injuries, degree of harm, or injury, causation, disease symptoms and progression, standard of care	Physical abuse, neglect, sexual assault
Treating physician	Medical history, identification of injury, disease symptoms and progression, care instructions provided to elder or caregiver, prescribed medications, tests ordered and results	Physical abuse, sexual assault, and neglect
Pharmacist, pharmacologist, toxicologist	Medication purpose, interactions, and effects	Physical abuse, sexual assault, and neglect
Pathologist, including medical examiner	Identification of injuries, harm caused, degree, cause and manner of death	Physical abuse, sexual abuse, and neglect
Nurse, including those specializing in wound care, in-home care, and geriatrics	Description of injury, treatment provided, progress with treatment, standard of care, wound care, evidence of inadequate or improper care, cause of injury	Physical abuse, sexual abuse, and neglect
Ophthalmologist, optometrist	Identification and cause of eye injuries or conditions	Physical abuse
Dentist	Identification and mechanism of force for injuries to mouth	Physical abuse, sexual abuse
SART/SANE	Examination and collection of evidence, description of injuries	Sexual abuse
Forensic accountant, tax attorney or investigator, banker, accountant	Accounting principles, fiduciary duty, victim and perpetrator's spending and assets, financial timeline, impact of financial issues and spending on tax laws and Medicare eligibility	Financial exploitation
Probate investigator or examiner	Prior accountings provided to court; information or training provided to guardian or conservator regarding duties and responsibilities	Financial exploitation
Elder or civil law attorney	Standard of practice, meaning of technical documents	

Modified from National Center for State Courts (2012) Prosecuting Elder Abuse Cases: Basic Tools and Strategies, pp. 17–21

Lack of professional training has consequences in the detection and reporting of elder abuse. Physicians may be the only person outside the family that an older adult sees regularly and as such, are uniquely positioned to recognize and report elder abuse. Health care providers who do not recognize elder abuse are ineffective at addressing the consequences of abuse in patient care [137].

Only a minority of health care providers ask about abuse [45] which delays earlier detection and identification. "Basing detection of abuse only on objective evidence means a high bar by which time people are, for example, bruised, dirty, or have pressure sores" [45, at p. 844].

Kennedy [90] surveyed nearly 400 family and internal medicine physicians and found that 63 % had never asked their patients about elder abuse and only 23 % believed elder abuse to be a significant problem for their patients [90]. Unpublished data from a 2013 pilot study conducted at the Durham Veterans Affairs (VA) Medical Center also showed poor baseline knowledge of elder abuse among health care professionals, including social workers, geriatric pharmacists, and internal medicine residents. Respondents also identified a lack of knowledge of how to intervene once elder abuse was detected as a critical need [164].

Rates of reporting suspected elder abuse by health care professionals are very low. According to an APS survey, healthcare professionals submitted only 11.1 % of elder abuse reports; physicians accounted for only 1.0 % of reported cases even though virtually all states mandate reporting of suspected elder abuse by health care professionals [92, 111]. Dong et al. [54] found a rate of physician reporting in Connecticut of 1.5 % over a 10-year period. Only 1.4 % of cases reported to APS come from physicians [152] and in a survey of APS workers, of 17 occupational groups physicians were among the least helpful in reporting abuse [23].

Many reasons have been offered for why professionals do not report abuse

- Lack of knowledge/understanding of what constitutes abuse [4, 46, 137]
- Uncertainty regarding how to ask people with dementia about abuse [46, at p. 847]
- Inability to recognize abuse or lack of knowledge regarding how to handle it [46, 137]
- Fear of a breakdown in therapeutic relationships [46]
- Fear of causing offense [46]
- Fear of recrimination [46]
- Fear of being wrong (reluctance to act without strong evidence) [46]
- Empathy with the perpetrators [46]
- Belief that procedures designed to deal with the offense are inappropriate and punitive [45, at p. 847]
- Lack of knowledge of state laws requiring reporting [53]
- Fear of angering perpetrators [53]
- Skeptical of investigative follow up [53]
- Lack confidence in social services [53]

This part of the chapter has highlighted problems associated with the role of experts in identifying and reporting suspected elder abuse for it can be addressed by the legal, health care, mental health, and social services systems. In particular, this segment described the many kinds of experts who are needed to identify elder abuse and assess its victims and (sometimes its) perpetrators, training and education challenges, and lack of professional reporting. Taken together they paint a bleak picture.

Rather than ending on such a sobering picture, Part V "Collaboration" concludes this chapter highlighting several promising practices and approaches for enhancing the identification of elder abuse using forensic markers, and the assessment of capacity by qualified experts, and the development of targeted and tailored professional training.

18.11 Part V "Collaboration"

"Elder abuse and neglect cases often pose multiple, complex issues that may be social, medical, ethical, legal, and financial in nature, and which require expertise beyond that available from any single discipline" [55, p. 430]. "Few professionals who work for these agencies and systems have specialized training on how to recognize and respond to elder abuse cases…" [161, at p. 73].

Improved response requires

- Development of specialized training for experts and attorneys handling elder abuse matters so each has the required technical skills to handle cases within their area of practice;
- Availability of experts to provide technical assistance; and
- Development of community-based responses that best use those skills and expertise

18.11.1 Training Initiatives

Those working with elders who have been abused or neglected must rely on forensic markers. Unfortunately, caregivers, Adult Protective Services agencies, and doctors are often not trained to distinguish between injuries caused by mistreatment and those that are the result of accident, illness, or aging [109]. "Training and education are critical to improving the knowledge and skills of criminal justice professionals enabling them to handle elder abuse cases effectively. These efforts have been at the federal, state, and local levels" [71, at p. 86].

Table 18.5 highlights some of the specialized training that has been developed in recent years. It is not an all-inclusive list.

18.11.2 Multidisciplinary/Interdisciplinary Responses

Preventing, identifying, and responding to elder abuse requires a multifaceted approach because abuse does not fit a single pattern. Elder abuse is a "complex cluster of distinct but related phenomena" that involves health, legal, social service, public safety, and financial issues, and therefore calls for a coordinated and sustained response across multiple disciplines [166]. And because older adults are a richly diverse heterogeneous group, each elder and each case presents unique medical, social, cultural, religious, and economic circumstances.

One of the most important initiatives in addressing elder abuse has been the development of multidisciplinary/interdisciplinary collaborations. First used in child abuse, "the use of interdisciplinary or interprofessional teams, also referred to as multidisciplinary teams in the context of elder abuse, has emerged as one of the intervention strategies to address the complex and multidimensional needs and problems of victims of elder abuse, and such teams are an important resource for physicians" [96, at p. 1947]. This model reflects a "one-stop-shop" where the "consumer" is an agency with a complex elder abuse case who requests the assistance of other agencies with expertise in elder abuse [158]. Data suggests that teams improve efficiency, coordination, and professional support among team members [95].

Team membership can mirror the diverse and varied circumstances of the elder abuse cases they address. Not only are teams comprised of a variety of professionals and disciplines, but their members may come from the same minority cultural and religious communities as the victims allowing for a more nuanced understanding of the context in which abuse may be occurring, but may be able to develop more culturally acceptable remedies and interventions.

Professionals working on elder abuse cases within an IDT also relate better outcomes. For example, in one study, 97 % of those who referred cases to an elder abuse IDT indicated that the team was helpful in confirming abuse, documenting impaired capacity, reviewing medications and medical conditions, facilitating the conservatorship process, persuading the client or family to take action, and supporting the need for law enforcement involvement [113, 158].

These interdisciplinary efforts result in the diverse professionals critical to investigating and assessing cases already knowing one another, having experience with the issues that may arise, being committed to the effort, and having each gathered information relevant to the decision to be made. Investigators will have spoken to witnesses, obtained critical medical, financial and other records, conducted laboratory and other expert evaluations. The medical team may have cared for the patient/victim, but also reviewed medical and pharmacy records, conducted medical, social, functional, and mental health assessments, and in some cases, conducted home visits. Each will have sought out advanced directives and statements of life preferences. As a team, and subject to local laws on information-sharing and confidentiality, will have all of these materials to best assess and understand the critical legal and medical issues.

Collaborations have taken the form of teams, family justice centers, and forensic centers. They have developed to benefit from the varied experience, knowledge, training, and resources available to members.

18.11.2.1 Teams[9]

Elder abuse medical management teams were first formed in Massachusetts at Beth Israel Hospital. In 1998, Mount Sinai Hospital in New York began its team. Subsequently, teams have formed in Minnesota, New Jersey, California, and Texas [55]. One of the first, the Texas Elder Abuse and Mistreatment Team (TEAM),[10] was a collaborative effort of the Baylor College of Medicine Geriatrics Program, local county hospital, and local Adult Protective Services office to strengthen and expand clinical relationships and improve identification of elder abuse and neglect. These teams and those that have since developed are able to draw from an array of medical professionals with varying expertise to improve the identification of elder abuse cases.

In Southern California, regional medical centers have partnered with local agencies to improve geriatric assessments. These teams can provide both medical and capacity assessments for suspected elder abuse victims and provide important investigative information, testimony, and declarations for use in protective conservatorship (guardianship), and criminal cases [159].

Medical management teams are better able to conduct comprehensive geriatric assessments (CGA), the gold standard for assessing the health and well being of older adults. CGAs often incorporate the physical health, mental health, and social and cognitive domains important for quality of life and protection from elder abuse [55, 64] and use an interdisciplinary approach since no single professional possesses all of the skills to meet the needs of frail older persons [55].

CGAs are not suited for brief clinical visits; they are lengthy and require the participation of several disciplines. Therefore, family physician practices, non-geriatric specialists, and emergency departments are not likely to perform CGAs, suggesting the need for alternative approaches such as referrals to local geriatric medical teams which are trained in CGA and accustomed to completing some combination of these assessments [31].

Specialty multidisciplinary/interdisciplinary teams have formed to focus on specific kinds of cases. These include Fiduciary/Financial Abuse Specialist Teams ("FAST")

[9]For a more complete look at Teams and Collaborations, see Table 6.1. Examples of Collaboration Types, in Brandl et al. [26, at pp. 111–114].
[10]More information is available at http://www.uth.tmc.edu/schools/med/imed/divisions/geriatrics/team-institute.html.

Table 18.5 Training initiatives

Discipline or profession	Details of training
Medical examiners and coroners	The University of California at Irvine Program in Geriatrics and Forensic Center developed an elder death review investigation course for medical examiners and coroners which is now approved by the state accreditation agency, the Commission on Peace Officer Standards and Training (POST). A sample agenda is available at http://www.centeronelderabuse.org/docs/ElderDeathInv_SampleSched2007.pdf
Nurses, forensic nurses	The International Association of Forensic Nurses curriculum "Nursing Response to Elder Mistreatment Curriculum" and available at http://www.forensicnurses.org/?page=ElderMistreatment
Dentists	UCLA School of Dentistry has developed a curriculum on aging and elder abuse and neglect that can be infused in preprofessional and existing dental school courses with the goal of increasing awareness of elder abuse and understand reporting responsibilities and increase skill and comfort with recognizing and reporting elder abuse and neglect
Paramedics and emergency medical technicians	San Francisco City College has developed curricula on elder abuse and neglect which includes the recognition and identification of elder abuse and reporting responsibilities
Pharmacy and medical students	Several courses, including basic overview; law for second and third year students; pharmacy practice experiences and geriatric ambulatory care rotations. See: http://www.centeronelderabuse.org/Kaiser_Pharmacy.asp
Judges/judicial officers	The US Department of Justice, Office on Violence Against Women (OVW) oversees the Enhanced Training and Services to End Violence and Abuse of Women Later in Life Grants Program which has funded the creation of national curricula on elder abuse for judicial officers. Focusing on making informed decisions in elder abuse matters. Medical and capacity subjects are included. Open to non-grantee judicial officers. www.ncjfcj.org
Prosecutors	California District Attorneys Association National Symposium on Elder Abuse, held each December, addresses many aspects of elder abuse identification, response and prosecution, including role of medical, mental health, accounting, and other forensic experts www.cdaa.org National Institute for the Prosecution of Elder Abuse annual course on prosecuting elder abuse, working with medical and mental health experts, and trial-focused subjects. Part of the (OVW) Enhanced Training and Services to End Violence and Abuse of Women Later in Life Grants Program but open to non-grantee prosecutors. www.ncall.us
Legal services attorneys	The US Department of Justice, Office for Victims of created four modules on elder abuse for legal services providers. Modules cover *What Every Legal Services Lawyer Needs to Know About Elder Abuse' Practical and Ethical Strategies, Domestic Violence and Sexual Assault, and Financial Exploitation. See* https://www.ovcttac.gov/views/dspLegalAssistance.cfm?tab=1#onlinetraining
Court officials	The National Center for State Courts (NCVC) created an online training program on elder abuse which includes The Physiology of Aging, Identifying Elder Abuse and Neglect, and Crafting. See http://www.eldersandcourts.org/Training/Elder-Abuse-Curriculum.aspx
Law and medical and dental students	The University of California at San Francisco, a medical, nursing, dental, and other health care professionals has created the Consortium on Law, Science and Health Policy, with the University of California's Hastings College of the Law. The Consortium connects medical and legal professionals; students can take courses at either University campus for the purpose of supporting interdisciplinary collaboration at "the intersection of law, science, and health policy" in the areas of education, research, and clinical training and service. See www.ucconsortium.org

which focus on financial abuse cases and typically include medical and mental health professionals along with experts in financial transactions such as financial planners, forensic accountants, real estate, stocks and bonds, and annuities to assist with understanding the transactions and in assessing relevant capacity issues.[11]

Another specialized team, the Death/Fatality Review Team, evaluates elder death cases and assesses medical evidence and forensic markers to identify elder abuse related deaths from others.

18.11.2.2 Forensic Centers

Beginning in 2003, a new form of multidisciplinary/interdisciplinary team was formed, the forensic center [169]. "Forensic centers are a new tool in the field of elder abuse. They grew out of a need to have a responsive group of professionals (from social services, criminal justice, and health care fields) advise and assist in cases of abuse and neglect." [136, at pp. 255–256]. Forensic center teams provide support to APS and law enforcement investigators. Members include experts in geriatric medicine, civil and criminal law, neuropsychology, advocates for persons with developmental disabilities and residents of long-term care facilities. Team members may conduct home visits and assessments, provide consultation, accept referrals for services, and testify in legal proceedings [121, 122]. Early data from the Los Angeles County Forensic Center suggests that cases handled by the forensic center improve the likelihood the case will be prosecuted [119]

- A ten and a half times greater likelihood of getting an APS case submitted to the DA, when the Center is involved.
- Just over an 8 times greater likelihood of a case having charges filed when case reviewed by forensic center members than only investigated by
- Nearly 9 times greater likelihood of establishing guilt, defined as pleas and convictions, when case reviewed by Forensic Center members [120].

These findings were further analyzed, including costs associated with case processing by a forensic center [151]. Conclusions include:

- Cases reviewed at the Forensic Center were significantly more likely to be submitted to the district attorney than ones only handled by Adult Protective Services and then referred to the district attorney
- Proportion of cases in which charges filed by district attorney did not vary significantly between the two groups
- Proportion of cases with successful plea or conviction did not vary significantly
- Cases reviewed by the forensic center significantly more likely to be referred to the Public Guardian's Office though no significant difference in number of cases that needed conservatorship (guardianship)
- The recurrence of elder abuse was significantly reduced in Forensic Center cases, (from 42.7 to 24.6 %). By contrast, usual care APS cases actually showed a small but nonsignificant increase in recurrence (from 16.7 to 20.3 %).
- Cases heard by the forensic center on average took longer compared to cases just handled by APS (Just over 10 h vs. just under 4 h)
- Forensic center processing costs significantly higher than usual care APS cases ($1408.58 vs. $153.30)
- 20 % of cases reviewed by the Forensic Center were referred to the district attorney's office for filing of charges; 100 % of these cases resulted in charges being filed vs. none of the 39 usual care APS cases which were never sent to the district attorney's office
- When the Forensic Center model is adopted, the average additional cost per case is
    - Successful prosecution = $8,731.40
    - Referral to the Public Guardian = $4,485.97
    - Referral to the Public Guardian resulting in conservatorship = $6,691.93.

This is the first rigorous analysis of the cost-effectiveness of an Elder Abuse Forensic Center. While costs are significantly higher when cases are processed at a Forensic Center, the Forensic Center approach resulted in better outcomes than the usual care APS system. The researchers characterized the incremental costs associated with the Forensic Center "modest" when compared to health intervention costs. These findings suggest that the forensic center model shows promise in handling complex elder abuse cases more comprehensively while reducing recidivism, and in the longer run, may be cost neutral or cost effective.

18.11.2.3 Family Justice Centers

Family Justice Centers began in the domestic violence/intimate partner violence arena in San Diego in 2002 and have expanded across the United States and into other nations. Their goal is to be a "one-stop" for victims of domestic violence where a victim can obtain help from numerous community agencies, such as legal assistance with civil protection orders and other legal services, medical evaluation and documentation, counseling, housing, law

[11]For more information on FAST and fatality review teams, please see Brandl et al. [26].

enforcement, child protective agencies, etc. More recently, some centers have added specific agencies and services for older victims of family violence and elder abuse, including Adult Protective Services. The victim can meet a case detective, work with an advocate, discuss the matter with APS, get help with a restraining order, and talk with a faith leader. At the same time, the victim's injuries can be forensically documented. While not all centers provide the same services, some conduct forensic interviews for older adults and adults with cognitive disabilities.

All of these collaborative efforts share a commitment to bringing together professionals from diverse disciplines to focus efficiently on the forensic needs of elder abuse cases to assure that cases are properly identified and assessed, using evidence-based standards.

18.12 Conclusion

Elder abuse is still a "young field." Its evolution from decision-making based on anecdotal experience to decisions that are evidence-based will take time, energy, and a commitment of significant resources. Many authors have noted that elder abuse research has lagged far behind child abuse and intimate partner violence due to a historical lack of a national commitment and dollars for research.

In recent years the picture has begun to change and change dramatically, with many new and innovative efforts underway. The changes are due, in no small part to the passage of the Elder Justice Act in 2010, the Roadmap Project developed consensus in the field about the nature, extent, and elements of elder abuse, and created national priorities to address it, and the 2015 White House Conference on Aging which further highlighted national priorities and recently undertaken projects.

The Elder Justice Act, passed in 2010, as part of the "Patient Protection and Affordable Care Act" (Public Law 111-148), created the Elder Abuse Coordinating Council[12] comprised of representatives from 12 federal agencies. Chaired by the Secretary for Health and Human Services in consultation with the Attorney General, the Council is responsible for coordinating activities related to elder abuse, neglect, and exploitation across the federal government [42]. The Council is required to report every 2 years to Congress on its recommendations. Among the recommendations in the 2014 Report are the development of a coordinated federal elder justice research agenda to identify best practices for prevention of and intervention in elder abuse and elder financial exploitation. (Recommendation 4); Develop cross-disciplinary training to educate stakeholders across multiple sectors and disciplines on preventing, detecting, intervening in, and responding to elder abuse, neglect, and exploitation (Recommendation 6)' and to improve screening for dementia, cognitive capacity, financial capacity, and financial exploitation and the ability of APS and first responders to screen for diminished capacity, diminished financial capacity, and vulnerability to or victimization of financial exploitation (Recommendation 8) [162].

The Elder Justice Act also supports the creation of forensic centers and the development of forensic markers and forensic expertise by requiring the Secretary of Health and Human Services, in consultation with the Attorney General, to award grants for stationary and mobile forensic centers to develop expertise on elder abuse, neglect, and exploitation. Grantees are to use funds to develop forensic markers and methodologies to determine whether abuse, neglect, or exploitation or a crime has occurred; develop forensic expertise regarding elder abuse, neglect, and exploitation to provide medical and forensic evaluation, therapeutic intervention, and victim support and advocacy; and develop the capacity of geriatric health care professionals and law enforcement to collect forensic evidence. Forensic centers are also required to conduct research on forensic markers and methodologies for determining when and how health care, emergency services, social and protective services, and legal service providers should intervene in a case, and when reports should be made to law enforcement officials.

Other actions which have evolved from the Elder Justice Act include grants made by the National Institute of Health/National Institute on Aging including a scientific investigation about the social and neural bases of vulnerability to financial fraud and a research study on the neurological basis of financial decision-making errors which render people with Alzheimer's disease and frontotemporal dementia vulnerable to financial exploitation [162].

The Department of Justice has created an elder justice website (www.justice.gov/elderjustice) which serves a resource for elder abuse prosecutors, researchers, practitioners, as well as victims of elder abuse and their families. It currently houses resources, pleadings, and research material of particular import to attorneys and researchers.

The Elder Justice Roadmap Project synthesized information from 750 practitioners and subject matter experts from around the country through a concept mapping approach. With this information the Project identified priorities and strategies for public and private engagement at the local, state and federal levels to provide a resource for strategic planning to combat elder abuse (National Center on Elder Abuse). The Roadmap identified priority areas, several of which are germane to this chapter. These include

[12]The Coordinating Committee was created by Title XX of the Social Security Act, Subtitle B, the Elder Justice Act of 2009.

- **Geriatric experts**: Develop more health professionals with expertise in aging and elder abuse by providing additional training to existing professionals and recruiting students into the field. Such professionals also should learn about local multidisciplinary teams that address legal, social service, or financial issues, and, where appropriate, participate in such teams. Training for some also should include cross-training in geriatrics and forensic pathology. These experts need to know how to detect suspicious signs and report elder abuse cases (when appropriate) so that they can assist older adults to prevent, ameliorate, or end elder abuse (page 20).
- **Multidisciplinary responses**: Develop and support multidisciplinary responses to elder abuse. Encourage participants involved in multidisciplinary teams to collect data about their practice and to describe their successes and challenges in ways that can inform others engaged in similar efforts (page 26–27).
- **Partnerships with related fields**: Develop collaborations between the elder justice field and other allied fields involved with older adults, including aging, caregiving, civil, legal, domestic violence and sexual assault, mental health, substance abuse, and trauma (page 20).
- **Coordination and Multidisciplinary Approaches**: Encourage coordination and the development of multidisciplinary approaches (page 27).
- **National research agenda**: Develop a focused research agenda to get the most information from limited funding. Priorities to consider include: Cognitive Impairments ▪ Develop better instruments and methods to assess whether potential victims have cognitive impairments (page 27).
- **Risk Factors and Forensic Markers:** Identify forensic markers to assist in the detection of elder abuse (page 28).
- **Brain Health and Functioning** of Potential Victims: Expand knowledge and improve integration of cognitive capacity and mental health issues as they relate to elder abuse. Some older victims may experience mental health issues, such as depression and posttraumatic stress disorder—especially those who have experienced ongoing, long-term trauma related to the elder abuse. We need additional research to understand how to evaluate cognitive capacity and mental health issues within the context of elder abuse and how to protect and provide a range of effective services to those with cognitive impairments and/or mental health issues (page 26–27).
- Brain health of perpetrators (page 27).

Subsequently, the 2015 White House Conference on Aging embraced many of these same themes and priorities. Moving forward, the forensics of elder abuse will continue to need

- Sound research
  - To identify forensic markers of elder abuse and ways to differentiate elder abuse from other causation;
  - Brain function and capacity
- Professional education and training, including creation of interdisciplinary college and graduate programs where law and the sciences work together
- Enhanced interaction across legal, medical, protective services, law enforcement, social services focused in elder abuse
- Validated tools for assessing capacity in various contexts and settings and which are also relevant for use with older members of minority communities
- Centers of Excellence to develop and test modes for interdisciplinary collaboration and disseminate findings
- Funding to accomplish these tasks.

Together these laws, priorities, and actions create a blueprint for future action. If undertaken they herald a future marked by enormous strides in the ability to identify abuse and neglect, intervene, and reduce human suffering. All this is possible when law and science tare able to make an effective and compelling "forensic intersection."

Acknowledgments The author wishes to acknowledge the assistance of Dr. Dean Hawley of the Indians Indiana University School of Medicine, Dr. Diana Homeier of the University of Southern California, Keck School of Medicine, and Mr. Randy Thomas South Carolina State Law Enforcement Academy (retired) and thank them for their guidance, careful review, and suggestions.

References

1. Aamodt WW, Terracina KA, Schillerstrom JE. Cognitive profiles of elder adult protective services clients living in squalor. J Elder Abuse Negl. 2015;27(1):65–73.
2. Agarwal S, Driscoll J, Gabaix X, Laibson D. The age of reason: financial decisions over the life cycle and implications for regulations. Washington, DC: Brookings Institution; 2009. http://www.brookings.Edu/~/media/Projects/BPEA/Fall%202009/2009b_bpea.
3. Alliance for Health Care Reform. Health care workforce: future demand v. supply. 2011. http://www.integration.samhsa.gov/images/res/Workforce,%204.22.pdf. Accessed 12 Dec 2015.
4. Alt K, Nguyen A, Meurer L. The effectiveness of educational programs to improve recognition and reporting of elder abuse and neglect: a systematic review of literature. J Elder Abuse Negl. 2011;23(3):213–33.
5. American Bar Association. Module rules of professional conduct. 2013. http://www.americanbar.org/groups/professional_responsibility/publications/model_rules_of_professional_conduct/model_rules_of_professional_conduct_table_of_contents.html.
6. American Bar Association and American Psychological Association. Assessment of older adults with diminished capacity: a handbook for lawyers. 2005. http://www.apa.org/pi/aging/resources/guides/diminished-capacity.pdf.

7. American Bar Association Commission on Law and Aging & American Psychological Association. Assessment of older adults with diminished capacity: a handbook for psychologists. 2008. http://www.apa.org/pi/aging/programs/assessment/capacity-psychologist-handbook.pdf.
8. American Bar Association, American Psychological Association, and National College of Probate Judges. Judicial determination of capacity of older adults in guardianship proceedings: a handbook for judges. 2006. www.abanet.org/aging/docs/judges_book.
9. American Board of Forensic Odontology. Guidelines for bite mark analysis. J Am Dental Assoc. 1986;112:383–6.
10. American Psychiatric Association. "Hoarding Disorder" diagnostic and statistical manual of mental disorders. 2014. http://www.dsm5.org/Documents/Obsessive%20Compulsive%20Disorders%20Fact%20Sheet.pdf.
11. American Psychological Association. Cognitive problems. 2015. http://www.apa.org/pi/about/publications/caregivers/practice-settings/assessment/tools/cognitive-problems.aspx. Accessed 2 Jan 2016.
12. Anonymous. Protecting older americans: a history of federal action on elder abuse, neglect, and exploitation. J Elder Abuse Negl. 2002; 14(2/3):9–85.
13. Appelbaum PS. Assessment of patients' competence to consent to treatment. N Engl J Med. 2007;357:1834–40.
14. ASCP (American Society of Consultant Pharmacists). What is a consultant pharmacist? 2014. https://www.ascp.com/articles/what-consultant-pharmacist). 2015. ASCP fact sheet. https://www.ascp.com/articles/about-ascp/ascp-fact-sheet.
15. Asp E, Manzel K, Koestner B, Cole CA, Denburg NL, Tranel D. A neuropsychological test of belief and doubt: damage to ventromedial prefrontal cortex increases credulity for misleading advertising. Front in Neurosci. 2012;6:1–9.
16. Bardach, S.H. & Rowles, G.D. Geriatric Education in the Health Professions: Are We Making Progress?. The Gerontologist. 2012 Oct 52(5): 607–618. http://www.ncbi.nlm.nih.gov/pmc/articles/PMC3463419. Accessed 12 Dec 2015.
17. Bartlett S. Autopsy cutbacks reveal 'Gray Homicides.' Part of the series: NPR news investigations: post mortem: death investigation in America. Co-published on broadcast media and web distribution by NPR(National Public Radio) All Things Considered, and PBS Frontline, Feb. 5, 2011. www.npr.org. Accessed 24 May 2011.
18. Bates DW, Cullen DJ, Laird N, Petersen LA, Small SD, Servi D, Laffel G, Sweitzer BJ, Shea BF, Hallisey R, Vliet MV, Nemeskal R, Leape LL, for the Bardach SH, Rowles GD. Geriatric education in the health professions: are we making progress?" Gerontologist. 2012;52(5):607–618. http://www.ncbi.nlm.nih.gov/pmc/articles/PMC3463419. Accessed 12 Dec 2015.
19. Bell-McGinty S, Podell K, Franzen M, Baird AD, Williams MJ. Standard measures of executive function in predicting instrumental activities of daily living in older adults. Int J Geriatr Psychiatry. 2002;17(9):828–34.
20. Berlowitz DR, Brandeis GH, Anderson JJ, Ash AS, Kader B, Morris JN, Moskowitz MA. Evaluation of a risk-adjustment model for pressure ulcer development using the minimum data set. J Am Geriatrics Soc. 2001;49(7):872–6.
21. Berry SD, Kiel DP. Falls. In: Durso SC, Sullivan GM, editors. Geriatrics review syllabus: a core curriculum in geriatric medicine. 8th ed. New York: American Geriatrics Society; 2013. p. 261–9.
22. Billioti de Gage S, Begaud B, Bazin F, Verdoux H, Dartigues JF, Peres K, Kurth T, Pariente A. Benzodiazepine use and risk of dementia: Prospective population based study. BMJ (Clin Res Ed). 2012;345:e6231.
23. Blakely BE, Dolon R. Another look at the helpfulness of occupational groups in the discovery of elder abuse and neglect. J Elder Abuse Negl. 2003;13:1–23.
24. Blum B. Forensic evaluations: testamentary capacity. Psychiatric Times. 2015. http://www.psychiatrictimes.com/geriatric-psychiatry/forensic-evaluations-testamentary-capacity.
25. Bowden ML, Grant ST, Vogel B, et al. The elderly, disabled and handicapped adult burned through abuse and neglect. Burns Incl Thermal Inj. 1988;14(6):447–50.
26. Brandl B, Dyer CB, Heisler CJ, Otto JM, Stiegel LA, Thomas RW. Elder abuse detection and intervention: a collaborative approach. New York: Springer; 2007.
27. Brown K, Streubert GE, Burgess AW. Effectively detect and manage elder abuse. Nurse Pract. 2004;29(8):22–7.
28. Brown AS. Patterns of abuse among native American elderly. In: Tatara T, editor. Understanding elder abuse in minority communities (ch. 10, pp. 143–159). Philadelphia: Brunner/Mazel; 1999.
29. Burgess AW, Hanrahan NP, Baker T. Forensic markers in elder female sexual abuse cases. Clin Geriatr Med. 2005;21:399–412.
30. Burgess A, Ramsey-Klawsnik H, Gregorian S. Comparing routes of reporting in elder sexual abuse cases. Elder Abuse Negl. 2008;20:336–52.
31. Burnett J, Achenbaum WA, Murphy KP. Prevention and early identification of elder abuse. Clin Geriatr Med. 2014;30:743–59.
32. Burnett J, Mitchell RA Jr, Cloyd EA, et al. Forensic markers associated with elder mistreatment and self-neglect: a case-control study. Acad Forensic Pathol. 2013;3(4):458–67.
33. California Courts. Elder abuse in tribal communities: a guide for California state judges. 2014. http://www.courts.ca.gov/documents/Elder_Abuse_Tribal_Communities.pdf.
34. California Courts. Definitions of elder abuse and settings in which abuse occurs, Chapter 2, abuse in later life bench guide. 2015. In press.
35. Campbell N, Boustani M, Limbil T, Ott C, Fox C, Maidment I, Schubert CC, Munger S, Fick D, Miller D, Gulati R. The cognitive impact of anticholinergics: a clinical review. Clin Interv Aging. 2009;4:225–33.
36. Carriere I, Fourrier-Reglat A, Dartigues JF, Rouaud O, Pasquier F, Ritchie K, Ancelin ML. Drugs with anticholinergic properties, cognitive decline, and dementia in an elderly general population: the 3-city study. Arch Int Med. 2009;169(14):1317–24.
37. Carson DK, Hand C. Dilemmas surrounding elder abuse and neglect within Native American communities. In: Understanding and combatting elder abuse in minority communities. Archstone Foundation; 1998. pp. 87–96.
38. Chang AL, Wong JW, Endo JO, et al. Geriatric dermatology Part II. Risk factors and cutaneous signs of elder mistreatment for the dermatologist. J Am Acad Dermatol. 2013;68(4):533.e1–10.
39. Collins KA, Bennett AT, Hanzlick R. The autopsy committee of the college of american pathologists. Elder Abuse Negl. Arch Intern Med. 2000;160:1567–69.
40. Collins KA, Presnell SE. Elder neglect and the pathophysiology of aging. Am J Forensic Med Pathol. 2007;28(2):157–62.
41. Collins KA. Elder maltreatment: a review. Arch Pathol Lab Med. 2006;130:1290–6.
42. Connolly MT, Brandl B, Breckman R. The elder justice roadmap: a stakeholder initiative to respond to an emerging health, justice, financial and social crisis. 2014. http://ncea.acl.gov/Library/Gov_Report/docs/EJRP_Roadmap.pdf. Accessed 7 Jan 2016.
43. Connolly MT. Where Elder abuse and the justice system collide: police power, parens patriae, and 12 recommendations. J Elder Abuse Negl. 2010;22(1/2):37–93.
44. Cooney LM, Kennedy GJ, Hawkins KA, et al. Who can stay at home? Assessing the capacity to choose to live in the community. Arch Int Med. 2004;164:357–60.

45. Cooper C, Livingston G. Mental health/psychiatric issues in elder abuse and neglect. Clin Geriatr Med. 2014;30:839–50.
46. Cooper C, Selwood A, Livingston G. Knowledge, detection and reporting of abuse by health and social care professionals: a systematic review. Am J Geriatr Psychiatry. 2009;17:826–38.
47. Cosman F, de Beur SJ, LeBoff MS, Lewiecki EM, Tanner B, Randall S, Lindsay R. Clinician's guide to prevention and treatment of osteoporosis. Osteoporosis Int. 2014;25(10):2359–2381, viewed December 28, 2015. http://www.ncbi.nlm.nih.gov/pmc/articles/PMC4176573/.
48. Crane J. Injury interpretation. In: Stark MM, editors. Forensic science: a physician's guide to forensic medicine. Totowa: Humana Press.
49. Del Carmen T, LoFaso VM. Elder neglect. Clin Geriatr Med. 2014;30:769–77.
50. Denburg NL, Cole CA, Hernandez M, Yamada TH, Tranel D, Bechara A, Wallace RB. The orbitofrontal cortex, real-world decision making, and normal aging. Ann NY Acad Sci. 2007;1121:480–98.
51. de Vries OJ, Peeters G, Elders P, Sonnenberg C, Muller M, Deeg DJ, Lips P. The elimination half-life of benzodiazepines and fall risk: Two prospective observational studies. Age Ageing. 2013;42(6):764–70.
52. Dong X. Elder abuse in chinese populations: A global review. J Elder Abuse Negl. 2015;27(3):196–232.
53. Dong X. Medical implications of elder abuse and neglect. Clin Geriatr Med. 2005;21:293–313.
54. Dong X, Lachs MS, Tinette ME. Reporting patterns of elder abuse and neglect in connecticut: an analysis of statewide database from 1992 to 2001. J Am Geriatr Soc. 2002;50:147.
55. Dyer CB, Heisler CJ, Hill CA, Kim LC. Community approaches to elder abuse. Clin Geriatr Med. 2005;21(2):429–47.
56. Dyer CB, Goodwin JS, Vogel M, et al. Characterizing self-neglect: a report of over 500 cases of self-neglect seen by a geriatric medicine team. Am J Public Health. 2007;97:1671–6.
57. Dyer C, Connolly M, McFeeley P. The clinical and medical forensics of elder abuse and neglect. In: Bonnie RJ, Wallace RB, editors. Elder mistreatment: abuse, neglect, and exploitation in an aging America. Washington, DC: National Academies Press; 2003. p. 339–81.
58. Falk E, Hoffman N. The role of capacity assessments in elder abuse investigations and guardianships. Clin Geriatr Med. 2014;30:851–68.
59. Falk E, Mosqueda L, Schneider DC, Bernatz S, Wood S. Geriatricians and psychologists: essential ingredients in the evaluation of elder abuse and neglect. J Elder Abuse Negl. 2010;22(3/4):281–290.
60. Faugno D, Waszak D, Strack GB, et al. Strangulation forensic examination: best practice for health care providers. Adv Emerg Nurs J. 2013;3(4):314–27.
61. Fick DM, Semla TP. American geriatrics society beers criteria: New Year, new criteria, new perspective. J Am Geriatr Soc. 2012;60(4):614–5.
62. Fried LP, Tangen CM, Walston J, Newman AB, Hirsch C, Gottdiener J, Seeman T, Tracy R, Kop WJ, Burke G, McBurnie MA. Frailty in older adults: evidence for a phenotype. J Gerontol A Biol Sci Med Sci. 2001;56:M146–56.
63. Friedman LS, Avila S, Tanouye K, et al. A case-control study of severe physical abuse of older adults. J Am Geriatr Soc. 2011;59 (3):417–22.
64. Fulmer T, Guadagno L, Dyer CB, et al. Progress in elder abuse screening and assessment instruments. J Am Geriatr Soc. 2004;52:1–8.
65. Gibbs LM. Understanding the medical markers of elder abuse and neglect: physical examination findings. Clin Geriatr Med. 2014;30:687–712.
66. Gibson SC, Greene E. Assessing knowledge of elder financial abuse: a first step in enhancing prosecutions. J Elder Abuse Negl 2013;25(2):162–182.
67. Gill JR, Cavalli DP, Ely SF, Stahl-Herz J. Homicidal neck compression of females: autopsy and sexual assault findings homicidal neck compression of females: autopsy and sexual assault findings. Acad Forensic Pathol. 2013;3(4):454–7.
68. Greenbaum AR, Horton JB, Williams CJ, et al. Burn injuries inflicted on children or the elderly: a framework for clinical and forensic assessment. Plast Reconstr Surg. 2006;118:46–8.
69. Greenbaum AR, Donne J, Wilson D, Dunn KW. Intentional burn injury: an evidence-based, clinical and forensic review. Burns. 2004;30(7):628–42.
70. Hansberry MR, Chen E, Gorbien MJ. Dementia and elder abuse. Clin Geriatr Med. 2005;21:315–32.
71. Heisler CJ. Elder abuse and the criminal justice system: an uncertain future. Generations. 2012;36(3):83–8.
72. Hudson MF, Carlson J. Elder abuse: its meaning to caucasians, African Americans, and Native Americans. In: Tatara T, editor. Understanding elder abuse in minority communities, chapter 12. Philadelphia: Brunner/Mazel; 1999. pp. 187–204.
73. Griffith HR, Belue K, Sicola A, et al. Impaired financial abilities in mild cognitive impairment: A direct assessment approach. Neurology. 2003;60:449–57.
74. Harning AT Initial findings in stargulation injury aren't indicative of outcome. J Emerg Med Serv. 2015. http://www.jems.com/articles/print/volume-41/issue-1/departments-columns/case-of-the-month/initial-findings-in-strangulation-injury-aren-t-indicative-of-outcome.html. Accessed 28 Dec 2015.
75. Hawley DA Death by strangulation or suffocation (chapter 6) in the investigation and prosecution of strangulation cases. Training Institute on Strangulation Prevention and California District Attorneys Association; 2013.
76. Hawley DA, McClane G, Strack GB. A review of 300 attempted strangulation cases part III: injuries in fatal cases. J Emerg Med. 2001;21:317–22.
77. Hendrix LR. Ethnogeriatric curriculum module: health and health care of American Indian and Alaska native elders. www.stanford.edu/group/ethnoger/americanindian.html.
78. Homeier D. Aging: physiology, disease and abuse. Clin Geriatr Med. 2014;30:671–86.
79. Howe A, Collins KA, King PS, Yeoman C. Investigation of elder deaths. Acad Forensic Pathol. 2014;4(3):290–304.
80. Institute of Medicine. Risk and Protective Factors and Interventions: Health and Medical Factors. In: Dan G. Blazer, Kristine Yaffe, and Catharyn T. Liverman, editors. Cognitive Aging: Progress in Understanding and Opportunities for Action, Chapter 4B. Washington, DC: The National Academies Press; 2015. p. 149–186. https://www.nap.edu/download/21693.
81. Iserson KV. Strangulation. A review of ligature, manual, and postural neck compression in juries. Ann Emerg Med. 1984;13:179–85.
82. Johannesen M, LoGiudice D. Elder abuse: a systematic review of risk factors in community-dwelling elders. Age Ageing. 2013;42:292–8.
83. Johnson SC. Traumatic brain injury, Chapter 68. In: Halter JB, Ouslander JG, Tinetti ME, et al., editors. Hazzard's geriatric medicine and gerontology. 6th ed. New York: McGraw-Hill; 2009.
84. Johnson K. Financial crimes against the elderly. Problem-oriented guides for police. Guide number 20. 2004. http://www.popcenter.org/problems/crimes_against_elderly/.
85. Kalisch Ellett LM, Pratt NL, Ramsay EN, Barratt JD, Roughead EE. Multiple anticholinergic medication use and risk of hospital admission for confusion or dementia. J Am Geriatr Soc. 2014;62(10):1916–22.

86. Kane R, Goodwin J. Pathologic fractures of the long bones in nursing home patients. Am J Med. 1991;90:263–6.
87. Karch D, Nunn KC. Characteristics of elderly and other vulnerable adult victims of homicide by a caregiver: national violent death reporting system-17 US States, 2003–2007. J Interpers Violence. 2011;26(137):137–57.
88. Karlsson MK, Magnusson H, von Schewelov T, et al. Prevention of falls in the elderly—a review. Osteoporos Int. 2012. http://dx.doi.org/10.1007/s00198-012-2256-7.
89. Karp N. Protecting older investors: the challenge of diminished capacity. Generations. 2012;36(2):33–8.
90. Kennedy R. Elder abuse and neglect: the experience, knowledge, and attitudes of primary care physicians. Fam Med. 2005;37:481–5.
91. Kim L, Mitchell S, Dyer C. Do medical examiners determine elder mistreatment as a cause of death? Forensic Sci Med Pathol. 2007;3:9–13.
92. Koenig R, DeGuerre C. The legal and governmental response to domestic elder abuse. Orlando: Elsevier Saunders; 2005. p. 383–98.
93. Krauss D, Cassar D, Strother A. The admissibility of expert testimony in the united states, the commonwealth, and elsewhere. In: Krausee D, Lieberman J, editors. Psychological expertise in court. Burlington: Ashgate Publishing; 2009. p. 1–24.
94. Kuter DJ. Senile Purpura. Merck Manual, Professional Version. 2014. http://www.merckmanuals.com/professional/hematology-and-oncology/bleeding-due-to-abnormal-blood-vessels/senile-purpura. Accessed 29 Dec 2015.
95. Lachs MS, Pillemer KA. Elder abuse. New Engl J Med. 2015;373:1947–56.
96. Lachs M, Pillemer K. Abuse and neglect of elderly persons. N Engl J Med. 1995;332:437–43.
97. Lezak M, Howieson DB, Loring DW. Neuropsychological assessment. 4th ed. New York: Oxford University Press; 2004. p. 611.
98. Li J, Brown J, Levine M. Mild head injury, anticoagulants, and risk of intracranial injury. Lancet. 2001;357:771.
99. LoFaso VM, Rosen T. Medical and laboratory indicators of elder abuse and neglect. Clin Geriatr Med. 2014;30:713–28.
100. Lusardi A. Financial literacy and financial decision-making in older adults. Generations. 2012;36(2):25–32.
101. Lyder CH. Pressure ulcer prevention and management. JAMA. 2003;289:2.
102. Merriam Webster Dictionary (ND) "Forensic. http://www.merriam-webster.com/dictionary/forensic. Accessed 9 Dec 2015.
103. Marson DC. Clinical and ethical aspects of financial capacity in dementia: a commentary. Am J Geriatr Psychiatry. 2013;21(4):390–2. doi:10.1097/JGP.0b013e31826682f4.
104. Marson DC, Heber K, Solomon A. Assessing civil competencies in older adults with dementia: consent capacity, financial capacity, and testamentary capacity. In: Larrabee GJ, editor. Forensic neuropathology: a scientific approach. 2d ed. New York: Oxford University Press; 2011. p. 401–37.
105. Marson DC, Sabantino CP. Financial capacity in an aging society. Generations. 2012;36(2):6–11.
106. Marson DC, Sawrie SM, Snyder S, et al. Assessing financial capacity in patients with Alzheimer Disease: a conceptual model and prototype instrument. Arch Neurol. 2000;57(6):877–84. doi:10.1001/archneur.57.6.877.
107. Marson DC, Earnst KS, Jamil F, Bartolucci A, Harrell LE. Consistency of physicians' legal standard and personal judgments of competency in patients with Alzheimer's Disease. J Am Geriatr Soc. 2000;48(8):911–8.
108. McClane G, Strack GB, Hawley DA. A review of 300 attempted strangulation cases part II: non-fatal assaults. J Emerg Med. 2001;21:311–5.
109. McNamee CC, Murphy MB. Elder abuse in the United States. NIJ J. 2001;255. http://www.nij.gov/journals/255/pages/elder_abuse.aspx.
110. Moskowitz S. Filial responsibility statutes: legal and policy considerations. J Law Policy. 2001;9(3):709–36.
111. Mosqueda L, Dong X. Elder abuse and neglect, "I don't care anything about going to the doctor, to be honest. JAMA. 2011;306:532–40.
112. Mosqueda L, Burnight K, Liao S. The life cycle of bruises in older adults. J Am Geriatr Soc. 2005;53(8):1339–43.
113. Mosqueda L, Burnight K, Liao S, et al. Advancing the field of elder mistreatment: a new model for integration of social and medical services. Gerontologist. 2004;44(5):703–8.
114. Moye J. Clinical frameworks for capacity assessment. In: Qualls S, Smyer M, editors. Changes in decision-making capacity in older adults: assessment and intervention. Hoboken: Wiley; 2007. p. 177–89.
115. Moye J, Marson D. Assessment of decision-making capacity in older adults: an emerging area of practice and research. J Gerontol B Psychol Sci Soc Sci. 2007;62(1):3–11.
116. Naik AD, Lai JM, Kunik ME, et al. Assessing capacity in suspected cases of self-neglect. Geriatric. 2008;63:24–31.
117. Nasreddine ZS, Phillips NA, Bédirian V, Charbonneau S, Whitehead V, Collin I, Cummings JLC, Chertkow H. The montreal cognitive assessment, MoCA: a brief screening tool for mild cognitive impairment. J Am Geriatr Soc. 2005;53:695–9.
118. National Research Council. Elder Mistreatment: abuse, neglect, and exploitation in an aging America. In: Bonnie RJ, Wallace RBRB, editors. Washington, DC: National Academies Press; 2003.
119. Navarro AE, Gassoumis Z, Wilber K. Holding abusers accountable: an elder abuse forensic center increases criminal prosecution of financial exploitation. Gerontologist. 2013;53(2):303–12.
120. Navarro AE. Improving outcomes for victims of financial exploitation: the effect of an elder abuse forensic center, dissertation. 2011. http://www.academia.edu/1903264/Improving_outcomes_for_victims_of_financial_exploitation_The_effect_of_an_elder_abuse_forensic_center. Accessed 12 Dec 2015.
121. Navarro AE, Wilber KH, Yonashiro J, Homeier DC. Do we really need another meeting? Lessons from the Los Angeles county elder abuse forensic center. Gerontologist. 2010;50(5):702–11.
122. Nerenberg L, Davies M, Navarro A. In pursuit of a useful framework to champion elder justice. Generations. 2012;36(3):89–96.
123. Nusbaum NJ, Cheung VM, Cohen J, Keca M, Malley B. Role of first responders in detecting and evaluating elders at risk. Arch Gerontol Geriatr. 2006;43:361–7.
124. O'Connor D, Hall MI, Donnelly M. Assessing capacity within a context of abuse or neglect. J Elder Abuse Negl. 2009;21(2):156–69.
125. Payne BK, King PS, Manaois A. Training police officers about elder abuse: training needs and strategies. Int Perspect Victimol. 2009;4(2):40–9.
126. Plattner T, Bolliger S, Zollinger U. Forensic assessment of survived strangulation. Forensic Sci Int. 2005;153:202–7.
127. Policastro C, Payne BK. Assessing the level of elder abuse knowledge preprofessionals possess: implications for the further development of university curriculum. J Elder Abuse Negl. 2014;26(1):12–30.
128. Powers JS. Common presentations of elder abuse in health care settings. Clin Geriatr Med. 2014;30:729–41.
129. Prahlow JA. Investigation of deaths of chronically disabled persons and institutionalized persons. Acad Forensic Pathol. 2014;4(3):262–89.

130. Rathbone-McCuan, Bricker-Jenkins. Self-neglect and adult protective services in social counselor certification resource handbook. Nashville, TN Department of Social Services; 1989. 301 (cited in Longres, Self-neglect among the elderly. J Elder Abuse Negl. 1995;7(1):69–86).
131. Reyes-Ortiz CA, Burnett J, Flores DV, Halphen JM, Dyer CB. Medical implications of elder abuse: self-neglect. Clin Geriatr Med. 2014;30:807–23.
132. Royall DR, Chiodo LK, Polk MJ. An empiric approach to level of care determinations: the importance of executive measures. J Gerontol A Biol Sci Med Sci. 2005;60A:1059–64.
133. Safarik ME, Jarvis JP, Nussbaum KE. Sexual homicide of elderly females: linking offender characteristics to victim and crime scene attributes. J Interpersonal Violence. 2002;17:500–25.
134. Samanez-Larkin GR, Levens SM, Perry LM, Dougherty RF, Knutson B. Frontostriatal white matter integrity mediates adult age differences in probabilistic reward learning. J Neurosci. 2012;32(15):5333–7.
135. Samton JB, Ferrando SJ, Sanelli P, et al. The clock drawing test: diagnostic, functional, and neuroimaging correlates in older medically ill adults. J Neuropsychiatry Clin Neurosci. 2005;7:533–40.
136. Schneider DC, Mosqueda L, Falk E, Huba GJ. Elder abuse forensic centers. J Elder Abuse Negl. 2010;22(3/4):255–74.
137. Schmeidel A, Daly J, Rosenbaum M, et al. Health Care professionals' perspectives on barriers to elder abuse detection and reporting in primary care settings. J Elder Abuse Negl. 2012;24(1):17–36.
138. Shany-Ur T, Poorzand P, Grossman SN, Growdon ME, Jang JY, Ketelle RS, Miller BL, Rankin KP. Comprehension of insincere communication in neurodegenerative disease: lies, sarcasm, and theory of mind. Cortex. 20121;48:13329–1341. http://www.sscnet.ucla.edu/polisci/faculty/chwe/austen/shany-ur.pdf. Accessed 16 Dec 2015.
139. Sherod MG, Griffith HR, Copeland J, Belue K, Krzywanski S, Zamrini EY, Harrell LE, Clark DG, Brockington JC, Powers RE, Marson DC. Neurocognitive predictors of financial capacity across the dementia spectrum: normal aging, mild cognitive impairment, and alzheimer's disease. J Int Neuropsychol Soc. 2009;15(2):258–67.
140. Shields L, Hunsaker D, Hunsaker J. Abuse and neglect: a ten-year review of mortality and morbidity in our elderly in a large metropolitan area. J Forensic Sci. 2004;49(1):122–7.
141. Simpson AR. Cultural issues and elder mistreatment. Clin Geriatr Med. 2005;21:355–64.
142. Smith DJ, Mills T, Taliaferro EH. Frequency and relationship of reported symptomology in victims of intimate partner violence: the effect of multiple attempted strangulation attacks. J Emerg Med. 2001;21:323–9.
143. Stahl S. Building consensus on research priorities in elder mistreatment. 2015. http://www.justice.gov/elderjustice/research/resources/Building_Consensus_On_Research_Priorities_In_Elder_Mistreatment.pdf. Accessed 7 Jan 2016.
144. Stapczynski JS. Strangulation injuries. Emerg Med Rep. 2010;31(17):193–203.
145. Stiegel L, Klem E, Turner J. Neglect of older persons: an introduction to legal issues related to caregiver duty and liability. 2007. Neglect. Retrieved from http://www.americanbar.org/content/dam/aba/migrated/aging/about/pdfs/neglect_of_older_persons.authcheckdam.pdf.
146. Stiegel L. The changing role of the courts in elder abuse cases. Generations. 2000;24(11):59–64.
147. Strack GB, McClane G, Hawley DA. A review of 300 attempted strangulation cases part I: criminal legal issues. J Emerg Med. 2001;21:303–9.
148. Suffla S, Seedat M. The epidemiology of homicidal strangulation in the city of Johannesburg, South Africa. J Foren Legal Med. 2016;37:97–107.
149. Talamantes M, Aranda M. Cultural competency in working with latino caregivers. National Center on Caregiving; 2004.
150. Tannenbaum C, Paquette A, Hilmer S, Holroyd-Leduc J, Carnahan R. A systematic review of amnestic and non-amnestic mild cognitive impairment induced by anticholinergic, antihistamine, gabaergic and opioid drugs. Drugs Aging. 2012;29(8):639–58.
151. Taylor T, Mulford C. Evaluating th Los Angeles County elder abuse forensic center. 2015. http://www.nij.gov/journals/276/Pages/elder-abuse-forensic-center.aspx.
152. Teaster PB, Dugar TA, Mendiondo MS, et al. The 2004 survey of state adult protective services: abuse of adults 60 years and older. Report prepared by The National Committee for the Prevention of Elder Abuse and The National Adult Protective Services Association. Washington, DC: National Center on Elder Abuse; 2007.
153. Terracina KA, Aamodt WW, Schillerstrom JE. Executive function impairment and recidivism in adult protective services clients referred for a decision making capacity assessment. J Elder Abuse Negl. 2015;27(2):91–9.
154. Tisdale M. Biology of cachexia. JNCI J Natl Cancer Inst. 1997;89(23):1763–73. Retrieved 9 Jan 2016 from http://jnci.oxfordjournals.org/content/89/23/1763.full.
155. Triebel KL, Martin R, Griffith HR, Marceaux MA, Okonkwo OC, Harrell L, Clark D, Brockington J, Bartolucci A, Marson DC. Declining financial capacity in patients with mild cognitive impairment: a one-year longitudinal study. Neurology. 2009;73:928–34. http://www.ncbi.nlm.nih.gov/pmc/articles/PMC2754335/.
156. Triebel KL, Marson DC. The warning signs of diminished financial capacity in older adults. Generations. 2012;36(2):39–45.
157. Tronetti P. Evaluating abuse in the patient with dementia. Clin Geriatr Med. 2014;30:825–38.
158. Twomey MS, Weber C. Health professionals' roles and relationships with other agencies. Clin Geriatr Med. 2014;30:881–95.
159. Twomey MS, Jackson G, Li H, Marino T, Melchior LA, Randolph JF, Retselli-Deits T, Wysong J. The successes and challenges of seven multidisciplinary teams. J Elder Abuse Negl. 2010;22(3/4):291–305.
160. Uekert BK, Keilitz S, Saunders D, Heisler CJ, Ulrey P, Baldwin EG. Prosecuting elder abuse cases: basic tools and strategies. National Center for State Courts; 2012.
161. Ulrey P, Brandl B. Collaboration is essential: king county's response to a case of elder abuse and exploitation. Generations. 2012;36(3):73–8.
162. US Department of Health and Human Services & Elder Justice Coordinating Council. Report to congress. 2012–2014. http://www.aoa.acl.gov/AoA_Programs/Elder_Rights/EJCC/docs/EJCC-2012-2014-report-to-congress.pdf. Accessed 7 Jan 2016.
163. US Legal. Preponderance of the evidence. 2015. http://courts.uslegal.com/burden-of-proof/preponderance-of-the-evidence/. Accessed 28 Dec 2015.
164. Vognar L, Gibbs LM. Care of the patient. Clin Geriatr Med. 2014;30:869–80.
165. Warren L, et al. The burden and outcomes associated with dehydration in the elderly, 1991. Am J Public Health. 1994;84:1265–9.
166. White House Conference on Aging. Final report. 2016. http://www.whitehouseconferenceonaging.gov/2015-WHCOA-Final-Report.pdf.
167. Widera E, Steenpass V, Marson D, et al. Finances in the older patient with cognitive impairment 'he didn't want me to take over'. JAMA. 2011;305(7):698–706.

168. Wiglesworth A, Austin R, Corona M, et al. Bruising as a marker of physical elder abuse. J Am Geriatr Soc. 2009;57:1191–6.
169. Wiglesworth A, Mosqueda L, Burnight K, Younglove T, Jeske D. Findings from an elder abuse forensic center. Gerontologist. 2006;46:277–83.
170. Wilbur L, Higley M, Hatfield J, et al. Survey results of women who have been strangled while in an abusive relationship. J Emerg Med. 2001;21(3):297–302.
171. Wolf RS. Introduction: the nature and scope of elder abuse. Generations. 2000;24(11):6–12.
172. Wolfe DA. Elder abuse intervention: lessons from child abuse and domestic violence interventions. In: Bonnie RJ, Wallace RB, editors. Elder mistreatment: abuse, neglect, and exploitation in an aging America. Washington, DC: National Academies Press; 2003. p. 501–25.
173. Xue Q. The frailty syndrome: definition and natural history. Clin Geriatr Med. 2011;27(1):1–15. doi:10.1016/j.cger.2010.08.009.
174. Young LA. Elder physical abuse. Clin Geriatr Med. 2014;30:761–8.
175. Zelazo PD, Craik FI, Booth L. Executive function across the life span. Acta Psychol. 2004;115(2–3):167–83.
176. Ziminski CE, Phillips LR, Woods DL. Raising the index of suspicion for elder abuse: cognitive impairment, falls and injury patterns in the emergency department. Geriatr Nurs. 2012;33(2):105–12.

Cases

177. Berger v. United States (1935) 295 U.S. 78.
178. Daubert v. Merrell Dow Pharmaceuticals (1993) 509 US 579, 113 S. Ct. 2786.
179. Frye v. United States (DC, 1923) 293 F. 1013.
180. Glage v. Hawes Firearms Co. (CA, 1990) 226 Cal.App.3d 314, 276 Cal.Rptr. 430.
182. In re Angelia P. (CA, 1981) 28 Cal.3d 908, 171 Cal.Rptr. 637, 623 P.2d 198.
182. People v. Heitzman, (CA, 1994) 9 Cal. 4th 189, 37 Cal. Rptr. 2d 236, 886 P. 2d 1229.
183. People v. Miller (CA, 1916) 171 Cal. 649, 154 P. 468.
184. California Criminal Jury Instructions (CALCRIM) 220.
185. California Penal Code §1096.
186. California Penal Code §1096a.
187. Public Act 111–148, Title VI, Subtitle H—the Elder Justice Act, Subtitle B "Elder Justice", Section 2011(18), available at http://www.ncea.aoa.gov/Resources/Publication/docs/ELDER_JUSTICE_ACT_2010.pdf.

19 Elder Abuse Multidisciplinary Teams

Georgia J. Anetzberger

Multidisciplinary teams (M-teams) have a long history in the field of elder abuse, beginning with the inception of adult protective services at mid-twentieth century. However, as the disciplines and systems interested in this problem have grown, and, with them, competing laws and philosophies, so too has the belief that M-teams are critical for effectively addressing elder abuse. Recent examples of this viewpoint are many, and include the *Elder Justice Roadmap* funded by the US Department of Justice with support from the US Department of Health and Human Services, which prioritized the development of "more multidisciplinary teams throughout the country that have adequate support for facilitators and operations" [17, p. 10]. In addition, two documents surrounding the 2015 White House Conference on Aging underscore the importance of elder abuse M-teams. The "Elder Justice" policy brief acknowledges, "with so many entities playing a role, there is growing recognition of the need for multidisciplinary collaboration" [84, p. 3]. Moreover, in a special issue of *The Gerontologist* on the event, there was a call made for a coordinated response to elder abuse: "Multidisciplinary teams (MDTs) have emerged as an effective response to coordinating care and reducing fragmentation, leveraging resources, increasing professional knowledge, and improving outcomes" [64, pp. 324–325].

This chapter examines M-teams as an intervention model for elder abuse in large part through review of literature on the subject both historic and current. It describes the various facets of M-teams in six sections. "Overview" considers their rationale, definition, and functions. "Onset" gives the evolution of M-teams over time, along with present types and legal basis. "Organization" examines M-team formality, auspice, policies, membership, and coordination. "Operations" explores leadership, member roles, member training, case selection criteria, and case review process of M-teams. "Obstacles" begins by delineating the benefits of M-teams before identifying the many challenges they can face. "Outcomes" summarizes evaluative research on M-teams. Finally, "Outlook" considers the future for M-teams as an elder abuse intervention. Throughout this chapter, Ohio elder abuse M-teams are used for illustration. This is appropriate, because among the earliest collaborative efforts in elder abuse, including M-teams, occurred in Ohio. Furthermore, the commitment to this approach continues, exemplified by recent legislation to expand and structure M-teams statewide.

19.1 Overview

The field of elder abuse is infamous for an inability to achieve consensus on such fundamentals as "how should elder abuse be defined" and "what forms does it take" [2, 65]. Consequently, it may be surprising to learn there is near universal agreement that problem prevention and intervention require a multidisciplinary approach (e.g., [36, 41, 55]). Increasingly the preferred one is a clinical or case consult team (e.g., [20, 22]).

19.1.1 Rationale for M-Teams

The rationale for M-teams is found in the complexity and scope of elder abuse itself, and therefore the many different laws and services that may be required to address it. Indeed, elder abuse has properties of an amoeba. It seems to lack definite shape. Rather, it is in a constant state of movement, change, and absorption. For example, earliest recognition of the problem had limited sights on what we now label "self-neglect," with the potential of "exploitation" [31]. Over time other forms came into view and were included in the conceptualization of elder abuse, as researchers, practitioners, and advocates tried to give structure to the myriad examples of harm inflicted on older adults [45, 48]. These

G.J. Anetzberger (✉)
Department of Medicine, Case Western Reserve University, 1105 Hillrock Drive, 44121 South Euclid, OH, USA
e-mail: g.anetzberger@csuohio.edu

X. Dong (ed.), *Elder Abuse*, DOI 10.1007/978-3-319-47504-2_19

forms ranged from physical abuse to emotional abuse to abandonment. Similarly, perpetrators of elder abuse have been found to vary, from the victim him/herself (as with self-abuse and self neglect) to such "trusted others" as family members and formal caregivers to even strangers and acquaintances. Finally, the settings wherein elder abuse occurs are many, including private homes, adult day service centers, and nursing facilities. Adding to the complexity can be polyvictimization, where victims experience multiple forms or multiple perpetrators within or across types of settings [69]. This variety of forms, perpetrators, and settings has implications for which laws and systems might be relevant in given situations of elder abuse along with which discipline perspectives and procedures might best remedy them. Further complicating the selection is the fact that no one system or discipline is seen as dominating the field, although some "jockeying for power" has occurred, especially with the recent availability of more federal funding to better understand and address the problem [3].

19.1.2 Definition of M-Teams

Multidisciplinary teams can be defined as groups of persons representing different professional disciplines or service systems assembled for problem identification and treatment recommendation [4]. Their focus is on the older adult who has been victimized by elder abuse or is at risk of the same. To a lesser extent, but still important, teams may consider the problems and needs of caregivers, perpetrators, or other involved parties in abuse situations in order to prevent further abuse occurrence.

The terms "multidisciplinary" and "interdisciplinary" often are used interchangeably in the field of elder abuse (e.g., [22, 47]). However, they differ with respect to locus of decision-making, with M-teams delegating the responsibility to one member and interdisciplinary teams requiring each member's participation. M-teams also are distinguishable from elder abuse networks, alternatively called coalitions, councils, or task forces. Although some sources collapse teams and networks together [10, 46], they actually differ from one another in three ways: focus, purpose, and membership. Unlike teams, networks are not focused on individual cases, but rather on systems, communities, or in some instances even regions and states. Their intent is to identify gaps or inadequacies in elder abuse detection, prevention, and treatment and then to facilitate required changes to remedy them. Because of their particular focus and purpose, networks have change agents as members, be they community planners, policy makers, government officials, agency leaders, or media representatives. In contrast, members of M-teams are clinical experts with practice involvement. Finally, teams and networks can be interrelated, with networks forming teams for case handling and teams identifying issues for system or community change. This interrelationship is illustrated in Box 1, which describes the Clinical Consultation Team as a standing committee of the Protective Services Consortium for Older Adults of Cuyahoga County, Ohio.

19.1.3 Functions of M-Teams

Twomey et al. [83] summarize the functions of M-teams as advice, resources, and new perspectives. These functions are evident in results from a national survey of 31 such teams, which found that 80 % or more fulfilled each of the following tasks [82]:

- Providing expert consultation to service providers
- Identifying service gaps or problems
- Updating members on services, programs, and policy
- Advocating for change
- Planning and implementing training events
- Planning and facilitating coordinated investigations and service delivery.

In addition, M-teams also may engage in activities aimed at achieving desired outcomes, like insuring offender accountability or increasing offender prosecution [49, 52]. They can serve to support the case referent, struggling with clinical and ethical issues endemic to elder abuse situations [30]. In this light, it should not be surprising that most M-teams tackle only difficult or complex cases, those which present no easy solutions or where remedies transcend agencies or systems [44]. Examples of qualifying cases seen by the Interdisciplinary Team of the Adult Protective Collaborative in Cuyahoga County, Ohio are identified in Box 2. Collectively they suggest elder abuse situations challenging to assess and treat effectively without the benefit of multiple professional perspectives and categories of practice. Even then, remedy can be elusive, a subject examined later in this chapter under "Outcomes."

19.2 Onset

The antecedent to elder abuse M-teams can be found in the beginning formation of adult protective services well over a half century ago. It started during the 1950s with conversations among service providers in urban centers, who were seeing a growing number of older adults living alone without nearby family support, but incapable of managing their personal affairs or assets because of frailty or incapacity. Ultimately these service providers came to believe that a new intervention model was required to insure the safety and well-being of this population. At Cleveland's Welfare Federation the general consensus favored one that was "multidisciplinary in character" [7, p. 1].

By the early 1960s these community dialogues were elevated to national forums on "protective care or services [which should] represent a constellation of services, preventive or supportive in nature" [26, p. xii] and assume "an interdisciplinary approach" [60, p. 124]. Social work, law, and medicine were seen to be the key disciplines in this approach, with social work having the leadership role [31].

Protective service demonstrations followed during the period 1964–1970. Their aim was to develop and evaluate protective services as an intervention model as well as to delineate its service population. There were seven such demonstrations in places like San Diego and Philadelphia. Their evaluation findings suggested the necessity of protective services being able to access a broad range of services and to establish protocols for multidisciplinary diagnosis and referral. Although social work continued to guide service organization and delivery, it was recognized that other disciplines should be represented on staff or as consultants, particularly law, psychiatry, and medicine [70]. However, when Horowitz and Estes [32, p. 10] examined the multidisciplinary responses among the demonstrations, they found that most employed "consultants only on the request of the program's social workers." For instance, with ample revenues on hand to purchase outside ancillary services, social workers at the Cleveland Benjamin Rose Institute demonstration (described in Box 3) used this funding for medical evaluation in one-half of the cases and psychiatric or legal consultation in one-fifth of the cases [9]. Still, the result hardly could be considered an M-team, more like contracted professional service provision. This approach dominated adult protective services during the 1970s, as Title XX of the Social Security Act led to its spread nationwide along with the availability of funds for purchasing supportive services [13].

19.2.1 Types of M-Teams

The 1980s witnessed the emergence of the many types of elder abuse M-teams with which we are familiar today. This emergence was sparked by growing recognition and concern about elder abuse in American society, with communities struggling to address individual situations effectively amid the passage of various intersecting laws and increasing numbers of implementing service systems [16]. The emergence of such M-teams also reflected elder abuse's general tendency to borrow what works in other fields, rather than create its own. Typically borrowing has been from the other aspects of family violence, and can be illustrated by modeling most adult protective services laws after child protective services laws [87] and often adopting child abuse and spouse abuse theory to explain elder abuse [63]. In this context, although some types of M-teams had their origins with other aspects of family violence, such as fatality review teams, other types like Fiduciary Abuse Specialist Teams, uniquely belong to elder abuse.

The literature suggests there may be as many as seven common or emerging elder abuse M-teams. Each is briefly described below:

- Geriatric or medical assessment team: This type is usually based in either a hospital or health care system where the focus is on clinical evaluation, report recommendation, and care management, including appropriate discharge, of elder abuse situations as complex cases [11, 61]. Geriatric assessment teams concerned with elder abuse emerged in the early 1980s. At their simplest they consist of physicians, nurses, and social workers, but teams also may include such other disciplines as therapists and chaplains [25]. Examples of these teams are Beth Israel Hospital Elder Assessment Team in Boston [30] and Texas Elder Abuse and Mistreatment (TEAM) [24].
- Community case consult teams: This team is generally under the auspice of an elder abuse network or cooperative partnership [8]. The latter is illustrated in Ohio though efforts by the state's Supreme Court to encourage county probate courts and adult protective services programs to cooperate in the formation local elder abuse coordinated action plans, including M-teams (see Boxes 4 and 5). Community case consult teams also tend to have among the largest and most diverse memberships of the various types of M-teams. This, in turn, results in a broad array of potential cases referred for review, necessitating very wide-ranging service and legal options. A long-standing example of such a team is found in San Francisco under the Institute on Aging, with over 50 participating organizations [10, 88].
- Adult protection team: This team is formed by a local adult protective services program, and sometimes required by state law or regulation. It includes other community partners that volunteer in efforts to address elder abuse situations. However, unlike community case consult teams, a clear purpose of an adult protection team is to assist adult protective services caseworkers in case assessment and resource securement. In addition, the team may promote connections between adult protective services programs and other community agencies, educate community agencies about the role and limitations of adult protective services work, and improve the image of the program, thereby fostering elder abuse reporting.

Illinois requires adult protective services programs to have M-teams [53], and Colorado strongly encourages their development [76].

- Financial Abuse Specialist Team (FAST): This is perhaps the best known type of elder abuse M-team. Begun in California in the early 1990s, FAST has spread to other states, the appeal to replicate bolstered with growing interest and activity related to financial exploitation. FAST is distinguished from other M-teams in four ways: (1) specialty in financial exploitation; (2) emphasis on early intervention, with some FAST including rapid or emergency response components [43]; (3) often membership from the private sector, including bankers, financial planners, accountants, or securities brokers [6]; and (4) frequent representation from state and federal law enforcement and regulatory agencies, where financial exploitation may fall under their jurisdiction [52].
- Fatality review team: The role of this team is to identify and prosecute elder abuse-related deaths that otherwise might be missed [54]. The team also often uncovers problems or conduct that can lead to death, making recommendations to improve service systems or professional behavior [10]. Unlike the deaths of children, adolescents, and younger adults, those of older adults typically are viewed as "natural" or "expected," and therefore not subject to scrutiny. Interest in this type of team emerged from highly publicized wrongful deaths in residential care facilities. Team members typically include professionals less often found in other M-teams, such as representatives from the coroner's office, state licensing agency, funeral homes, health maintenance organizations, and hospice agencies [51].
- Forensic center team: Elder abuse forensic center teams originated in California during the early 2000s with the broad mission of convening professionals to protect "vulnerable elders and dependent adults from abuse and neglect" through the application of "scientific knowledge" to [these] "legal problems" [50, pp. 703–704; 85]. Representatives from health care, justice, and adult protective services meet regularly toward case analysis, problem-solving, service provision, and prosecution in these teams [23]. Evaluation of the Los Angeles team demonstrated its effectiveness in increased prosecution over matched cases receiving usual care from adult protective services [49]. The earliest example of this type of team is found under the Geriatric Program at the University of California Irvine [42].
- Hoarding team: A multidisciplinary approach is regarded as the only successful one for dealing with hoarding cases [29, 62]. Not surprisingly, therefore, M-teams are increasingly used for older adults with mental health problems who exhibit hoarding behaviors, many situations of which qualify as "self-neglect" under state adult protective services laws [14]. Like other M-teams, hoarding team members represent a variety of agencies and disciplines. However, these teams are distinguished by the inclusion of code enforcement departments, public health officials, veterinarians, and animal control agencies. Hoarding teams focus on severe hoarding situations and "providing unduplicated services [that] can meet the multifaceted needs of the hoarder," with leadership changing depending on the most immediate issues presented [39, p. 63]. An example of a hoarding team is discussed in Box 6. The Enforced Harm Reduction Approach of the Hoarding Connection of Cuyahoga County, Ohio is a replication of a model that originated in Orange County, California.

19.2.2 Legal Basis for M-Teams

Several states have statutory language on elder abuse M-teams, typically as part of adult protective services law [18, 79]. They include California, Colorado, Florida, Iowa, Kentucky, Minnesota, and Nevada. Among these states, some mandate M-teams, others authorize them. The designated functions of M-teams vary considerably, with the following most common: case assessment of need, plan development, and service monitoring; service coordination; resource development; and community education. Likewise, diverse disciplines are named for representation on M-teams, with the following listed most often: medical or health care personnel, law enforcement officials, social workers, mental health service providers, and county attorneys. Research by Daly and Jogerst [18] suggests that elder abuse investigation rates for states having M-team statutory language are significantly higher than for states without it. In 2015 Ohio joined those states mandating the establishment of M-teams as a provision of adult protective services law, with state funding available to support this effort for successful applicant counties. This occurred one decade after the Ohio Elder Abuse Task Force recommended such action (see Boxes 7, 8, and 9).

19.3 Organization

Several elements comprise an elder abuse M-team, directing its operations and enabling it to function as an integrated whole. Each element offers options, ultimately creating variation among teams, even those of the same type.

19.3.1 Formality

The relationship among M-team members can be informal or formal. Informal relations tend to occur early in team formation, often evolving into formal relations over time [57]. They also are common among professionals who have a long history of working together [10], as often occurs in small or rural communities. Informal relations offer flexibility, but they can be forgotten or subject to reinterpretation. In contrast, formal relations among team members are characterized by written agreements, like contracts or memorandums of understanding, which delineate team member responsibilities and must be periodically renegotiated. Agreements provide clarity and specificity, but they can seem restrictive and fail to accommodate individual circumstance. Formal relations are necessary when M-teams must comply with state statutes and regulations, and naturally develop when teams become large. In their national survey of elder abuse M-teams, Teaster et al. [82] found that just over half required members to sign agreements. For instance, the Membership Agreement of the Cuyahoga County Adult Protective Collaborative's Interdisciplinary Team described in Box 2, requires members to agree to the following:

- Attend required training
- Participate in monthly meetings
- Provide professional expertise regarding resources
- Respect and maintain client confidentiality
- Engage in telephone consultations on an emergency basis, as time permits.

19.3.2 Auspice

Either a community or organization can be the auspice for an M-team, supporting its purpose and sponsoring some of its activities. A community is more appropriate when the M-team functions to address the collective concerns of many organizations or professionals in one locale. An organization is more suitable when the M-team serves the needs of a single agency or institution [3]. Community auspices include elder abuse networks and councils for older adults, and are illustrated in Box 10 by the Trumbull Advocacy and Protective Network of Trumbull County, Ohio. Organization auspices tend to be either hospitals or adult protective services agencies, like the Beth Israel Hospital Elder Assessment Team and the Illinois adult protective service teams discussed previously in this chapter.

An auspice can provide the M-team with such tangibles as meeting space and refreshments, access to copiers and other equipment, and staffing. They also offer such intangibles as legitimacy and continuity. In the later regard, an auspice can help anchor the M-team, providing the foundation required to sustain it in the face of changes in leadership, membership, or funding. The commitment of the auspice to the M-team tends to be strongest when the M-team is seen by the auspice as consistent with its mission and furthering its strategic goals.

19.3.3 Policies

Policies may be unwritten and implicit in informal M-teams, but they will be written and explicit in formal ones, and therein sometimes compiled into an operations manual (e.g., [35, 86]). Written or unwritten, policies must express the will of team members and be adopted through deliberation and consensus. Policies are essential to M-teams, enabling sound understanding among members, smooth operations, and consistency in practice over time. The topics covered by team policies may include the following [56, 78]:

- Name, jurisdiction, mission, and goals
- Membership criteria, selection process, and expectations
- Officers and their duties
- Team purpose and function
- Standing and ad hoc committees, if applicable
- Meeting location, frequency, length, and procedures
- Case review criteria, procedures, and recommendation format
- Record keeping, handling, and access, including forms
- Conflict resolution.

19.3.4 Membership

Just as the functions of an M-team primarily reflect its auspice, legal basis, and type, so, too, does its membership. More specifically, community teams tend to have larger memberships than organization teams do. M-teams governed by statute or regulation ordinarily have prescribed membership categories, sometimes with limited selection discretion based on local circumstance or discipline availability. This is illustrated in the elder abuse interdisciplinary teams described in Box 8. Finally, the membership composition understandably will differ between a FAST and a hoarding team, given their unique concerns.

Across M-teams, certain disciplines or service systems are commonly represented in membership. The most likely to be included are law enforcement, adult protective services, mental health programs, aging services, and domestic violence advocacy [82]. For instance, all of these are found within the memberships of four California forensic center teams [72]. However, given their particular functions, these teams also usually include a geriatrician, psychologist, and researchers. Moreover, most of these teams have some discipline or service system representation that is distinctive. In this regard, only the Los Angeles team has a member from legal services and only the San Diego team has a volunteer client advocate.

Other types of M-teams have somewhat different memberships. An early study of Illinois adult protection teams indicates that membership covered six disciplines besides adult protective services: mental health, medicine, law enforcement, religion, legal, and financial [34]. In contrast, membership on the Santa Clara County FAST is limited to representation from adult protective services, public guardian/conservator, district attorney office, and county counsel [43]. Finally, Twomey et al. [83] describe seven different M-teams in California funded by the Archstone Foundation Elder Abuse and Neglect Initiative. Although they represent various types of M-teams, all found it necessary to include the following service systems as members: adult protective services, long-term care ombudsman, law enforcement, and district attorney office. Beyond these, membership differs depending upon the team's goals, for example, with Ventura County and Solana County FASTs including private professionals, like bankers and financial planners.

Ultimately M-team memberships can be secured through prescription or self-selection, characterized as closed or open, or some combination of these. For example, the Executive Board of the Trumbull Advocacy and Protective Network has a membership that tends to be prescribed and closed, but its Clinical Committee is more open and based on self-selection (see Box 9). Using a reverse approach, the Hoarding Connection of Cuyahoga County has an open membership derived from self-selection, but the hoarding task force model it advocates for adoption by municipalities tends toward a prescribed, closed membership (see Box 6).

M-team membership can change over time. This happened to the San Francisco Consortium Multidisciplinary Team, which modified its composition based upon new interests and grew its numbers as information was needed from other disciplines [57]. It also occurred with the Cuyahoga County Adult Protective Collaborative's Interdisciplinary Team described in Box 2, when the Team decided to seek representation from financial institutions with mounting concern about exploitation and when it saw membership expand as enthusiasm about Team participation spread.

19.3.5 Coordination

Multidisciplinary team coordination can be achieved though staff hired and paid to fulfill the role or individuals who undertake it as an ongoing in-kind contribution of the auspice organization or a member agency. Alternatively, the varied tasks of the team coordinator can be completed without dedicated personnel, simply on an ad hoc volunteer basis by team members. The tasks of team coordination are wide-ranging and may include any of the following [12, 34, 61, 82, 83]:

- Recruiting and orienting members, negotiating agreements
- Planning and organizing meetings, including sending out announcements, developing agendas, and producing minutes
- Selecting and preparing cases for review, tracking and recording team discussions during reviews, and insuring follow-up to case recommendations
- Serving as a resource for and liaison between members
- Answering questions and providing information on the work of the team
- Preparing forms and other materials, like manuals
- Collecting and compiling case data for periodic team reports
- Obtaining and administering grants to fund team operations.

There is increasing recognition of the importance in having paid staff coordinate M-teams, and with it, efforts to stimulate designated funding [12, 17]. This recognition comes from awareness of the specific knowledge and skills required for team coordination, along with the importance of the role for effective team operations, desired outcomes, and sustainability.

19.4 Operations

There are five essential components for the operations of an elder abuse M-team: leadership, member roles, member training, case selection criteria, and case review process. Each is discussed separately below. Although there are variations among the different types of teams with respect to these components, their commonalities are emphasized.

19.4.1 Leadership

The M-team leader is the person(s) who champions the concept of multidisciplinary collaboration, rallies others in establishing the M-team, and often remains the "point person" for the team, at least for a while after its formative phase. The ideal person should have professional credibility, knowledge of community resources, systems thinking, group leadership skills, a democratic style, and the time and energy for the job [8]. The leader also should respect the differing philosophies and perspectives of professional disciplines and service systems as well as understand the value of their linkage in responding to individual elder abuse situations. The ideal person further must have the power of persuasion, able to get buy-in for the concept, and belief that the team will be a community asset [12]. The leader can come from any discipline or agency as long as he/she is "enthusiastic, persevering, and work[s] well with others" [83, p. 296].

For the various Ohio M-teams highlighted in the chapter boxes, the leaders have been community planners, probate court judges, adult protective services administrators, and public health officials. Besides having the characteristics already discussed, all were visionaries, locally recognized elder abuse experts, and passionate about collaboration. All also created the foundation for others to sustain the team after the leader no longer had that role, and sometimes had left the team entirely.

19.4.2 Member Roles

The strength of the M-team—essentially its ability to assess and intervene effectively in individual elder abuse situations—comes from the expertise and resources of its members. This means having the right representation of disciplines and service systems on the team, members who have the knowledge, experience, and position within their organizations to participate meaningfully in case reviews and provide or secure needed services for case recommendation implementation. M-team membership composition and selection were discussed earlier in this chapter under "Organization." Here the focus is on member roles and responsibilities, in other words, the particular contributions that a professional discipline or service system offers to team operations. The literature on elder abuse M-teams includes many such descriptions (e.g., [1, 4, 10, 19, 34, 53, 61]). Among those described, the most commonly listed service systems are the six identified below. Although sometimes given other names (e.g., "Health care" may be called "medical" or "physician."), each service system provides unique perspective and resources for team functioning. Service systems can assume many roles and responsibilities. However, only those most important to addressing elder abuse are named.

- Aging services represent the vast network of supportive, clinical, and life-enhancing services targeting older adults and offered through such settings as offices on aging and senior centers. These services may include congregate and home-delivered meals, home care, transportation, and home maintenance or repairs. Available, too, may be services for family caregivers, like respite, counseling, and peer support. Aging services can help elder abuse victims manage at home without an abusive caregiver or self-neglect. They also provide reassurance, support, and service access for older adults who are socially isolated or otherwise at risk of elder abuse.
- Adult protective services programming is authorized under state law, which varies nationwide. It operates through state or local governments and typically under either human services or aging services agencies. The responsibilities of the program are to receive and investigate reports of the abuse, neglect, exploitation of older adults (and usually vulnerable younger adults) and assess the victims' service needs and capacity to give consent to intervention. Adult protective services can provide or arrange for services to correct or discontinue the elder abuse and prevent its reoccurrence, with the victim's voluntary agreement, if the person is able to give such, and only through court order, if not.
- Civil justice is concerned with individual legal rights and obligations, and in the case of elder law, focused on older adults. Civil attorneys in private law firms, legal services organizations, and government agencies may handle cases of guardianship or conservatorship, mental health commitment, or involuntary protective services affecting elder abuse victims. They may bring lawsuits against those who fail to fulfill their mandatory reporting responsibilities. They also can advise older adults about estate planning and assist with legal document preparations in the event of decision-making incapacity.
- Criminal justice acts to protect the public and address violations of law. Peace officers, like municipal police and county sheriffs, investigate elder abuse situations that reflect criminal conduct and have the authority to arrest perpetrators. They also can enforce restraining and other court orders, support the work of adult protective services, respond to many types of crises (such as elder abuse likely to be life-threatening or to result in irreparable harm), and provide "wellness" checks to determine the status of vulnerable older adults. Prosecutors initiate charges against elder abuse perpetrators who violate criminal law, prosecute these cases, and obtain convictions against the perpetrators. They also obtain various court orders. Collectively those in the criminal justice system signal that elder mistreatment represents unacceptable behavior and is a violation against society.
- Health care represents the various hospitals, clinics, practitioner offices, mental health agencies, long-term care facilities, and other settings where personnel, like physicians and therapists, aim to diminish illness, disability, and suffering, including providing emergency and

ongoing treatment for physical harm and mental disorder caused by elder abuse. Health care providers are critical to abuse detection and service referral, because older adults frequent health care settings more than other age groups and they tend to have greater trust and confidence in physicians and other health care providers, including revealing elder abuse when it occurs. Through patient histories, physical and mental examinations and tests, physicians, dentists, psychologists, and others diagnose, assess, and then provide or recommend interventions that not only can address the effects of elder abuse but also may improve the health and functioning of older adults, rendering them less vulnerable to future abuse occurrence.
- Victim advocacy is integral to domestic violence programs, sexual assault centers, and victim witness assistance agencies, which work to insure safety for victims and to hold perpetrators accountable for their abusive behavior. Emphasis is placed on confidentiality and empowering victims to voluntarily seek help. Across types of settings, this means offering victims crisis intervention, information and referral, counseling, and support. In addition, domestic violence programs usually provide emergency shelters, transitional housing, safety planning, help in obtaining court orders, and peer support groups. Sexual assault centers typically offer accompaniment to medical and court appointments, self-defense programs, and peer support groups. Victim witness assistance agencies help in obtaining legal benefits, court orders, and transportation to court. Further, they try to make the criminal justice process more understandable to victims and help victims prepare for court appointments and offer to accompany them there.

19.4.3 Member Training

Training is fundamental to elder abuse M-team functioning and member development. Therefore, it tends to be an essential part of team operations, where there may be three categories of training experiences for members. Membership orientation is the first, offered to new team members and often facilitated by the team coordinator, if present. It covers the team's background and operations, including membership expectations, forms, and case selection, presentation, and consultation. The second training category may be a regular or periodic part of team meetings. It is typically brief and presented either by a team member or outside visitor with expertise in the subject of interest [10, 35, 73]. Topics covered generally can be classified threefold:

- Overview of a particular member service system, discipline, organization, or program
- Description of recent research, new statutes or regulations, or emerging best practices related to elder abuse or a team service system
- Techniques for improving team operations or member relations

Finally, the team meeting agenda may include announcement of relevant outside training and educational offerings, such as upcoming webinars and conferences.

19.4.4 Case Selection Criteria

Elder abuse M-teams generally find challenging cases compelling and select them for review. Such cases are challenging for any number of reasons [12, 24, 56]:

- The victim experiences multiple forms of elder abuse.
- Coordination across systems or disciplines is required to meet complex service needs.
- There is a lack of role clarity among service providers involved in the case.
- Ethical or clinical concerns confound problem resolution.

Beyond such challenges, case selection criteria may reflect answers to such questions as the following [10, 53, 82]:

- Can only team members propose cases for review, or can nonmembers, even the public, also propose cases?
- Should only cases be selected that have received initial investigation or evaluation, or can the team assist in this sometimes?
- Must cases be open and active to be selected for review, or can closed cases be reviewed as well?
- Must the victim always be an older adult, however that is defined, or can cases receive review where vulnerable younger adults are victimized?
- Must all victims be community-dwelling, or can those in residential care also have their cases selected for review?
- Should case review be limited to a specific elder abuse form, or should all forms be eligible for review?

19.4.5 Case Review Process

As with member roles and case selection criteria, much literature on elder abuse M-teams is devoted to delineating the case review process (e.g., [10, 24, 30, 50, 56, 73, 76].

The process as described can be divided into three meeting phases: preparations, essential components, and optional aspects.

Preparations involve determining the meeting schedule and location. Teams typically are convened either weekly or monthly on the same day and time. The place ordinarily is the team auspice or a member organization. Meetings tend to last 1–2 hours and are facilitated by the team coordinator, who also assures that the meeting announcement, agenda, and any advance materials are sent.

Essential meeting components focus on the key steps for case review and accountability. They are listed below in the order of their usual occurrence.

- Case presentation: The case manager or team member who asked to present the case describes the elder abuse situation of concern verbally and distributes written copy of it, unless this was sent earlier with the meeting announcement. Sometimes more than one person makes the case presentation. This happens when already there are multiple disciplines and service systems involved in assessing or addressing case dynamics. The case description includes information on victim demographics, elder abuse incidents and forms, living arrangements and supports, current problems, victim's wishes about interventions, interventions tried to date and the results, and questions for team consideration or desired information and help from the team.
- Information gathering: Team members ask questions and seek clarity on the information provided by the case managers and victim or family.
- Intervention recommendation: Team members dialogue, identifying and evaluating various intervention options, before recommending a course of action.
- Intervention plan development: The team outlines a coordinated intervention plan, determining the time table, responsible parties, and desired outcomes for each element.
- Intervention follow-up: The team decides on a date when the case will be discussed again, at which time the responsible parties in the intervention plan implementation will indicate progress made and identify any new issues for team consideration.
- Case summary: The coordinator or case manager summarizes the team discussion, its intervention plan and implementation strategy, and team monitoring.
- Case updates: Team members report on previous cases reviewed and scheduled for update at this time. Emphasis is placed on discussing progress made and obstacles encountered to achieving desired outcomes. Additional counsel and help are sought, where indicated. Dates are assigned for future updates, if needed.

Optional meeting aspects tend to be placed at the end of the agenda. These include announcements of new community resources, recently enacted laws, staffing and funding changes, and upcoming training events; team education presentations, discussed earlier in this section; and identification of services gaps, including activities required to fill them.

19.5 Obstacles

The primary benefits of elder abuse M-teams are derived from fulfilling their basic functions, as delineated in the "Overview" section of this chapter. Beyond these, M-teams help victims by providing a more holistic perspective on their situation than possible from a single discipline or system alone [5]. They also provide "checks and balances" to insure that the rights and interests of all parties involved in such situations are protected [53].

M-teams benefit individuals as members by offering mutual support and probable assistance in future cases [6]. They enhance knowledge and skills and keep individual members updated on community resources and developments. M-teams also can reduce worker burnout and make it difficult for perpetrators to retaliate against any particular one [10].

Member disciplines, organizations, and systems often find M-teams participation improves agency decision-making and reduces territorial disputes. M-teams can clarify roles and foster interagency understanding. They assure that no single discipline or agency has the lone responsibility in case handling. They avoid situations where there may be too few or too many service providers involved [88].

Finally, M-teams benefit communities by enhancing broader awareness and understanding about elder abuse as a societal concern. They promote a community-wide approach to problem assessment, prevention, and treatment. Through reduced service duplication, they also can cut intervention costs [10].

The many benefits of elder abuse M-teams do not negate the challenges teams can face from inception onward. Among the most common are the obstacles listed below:

- Personal conflicts: Individual team members may have a history of animosity that interferes with interpersonal relations and can adversely affect team functioning. They also may have been disappointed in prior interactions and therefore fail to believe that future ones would be better [11, 82].

- Geographic barriers: The reality of work in rural areas, with their typical sparse resources and long distances, can limit intervention plans and member participation. In contrast, the large number of cities or political jurisdictions in an urban county—Cuyahoga County, Ohio has nearly 60, for example—may mean lots of police departments and service agencies to complicate team member selections [19, 71, 72].
- Communication problems: The use of professional jargon may inhibit understanding by team members representing different disciplines. Disciplines also may have varying definitions and understanding about elder abuse, for instance, with law enforcement considering it a crime and APS, a social problem. Finally, there may be confusion across service systems regarding the legal requirements and limitations that affect them, such as provisions emphasizing self-determination for capacitated older adults contained in APS laws [10, 42].
- Inadequate support: There may be insufficient funding or in-kind contribution for M-team operations. There further may be a lack of participation in the work of the M-team by key disciplines or agencies, such as law enforcement and mental health services [12, 82, 83].
- Competition: Multiple teams may operate within a community, creating competition over cases. Other priorities may compete for team members' time and attention. Organizations may be threatened by the power they have assigned to the team. Finally, there may be concern about inequities of status and authority among the disciplines represented on the team [15, 38, 42].
- Logistic issues: Scheduling conflicts can limit some team members' meeting attendance. Team meeting frequency and distance can seem burdensome under the weight of work demands [3, 42].
- Resistance and distrust: Agencies may be used to working without assistance from others. There may be concern about client confidentiality or conflict of interest in case reviews and intervention plan development. Various disciplines or service systems may lack confidence in the others' intervention approach and follow through [3, 10, 82].
- Deficit involvement: Case referrals may decline. Certain agencies may not bring cases to the team for consideration. Some team members may fail to follow-up on tasks that they have agreed to do. Team members may feel that their time is not well-spent doing team activities [72, 83].
- Change: There may be high staff turnover, resulting in team membership changes or gaps. Agencies may experience service shortages due to funding cuts, limiting their contributions to case plan implementation [10, 83].

19.6 Outcomes

In 2015 three New York City centers convened a forum on "Elder Abuse Multidisciplinary Teams: Planning for the Future." Elder justice experts and funders met to consider the value of M-teams and how to replicate and sustain them nationwide. A major set of recommendations from the group concerned the need for more and better related research, with priority placed on the following: nationwide descriptive study, rigorous multi-site evaluations to identify best practices, nationally relevant cost–benefit analysis, and victim-centered investigations. Lamented Sidney Stahl, PhD, consultant to the US Department of Justice, "Unfortunately, there is no compelling body of research on whether or not multidisciplinary teams are effective in any context" [12, p. 14].

Neither obstacles encountered in M-teams work nor scarcity of research demonstrating positive effects [27, 66] have dampened general enthusiasm for this intervention model. There remains steadfast belief in the virtue of M-teams, without the desired compliment of persuasive research findings.

Perhaps the earliest published evaluation of an elder abuse M-team was done by Wolf and Pillemer [88]. They conducted in-depth interviews with project personnel and staff members of the sponsoring organization before designating the San Francisco Multidisciplinary Team one of four best practices in elder abuse programming. This initial research failed to spark further interest in M-team evaluations, however. A decade later Teaster and Nerenberg [81] submitted their final report on the national survey on elder abuse M-teams and had identified none reporting evaluation findings. As recently as 2011, in a report for the National Center on Elder Abuse on the use of evidence-based practices for elder abuse projects, Teaster identified M-teams as a promising practice, but one with little actual evidence indicating their effectiveness [80].

Most research on M-teams to date has focused on member satisfaction and outputs, both of which tend to receive high marks. For example, nine of ten members completing the evaluation of the Cuyahoga County Adult Protective Collaborative, described in Box 5, were satisfied with the team. Similarly, members of the Trumbull Advocacy and Protective Network, discussed in Box 10, perceived greater team accomplishment over time.

In California Huba et al. [33] evaluated the Archstone Foundation Elder Abuse and Neglect Initiative from 2006 to 2008, including four forensic centers [72] and seven other types of M-teams [83]. Reported "outcomes" actually represented team efforts, such as number of infrastructure meetings, media events, assessments, and formal presentations. Nowhere was there mention of the effects of these activities on victims, member organizations, or communities. Likewise, Navarro et al. [50] reports "process outcomes" for the Los Angeles County Elder Abuse Center in comparable activity areas. Although these outputs are important indication of team engagement and productivity, they say little about its impact. Finally, a study of the Elder Abuse Forensic Center in Orange County, California examined case handling during 1 year of team operations. Team members found that working together to manage and process elder abuse cases enhanced efficiency and effectiveness [85]. This was the members' perception at least. There was no evidence presented that these were team outcomes.

Part of the challenge in evaluating any intervention is deciding what to measure and what constitutes a positive outcome. Opinions can differ widely among team members representing various disciplines and service systems, victims whose situations are subjected to case review, and other involved parties. Still, a small but growing body of research has emerged in the past few years which applied more rigorous methods to determine whether or not elder abuse M-teams "make a difference." An illustration of this research is offered by Ernst and Smith [28], who examined case handling effectiveness, comparing a social worker acting alone and a social worker/registered nurse team, considering 869 elder abuse cases seen in two Maryland counties. The results were mixed. The lone social worker had better success at confirming mistreatment and represented a more cost-effective approach. However, the team was better at risk reduction. Perhaps the most interesting research on M-team outcomes is concentrated on the Los Angeles County Elder Abuse Forensic Center. More specifically, comparing matched financial exploitation cases handled by the Center's M-team with those receiving usual care through adult protective services found that there were ten times more cases submitted to the district attorney for prosecution by the team than by adult protective services [49]. Using a similar study design, Yonashio-Cho et al. [89] found that team involvement increased the odds of conservatorship (guardianship in many other states) petition five times. Of course, whether or not outcomes like prosecution and conservatorship are positive can be "in the eye of the beholder." Prosecution may hold perpetrators accountable for their elder abuse crimes and help protect society, but some elder victims may prefer not to prosecute their abusers, especially when they are family member. Conservatorship can offer surrogate decision-making for older adults with diminished mental capacity, but it also represents a very restrictive legal intervention, denying basic rights to some older adults who prefer to live with risk rather than lose them. Finally, again using a similar study design, Nichol et al. [58] found that despite more successful prosecutions and more granted conservatorships, the Center's team incurred greater case processing costs than did adult protective services usual care by sevenfold.

19.7 Outlook

It is impossible to imagine an elder abuse response future without the presence of M-teams. The rationale for their existence will be no less evident in 2065 than it was a century before, when the protection of vulnerable older adults first was seen to require a constellation of services and therefore an interdisciplinary approach. Indeed, the existence of M-teams may become more important over time, particularly if the concept of elder abuse continues to expand and laws addressing it multiply, engulfing new disciplines and systems. The effect of these trends is illustrated in recent activities of the North American Securities Administrators Association, as it grapples with financial exploitation affecting older investors with diminished capacity. A committee of the Association has developed model state legislation which would provide direction for broker-dealers, investment advisors, and their qualified employees in reporting the problem, delaying account disbursements, and turning over records to authorities. Such financial professionals initially were excluded as mandatory reporters when the initial elder abuse reporting and adult protective services laws were enacted. Likewise, they typically were absent from early M-teams. However, in a time when retirement income is more likely to be based on personal savings and investments than employer pensions and thus even more at potential risk of financial exploitation by trusted others and strangers than previously, their involvement is needed.

Still, if elder abuse M-teams are to endure, they must be seen as effective and efficient. To date, there is no compelling evidence of M-team effectiveness. Worse, there is no consensus on the goals and desired outcomes for M-terms. Both are required for evaluative research, the findings from which will promote sound practice and can help advocacy for supportive M-team public policy and funding. The recent New York City's "Elder Abuse Multidisciplinary Teams: Planning for the Future" was a laudable beginning, but more specificity on M-team goals and desired outcomes from a broader representation of stakeholders is required for moving forward. A national forum on the subject seems indicated, as has occurred for a variety of other elder abuse concerns in the past, such as research (National Research Council's Panel to Review Risk and Prevalence of Elder Abuse and Neglect) and policy (National Center on Elder Abuse's National Policy Summit on Elder Abuse). In fact, the processes that proved useful for them may have application for a national forum on M-teams as well.

Elder abuse M-teams also often are considered inefficient. Complaints include the number and length of case reviews, cost of travel and lost work time, and competing and duplicative teams in a given geographic area. Attention must be directed at increasing M-teams efficiency, with consideration given to the use of case prioritization through risk assessment tools, adherence to established meeting aims and formats, distance communication technology, and team consolidation processes. No less can be expected, as service providing organizations everywhere more and more frequently deal with increasing workloads, declining staffs, and advancing productivity standards.

Box 1
Clinical Consultation Team,
Protective Services Consortium for
Older Adults of Cuyahoga County (Ohio)

The oldest continuously operating elder abuse network in the United States was formed in 1980 by the Council on Older Persons of Cleveland, Ohio. Its initial tasks were to draft legislation, advocate for its passage, and then provide professional awareness and education on what would become Ohio's Adult Protective Services Law. By 1984 the group reorganized and expanded into a formal membership association. Originally called the Protective Services Consortium for Older Adults of Cuyahoga County (now the Consortium Against Adult Abuse), its purpose was to develop an effective community-wide response system for meeting the needs of older adults who suffer from or are at risk of abuse or neglect. One of the Consortium's standing committees was the Clinical Consultation Team. Meeting monthly and comprised of persons from multiple disciplines and systems, the Team offered case review and advice to members upon request. According to its Chair, Elizabeth Lau [40, p. 80], the Team also developed "guidelines for the receiving and management of representative categories of adult protective cases…[and suggested] ways in which current system procedures can be changed to assure higher quality, more effective service delivery to adult protective cases."

Box 2
Interdisciplinary Team,
Cuyahoga County (Ohio) Adult Protective Collaborative

The Interdisciplinary Team of the Cuyahoga County (Ohio) Adult Protective Collaborative meets monthly to provide case consultations and promote best practices, validate the efforts of case workers, and foster an interdisciplinary perspective to problem-solving. With about three dozen member agencies, examples of case scenarios typically reviewed by the Team follow:

- Undecided case dispositions
- Ethical dilemmas, such as the right of self-determination
- Clients refusing help and remaining at high risk
- Capacity issues
- Seeking involuntary intervention through the court
- Limited access that impedes successful intervention
- Case closure that presents concern for the case worker or service agency.

Box 3
Adult Protective Services Demonstration Project,
The Benjamin Rose Institute
Cleveland, Ohio

The Benjamin Rose Institute of Cleveland, Ohio was one of the original demonstration sites for the development, implementation, and evaluation of protective services for community-dwelling older adults, both mentally incapacitated and unable to maintain self-care. Plans for the project began in 1962, with the 2-year demonstration and 1-year follow-up commencing in 1963. When the final report on the project was published a decade later, it recognized social work as having the central role in case management, primarily because the social treatment model dominated interventions at the time. However, it also acknowledged that "intervention in protective cases often results in complex interdisciplinary role relations" [9], with consultation from physicians, psychiatrists, or attorneys utilized in case assessment, planning, and implementation.

Box 4
Ohio Summit on Aging

Failing to pass state legislation that would mandate county multidisciplinary teams by 2010, the Supreme Count of Ohio's Subcommittee on Adult Guardianship that year held the Ohio Summit on Aging. The objective of the Summit was to enhance the safety and well-being of older Ohioans by focusing on elder abuse and guardianship issues as the two greatest challenges faced by probate courts statewide working with an aging population. Each county's probate judge was invited to attend and to bring along representatives of stakeholder agencies concerned about these problem areas. A key summit tenet was "when county members collaborate on challenging issues, better results are achieved." To realize this, attending county teams were asked to develop a coordinated action plan (including multidisciplinary team) and given a self-assessment tool to facilitate creation [59]. Of attending counties, an estimated half developed plans having multidisciplinary teams. Post-Summits held in 2011 and 2012 provided opportunities for counties to share successes and barriers to action plans being refined and implemented. Among barriers identified were the sometimes lack of involvement of financial institutions on multidisciplinary teams and cases of financial exploitation coming to probate court too late for effective judicial action.

Box 5
Cuyahoga County (Ohio) Adult Protective Collaborative

One of the multidisciplinary teams that emerged from the Ohio Summit on Aging was the Cuyahoga County Adult Protective Collaborative. A joint effort of adult protective services and the probate court locally, the Collaborative was launched in 2011. It has a Steering Committee to design, oversee, and assess Collaborative work as well as an Interdisciplinary Team to provide case consultation, promote best practices, and identify needed resources. The Team process is formalized with ground rules, required forms, and procedures. It also was evaluated in 2013 by the Benjamin Rose Institute on Aging through a self-administered, structured survey completed by Committee and Team members [67]. The response rate was 75 % among 57 respondents. Respondents gave highest marks for adequacy of information about the Team (95 %) and satisfaction with the Team (88 % or higher across four identified dimensions). They gave lowest marks for existing organization barriers to Team success (54 %) and impact on client outcomes (56 %).

Box 6
Enforced Harm Reduction Approach,
Hoarding Connection of Cuyahoga County (Ohio)

The mission of the Hoarding Connection of Cuyahoga County is to educate the community about the need for a coordinated effort to effectively help individuals who hoard and those working with individuals who hoard. Although more than 20 organizations comprise the association, only three are sponsors, one of them The Benjamin Rose Institute on Aging. The Institute's interest stems from its history in adult protective services, current mental health programs for older adults, and consequent recognition that many older persons with mental health problems hoard and self-neglect [21, 75, 77]. The Hoarding Connection recommends to and assists local municipalities in the use of the Enforced Harm Reduction approach to impact individual hoarding situations. The approach originated with the Orange County, CA Hoarding Task Force. It uses a multidisciplinary team composed of the consumer (if able), a helper (someone who has the confidence of the consumer), housing inspector, housing court (if needed), and representatives of community agencies (like mental health services and animal control). The approach includes clear housing codes and regulations, long-term perspective on problem management (rather than resolution) as the goal, and integrated planning.

Box 7
Ohio Elder Abuse Task Force

In the aftermath of the National Policy Summit on Elder Abuse, which recommended a state-by-state response, the Ohio Attorney General and Ohio Department on Aging Director convened the Ohio Elder Abuse Task Force in 2003 to study and make recommendations regarding the state's elder abuse programs and systems. The Task Force was comprised of subject experts from across Ohio, such as academicians, advocates, and service professionals. To conduct its work the Task Force established three committees that collectively promulgated 21 recommendations, contained in a final report released in 2005. The major product of the Coordination Committee was draft legislation mandating a memorandum of understanding in each county which would create an interdisciplinary team (I-Team) to improve community response to elder abuse. "The I-Team will be comprised of a group of professionals from a variety of disciplines who will meet regularly to discuss and provide consultation on specific cases of elder abuse… The remedy for elder abuse transcends disciplines and requires a joint effort to aid in the protection of a vulnerable population" [37, p. 13].

Box 8
Ohio Adult Protective Services Funding Workgroup

In the state budget for fiscal year 2015 the Ohio General Assembly appropriated $10 million for adult protective services (APS). The amount was twenty times the annual state appropriation for the program in recent years. As a result, the General Assembly also established the APS Funding Workgroup to investigate gaps in the APS system, identify county-level best practices, determine overlap and linkages, and identify a distribution method for the $10 million. After meeting nearly 6 months, the Workgroup released its report, which concluded that lacking a statewide APS system, APS reform should be comprehensive, multidisciplinary, and accountable. Interdisciplinary teams were found to be a best practice for organizing access to comprehensive services. Therefore, the Workgroup recommended that a portion of the funds be used to enable individual counties the opportunity to develop and implement functional interdisciplinary teams, with formal agreements from partnering organizations involved in elder abuse work. Ultimately $3 million was divided among 22 counties to create partnerships for programs aimed at filling service gaps in innovative ways and $1.5 million was distributed among 52 counties in order to build capacity to meet APS requirements often through "work with community partners on prevention and intervention services" [68].

Box 9
Ohio Statutory Mandate for the Establishment of Elder Abuse Interdisciplinary Teams

In 2015 Ohio was added among those states with M-team language as part of its adult protective services law. The amendment passed the Ohio General Assembly as part of the 2016–2017 state biennium budget, and reflects the legislative changes recommended by the Ohio Adult Protective Services Funding Workgroup, discussed in Box 7. The revised law requires each county department of job and family services (responsible for adult protective services programming locally) to "establish an interdisciplinary team to coordinate prevention, reporting, and treatment activities designed to address elder abuse, neglect, and exploitation." A related "memorandum [of understanding] shall describe the roles and responsibilities of each team member." The memorandum must be signed by seven local government officials (such as the county sheriff and county coroner) and may be signed by other persons or entity representatives "whose participation furthers the goals of the memorandum of understanding" (like the regional long-term care ombudsperson and representative of the county health department).

Box 10
Trumbull Advocacy and Protective Network
Trumbull County, Ohio

Planning to establish the Trumbull Advocacy and Protective Network began in 2002, when various agencies in Trumbull County, Ohio recognized a need for better communication and coordination among existing systems to address complex, high risk situations involving older adults. It became incorporated as a private, not-for-profit organization 4 years later and has received support from multiple sources, like foundation and senior citizen levy grants. A formal evaluation of the Network conducted in fall 2007 and fall 2008 found that members perceived significant greater accomplishment over time, particularly in such areas as addressing the special needs of older adults and centralizing advocacy for required resources [74]. The Network's structure has four key components:

- Full Network: meets quarterly, consists of leaders from approximately thirty member agencies serving older adults, focuses on system issues.
- Executive Board: meets monthly, consists of leaders from 11 mostly public agencies, maintains direction and goal administration set by the Full Network.
- Clinical Committee: meets monthly, includes individuals with casework involvement from member agencies, provides the forum for addressing challenging cases.
- Executive Director: part-time, handles day-to-day operations, functions under the direction of the Executive Board.

References

1. Allen JV. Financial abuse of elders and dependent adults: the FAST (Financial Abuse Specialist Team) approach. J Elder Abuse Negl. 2000;12(2):85–91.
2. Anetzberger GJ. An update on the nature and scope of elder abuse. Generations. 2012;36(3):12–20.
3. Anetzberger GJ. The evolution of a multidisciplinary response to elder abuse. Marq Elder's Advis. 2011;13(1):107–28.
4. Anetzberger GJ, editor. The clinical management of elder abuse. Binghamton, NY: The Harworth Press; 2005.
5. Anetzberger GJ, Dayton C, Miller CA, MeGreevey JF, Schimer M. Multidisciplinary teams in the clinical management of elder abuse. Clin Gerontol. 2005;28(1/2):157–71.
6. Aziz SJ. Los Angeles county fiduciary abuse specialist team: a model for collaboration. J Elder Abuse Negl. 2000;12(2):79–83.
7. Barry MC. Responsibility of the social welfare profession in providing guardianship and protective services. Paper presented at the Arden House Seminar on Protective Services for Older People, Harriman, NY; 1963.
8. Bernatavicz F. Improving protective services for older Americans: community role. Portland, ME: University of Southern Maine, Human Services Development Institute; 1982.
9. Blenkner M, Bloom M, Nielson M, Weber R. Final report: protective services for older people. Cleveland, OH: The Benjamin Rose Institute; 1974.
10. Brandl B, Dyer CB, Heisler CJ, Otto JM, Stiegel LA, Thomas RW. Elder abuse detection and intervention: a collaborative approach. New York: Springer; 2007.
11. Breckman RS, Adelman RD. Strategies for helping victims of elder mistreatment. Newbury Park, CA: Sage; 1988.
12. Breckman R, Callahan J, Solomon J. Elder abuse multidisciplinary teams: planning for the future. New York: New York City Elder Abuse Center, Brookdale Center for Healthy Aging, and The Harry and Jeanette Weinberg Center for Elder Abuse Prevention at the Hebrew Home at Riverdale; 2015.
13. Burr JJ. Protective services for adults: a guide to exemplary practice in states providing protective services to adults in OHDS programs. Washington, DC: US Department of Health and Human Services; 1982.

14. Chapin RK, Sergeant JF, Landry ST, Koenig T, Leiste M, Reynolds K. Hoarding cases involving older adults: the transition from a private matter to the public sector. J Gerontol Soc Work. 2010;53:723–42.
15. Conley DM. Developing a comprehensive approach: the key for the future. In: Galbraith MW, editor. Elder abuse: perspectives on an emerging crisis. Kansas City, KS: Mid-America Congress on Aging; 1986. p. 177–88.
16. Connolly MT. Where elder abuse and the justice system collide: police power, parens patriae, and 12 recommendations. J Elder Abuse Negl. 2010;22(1/2):37–93.
17. Connolly MT, Brandl B, Breckman R. The elder justice roadmap: a stakeholder initiative to respond to an emerging health, justice, financial and social crisis. Washington DC: US Department of Justice and US Department of Health and Human Services; 2014.
18. Daly JM, Jogerst GJ. Multidisciplinary team legislative language associated with elder abuse investigations. J Elder Abuse Negl. 2014;26:44–59.
19. Decalmer P, Marriott A. Multidisciplinary assessment of clients and patients. In: Decalmer P, Glendenning F, editors. The mistreatment of elderly people. London: Sage Publications; 1993. p. 117–35.
20. Dong X. Elder abuse: research, practice, and health policy. The 2012 GSA Maxwell Pollack Award Lecture. The Gerontologist. 2014;54(2):153–62.
21. Dong X, Simon MA, Mosqueda L, Evans DA. The prevalence of elder self-neglect in a community-dwelling population: hoarding, hygiene, and environmental hazards. J Aging Health. 2012;24 (3):507–24.
22. Dyer C, Heisler C, Hill C, Kim L. Community approaches to elder abuse. Clin Geriatr Med. 2005;21(2):429–47.
23. Dyer CB, Connolly MT, McFeeley P. The clinical and medical forensics of elder abuse and neglect. In: Bonnie RS, Wallace RB, editors. Elder mistreatment: abuse, neglect, and exploitation in an aging America. Washington, DC: The National Academies Press; 2003. p. 339–81.
24. Dyer CB, Goins AM. The role of the interdisciplinary assessment in addressing self-neglect of the elderly. Generations. 2000;24 (2):23–7.
25. Dyer CB, Barth J, Portal B, Hyman DJ, Pavlik VN, Murphy K, Gleason MS. A case series of abused or neglected elders treated by an interdisciplinary geriatric team. J Elder Abuse Negl. 1999;10 (3/4):131–9.
26. Eckstein R, Lindsey E, editors. Seminar on protective services for older people. Washington, DC: National Council on the Aging; 1963.
27. Erlingsson CL. Searching for elder abuse: a systematic review of database citations. J Elder Abuse Negl. 2007;19(3/4):59–78.
28. Ernst JS, Smith CA. Assessment in adult protective services: do multidisciplinary teams make a difference? J Gerontol Soc Work. 2012;55(1):21–38.
29. Frost RO, Steketee G, Williams L. Hoarding: a community health problem. Health Soc Care Commun. 2000;8:229–34.
30. Fulmer TT, O'Malley TA. Inadequate care of the elderly: a health care perspective on abuse and neglect. New York: Springer; 1987.
31. Hall GH. Protective services for adults. In: Morris R, editor. Encyclopedia of social work, vol. 2. Washington, DC: National Association of Social Workers; 1971. p. 999–1007.
32. Horowitz G, Estes C. Protective services for the aged. Washington, DC: US Department of Health, Education, and Welfare; 1971.
33. Huba GJ, Melchior LA, Philyaw ML, Northington KR. The archstone foundation elder abuse and neglect initiative: outcomes and lessons learned in three years from 2006 to 2008. J Elder Abuse Negl. 2010;22(3/4):231–46.
34. Hwalek M, Williamson D, Stahl C. Community-based M-teams roles: a job analysis. J Elder Abuse Negl. 1991;3(3):45–62.
35. Illinois Department on Aging. Multidisciplinary team member handbook. Springfield: Illinois Department on Aging; 2006.
36. Jackson SL, Mulford CF. Re: the complexity of responding to elder abuse demands the use of multidisciplinary teams (National Council on Crime and Delinquency Blog). 2013. Retrieved from http://www.nccdglobal.org/blog/the-complexity-of-responding-to-elder-abuse-demands-the-use-of-multidisciplinary-teams.
37. Jim Petro Attorney General, State of Ohio. Ohio elder abuse task force report. Columbus, OH: State of Ohio; 2005.
38. Johnson TF. Ethics and elder mistreatment: uniting protocol with practice. In: Johnson TF, editor. Elder mistreatment: ethical issues, dilemmas, and decisions. New York: The Haworth Press; 1995. p. 1–18.
39. Koenig TL, Leiste MR, Spano R, Chapin RK. Multidisciplinary team perspectives on older adult hoarding and mental illness. J Elder Abuse Negl. 2013;25:56–75.
40. Lau EE. Inpatient geropsychiatry in the network of elder abuse services. In: Galbraith MW, editor. Elder abuse: perspectives on an emerging crisis. Kansas City, KS: Mid-America Congress on Aging; 1986. p. 65–80.
41. Levitt SJ, O'Neill RJ. A call for a functional multidisciplinary approach to intervention in cases of elder abuse, neglect, and exploitation: one legal clinic's experience. Elder Law J. 1997;5(1):195–212.
42. McNamee C, Mulford C. Innovations assessment of the Elder Abuse Forensic Center of Orange County, California. Washington, DC: National Institute of Justice; 2007.
43. Malks B, Buckmaster J, Cunningham L. Combating elder financial abuse—a multi-disciplinary approach to a growing problem. J Elder Abuse Negl. 2003;15(3/4):55–70.
44. Mixson P, Chelucci K, Heisler C, Overman W, Sripada P, Yates P. The case of Mrs. M.—a multidisciplinary team staffing. J Elder Abuse Negl. 1991;3(4):41–55.
45. National Center on Elder Abuse. Frequently asked questions. 2015a. Retrieved on April 6, 2015 from http://www.ncea.aoa.gov/faq/index.aspx.
46. National Center on Elder Abuse. Local coalitions: list of more than 100 local elder justice coalitions in the United States. 2015b. Retrieved on July 15, 2015 from http://www.ncea.aoa.gov/Stop_Abuse/Teams/Local/index.aspx.
47. National Center on Elder Abuse. Bibliographics: multidisciplinary and collaborative approaches in responding to elder abuse (Electronic listserve message). 2006. Retrieved from http://www.elderabusecenter.org/default.cfm?p=CANE_MulitdisciplinaryAndCollaborativeApproaches.cfm.
48. National Research Council. Elder mistreatment: abuse, neglect, and exploitation in an aging America. In: Bonnie RJ, Wallace RB, editors. Panel to review risk and prevalence of elder abuse and neglect. Washington, DC: The National Academies Press; 2003.
49. Navarro AE, Gassoumis ZD, Wilber KH. Holding abusers accountable: an elder abuse forensic center increases criminal prosecution of financial exploitation. The Gerontologist. 2013;53 (2):303–12.
50. Navarro AE, Wilber KH, Yonashiro J, Homeier DC. Do we really need another meeting? Lessons from the Los Angeles County Elder Abuse Forensic Center. The Gerontologist. 2010;50(5):702–11.
51. Nerenberg L. Elder abuse prevention: emerging trends and promising practices. New York: Springer; 2008.
52. Nerenberg L. Communities respond to elder abuse. J Gerontol Soc Work. 2006;46(3/4):5–33.
53. Nerenberg L. Multidisciplinary elder abuse prevention teams: a new generation. NCEA Newslett. 2003;5(12):4.

54. Nerenberg L. A new generation of multidisciplinary teams. Nexus, 2001; 6.
55. Nerenberg L. Developing a service response to elder abuse. Generations. 2000;24(2):86–92.
56. Nerenberg L. Building partnerships: a guide to developing coalitions, interagency agreements and teams in the field of elder abuse. Washington, DC: National Center on Elder Abuse; 1995.
57. Nerenberg L. The San Francisco Consortium Multidisciplinary Team: another perspective. J Elder Abuse Negl. 1991;3(3):66–71.
58. Nichol MB, Wu H, Gassoumis ZD, Yonashiro-Cho J, Wilber KH. Access cost effectiveness of the multidisciplinary approach to elder abuse: economic evaluation of elder abuse forensic center model. Poster presented at the annual meeting of the American Public Health Association, Chicago; 2015.
59. Ohio Summit on Aging. Presentation materials. Columbus, OH: Supreme Court of Ohio; 2010.
60. O'Neill V. Protecting older people. Public Welf. 1965;23(2): 119–27.
61. Parkins SM. Hospital response to elder abuse: the adult protection team. In: Baumhover LA, Beall SC, editors. Abuse, neglect, and exploitation of older persons: strategies for assessment and intervention. Baltimore: Health Professions Press; 1996. p. 163–83.
62. Patronek GJ, Loar L, Nathanson JN. Animal hoarding: structuring interdisciplinary responses to help people, animals and communities at risk. Boston, MA: Hoarding of Animals Research Consortium; 2006.
63. Pedrick-Cornell C, Gelles R. Elder abuse: the status of current knowledge. Fam Relat. 1982;31(3):457–65.
64. Pillemer K, Connolly MT, Breckman R, Spreng N, Lachs MS. Elder mistreatment: priorities for consideration by the White House Conference on Aging. The Gerontologist. 2015;55(2): 320–7.
65. Pillemer K, Breckman R, Sweeney CD, Brownell P, Fulmer T, Berman J, Lachs MS. Practitioners' views on elder mistreatment research priorities: recommendations from a research-to-practice consensus conference. J Elder Abuse Negl. 2011;23(2):115–26.
66. Ploeg J, Fear J, Hutchinson B, MacMillan H, Bolan G. A systematic review of interventions for elder abuse. J Elder Abuse Negl. 2009;21(3):187–210.
67. Primetica B, Bukach A, Bass D. Evaluation of the Cuyahoga County adult protective services interdisciplinary team: final report. Cleveland, OH: The Benjamin Rose Institute on Aging; 2013.
68. Pyle E. State's $10 M set-aside goes to programs to protect elderly from abuse. The Plain Dealer. 2015.
69. Ramsey-Klawsnik H, Heisler C. Polyvictimization in later life. Victim Elder Disabl. 2014;17(1):3–6.
70. Regan JJ, Springer G. Protective services for the elderly: a working paper. Prepared for the Special Committee on Aging, US Senate. Washington, DC: US Government Printing Office; 1977.
71. Schimer MR, Anetzberger GJ. Examining the gray zones in guardianship and involuntary protective services laws. J Elder Abuse Negl. 1999;10(3/4):19–38.
72. Schneider DC, Mosqueda L, Falk E, Huba GJ. Elder abuse forensic centers. J Elder Abuse Negl. 2010;22(3/4):255–74.
73. Sekora D. The Montana adult protective service teams: a rural perspective. J Elder Abuse Negl. 1991;3(3):62–6.
74. Slivinske LR, Slivinske JD, Causey LA, Wyant KA. Evaluating the effectiveness of the Trumbull Advocacy and Protective Network: a formative evaluation. J Appl Gerontol. 2011;30(2):254–66.
75. Snowdon J, Shah A, Halliday G. Sever domestic squalor: a review. Int Psychogeriatr. 2007;19(1):37–51.
76. Spinale R. Adams County community adult protection multidisciplinary team. Victim Elder Disabl. 2005; p. 51, 62.
77. Steketee G, Frost RO, Kim H-J. Hoarding by older people. Health Soc Work. 2001;26(3):176–84.
78. Stiegel LA. Elder abuse fatality review teams: a replication manual. Washington, DC: American Bar Association Commission on Law and Aging; 2005.
79. Stiegel LA, Klem E. Multidisciplinary teams authorizations or mandates: provisions and citations in adult protective services laws, by state. Washington, DC: American Bar Association Commission on Law and Aging; 2007.
80. Teaster PB. The use of evidence-based practices for elder abuse programs. Washington, DC: National Center on Elder Abuse; 2011.
81. Teaster PB, Nerenberg L. A national look at elder abuse multidisciplinary teams: report for the National Committee for the prevention of elder abuse, partner in the National Center on elder abuse. Washington, DC: National Committee for the Prevention of Elder Abuse; 2005.
82. Teaster PB, Nerenberg L, Stansbury KL. A national look at elder abuse multidisciplinary teams. J Elder Abuse Negl. 2003;15 (3/4):91–107.
83. Twomey MS, Jackson G, Li H, Marino T, Melchior LA, Randolph JF, Wysong J. The successes and challenges of seven multidisciplinary teams. J Elder Abuse Negl. 2010;22(3/4):291–305.
84. White House Conference on Aging. Elder justice. 2015. Retrieved from http://www.whitehouseconferenceonaging.gov/blog/policy/post/elder-justice-policy-brief.
85. Wiglesworth A, Mosqueda L, Burnight K, Younglove T, Jeske D. Findings from an elder abuse forensic center. The Gerontologist. 2006;46(2):277–83.
86. Wisconsin Department of Health and Family Services. Elder abuse interdisciplinary team manual. Madison: Author; 2006.
87. Wolf RS. Elders as victims of crime, abuse, neglect, and exploitation. In: Rothman MB, Dunlop BD, Entzel P, editors. Elders, crime, and the criminal justice system. New York: Springer; 2000. p. 19–42.
88. Wolf RS, Pillemer K. What's new in elder abuse programming? Four bright ideas. The Gerontologist. 1994;34(1):126–9.
89. Yonashiro-Cho JM, Gassoumis ZD, Wilber K. Conservatorship characteristics among forensic center and adult protective services clients. Poster presented at the Annual Scientific Meeting of the Gerontological Society of America, Washington, DC; 2014.

20 Elder Abuse Prevention Interventions

Karen Stein

20.1 The Important Question: What "Works?"

> There are a plethora of "best practice" models for increasing the effectiveness of prevention and treatment efforts within service delivery agencies. However, without an evaluation of our current...systems...we do not have a valid basis upon which to institute these practice models. We still lack reliable knowledge of what types of programs and delivery systems function effectively given different sets of conditions and circumstances. In essence, we still need to determine what "works" and what doesn't "work." Given a more complete state of knowledge of the effectiveness of prevention and treatment programs and systems, we can: Better determine the roles and responsibilities of the different systems involved in treatment modalities; reduce the frustration level of social service personnel, leading to more effective functioning; have a better basis for advocating particular programs to the public and to funding agencies; and better design programs for the future, as much of this knowledge may be transferable to other systems... Given that many intervention programs and systems may involve high costs, it is most important that we have a true indication of their effectiveness for different types of people under a variety of circumstance [100].

That statement was written a quarter of a century ago. In the intervening time, we have had 25 years of intervention funding for a host of organizations and services ranging from protective services to multidisciplinary coalitions to national resource centers; 25 years of training programs developed for almost every conceivable profession interacting with older people from hairdressers to mail deliverers to gas meter readers to prosecutors and judges to allied health professionals to financial planners and bankers; and 25 years of public education and awareness efforts with international recognition of World Elder Abuse Awareness Day, United Nations Proclamations, and continuous funding for a National Center on Elder Abuse.

Given this, one could and should reasonably expect that our state of both knowledge and practice regarding effective prevention and intervention efforts would be immeasurably improved: that, unlike in 1991, we now would know what "works" and does not "work." In 2014, the U.S. Departments of Justice and Health and Human Services commissioned an initiative to set strategic priorities to advance elder justice. The result was the Elder Justice Roadmap [22], designed to be a "strategic planning resource to guide federal, state and local actions to advance collective efforts to prevent and combat elder abuse ([22], p. 2)." To generate this Roadmap, 750 stakeholders were asked to complete the statement "to understand, prevent, identify or respond to elder abuse, neglect or exploitation, we need....". From these responses, over 35 subject matter experts and 21 federal participants identified the field's most urgent needs and offered recommendations for the highest priority action items. Intervention and Prevention was identified as a priority area. As an illustration of how our state of knowledge may (or may not) have changed over the last quarter-century, Table 20.1 compares the 2014 Elder Justice Roadmap recommendations with those cited in the 1991 national research agenda report.

The 1991 report indicates what we did not know at that time. The recommendations from the 2014 report indicate that prevention and intervention efforts still lack testing and evaluation. In essence, several decades later, the strategic questions and quest for knowledge have not radically changed. What has changed, however, is the increased amount of research, practice, and service efforts devoted to elder abuse prevention and intervention.

K. Stein (✉)
School of Public Policy and Administration,
University of Delaware, 298 C, Graham Hall
184 Academy Street, 19716 Newark, DE, USA
e-mail: kstein@udel.edu

X. Dong (ed.), *Elder Abuse*, DOI 10.1007/978-3-319-47504-2_20

Table 20.1 Recommendations for prevention and intervention: 2014 and 1991

2014 Elder justice roadmap[a]	1991 Elder abuse and neglect: a National Research Agenda[b]
Determine what messages are effective in reaching critical audiences	What is the impact of public education and awareness?
Determine what causes elder abuse, determine what theoretical models explain it, and develop and evaluate interventions to test the theoretical models	What theoretical frameworks offer the best explanation for elder abuse? Does the framework differ for different types of abuse? How do we measure the effectiveness of interventions?
Test and evaluate the efficacy of various types of multidisciplinary responses to elder abuse	What is the effectiveness of interagency coordinating mechanisms (multidisciplinary teams, state units, community organizations, etc.)?
Evaluate the efficacy of programs designed to address elder abuse, such as adult protective services	What are the factors related to effective adult protective services? What are the appropriate outcomes of APS?
Evaluate the effectiveness of laws and legal interventions in preventing and stopping elder abuse	What is the effect of the criminal justice system, including law enforcement, in prevention/treatment of elder abuse? For example, does arrest deter future incidents?
Create and test intervention strategies that are designed to enhance strengths and ameliorate risks for elder abuse	How do we measure the effectiveness of intervention? For example, at what threshold point along the dimensionality continuum is early intervention effective for different types of abuse and for clients at different stages of functioning and competency? At what threshold points will intervention not matter?
Evaluate the availability of victim service options for older victims. Evaluate existing services to determine which models best meet older victims' needs and preferences	What programmatic and individual interventions are effective in dealing with each form of abuse (e.g., respite programs, day care, counseling, education, support groups?)

[a]Connolly et al. [22], pp. 23–24
[b]Stein, Elder Abuse and Neglect: A National Research Agenda (1991, pp. 20–22)

20.2 Conceptual and Definitional Frameworks of Prevention and Intervention

There is no general agreement in the literature or in practice arenas as to whether the terms "prevention" and "intervention" represent two distinct categories of actions or are continuums of each other. The Institute for Work and Health, for example, takes the view that all interventions are various forms of either primary, secondary, or tertiary preventions [56], differing by the stage of the adverse condition addressed by the preventive action. This view, based on the early work of Robert Caplan [18], is most common in the public health field. The Substance Abuse Mental Health Services Administration and the National Institute for Mental Health take the view that prevention differs from interventions, inasmuch as prevention efforts are targeted to the general population who may or may not be at risk for a particular condition and are designed to eliminate or reduce new cases, while interventions are specifically designed to assist those who are at some degree of risk [34, 108]. In this latter view, interventions are classified as universal, selective, or indicated, differing by a target population's degree of vulnerability to risk.

20.3 Primary, Secondary, and Tertiary Prevention

Primary prevention efforts are aimed at a general population designed to inform and educate people about risky or dangerous behaviors (such as drunk driving or smoking) or about healthy and safe practices to reduce risk (such as immunizations and cancer screenings). These types of prevention efforts would include education and awareness initiatives such as public service announcements, posters, billboards, media stories, and walk–run events. They are designed to raise social awareness of a problem or of a good practice, without consideration of the audience's specific potential to be impacted by the problem or practice.

Secondary prevention efforts are aimed at individuals who are already at risk or who are identified as being potentially at risk for a particular adverse condition. The goal of these efforts is early identification, so that the adverse impacts can be reduced or eliminated at an early stage before significant injury occurs. Examples of secondary prevention efforts would be diet modifications for people with high cholesterol levels, and more frequent regularly scheduled mammograms for people with a family history of breast cancer.

Tertiary prevention efforts are aimed at people who are diagnosed with or suffering from a particular illness, injury, or adverse condition that impacts their quality of life. The goal of these preventions is to help manage the condition as best as possible to maintain an acceptable quality of life, to delay the onset of even further damage, and to offer an individual some sense of control. Examples of these efforts would be physical rehabilitation programs, self-management of chronic diseases, and psychosocial strategies such as ongoing counseling/support meetings.

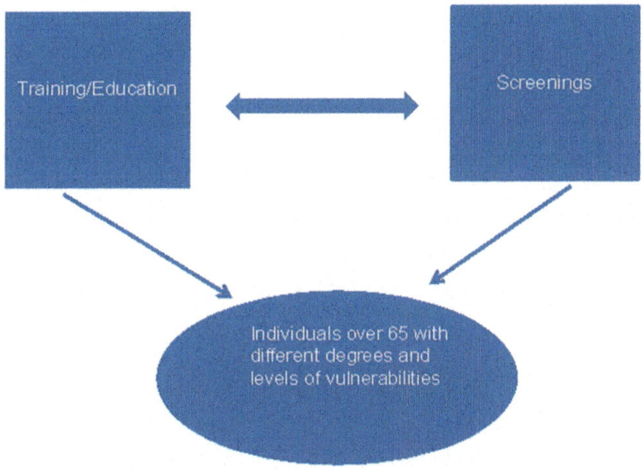

Fig. 20.1 Examples of selective prevention interventions: short-term strategies to identify those at elevated risk for elder abuse or neglect

20.4 Institute of Medicine Model of Preventive Interventions

The Institute of Medicine Model of interventions is based on work first introduced by Robert Gorden in 1983 [47]; Institute of Medicine [57]; Springer and Phillips [98]. This model assumes that different subpopulations within any targeted population are at different levels of risk for developing a behavioral or health problem. Consequently, preventive interventions are designed to address a target population's vulnerability to risk and are classified as either universal, selective, or indicated preventive interventions.

Universal preventive interventions are identical to primary prevention efforts. These are strategies that are focused on education and awareness, delivered across population groups. As the susceptibility to risk is not a factor, these interventions are not targeted toward any subgroup of the population. Strategies include media campaigns, all forms of public awareness campaigns, educational programs, advocacy, and community outreach programs.

Selective prevention interventions, like secondary preventions, are aimed at subgroups within a target population who either are at risk, or have a vulnerability or characteristic that increases their probability of becoming at risk. These interventions are usually short term and are focused on identifying the degree of vulnerability. Strategies include screenings, clinical assessments, gatekeeper programs, and training programs for professionals and caregivers (Fig. 20.1).

Indicated prevention interventions target high-risk individuals within a subgroup who exhibit early danger signs or potential symptoms of a condition. The goal of these interventions is to involve them in special programs or services that may delay or eliminate the onset of the condition. Strategies include counseling programs, support groups, and wrap-around community services.

20.5 Prevention Interventions Versus Treatment Interventions

The National Research Council and Institute of Medicine distinguish between interventions that are part of prevention and those interventions that are actually considered treatments (National Research Council [76] and Institute of Medicine (US) Committee on the Prevention of Mental Disorders and Substance Abuse Among Children, Youth, and Young Adults, 2009). Prevention interventions are appropriate before the full onset of a condition and are designed to reduce risk. When individuals have passed the stage of being "at risk," and are already in need of services to address or ameliorate an existing adverse condition, prevention is no longer an option. The need passes from preventive interventions to treatment interventions. These interventions may be of either immediate, short- or long-term duration. Indicated treatments include legal services and criminal justice processes, protective services, shelters, support groups, interagency and community coordinated services, and mental health services. In this sense, tertiary interventions would be considered treatments, not prevention.

20.6 Prevention Interventions in the Context of Elder Abuse

There are a plethora of selective and indicated strategies and services available to assist in identifying elders at moderate and high risk for mistreatment, services ("treatments" in the Institute of Medicine model) available for those who are identified as abused and neglected, and far-ranging but uncoordinated universal awareness and education activities and initiatives mostly mounted at local levels. In essence, the field does not lack for prevention and intervention action, programs, and services.

However, unlike the public health and mental health fields that have widely adopted the Institute of Medicine framework of prevention interventions, the elder abuse field has not yet agreed upon a singular way of defining and delivering interventions, nor is there agreement about the need or desirability of delineating prevention from treatment interventions. Anetzberger [7] notes that elder abuse researchers, since the early 1980s, have categorized interventions for victims of elder abuse by either service type (such as legal or medical services), targeted group (such as victim or abuser), response level (such as community or professional), or by duration (such as emergency or long term). She suggests an integrative model of intervention that simultaneously considers approach or purpose (such as protection or advocacy), target (such as victim–perpetrator dyad or family system), and basic intervention function or response including but not limited to support, prevention, or emergency services [7, 26]. In these various frameworks, there is no differentiation between prevention and treatment interventions.

20.7 Conceptualizing a New Prevention Intervention Framework for Elder Abuse

20.7.1 Framework Characteristics

Knapp provides a basis for differentiating universal, selective, and indicated prevention interventions from treatments by the characteristics of threshold, risk population, target case, caseness, modality, timing, provider, dose, attrition, and outcomes [34]. While Knapp's framework was developed to illustrate the characteristics of mental health interventions for children at risk, many of these same characteristics can be adapted and applied to a conceptual framework for organizing elder abuse and neglecting prevention interventions.

20.7.1.1 Threshold

Threshold refers to the degree of direct effects or impact upon the subject of the intervention. In the context of elder abuse, universal prevention interventions, aimed at the general population, have low individual impacts but the potential for very wide reach. These interventions aim to generate societal changes in behaviors and attitudes, a process that requires sustained reinforcement over time. Examples of these interventions include public awareness and education, community outreach, and advocacy.

Selective prevention interventions, aimed at those over a certain age without regard to susceptibility to risk are classified as having medium personal impacts. These interventions aim to increase the identification of those with higher than average risk for abuse and neglect but who are not yet vulnerable. Examples of these interventions include screenings, professional training and education programs, and gatekeeper programs.

Indicated prevention interventions, delivered to those with early warning signs or potential symptoms of abuse, neglect, and self-neglect have the potential for high personal impacts. Examples of these interventions are counseling programs including a variety of social-psychological supports, forensic multidisciplinary teams, home visits, and case management. A unique feature of these indicated prevention interventions is that they may target the vulnerable elder and his/her caregivers and perpetrators.

20.7.1.2 Target Population

Target population refers to the specific audience for whom the intervention is designed. In the context of elder abuse, universal prevention strategies would be targeted to the general public, selective prevention interventions would be targeted to those of a certain age such as 60 and older, and indicated prevention strategies would be targeted to those exhibiting potential or early symptoms of elder abuse, neglect or self-neglect.

20.7.1.3 Timing

Timing refers to when the intervention is first applied to the target population, and the duration of the intervention. In the context of elder abuse, universal prevention interventions, to have a lasting societal impact upon a general public, should be extended and sustained over time; selective prevention interventions are usually of short-term duration focused on early identification; and indicated prevention strategies occur after a diagnosis of being "at risk" but before abuse or neglect is substantiated and may be of limited or continuing duration depending upon the type and level of need.

20.7.1.4 Provider

Provider refers to systems, individuals, groups, and professionals who are capable of delivering the intervention. In the context of elder abuse, societal institutions and community groups may be the prime providers of universal prevention interventions; selective prevention interventions are most usually delivered by professionals in the field who are likely to come into contact with the target population but may also be provided by community members; and indicated prevention strategies are most usually delivered by professional and/or community organizational support systems. Targeted populations served by providers may include the older adult, caregivers, and perpetrators. Cultural issues and preferences may impact the effectiveness of the provider.

20.7.1.5 Attrition and Dosage

Attrition refers to the reasons why the target population drops out of participating in the intervention, and dosage refers to the amount of exposure needed for an intervention to be effective. In the context of elder abuse, whether or not a member of the target population remains engaged in a universal prevention intervention is influenced by the power and duration of the messaging. Dosage usually needs to be sustained over time to make a difference on a personal and societal level. A member of a targeted group for selective prevention interventions may discontinue participation because a short-term dosage of the intervention is felt to be sufficient, or because the member does not feel himself or herself in need of the intervention. A member of a targeted group for indicated prevention interventions may discontinue participation because the intervention is not acceptable or because the treatment may not be bringing about the desired level of change or improvement. In the case of both selected and indicated interventions, attrition may be impacted by lack of sensitivity to cultural issues and self-perceptions of autonomy; and the "sufficient dosage" for producing change or improvement may be unknown, exacerbating feelings of frustration on the part of providers and clients.

20.7.1.6 Outcomes

Outcomes refer to the desired impacts of the intervention upon the member of the targeted population, and may be defined by providers and/or the subjects of the intervention. In the context of elder abuse, outcomes of effective universal prevention interventions would be changes in societal attitudes and behaviors such as increased sensitivity to the issue of elder abuse, the growth of advocacy movements, and laws and regulations. Examples of outcomes of effective selective prevention interventions are increased recognition of those at risk or in need of services through means such as screening, gatekeeper reports, or professional training and education. Successful indicated prevention interventions may be measured by reductions in vulnerability or symptoms that lessen the probability of abuse. The ability to achieve successful outcomes may be impacted by cultural influences including client and community perceptions of what constitutes abusive behavior and barriers to accepting services; client self-perceptions of need and autonomy; the availability, involvement, and cooperation of appropriate community, professional, and legal resources; perpetrator and/or family dyad involvement or cooperation in the intervention; and the acceptability of the intervention to the client [28, 29, 30, 46, 61, 67, 97].

20.7.2 Why This Conceptual Framework Moves the Field Forward

What would the elder abuse field gain by providing clarity and consistency in formulating a prevention framework that differentiates interventions as universal, selective, and indicated, and considers tertiary interventions to be the treatment and not prevention? First and perhaps most important, distinguishing between prevention and treatment interventions clarifies priorities as measured by funding decisions. Second, delineating among the different forms and stages of intervention, and separating prevention from treatment, refines both research questions and methodologies, encouraging evaluation studies of effectiveness that differ by expected outcomes. Third, definitional differences between types of prevention are necessary to measure the impacts of different preventive approaches. Fourth, adopting and using a tested and valid prevention framework that is already widely accepted in allied fields integrates elder abuse into a larger network of social systems (such as public health) and movements (such as justice, interpersonal violence), and increases funding and collaborative opportunities for both researchers and practitioners. Fifth, an accepted theoretical perspective can help the field understand the external conditions and internal behavioral characteristics that can impact the effectiveness of a particular strategy, improving the probability of achieving defined goals [73].

20.7.3 Applicability of the Framework

Because this framework is organized by types of prevention interventions instead of by types or definitions of abuse, it offers wide applicability. The framework's characteristics can be applied to prevention intervention strategies designed to address any form of abuse including polyvictimization, neglect, or self-neglect regardless of how a particular culture or society defines abuse and neglect. Given that definitions to a large extent may be cultural based and that many international, diverse cultures are in the first stages of conceptualizing and understanding the meaning and extent of elder abuse [11, 61, 71, 84, 121], this framework has the advantage of applicability to prevention interventions in the absence of global definitional standardizations. It considers that culture and the ethnicity of a member of the targeted population may impact the effectiveness of the provider, attrition rates, and the formulation of desired outcomes [24, 35, 52, 54, 70]. It recognizes that the affected elder's self-perceptions of vulnerability, safety, and autonomy, as well as the perceptions of professionals, community, and family, impact outcomes, dosage, and attrition [24, 35, 54, 70]. Additionally, the framework characteristics can apply to the analysis of elder abuse and neglect prevention interventions in countries other than the United States. While Table 20.2 examples used to illustrate threshold levels are those that predominate in the United States, the framework recognizes that while different prevention interventions may be more prevalent and appropriate in other developing and developed countries [63], they all share the same characteristic of low, medium, and high thresholds.

The following sections of this chapter explore this framework more fully. Within each category of universal, selective, and indicated prevention interventions, we examine the literature, policies, and practices that attest to what is known about the effectiveness, or ineffectiveness, of elder abuse and neglect prevention interventions. The chapter concludes with identifying the methodological and ethical challenges in conducting elder abuse prevention intervention research, and recommends paths forward for increasing our knowledge base of prevention interventions that work.

20.8 Public Awareness Campaigns

20.8.1 Universal Prevention Interventions

Public awareness campaigns have become part of our culture in a way that few modes of messaging can. For example, the tagline, "Friends don't let friends drive drunk," the slogan from the drunk-driving campaign developed by the Ad Council more than 30 years ago, was familiar to 90 % of adults surveyed in 2002 ([4], p. 20). But more than simply being memorable, there are numerous case studies of a variety of national public awareness campaigns that have resulted in long-term individual behavioral change [55, 115] as well as lasting social change [4, 83]. Two examples: an evaluation of the drunk-driving campaign reported that over 62 % of a national sample of respondents attempted to stop someone from driving while under the influence and that 15 years after the start of the campaign, alcohol induced auto fatalities had decreased from 60 to 40 % ([4], p. 21); and the current public awareness campaign to encourage adoption of children in foster care, begun in 2004 with the consistent message of "You don't have to be perfect to be a perfect parent," resulted in over 20 million visits to the AdoptUSKids website, over 218,000 inquiries, and more than 20,700 children being adopted from foster care [3]. All of these successful campaigns shared similar characteristics: coordinated messaging, sustained efforts over time, and clear goals with target outcomes. In essence, "the ability to create discussion (through consistent messaging), penetrate the intended environment, and eventually provoke true behavioral change is the sign of a successful public awareness campaign with measurable impacts" [107].

20.8.2 Elder Abuse National Media Initiatives

While public awareness initiatives can be implemented at all levels of exposure, Faccinetti [41] posited that the field of elder abuse prevention requires the cohesiveness and consistency of a national campaign with a consistent goal and singular message if elder abuse is to be placed on the public agenda for awareness and action. A lack of data confirming the impact of national elder abuse public awareness as a universal prevention intervention has not stopped the field from engaging in, and committing considerable resources to, these efforts.

In the winter of 2001, a National Policy Summit on Elder Abuse was convened with the intent to develop a National Action Agenda on Elder Abuse. All Summit participants agreed that implementing a national media campaign to increase awareness of elder abuse should be at the top of the agenda [74].

In 2009, a University of Delaware report for the National Center on Elder Abuse set forth a strategic blueprint that described and analyzed the essential elements needed to successfully plan and implement a public communication campaign at the national level focused on elder abuse. Chief among those elements was to position elder abuse as a highly important personal and social problem in our communities, making elder abuse an issue of personal relevance emphasizing the collective social responsibility and efficacy to act and succeed [104].

Also in 2009, partly in response to the University of Delaware report, the U.S. Administration on Aging contracted with a private social marketing firm, Reingold, Inc., to determine the feasibility of a social marketing campaign addressing elder abuse. After a nearly year-long effort, Reingold concluded that a public awareness campaign with consistent messaging is needed [38], Appendix B2, pp. 54–54; Stein, private notes, [105].

In 2011, a University of Delaware report for the National Center on Elder Abuse noted that over 500 public awareness materials produced by local, state, and regional entities were documented in the Clearinghouse on Abuse and Neglect of the Elderly. However, there was no consistent message nor branding among them that positioned elder abuse and neglect as a public issue [107].

In 2013, the Elder Justice Coordinating Council, authorized through the Affordable Care Act to coordinate activities

Table 20.2 Characteristics of universal, selective, and indicated prevention interventions versus treatments: a context for elder abuse

Characteristic	Universal prevention intervention	Selective prevention intervention	Indicated prevention intervention	Treatments
Threshold	Low examples: public awareness, public education, advocacy, community outreach	Medium examples: screenings, professional training and education programs, gatekeeper programs	High examples: counseling programs including mental health, support groups, forensic multidisciplinary teams, community services, home visits, case management	Very high examples: adult protective services, legal protections, shelters, emergency services, criminal justice processes, support groups, interagency and community coordinated services, mental health services
Target population	General public	Those over a certain age, usually a threshold of 60	Those exhibiting potential symptoms or early warning signs of abuse or neglect or self-neglect May also include informal caregivers and abusers within the family dyad	Abused and neglected elders May also include informal caregivers and abusers within the family dyad
Timing	Extended and sustained over time	Short term. Before symptoms appear	After risk assessed but before "diagnosis" of abuse or neglect or self-neglect is substantiated May be of limited or continuing duration to avoid or delay onset of abuse, neglect, self-neglect	After determination of substantiated elder abuse or neglect or self-neglect or high levels of danger
Provider	Public communication and education systems at national or community levels Community members with or without special training but with concern for issue.	Professionals in fields likely to come into contact with target population (examples: health system, legal/justice system, social services system). May also be provided by community members Cultural issues and preferences and client self-perceptions of need and autonomy may impact the effectiveness of the provider	Support systems usually community based. May be a team of professionals, usually with special training Services may be focused on vulnerable adult and on caregivers and abusers Cultural issues and preferences and client self-perceptions of need and autonomy may impact the effectiveness of the provider	Social services systems, legal systems, adult protective services systems, health systems including mental health services, criminal justice systems Services may be focused on vulnerable adult and on caregivers and abusers Cultural issues and preferences and client self-perceptions of need and autonomy may impact the effectiveness of the provider
Attrition and Dosage	Influenced by strength and duration of messaging Dosage needs to be sustained over time to make an impact	May be due to early success or client resistance or refusal May be impacted by lack of sensitivity to cultural issues and client self-perceptions of need and autonomy Sufficient dosage for producing improvement may be unknown	May be due to treatment not acceptable to client or client perception that treatment not bringing desired level of change or improvement May be impacted by lack of sensitivity to cultural issues and client self-perceptions of need and autonomy Sufficient dosage for producing improvement may be unknown	May imply services or treatments not acceptable to client, client feels treatment not bringing desired level of change or improvement, or client not able to participate in services/treatments May be impacted by lack of sensitivity to cultural issues and client self-perceptions of need and autonomy Sufficient dosage for producing improvement may be unknown

(continued)

Table 20.2 (continued)

Characteristic	Universal prevention intervention	Selective prevention intervention	Indicated prevention intervention	Treatments
Outcomes	Increased sensitivity to elder mistreatment as a societal issue of salience; alteration of individual and societal attitudes, behaviors; laws and regulations	Increased effectiveness in recognizing those within a target population who may be in need of services or assistance Successful outcome may be influenced by knowledge of what constitutes risk for abuse/neglect, ability to screen appropriately, sensitivity to cultural influences, and perceptions of vulnerability, autonomy, and safety	Vulnerability reduction or symptom elimination that lessens probability of abuse or neglect Successful outcome may be defined by provider or by client Outcomes individualized to client may reduce attrition and increase probability of improved condition Sensitivity to cultural influences, and perceptions of vulnerability, autonomy, and safety will impact ability to attain outcomes	Improved life condition; removal from abusive or neglectful situation; reduced vulnerability to or degree of severity of elder abuse or neglect; reduced ancillary conditions such as depression or other forms of mental illness Successful outcome may be defined by provider or by client Outcomes individualized to client may reduce attrition and increase probability of improved condition Sensitivity to cultural influences, and perceptions of vulnerability, autonomy, and safety will impact ability to attain outcomes

Format and characteristics from Penny Knapp, Program Director, Infant Preschool Family Mental Health Initiative; Medical Director, California Department of Mental Health, "Characteristics of universal, selective and indicated interventions" (Doyle [34], p. 10)

related to elder abuse, neglect, and exploitation across the Federal government, developed a set of eight recommendations for increased federal involvement and actions to address elder abuse, neglect, and exploitation. Recommendation #5, made 12 years after the National Policy Summit, was to "Develop a comprehensive, strategic, and broad-based national public awareness campaign, with clear and consistent messaging to raise awareness and understanding of elder abuse, neglect, and exploitation" [39].

While the identification of the need for a national elder abuse public awareness campaign and the recommendation to take action spans more than a decade, the closest we have come to that was a 2009 public service announcement shown in 694 screens in 25 major cities and metropolitan areas with 2 million views over a 4-week period.[1] While the in-theater advertisements over a period of 4 weeks was a cost-effective mode for an elder abuse public communications campaign, and resulted in a 38 % increase in public inquiries to the National Center on Elder Abuse during its showing [107], it did not generate the required level of public attention and action that sustains the movement of a social issue onto the public agenda.

There are no examples of "one-shot" national campaigns that moved any issue onto the public agenda. To the contrary, the social marketing literature makes it clear that campaigns need to be sustained over time, using a variety of dissemination mediums that consistently maximize exposure to the message [41, 83, 91, 92]. In this sense, sustainability is closely related to cost-effectiveness with sustained efforts being more expensive but also more cost-effective: they are much more likely to produce the desired results than intermittent or one-time only activities.

20.8.3 Word Elder Abuse Awareness Day: A Sustained (but Intermittent) National Campaign[2]

World Elder Abuse Awareness Day (WEAAD) began in 2006 as an initiative of the International Network for the Prevention of Elder Abuse (INPEA) and the World Health Organization (WHO) for the express purpose of raising community-level awareness of elder abuse and neglect. It has grown from a relatively small initiative to one that now involves hundreds and perhaps thousands of national and international communities, professional and civic organizations, media outlets,

[1]The 15 second spot was produced by the University of Delaware in its capacity as co-manager of the National Center on Elder Abuse. The negotiated price for placement was $35,000 for a cost of reach of 1.22 cents a view. Actor William Mapother donated his time and production costs. The branded message was "Why Should I Care?"

[2]Although originally written specifically for this chapter, this section was incorporated into another manuscript that was subsequently published prior to the publication of this book [102].

and governments in a wide range of activities ranging from seminars to walk–runs to coffee cup messages to chat rooms to government proclamations to theater pieces to international global summits [68]. The National Center on Elder Abuse indicates that, in 2015, elder abuse awareness and education events occurred in more than 40 of the 50 United States [75]; INPEA notes WEAAD-related events sponsored by eight countries across the globe [58]. Recent years have seen United Nations observances, World Conferences, U.S. Presidential Proclamations recognizing June 15 as World Elder Abuse Awareness Day, and web-based sharing of photos, videos, podcasts, and blogs.

Without doubt, for 10 years WEADD has been the elder abuse field's most widely recognized and participatory national and international public awareness and education campaign, centered in community outreach and advocacy. There is no record of the amount of resources—human and financial—involved in this campaign but, given the scope and variety of activity and materials, it would not be unreasonable to assume that the costs are substantial, albeit widely distributed among hundreds or thousands of individual entities.

WEADD is a sustained over time universal preventive intervention. However, given the substantial investment in WEADD, the logical question to ask is "Is WEADD an effective universal preventive intervention?" We do not know. The National Center on Elder Abuse, a strong advocate of WEAAD community activities, tracks the number of events that are reported to it, but that is an output measure, not an evaluative outcome. The Elder Justice Coordinating Council who in its 2014 report to Congress cites WEAAD as evidence of its strength in promoting national recognition of elder abuse and neglect prevention [38], does not provide any evidence or effort toward evaluating the outcomes of WEAAD as prevention.[3]

20.8.3.1 A Logic Model to Evaluate the Outcomes of WEAAD

Purtie and Roman [90] indicate that the lack of evaluation of "Awareness Days" as a preventive intervention is not uncommon, particularly as many of these types of events are organized by community members without any particular expertise or motivation beyond concern for a particular cause. Guidance beyond "WEAAD serves as a call-to-action for individuals, organizations, and communities to raise awareness about elder abuse, neglect, and exploitation ([38] p. 10)" is needed so that involved organizations understand and can implement WEAAD as an outcomes-based prevention intervention. With a template that is incorporated into all WEAAD planning activities that clearly identifies the national goal and state and community-level personalizable objectives, programs can be designed to meet specific, identified, universal outcomes that include appropriate evaluation strategies ([90], p. 1064).

Examples of such outcomes could include short and long-term changes in knowledge of elder abuse (as a social problem, causes, extent, etc.); continued participation in elder abuse awareness related community activities; number of visitors to WEAAD website pages that showcase community involvement opportunities during and at 3-, 6-, 9-month follow-ups[4]; number of calls to elder abuse reporting helplines during and at 3-, 6-, 9-month follow-ups; personal screening for risk factors with follow-ups; identification of participants in need of treatment with follow-ups; media coverage during and at 6-month follow-up; legislation or placements on policy agendas that result from government proclamations recognizing WEAAD; formation of support groups that persist over time; and fundraising that is reinvested in future elder abuse prevention activities. Table 20.3 offers an example of a community-level logic model that has the potential to increase the effectiveness of WEAAD activities as a nationally coordinated universal prevention intervention.

20.9 Public Awareness Information and Education

In the context of universal prevention, information and education programs are targeted to the general public without regard for any individual susceptibility to risk. There is mixed evidence that information, alone or in combination with other forms of educational interactions, can be effective in changing individual beliefs, behavior, and attitudes. Finseraas and Jakobsson [43] randomly assigned 3000 individuals to a treatment group and a control group to investigate whether or not the provision of written information describing a government reform in a pension system led people to believe that the reform was beneficial at the consumer level. Results indicated that those who read the informational brochure were more likely to believe that the reform made the pension system easier to understand. Another randomized controlled group study found that the impact of information to encourage behavior change was

[3]The value of WEAAD goes beyond its impact as a prevention measure. WEAAD and its myriad events "reinforce the concept that elder abuse is a universal problem experienced by a diverse and vast audience, and also serve to generate a sense of inclusiveness for those working to address the issue ([68], p. 346)." This, alone, makes WEAAD a powerful social event, as well as a continuing motivation for those who work to better the lives of abused and neglected elders and who, more often than not, face frustrations on a daily basis.

[4]These time periods were chosen with the assumption that new and/or continuing WEAAD activities would commence in month 12, if this continues to be an annual event. Thus, evaluation would be continuous and sustained over a period of years.

Table 20.3 Example of logic model for outcomes of community WEAAD

Inputs	Outputs: activities/participation	Outcomes: short (immediately after)	Outcomes: medium (3–6 months after)	Outcomes: long term (9–12 months after)
Community organizations, media, government leaders with interest in elder abuse Physical place for Fair Supplies and equipment Expertise to produce publicity Volunteers and professionals to staff booths and programs Booths, tables, display spaces Funds to mount event	Community Fair 10 risk assessment booths manned by 10 professionals Organization membership drives 2500 copies of printed information distributed 15 educational workshops attended by 300 people Launch of WEAAD website Media coverage by 3 TV stations and 2 newspapers 1500 individual attendees at Fair 100 risk assessments completed	Increased knowledge/awareness of risk factors, types of elder abuse and neglect Increased knowledge/awareness of community services and volunteer opportunities Sign-ups to participate in elder abuse awareness related community activities Visitors to WEAAD website Increased calls to elder abuse reporting hotlines New identifications of those at risk or in risk in need of interventions or treatments Government proclamations recognizing benefits of WEAAD Fundraising activities planned	Increased participation in elder abuse awareness related community activities Visitors to WEAAD website who click to volunteer in community activities Increased calls to elder abuse reporting hotlines Those identified at risk or in risk are provided with appropriate services Media coverage continues with consistent information Policy/legislative sessions considering new protections for elder abuse potential and current victims Formations of support groups Donors and community support for elder abuse prevention activities	Continuing participation in elder abuse awareness related community activities Increased calls to elder abuse reporting hotlines Improved conditions for those identified at risk or in risk Regularly appearing media stories/columns in a variety of formats Legislation and regulations affording greater protections and avenues of redress Support groups persist over time with increasing membership Fundraising invested in future elder abuse prevention awareness

National Goal WEAAD serves as a call-to-action for individuals, organizations, and communities to raise awareness about elder abuse, neglect, and exploitation

Community XYZ Goals Hold WEAAD Community Fair to: Increase community awareness of elder abuse and neglect, engage community members in efforts to combat elder abuse, identify people who are at risk in our community, and connect people with services

strong immediately after the intervention, but had essentially no effect on behavior change after a 2-year period [99]. A similar result was found by Brug [15] who concluded that information may be essential for behavioral change but, in and of itself, does not cause lasting changes in behavior. Other studies have shown that the impact of information alone, without person-to-person contact, had little or no impact upon retention, behavior change, or decision-making [6, 36, 65] or, at the very least, that a combination of technological and face-to-face delivery increased the likelihood that some behavioral change may occur [64].

20.9.1 Elder Abuse Information and Education Marketed to the General Public

There is no lack of public awareness information materials produced by public, nonprofit, and private organizations. For example, The Office of Financial Protection for Older Americans in the Office of Consumer Protection distributed nearly 600,000 copies of just two public education guides in 2013–2014 [38], and held 225 workshops attended by more than 9000 people [38]. The Federal Trade Commission produced a series of public information materials as part of its 2014 "Pass It On" campaign. In its first month of availability, over 2500 copies were distributed in 49 states [38]. The website of the federally funded National Center on Elder Abuse Information Clearinghouse (National Center on Elder Abuse, NCEA Publications) managed by the Keck School of Medicine of the University of Southern California lists 17 public awareness, education, and outreach materials, ranging from fact sheets to postcards to elevator posters all available for free downloads and reproduction.

Federal agency information efforts are also joined by those in the private sector. One of the more novel efforts is the July 2015 "On the Road to End Elder Financial Abuse" campaign by Wells Fargo, a cross-country bus tour to distribute information to help older people and their families recognize and avoid financial exploitation [118]. The 2009 and 2011 MetLife studies of the extent and costs of financial exploitation [69] were a springboard for a myriad of articles in the popular press and media, including CNN, Consumer Reports, Money Magazine, and Forbes.

In addition to these examples, a search of "public awareness" in the Clearinghouse on Abuse and Neglect of the Elderly yields descriptions of over 700 materials ranging from posters to one-page fact sheets to brochures to menu templates. A Google search of "elder abuse information booklet" produces 97,100 citations. If even only 10 % of these materials were appropriate and available for dissemination to and by the general public, one could conclude that there is no lack of information resources. Recognizing that many community organizations, particularly as part of World Elder Abuse Awareness Day, produce their own materials that never find their ways into databases or beyond community dissemination, it is safe to say that it is literally impossible to know the extent of elder abuse universal prevention information resources that have been created, printed, downloaded, and/or disseminated as part of public, nonprofit, and private organizational information and education efforts. Despite the significant investment of resources in elder abuse information and education, we have no studies that validate the long-term impacts of public awareness materials on changed behavior.

20.9.2 Elder Abuse Education for Pre-professionals

While the purpose of public awareness information materials is to educate the general public, we should also consider a special target of elder abuse education: college students who, in their professional careers, may be likely to encounter and/or serve older people. Unlike training initiatives aimed to increase specific practice competencies of targeted professionals such as those in law enforcement or health care, elder abuse education for college students has the same goal as elder abuse information/education marketed to the general public: increased awareness and recognition of the phenomenon of elder abuse as the first step in prevention.

The earliest study to investigate the extent of elder abuse and neglect content in 211 gerontology programs in higher education found, perhaps unsurprisingly given the small degree of societal attention given to elder abuse over 30 years ago, that less than 5 % of the total content area in aging included any aspect of elder abuse and neglect [104]. When content was included, those topics addressed most frequently were the types of abuse (definitional) and causes of abuse. Those topics addressed least frequently dealt with case assessment and service delivery, and intervention and prevention. Of four serious issues facing older people, elder abuse was rated by the respondents, who were either department heads or course instructors, as the least important by a 2–1 margin.

In the intervening years, there have been several studies attesting to the need for professional training (addressed in this chapter's section on Selective Prevention Strategies), but little attention paid to the education of pre-professionals until two recent studies. Policastro [89] surveyed 202 students enrolled in required health and human sciences classes at one university to determine whether students majoring in social work, nursing, health professions, or criminal justice had different levels of, and perceived need for, elder abuse awareness and knowledge. Students majoring in social work indicated they had the most knowledge about several aspects of elder abuse awareness and good professional practices, followed by human services and health sciences majors, followed by criminal justice majors who indicated the least exposure. However, most students, regardless of major, reported that they lacked sufficient knowledge about elder abuse and neglect in general, and particularly regarding identification, dynamics, and the special needs of victims.

Noting the role that ageism plays in our society, and particularly among young people, Hayslip et al. [50] investigated whether limited exposure to elder abuse information and education could impact their attitudes toward older people and their tolerance for abusive or neglectful behaviors. Students in an Elder Abuse Education and Aging Education treatment group participated in group discussions with an instructor, viewed videos, and received and discussed elder abuse-related educational materials over a course of four evenings. Compared to students who participated in three other aging-issue-related treatment groups without elder abuse content, these students, as measured by a series of pretests and posttests immediately following the educational treatment intervention, demonstrated less tolerance for abuse-related attitudes and behaviors. However, unique among such studies, Hayslip retested the students in the Elder Abuse Education and Aging treatment group 1 month after the initial intervention. The differences observed in the immediate posttest were no longer significant, and students had basically retreated to the attitudes and behaviors exhibited pretreatment.

20.10 Are Elder Abuse Public Awareness and Education Effective Universal Prevention Strategies?

Awareness and education are necessary ingredients for bringing attention to a social issue or problem, but in and of themselves are not sufficient. Effective national campaigns, capable of producing changes in attitudes and behaviors, share similar characteristics: coordinated messaging, sustained efforts over time, and clear goals with target outcomes. Nearly a quarter of a century after the question "what is the impact of public education and awareness on elder abuse prevention" was first raised [101], we still do not know the answer. The characteristics of effective national campaigns are lacking in current elder abuse public awareness and education efforts. The evidence-based outcomes of WEAAD and all other elder abuse public awareness initiatives as a universal preventive intervention have yet to be evaluated. While the elder abuse field abounds in the production and dissemination of information designed to both increase awareness and educate, studies indicate that education and information, alone, do not result in sustained behavioral and attitude changes that persist over time. Still, a lack of data confirming the impact of public awareness and education as universal prevention interventions has not stopped the field from engaging in, and committing considerable resources to, these efforts.

20.11 Selective Prevention Interventions

Selective prevention interventions are targeted toward subgroups within a population who may be at elevated risk because of a vulnerability or characteristic. These interventions are usually short term and center on identifying the degree of risk within a particular group. As elder abuse and neglect can happen to anyone, with maltreated and neglected elders found at all socioeconomic levels, it would be difficult to state with absolute certainty that anyone is completely risk-free. In this sense, merely being of a certain age would place one within the subgroup of "elderly" persons who could be targeted for selective prevention interventions. These interventions could be applied to the individual or to those who come in contact with the individual, usually through the provision of services. The objective of these interventions is to identify an individual's degree of risk—which could range from none to high—for abuse and/or neglect.

Selective prevention interventions recognize that not everyone within the subgroup has the same degree of risk or level of risk [98]. For example, the targeted subgroup of "people over the age of 65," can be further classified into smaller subcategories based upon vulnerabilities such as geographic isolation, drug or alcohol abuse, living with a substance abuser, social isolation from friends and family, mental and/or physical impairments, or advanced age. Those with greater vulnerabilities, even though they all belong to the same subgroup of "over 65," can face higher degrees of risk. At the same time, even within these subcategories, people with the same vulnerabilities can be at different levels of risk.

Within the elder abuse field, predominate selective prevention interventions include screenings and training and education for professionals and allied service providers. These interventions may also be applied in combination with each other, and often the effectiveness of one may depend upon the effectiveness of the other. For example, the effectiveness of screening to detect vulnerabilities may be impacted by the screener's knowledge of available services and resources, an awareness of cultural influences upon client or caregiver responses, and a sensitivity to the elder's own perceptions of vulnerability, autonomy, and safety.

20.11.1 Screening

We have uncovered no sound research or study that demonstrates that it is usual for older people to take the initiative to identify themselves as being abused or neglected. Yet, identification is a necessary first step toward intervention, and screening tools for use by professionals who come into contact with older people, have long been advocated as a means for early detection [19, 44].

As with public information/education materials, the field does not lack for elder abuse screens. Pisani and Walsh [87] undertook a systematic review of validation studies of elder abuse screens used by health service providers, and noted four that relied on clinician assessments (IOA—Indicators of Abuse; EAI—Elder Assessment Instrument; BASE—Brief Abuse Screen for the Elderly; and MDS-A—Minimum Data Set Abuse Screen), five that asked questions of the older adult (AMA—American Medical Association Diagnostic and Treatment Guidelines; HS-EAST (S)—Hwalek-Sengstock Elder Abuse Screening Test Short; EASI—Elder Abuse Suspicion Index; CTS2S—Conflict Tactics Scale 2 Short; and VASS—Vulnerability to Abuse Screening Scale) and two screens that asked questions of nonprofessional caregivers (CASE—Caregiver Abuse Screen; M-CTS—Modified Conflict Tactics Scale). In addition to these, Fulmer et al. [44] identified four other screening tools in the published literature that are primarily used in clinical settings. These tools, some of which document psychometrics, range from brief to extensive questioning. More recently, practitioners are using or adapting screening tools that have been designed to detect risk other than abuse and neglect. For example, the Identification of Seniors at Risk (ISAR) screen has traditionally been used to assess for physical functional decline and a pilot study indicates that the use of this very brief and easily administered screen in Emergency Departments can be particularly helpful in identifying older people whose physical difficulties may increase their vulnerability to abuse or neglect [40]. A pilot project is evaluating the impact of co-locating adult protective services specialists within clinics to provide training on using the EASI screening tool, assist screeners in interpreting the results to identify risk levels, and educate screen administers and clinic personnel on available resources and services for those at varying degrees of risk [80].

There is also movement toward screening tools that are self-administered by the target group. Results indicate that self-administered screens are as valid as clinician administered screens [49] and are more likely to be fully and more honestly completed by the respondents when compared to face-to-face questioning [66, 114]. Yaffe et al. [120] developed a self-administered written version of the Elder Abuse Suspicion Index which was taken by over 200 older people in a doctor's waiting room. Less than 5 % of those approached to take the survey refused, and all those who did participate answered all questions. Preliminary results indicate that this method increased people's awareness of abuse and neglect, with some risk factors emerging for potential mistreatment.

Computerized self-assessments are also gaining traction. While many studies have investigated computerized self-screens in non-elderly populations [23, 59], there is emerging evidence that this mode of screening also holds promise for better detection of potential abuse and neglect. A study that compared traditional in-person interviewing with audio computer-assisted self-interviewing found that the computer-assisted mode resulted in twice as much identification of financial and psychological mistreatment [10]. While the home is a usual setting for computer-assisted self-interviewing, this technology is also portable, increasing the possibility of reaching older people who may not have home computer technology. While waiting to be seen in a public dental clinic, nearly 140 people over the age of 60 agreed to take the Hwalek-Sengstock Elder Abuse Screening Test, reformatted as an audio computer-assisted self-interview. The scores of 48 % of the participants indicated that they were at risk for elder maltreatment, a risk that may never have been otherwise identified as elder abuse screening is not the usual practice in dental offices [95]. Despite numerous limitations noted by the authors of these studies that prevent generalizations based on the results, preliminary evidence indicates that older people may be willing to self-screen in a variety of settings, thereby increasing the likelihood of early identification.

20.12 Is Screening an Effective Selective Prevention Strategy?

It makes logical sense that a necessary component of prevention is to identify the degree of risk that may be present in a subgroup of a population, so that prevention resources can be efficiently targeted toward those whose risk of becoming abused or neglected is above average. Screening can accomplish that purpose. But there are still serious questions and concerns surrounding the accuracy and consistency of screening instruments and resultant assessments, given influences on the target subpopulations responses, the ability of professionals to accurately administer the screen and interpret the results, and inconsistencies in the instruments themselves.

The responses to screening questions, whether by the elder, a caregiver, or family member can be affected by: the setting, the trust in the interviewer, privacy considerations, interpretations of what constitutes maltreatment on the part of the respondent, cultural influences that impact understanding of the questions, and respondent emotions ranging from fear of possible consequences, discomfort, or anger at being asked questions that could seem an invasion of privacy or relief that someone who could provide help may finally be paying attention.

The use and interpretation of screens can be affected by the ability of professionals to: understand the range of potential risk factors and the complexity and interrelationships among numerous forms of abuse and neglect, recognize that vulnerabilities may be well hidden, respect the need for privacy and discretion in conducting the interview, appreciate the need of some clients to first form a trusting relationship, be sensitive to cultural considerations that can influence the understanding and interpretation of responses, balance a tendency toward professional objectivity with respect for client autonomy, and recognize the strengths and limitations of the various instruments (such as training vs. easy administration, quick and brief vs. in-depth interviewing) in order to choose that instrument that is more likely to be actually used within the particular professional or service setting.

Finally, an evaluation of screening as an effective selective prevention intervention is complicated by the fact that the instruments, themselves, have limitations [44]. Measurement scales are not standardized across screening tools so that a score that might indicate a high degree of risk on one instrument might indicate an average degree of risk on another instrument. Screens that are administered only to clients or only to their caregivers or only to their family members may reveal very different data than screens that are administered to all members in the relationship. The form and format of the tool can impact the consistency by which it is administered and the quality and completeness of the data that is collected. For example, brief screens may be all that emergency room workers have time to use, but may not give the respondent enough time or privacy to answer completely and honestly. But perhaps that brief screen *is* sufficient to accurately recognize those with above average risk—which brings us to the summary point: We do not know the effectiveness of screening as a selective prevention intervention. To date, there are no comprehensive empirical tests of the ability of screening to achieve the long-term outcome of accurately identifying older people who have an above average risk for maltreatment.

20.13 Training and Education

The previous section noted that it is important for professionals and service providers who are likely to come into contact with older people to have knowledge of elder abuse and neglect. Without such knowledge, it would be virtually impossible for them to identify their clientele's degree of vulnerability to an above average risk of maltreatment. In that sense, training for professionals and service providers is a selective prevention intervention.

20.13.1 Professional Training and Education

Just as there is no lack of educational materials aimed at the general public, and no lack of screening instruments, there is no lack of training and educational materials developed for specific professionals and occupational groups. The Center of Excellence on Elder Abuse at the University of California-Irvine (http://www.centeronelderabuse.org/education_overview.asp) makes available dozens of training curricula, webcasts, and handbooks specifically tailored for those in the judiciary, law enforcement, law, medicine, nursing, pharmacy, and social services. The American Bar Association Commission on Law and Aging produces and widely disseminates training and educational materials specifically for elder law attorneys, the judiciary, and advocates. In cooperation with the Investor Protection Trust and Investor Protection Institute, the Commission has recently begun to develop a model national continuing education curriculum for practitioners in a wide variety of legal specializations [37]. The CFP Board approves over 48 continuing education courses for its certified financial planner members (http://www.cfp.net/for-cfp-professionals/continuing-education/ce-resources/find-ce-program/Results/#/Results/name/1). The American Medical Association website publishes the Physicians' Obligations in Preventing, Identifying, and Treating Violence and Abuse (http://www.ama-assn.org/ama/pub/physician-resources/medical-ethics/code-medical-ethics/opinion202.page), and more than 7800 doctors and health care professionals have participated in 86 continuing medical education programs as part of the Elder Investment Fraud and Financial Exploitation Prevention Program Medical [37]. The International Association of Forensic Nurses publishes an elder abuse curriculum (http://www.forensicnurses.org/?page=eldermistreatment), as does the Nursing League for Nursing (http://www.nln.org/professional-development-programs/teaching-resources/aging/ace-s/teaching-strategies/aces-knowledge-domains/complexity-of-care/elder-abuse-in-the-united-states-a-teaching-strategy-for-nurses). The National Institute on the Prosecution of Elder Abuse is a 3.5-day course designed to train prosecutors in best practices for prosecuting elder abuse cases. For breadth, look no further than Google. A search of "elder abuse training for…." produces 267,000 resources for law enforcement; 310,000 for banks; 5,950,000 for all health care providers; 395,000 for the judiciary; 767,000 for dentists, and 318,000 for pharmacists. Of course, by no means could we imagine that the vast majority of these would be useful for professional training. Yet, even if we assumed that only one-tenth of one percent (0.1 %) would have educational value, that would still mean the availability of 7651 training materials and resources addressing elder abuse and neglect directed toward professionals and service providers.

Is continuing education and training needed? Studies indicate that educational interventions are more effective than years in practice when it comes to knowledge and awareness of elder abuse and neglect [109]. This may be at least partially due to the paucity of elder abuse education in professional training programs [89]. A study by Tildon and colleagues revealed that elder abuse educational content in their professional training programs could be recalled by only 27 % of the 1516 professionals in their sample, with oral care providers indicating receiving (or retaining) the least content in their professional preparations. However, those who did receive elder abuse education were statistically significantly more likely to commonly suspect physical abuse among their clients, compared to those without exposure to elder abuse education [113].

Does the format of delivery make a difference? Some studies indicate that in-person education sessions designed for professionals and paraprofessionals working with older people are more effective than written materials alone in increasing knowledge and awareness, as well as familiarity with reporting requirements, and that this holds true regardless of the length of the educational intervention [93, 109]. Studies of this type based their conclusions almost exclusively on changes in knowledge based on tests administered just before and fairly immediately after the intervention. We have found no methodologically sound studies that evaluate changes in behavior over time due to the educational intervention.

20.13.2 Gatekeepers

Gatekeepers constitute another audience for education and training. First developed by the Spokane Mental Health Elder Services Program in Washington State; the model of training employees who would not traditionally have older people as their specific clientele has been replicated in various forms in communities across the country. The theory is that people who deliver the mail and packages, who read meters, who take care of lawns, who are apartment building doormen or maintenance workers, often have opportunities to talk to or observe older people in the course of providing their services. With training, they are in a position to recognize increased vulnerabilities or warning signs of distress that could indicate the need for assistance, and in this sense, behave as a "personal screen" for identifying people with a more than average risk of maltreatment or neglect. There is no national data on the number of gatekeepers trained, although anecdotal evidence from even a few communities would indicate that it is substantial.[5]

20.14 Is Continuing Education and Training an Effective Selective Prevention Strategy?

Selective prevention interventions are targeted toward subgroups within a population who may be at elevated risk because of a vulnerability or characteristic. These interventions are usually short term and center on identifying the degree of risk within a particular group. It would be illogical to assume that one could identify the degree of risk within a particular group if one has no knowledge of the condition, risk factors, or means of identifying or assessing vulnerabilities that could indicate above average risk. Education and training interventions, therefore, would seem to be necessary for effective selective prevention. For example, we might assume that increased knowledge leads to more competent practices which lead to behavioral changes that last over time. Is that true? Published studies more usually evaluate single programs with convenience samples, and measure immediate gains in knowledge; or measure outputs in terms of how many people participated in an educational program. Similarly, despite a plethora of training curricula, many of which are targeted toward the same professional or service provider groups with little differentiation in content or format, we have found no studies that reliably test outcomes over time to gain knowledge of differentiated design or implementation factors, if any, that facilitate improved competencies that lead to behavioral change. The field lacks systematic and methodologically sound studies to measure and evaluate the long-term impacts of education and training.

20.15 Indicated Prevention Interventions

Indicated prevention interventions target high-risk individuals within the elderly population subgroup who exhibit early danger signs of potentially falling victim to abuse or neglect. Indicated interventions are applied to a person not entered into the adult protective services system with a substantiated case of abuse or neglect, and usually consist of longer term provision of services or programs that could involve the potential victim, the potential abuser, the complete family system, or everyone involved in the caregiving dyad. The goal of these interventions is to eliminate, or at the least delay, the full onset of abuse and neglect.[6] Assessing and identifying the degree and level of vulnerabilities within the subgroup through selective prevention interventions can facilitate the design and application of programs and services that constitute indicated prevention interventions. However, there is not always a straight line relationship; selected preventions are not a prerequisite to indicated preventions and people can enter the prevention intervention stage at any point.

Within the elder abuse field, indicated prevention interventions include home care and case management services, multidisciplinary/forensic team[7] approaches to providing coordinated and comprehensive community services and programs, and individualized counseling. Many of these interventions are psychosocial in nature, intended to change behaviors and/or attitudes of those involved in the family dyad, including vulnerable elders, abusers, and caregivers.

Selected and indicated prevention interventions can be combined to improve overall effectiveness and client acceptability. For example, the ability of multidisciplinary teams to deliver a coordinated package of community services that are acceptable to an at-risk elder may be enhanced by an array of clinical screens and assessments. The ability of multidisciplinary teams to deliver a coordinated package of community services that are acceptable to an at-risk elder may be enhanced by counseling and psychosocial support services that are focused on identifying outcomes important to the client. While it is possible that any one indicated prevention intervention can be delivered independently of any other, a combination of these interventions are often part of a coordinated service plan and, in many cases, are inseparable, as illustrated in Fig. 20.2 and as described in the following section's examples of programs.

[5]For example, Colorado Senior Reach, in its first 28 months, trained 5561 community partners who identified 478 people in need of, and eligible for, assistance. Mid Kansas Senior Outreach in its first 32 months trained 13,992 community partners who identified 483 people in need of and eligible for assistance [9].

[6]As explained earlier in this chapter, once elder abuse or neglect is substantiated, interventions are no longer preventive, but consist of treatments.

[7]The forensic team concept was launched at the University of California at Irvine in 2003, in which professionals from the justice system, health care, protective services, and mental health would meet regularly to engage in multidisciplinary consultation, case examination, action recommendations, and service delivery. A key feature is that these forensic teams would meet regularly under one roof, called a Forensic Center [78]. Due to their similarity in function and concept, this chapter uses the term "multidisciplinary team" to include forensic teams.

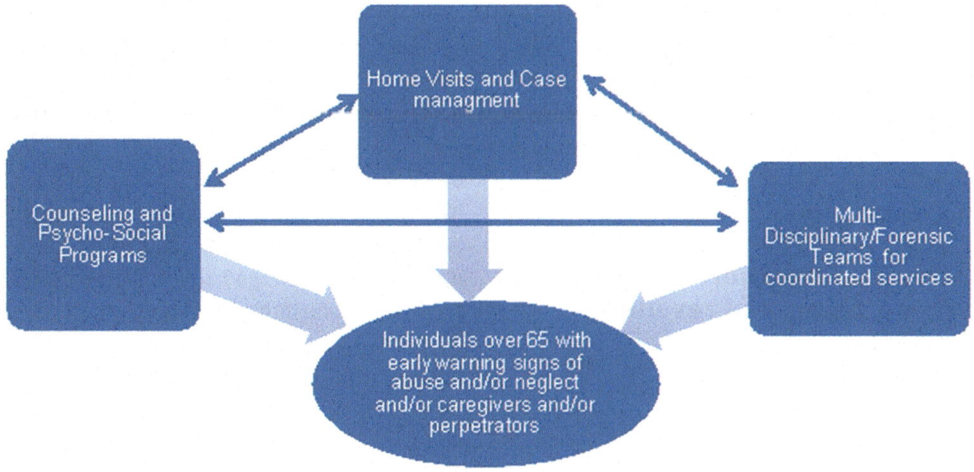

Fig. 20.2 Examples of Indicated Prevention Interventions: Longer term strategies to target individuals with very high risk of being abused or neglected, and who may already be exhibiting some early warning signs of being in an abusive or neglected condition. These interventions may also be applied to others in the family dyad, such as caregivers and perpetrators

20.15.1 Program Examples of Coordinated and Combined Strategies[8]

20.15.1.1 The Elder Services Case Management Prevention Intervention

The Elder Services Case Management Prevention Intervention implemented by the Alaska Division of Senior and Disabilities Services targets high-risk vulnerable adults and their caregivers using the Critical Time Intervention case management model [81]. In this model, home visits, case management, client counseling, and coordination of wrap-around community services are all integral components. During the transition phase of the model, case managers work with clients to formulate client-centered goals, and coordinate with community services to provide critical needs that allow the elder to stay in the home. During the second phase (Try-Out), the case manager and the client identify ongoing formal and informal support needs and transfer more responsibility for working with the service providers to the client and caregiver. During the final phase of Transfer, the case manager transfers care to the long-term support system created for the client.

Preliminary evaluations indicate that the program is successful in keeping clients, who have not yet experienced abuse or neglect but who have high levels of risk, out of the APS system. Key to the success is regular community partner meetings which operate similar to a multidisciplinary team of service providers; and the involvement of the clients themselves in determining needs and desired outcomes.

[8]The first three program examples from Alaska, University of Southern California, and New York were chosen, as they were, at the time of this writing, three of the five projects most recently funded by the U.S. Administration on Aging to test and evaluate prevention interventions.

20.15.1.2 Take AIM Against Elder Abuse

The Take AIM Against Elder Abuse Intervention–Prevention Model developed by the University of Southern California Kerck School of Medicine targets older adults with dementia and their caregivers/families. Selected and indicated interventions are combined to administer baseline screens and follow-up risk assessments, target referrals for services from among team members in nine multidisciplinary collaborating organizations, and conduct 3 months of home visits [51]. A key feature of the intervention is that the wide array of coordinated multidisciplinary team members involved in the intervention encourages simultaneous interventions at multiple risk points, linking both the care recipient and the caregiver/family members to appropriate supports and services, with the goal of preventing a difficult care situation turning into an abusive relationship.

20.15.1.3 Enhanced Multidisciplinary Teams

The New York State Office for the Aging is piloting an Enhanced Multidisciplinary Teams (E-MDTs) intervention, incorporating the services of a forensic accountant and a geriatric psychologist to join the more usual team members drawn from aging and social services, law enforcement, advocacy, and community care organizations [48]. While the primary goal of the E-MDT is to protect the elder's assets and to prevent future occurrences, the team also recognizes that many of their clients are high risk for other forms of elder abuse and so prepares client-centered coordinated community care plans based, partly, on needs indicated on medical and/or mental assessments.

20.15.1.4 Eliciting Change in At-Risk Elders

The Eliciting Change in At-Risk Elders (E-CARE) project [67] has elements common to the programs previously described, including home visits, client and caregiver/family counseling, case management, and multidisciplinary teams of outreach specialists who connect elders to community services and resources that support in-home care and reduce the level of risk of maltreatment. Similar to the Alaska program, a key concept is that the high-risk elder is not simply someone to be protected or someone who receives services, but someone with rights and responsibilities for determining his/her desired outcomes and taking actions to achieve those outcomes. Unique to this program, the counseling function is central to the intervention and consists of motivating clients to make changes themselves and for themselves that would result in safer environments and greater autonomy. Rather than a strict template, the change model was individualized for each client to facilitate movement from desire to change to ambivalence about change, to preparing to change, to making change, to following through with change over time. Bivariate and anova analyses indicated a reduction in risk factors, the majority of vulnerable elders in the program making some progress toward achieving their self-defined outcomes, and somewhat less than half actively taking and maintaining actions to change their life conditions.

20.16 Are Multidisciplinary Teams, Case Management, and Psychosocial Programs Aimed at Changing Attitudes or Behaviors Interventions, Effective Indicated Prevention Strategies?

20.16.1 Multidisciplinary Teams

One common characteristic of these programs is the employment of some form of multidisciplinary team or approach. Multidisciplinary teams have been recognized and advocated as effective interventions for several decades [5, 7, 8, 42, 79, 111], even though studies have been primarily descriptive. The majority of studies that attempted to evaluate the impacts of these teams have been hampered with methodological limitations, including small samples, convenience sampling, and the use of relatively simple bivariate analyses [88]. Among those fewer studies using regression and multivariate analyses to evaluate outcomes, Navarro [78] examined complaints of financial exploitation and found that the strongest predictor of case review, court filing for prosecution and conviction was whether or not the case was first examined by a Forensic Center before going to the District Attorney's office. A follow-up study comparing outcomes for clients referred to the Forensic Center to outcomes for clients with similar conditions referred to Adult Protective Services, found the Forensic Center intervention to be more cost-effective [82]. Rizzo [94] examined a multidisciplinary social work-lawyer indicated prevention intervention program and found that clients using these combined services were more likely to have reduced risks for maltreatment compared to clients who only used social work services.

These results give greater credence to the possibility that multidisciplinary teams may be an effective intervention. However, the results were generated from studies of a specific program in a specific city and thus are not generalizable to elder mistreatment interventions.

20.16.2 Psychosocial Supports for Clients and Abusers

The other characteristic shared among these programs is the provision of psychosocial supports such as individualized client-centeredness counseling and case management that emphasizes client determination and identification of desired outcomes over professional assessments. Numerous studies indicate that cognitive, at-risk elders are more likely to accept services if they feel themselves to be partners in the decision-making processes, with autonomy to determine their own goals [33, 67, 97, 106, 117] and it is becoming increasingly recognized that what constitutes "successful" outcomes, and thus indicators of success, can vary by client [16].

Literature is more mixed concerning the effectiveness of psychosocial support systems for abused elders. A control group study of a psychoeducational support group intervention for older women victims of family mistreatment found no difference in outcomes between women who underwent the intervention and those who did not [14]. A small control group study of Iranian abusers and abused family members found that a family-based cognitive behavioral social work intervention resulted in reduced emotional neglect, care neglect, financial neglect, curtailment of personal autonomy, psychological abuse, and financial abuse but there was no statistically significant difference in physical abuse before and after the intervention [60]. A review of 473 strategies employed in 83 cases revealed that empowerment strategies including support groups and counseling for abused elders was the fourth of ten most accepted and successful interventions [72].

While there is some doubt as to the effectiveness of psychosocial programs as an indicated prevention intervention for abused elders, the literature regarding successful interventions for perpetrators more strongly indicates that psychosocial and educational interventions can be effective for perpetrators within the family dyad [72, 96]. Campbell Reay and Brown's [17] study of an anger management and education program for those who physically abused and for those who neglected their older dependents found both groups showed reductions in strain, depression, and anxiety after the educational intervention, with further reductions evidenced after subsequent participation in the anger management program. Further, the perpetrators of physical abuse were found to have engaged in fewer conflicts with the dependent elder at a 6-month follow-up period. Psychosocial behavioral interventions with perpetrators of domestic violence and child abuse also found therapeutic interviews, anger management and education to be effective indicated prevention interventions [27, 62, 119], lending further credence to the apparent effectiveness of these interventions aimed at perpetrators.

20.16.3 What can We Conclude?

The same criticisms that applied to the study of multidisciplinary teams apply to these studies of psychosocial prevention interventions designed to induce behavioral and/or attitudinal change. Most are primarily descriptive. While some employed an experimental design with a control group, they also had small sample sizes and, consequently, results are not generalizable.

The broader question would really refer to all indicated prevention strategies. The short answer, as it was for universal and selected prevention strategies, is that we do not know which, if any, indicated prevention strategies are effective. Although many of the illustrated programs in this chapter were funded specifically to evaluate outcomes of prevention services, we cannot discern (at least at this stage) whether impacts are due more to the characteristics of the agency and its personnel than to the intervention [77]. Studies that assert to test outcomes usually evaluate a single program, often with small samples. Descriptive, bivariate statistical analyses are primarily used which may reveal associations, but do not allow us to make causal conclusions about significant relationships. As a summary statement, the field lacks systematic and methodologically sound studies to measure and evaluate the long-term impacts of indicated prevention interventions.

20.17 Prevention Interventions: Ethical Issues and Challenges

At this time, we have little or no evidence of the long-term efficacy of the many different strategies and services currently employed to reduce the occurrence or the severity of elder abuse and neglect through prevention or even through treatment. A 2009 review of the effectiveness of elder abuse and neglect interventions found that few published studies used valid and reliable methods to evaluate the impact of the intervention when interventions were evaluated at all, and that there is not sufficient evidence to attest to the effectiveness of any intervention targeting clients, perpetrators, or even professionals [77, 88]. A 2016 review of the literature confirms this conclusion and further notes the lack of data relating to the total costs of any prevention intervention [86].

Without a valid body of outcomes-based evidence, informed by well-designed and sound methodological research, we do not know if the investment in our current prevention programs and services has any positive payoffs in terms of improved individual or societal well-being. Lacking longitudinal studies, we do not know the dosage impacts of current prevention programs; that is, the threshold amount of exposure to an intervention necessary for it to have a lasting effect. Perhaps most dangerous, we do not know if we are doing more harm than good.

Why has the field lagged in conducting rigorous studies of prevention interventions engaging to a much greater degree in activities with unproven or uncertain results that do not address our "real need of reliably knowing what works, for whom, under what conditions and what settings [45]"? Teaster posits that practitioners and researchers may be so vested in delivering and advocating an intervention that they believe to be valuable, that they fear that evaluations might cause them to lose resources or stop services [112]. Another explanation lies in the fact that despite a recognition for the need to conduct large-scale experimental design and/or randomized control trials to evaluate whether an intervention has positive, neutral, or negative impacts [86, 88], the nature of elder abuse and neglect presents ethical challenges to research design and implementation in general and to experimental research design specifically that mitigate against its use. These barriers include: obtaining consent, as high at-risk elders may suffer from psychological distress, poor mental health and depression; human subject protection rules that mitigate against experimental designs that withhold the intervention to vulnerable groups or concern that the intervention could increase vulnerabilities or cause further harm; concerns or fear over mandatory reporting requirements that may cause elders and their families to hide information; participant access, recruitment, and retention as elders may be reluctant to admit to their situations, and may drop out because of feelings of lack of control, loss of autonomy, or finding the outcomes unacceptable; and lack of sufficient agency and community resources to assist newly identified at-risk or high-risk elders [20, 94, 97].

In addition to these barriers related to the actual conduct of the research, researchers themselves face ethical dilemmas in designing experimental and randomized control studies [1]. How does one maximize the benefits to society of more reliably knowing the cost-effectiveness of elder abuse prevention interventions, while minimizing the harm to any individual subject who may be subject to abuse and neglect, but not receive any intervention in a randomized control study? What protocols must be put in place to continuously monitor unanticipated risks to participants? What level of negative effects upon a treatment group or an individual would necessitate stopping the study if, for example, indications were that a specific intervention strategy was causing increased distress or exposure to abusive conditions? In the event of early indications of negative or positive effects, how does one determine the appropriate dosage of the intervention to ensure that participants have sufficient exposure for sustained impact? Should researchers determine, prior to the intervention, that there are systems in place to continue providing successful interventions once the study is completed?

Given the complex ethical concerns that should be addressed before implementing large-scale experimental or randomized control treatment studies, it is tempting to say that the field cannot wait that long to offer prevention interventions to people in need of services. Rather, that the more practical way forward to knowing "what works and what does not work" requires more money, more training, more demonstration studies—more of the usual suspects to do more of what we have been primarily doing for at least the past 25 years. But if all these past efforts have not led us to answer the questions first posed in 1991 that opened this chapter, why would we expect that doing more of the same will give us those answers?

20.18 Paths Forward

Members of a panel of researchers at a 2015 National Institute of Health workshop on Multiple Approaches to Understanding and Preventing Elder Abuse identified several new approaches and actions for building a body of reliable and valid prevention intervention research that emphasizes experimental design, sophisticated data analysis, and rigorous evaluation. The remainder of this chapter states and further discusses their recommendations to establish standards for large-scale experimental design studies, address Institutional Research Board concerns, develop outcomes methodologies to capture individualized change, and place funding priorities upon rigorously designed experimental studies.[9] The remaining suggestions for advancing the field are those of the chapter author.

[9]These specific recommendations are from the remarks of Mark Lachs, Weill Cornell Medicine, Cornell University; Richard Gelles, University of Pennsylvania; Karl Pillemer, Cornell University; David Burns, University of Toronto; and Laura Mosqueda, University of Southern California.

20.18.1 Establish Methodological and Ethical Standards to Advance Large-Scale Experimental Studies

NIH Participant(s) Recommendation. Recognizing the barriers and ethical issues that present challenges to elder abuse and neglect research, a key action for moving forward effectively is the formulation of policies and practices to guide and advance experimental and/or randomly controlled treatment large-scale research design, implementation, and data analysis.

Expansion and Discussion. Key to these discussions is the development of a set of ethical principles and guidelines that address the previously identified barriers and ethical challenges inherent in elder abuse research while adhering to accepted research ethical standards of respecting the autonomy, safety, privacy, and welfare of the research subjects. Particularly important is developing criteria for assessing the risks and benefits of participation, recognizing that in randomized control trials, some people at risk for, or suffering from, elder abuse may not receive any intervention.

20.18.2 Address Institutional Research Board Concerns, Particularly Regarding Intervention Fidelity

NIH Participant(s) Recommendation. Recognizing that Institutional Research Boards (IRBs) are often an impediment to approving experimental designs, there is a need to develop guidelines and principles for standardizing language in elder abuse research proposals to IRBs. Relatedly, with a small number of investigators conducting rigorous elder abuse research, there is a paucity of proposal reviewers who understand the importance of elder abuse research or the methods that need to be employed, given barriers to participation and retention of subjects. Funding agencies, and IRBs, need to be made aware that there are ethical ways to conduct elder abuse and neglect research that do not necessarily follow traditional methods.

Expansion and Discussion. It may be particularly pertinent, given the complex ethical concerns in delivering interventions to a vulnerable population, that proposals specifically address intervention fidelity by standardizing guidelines for procedures and policies that ensure an intervention is delivered as intended [12] and that procedures for addressing social threats to internal validity are standardized. Two particular social threats, identified by Horner et al. [53], may predominate in elder abuse research. First, that subjects assigned to a control group become aware of the intervention given to the treatment group and may become resentful or discouraged about their own situation, leading to worse outcomes than they would normally have. Second, subjects or their family members might implore researchers to assign them to a different group than their random assignment either out of a desire for the intervention if randomly assigned to the control group, or a fear or distrust of an intervention if randomly assigned to the treatment group. Without researcher-accepted protocols in place, individual researchers may respond differently to these demands, jeopardizing internal validity and, consequently, results of the study [53].

Relatedly, the inclusion of a RE-AIM[10] framework that is focused on the organizations and staff who are intended to deliver the evidence-based interventions can assist IRB's in assessing intervention fidelity [85] as well as external validity. As large-scale experimental research studies of elder abuse interventions are likely to involve multiple partners from a variety of organizations and may involve multiple levels of implementation, RE-AIM can assist researchers, and thus IRBs, from the onset in understanding and determining the implementation issues that may arise from evaluating the interventions [110].

20.18.3 Develop Outcome Methodologies to Capture Individualized Change that is also Sustainable and Culturally Acceptable to the Community

NIH Participant(s) Recommendation. Research design is often stymied because the field does not have a sense of what constitutes a successful outcome or of the metrics to evaluate the success of a prevention intervention. However, it may be more fruitful to consider that outcomes and indicators of success can vary by client and to develop methodologies that capture individualized change. While generalization of results is the goal of prevention intervention research, we should recognize that standardization of interventions may not be possible or desirable. Generalization of results should lead us to understand that any one particular intervention cannot be applied to all cases, but any one particular intervention can be applied to serve a similar need.

Expansion and Discussion. An insensitivity to cultural and community differences can further complicate the effectiveness of even a well-documented evidence-based prevention intervention to the extent that any one particular intervention should not be applied to serve a similar need. Given this, the adoption of a community-based participatory research approach (CBPR) can be useful in formulating and achieving outcomes that are likely to be sustainable and acceptable to the targets of the prevention interventions [13, 31, 32]. A full partnership among academic researchers, community organizations, and key community stakeholders could result in developing a methodology that better accounts for the needs, challenges, infrastructure, and potential barriers, most significantly recruitment and cultural acceptability, that could otherwise negatively impact the desired outcomes of the proposed prevention intervention [28, 63].

20.18.4 Use the Results of Outcomes Methodologies to Assess Effectiveness of Nonexperimental Prevention Intervention Programs

While the majority of this section advocates that the path forward for elder abuse prevention research rests with large-scale experimental designs and controlled randomized treatments, it is recognized that there will be a continuing body of pilot projects, demonstration projects, and community/agency-level intervention practices that are of low cost, small scope, and do not adhere to the methodologies of experimental/randomized control treatments. For example, despite acknowledging the lack of effectiveness data, Pillemer et al. [86] identified caregiver interventions, money management programs, helplines, emergency shelters, and multidisciplinary teams as promising prevention intervention practices.

Two evaluation tools readily available that can generate evidence-based assessments of even nonexperimental design program impacts and effectiveness and contribute to intervention fidelity are RE-AIM and Logic Models. The RE-AIM framework has traditionally been used to evaluate the impacts of different approaches to health promotion interventions in areas such as cancer screening, dietary change, physical activity, medication adherence, health policy, environmental change, chronic illness self-management, and women's health [116]. To the extent that elder abuse prevention can be considered a public health issue [21], this framework is particularly applicable to elder abuse and neglect prevention intervention programs, yet the published literature does not indicate its use in elder abuse intervention

[10]The RE-AIM framework has primarily been used in translational research in the public health arena to help improve the sustainable adoption and implementation of effective, generalizable, evidence-based interventions. Sweet et al. [110] describes the five assessment points as: reach (percentage and characteristics of people from a given population who participate—as subjects or as staff—in the intervention); effectiveness, (positive and negative outcomes of the intervention); adoption (the percent of possible organizations and staff that have agreed to participate in the intervention); implementation (the extent to which the program was delivered as intended and its cost); and maintenance (outcomes sustained at the individual level for at least 6 months, and that intervention or practice or policy is institutionalized at the organizational level).

programs. Similarly, logic models are used as part of a program's design prior to implementation to develop logical connections between goals, capabilities (inputs), activities (outputs), and outcomes. Given the requirement of some funders for proposals to include a logic model, it is possible that organizational applicants may have developed logic models as descriptions of their planned intervention. However, we have found no published research in the elder abuse arena that demonstrates that the results of these evaluation tools have been specifically used for determining outcomes effectiveness of an elder abuse prevention intervention. The use of low-cost evaluation measures to guide program evaluation and improvement is necessary to begin building a body of evidence-based documented effectiveness for even nonexperimental design interventions.

20.18.5 Conduct Externality Analyses to Determine Total Costs of Interventions

The efforts and resources devoted to universal, selective, and indicated prevention interventions are considerable. We replicate and engage in new variations of prevention interventions such as screenings, public education, and multidisciplinary teams at substantial costs, without knowing if their impacts are positive, neutral, or actually harmful. No research studies have measured the direct costs of these programs [86], let alone the costs of unintended effects that may fall upon those who are not part of the targeted population subject to the intervention but may still be affected. Employing an externality analysis would identify and measure the intended direct costs and benefits and the unintended social costs or benefits of preventive interventions. Given that one of the few studies to use an experimental design found that those who were randomly assigned to receive the intervention actually had their abusive condition worsened [25], the importance of knowing the actual impacts of interventions upon those they are intended to help, of knowing the private costs and benefits of delivering these interventions, and of knowing the social costs and benefits, becomes vital. These measures of private and social costs and benefits provide documentation for the efficient allocation of prevention intervention resources.

20.18.6 Make Funding Decisions that Drive Rigorous Research and Evaluations

NIH Participant(s) Recommendation. Funders of elder abuse research have a leading role in promoting, by their funding decisions, prevention research that is characterized by rigorous research and evaluative designs.

Expansion and Discussion. The Administration for Community Living is implementing a requirement for evidence-based research as a condition for receiving Disease Prevention and Health Promotion Services (Title III-D), effective from October 1, 2016. To meet the requirement, programs must: "demonstrate through evaluation to be effective for improving the health and well-being or reducing disease, disability and/or injury among older adults; and (be) proven effective with older adult populations, using experimental or quasi-experimental design; and (publish) research results in a peer review journal. [2]." While directed at states and Area Agencies of Aging, this new policy will necessarily forge new partnerships between practitioners and researchers. Meeting journal publication standards will subject these practices to systematic evaluation. The requirement of at least quasi-experimental designs will elevate the reliability of findings and lessen the probability of good money going toward unproven or bad practice.

Similarly, the National Institute of Justice, in noting that none of the 30 elder abuse research projects it has funded over the past 10 years used a rigorous scientific design to test a universal or selected prevention intervention, issued a 2016 request for proposals that will use a rigorous design, such as a randomized control trial, propensity score matching, or regression discontinuity, to test the impacts of a multiyear demonstration project to prevent abuse, neglect, and/or financial exploitation among community-residing elderly individuals identified to be at risk for elder mistreatment.

20.18.7 Concluding Statement: Policy Drives Research that Drives Practice

It is an axiom that budgets should not drive priorities, but budgets reveal priorities. To the extent that funding dollars specifically for elder abuse prevention intervention programs continue to be awarded to pilot programs, demonstration projects, and resource centers without requiring scientifically sound rigorous methodologies for evaluating outcomes, our answer to the question of "what prevention interventions work and don't work?" will be we still do not know.

References

1. Adams LC. Research ethics. Retrieved February 25, 2016, from ETHICS IN MEDICINE University of Washington School of Medicine. 2014. https://depts.washington.edu/bioethx/topics/resrch.html.

2. Administration for Community Living. (n.d.). Disease Prevention and Health Promotion Services. Retrieved November 12, 2015, from http://www.aoa.acl.gov/AoA_Programs/HPW/Title_IIID/index.aspx.
3. Advertising Council. Adoption from Foster Care. Retrieved October 28, 2015, from Ad Council. 2015. http://www.adcouncil.org/Impact/Case-Studies/Adoption-from-Foster-Care-2013.
4. Advertising Council. Public Service Advertising that Changed a Nation. Retrieved October 3, 2015, from http://www.adcouncil.org/Impact/Research/Public-Service-Advertising-that-Changed-a-Nation.
5. Alon S, Berg-Warman A. Treatment and prevention of elder abuse and neglect: where knowledge and practice meet-a model for intervention to prevent and treat elder Abuse in Israel. J Elder Abuse Negl. 2014;26:150–71.
6. Alt K, Nguyen A, Meure L. The effectiveness of educational programs to improve recognition and reporting of elder abuse and neglect: a systematic review of the literature. J Elder Abuse Negl. 2011;23(3):213–33.
7. Anetzberger G. The clinical management of elder abuse. New York, New York: The Haworth Press; 2005.
8. Anetzberger G, Dayton C, Miller C, McGreevey J, Schimer M. Multidisciplinary teams in the clinical management of elder abuse. Clin Gerontol. 2006;28:157–71.
9. Bartsch D, Rodgers V, Strong D. Outcomes of senior reach gatekeeper referrals: comparison of the spokane gatekeeper program, colorado senior reach, and mid-kansas senior outreach. Care Manag J. 2013;14(1):11–20.
10. Beach S, Schulz R, Degenholtz H, Castle N, Rosen J, Fox A, et al. Using audio computer-assisted self-interviewing and interactive voice response to measure elder mistreatment in older adults: feasibility and effects on prevalence estimates. J Off Stat. 2010;26(3):507–33.
11. Bhattarai L. Neglect and abuse of older people in nepal: a commentary on a baseline study on reported cases of elder abuse in Nepali Press. J Elder Abuse Negl. 2014;26(3):333–6.
12. Borrelli B. The assessment, monitoring, and enhancement of treatment fidelity in public health clinical trials. J Public Health Dent. 2011;71:S52–63.
13. Brossoie N, Roberto K. Community professionals' response to intimate partner violence against rural older women. J Abuse Negl Elder. 2015;27(4–5):470–88.
14. Brownell P, Heiser D. Psycho-educational support groups for older women victims of family mistreatment. J Gerontol Soc Work. 2006;46(3):145–60.
15. Brug J. Determinants of health eating: Motiation, abilities and environmental opportunities. Fam Pract. 2008;25:50–5.
16. Burnes D. Novel intervention and presentation strategies presentation, NIH workshop of multiple approaches to understanding and preventing Elder Abuse. Bethesda, MD; 2015.
17. Campbell Reay A, Browne K. The effectiveness of psychological interventions with individuals who physically abuse or neglect their elderly dependents. J Interpers Violence. 2002;17(4):414–31.
18. Caplan G. Principles of prevention psychiatry. Oxford, England: Basic Books; 1969.
19. Choi N, Mayer J. Elder abuse, neglect and exploitation: risk factors and prevention strategies. J Gerontol Soc Work. 2000;33(2):5–25.
20. Connolly M. Elder self-neglect and the justice system: an essay from an interdisciplinary perspective. J Am Geriatr Soc. 2008;56:S244–52.
21. Connolly MT. II.2, Seven policy priorities for an enhanced public health response to elder abuse. Elder Abuse and Its Prevention: Workshop Summary. In Forum on Global Violence Prevention; Board on Global Health; Institute of Medicine; National Research Council. Washington, DC: National Academies Press; 2014.
22. Connolly M, Brandl B, Breckman R. The Elder Justice Roadmap. Retrieved July 10, 2015, from USDOJ elder justice and prosecution. 2014. www.justice.gov/elderjustice/research/roadmap.html.
23. Corkrey R, Parkinson L. Interactive voice response: review of studies 1989–2000. Behav Res Methods Instrum Comput. 2002;34(3):342–53.
24. Dakin E, Pearlmutter P. Older women's perceptions of elder maltreatment and ethical dilemmas in adult protective services: a cross-cultural, exploratory study. J Elder Abuse Negl. 2009;21(1):15–57.
25. Davis R, Medina-Ariza J. Results form an elder abuse prevention experiment in New York city. National Institue of Justice Research Brief; 2001.
26. Department of Economic and Social Affairs, Division for Social Policy and Development. Neglect, abuse and violence against older women. New York: United Nations; 2013.
27. Deschner R, McNeil J. Results of anger control training for battering couples. J Fam Viol. 1986;1(2):111–20.
28. Dong X. Addressing health and well-being of U.S. Chinese older adults through community-based participatory research: introduction to the PINE Study. AIMS Med Sci. 2015;2(3):261–70.
29. Dong X. Elder abuse in chinese populations: a global review. J Abuse Negl. 2015;27(3):196–232.
30. Dong X. Elder abuse: systematic review and implications for practice. J Am Geriatr Soc. 2015;63(6):1214–38.
31. Dong X, Chang E, Wong E, Simon M. Perceived effectiveness of elder abuse interventions in psychological distress and the design of culturally adapted interventions: a qualitative study in the Chinese Community in Chicago. J Aging Res. 2013;845425:8.
32. Dong X, Chang E, Wong E, Wong B, Simon M. How Do U.S. Chinese older adults view elder mistreatment? Findings from a community-based participatory research study. J Aging Health. 2011;23(2):289–312.
33. Doyle S. The impact of power differentials on the care experiences of older people. J Elder Abuse Negl. 2014;26:319–32.
34. Doyle J. Prevention and early intervention. Retrieved September 21, 2015, from EMQ Families First. 2006. http://emqff.org/wp-content/uploads/Prevention-and-Early-Intervention-Issue-1-Addendum-03-07-06.pdf.
35. Doyle J. Prevention and early intervention, Issue 1 Addendum: Definitions. Retrieved September 30, 2015, from http://emqff.org/wp-content/uploads/Prevention-and-Early-Intervention-Issue-1-Addendum-03-07-06.pdf.
36. Elder JP-M. Interpersonal and print nutrition communication for a Spanish-dominant Latino population: Secretos de la buena vida. Health Psychol. 2005;24:49–57.
37. Elder investment fraud and financial exploitation prevention program–legal. Bifocal. 2014;35(6):175–176
38. Elder Justice Coordinating Committee. The Department of Health and Human Services Elder Justice Coordinating Council 2012–2014 Report to Congress; 2014.
39. Elder Justice Coordinating Council. Eight Recommendations for Increased Federal Involvement in Addressing Elder Abuse, Neglect and Exploitation. Retrieved September 13, 2015, from Elder Justice Coordinating Council. 2013. http://www.aoa.gov/AoA_programs/Elder_Rights/EJCC/index.aspx.
40. Eulitt P, Tomberg R, Cunningham T, Counselman F, Palmer R. Screening elders in the emergency department at risk for mistreatment: a pilot study. J Elder Abuse Negl. 2014;26(4):424–35.

41. Facinetti J. Making strategic commiunications work to prevent elder abuse. J Elder Abuse Negl. 2002;14(4):11–20.
42. Filinson R, Ingman S. Elder abuse practice and policy. New York: Human Sciences Press; 1989.
43. Finseraas H, Jakobsson N. Does a simple information intervention change the perception of reform? Appl. Econ. Lett. 2014;21 (18):1266–8.
44. Fulmer T, Guadagno L, Dyer C, Connolly M. Progress in elder abuse screening and assessment instruments. J Am Geriatr Soc. 2004;52:297–304.
45. Gelles R. Novel intervention and presentation strategies presentation, NIH workshop of multiple approaches to understanding and preventing elder abuse. Bethesda, MD; 2015.
46. Gil A, Kislaya I, Santos A, Nunes B, Nicolau R, Fernandes A. Elder abuse in portugal: findings from the first national prevalence study. J Elder Abuse Negl. 2015;27(3):174–95.
47. Gordon R. An operational classification of disease prevention. In: Steinberg J, Silverman M, editors. Preventing mental disorders. Rockville, MD: Department of Health and Human Services; 1987. p. 20–6.
48. Hafford C, Nguyen K, Henning S. New york state office for the aging: enhanced multi-disciplinary teams. Elder Abuse prevention intervention program. Assistant Secretary for Planning and Evaluation, U.S. Department of Health and Human Services: NORC at University of Chicago; 2015.
49. Harris S, Knight J, Van Hook S, Sherritt L, Brooks T, Kulig J, et al. Adolescent sustance use screening in primary care: validity of computer self-administered versus clinician-administered screening. Substance Abuse; 2015
50. Hayslip B, Reinberg J, Williams J. The impact of elder abuse education on young adults. J Elder Abuse Negl. 2015;27:233–53.
51. Henning S, Hafford C, Nguyen K. Take AIM against elder abuse: the abuse intervention-prevention model. Elder abuse prevention intervention program. Assistant Secretary for Planning and Evaluation, U.S. Department of Health and Human Services: NORC at University of Chicago; 2015.
52. Hernandez-Tejada M, Amstadter A, Muzzy M, Acierno R. National elder mistreatment study: race and ethnicity findings. J Elder Abuse Negl. 2013;25(4):281–93.
53. Horner S, Rew L, Torres R. Enhancing intervention fidelity: a means of strengthening study impact. J Spec Pediatr Nurs. 2006;11:80–9.
54. Horsford S, Parra-Cordona J, Post L, Schiamberg L. Elder abuse and neglect in African American families: informing practice based on ecological and cultural frameworks. J Abuse Negl Elder. 2010;23(1):75–88.
55. Huhman M, Potter L, Nolin M, Piesse A, Judkins D, Banspach SW. The influence of the VERB campaign on children's physical activity in 2002–2006. Am J Public Health. 2010;100(4):638–45.
56. Institute for Work and Health. Basic concepts in prevention, surveillance and health promotion. Retrieved July 19, 2015, from AFMC Primer on Population Health. 2009. http://phprimer.afmc.ca/Part1-TheoryThinkingAboutHealth/Chapter4BasicConceptsInPreventionSurveillanceAndHealthPromotion/Thestagesofprevention.
57. Institute of Medicine, Committee on Prevention of Mental Disorders, Division of Biobehavioral Sciences and Mental Disorders. In: Mrazek P, Haggerty RJ, editors. Reducing risks for mental disorders: frontiers for preventive intervention research. Washington, DC: National Academy Press; 1994.
58. International Network for the Prevention of Elder Abuse. 10th WEAAD International Events 2015. Retrieved October 23, 2015, from http://www.weaad.com.
59. Kepple N, Freisthler B, Johnson-Motoyama M. Bias in child maltreatment self-reports using interactive voice response. Child Abuse Negl. 2014;38(10):1694–705.
60. Khanla Z, Maarefva M, Biglaria A, Heravi-Karimo M. The effect of a family-based intervention with a cognitive-behavioral approach on elder abuse. J Elder Abuse Negl. 2016;28(2):114.
61. Killick C, Taylor B, Begley E, Anand J, O'Brien M. Older people's conceptualization of abuse: a systematic review. J Elder Abuse Negl. 2015;27(2):100–20.
62. Kohn N. Second Childhood: What child protetion systems can teach elder protection systems. Stanford Law Pol Rev. 2003;14:175.
63. Krug E, Dahlberg L, Mercy J, Zwi J, Lozano R. World report on violence and health. Geneva: World Heath Organization; 2002.
64. Lau PW. A systematic review of information and communication technology-based interventions for promoting physical activity behavior change in children and adolescents. J Med Internet Res. 2011;13(3):e48.
65. Lee T, Pearson S, Johnson P, Garcia T, Weisberg M, Guadagnoli, et al. Failure of information as an intervention to modify clinical management. A time-series trial in patients with acute chest pain. Ann Intern Med. 1995;122(6):434–7.
66. MacMillan H, Wathen C, Jamieson E, Boyle M, McNutt L, Worster A, et al. Approaches to screenings for intimate partner violence in health care settings: a randomized trial. J Am Med Assoc. 2006;296(5):530–6.
67. Mariam L, McClure R, Robinson J, Yang J. Eliciting Change in At-Risk Elders (ECARE): evaluation of an elder abuse intervention program. J Abuse Negl Elder. 2015;27(1):19–33.
68. Merriman-Nai S, Stein K. World Elder Abuse awareness day: the concept, the reality, and the promise. J Elder Abuse Negl. 2014;26(3):345–9.
69. MetLife. (n.d.). The MetLife Study of Elder Financial Abuse. Retrieved June 6, 2015, from MetLife: https://www.metlife.com/mmi/research/elder-financial-abuse.html#key%20findings.
70. Moon A, Benton D. Tolerance of elder abuse and attitudes toward third-party intervention among African American, Korean American, and White Elderly. J Multicult Soc Work. 2000;8(3–4): 283–303.
71. Mysyuk Y, Westendorp R, Lindenberg J. Older persons' definitions and explanations of elder abuse in the Netherlands. J Elder Abuse Negl. 2016;28(2):95–113.
72. Nahmiash D, Reis M. Most successful intervention strategies for abused older adults. J Elder Abuse Negl. 2001;12(3–4):53–70.
73. Nation M, Crusto C, Wandersman A, Kumpfer K, Seybolt D, Morrissey-Kane E, Davino K. What works in prevention: principles of effective prevention programs. Am Psychol. 2003;58:449–56.
74. National Center on Elder Abuse. The National Policy Summit on Elder Abuse: Creating the Action Agenda-Proceedings. Report submitted to the U.S. Administration on Aging, Department of Health and Human Services; 2002.
75. National Center on Elder Abuse. World Elder Abuse Awareness Day. Retrieved October 2, 2015, from http://www.acl.gov/NewsRoom/Observances/WEAAD/Events/Event-Lookup.aspx.
76. National Research Council (US) and Institute of Medicine (US) Committee on the Prevention of Mental Disorders and Substance Abuse Among Children, Youth, and Young Adults. In: O'Connell M, Boat T, & Warner K, editors. Research advances and promising interventions. Washington: National Academies Press; 2009.
77. National Research Council (US) Panel to Review Risk and Prevalence of Elder Abuse and Neglect. Evaluating interventions. In Bonnie R, Wallace R, editors. Elder mistreatment: abuse,

neglect, and exploitation in an aging America. Washington: National Academies Press; 2003.
78. Navarro A, Gassoumis Z, Wilber K. Holding abusers accountable: an elder abuse forensice center increases criminal prosecution of financial exploitation. Gerontologist. 2012;53:303–12.
79. Nerenberg L, D M, Nava A. In pursuit of a useful framework to champion elder justice. Generations. 2012;36(3):89–96.
80. Nguyen K, Hafford C, Henning S. Elder services case management prevention intervention. Elder Abuse Intervention Program. Assistant Secretary for Planning and Evaluation, U.S. Department of Health and Human Services: NORC at University of Chicago; 2015b.
81. Nguyen K, Hafford C, Henning S. Use of the Elder Abuse Suspicion Index Screening Tool and Adult Protective Services Specialists in a Clinical Setting. Elder Abuse Prevention Intervention Program. Washington, D.C.: Assistant Secretary for Planning and Evaluation, U.S. Department of Health and Human Services: NORC at University of Chicago; 2015a.
82. Nichol M, Wilber K, Wu J, Gassoumis Z. Evaluating the cost effectiveness of the elder abuse forensic center model. U.S. Department of Justice. The National Institute of Justice; 2015.
83. Noar S. A 10 year retrospective of research in health mass media campaigns: where do we go from here? J Health Commun. 2006;11:21–42.
84. Oveis S, Karimi R, Mahra M. Note from iran: self-reported elder abuse in Qazvin, 2012. J Abuse Negl Elder. 2014;26(3):337–40.
85. Payne JM, F K. RE-AIM evaluation of the alcohol and pregnancy project: educational resources to inform health professionals about prenatal alcohol exposure and fetal alcohol spectrum disorder. Eval Health Prof. 2011;34:57–80.
86. Pillemer K, Burnes D, Riffin C, Lachs M. Elder abuse: global situation, risk factors, and prevention strategies. Gerontologist. 2016;56(S2):S194–205.
87. Pisani L, Walsh C. Screening for elder abuse in hospitalized older adults with dementia. J Elder Abuse Negl. 2012;24(3):195–215.
88. Ploeg J, Fear J, Hutchison B, MacMilllan H, Bolan G. A systematic review of interventions for elder abuse. J Elder Abuse Negl. 2009;21(3):187–210.
89. Policastro C, Payne B. Assessing the level of elder abuse knowledge preprofessionals possess: implications for the Further Development of University Curriculum. J Elder Abuse Negl. 2014;26(1):12–30.
90. Purtie J, Roman L. Health awareness days: sufficient evidence to support the craze? Am J Public Health. 2015;105(6):1061–5.
91. Randolf W, Viswanath K. Lessons learned from public health mass media campaigns: marketing health in a crowded media world. Annu Rev Public Health. 2004;25:419–37.
92. Rice R, Adkin C. Public communication campaigns. Thousand Oaks, CA: Sage; 2001.
93. Richardson B, Kitchen G, Livingston G. The effect of education on knowledge and management of elder abuse: a randomized controlled trial. Age Ageing. 2002;31:335–41.
94. Rizzo V, Burnes D, Chalfy A. A systematic evaluation of a multidisciplinary social-work-lawyer elder mistreatment intervention model. J Abuse Negl Elder. 2015;27(1):1–18.
95. Russell S, Fulmer T, Singh G, Valenti M, Vermula R, Strauss S. Screening for elder mistreatment in a dental clinic population. J Elder Abuse Negel. 2012;24:326–39.
96. Sethi D, Wood S, Mitis F, Bellis F, Penhale B, Marmolejo I, et al. European report on preventing elder maltreatment. Geneva: World Health Organization; 2011.
97. Sirey J, Berman J, Salamore A, DePasquale A, Halkett A, Raeifar E, et al. Feasibility of integrating mental health screening and services into routine elder abuse practice to improve client outcomes. J Elder Abuse Negl. 2015;27(3):254–69.
98. Springer F, Phillips J. The IOM model: a tool for prevention planning and implementation. Retrieved June 30, 2015, from Prevention Tactics. 2006. http://www.cars-rp.org/publications/Prevention%20Tactics/PT8.13.06.pdf.
99. Stadler G, Oettingen G, Gollwitzer P. Intervention effects of information and self-regulation on eating fruits and vegetables over two years. Health Psychol. 2010;29(3):274–83.
100. Stein K. A national agenda for elder abuse and neglect research. J Elder Abuse Negl. 1991;3(3):91–108.
101. Stein K, Merriman-Nai S, Petrak C. A Strategic Blueprint for Mounting a National Communication Campaign on Elder Abuse. University of Delaware, National Center on Elder Abuse, Report submitted to the U.S. Administration on Aging, Department of Health and Human Services, Washington DC; 2009.
102. Stein K. Elder abuse and neglect content in higher education programs on aging. Clearinghouse on abuse and neglect of the Elderly, University of Delaware. Research report submitted to the U.S. Administration on Aging, Department of Health and Human Services, Washington. DC; 1992.
103. Stein K. Elder abuse and neglect: a National Research Agenda. Washington: National Aging Resource Center on Elder Abuse; 1991.
104. Stein K. Private notes, Reingold contract; 2009.
105. Stein K Merriman-Nai S, Brendza G. A report to senior victim services: client satisfaction and outcomes evaluation; 2009.
106. Stein K, Merriman-Nai S, Petrak C, Siegal L. Raising National Public Awareness of Elder abuse: a meta analysis of existing elder abuse public awareness materials, a case study analysis of effective social marketing strategies, and a strategic blueprint for mounting a national communication campaign on elder abuse. National Center on Elder Abuse, Research report submitted to the U.S. Administration on Aging, Department of Health and Human Services, Washington DC; 2011
107. Stein K. Rosalie Wolf Memorial Lecture: a logic model to measure the impacts of World Elder Abuse Awareness Day. J Elder Abuse Negl. 2016;28(3):127–133.
108. Substance Abuse and Mental Health Administration. Risk and protective factors. Retrieved October 21, 2015, from SAMHSA. 2015. http://www.samhsa.gov/capt/practicing-effective-prevention/prevention-behavioral-health/risk-protective-factors.
109. Sugita J, Garrett M. Elder abuse and oral health care providers: an intervention to increase knowledge and self-perceived likelihood to report. J Elder Abuse Negl. 2012;24(1):50–64.
110. Sweet S, Ginis K, Esterbrooks P, Latimer-Cheung A. Operationalizing the RE-AIM framework to evaluate the impact of multi-sector partnerships. Implement Sci, 9(74); 2014.
111. Teaster P, Wangmo T. Kentucky's local elder abuse coordinating councils: a model for other states. J Elder Abuse Negl. 2010;22 (1/2):191–206.
112. Teaster P, Vorsky F, Wangmo T. The Use of Evidence-Based Practices for Elder Abuse Programs. Report to U.S. Administration on Aging; 2011.
113. Tilden VP, Schmidt TA, Limandri BJ, Chiodo GT, Garland MJ, Loveless PA. Factors that influence clinicians' assessment and management of family violence. Am J Public Health. 1994;84:628–33.
114. Tourangeau R, Yan T. Sensitive questions in surveys. Psychol Bull. 2007;133(5):859–83.
115. Vega M, Roland E. Social marketing techniques for public health communication: a review of syphilis awareness campaigns in 8 US cities. Sex Transm Dis. 2005;32:S30–6.

116. Virginia Tech. What Is RE-AIM (n.d.). Retrieved 2017, from About RE-AIM: http://www.re-aim.hnfe.vt.edu/about_re-aim/what_is_re-aim/index.html.
117. Vladescu DE. An evaluation of a client centered case management program for elder. J Elder Abuse Negl. 1999;11(4):5–22.
118. Wells Fargo Will Hit The Road To End Elder Financial Abuse. Retrieved October 31, 2015, from Wells Fargo Advisors. 2015. https://www.wellsfargoadvisors.com/about-wells-fargo-advisors/newsroom/2015-elder-financial-abuse.htm.
119. Wolfe D. Elder abuse intervention: lessons from child abuse and domestic violence initiatives. In Bonnie R, Wallace RE, editors. Elder mistreatment: abuse, neglect and exploitation in an aging America. Washington: National Academies Press; 2003.
120. Yaffe M, Weiss D, Lithwick M. Seniors' self-administration of the Elder Abuse Suspicion Indix (EASI): a feasibility study. J Abuse Negl Elder. 2012;24(4):277–92.
121. Yan E. Elder abuse in Asia—an overview. In Forum on Global Violence Prevention; Board on Global Health; Institute of Medicine; National Research Council. Elder abuse and its prevention: workshop summary. Washington: National Academies Press; 2014, p. II.10.

Part V

Elder Abuse and Culture: Anthropological and Ethnographic Experiences

Elder Abuse and Culture: Africans and African Americans

21

Charles P. Mouton and Janet H. Southerland

Older adults are the fastest growing segment of the population worldwide [1, 2]. Globally, the number of persons aged 60 years or over is expected to almost triple within the next few decades, from 672 million in 2005 to nearly 1.9 billion by 2050 [2]. The population in the very old group—aged 80 and over—will increase even faster. These "oldest old" are especially vulnerable and at risk for being abused. For example, in the United Kingdom by 2025, the number of people over the age of 80 years is expected to have increased by almost 50 % and the number of people over 90 years is expected to have doubled [3]. This exploding older population makes elder abuse an emerging issue for those responsible to care for the population.

While elder abuse is not a new phenomenon, the speed of population aging world-wide is likely to lead to an increase in its incidence and prevalence [4, 5]. Elder abuse has devastating consequences for older persons leading to poor quality of life, psychological distress, and loss of property and security. Elder abuse is also associated with increased mortality and morbidity [6]. Elder abuse is a problem that manifests itself in both developed and developing countries and at all levels of society, both rich and poor [4].

Elder abuse and mistreatment has been increasingly identified as a problem for older adults since it was first described as "granny battering" over 35 years ago [7]. With the growing population of older adults and the increasing numbers living into the oldest ages, elder abuse, and mistreatment unfortunately will continue to be a problem that healthcare providers will need to recognize and manage. While the abuse of older people was first described in British scientific journals in 1975 [7, 8], scientific and legal action was first developed in the US. In 1990, the first, and to date only, population prevalence study on elder abuse was published in the United Kingdom [9]. More well-designed epidemiologic research is needed to address this emerging problem.

Elder abuse, a very complex issue with diverse definitions and names, has been very slow to capture the public eye and public policy. Information on the prevalence of elder abuse is based on a small number of population-based studies that have been conducted in developed countries. These studies suggest that between 4 and 6 % of older persons have experienced some form of abuse in the home.

These prevalence rates or estimates exist only in selected developed countries—ranging from 1 to 10 %. At this point, there are no well-designed prevalence studies of elder abuse in the developing world. Although the extent of elder mistreatment is unknown, its social and moral significance is obvious. As such, it demands a global multifaceted response, one which focuses on protecting the rights of older individuals.

Even in the US, well-designed overall prevalence data is lacking. For the US minority population, the data is even sparser. Available data suggest 10 % of US elders experience abuse [10]. Approximately 820,000–1.9 million older individuals experience maltreatment annually [11]. Women are identified as victims in two-third of reported elder abuse cases. Only in abandonment case do men clearly predominate. In a community-based sample of older adults, Pillemer showed the prevalence of abuse in older adults to be 3.2 %, much lower than the other non-community-based estimates [12]. More recently, the National Elder Abuse Incidence Study (NEAIS) showed that approximately 450,000 older adults were abused and/or neglected during 1996 [13]. In this study, women were victims in 76.3 % of reports of emotional/psychological abuse, 71.4 % of physical abuse, 63.0 % of financial/material exploitation, and 60.0 % of neglect. Both studies detected abuse in functionally dependent older adults receiving care. Few studies have focused

C.P. Mouton (✉)
Family and Community Medicine, School of Medicine, Meharry Medical College, Nashville, TN 37208, USA
e-mail: cmouton@mmc.edu

J.H. Southerland
Oral and Maxillofacial Surgery, School of Dentistry, Meharry Medical College, Nashville, TN, USA

X. Dong (ed.), *Elder Abuse*, DOI 10.1007/978-3-319-47504-2_21

on abuse in functionally independent adults. Mouton et al. showed that 11.1 % of functionally independent older women were abused in the past year with a 5 % 3-year incidence [6]. Fisher and Regan reported even higher rates, with 47 % of women over 60-years old reporting abuse since age 55 [14]. While there is an emerging body of scholarly literature on elder abuse and mistreatment, relatively little data is available on elder abuse in the certain subpopulations, particularly individuals from the African Diaspora. In this chapter, we will review elder abuse in various populations of African origin, namely the sub-Saharan African Continent, the Caribbean, and starting with the US. To do so, we will provide a brief review of the history of African American in the US as it pertains to elder abuse.

21.1 History of African Diaspora

The African Diaspora began with the capture, exploitation, and exportation of Africans, mainly from the Western coast, by the Portuguese, Spanish, British, and French. African Americans have been part of the US historical fabric since the time of Columbus' arrival. With the advent of chattel slavery, African slaves were imported to America beginning in 1619. This process of importing Africans, most from the west coast of Africa, involved the process of the "middle passage" where captured Africans were herded onto ships and transported across the Atlantic Ocean to the Americas. It has been estimated that over that 6-month journey over 10 million African lives were lost.

Chattel slavery was uniquely harsh in the Americas. During colonial times, captured Africans worked alongside white indentured servants. The plantation system required lifetime slaves for its economy transforming slavery in the Americas. The importation of African slaves to the Americas became the backbone of the economy for the southern US and many Caribbean countries. It fueled what was known as the "triangle trade" where African slaves were brought to the Caribbean, sugar sent to US and Rum to Africa. Another aspect of the slave trade was to continue the subjugation of these captured Africans, their white "owners" required physical and psychological techniques of oppression, supported by the legal system here in the US. These techniques included wiping, beating, traumatic amputation, castration, and grueling physical labor. Many of these punishments were metered out publically to instill fear in the other slaves. The psychological "scars" have been transgenerational and remnants can still be seen in the African American community.

Also since African slaves were considered "property," slave owners did not support the establishment of familial bonds. Husbands were separated from wives, children separated from parents. If fact, disruption (or threat of disruption) of familial or supportive social bonds were used as a form of psychological abuse to control slaves' behavior. This psychosocial abuse may have an influence on familial structure and relationships seen in current African American families. During this period of slavery, the majority of African Americans were located in the Southern US and provided forced labor on plantations. By 1850, over 4 million people were enslaved, 12 % of the total US population. This harsh treatment of enslaved African Americans continued for 246 years until the passage of the 13th amendment in 1865. This proclamation banned slavery in the southern states and freed the enslaved African Americans.

After a brief period of reconstruction that ended in 1877, federal troops protecting the newly freed slaves were remove from the former confederate states and their former white oppressors were re-enfranchised and in control of the governmental structures in the South. Subsequently, African Americans were subjugated to variety of governmentally sanctioned infringements of their civil rights, e.g. Jim Crow laws. Also, the rise of vigilante groups, such as the Ku Klux Klan and lynch mobs, terrorized the newly freed African Americans and were publicly supported by much of white southern society. In addition, the US Supreme Court's Plessy vs Ferguson ruling allowed for segregation of public services, effectively sanctioning and legally protecting discrimination against African Americans. Over the next 77 years, segregation allowed African Americans to be provided substandard and restricted housing, education, healthcare, and economic opportunities. African American elders over 62-years old have spent at least some part of their lives in this period. It was not until another 11 years that African Americans were given full enfranchisement with the passage of the voting right act of 1965. In the 51 years since its passage, African Americans have continued to struggle against the racism that underpinned the system of chattel slavery and segregation in the US. It is against this historical backdrop that one must view the problem of elder mistreatment in the African diaspora. It is this history of African Americans in the US that influence attitudes and behaviors regarding abuse and mistreatment.

21.2 Elder Abuse in US African Americans

As with other populations, older African Americans are exposed to various forms of abuse and mistreatment. Hudson showed in a sample of 944 community-dwelling adults (318 African Americans) that 9.2 % of those over 65-years old reported experiencing physical abuse [15]. In a study of Chicago residents, 24.9 % of older African American participants reported abuse exposure [16]. Mouton showed that among African American women, age 50–79 years, from a nationally representative sample 0.7 % reported exposure to Physical Abuse, 8.5 % reported exposure to Verbal Abuse, and 1.8 % reported both physical and verbal abuse [17]. In a prospective population-based study from Chicago, African Americans were more likely to experience elder abuse than whites (89 vs 56 %) but less likely to have a hospitalization associated with abuse (RR 0.81) [18]. Thus, with regard to physical and verbal abuse, African Americans report similar or higher levels of abuse exposure.

Others report that African Americans are 1.77–8.57 times more likely to experience financial abuse [19, 20]. If fact, this supports earlier research showing financial abuse to be the most common abuse in African Americans, from both urban and rural areas. Also, African Americans 2.18–2.30 times more likely to experience psychological abuse (Beach SR). These levels of financial abuse in African Americans are even more disturbing given that African Americans tend to have lower financial resources and higher levels of poverty than their White counterparts.

Also, exposure to abuse in US African Americans adds to the already high levels of stress this population is exposed to through both the environment and personal circumstances. Older African Americans are more likely to live in neighborhoods that are poor, underresourced, and plagued by violent crime. The violence in the neighborhoods exposes elderly African Americans to violence-related stressors at greater levels than those experienced by their White counterparts.

Also, exposure to racism and segregation over their lifetimes adds to the accumulated stress experienced by US African Americans. Accumulated stressors are shown to have a substantial impact on overall health and increase the risk of several chronic diseases. In fact, the greater accumulation of stress has been suggested as one of the contributors to the health disparities seen in this population of older adults. US African American have an overall shorter life expectancy after age 65 and higher rates of cardiovascular disease, diabetes, cancer, and dementia. Older African Americans have 1.3–1.8 times rates of stroke, 60 % higher risk of diabetes and twice as likely to have Alzheimer's disease as Whites. Older African Americans also live more years with chronic disability. These factors tend to make older African Americans more vulnerable and at risk for elder abuse.

21.2.1 Risk Factors for Elder Abuse in US African Americans

Several factors have cited as predisposing risks for elder abuse. Elders with dementia or cognitive impairment who exhibit disruptive behavior are at increased risk of physical abuse. Elders who suffer from depression, other serious mental health issues, or physical incapacity are more likely to suffer from neglect. Elders who have poor mental and physical health and social isolation are more likely to become a victim of financial abuse. Perpetrators of elder abuse are more likely to suffer from mental illness or substance abuse disorders or are dependent (usually financially) on the victim. Any history of violence in the past with the spousal or familial relationship can precipitate abuse. Each of these risk factors has a higher rate in US African Americans.

US African Americans have high rates of Alzheimer's dementia and vascular dementia, with estimates for Alzheimer's disease of 14–100 % higher. African American elders also have rates of depression similar to Non-Hispanic Whites but are 20 % more likely to report serious psychological distress. African Americans are also less likely to receive treatment for mental health concerns (8.7 vs. 16 % for Non-Hispanic Whites). Williams et al. showed that for chronic depression the rates were highest in African Americans at 56.5 % followed Caribbean Blacks at 56 % and Non-Hispanic Whites at 38.6 % [21].

In African American elders, contextual issues affecting both elders and caregivers can have an important role [22]. The legacies of slavery and racism have led to anger and hopelessness and have resulted in economic and health disparities. Also, many caregivers are economically dependent on the elders they care for. This economic dependency perpetuates anger and frustration due to a higher level of cognitive dissonance. Caregivers feel they should be taking care of their older parents but instead are dependent on them for economic support. Moreover, some African American caregivers face barriers in developing the necessary skills for competent caregiving [22].

Older US African Americans have a unique shared history that may have an adverse impact and leads to a greater risk of abuse. This slavery legacy has overlaid African Americans with a shared experience of racism, racial discrimination, and structural segregation. This shared experience is compounded by the anger and hopelessness associated with socioeconomic deprivation, poor health status, and health disparities. Also, this shared history along with experiences like the Jim Crow laws and police brutality causes African Americans to distrust governmental authority and institutions. This mistrust also spills over to medical institutions. Furthermore, medicine has its own legacy of mistreatment of African Americans, such as the Tuskegee Experiment. These historically exploitive practices reinforce the opinion of some African Americans that public and healthcare institutions cannot be trusted [23]. Thus, African American elders and their caregivers will avoid seeking outside help even when needed. Caregivers may be unaware or wary of social support services, particularly those services from governmental agencies.

Moreover, the legacy of slavery has some transgenerational effects that influence how older African Americans perceive and respond to physical and psychological abuse, even at the cellular and molecular level [24]. Transgenerational epigenetics has been recently recognized and has received increasing attention. This field has significant implications for elder abuse, particularly African American given the aforementioned history of slavery and discrimination. Children of women abused during pregnancy have high rates of methylated glucocorticoid receptor genes resulting in a greater susceptibility to anxiety in response to stressful events [25] Rodger et al. and Bohauk and Mansay in separate studies demonstrated that RNA in sperm can transmit the transgenerational effects of trauma leading to an altered stress response in their offspring [26, 27] These studies and others suggest that exposure to psychological and social stressors can be transmitted across generations and this transmission may be through epigenetic modification at the cellular and subcellular level [28]. The impact of these transgenerational factors has not been fully elucidated in humans and not clearly understood with regard to aging. The elucidation of these effects is ongoing focusing on both the attenuation and blunting of responsiveness to abuse-related stressors. Future research may clarify the role of transgenerational factors on vulnerability and risk for abuse in older African Americans.

Coping with the stress of caregiving may be another factor that presents a risk for elder abuse in older African Americans. A modification of John Henryism theory may also be seen in African Americans exposed to abuse. John Henryism describes a coping mechanism by African Americans in response to prolonged exposure to stressors that describe a process where African Americans expend a high level of effort to overcome the stressor which in turn results in greater psychological costs. This psychological cost may be manifested in higher levels of caregiver stress with resulting burnout. This cost may also explain why older adults in a shared living situation find themselves at greater risk for abuse than those living alone [29]. As the burden of caregiving increases, African Americans will continue to just work harder and utilize the available resources, such as respite services. Moreover, since African Americans are more likely to be living with another relative/friend, there may be weaker social ties (nonfamily member) and more susceptible to caregiver stress.

The research on the risk of abuse and an elder's living situation has been mixed. Older adults in a non-spousal shared living situation are at greater risk for abuse than those living alone [29]. This finding has implications for US African American elders. African American elders more likely to be living with another relative/friend. In these settings, the perpetrator is more likely to be female. However, other research has found that the risk of abuse is greater for those who are socially isolated, have poor social networks, or have low social support [10]. These differences may reflect the varying dynamics of abuse in supportive, caring social environments compared to dysfunctional, codependent caring environments.

Alcohol abuse and exposure to previous traumatic events [10] place older adults at risk for abuse. Chronic alcoholism exacerbates the vulnerability of older adults and worsens decision-making regarding self-protection. Moreover, for African Americans, alcohol/drug problems are more likely associated with the perpetrators of abuse. While their overall rate of alcoholism is lower than in Non-Hispanic Whites, African Americans have a higher rate of high-risk alcohol use as well [30].

In addition to living arrangements and the social environment, US African American elderly are aging during a time of shifting social roles and expectation of behavior. These shifting roles not only lead to conflict between older adults and their younger children as caregivers but may lead to stress in with their spousal caregiving. Research by Mouton el al. showed that US African Americans have certain social expectation that may put them at risk for abuse [31]. This study found that both males and females are expected to adhere to traditional gender-defined roles, such as men doing the outdoor yardwork while women do the cooking and household cleaning. Also, filial obligations for African Americans take precedence over personal needs. Thus, if it protects members of the family, African American elders will tolerate an abusive situation. This filial obligation also leads to a reluctance of African American elders to acknowledge abusive behaviors and to report abuse. Moreover, identifying and reporting abuse reflects poorly on the family. Family loyalty is used to justify abuse, justify living in an abusive situation to have the family together, and refusal to seek help to remedy abuse.

Social expectations concerning family's role as primary caregiver hinders African Americans' willingness to seek professional help in caregiving. As mentioned above, this underutilization of resources may put African American caregivers under undo stress and precipitate abusive behaviors. Traditional attitudes that tend to rely upon informal caregiving, through friends and extended family, may pose a significant risk for neglect or abuse. Numerous community-based interventions have been successful in changing these traditional attitudes. But while these attitudes are rapidly changing with each successive generation, some African American communities still demonstrate an underutilization of professional caregiving services. This underutilization can increase the stress in households and thus increase the risk for abuse.

In addition to the social environment and attitudes, culturally based reactions to interactions between caregivers and older African Americans can shape attitudes to or even precipitate abuse. Mouton et al. showed that African Americans perceive caregiving situations where the older adult refuses care to be especially problematic and the use of force is acceptable in those cases. This aggressive posture may be particularly true regarding forcing an elder to accept what is perceived to be beneficial, e.g., medications. Altruism and beneficence seem to trump personal preferences when dealing with African Americans and their caregivers. Also, combative elders should expect physical abuse to be a response to any violent outburst. This retaliatory mindset is a potential caregiver response to combative, violent behaviors by African American elders. Often there is an element of "victim blaming" by caregivers in relation to abuse of older African Americans. African Americans elders and caregivers also viewed that abuse must have an element of intentionality to be considered problematic. In some situations, use of physical restraints is often seen as appropriate by some caregivers. These culturally bound attitudes may put African American elders at risk for traditionally defined mistreatment and contribute to its underreporting.

21.3 Elder Abuse in Sub-Saharan Africa

Africa is the second largest and the second most populous continent in the world. With its tremendous size sub-Saharan Africa has enormous diversity that is apparent in its physical geography and climate, its plurality of cultural heritages, official and native languages, traditions, beliefs, religions, and value systems, in its modes of production and levels of economic development, and in its diverse social and political structures. Thus, the older populations in Africa will tend to have the same type of geographic, cultural and economic diversity. Because of its size and diversity, discussing elder abuse in the sub-Saharan African context as a whole will be difficult and arguably inappropriate, but we will cover it in broad general areas.

In fact, even what it means to be "older" or "elderly" is different across Africa. Chronological age—which in any event may not even be known in sub-Saharan Africa—may be a poorer indicator of being elderly than social standing. Many older Africans, particularly in rural areas may not have birth certificates and be unable to accurately delineate their chronological age. "Elder" may be interpreted as a member of the community who has good judgment and wisdom and whom people look up to for decision-making. Thus being elderly may have a different meaning from chronological age. Also, chronological age may differ markedly from functional age, which can be the most important dimension of aging in a rural subsistence agricultural context. In general, it is important to recognize that in some sub-Saharan African areas, individuals younger than 60 may be considered "old" because they exhibit morbidity profiles and take on status roles more usually associated with the elderly.

Sub-Saharan Africa also faces a greater set of development challenges than any other major region of the world, with an average per capita income that is now lower than it was at the end of the 1960s. In industrialized countries, economic support for the elderly comes to a great extent from large public or private pensions and health systems. By contrast, throughout most of sub-Saharan Africa, providing support for the older population is still primarily a family responsibility. Those fortunate enough to receive pension benefits are former employees of the formal workforce which accounts for less than 10 % of the population in sub-Saharan Africa. Traditionally in sub-Saharan Africa, [mudaire] the main source of support has been the household and family, supplemented by other informal mechanisms, such as kinship networks, extended family, and mutual aid societies. With the notable exceptions of Botswana, Mauritius, Namibia, and South Africa, formal pensions or other social welfare systems are virtually nonexistent. The systems that are functional tend to pay minimal benefits and cover only a small fraction of the needs of the elderly population.

The profound economic and social changes in Africa are also associated with increasing development and modernization. In sub-Saharan Africa, older people have traditionally been viewed in a positive light, as repositories of information and wisdom. Families valued their wisdom in decision-making and respected their position in the family and community. Also, sub-Saharan African families have shown a great deal of resilience and are generally still intact. The changes associated with development and modernization can, however, combine to weaken traditional social values and networks that stress the important role of older people in society. The changes dismantle the traditions of intergenerational exchange and reciprocity. These changes include increasing formal education and the migration of young people from rural to urban areas, leaving older family members behind. This rural to urban migration results in separating family members and weakening the economic forces in the family and community that are available to support the elderly left behind. Modernization and development have led to broad social and economic changes that put in doubt the continued viability of traditional arrangements for the care and support of older people. For example, formal education and modernization are generally associated with weakening traditional social ties and obligations as well as greater independence and autonomy. These are factors that also tend to undermine traditional extended family systems. Similarly, economic development is associated with young people migrating from rural to urban areas, leaving older family members geographically isolated. Once established in urban areas, migrants tend to form new nuclear households. These changes, accompanied the growing older African population lends to the possibility of mistreatment of vulnerable elders.

It is in the setting of the erosion of traditional family values that elder abuse occurs throughout the African diaspora. As the older population continues to grow on the African continent, elder abuse will begin to emerge as well. Additionally, the process of modernization and urbanization in sub-Saharan Africa has begun to erode traditional value systems that emphasize respect for the elderly as well as destroys the traditional social welfare system of the family. [32]

21.3.1 Epidemiology

Although the data is sparse, elder abuse does occur on the sub-Saharan African continent. The prevalence of elder abuse varies from region to region, even within different countries. In one of the few prevalence studies, Bigala et al. reports that in South Africa 64.3 % of older men and 60.5 % of older women experiences elder abuse [33]. In a study in Kenya, 81.1 % of the elderly experienced abuse [34]. In Nigeria, Akpin showed 47 % experience physical abuse and 37 % experienced theft (Akpin). In Lagos, Nigeria's largest city, Asogua found a population-base rate of physical abuse in the elderly of 7.8 % but 88 % reported being "denied freedom" and 73 % experienced verbal abuse (Asogua). In these data, women were more likely to experience abuse that men. In an Ekiti study, over 58 % of elders experienced some form of abuse with abandonment and neglect in 60.9 %, financial abuse in 41.6 %, physical abuse in 37.2 % and sexual abuse in 32.1 %.

21.3.2 Risk Factors in Sub-Saharan Africa

Many of the same risk factors for abuse and mistreatment in the Caucasian/European population also exist for the African population. However, there are some risks that are unique in the developing world particularly sub-Saharan Africa. These risks may be part of certain structural factors or cultural factors that are unique in the African Diaspora to sub-Saharan Africa.

21.3.3 Structural Factors

In Africa, the traditional extended family had the potential to adequately care for its older members because of the large number of familial and social relations and the frequency of interactions among family members. The nature of daily interactions in the local community reinforced the care provided to these elders. Also, the culturally well-defined roles and responsibilities have been established for and inherently understood by different age groups. However, as mentioned previously, given the modernization and urbanization of sub-Saharan Africa, the traditional social welfare role played by the extended family has begun to erode. The migration and forced displacement of various populations has also contributed to the erosion of the family. This erosion is seen most acutely in countries with rapid development and displacement of the population to the urban business centers. This erosion is leading to a population of older adults who are vulnerable both socially and economically as well as having a negative impact on health and self-esteem [32]. This increased vulnerability sets the stage for elder abuse and neglect.

As this modernization continues, society is showing less respect for the elderly, which results in poorer treatment and abuse. This lack of respect is fueled by the lack of formal education and a lack of economic resources afforded to older adults. Also, the majority of elder sub-Saharan Africans, especially women, are un- or under-educated with many having no formal education. Thus, their ability to identify limited resources is diminished as is their ability to generate income to support themselves. This inability to economically support themselves put older African women at especially high risk of abuse.

Older Africans also risk being vulnerable due to the impact of HIV on young adults who were their potential caregivers. HIV/AIDS causes young adults to leave the workforce due to illness thus leaving older adults with a loss of economic support and having to provide caregiving support to those young adults. When these young adults succumb to the disease, older Africans with any economic funds must care and support orphaned grandchildren. The ravages of HIV/AIDS has led to older adults facing economic hardships as they lose the economic support of their infected children and then having to support these sick children and grandchildren [35].

In sub-Saharan Africa, other structural causes of elder mistreatment are related to poverty, alcoholism, drug abuse, lack of governmental programs and support for the aged [36]. Sub-Saharan African countries have limited social welfare systems. Few countries have defined benefit programs that support older adults. The lack of these programs and the overall rates of poverty in these developing countries limit the ability to support older adults. In 2012, 42.7 % of the population in sub-Saharan Africa lived in poverty (improved from 56.8 % in 1990). Central African countries of the Democratic Republic of Congo, Central African Republic, Zambia, Malawi, Mozambique and Madagascar having the highest rate (81.76 % in Madagascar). Their rates compare to the Caribbean at 5.6 % and the overall global rate of 12.7 %. Compared to the US and Europe, alcoholism in sub-Saharan Africa is generally low. However, episodic heavy drinking was found in 40–52 % of the Nigerian population and 17.6–46 % of the Ugandan populations [37]. These episodes of heavy drinking may not reflect the consumption of other fermented beverages or local "home brews" that may be used during celebrations or other rituals. These structural problems coupled with a lack of formal social support structures may set the stage for elder abuse.

21.3.4 Cultural Factors/Variations

In African societies, the socioeconomic roles of the elderly remain very important within the family. However, they are becoming unrewarded and undervalued [35]. Older adults are often the caregivers for young children while their adult parents are out of the home or at work [35]. In this traditional setting, older adults were well integrated into the family and shared help in childrearing. However, with the breakdown of traditional families' structure, older Africans face social isolation and the erosion of intergenerational bonds both of which put them at risk for abuse. As African family structure changes, fewer adults are willing to care for older family members. In fact, HelpAge International reports that at one hospital in Kenya, 3 of 10 older adults are abandoned; sometimes due to the fees at the hospital. Some elders report that they are sometimes turned away from the hospital by staff who says they are not sick, just old. Some hospital workers in the Kiambu District hospital reported elderly being slapped, pushed, verbally abused, and being denied medication by health workers. In one hospital, 60–70 % of abandoned patients were male and males were treated worse. These rates of abuse indicate a changing cultural view of the elderly.

These sociocultural issues that may lead to abuse are related to the decline in respect for older adults, beliefs in magic and witchcraft, and expectation that the local community cares for its members [36]. Traditionally, African families develop strong bonds, often with multiple generations in one household. Also, older Africans begin to be viewed as weak, frail, and dependent, requiring care like that for small children. Older Africans lose their standing as wise leaders of the family and lose decision-making power. In this new setting, older Africans lose autonomy and receive childlike treatment. These elders' wishes are often ignored and their independence restricted. This infantilization also puts older Africans at risk for abuse.

Older African women are especially vulnerable to abuse due to sociocultural factors. Traditionally, African women have an inferior status in many countries, facing discrimination in inheritance rights and land distribution. Widowhood makes them especially vulnerable and creates opportunities for abuse. Mourning rites of passage for widows may include sexual violence, forced levirate marriages (where a man is obliged by custom to marry the childless widow of his brother) and expulsion from their homes. Older widows are often abandoned and may even have their property seized. Many elderly, especially widows, are isolated in rural areas and separated from family which sets the stage for them to experience sexual abuse. One report from Nigeria in 2011 indicated a raping spree where in one region widows 60–80 years were raped en masse with no prosecution of these rapists.

In many parts of sub-Saharan Africa, older women are often accused of witchcraft, which results in their further isolation, abandonment, and in some cases physical abuse. Accusations of witchcraft, often connected with unexplained events in the local community, such as a death or crop failure, are directed at isolated, older women. It is often easy to blame natural disasters or societal problems on the most vulnerable. In this case, older African women become dehumanized by the accusation of witchcraft and become acceptable victims of violence. In the United Republic of Tanzania, an estimated 500 older women accused of witchcraft are murdered every year.

21.4 EM in Afro-Caribbean

EM occurs in the Afro-Caribbean diaspora. However, there have been no systematic epidemiologic studies to determine the prevalence or incidence of elder abuse in this region. Only anecdotal reports have been presented about this problem.

21.4.1 Risk Factors

As for the risk factors for abuse, we see similar factors to the sub-Saharan African elder population. In the Caribbean region, the respect that has been traditionally shown to older adults has begun to decline as well. There are many newspaper accounts of the elderly being robbed, abused, sexually assaulted, and violated. There are also a number of growing negative stereotypes about the elderly and their way of life. These reports make life sometimes very frustrating and extremely difficult for older adults. Despite the growing elderly populations, these stereotypes of frailty, diminished mental capacity, and a burden on family have not changed. Therefore, for many older persons especially the less financially able and the more vulnerable, growing older can be especially challenging and create varying degrees of vulnerability and isolation.

21.4.2 Cultural Factors/Variations

In the Trinidadian study [38], older adults reported that loneliness for them was one of the most significant concerns. In that study, 33 % of the 845 elderly men and women reported feelings of loneliness. While many participants reported loneliness, only 16 % lived alone. This high level of "loneliness" speaks to the need to examine the relationship between older persons and those with whom they live, with a view to improving intergenerational interactions. The majority (70 %) of those who reported that they were lonely stated that their family and friends were too busy to spend time with them, prompting feelings of neglect. Interestingly enough, more men than women in that study reported "feeling lonely." Not only were these older people lonely, but some also stated that they were especially unhappy because they had to 'eat alone'. Eating alone, some stated felt 'like punishment' and a form of psychological abuse. More than a third of the sample (35 %) 'ate alone.' This sense of isolation and loneliness, as with other African populations, can lead to willingness to tolerate abuse and reluctance to report abuse.

21.5 Intervention

21.5.1 Prevention

Interventions for elder abuse are important to consider as strategies to address the growing risk. Addressing prevention of elder abuse and mistreatment has typically focused on identifying and mitigating these risk factors. For elders from the African diaspora, targeted interventions may be appropriate to mitigate abuse. Caregivers, the general population, and older adults themselves should be considered the "target audience" for these interventions. Avoiding social isolation, identifying and treating substance abuse in caregivers, and providing support to dependent elders are some general approaches to prevent the occurrence of elder abuse and mistreatment.

Prevention of elder abuse requires the involvement of multiple sectors of society. Appropriate interventions for preventing elder abuse could include legislation, education, respite, social support, batterer interventions, and money management programs. According to the National Research Council [39] no efforts have yet been made to develop, implement, and evaluate interventions to prevent elder abuse. They also indicate that no systematic research has been conducted to measure and evaluate the effects of existing interventions.

Prevention of elder abuse also requires the involvement of multiple sectors in the community: (1) legislation, (2) Respite services, (3) Social services, (4) Batterers support, (5) Money management, etc.

21.5.1.1 Legislation

All governments have a responsibility to protect the vulnerable among its citizens. The World Health Organization recognizes this responsibility in its plan for global health improvement [1]. These responsibilities include providing for a safety environment for older adults, particularly to vulnerable elderly, to spend their final years. The African Union has understood this need as it has begun a health initiative for the African Diaspora that includes many of its sub-Saharan African partners. It incorporates an acknowledgement about the importance of health for all its citizens.

In the US, forty-four states and the District of Columbia have laws providing that individuals who assume the care or custody of older people are considered mandatory reporters, and 38 statutes specify a penalty for mandatory reporters who do not report abuse or suspected abuse. Higher abuse investigations rates are associated with a mandatory reporting requirement in the law. While quantitative figures are absent, more countries in sub-Saharan African and the Caribbean are enacting or discussing legislation to foster protections for the elderly.

21.5.1.2 Education

Many advocates indicate that education of professional and lay caregivers as well as the general public is an important part of preventing elder abuse. Studies vary in which education interventions are the most efficacious. Education and dissemination of information are vital for healthcare professionals and for the general public. Educational interventions can help shift cultural attitudes to the elderly and mitigate the risk of abuse. Unfortunately; only 14 elder abuse intervention studies have been conducted, with the majority focused on education interventions for caregivers. None were conducted specifically for African or African American caregivers.

Educational interventions range from 1 to 8 h and are taught by many different methods, such as one-on-one instruction, in a classroom or at a conference, or with group support. Improvements after educational interventions were noted by increased knowledge, use of assessment tools, improved job performance, and declines in reports of abusive actions of staff. Tailoring the message and the location of the intervention for African and African American communities is the next step.

21.5.1.3 Respite

Many studies have shown the usefulness of respite care in relieving the burden of caregiving. A meta-analysis of respite intervention studies was conducted to determine its effect on caregivers [40]. Twenty-nine studies were usable for analysis but because of the variety of respite interventions offered, a true meta-analysis was not possible. It was determined that "although caregivers often exhibit improvements in well-being during respite periods, these gains are short-lived," suggesting the respite does not provide a long-term social support system 40. For some US African American populations and well as many of the populations in the African Diaspora, developing cultural acceptance and trust with professional caregiving will be a major step to broader utilization of respite care services. In fact, public information sessions sponsored by trusted sources have been a major factor in helping African American communities to accept respite services. Continuing to work with communities in the African Diaspora to raise awareness and gain acceptance of respite services is needed to move these programs forward.

21.5.1.4 Social Support

While a lack of social support is a risk factor, increasing social support has a protective effective against elder abuse. In fact, increased social support and social interactions have been a few of the factors that promote a greater quality of life in older adults. A meta-analysis of 18 studies providing interventions for caregiver distress demonstrated that respite services and individual psychosocial interventions were moderately effective, and group psychosocial interventions were slightly effective. For elders from the African diaspora, increased social support offers an opportunity to decrease elder abuse risk.

21.5.1.5 *Batterer Intervention*

Programs to address the perpetrators of abuse have begun to emerge as a strategy to address elder abuse. The US Department of Justice reports that 88 % of the 34 programs offering cognitive-behavioral therapy for abuse perpetrators, the re-offense rates were significantly lower in the treatment groups when compared with groups receiving no treatment. As the programs become more broadly disseminated, their impact on elder abuse may become more apparent.

21.5.1.6 Money Management Programs

There has been a growing recognition of the problem of financial abuse. Guardianship and conservatorship services have been designed and utilized to assist vulnerable elders to retain their financial assets and avoiding loss of financial independence. These services have varying degrees of effectiveness in preventing financial abuse. On study of 63 community-dwelling adults ages 60–96 were assigned to usual customary screening or to money management groups. After 12 months of intervention, no significant differences in rates of conservatorship were found between the groups, suggesting the individuals who require conservatorship may be different from those who need only money management services. Other interventions attempted were support groups for caregivers, which did not alleviate stress [41], and daily money management programs for the older adults to hinder financial exploitation, which did not lessen financial exploitation.

21.5.2 *Secondary Prevention* (Post Abuse)

In addition to interventions to prevent elder abuse occurrence or to diminish the risk of abuse, interventions are needed to help older adults cope with the experience of abuse. These strategies can help the older adult recover from and adapt to the abuse event and possibly avoid any long-term sequel from abuse.

21.5.2.1 Social Support

High levels of social support also have a favorable effect on psychological outcomes in victims of abuse [42]. High levels of abuse are correlated with a lack of social support in battered women. Moreover, high social support mitigates the adverse mental health effects of abuse exposure (RR 0.5 vs. low social support). Importantly, older adults may have a greater opportunity for forming social networks over time than their younger counterparts. These networks are available to be mobilized to help older adults cope with the experience of abuse.

Health providers need to be aware of and have the ability to activate social services for their elderly patients. Referral to case management, home health care, inpatient and home respite services, and home maker services are just a few of the support services that can help a dependent elders avoid problems of neglect or self-neglect. Many disease-specific support groups, such as the Alzheimer's Association, are available to provide support and education to caregivers as well as provide services to demented victims of elder abuse and neglect.

21.5.2.2 Resilience

Coping with the stress of violence may be a key factor contributing to the mental health effects of violence in older adults. Resilience of older adults mitigates the negative impact of stressors, such as abuse [43–45]. Greater life experiences provide a perspective that allows one to look forward to a better future. This optimistic view is one of the key elements in resilience following a traumatic life event and is important for psychological well-being [46–49]. Also, low optimism is correlated with depression ($r = -0.42$), lack of religion ($r = 0.22$), and alcohol use ($r = -0.11$) [49]. Several psychological techniques, including cognitive-behavioral therapy and group therapy, have been useful in increasing resilience in older adults.

21.6 Interventions in African American Community

Interventions to address elder abuse across the African Diaspora must utilize strategies that reflect the unique experiences of this population. Policy planners and other interested in intervention programs must engage the specific target communities in identifying and tailoring these strategies. Engaging these communities helps to identify the particular factors that would have the greatest impact is an essential element in planning an intervention strategy. This community-engagement focus may draw from a variety of strategies to reduced overall violence in communities. Programs that emphasize a trauma-informed community approach with strong community-based input are necessary for effective intervention programs.

Elder abuse intervention in these settings can be developed as an extension of the intimate partner violence intervention program. These programs understand the ecology of abuse and interventions must address abuse in this context. The engagement of the community in these programs allow them to address the broader context of the local community and society that under pin the problems with the individual elder and the relationship with the trusted caregiver (Fig. 21.1).

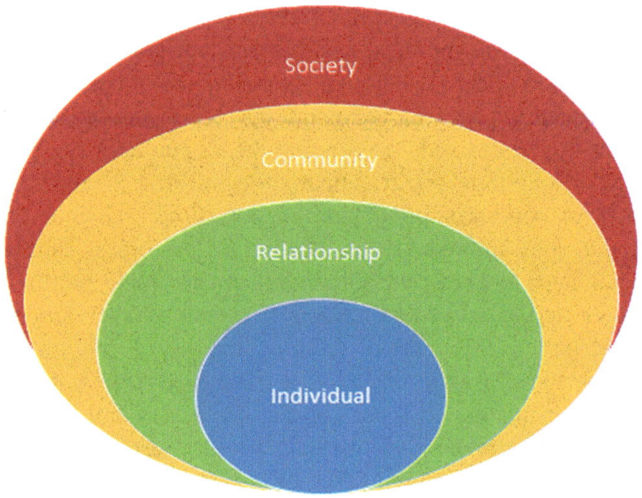

Fig. 21.1 Interventions in African American Community

Interventions to prevent elder abuse and its untoward effects need to be modeled after successful prevention strategies in the African American community. Several studies have demonstrated the effectiveness of community education in cancer prevention and screening, hypertension detection and management, diabetes detection and treatment, as well as HIV prevention, screening, and treatment. These programs have used barber shops, beauty salons, and local churches as a focus of prevention strategies. These sites may also serve as a focus of a community-based education strategy for abuse prevention. We have not identified any study focusing on preventing elder abuse in the African American communities that utilize these sites but one study found that Black church officials were willing to have speakers on issues affecting the elderly [50]. These venues may provide a welcoming environment for various elder abuse prevention strategies.

In addition of education and prevention strategies, other opportunities for community-based interventions are available to address elder abuse. Respite programs to support lay caregivers may be organized by churches, community centers, community-based organizations and nonprofits. Other community organizations are available for social support in the African American communities such as the black sororities and fraternities, social and pleasure clubs and college alumni associations. These particular networks are unique in the African American community and were utilized by older African Americans during times of forced segregation. These organizations not only provided a means of social interaction and social support but were also a trusted source for investments, life insurance, mortgages, and other business matters. African American elders often find these informal networks more helpful than formal social service agencies [51].

Communities can also provide services to support caregiving and prevent elder abuse. While there are numerous examples in several African American communities, one program that can be considered a model is Newark, New Jersey's New Community Corporation. Established in the aftermath of the 1968 riots, New Community Corporation was founded by a group of civic-minded community leaders to provide low income and senior housing. It grew to provide a comprehensive approach to care for the underserved and elder populations in Newark. As one of President George HW Bush's Thousand Points of Light, New Community Corporation has adult day care services, long-term care facilities, respite services and hospice care. It also provides a training program for professional caregiver through its award-winning practical nursing program. Many of this program graduates were also residents of New Community's apartments for the homeless program. New Community Corporation is one example of what can be done in African American communities. Other organizations sponsor community-based caregiver training programs; unfortunately they are underutilized in the African American community.

Conflict resolution for families at risk has been shown to be effective in the African American Community. Strategies that provide a safe, stable forum to discuss areas of family conflict may be essential for restoring family harmony. Extending these services, especially in minority communities, may be an essential resource component to prevent elder abuse. For financial abuse, strategies to protect elder have included guardianship services and the Black Chamber of Commerce may be recruited to develop targeted programs for their constituents.

21.7 Interventions Internationally in the African Diaspora

As the problem of elder abuse grows throughout the Africa Diaspora, several governmental and nongovernmental organizations (NGOs) have begun to develop strategies and programs to address elder abuse. Sub-Saharan Africa has seen several new advocacy groups formed to address the need to educate the community and helps victims of abuse. The Nigerian Coalition on the Prevention of Elder Abuse has begun program in both urban and rural Nigeria to help develop better attitudes and caregiving practices. As an arm of the International Network for the Prevention of Elder Abuse (INPEA), the coalition is working through education to help provide better resources to care for the elderly. Also, the new African Platform for Social Protection will be a new advocacy organization striving to elder abuse in sub-Saharan Africa. Although there is no quantitative data on the effectiveness of these programs, both are having an impact on redefining cultural stereotypes and traditions in sub-Saharan African while providing support and training for health workers and lay caregivers.

INPEA has been a major on the world stage highlighting the problem of elder abuse and helping develop program to address this problem. It has developed tool kits to help governments and NGOs raise awareness of the problem of elder abuse, has helped promote the UN Convention of the rights of older persons, and hosts World Elder Abuse Awareness Day annually. Working in cooperation with other advocacy groups, INPEA is helping to develop legislative initiatives to codify appropriate treatment of older adults.

21.8 Outcomes of Abuse Exposure in African Americans

As with the risk factors for abuse, the shared legacy of older US African American may impact the outcomes from abuse exposure. As mentioned African American elders already suffer from untoward health outcomes due to a history of slavery and forced segregation. The continuation of these lifelong stressors amplifies the effect of great environmental and interpersonal violence in their communities. Living in these underresourced environments adds to the burden of violent stress the African American elders face and would be expected to lead to greater mental and physical health problems in abused African American elders. However, it is unclear if late life abuse has the same mental health effects as abuse in younger victims. Coker reports that victims age 18–65 years report a number of health effects including depressive symptoms, alcoholism, drug use, greater chronic disease burden and poorer overall health [44, 45]. Mouton showed similar findings with older women who suffered abuse having poorer overall physical and mental health. In Africa, Mudiare reports how elder victims of abuse live in fear and suffer mental and physical incapacitation [52].

Dong and Simon [18] showed in a multiethnic group of elder from Chicago that elder abuse resulted in a twofold higher rate of hospitalization. Rovi et al. [53] showed that patients with elder abuse had longer hospital stays and those with neglect had the highest hospital charges. Roepke-Buehler et al. [16] also showed that elder abuse was associated with a twofold rate of depressive symptoms.

21.9 Conceptual Framework

The Institute of Medicine has proposed a theoretical framework to understand the problem of elder abuse. The framework describes on the left a set of social, psychological and physical attributes that put older adults at risk for elder abuse. On the right, the framework describes a set of social, psychological, and physical attributes that identify characteristics of individuals in a "trusted relationship" with the elder who can potential become perpetrators of abuse. The middle set of boxes describe the interaction of these two individual-level factors and that define the level of social and/or economic dependence (status inequality), the type of social relationship between the older adult and trusted other, the differences in normative expectations held be different stakeholders and the power dynamics operating in the caregiving relationship. The model also includes social embeddedness which refers to the sets of people in the social networks of these individual that can be drawn on for support.

For those of African descent, this framework must be understood in the historical, social, economic, and psychological context of the African diaspora (Fig. 21.2). This history influences the impact of each of these factors and magnifies the degree of their influence on the model and each other. The key concepts of this framework from social embeddedness, individual-level factors to status inequality. In African Americans, social embeddedness moves beyond the traditional family to include caring others such as church members, fraternity/sorority members, and other social cubs. Also, African Americans are more likely to have non-kin household members or greater networks of "trusted others." The development of these social non-kin communities has its origins in the slavery and segregation legacy of African Americans. Research on elder abuse in the African American community should consider the role of these varying networks and the degree of social embeddedness of the target population.

This "slavery legacy" also has an impact on several of the individual-level factors discussed in the framework. Clearly, discrimination has led substantially inequities in wealth, physical health, and mental health. This shared historical experience has led to lack of access to health care, unequal treatment but governmental authorities, socioeconomic deprivation with the consequence of greater chronic diseases, and fewer opportunities to use preventive measures. Also, since many of the preventive measures are institutionally based, the slavery legacy creates some hesitation and distrust in African Americans to use those services. This distrust leads African Americans to accept an overburdened familial caregiver network with its associated increase in caregiver stress or an overwhelmed caregiver network that cannot provide care when needed. Also, the legacy of discrimination leaves some African American neighborhoods that are deprived of services or economic opportunity. This economic vacuum allows the illegal criminal economic system to flourish. As the judicial systems addresses the criminal system, some African American face the separation caregivers from families and/or the separation of the main economic provider from the family. For African American elders in these environments, the stress the face as well as that of their caregivers can be overwhelming. The factors also influence the various components of the framework when it is applied to African American.

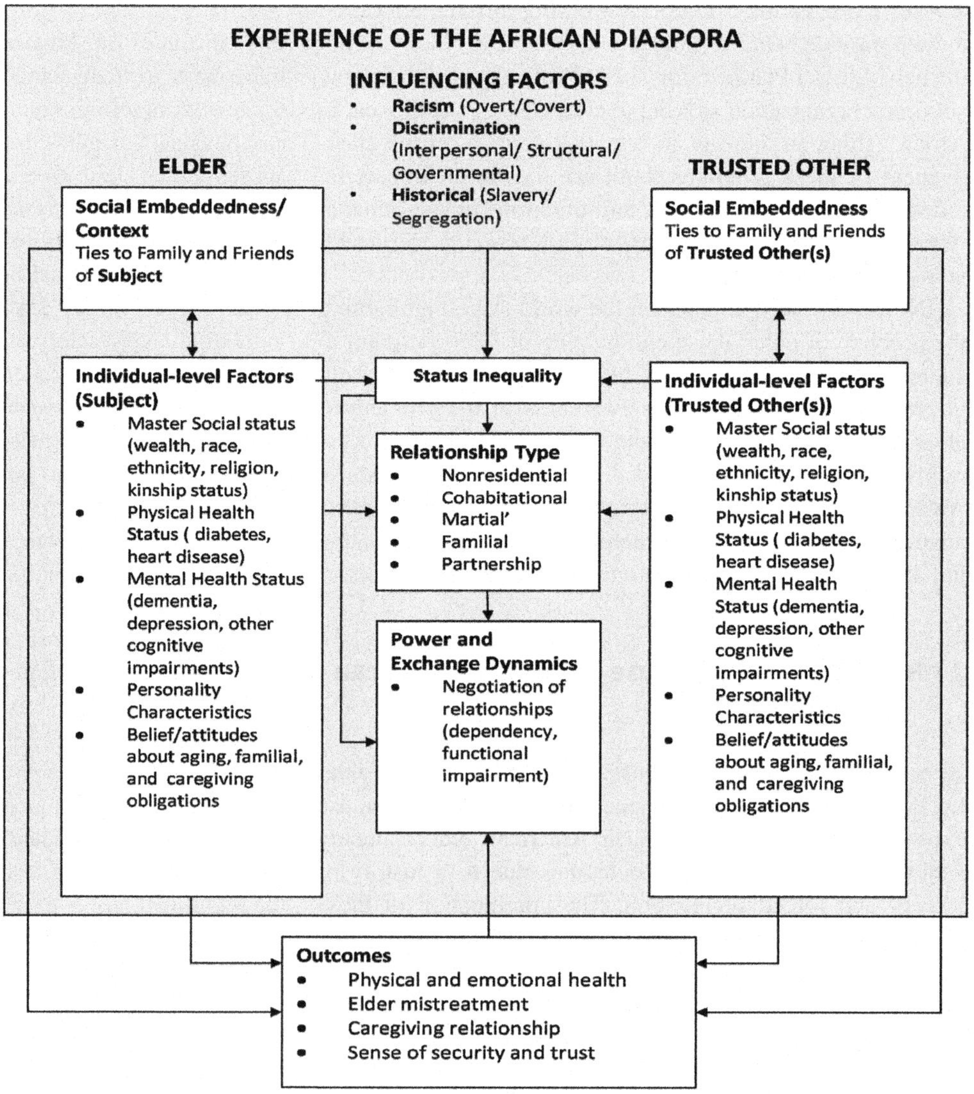

Fig. 21.2 Experience of the African diaspora

21.10 Future Directions

Future directions for the field of elder abuse research and prevention in the African diaspora need to address a number of important areas. First, continued high-quality epidemiological studies need to be done to define the problem, the extent of abuse across the African diaspora, its demonstrated risk factors, and its effects on the population. Second, ongoing monitoring through large population-based surveys need to be established to track the problem in this population and support the planning efforts for prevention and intervention. Use of ongoing epidemiologic studies are needed to monitor rates of abuse in populations of African descent. Third, governments and policy organizations need to engage communities that are affected by elder mistreatment in developing trauma-informed communities and abuse-free environments that support health aging and value older adults. Also, social support and social welfare programs need to be developed to provide care for older persons of African descent who have no family or other caregivers. Testing the effectiveness of these programs in addressing the needs of this elder community and fully evaluating their success will allow for broader implementation across the African diaspora, backed by the evidence. Fourth, collaborative models of research and community-engagement need to be encouraged to provide a continued focus on this problem. An annual/biannual international conference should be sponsored to allow the dissemination of the best research and best practices in addressing elder abuse in the African diaspora. This conference should highlight the collaboration between governments, NGOs, communities and researchers to address elder abuse. The WHO, perhaps through INPEA, or NIH should provide a annual report highlighting the progress made in addressing elder abuse across the African diaspora.

21.11 Policy Implications

Prevention of elder abuse demands governmental and public policy attention. If it is true that civilized society is judged by how it cares for the most vulnerable citizens then public policies must address the potential victims of elder abuse, particularly those from the African diaspora. Clearly, a variety of public and governmental programs can be launched to address each area of risk mentioned above and funding through grants encourages the development and implementation of these programs. Also, funding is needed to fully elucidate the epidemiology and risk factors of elder abuse in the African diaspora. However, a broad scope of programs with a unique focus in the African American communities and communities across the African Diaspora need to be considered.

Many African American communities have been designed as economic empowerment zones or economic development zones. This designation allows entrepreneurs to receive low interest (often government backed) loans and grants to redevelop these neighborhoods. Each of these projects should place restrictions and require 20 % of the housing units to provide low income senior housing and 20 % of the retail space to provide low (or no) rent venues for community benefit programs. These programs could be (1) adult learning programs for caregiver education, (2) community-based adult day care (and respite) services, (3) workforce re-entry and job training for seniors, and (4) guardianship and/or financial management services for older adults. These programs would begin to redevelop communities and increase the opportunities to build healthy environments for older African Americans.

In additional to utilizing the empowerment zone, expanding Department of Justice Program's effort around child abuse and intimate partner violence to include more programs with a specific focus on elder abuse in minority communities. Expanding the Department's Violence Prevention Program to provide "one-stop shopping" for older adults seeking medical care, dental care, and mental health services could be extremely helpful. Providing caregiver support, victim support services, guardianship and financial service, and identification and linkage with other social services would provide an ideal program to mitigate the risks of elder abuse.

21.12 Summary

In this chapter, the prevalence of elder abuse in those from the African Diaspora has been highlighted. While they share similar risk for abuse as their White counterparts, unique risks for elder abuse are present in the African American community and those from the African Diaspora. These unique risks present new opportunities for interventions to prevent and potentially eliminate the effects of elder abuse in this population.

References

1. Active ageing: a policy framework. Geneva: World Health Organization; 2002 (WHO/NMH/ NPH/02.8).
2. World population prospects: the 2004 revision highlights. New York: United Nations; 2005.
3. National service framework for older people. London: Department of Health; 2001.
4. Bennett G, Kingston P. Elder abuse, concepts, theories and interventions. London: Chapman & Hall; 1993.
5. Carney MT, Kahan FS, Paris B. Elder abuse: is every bruise a sign of abuse? Mt Sinai J Med. 2003;70:69–74.

6. Mouton CP, Rodabough RJ, Rovi SL, Hunt JL, Talamantes MA, Brzyski RG, Burge SK. Prevalence and 3-year incidence of abuse among postmenopausal women. Am J Public Health. 2004;94:605–12.
7. Baker AA. Granny battering. Mod Gerlatr. 1975;5:20–4.
8. Burston G. Do your elderly relatives live in fear of being battered? Mod Geriatr. 1977;7:54–5.
9. Ogg J, Bennett G. Elder abuse in Britain. Br Med J. 1992;305:998–9.
10. Acierno R, Hernandez MA, Amstadter A, Resnick HS, Steve K, Muzz W, Kilpatrick DG. Prevalence and coreelate of emotional, physical, sexual, financial abuse and potential neglect in the United States: the National Elder Mistreatment Study. Am J Public Health 2010;100(20): 292–7.
11. Tatara T, Toshio T, Kuzmeskus L. Summaries of statistical data on elder abuse in domestic settings for FY 95 and FY 96. Washington: National Center on Elder Abuse; 1997.
12. The National Center on Elder Abuse. The national elder abuse incidence study. Final report. Washington: Administration for Children and Families and the Administration on Aging, DHHS; 1998 Sept.
13. American Medical Association Diagnostic and Treatment Guidelines on Domestic Violence. Arch Fam Med 1992;1(1):39–47.
14. Fisher BS, Regan SL. The extent and frequency of abuse in the lives of older women and their relationship with health outcomes. The Gerontologist. 2006;46(2):200–9.
15. Hudson MF, Armmachain WD, Beasley CM, Carlson JR. Elder abuse: two Native American Views. Gerontologist 1998;38 (5):536–8.
16. Roepke-Buehler SK, Simon M, Dong X. Association between depressive symptoms, multiple dimensions of depression, and elder abuse: a cross-sectional, population-based analysis of older adults in urban Chicago. J Aging Health. 2015;1–23.
17. Mouton CP. Partner violence and health status among older women. Violence against women. 2003;9(12):1465–78.
18. Dong X, Simon MA. Elder abuse as a risk factor for hospitalization in older persons. JAMA Intern Med. 2013;173(10):911–7.
19. Beach SR, Schulz R, Castle NG, Rosen J. Financial exploitation and psychological mistreatment among older adults: differences between African Americans and non-African Americans in a population-base survey. Gerontologist. 2010;50(6):744–57.
20. Laumann EO, Leitsch SA, Waite LJ. Elder mistreatment in the United States: prevalence estimates from a Nationally Representative Study. J Gerontol Ser B Psychol Sci Soc Sci. 2008;63 (4):5248–54.
21. Williams DR, Gonzalez HM, Neighbors H, Messe R, Abelson JM, Sweetman J, Jackson JS. Prevalence and distribution of major depressive disorders in African Americans, Caribbean Blacks and NonHispanic Whites. Arch Gen Psychiatry. 2007.
22. Horsford SR, Parra-Cardona JR, Pose LA, Schamberg L. Elder abuse and neglect in African American families: informing practice based on ecological and cultural frameworks. J Elder Abuse Negl. 2011;23:75–88.
23. Bernier BL. Class, race, and poverty. Medical technologies and sociopolitical choices. Harv Black Lett J. 1994;11:115–44.
24. Sullivan S. Inheriting racist disparities in health: epigenetics and the transgenerational effects of White Racism. Crit Philos Race. 2013;1(2):190–218.
25. Radke KM, Ruf M, Gunter HM, Dohrmaun K, Schauer M, Meryer A, Elbert T. Transgenerational impact of intimate partner violence on methylation in the promoter of the glucocorticoid receptor. Transl Psychiatry. 2011;21.
26. Bohauk J, Mansay IM. Epigenetic inheritance of disease and disease risk. Neuropsychopharmacology. 2013;38(6):220–36.
27. Rodgers AB, Morgan CP, Bronson SL, Revello S, Bale TL. Paternal stress exposure alter sperm microRNA content and reprograms offspring HPA stress axis regulation. J Neurosci. 2013;33(21):9003–12.
28. Thayer ZM, Kuzawa CW. Biological memories of past environments: epigenetic pathways to health disparities. Epigenetics. 2011;6(7):1–6.
29. Pillemer K, Finkelhor D. The prevalence of elder abuse: a random sample survey. Gerontologist. 1988;28:51–7.
30. Sacco P, Bucholz KK, Spitznagel EL. Alcohol use among older adults in the National Epidemiology Survey on alcohol and related conditions: a latent class analysis. J Stud Alcohol Drugs. 2009;70 (6):829–38.
31. Mouton C, Larme A, Alford C, McCorkle R, Talamantes M, Burge S. Multiethnic perspectives on elder mistreatment. J Elder Abuse Negl. 2005;17(2):21–44.
32. Mba CJ. Elder abuse in parts of Africa and the way forward. Gerontechnology. 2007;6(4):230–5.
33. Bigala P, Ayiga N. Prevalence and predictors of elder abuse in Mafikeng local municipality in South Africa. Afr Popul Stud. 2014;28(1):463–74.
34. Kabole AL, Kioli FN, Onkware K. The social context of abuse of elderly people in Emuhaya District, Kenya. Sociol Anthropol. 2013;1(2):76–86.
35. HelpAge International (Nhongo T, editor) Kenya elder abuse in the health care services in Kenya. Sept 2001.
36. Keikelame J, Ferreira M. Mpathehombi, ya Bantu Abadala: elder abuse in black townships on the Cap Flats. 2000.
37. Obot IS. Africa faces a growing threat from neo-colonial alcohol marketing. Addiction 2011;106(11):1894–5.
38. Rawlins JM, Simeon DT, Ramdath DD, Chadee DD. The elderly in Trindad: health, social, and economic status and issues of loneliness. West Indian Med J. 2008;57(6):589–95.
39. National Research Council. Aging in Sub-Saharan Africa: recommendations for furthering research. Panel on policy research and data needs to meet the challenge of aging in Africa. In: Cohen Barney, Menken Jane, editors. Committee on population, division of behavioral and social sciences and education. Washington: The National Academies Press; 2006.
40. McNally S, Ben-Shiomo Y, Newman S. The effects of respite care on informal carers' well-being: a systemic review. Disabil Rehabil. 1999;21(1):1–14.
41. Hsieh HF, Wang JJ, Yen M, Liu TT. Educational support group in change caregivers' psychological elder abuse behavior toward caring for institutional elders. Adv Health Sci Educ Theory Pract. 2009;14(3):377–86.
42. Scheier M, Carver C, Bridges M. Distinguishing optimism from neuroticism (and trait anxiety, self-mastery and self-esteem): a reevaluation of the life orientation test. J Pers Soc Psychol. 1994;67:1078.
43. Jaffe P, Wolfe D, Wilson S, Zak L. Emotional and physical health problems of battered women. Can J Psychiatry. 1986;31:625–54.
44. Coker A, Smith P, Thompson M, McKeown R, Davis K. Social support protects against the negative effects of partner violence on mental health. J Women's Health Gender Based Med. 2002;11:465–76.
45. Coker AL, Davis KE, Arias I, Desai S, Sanderson M, Brandt HM, Smith PH. Physical and mental health effects of intimate partner violence for men and women. Am J Prev Med. 2002;23(4):260–8.
46. Baltes PB, Baltes MM. Psychological perspectives on successful aging: the model of selective optimization with compensation. In: Baltes PB, Baltes MM, editors. Successful aging: perspectives from the behavioral sciences. Cambridge: Cambridge University Press; 1990.

47. Bowen DJ, Morisca AA, Meischke H. Measures and correlates of resilience. Women Health. 2003;38(2):65–76.
48. Ryff CD, Singer B, Love GD, Essex MJ. Resilience in adulthood and later life: defining features and dynamic process. In: Lomranz J, editor. Handbook of aging and mental health: an integrative approach. New York: Plenum Press; 1998. p. 69–96.
49. Taylor JY. Moving from surviving to thriving: African American women recovering from intimate male partner abuse. Res Theory Nurs Pract. 2004;18(1):35–50.
50. Chadiha L, Morrow-Howell N, Darkwa O, McGillick J. Targetign the black church and clergy for disseminating knowledge about Alzheimers disease and caregiver support services. Am J Alzheimer's Care Relat Disorders Res. 1994;9:17–20.
51. Williams OJ, Becker RL. Domestic partner abuse treatment programs and cultural competence: the results of a national survey. Violence Vict. 1994;9:287–96.
52. Mudiare PEU. Abuse of the aged in Nigeria: elder also cry. Am Int J Contemp Res. 2013;3(9):79–87.
53. Rovi S, Chen PH, Vega M, Johnson MS, Mouton CP. Mapping the elder mistreatment iceberg: US hospitalizations with elder abuse and neglect diagnoses. J Elder Abuse Negl. 2009;21:346–59.

Elder Abuse and Neglect in Asia

22

Elsie Yan and Gracy Fang

The population of Asia is aging at an unprecedentedly fast pace. It is expected that Asian population aged 60 or above would reach 24 % by 2050 [80]. The growth will be particularly acute among the old–old with the percentage of those older than 75 years rise to 27 % by 2050 [80].

Over the past three decades, various studies have been conducted on the subject of elder abuse in Asian societies. This article summarizes cultural considerations relevant for understanding the phenomenon in Asia. Attempts are made to examine cultural values in three major areas: (1) new interpretations of filial piety and changing intergenerational relationships, (2) gender roles and patriarchal society, and (3) changing demographics and social structure.

22.1 Cultural Considerations Regarding Elder Abuse in Asia

Interpersonal relationships are culturally constructed. This is especially true for intergenerational relationships. Cultural values govern what the aging experience is like for an older person, how intergenerational relationships play out, and the social expectations of the young and the old. In most parts of Asia, e.g., China, Korea, Vietnam and Japan, intergenerational relationships and exchange are guided by Confucian teachings. The notion of filial piety prescribes that parents take care of their children when they are young, and that adult children, in return, are to obey, respect, care for, and support their older parents both emotionally and financially [37, 127, 158, 157].

E. Yan
Department of Applied Social Sciences, Hong Kong Polytechnic University, Hong Kong, Hong Kong

E. Yan (✉) · G. Fang
Department of Social Work and Social Administration, University of Hong Kong, 5th Floor, Jockey Club Tower, Centennial Campus, Hong Kong, Hong Kong
e-mail: elsie.yan@polyu.edu.hk

Research shows that older parents continue to have filial expectations of their children, who in turn generally accept such expectations [123]. That said, a more recent study has suggested that young people today interpret filial piety differently than their parents. Whilst most still consider it virtuous to adhere to cultural traditions and reciprocate parental care and love, many believe the actual exercise thereof should depend on their life circumstances [210].

Filial piety also prescribes sons' obligation to maintain the continuity of family life, preserve family integrity and harmony, and to perform the ritual duties related to ancestor worship [82]. In many Asian societies, it is the responsibilities of the elder son and daughter-in-laws to provide care to the aging parents. All these are typical of the patrilineal systems. The patrilineal systems emphasize kinship and intergenerational harmony [111]. The cultural virtue of collectivism, which stipulates the prioritization of other family members' needs over one's own desires, also affects upon intergenerational relationships among Asians [183]. These institutionalized rules have provided a solid moral basis for intergenerational co-residence, whereby family resources are shared and older parents are guaranteed care and respect from their children [68]. However, this type of living arrangement is highly susceptible to intergenerational conflict in the contemporary Asian context, due to differing views on everyday matters between generations [201].

Furthermore, social development ushered in by westernization, urbanization, and industrialization has not only altered young people's interpretation and practice of filial piety [229], but also resulted in demographic and social changes that further erode intergenerational support. For examples, labor-related migration has created geographical segregation among generations, which has further loosened intergenerational exchange and reciprocal support [230]. Women's participation in the workforce has also limited their availability to provide care to elders in the family [211]. Besides increasingly inadequate family care, the formal social support provided to older people is inadequate, due to

X. Dong (ed.), *Elder Abuse*, DOI 10.1007/978-3-319-47504-2_22

the prevailing assumption that the family should bear the primary responsibility for elderly care [169]. In view of these sociocultural transitions, we can no longer assume that older Asians are immune from abuse and neglect.

The following section provides an in-depth discussion of the changing values and social demographics in major Asian societies relevant to understanding elder abuse.

22.1.1 Chinese Societies

22.1.1.1 Changing Intergenerational Relationships

In Chinese societies (People's Republic of China, Hong Kong, Taiwan), where Confucian teachings prevail, filial piety has long been emphasized as a fundamental social norm guiding parent–child interactions and family relationships. Traditionally, children are inculcated to respect, support, and obey their parents [36]. However, modernization and westernization in recent decades have resulted in reconstructed and broadening definitions of filial piety in the younger generation [51]. For example, unlike the older cohorts, younger Chinese in both Hong Kong and Taiwan tend to interpret filial piety as various forms of repayment based on mutual affection and parent–child equality, rather than absolute obedience and a responsibility to provide direct care to their parents [229]. As a result, more and more young people in Hong Kong and Taiwan are performing their filial duties by paying for parents' institutional care or home care services, a practice sometimes seen by older Chinese as abandonment and unfilial [38, 233]. Young people today also demand greater equality in intergenerational interactions and tend to speak less respectfully to their parents [231], using language often considered verbal abuse by elders [204]. In contrast, in the PRC, filial piety is still characterized by parental authority and absolute submission [42]. "Talking back" to parents is viewed as a serious offense [46].

22.1.1.2 Gender Roles

The Chinese family has also been characterized as patriarchal, patrilocal and patrilineal, a nexus in which roles are strongly gendered [60]. Females are expected to obey their fathers, husbands, and, later, their adult sons [46]. Reflecting this imbalanced distribution of power is the preponderance of older females suffering from domestic violence [48, 49]. Paradoxically, younger Chinese women are at an increased risk of becoming abusers. According to tradition, daughter-in-laws are supposed to reside with their husbands' families and, until they succeed in continuing the family lineage by producing a son, are frequently considered "temporary or outside" family members [43]. However, modern women, influenced by the western values of individuality and independence, have become less devoted to the patriarchal system [76]. Divergent intergenerational views regarding women's family roles have become a noteworthy factor in elder abuse committed by daughters-in-law [3].

In the PRC, another prominent factor contributing to elder abuse involving daughters-in-law is the distribution of money [231]. In most cases, parents receive regular financial support from their son and his wife. The wives' parents, however, are only subsidized if they help with childcare or if the husband's parents are dead [191]. This practice survived until the implementation of the one-child policy, which forced some parents to depend on their daughter [231]. In-law conflicts can occur if the husbands' parents disagree with the couple's decision to provide financial help to the wives' parents [23]. Frustration experienced by daughters-in-law may also transform into violence.

Hong Kong is similar to the PRC in that family obligations are transforming, abandoning a duty-bound for a spontaneous approach within kinship networks [159]. As women's social roles and employment status change, male family members are no longer expected to assume all family expenses and responsibilities [33]. Women are expected to simultaneously fulfill their newly defined role of breadwinner and traditionally assigned role of family caregiver to older parents or parents-in-law [83]. Such dual responsibilities impose significant stress and burden on women, which may turn into aggression toward their older family members.

In Taiwan, a new type of "quasi-co-residence" arrangement known as "rotation" has emerged. It allows adult siblings to rotate take turns in taking on the responsibility to host and provide meals to their older parents [34]. However, some elders criticize this living arrangement as improper treatment due to the violation of their wish to live with a particular child and the inconvenience caused by moving around [128].

22.1.1.3 Changing Demographic and Social Structure

Researchers have noted the declining social status of the elderly in the family as early as the 19,902 [208]. Social exclusion and discrimination against older people have become risk factors leading to elder abuse and neglect [24]. Another factor leading to increased risk of elder abuse is the lack of a social safety net provided for the elderly, only 4.67 % retirees in Hong Kong receive a pension [74]. The majority of older Chinese depends entirely on their adult children for financial assistance, which increases their vulnerability to abuse [225].

Traditionally, older persons prefer to reside with their adult children. Intergenerational co-residence represents an ideal virtue of collectivism that symbolizes family prosperity and harmony, and is therefore highly encouraged [208]. Co-residing with older parents and providing them with daily care enables adult children to fulfill the filial obligations [234]. Parent–child co-residence has thus become a strategy for adult children to satisfy their older parents' needs of instrumental help, physical care, companionship, and financial support. Altruism and collectivism demand that the whole family should work together to maximize resources and allocate them equitably to ensure every family member's well-being, and these objectives can best be realized by intergenerational co-residence [142]. Rising housing prices and housing shortages in urban China also mean that many young people are forced to live with their parents even after joining the workforce, due to their financial incapacity to purchase or rent a house on their own [145]. It is estimated that 59.9–67 % of older adults co-reside with their adult children in the PRC [46, 234].

This is changing in the PRC, the massive flow of rural-to-urban migration over the past two decades has led to significant changes in the relationship between young labor in urban areas and their left behind older parents in rural areas. Migrant children are no longer available to provide direct physical care due to their limited physical contact with their parents [142]. Younger workers are relatively less mobile in Hong Kong. However, increasing numbers of adult children are still opting to place their older parents in long-term care facilities, probably due to the shortage of housing [1].

Even the multi-generational households, the increasing demands of workplace have limited children's ability to provide physical care for their parents [116]. This is especially true in urban areas. Increasingly, paid domestic help has become the primary source of care in daily caregiving tasks for the elderly in the PRC, Hong Kong, and Taiwan. As Chinese parents place great value on children's moral obligations to attend to parental needs, the failure of adult children to provide hands-on care is frequently considered as neglect or abandonment [114, 226].

It is expected that proximate intergenerational contact as a result of co-residence gives rise to intergenerational conflicts, due to differences between young people and the older generations in terms of lifestyle, social activities, financial matters, role expectations, etc. [10]. Adult children who are not able to resolve conflicts with their older parents via positive coping strategies may resort to maladaptive and aggressive behaviors, the worst-case scenario being elder abuse [216]. In this light, elders co-residing with their adult children may be subject to a higher risk of abuse. However, elder abuse occurring in the co-residing environment tends to remain hidden, in part due to the private nature of the home.

Intergenerational exchange of support seems more common in rural areas of the PRC [45]. Intergenerational relationships in rural Chinese families indicate a bidirectional pattern represented by the exchange of resources [190]. Most parents' motivation to provide grandchild care is determined by their expectations that their children will reciprocate financially [125]. Although most elders describe their grandparenting experience as a strategic investment to increase intergenerational emotional closeness and financial security [125], some are reluctant to assume the grandchild caregiving role or even consider it unfilial and an exploitation of labor [45, 142].

22.1.1.4 Cultural Specific Examples and Attitudes Toward Elder Abuse

The filial tradition that older parents should receive not only financial support, but also love, care, and attention from their adult children has deep roots in Hong Kong. It is therefore hardly surprising that "being treated as if transparent" is often considered a severe and common form of abuse by older Chinese in Hong Kong [84].

Given the above, it is not surprising that many Chinese people regard elder abuse as a private family matter into which a "third party" from outside the family should not intervene, a notion that makes victims reluctant to seek help [48, 49]. Furthermore, many older Chinese cultivate the belief that it is improper to involve themselves in others' family matters, which makes them reluctant to offer advice or concrete help to victims of elder abuse. Moreover, in the majority of cases, the victims fear that they will create domestic conflict and jeopardize the family's reputation if they admit to being abused [224]. Victims' acknowledgement of abuse also entails admission of their children's failure to fulfil their filial obligation to respect and obey them, which is often perceived as a result of poor parenting, and can lead to a loss of face [32, 37, 197]. In Chinese cultures, the acknowledgement of abuse is therefore a source of shame for the victims. As a result, older Chinese are generally comparatively tolerant of elder abuse. Instead of protecting older Chinese from abuse, filial piety may be a hurdle to the reporting and investigation of abuse [224].

22.1.2 South Korea

According to traditional Korean culture, the family serves as the basis of the self and has priority over all other social relationships [109]. Children are conceived as an important part of the completeness of life [163]. For Koreans, the concept of past and future is relationally based, rather than a mere abstract idea, and children are considered the future of the family [184]. Therefore, considerable financial, emotional, and social investments are made in them [109]. Indulgence, devotion, and sacrifice are considered as parents' basic duty, as children are viewed as the extension of their parents' life [167].

22.1.2.1 Changing International Relationship

South Korea is at the transitional stage of social development, where traditional interpretations and contemporary values of filial piety coexist [39]. The younger generation has interpreted filial piety as providing support to aging parents where feasible and according to their needs, rather than an obligation to care for them [169]. However, many older Koreans still expect their adult children to provide them with unconditional emotional support and hands-on care, and legitimize their expectation with reference to the tradition of filial piety [124]. Conflicts associated with different interpretations of filial piety and ways of providing support are observed in Korean parent–child dyads [169]. Intergenerational conflicts and separation have been identified as prominent factor leading to elder abuse and neglect [215].

22.1.2.2 Gender Roles

Another salient cultural characteristic in Korea is patriarchy and family centeredness, which prescribes the exclusive authority of the older male to control other family members [168]. Although the Civic Codes have abolished the traditional system of patrilineage and instituted the married couple as a family unit [170], the Korean family system remains highly gendered, primarily manifested in the unequal husband–wife relationship, inheritance skewed in favor of adult sons, and the dominant power of male family heads [169]. The inferior statuses of women in the family may put them in a vulnerable position open to abuse or manipulation, as reflected in increasing numbers of older female victims of domestic abuse [122].

The Confucian value of filial piety has maintained this patriarchal and conservative structure in Korean families and society [109]. Filial obligations are highly stratified by gender in Korea. An adult son and his wife, rather than a daughter, are obliged to provide primary support to older parents [163]. This means in practice that in most cases, women are expected to provide instrumental support to their parents-in-law rather than their own parents [61]. Therefore, it is frequently observed that the husband's parents receive sufficient support whereas the needs of the wife's parents are neglected [109]. However, the wife's parents generally tolerate such financial neglect. Having internationalized the patrilineal tradition [120], most perceive it to be a cultural custom of intergenerational exchange [64].

22.1.2.3 Changing Demographic and Social Structure

Although social changes brought on by modernization and urbanization have undermined young people's adherence to traditional values and prompted a desire for an autonomous life away from the parental home, intergenerational co-residence still prevails in Korea [108]. First, the normative force of familism serves as the primary motivation encouraging young people to live with their parents [109]. Second, marginal social welfare benefits and poor post-retirement economic statuses limit older Korean adults' capacity to live independently [90], thus increasing their need of family support and geographical proximity to their children [168]. Although co-residence can significantly facilitate the transmission of resources and the exchange of material and emotional support between generations [124], intensive interactions between parents and children who have sharp differences in terms of lifestyle and values may increase the likelihood of intergenerational conflict, which is a significant predictor of elder abuse.

22.1.2.4 Cultural Specific Examples and Attitudes Toward Elder Abuse

A lack of respect and care and inappropriate treatment by family members are regarded by older Korean adults as major forms of abuse [35]. Associated with the patriarchal traditions, older Koreans consider insufficient attention paid to them by their daughter-in-law as a form of abuse [35]. Other examples of abuse by daughters-in-law include "failure to acknowledge the elder when he or she arrives at or leaves the residence," "failure to use certain words or phrases in the Korean language that denote respect," and "direct expression of disagreement with mother-in-law" [35]. In one survey of 587 older community dwellers in South Korea, 58.9 % of the respondents believed that Korean elders did not receive sufficient respect [107]. The respondents identified neglect as the most severe form of elder abuse, followed by verbal abuse. Another example reflecting Korean parents' relational orientation is the culture of inheritance [109]. It is culturally accepted that family wealth flows from one generation to the next. As a result, many Korean children consider it their rights to manipulate their parents' economic resources, whereas parents tend to tolerate such financial exploitation [121]. More recent empirical evidence consistently indicates that although many Korean parents provide generous support to their adult children, the latter tend to take it for granted and do not reciprocate [65].

Similar to Chinese, most older Koreans are reluctant to report elder abuse [118]. Previous studies noted that over one-third (36 %, $n = 45$) of Korean elders indicated no intention to seek help when presented with a hypothetical situation of abuse. Reasons given included the perception of elder abuse as a family issue, appeasement, victim blaming, a desire to preserve family honor, and mistrust of "third-party intervention" [121]. Older Koreans also have a propensity to blame the victim and lack help-seeking intention and behavior [151]. Most consider elder abuse an immoral misconduct that violates the virtue of filial piety [151]. Acknowledging it thus equals admitting that one's children have not fulfilled their filial obligation, which can be seen as a result of poor parenting [121]. Third-party intervention is generally rejected, primarily because discussing such negative family matters with outsiders is considered a stain on family honor [121].

22.1.3 Japan

In terms of managing interpersonal relationships in family settings, Japanese people tend to deliberately avoid confrontation in order to preserve harmony and face [133]. A lack of verbal communication and suppression of emotions can further result in deepening resentment in the conflicting parties, which is a major cause of filial violence in Japan [113].

22.1.3.1 Changing Intergenerational Relationships

Intergenerational relationships in Japan are also characterized by closeness between mothers and sons [202]. In Japanese culture, mothers are shown respect for successfully raising their sons to take over family responsibilities [218]. As a result, of this strong mother–son attachment, most mothers continue to care for their sons even after they are married. It is common for mothers to interfere with their sons' marriage and to expect their daughters-in-law to obey their sons totally [193]. In most cases, sons tend to be nonchalant about their mothers' interference in their marriage, perhaps due to their gratitude for the sacrifices their mothers have made for them [193]. Parental interference, and the son's indifference to it, can foster negative feelings in the son's wife, potentially contributing to conflict-prone or abusive in-law relationships.

22.1.3.2 Changing Demographics and Social Structure

Perhaps in consideration of reducing in-law conflicts and due to the influence of western values, an increasing proportion of newly married Japanese couples are opting to establish new families and live independently, away from their parents' households [209]. Increased public support for the elderly, such as healthcare and a universal pension system, have also reduced children's burden to support their parents, which allows them greater opportunities to pursue an autonomous life and personal development [202]. The traditional intergenerational co-residing family in Japan has gradually been replaced by "intimacy at distance" [168]. However, geographical segregation inevitably limits children's availability to fulfill their filial duty of providing daily care and emotional support to older parents, which increases the likelihood of psychological neglect.

22.1.3.3 Gender Roles

Under the influence of Confucian teachings, the traditional family structure in Japan has remained patriarchal, emphasizing the authority of the father and the continuity of the family lineage [211]. The family system also prescribes strict expectations of hierarchic and gender roles [203]. Due to the cultural expectations of filial piety in Japan, it is obligatory for a married couple to co-reside with the husband's family [100]. The wife is expected to conform to the lifestyle of her parents-in-law and provide them with daily care [201]. However, due to the changes the family institution has undergone in the last few decades, women with a better education have started to show a desire to express their own feelings and opinions, rather than submit totally to their parents-in-law and husband [132]. Differing opinions between daughters-in-law and parents-in-law regarding everyday matters may turn into in-law conflicts, which may further lead to poor in-law relationships [132]. Influenced by a stereotypical gendered division of labor, most husbands do not attempt to mediate in-law conflicts or to preserve family harmony. Such indifference can allow in-law conflicts to escalate [193], potentially resulting in elder abuse that jeopardizes aging parents' well-being. In fact, research reveals that daughters-in-law are the most common abusers in Japan, responsible for 38.5 % of the elder abuse cases occurring in domestic settings [100]. Another culturally specific reason for elder abuse by daughters-in-law relates to conflicts between women's traditional family roles and the new demands of work [203]. Women are expected to fulfill the multiple roles of obligatory caregiver for parents-in-law and secondary earner for supplementary family income [211]. The imposition of these conflicting expectations creates high levels of stress and frustration among women. Additionally, as increasing numbers of women define their identity as a daughter and wife, rather than as a daughter-in-law, caring for parents-in-law is often deemed an additional burden rather than a personal duty [133]. Furthermore, though daughters-in-law assume the majority of caregiving tasks, they are not entitled to any inheritance [119]. Tremendous stress, negative caregiving motivations, a sense of injustice, and in-law conflicts may lead to improper elderly care or even abuse directed at parents-in-law [193].

Similar to observations made in Korea, gender difference is also observed in older Japanese victims. Older women represent the majority (75 %) of abuse victims in Japan [100], which can in part be attributed to the unequal gender relationships of the older generation and women's traditionally submissive role.

22.1.3.4 Cultural Specific Examples and Attitudes Toward Elder Abuse

An example of culturally specific elder abuse can be found in Japanese culture. Older Japanese consider "blaming" an extreme case of abuse, such as being blamed by their adult children for their problems [11].

Historically, Japanese society was ruled by a totalitarian regime under which violence was internalized as a justified approach to conflict resolution and punishment [164]. It is therefore not surprising that rates of physical abuse against older Japanese range from 35.3 % to as high as 50 % [9, 11]. Furthermore, the investigation and prosecution of sexual abuse remain problematic in Japan [67]. Culturally, Japanese people consider sex a taboo that should not be discussed in public. Incidents of sexual abuse against the elderly are usually kept secret due to their association with humiliation and shame [113]. Even the mass media employs euphemisms to refer to sexual abuse. Some important examples include referring to rape as a "violent act" and molestation as a "mischievous act" [67]. As these euphemistic terms cannot accurately convey the seriousness of these sexual misconducts and their detrimental consequences, they may cause confusion in the investigation of sexual abuse cases.

There is also the tradition of family secrecy and shame [189]. Similar to their counterparts in other Eastern Asian societies, older Japanese comply strictly with traditional sociocultural norms and scorn deviancy. They purposefully avoid engaging in or talking about deviant behaviors that could bring shame on their families [189]. Domestic violence, especially elder abuse, is viewed as a serious deviant misconduct that should not be disclosed to people outside the family [113]. Believing in the importance of family secrecy, many older victims tend to tolerate abuse and continue to co-reside with their family abusers [100], which may place them at a high risk of repeated victimization.

22.1.4 India

Family structure in traditional Hindu society is characterized by the patriarchal system, intergenerational co-residence, and the caste system [21]. Old age is traditionally valued in India for it is associated with wisdom, reverence, and spiritual growth [30]. Veneration of one's own parents is an important virtue in Indian culture, as proclaimed by the Hindu scripture "Mathru Devo Bhava, Pithru Devo Bhava" (*revere mother as god, revere father as god*) [21]. Caring for aging parents is thus considered a sacred duty and the failure to do so is believed to result in dire consequences in the afterlife [30].

22.1.4.1 Changing Intergenerational Relationships

Consistent with the family care practice in many other Asian societies, sons' obligatory duty of parental care is usually realized through instrumental support provided by daughters-in-law [172]. Both sons and daughters-in-law are obliged to submit to parental authority without condition [30]. However, urbanization and modernization have gradually eroded these traditional values and institutions, leading to the weakening of family bonding and togetherness [96]. Working children now usually have an economic advantage over their parents who are lifelong agricultural labors, which contradicts the prescribed family hierarchy [98]. This economic imbalance has been identified as accounting for the erosion of parental authority and the emergence of intergenerational conflict [115]. Meanwhile, the increasing numbers of dual-career couples have led to inadequate family care for aging parents, which creates tension with regard to renegotiation of caregiving arrangements and reciprocal intergenerational exchange [17]. With these socioeconomic and cultural developments, older Indians are no longer guaranteed care or deference from their children. Increasing intergenerational tension, loss of economic advantage, and the weakening of their prestige in the family have increased older Indians' vulnerability to abuse [40].

Intergenerational co-residence is extremely common in India. Indians have upheld the strong social stigma associated with the elderly living alone, partly due to its association with the disruption of familial harmony and the failure of children to perform their filial duty, which is viewed as shameful [98]. The lack of social welfare benefits also weakens older persons' ability to live independently [143]. It is therefore not surprising that over 93 % of older Indians co-reside with their adult children [21]. Intergenerational co-residence unavoidably generates intergenerational tension because of differing attitudes toward power distribution and traditional values, which is a salient predictor of elder abuse [97]. Even so, Indian elders are reluctant to live in care facilities, primarily due to the social stigma attached to it. They generally consider such living arrangements as equivalent to abandonment and a violation of tradition [126].

22.1.4.2 Changing Demographics and Social Structure

Similar to many neighboring countries, India has witnessed a large flow of rural-to-urban migration over the last three decades [98]. However, most Indian elders prefer to follow their children to urban areas rather than be left behind in their rural home [195]. The high costs of urban living, the absence of a social security net, and inadequate support from their children have forced many older people to continue working to an advanced age. With their obsolete knowledge and experience, many older Indians suffer from various forms of improper treatment in the workplace, such as long working hours and lower-than-average wages [21]. In sum, material shortage, social discrimination, and loss of family authority have placed older Indians in a disadvantaged position, increasing the risk of elder abuse.

22.1.4.3 Cultural Specific Examples and Attitudes Towards Elder Abuse

Indian elders consider "disrespect and lack of dignified living conditions" a major form of abuse [78, 154]. Other examples of abuse commonly raised by older Indians include "being used as additional domestic help," "being taken for granted," and "not being appreciated for contributions made to domestic chores" [185]. In many cases, the fact that young people lead a lifestyle that deviates significantly from their parents' expectations is a major factor contributing to abuse [154]. Although Indian elders consider disrespect a serious form of abuse, they seem to be highly tolerant of financial exploitation. For instance, many Indian elders adhere to the traditional notion that worldly possessions should be forsaken in exchange for one's next reincarnation. Many act according to this belief and make all their financial resources available to their offspring, which often puts them at a high risk of financial exploitation. It is therefore not surprising that half of the financial abuse cases in Delhi are related to inheritance disputes [185]. It should also be noted that many Indian elders are reluctant to report abuse, possibly due to the social stigma attached to it. One recent study in India showed that as many as 55 % of all older victims do not report abuse. Among these, 80 % do not do so because of concerns of family honor [80].

Many older Indians are reluctant to report abuse, perhaps due to their desire to preserve the family honor (79). Chokkanathan, Natarajan, and Mohanty [41] conducted a qualitative study examining what hinders older Indians' help-seeking behaviors for abuse. Reasons given by older victims included the attribution of abuse to past sin, the fear of losing socioeconomic support, the worry of disturbing the family equilibrium, a propensity toward self-blame, as well as the fear of not realizing salvation if one's son is absent from one's funeral rites. Tolerating abuse and keeping it secret may result in repeated victimization, which can be seriously detrimental to older victims' well-being.

22.1.5 Singapore

In Singapore, traditional Confucian ethics emphasize familism, which advocates that all family members should work together for the family's continuity, prosperity, integrity, and honor [57]. A foundational cultural virtue internalized in familistic ethics is filial piety, prescribing children's submission and obedience to parental authority [82]. Under the influence of these ideological concepts, adult children have traditionally been the primary source of emotional and financial support for older people in Singapore [207]. Traditionally, intergenerational co-residence is a preferred living arrangement by which children exercise their filial obligations [191]. However, as with other Asian societies, industrialization and modernization have had a significant influence on the younger generation's interpretation and exercise of traditional values. Although filial piety remains an ethical principle guiding parent–child interactions in Singapore, many young people adhere less closely to the absolute norms stipulated by filial principles [179]. For instance, as aspiration for an autonomous and independent lifestyle increases, many younger Singaporeans prefer to live apart from their parents, leading to a reduction in the frequency of child-to-parent physical care and intergenerational interaction [207]. However, older Singaporeans have criticized institutional placement as an immoral option, partly because of Singaporean elders' strong emphasis on intergenerational support [57, 232]. A compromise, "vicinity care," has emerged as a means for young people to fulfill their duty to provide parental care [57]. Children who reside within a short distance of their parents can feasibly provide necessary assistance to the latter. However, some older persons consider this offensive too, as it can deprive them of the emotional comfort and natural intimacy that can only be achieved in intergenerational co-residence households [57].

22.1.6 Israel

Israel is experiencing a notable transition from traditionalism to modernization [101]. Traditionally, older people are viewed as the linkage between the past and the present, as well as the primary channel for the transmission of values and experiences [187]. The shorter life expectancy of Israelis in the past has also led to the relative rarity of elders and the overestimation of their expertise and wisdom [44]. Therefore, it is a commonly shared assumption that this traditional society should be immune from elder abuse, due to its emphasis of veneration of the elderly [140].

22.1.6.1 Changing Intergenerational Relationships

Arabs and Jews constitute the two major ethnic groups in Israel. Both cultures place considerable emphasis on collectivism, patrilineality and familism, which promote mutual support among family members and total submission to patriarchal authority [101]. Many older Israelis therefore have a normative expectation of instrumental and financial support from younger family members [192]. However, increasing exposure to the western values of individualism and freedom has weakened younger adults' adherence to traditional familistic values [102]. The geographical mobility brought by urbanization has further limited family members' availability to provide hands-on care to senior relatives [131]. Furthermore, the recent emergence of "instrumentalized kinship" implies that the provision of elderly care has transformed from a traditional obligatory commitment to an instrumental calculation based on family members' availability and elders' pragmatic needs [6]. The rising modern concept of individual development has also affected people's desire to care for the elderly. A vivid example to illustrate this point is that Arabs dwelling in modern, urban areas have been found to be less willing to care for their older relatives than their rural counterparts living a nomadic lifestyle [147]. Changes in the patterns of intergenerational exchange have led to the loss of entitlement to care and a safety net among older adults, which increases their vulnerability to abuse and emotional distress [131]. Probably due to gender bias in social status, female family members seem to be more vulnerable to abuse, accounting for 83 % of the identified victims [103].

22.1.6.2 Changing Demographics and Social Structure

Modernization brought on by social changes over the last few decades has had a tremendous effect on the lives of older Israelis [181]. For instance, technological advances have reduced the value of older workers with obsolete knowledge and skills. As a result, many of them are obliged to take up jobs with low pay, subjugated to diminished occupational status and economic strain [134]. Additionally, as modern schools and courts emerged, older Israelis could no longer perform their historical social roles as educators, mediators, and arbitrators [187]. The rise of nuclear families with fewer children has further reduced their function as caregivers to grandchildren [105]. The decline in the social functions of the elderly has unavoidably contributed to changes in their roles and power distribution within families [56]. The older father, who once upheld absolute authority and economic power in the family, has become increasingly dependent on his children or the state for support [85]. Social marginalization, loss of familial power advantages, and the difficulties of adapting to modern life have contributed to older Israelis' vulnerability to abuse [154].

Intergenerational co-residence remains prevalent in Arab populations in Israel: over 68 % of older Arabs living with their adult children [26]. A shared living environment allows for the fulfillment of filial responsibility and kinship-based mutual support as prescribed by traditional social norms [138]. However, the experience of social change often causes anxiety and discord in multigenerational households, mainly due to the consequent discontinuity of solidarity, stability, and trust that were previously maintained by traditional familistic obligation [117]. For instance, intra-household conflicts can be triggered by the process of modernization, due to differing levels of acceptance of modern ideology and adjustment to modern lifestyles among different generations [135]. In times of conflict, older persons often become convenient targets for abuse and exploitation, because of their frailty and inability to defend themselves [130]. At the same time, modernization processes can greatly loosen intergenerational solidarity and the emotional closeness among family members under the same roof, which undermines their capability to stand together to cope with adversity or transition [139]. When faced with unexpected family crises that exceed the family's resources and ability to cope, family members vent their frustration on their older relatives [148, 149]. Israeli data reveal that spouses (45 %) and adult children (41 %) are the most common perpetrators of elder abuse, and that most cases involve significant and taxing family transitions [103].

In societies undergoing transition from an agrarian to an industrial economy, a significant determinant of potential abuse is the level of the social network in which an older person is embedded [137]. Unlike traditional culture, which usually involves extensive social networks and mutual aid, diffuse social ties characterize modern culture [77]. Rural-to-urban migration as a by-product of modernization has dramatically changed the previous communal life of Israeli elders, diminishing their number of social contacts and the size of their social network [136], which predicts an increased risk of social isolation [62]. Social isolation is consistently identified as a prominent risk factor for substantiated and reported elder abuse in many ethnic groups [50, 88]. Conversely, an extensive social network seems to protect against elder abuse. This has received empirical support from Sharon and Zoabi [187], according to whom abuse is less serious in rural areas, where villagers lead a communal lifestyle with frequent social contact.

An estimated 16 % of Jewish and 30 % of Arab older Israelis are living with disabilities and geriatric diseases [29]. This frail group is expected to grow, given the unprecedented pace of population aging [25]. Aging and morbidity trends will result in increased numbers of elders in need of intensive care, which will impose a considerable burden on caregivers [53]. An increasing body of literature consistently proposes that elder abuse is derived from a combination of care recipient dependency and caregiver burden [44, 131].

22.1.6.3 Cultural Specific Examples and Attitudes Towards Elder Abuse

Ethnic heterogeneity in multicultural Israel should also be noted. It is anticipated that the perceived needs of family care and the perception of elder abuse can differ greatly between Jewish and Arab societies, due to different religious norms and subcultural values in these two ethnic groups. Jewish society has a higher level of westernization and looser familial solidarity than Arab society [129]. It is interesting to note that the receipt of excessive care from family members is sometimes deemed offensive by older Jewish Israelis, probably due to the unwanted dependency and intrusion upon personal autonomy that support may imply [177]. Apart from informal care received from families, Jewish society also reinforces social responsibility in the provision of care for the elderly [192]. The failure to obtain formal support from the state can lead to a sense of deprivation or abuse among Jewish Israeli elders [47, 192]. Older Jews are also frequent users of community facilities and formal care services [18]. Insufficient support and improper care received from formal caregivers, such as insufficient assistance in ADLs and failure to provide timely responses to warnings of disease, are considered significant forms of abuse [19, 217]. In comparison, Arab Israeli elders make less frequent use of formal services and rely more on informal family care. They thus consider the failure of adult children to provide direct care or financial aid a serious form of abuse [141, 192].

22.1.7 Turkey

Intergenerational relationships in Turkey are mutually influenced by normative values and socioeconomic conditions [155]. Historically, the hierarchical system entitles old people to supreme authority in both domestic and public spheres. Accordingly, young people are expected to respect and obey senior family members [66]. This tradition is reflected in customs such as kissing an elder's hand or placing one's hand upon an elder's forehead [220]. Turkish elders are also considered a source of knowledge and expertise, and an indispensable support in making major decisions [220]. They therefore enjoy reverence, prestige, and special protection in socioeconomic relationships in almost every sphere [166].

22.1.7.1 Changing Intergenerational Relationships

Rooted in the familial values of collectivism and interdependency, Turkish children are expected to embody economic and utilitarian values, by assisting with domestic chores, farming work, and providing elderly care [94]. Autonomy is not a desirable trait in children in such a familial system, because it presages an individualist lifestyle and separation from the family, which may endanger the survival and integrity of the entire family [95]. Therefore, obedience-oriented childrearing and strong parental control are upheld to secure intergenerational closeness and family stability [93]. Most Turkish elders, in turn depend on their adult offspring for financial, emotional, and instrumental support, due to the lack of an adequate social support network and institutional care systems [110].

During the process of urbanization and westernization, Turkish society has demonstrated patterns of both modernism and traditionalism [14]. Plausibly due to geographical proximity, European modernity has greatly influenced the consumption patterns and lifestyles of young Turkish people [155]. The "autonomous-related self," an idea which refers to identification with material independence, ideological autonomy, but nevertheless emotional interdependence in relation to one's family, has emerged in the familial context [95]. Although maintaining close emotional bonds, younger people no longer feel obliged to provide unconditional material and instrumental aid to their older relatives [212]. The replacement of extended households by nuclear households has further deprived older people of sufficient familial support [106]. Reduced parental authority and the increased autonomy of young people give rise to intergenerational conflict and leads to parental rejection [95]. Furthermore, worsening economic circumstances have imposed financial constraints upon many Turkish families, undermining their ability to provide proper care to older relatives [106]. All these changes in intergenerational relationships have increased the risk of elder abuse [106, 110].

22.1.7.2 Changing Demographic and Social Structures

Unlike other Asian countries, where co-residence is common, the majority of older Turks (63 %) live in their own home [221]. Although most adult children still have regular contact with and provide occasional support to their older parents, separate living has greatly reduced their physical availability to provide parents with sufficient care [52]. This situation has been exacerbated as increasing numbers of Turkish women, who used to be primary caregivers for older relatives, joined the workforce [223]. It is therefore not surprising that elderly abandonment, homelessness, and early nursing home placement have become increasingly common in Turkish society [221].

Only one-third of married Turkish couples co-reside with older relatives, the majority living with the husbands' parents, which reflects a cultural emphasis on the adult son's responsibility for parental care [196, 221]. Although co-residence facilitates the fulfillment of cultural expectations to consolidate family resources and provide mutual support, it can also lead to conflict in Turkey, as elsewhere in Asia [222]. Young Turkish people tend to embrace western values and prefer a modern lifestyle, but older parents usually find it difficult to adapt to sociocultural change [228]. Intergenerational attitudinal divergence and traditionalism can give rise to tension and discord, elder abuse being one of the potential consequences [152]. Additionally, the current older cohort, who grew up in a relatively closed environment, tends to be reluctant to talk about family problems within their household. Such emotional suppression is likely to incubate deeper misunderstanding and foment more intense conflict in the long term [63].

22.1.7.3 Gender Roles

Due to the concept of gender role differentiation, older parents tend to expect their daughters-in-law to take on the majority of the domestic chores, though most are now engaged in full-time employment [104]. In-law conflicts sometimes occur due to disputes over the division of household chores [99]. Intergenerational conflict in the domestic context can increase the risk of elder victimization, as cognitive, physical, and psychological factors usually undermine older people's capacity to defend themselves [216].

22.1.7.4 Cultural Specific Examples and Attitudes Toward Elder Abuse

A negative aging discourse has a strong impact in contemporary Turkey [99]. Being old is often associated with deficiency and worthlessness by Turkish elders themselves [146]. Turkish elders have reported higher level of loneliness, more negative attitudes toward aging, and lower satisfaction with life than their western counterparts [146]. They also stereotypically associate old age with life struggles and health problems [144]. Negative attitudes and psychological resistance to aging have enhanced the likelihood of elder abuse and neglect in Turkey [221].

22.1.8 Iran

Older people have long been deemed as sources of wisdom and experience in Iran [150]. Quranic doctrines stipulate Muslims' obligation to respect and submit to their elders [200] and the value of venerating the elderly finds expression in religious literature and Persian poetry [73]. Older Iranians' supreme social status is reflected in daily intergenerational interactions. For instance, younger people are expected to use respectful language when talking to the elderly [198]. When older persons enter a room, younger people are expected to stand and offer their seat [75]. In almost every context, priority should be given to older people [71]. However, under the influence of social and economic transformation, many younger Iranians are opting for a secular lifestyle and adhere less closely to Muslim religious norms [86]. With the gradual erosion of religion's influence, older Iranians are no longer sure of securing care and respect from their family members [165]. Their loss of prestige within the family has contributed to experiences of loneliness, insecurity, future uncertainty, and increased risk of abuse among the elderly [188].

22.1.8.1 Changing Intergenerational Relationships

Hierarchy, interdependent family relationships, and strict intergenerational solidarity are important characteristics of the traditional Iranian household structure [200]. Family members prefer to live in geographical proximity and have frequent contact so as to maintain emotional bonds and provide mutual support [75]. This interactive pattern has been threatened by the increasing influence of the western values of independence and individualism [227]. Young people who adopt a modern lifestyle tend to be more focused on personal development and feel less obliged to respond to older relatives' needs [150]. Without timely care and necessary support, Iranian elders have become more vulnerable to abandonment, neglect, and abuse [165].

22.1.8.2 Changing Demographic and Social Structures

The pattern of socialization in Iran has been influenced significantly by a series of political events, including but not limited to the Iranian Revolution, the Iraq–Iran War, Islamic sovereignty, and the formation of a democratic government [227]. The current older Iranian cohort was born and raised under Islamic governance prior to the Revolution, when the concept of maintaining a simple, religious life was profoundly rooted [194]. This older generation therefore instinctively avoids luxuries [73]. However, the establishment of democratic governance in the 1990s signified a transformation from traditionalism to modernism [59]. The modern values of materialism and self-reliance introduced by sociopolitical transitions have created intergenerational difference in the social behaviors and communicative patterns between the young and the old [194]. For instance, in contrast to the older generation's disregard for material goods, younger people tend to be materialistic [73]. Differing attitudes toward materialism may sometimes put older people at risk of financial exploitation and financial neglect [188]. In a recent survey, a majority of adult sons (55.8 %) and daughters (63.4 %) were found not to assist their older parents financially [188]. Generational discrepancies in consumption patterns, demeanor, and lifestyle have led to communicational dissatisfaction and intergenerational conflict [73], which is a prominent predictor for elder abuse [188]. Additionally, younger Iranians tend to use less respectful language in daily discourse, which older people consider offensive [15].

22.1.8.3 Cultural Specific Examples and Attitudes Toward Elder Abuse

Elder abuse in Iran demonstrates significant gender variation, with women accounting for 54–63 % of victims of different kinds of abuse [165]. Many cases of elder abuse and neglect could be perpetual partner violence continuing into old age [81, 214]. The prevalence of spousal abuse perpetrated by husbands has been found to range between 38 and 80.8 %, depending on the duration of marriages and the forms of abuse [70, 72, 199]. Primarily due to social discrimination and *shari'a*-based marital laws [178], many battered women remain in abusive relationships for fear of losing child custody and cultural stigma [8]. Therefore, routine screening for domestic violence in obstetrics and gynecology settings is crucial for halting its progress into elder abuse in later years [58].

22.1.9 Bangladesh

Bangladesh remains one of the most rural and poverty-stricken countries in the world, in which familial relationships are dominated by traditional values such as agrarianism, collectivism, and independency [162]. Playing an important role in maintaining older people's well-being, parental support in Bangladesh is mainly based on filial obligation, kin bondage and social norms, rather than on real needs [174]. This form of intergenerational exchange usually comprises unidirectional and imbalanced supportive behaviors flowing from the younger to older generation, without expectation of reciprocation [174]. In view of the significant imbalance in the socioeconomic developments taking place in rural and urban Bangladesh over the past two decades [12], it is expected that patterns of change in intergenerational relationships will differ in these two areas.

22.1.9.1 Rural Bangladesh

A rigid differentiation of gender roles are observed in rural Bangladesh in terms of the division of labor, status, control of power, and social behavior [87]. According to the traditional norms of "purdah" and "virilocality", married Bangladeshi women are generally confined to their husband's household, and obliged to care for their parents-in-law [180]. Therefore, filial caregiving, which is subject to gender bias in the Bangladeshi context, is obligatory for sons and daughters-in-law, but optional for daughters [206]. Regarding the forms of family care, adult sons are obliged to provide financial aid, while daughters-in-law are expected to provide instrumental help and emotional comfort [87]. Rigorous compliance to "purdah" greatly limits a daughter-in-law's social contact with people outside her husband's family and reinforces her submission to her parents-in-law [162]. The ideal daughter-in-law is characterized by unconditional submission and diligent work to meet the requirements of her husband's family [161]. Unfair treatment and abusive behaviors directed toward daughters-in-law by parents-in-law are common in Bangladesh [161]. The status of a daughter-in-law only improves upon the death or frailty of her father-in-law, when her husband becomes the head of the family [180]. Elder abuse can occur when a daughter-in-law takes revenge for the improper treatment she receives from her parents-in-law [54], especially when her husband is absent [182]. Furthermore, it remains traditional for adult sons to inherit their parents' resources, property, and wealth in rural Bangladesh, and so they tend to consider appropriating or misusing their parents' fortune, land, and property as their right [12]. Bangladeshi elders tend to accept and tolerate such financially exploitative behaviors [205].

22.1.9.2 Urban Bangladesh

Urban Bangladesh has experienced a higher level of modernization than the rural areas, which has affected intergenerational solidarity, patterns of functional exchange, and the continuity of elderly care in many families [92]. Some recent findings imply that the nature of familial exchange seems to be changing from obligatory to utilitarian [28]. For instance, the quality of the son–parent relationship can be affected by the quality and quantity of care for grandchildren provided by elderly parents, and relationships that are more rewarding are usually observed between sons and older parents who help with grandchild care [27, 28]. In contrast, nonreciprocal parental care tends to cause caregiver stress and intergenerational tension [7, 112], which predicts a risk of elder abuse [153]. In addition, increasing public participation, economic self-reliance, and exposure to modernity have resulted in young women refusing passivity and acquiescence with family decisions, which may precipitate the occurrence of family tension [91]. The disruption of working women's engagement in domestic chores can further intensify in-law conflict [112]. One of the detrimental results of in-law conflict and intergenerational tension is elder abuse [206].

The consequences of abuse can be particularly threatening for female Bangladeshi elders [176]. Living in a society under male domination, Bangladeshi women have very limited opportunities to earn an income and rely entirely on their male relatives for financial support [175]. Abandonment by adult sons or husbands can leave older Bangladeshi women destitute and even at risk of mortality [173]. More recent findings have concluded that gender discrimination, widowhood, childlessness, and old age constitute the most significant factors for abuse and premature mortality among older women in Bangladesh [2, 153]. It has also been noted that many Bangladeshi women of middle and reproductive age are subject to long-term spousal abuse [89]. Without timely intervention, perpetual spousal violence may progress into elder abuse in the future. Unfortunately, older Bangladeshi women are generally unable to seek help for abuse, mainly due to their inferior social status, low educational level, and ignorance about available supportive resources [5].

22.1.10 Nepal

Nepalese social and economic development has remained stagnant over the last few decades [55]. Partly due to the geographical remoteness, slow social change, and limited international exposure of the country, many Nepalese families remain traditional, agrarian, and sexually biased [219].

The differentiation of gender roles is significant in Nepalese society, with women subjected to implicit and explicit discrimination in almost all domains of social interaction and economic relationship [20]. The customs of inheritance explicitly deprive women of the right to own productive resources, resulting in their financial dependence on male family members [13]. Due to the patrifocal residence system and patrilineal descent prescribed by Hindu religious norms, married women must co-reside with their husband's extended family and participate in the family production [16]. These cultural norms further lead to women's submission to their husbands' families throughout their life [171]. A clear gender division of labor is also observed in Nepali society. Women's activities are usually limited to unpaid domestic work in and around their husbands' household, such as handcrafts, farming, and housework. In contrast, men dominate the formal labor market and paid employment [4]. Such a gender bias in social production has contributed to an economic gap between genders, with men controlling the majority of social resources and family wealth [31]. Gender discrimination is also manifested in prejudiced investment in human capital: school admission rates for Nepalese boys and girls stand at 57 and 27 %, respectively [55]. Meanwhile, the patriarchal legacy of male authority and female obedience has further negated women's autonomy in decision-making and participation in activities outside the family unit [16]. Financial constraints, low educational levels, insufficient engagement in public activities, and lack of control over family resources leave Nepalese women vulnerable to unfair treatment and abuse [69]. Such gender-based abuse can persist over years and continue into old age, mainly because discriminatory social norms prohibit women from changing their traditionally assigned role or circumstances [55]. It is therefore not surprising that the majority of abuse cases in Nepal involve older women [22]. Another worrying issue regarding elder abuse in Nepal is its inheritable nature. Due to relatively closed living environments, the culture of inheritance is strengthened in Nepalese families, most obviously reflected in parental model effects and intergenerational transmission of ideologies and lifestyles [160]. It is therefore very likely that domestic violence against older women is transmitted from one generation to the next [160, 171].

22.2 Social Responses

The discussion of elder abuse remains a taboo across Asia. In recent years, however, Asian societies have begun to acknowledge the phenomenon and steps have been taken to assess the extent of the problem, as evidenced by the increasing number of cases recorded by social services agencies, greater coverage by the media, and policy reforms in relevant areas. Much progress has been made in various representative countries and regions in Asia, including the PRC, Hong Kong, India, Japan, and Singapore, in dealing with this public health and human rights issue [186]. Significant progress has also been made in combating elder abuse in Asian societies since the Second World Assembly on Ageing in 2002, which raised awareness of elder abuse issues in the international community and encouraged governments to develop and fund national strategies to detect, prevent, and intervene in cases of elder abuse [213]. Such proactive steps by the international community have prompted countries to give higher priority to elderly protection in their national agenda through raising public awareness, facilitating policy reform, and introducing societal interventions and support services to alter abusive environments that put older populations at risk [156]. More recently, a number of Asian countries and regions have started observing World Elder Abuse Awareness Day (WEAAD), an initiative of the International Network for the Prevention of Elder Abuse (INPEA) [186].

22.3 Discussion

Researchers around the world have produced a substantial amount of literature on elder abuse. A certain level of understanding has been acquired of the severity of the problem, its predictors and consequences. However, research on elder abuse in Asian societies remains comparatively underrepresented in the overall body of work. One possible reason is that Asian scholarship has not been adequately represented in mainstream English language journals. In light of the increasingly international nature of the academic readership in this area, Asian scholars should be encouraged to publish in English language journals in order to disseminate their findings and ideas on a global scale. It would be beneficial for international readers if articles written in Asian languages were supplemented by an English summary, which would allow readers to acquire a general understanding of the major findings.

Cultural sensitivity remains an essential issue for research on elder abuse in Asian societies. Aforementioned, older people in Asia tend to define elder abuse differently based on their cultural expectations. It is thus necessary to employ culturally sensitive instruments when examining culturally specific forms of abuse. Instruments that allow for cross-cultural comparisons while attending to cultural specific forms of elder abuse is much needed. Regarding Asian elders' common reluctance to disclose their experiences of abuse to people outside their family, efforts should be made to develop an affinity with older persons. Routine screening at medical care units, as well as in the community would be helpful in early detection and intervention of abuse. Another possibility to reach out to abuse victims would be through the persons' social network. As is evident, older Aisans are reluctants to disclose their abuse experience to people outside of their families but are generally trusting to people in their close social networks. Prevention and intervention efforts should thus target the community. Public education programs on the community levels that raise awareness of and sensitivity to elder abuse issues, coupled with effective mechanisms to report abuse, and support programs for victims and abusers are essential. For research purpose, obtaining data through indirect informants regarding incidents they have witnessed or heard of is a feasible alternative to traditional data collection that focuses on first-hand experiences.

Asian cultures share a number of common cultural values, the strong emphasis placed on filial piety and intergenerational support, respects for older persons, patriarchal family structure, etc. Despites these shared values, Asian cultures are very different due to the different history and cultural heiritage. Various Asian societies are also undergoing different levels of social changes and have very different levels of exposure to Western ideology. In researching elder abuse in Asian populations, it is important not to overgeneralize the similarity among Asian cultures. Even within the same ethnic group, say Chinese for an example, people living in rural and urban areas may be very different. Researchers interested in the association between cultural values and elder abuse will need to pay special attention to this. In future studies, every effort should be made to identify the common groups and similarity among different cultural groups in Asia while paying attention to their differences.

Furthermore, one should not overestimate the difference between the "east" and the "west", with advances in technology; globalization has impact on every aspects of our lives. People in Asia, young and old, can easily assess information from western societies. The influx of information, changes in lifestyles will narrow the gaps between Asian societies and the west. Closely related to globalization are the changing economic and political circumstances in Asia, economic development and government policies have important implications for the aging experience and elder care. Researchers interested in studying elder abuse in Asian societies will also need to consider this in formulating their research.

To conclude, elder abuse will be a prominent issue for global gerontology, given the large proportion of the older population relative to the international population. It is important for scholars, practitioners, policymakers, and other stakeholders to work together to address this important issue.

References

1. Abedin S. Living and care arrangements of the elderly in Bangladesh. In: Kabir M, editor. The elderly—contemporary issues. Dhaka: Dhaka Presidency Press; 2003. p. 100–7.
2. Aboderin I. Modernisation and ageing theory revisited: Current explanations of recent developing world and historical Western shifts in material family support for older people. Ageing Soc. 2004;24:29–50.
3. Acharya M, Bennett L. Women and the subsistence sector: economic participation and household decisionmaking in Nepal. World Bank Staff Working Paper, 526, Washington, D.C. 1983.
4. Ahmed SM, Tomson G, Petzold M, Kabir ZN. Socioeconomic status overrides age and gender in determining health seeking behavior in rural Bangladesh. Bull World Health Organ. 2005;83 (2):109–17.
5. Alhaj M. Kinship and modernization in developing societies: the emergence of instrumentalized kinship. J Comp Fam Stud 1995;26:311–328.
6. Amin I, Ingman S. Eldercare in the transnational setting: insights from Bangladeshi transnational families in the United States. J Cross Cult Gerontol. 2014;29:315–28.
7. Amin AF. Violence against women. Women's Participation Research Center of Kurdistan Province: Sanandaj, Islamic Republic of Iran; 2000.
8. Anetzberger GJ, Yamada Y. A telephone counseling program for elder abuse in Japan. Journal of Elder Abuse & Neglect. 1999;11 (1):105–12.
9. Apostolou M. Parental choice: what parents want in a son-in-law and a daughter-in-law across 67 pre-industrial societies. Br J Psychol. 2010;101:695–704.
10. Arai M. Elder abuse in Japan. Educ Gerontol. 2006;32:13–23.
11. Asadullah MN. Intergenerational wealth mobility in rural Bangladesh. J Dev Stud. 2011;48(9):1193–208.
12. Asian Development Bank. Women in Nepal. Country Briefing Paper. Manila: Asian Development Bank; 1999.
13. Aykan H, Wolf DA. Traditionality, modernity and household composition: parent–child coresidence in contemporary Turkey. Res Aging. 2000;22(4):395–421.
14. Azadarmaki T. Generational changing process: a meta analysis of study survey in Iran. Youth Intergener Relatsh. 2007;1:41–68.
15. Baker J. Women's health in Nepal: the neglected dimension. J Nepal Med Assoc. 1994;32(111):214–8.
16. Baldassar L. Transnational families and aged care: the mobility of care and the migrancy of ageing. J Ethnic Migr Stud. 2007;33 (2):275–97.
17. Ben NM, Ariela L. Study of factors that affect abuse of older people in nursing homes. Nurs Manag. 2010;17(8):20–4.
18. Ben NM, Lowenstein A, Eisikovits Z. Psycho-social factors affecting elders' maltreatment in long-term care facilities. Int Nurs Rev. 2010;57(1):113–20.
19. Bennett L. Gender, caste and ethnic exclusion in Nepal. World Bank. Unpublished; 2005.
20. Bhat AK, Dhruvarajan R. Aging in India: drifting intergenerational relations, challenge, and options. Aging Soc. 2001;21:621–40.
21. Bhattarai LPS. Neglect and abuse of older people in Nepal: a commentary on a baseline study on reported cases of elder abuse in Nepali press. J Elder Abuse Negl. 2014;26(3):333–6.
22. Bian F, Logan JR, Bian Y. Intergenerational relations in urban China: proximity, contact, and help to parents. Demography. 1998;35:115–24.

23. Biggs S, Haapala I. Elder mistreatment, ageism, and human rights. Int Psychogeriatr. 2013;25:1299–306.
24. Brodsky J, Shnoor Y, Be'er S. The elderly in Israel: statistical abstract. Jerusalem: Brookdale Institute; 2009.
25. Brodsky J, Shnoor Y, Be'er S. The elderly in Israel: statistical abstract. Jerusalem: Brookdale Institute; 2014.
26. Burholt V, Dobbs C. Caregiving and carereceiving relationships of older south Asians: functional exchange and emotional closeness. GeroPsych. 2010;23(4):215–25.
27. Burholt V, Wenger GC. Families and migration: Older people from South Asia. Final report to the Department for International Development, Project ESA315. Bangor: University of Wales, Centre for Social Policy Research and Development; 2003.
28. Central Bureau of Statistics. Statistical abstracts of Israel. Jerusalem: Author; 2009.
29. Chadha NK. Understanding intergenerational relationships in India. J Intergener Relatsh. 2004;2:63–73.
30. Chalise HN, Saito T, Takahashi M, Kai I. Relationship specialization amongst sources and receivers of social support and its correlations with loneliness and subjective well-being: a cross sectional study of Nepalese older adults. Arch Gerontol Geriatr. 2007;44:299–314.
31. Chan KL. Protection of face and avoidance of responsibility: Chinese men's account of violence against women. J Soc Work Pract. 2009;23:93–108.
32. Chan H, Lee RPL. Hong Kong families: at the crossroads of modernism and traditionalism. J Comp Fam Stud. 1995;26 (1):83–99.
33. Chang GL, Chang CO. Transitions in living arrangements and living preferences among elderly: an analysis from family values and exchange theory. J Popul Stud. 2010;40(1):41–90.
34. Chang J, Moon A. Korean American elderly's knowledge and perceptions of elder abuse: a qualitative analysis of cultural factors. J Multicult Soc Work. 1997;6:139–55.
35. Chappell NL, Kusch K. The gendered nature of filial piety: a study among Chinese Canadians. J Cross Cult Gerontol. 2007;22:29–45.
36. Cheng ST, Chan ACM. Filial piety and psychological well-being in well older Chinese. J Gerontol Psychol Sci. 2006;61B:262–9.
37. Cheung CK, Kwan YH. The erosion of filial piety by modernization in Chinese cities. Ageing Soc. 2009;29:179–98.
38. Chi I. Development in long term care for frail elderly people in Hong Kong. In M. Knapp, D. Challis, & A. Netten. (Ed.), Long term care: Matching resources and needs. U.K.: Gower Publishing, Ashgate. 2004.
39. Choi JS. Hanguk eui chogi sawheihak kwa kajok yungu, [Early studies on sociology and family in Korea]. Seoul: Iillji sa; 2002.
40. Chokkanathan S, Lee AE. Elder mistreatment in urban India: a community based study. J Elder Abuse Negl. 2005;17:45–61.
41. Chokkanathan S, Natarajan A, Mohanty J. Elder abuse and barriers to help seeking in Chennai, India: a qualitative study. J Elder Abuse Negl. 2014;26(1):60–79.
42. Chou RJA. Filial piety by contract? The emergence, implementation, and implications of the 'Family Support Agreement' in China. Gerontologist. 2011;51:3–16.
43. Chu CYC, Xie Y, Yu RR. Coresidence with elderly parents: A comparative study of southeast China and Taiwan. J Marriage Fam. 2011;73:120–35.
44. Cohen M, Shinan-Altman S. A cross-sectional study of nursing aids' attitudes to elder abuse in nursing homes. Int Psychogeriatr. 2011;23(8):1213–21.
45. Cong Z, Silverstein M. Intergenerational exchange between parents and migrant and nonmigrant sons in rural China. J Marriage Fam. 2011;73:93–104.
46. Deutsch FM. Filial piety, patrilineality, and China's one-child policy. J Fam Issues. 2006;27:366–89.
47. Diener E, Suh EM, Lucas RE, Smith HL. Subjective well-being: three decades of progress. Psychol Bull. 1999;125:276–302.
48. Dong X, Simon MA, Gorbien M. Elder abuse and neglect in an urban Chinese population. J Elder Abuse Negl. 2007;19(3–4):79–96.
49. Dong X, Simon MA, Gorbien MJ, Percak BA, Golden R. Loneliness in older Chinese adults: a risk factor for elder mistreatment. J Am Geriatr Soc. 2007;55:1832–5.
50. Dong XQ, Wilson RS, Mendes de Leon CF, Evans DA. Self-neglect and cognitive function among community-dwelling older persons. Int J Geriatr Psychiatry. 2010;26:798–806.
51. Du P. Intergenerational solidarity and old-age support for the social inclusion of elders in Mainland China: the changing roles of family and government. Ageing Soc. 2013;33:44–63.
52. Durgun B, Tümerdem Y. Urbanization and services for the elderly. Turk J Geriatr. 1999;2(3):115–20.
53. Dwyer JW, Folts WE, Rosenberg E. Caregiving in social context. Educ Gerontol. 1994;20:615–31.
54. Ellickson J. Never the Twains shall meet: aging men and women in Bangladesh. J Cross Cult Gerontol. 1988;3(1):53–70.
55. Emran MS, Shilpi F. Intergenerational occupational mobility in rural economy evidence from Nepal and Vietnam. J Hum Resour. 2010;46(2):427–58.
56. Even-Zohar A, Sharlin S. Grandchildhood: adult grandchildren's perception of their role towards their grandparents from an intergenerational perspective. J Comp Fam Stud. 2009;40 (2):167–85.
57. Fan R. Confucian filial piety and long term care for aged parents. HEC Forum. 2006;18(1):1–17.
58. Faramarzi M, Esmailzadeh S, Mosavi S. Prevalence and determinants of intimate partner violence in Babol City, Islamic Republic of Iran. Eastern Mediter Health J. 2005;11(5–6):870–9.
59. Fazeli N. Modern ya emruzi shodane farhange Irani [modernization or Contemporization of the Iranian Culture]. Tehran: Pazhooheshkadeye Motalaate Farhangi va Ejtemaee; 2008.
60. Fei X. From the soil: the foundations of Chinese society (G. G. Hamilton & W. Zheng, Trans.). Berkeley: University of California Press; 1992.
61. Feldman MW, Tuljapurkar S, Li S, Jin X, Li N. Son preference, marriage, and intergenerational transfers in rural China. Int Stud Popul. 2007;3:139–62.
62. Fernandez-Ballesteros R, Zamarron MD, Ruiz MA. The contribution of socio-demographic and psychosocial factors to life satisfaction. Ageing Soc. 2001;21:25–43.
63. Fingerman KL. Ageing mothers and their adult daughters: a study of mixed emotions. New York: Springer; 2001.
64. Fingerman KL, Gilligan M, VanderDrift L, Pitzer LM. In-law relationships before and after marriage: Husbands, wives, and their mothers-in-law. Res Hum Dev. 2012;9:106–25.
65. Fingerman KL, Cheng YP, Kim K, Fung HH, Han G, Lang FR, et al. Parental involvement with college students in Germany, Hong Kong, Korea, and the United States. J Fam Issues 2014;37:1384–1411.
66. Fiâek GO. A cross-cultural examination of proximity and hierarchy as dimensions of family structure. Fam Process. 1991;30:121–33.
67. Fujiwara T, Okuyama M, Izumi M. The impact of childhood abuse history, domestic violence and mental health symptoms on parenting behaviour among mothers in Japan. Child Care Health Dev. 2012;38:530–7.
68. Funk LM. Responsibility for aging parents: reconciling independence and obligation within filial relationships. Dissertation, Victoria: University of Victoria; 2007.

69. Gautam R, Saito T, Houde SC, Kai I. Social interactions and depressive symptoms among community dwelling older adults in Nepal: a synergic effect model. Arch Gerontol Geriatr. 2011;53:24–30.
70. Ghahhari S, Mazdarani S, Khalilian A, Zarghami M. Spouse abuse in Sari-Iran. Iranian J Psychiatry Behav Sci. 2008;2(1):31–5.
71. Ghazi-Tabatabaei M, Karimi Z. Socio-demographic, economic and structural correlates of intergenerational support of the elderly in Iran. Ageing Int. 2011;36:428–44.
72. Ghazizadeh A. Domestic violence: a cross-sectional study in an Iranian city. Eastern Mediter Health J. 2005;11(5):880–7.
73. Giles H, Khajavy GH, Choi CW. Intergenerational communication satisfaction and age boundaries: comparative Middle Eastern data. J Cross Cult Gerontol. 2012;27:357–71.
74. Giles J, Mu R. Elderly parent health and the migration decisions of adult children: evidence from Rural China. Demography. 2007;44(2):265–88.
75. Giles H, Noels KA, Williams A, Ota H, Lim TS, Ng SH, et al. Intergenerational communication across cultures: young people's perceptions of conversations with family elders, non-family elders, and same-age peers. J Cross Cult Gerontol. 2003;18:1–30.
76. Gu D, Vlosky AD, Zeng Y. Gender differentials in transitions and expected years spending in seven living arrangements among the oldest-old in China: a population-based decrement-increment life table analysis. In: Benninghouse HT, Rosset AG, editors. Women and aging: new research. New York: Nova Publisher; 2009. p. 539–75.
77. Haj-Yahia MM. Toward culturally sensitive intervention with Arab families in Israel. Contemp Fam Ther. 1995;17:429–47.
78. HelpAge India. Elder abuse in India: Summary of research reports. 2012. http://www.helpageindia.org/helpageprd/download.php?fp=aW1hZ2VzL3B1Ymxpc2hpbmc=&f=MTMwNzA4MDExMS5wZGY=.
79. HelpAge International. Aging in the 21st Century. HelpAge International, 2012.
80. HelpAge International. Global age watch. 2013. http://www.helpage.org/global-agewatch/.
81. Hightower J. Abuse in later life: when and how does gender matter? In: Gloria G, Charmaine S, editors. Aging, ageism and abuse. London: Elsevier; 2010. p. 17–29.
82. Ho DYF. Filial piety and its psychological consequences. In: Bond MH, editor. The handbook of Chinese psychology. Hong Kong: Oxford University Press; 1996. p. 155–65.
83. Holroyd EE. Chinese family obligations toward chronically ill elderly members: comparing caregivers in Beijing and Hong Kong. Qual Health Res. 2003;13(3):302–218.
84. Hong Kong Christian Service. Elder abuse in Hong Kong. 2004. http://www.swd.gov.hk/doc/family/eld_abuse_rep.pdf.
85. Hooyman NR, Kiyark HA. Social gerontology. Boston: Allyn and Bacon; 1991.
86. Irudaya RS, Sankara SP, Mishra US. Demography of Indian Aging. In: Phoebe SL, Irudaya RS, editors. An aging India: perspecitives, prospects and policies. Rawat: Jaipur; 2005. p. 2001–51.
87. Jesmin S, Salway S. Marriage among the urban poor of Bangladesh: instability and uncertainty. J Int Dev. 2000;12(5):689–705.
88. Jogerst GJ, Dawson JD, Hartz AJ, Ely JW, Schweitzer LA. Community characteristics associated with elder abuse. J Am Geriatr Soc. 2000;48:513–8.
89. Johnston HB, Naved RT. Spousal violence in Bangladesh: a call for a public-health response. Journal of Health, Population, and Population. 2008;26(3):366–77.
90. Jung K, Honig AS. Intergenerational comparisons of paternal Korean childrearing practices and attitudes. Early Child Dev Care. 2000;165:59–84.
91. Kabeer N. Conflicts over credit: re-evaluating the empowerment potential of loans to women in rural Bangladesh. World Dev. 2001;29:63–84.
92. Kabir MH. Family structure and composition and care of the elderly in Bangladesh. In: United Nations (ed.) Implications of Asia's population future for older people in the family. Asian Population Studies Series No. 145. New York, NY: UN Economic and Social Commission for Asia and the Pacific, 1996.
93. Kagîtçıbası Ç. Autonomy and relatedness in cultural context: Implications for self and family. J Cross Cult Psychol. 2005;36:403–22.
94. Kagîtçıbası Ç, Ataca B. Value of children and family change: a three-decade portrait from Turkey. Appl Psychol Int Rev. 2005;54:317–38.
95. Kagîtçıbası Ç, Ataca B, Diri A. Intergenerational relationships in the family: ethnic, socioeconomic, and country variations in Germany, Israel, Palestine, and Turkey. J Cross Cult Psychol. 2010;41:652–70.
96. Kalavar JM, Jamuna D. Aging of Indian women in India: the experience of older women in formal care homes. J Women Aging. 2011;23:1–24.
97. Kalavar J, Van WJ. Older Asian Indians resettled in America: narratives about households, culture and generation in. J Cross Cult Gerontol. 2005;20:213–30.
98. Kalavar JM, Zarit SH, Ferraccio BJ. Transnational support of Asian Indian elderly in India: examining patterns of exchanges. Care Manag J. 2015;16(3):141–9.
99. Kalaycıoglu S, Rittersberger-Tılıç H. Intergenerational solidarity networks of instrumental and cultural transfers within migrant families: a sample from Turkey. Ageing Soc. 2000;20:523–42.
100. Kasuga K. Changing family structure and elder abuse issues in Japan. Geriatr Gerontol Int. 2004;4(s1):S226–8.
101. Katz R. Intergenerational family relations and life satisfaction among three elderly population groups in transition in the Israeli multi-cultural society. J Cross Cult Gerontol. 2009;27:77–91.
102. Katz R, Lowenstein A. Solidarity between generations and elders' life satisfaction: comparing Jews and Arabs in Israel. J Intergener Relatsh. 2012;10(1):5–21.
103. Katzman B, Litwin H. Protection of elderly people and prevention of violence against them in Herzelia. Jerusalem: National Insurance Institute; 2002.
104. Kağıtçıbaşı C. Individualism and collectivism. In: Berry JW, Segall MH, Kağıtçıbaşı C, editors. Handbook of cross-cultural psychology. London: Allyn and Bacon; 1998. p. 1–49.
105. Kemp CL. Dimensions of grandparent–adult grandchild relationships: from family ties to intergenerational friendships. Can J Aging. 2005;24(2):161–78.
106. Keskinoglu P, Pýcakcýefe M, Bilgic N, Giray H, Karakus N, Ucku R. Elder abuse and neglect in two different socioeconomic districts in Izmir, Turkey. Int Psychogeriatr. 2007;19(4):719–31.
107. Kim HG. Aging of the population and the subsequent increase in the mistreatment of the elderly in Korea. Nurs Health Sci. 2002;4:A1–2.
108. Kim CS. Intergenerational family relationships of the elderly in Korea. Korea J. 2008;48(4):35–59.
109. Kim K, Zarit S, Fingerman K, Han G. Intergenerational exchanges of middle-aged adults with their parents and parents-in-law in Korea. J Marriage Fam. 2015;77:791–805.
110. Kissal A, Beşer A. Elder abuse and neglect in a population offering care by a primary health care center in Izmir, Turkey. Soc Work Health Care. 2011;50(2):158–75.

111. Kobayashi KM. Of the family tree: congruence on filial obligation between older parents and adult children in Japanese Canadian families. Can J Aging. 2010;29:85–96.
112. Koenig MA, Saifuddin A, Mian BH, Mozumder KA. Women's status and domestic violence in rural Bangladesh: individual- and community-level effects. Demography. 2003;40(2):269–88.
113. Kozu J. Domestic violence in Japan. Am Psychol. 1999;54:50–4.
114. Lam RC. Contradictions between traditional Chinese values and the actual performance: a study of the caregiving roles of the modern sandwich generation in Hong Kong. J Comp Fam Stud. 2006;37(2):299–312.
115. Lamb S. Independence, intergenerational uncertainty, and the ambivalent state: perceptions of old age security in India. South Asia J South Asian Stud. 2013;36:65–78.
116. Lan P. Subcontracting filial piety: elder care in ethnic Chinese immigrant families in California. J Fam Issues. 2002;23 (7):812–35.
117. Lavee Y, Katz R. The family in Israel: between tradition and modernity. Marriage Fam Rev. 2003;35:193–217.
118. Lee M. A path analysis on elder abuse by family caregivers: Applying the ABCX model. J Fam Violence. 2008;23:707–12.
119. Lee KS. Gender, care work, and the complexity of family membership in Japan. Gender Soc. 2010;24:647–71.
120. Lee YB. Intergenerational caregiving and conflict between daughters/daughters-in-law and their elderly parents/parents-in-law [in Korean]. Fam Cult. 2011;23:41–76.
121. Lee HY, Eaton CK. Financial abuse in elderly Korean immigrants: mixed analysis of the role of culture on perception and help-seeking intention. J Gerontol Soc Work. 2009;52:463–88.
122. Lee M, Kolomer SR. Caregiver burden, dementia, and elder abuse in South Korea. J Elder Abuse Negl. 2005;17:61–74.
123. Lee YR, Sung KT. Cultural differences in caregiving motivations for demented parents: Korean caregivers versus American caregivers. Int J Aging Hum Dev. 1997;44:115–27.
124. Lee JE, Zarit SH, Rovine MJ, Birditt KS, Fingerman KL. Middle-aged couples' exchanges of support with aging parents: patterns and association with marital satisfaction. Gerontology. 2012;58:88–96.
125. Li S, Feldman MW, Jin X. Children, marriage form, and family support for the elderly in contemporary rural China: the case of Songzi. Res Aging. 2004;26:352–84.
126. Liebig P. An aging India. Binghamton: Haworth Press; 2005.
127. Lin AH. Study of filial piety in Confucian thought. Taipei: Wen Jin; 1992.
128. Lin JP, Yi CC. A comparative analysis of intergenerational relations in East Asia. Int Sociol. 2013;28:297–315.
129. Litwin H. Intergenerational exchange and mental health in later-life—the case of older Jewish Israelis. Aging Mental Health. 2004;8(3):196–200.
130. Litwin H, Zoabi S. Modernization and elder abuse in an Arab-Israeli context. Res Aging. 2003;25(3):224–46.
131. Litwin H, Zoabi S. A multivariate examination of explanations for the occurrence of elder abuse. Soc Work Res. 2004;28 (3):133–42.
132. Long SO, Campbell R, Nishimura C. Does it matter who cares? A comparison of daughters versus daughters-in-law in Japanese elder care. Soc Sci Jpn J. 2009;12:1–21.
133. Long SO, Harris PB. Gender and elder care: social change and the role of the caregiver in Japan. Soc Sci Jpn J. 2000;3(1):21–36.
134. Lowell BL, Gerova SG. Immigrants and the healthcare workforce: profiles and shortages. Work Occup. 2004;31(4):474–98.
135. Lowenstein A. Solidarity-conflict and ambivalence: testing two conceptual frameworks and their impact on quality of life for older family members. J Gerontol Soc Sci. 2007;62:100–7.
136. Lowenstein A, Doron I. Times of transition: elder abuse and neglect in Israel. J Elder Abuse Negl. 2008;20(2):181–206.
137. Lowenstein A, Eisikovits Z, Band-Winterstein T, Enosh G. Is elder abuse and neglect a social phenomenon? Data from the first national prevalence survey in Israel. J Elder Abuse Negl. 2009;21 (3):253–77.
138. Lowenstein A, Katz R. Living arrangements, family solidarity and life satisfaction of two generations of immigrants in Israel. Ageing Soc. 2005;25(5):749–67.
139. Lowenstein A, Katz R. Intergenerational family relations in the multicultural society of Israel. J Intergener Relatsh. 2015;13 (1):1–5.
140. Lowenstein A, Katz R, Daatland S. Filial norms and intergenerational support in Europe and Israel: a comparative perspective. In: Silverstein M, Schaie KW, editors. Annual review of gerontology and geriatrics. New York: Springer; 2005. p. 200–14.
141. Lowenstein A, Katz R, Gur-Yaish N. Reciprocity in parent–child exchange and life satisfaction among the elderly: a cross-national perspective. J Soc Issues. 2007;63:865–83.
142. Luo B, Zhan H. Filial Piety and functional support: understanding intergenerational solidarity among families with migrated children in rural China. Ageing Int. 2012;37:69–92.
143. Mandemakers JJ, Dykstra PA. Discrepancies in parent's and adult child's reports of support and contact. J Marriage Fam. 2008;70:495–506.
144. Mandiracioglu A, Çam O. Problems of homes for older people employees and their views about older people. Turk J Geriatr. 2004;7(1):29–32.
145. Mao W, Chi I. Filial piety of children as perceived by aging parents in China. Int J Soc Welf. 2011;20:S99–108.
146. McConatha JT, Hayta V, Teiser-Danner L, McConatha D, Polat TS. Turkish and U.S. attitudes toward aging. Educ Gerontol. 2004;30:169–83.
147. Meir A, Ben-David Y. Welfare support for Israeli Negev-Bedouin elderly men: Adaption during spacioecologic transformation. Gerontologist. 1993;33:308–14.
148. Mitrani VB, Lewis JE, Feaster DJ, Czaja SJ, Eisdorfer C. The role of family functioning in the stress process of dementia caregivers. Gerontologist. 2006;46(1):97–105.
149. Mittelman MS. Preserving health of Alzheimer caregivers: impact of a spouse caregiver intervention. Am J Geriatr Psychiatry. 2007;15(9):780–9.
150. Mohseni-Tabrizi A, Homayunpoor H. Examining elderly people situation in Iran. Soc Secur J. 2001;2:191–208.
151. Moon A, Tomita SK, Jung-Kamei S. Elder mistreatment among four Asian American groups: an exploratory study on tolerance, victim blaming and attitudes toward third-party intervention. J Gerontol Soc Work. 2001;36:153–69.
152. Mottram SA, Hortacsu N. The effects of social change on relationships between older mothers and daughters in Turkey: a qualitative study. Ageing Soc. 2005;25:675–91.
153. Munsur AM, Tareque I, Rahman KMM. Determinants of living arrangements, health status and abuse among elderly women: a study of rural Naogaon District, Bangladesh. J Int Women's Stud. 2010;11:162–76.
154. Nagpaul K. Elder abuse among Asian Indians: traditional versus modern perspectives. J Elder Abuse Negl. 1998;9:77–92.
155. Nauck B, Suckow J. Intergenerational relationships and cross-cultural comparison: how social networks frame intergenerational relations between mothers and grandmothers in Japan, Korea, China, Indonesia, Israel, Germany, and Turkey. J Fam Issues. 2006;27(8):1159–85.
156. Nerenberg L. Communities respond to elder abuse. In: Mellor MJ, Brownell P, editors. Elder abuse and mistreatment: policy,

practice and research. Binghamton: The Haworth Press; 2006. p. 5–33.
157. Ng SH, Loong CSF, Liu JH, Weatherall A. Will the young support the old? An individual- and family-level study of filial obligation in two New Zealand cultures. Asian J Soc Psychol. 2000;3:103–82.
158. Ng ACY, Phillips DR, Lee WKM. Persistence and challenges to filial piety and informal support of older persons in a modern Chinese society: a case study in Tuen Mun, Hong Kong. J Aging Stud. 2002;16:135–53.
159. Ngan R, Wong W. Injustice in family care of the Chinese elderly in Hong Kong. J Ageing Soc Policy. 1995;79(2):77–94.
160. Niaz U. Violence against women in South Asia. Arch Women S Mental Health. 2003;6(3):173–84.
161. Nosaka A, Andrews BW. Institutionalized powerlessness in context: the static and dynamic nature of women's status in rural Bangladesh. J Int Women's Stud. 2004;6(1):149–68.
162. Nosaka A, Radheshyam B. Traditional roles, modern behavior: intergenerational intervention and contraception in rural Bangladesh. Hum Organ. 2008;67(4):407–16.
163. Ok SW. Continuity and change in patrilineal culture of Korean families. In: Korean Family Studies Association, editor. Korean families: Continuity and change. Seoul: Seoul National University Press; 2011. p. 1–18.
164. Okonogi K. Seishinbunsekiteki ni mita boryoku no shinri [Psychology of violence from psychoanalytic perspectives]. *Gendaino Esupuri [L'esprit d'aujourd'hui]* 1994; 320, 135–145.
165. Oveisi S, Karimi R, Mahram M. Note from Iran: self-reported elder abuse in Qazvin, 2012. J Elder Abuse Negl. 2014;26 (3):337–40.
166. Ozer M. A study on the life satisfaction of elderly individuals living in family environment and nursing homes. Turk J Geriatr. 2004;7(1):33–6.
167. Park YS, Kim U. Adolescent culture and parent–child relationship in Korea: indigenous psychological analysis. Seoul: Kyoyook Kwahaksa; 2004.
168. Park KS, Kim IK, Kojima H. Intergenerational coresidence and nearness in Korea and Japan: unbalanced aspects of family changes. Int J Jpn Sociol. 1999;8:93–115.
169. Park KS, Phua V, Mcnally J, Sun R. Diversity and structure of intergenerational relationships: Elderly parent-adult child relations in Korea. J Cross Cult Gerontol. 2005;20(4):285–305.
170. Park KS. Geographic proximity between elderly parents and their children in the United States and Japan: convergence of individualism and familism? Unpublished Ph. D. Thesis, Brown University; 1998.
171. Poudel GS. Domestic Violence against Women in Nepal. Gender Technology and Development. 2007;11(2):199–233.
172. Rabindranathan S. Intergenerational co-residence: conflict and resolution in familial contexts in India. Asian J Women's Stud. 2004;58:4–10.
173. Rahman O. The impact of coresident spouses and sons in elderly mortality in rural Bangladesh. J Biosoc Sci. 2000;32:89–98.
174. Rahman MO, Barsky AJ. Self-reported health among older Bangladeshis: how good a health indicator is it? Gerontologist. 2003;43:856–63.
175. Rahman O, Liu J. Gender differences in functioning for older adults in rural Bangladesh: the impact of differences in reporting. J Gerontol Med Sci. 2000;55:28–33.
176. Rahman O, Manken J, Kuhn R. The impact of family members on the self-reported health of older men in a rural area of Bangladesh. Ageing Soc. 2004;24:903–20.
177. Reinhardt JP, Boerner K, Horowitz A. Good to have but not to use: differential impact of perceived and received support on wellbeing. J Soc Pers Relatsh. 2006;23:117–29.
178. Reynolds NY. States of law and sexuality in the Middle East. J Women's Hist. 2015;27(2):182–93.
179. Rozario PA, Rosetti AL. "Many helping hands": a review and analysis of long-term care policies, programs, and practices in Singapore. J Gerontol Soc Work. 2012;55:641.
180. Ruhul A, Mariam AG. Son preference in Bangladesh: an emerging barrier to fertility regulation. J Biosoc Sci. 1987;19 (2):221–8.
181. Schiamberg LB, Gans D. Elder abuse by adult children: an applied ecological framework for understanding contextual risk factors and the intergenerational character of quality of life. Int J Aging Hum Dev. 2000;50:329–59.
182. Schuler SR, Hashemi SM, Riley AP, Akhter S. Credit program, patriarchy, and men's violence against women in rural Bangladesh. Soc Sci Med. 1996;43:1729–42.
183. Schwartz SJ. The applicability of familism to diverse ethnic groups: a preliminary study. J Soc Psychol. 2007;147:101–18.
184. Schwarz B, Trommsdorff G, Kim U, Park Y. Intergenerational support—psychological and cultural analyses of korean and german women. Curr Sociol. 2006;54:315–40.
185. Shah G, Veedon R, Vasi S. Elder abuse in India. J Elder Abuse Negl. 1995;6:101–18.
186. Shankardass MK. Addressing elder abuse: review of societal responses in India and selected Asian countries. Int Psychogeriatr. 2013;25(8):1229–34.
187. Sharon N, Zoabi S. Elder abuse in a land of tradition: the case of Israel's Arabs. J Elder Abuse Negl. 1997;8(4):43–58.
188. Sheykhi MT. Safety and security of older person in threat, Iran: a sociological appraisal of elder abuse. Int J Aging Hum Dev. 2010;71(2):139–52.
189. Shibusawa T, Kodaka M, Iwano S, Kaizu K. Interventions for elder abuse and neglect with frail elders in Japan. Brief Treat Crisis Interv. 2005;5(2):203–11.
190. Silverstein M, Cong Z. Parents' preferred care-givers in rural China: gender, migration and intergenerational exchanges. Ageing Soc. 2014;34:727–52.
191. Silverstein M, Cong Z, Li S. Grandparents who care for their grandchildren in rural China: benefactors and beneficiaries. In: Cook IG, Powell JL, editors. New perspectives on China and aging. New York: Nova Science; 2007. p. 49–71.
192. Silverstein M, Lowenstein A, Katz R, Gans D, Fan YK, Oyama P. Intergenerational support and the emotional well-being of older Jews and Arabs in Israel. J Marriage Fam. 2013;75:950–63.
193. Soeda A, Araki C. Elder abuse by daughters-in-law in Japan. J Elder Abuse Negl. 1999;11(1):47–58.
194. Sohrabzadeh M. Moghayeseye zehniyate nasli va beine nasli dar naslhaye daneshgahipas az enghelabe eslami [Comparison of generational and intergenerational mindset in college generations after Islamic revolution]. Faslnameye Tahghighate Farhangi [Cultural Research Quarterly]. 2010;2:263–94.
195. Sudha S. Intergenerational relations and elder care preferences of Asian Indians in North Carolina. J Cross Cult Gerontol. 2014;29:87–107.
196. Sunar D, Fiâek GO. Contemporary Turkish families. In: Roopnarine JL, Gielen UP, editors. Families in global perspective. Boston: Allyn & Bacon; 2005.
197. Sung KT. Elder respect among young adults: a cross-cultural study of Americans and Koreans. J Aging Stud. 2001;18:215–30.
198. Sung KT, Kim BJ. Respect for the elderly: implications for human service providers. Lanham: University Press of America; 2009.
199. Tabatabai GM, Tabrizi MAR, Marjai SH. Studies on domestic violence against women. Tehran: Office of Public Affairs,

Ministry of Interior. Center of Women and Family Affairs, Presidency of the Islamic Republic of Iran; 2004.
200. Tajvar M, Arab M, Montazeri A. Determinants of health-related quality of life in elderly in Tehran, Iran. BMC Public Health. 2008;8:1–8.
201. Takagi E, Silverstein M. Intergenerational coresidence of the Japanese elderly: are cultural norms proactive or reactive? Res Aging. 2006;28:473–92.
202. Takagi E, Silverstein M. Purchasing Piety? Coresidence of married children with their older parents in Japan. Demography. 2011;48(4):1559–79.
203. Takagi E, Silverstein M, Crimmins E. Intergenerational coresidence of older adults in Japan: conditions for cultural plasticity. J Gerontol Soc Sci. 2007;62:S330–9.
204. Tam S, Neysmith S. Disrespect and isolation: elder abuse in Chinese communities. Can J Aging. 2006;25:141–51.
205. Tareque I, Islam TM, Koshio A, Kawahara K. Economic well-being and elder abuse in Rajshahi district of Bangladesh. Res Aging. 2015;37(2):200–24.
206. Tareque MI, Islam TM, Rahman MM. Determinants of elder abuse in Rajshahi city corporation, Bangladesh: evidence from a micro-level survey. Indian J Gerontol. 2008;22:411–21.
207. Thang LL, Mehta K, Usui T, Tsuruwaka M. Being a good grandparent: roles and expectations in intergenerational relationships in Japan and Singapore. Marriage Family Rev. 2011; 47:548–70.
208. Ting KF, Chiu SWK. Leaving the parental home: Chinese culture in an urban context. J Marriage Fam. 2002;64:614–26.
209. Traphagan JW. Power, family, and filial responsibility related to elder care in rural Japan. Care Manag J. 2006;7:205–12.
210. Tsai HH, Chen MH, Tsai YF. Perceptions of filial piety among Taiwanese university students. J Adv Nurs. 2008;63:284–90.
211. Tsutsui T, Muramatsu N, Higashino S. Changes in perceived filial obligation norms among coresident family caregivers in Japan. Gerontologist. 2013;54:797–807.
212. Tıktık A. Türkiye'de yaşlıların durumu ve ulusal eylem planı. Sosyal Sektörler ve Koordinasyon Genel Müdürlüğü. 2007. http://www.sp.gov.tr/documents/TurkiyedeYaslilarinDurumuveYaslanmaEylemPlani.pdf.
213. United Nations. Political declaration and Madrid international plan of action on ageing. New York: United Nations; 2002.
214. Vakili M, Nadrian H, Fathipoor M, Boniadi F, Morowatisharifabad MA. Prevalence and determinants of intimate partner violence against women in Kazeroon, Islamic Republic of Iran. Violence Vict. 2010;25(1):116–27.
215. VandeWeerd CV, Paveza GJ. Verbal mistreatment in older adults: a look at persons with Alzheimer's disease and their caregivers in the state of Florida. J Elder Abuse Negl. 2006;17 (4):11–30.
216. VandeWeerd C, Paveza GJ, Walsh M, Corvin J. Physical mistreatment in persons with Alzheimer's disease. J Aging Res. 2013;2013:1–10.
217. Winterstein TB. Nurses' experiences of the encounter with elder neglect. J Nurs Scholarsh. 2012;44(1):55–62.
218. Winther J. Household enumeration in national discourse: three moments in modern Japanese history. Soc Sci Hist. 2008;32:19–46.
219. World Bank (2006) Resilience amidst conflict. An assessment of poverty in Nepal, 1995–1996 and 2003–2004. Report No. 34834-NP. Washington: The World Bank.
220. Yalçinkaya A. Family violence in Turkey. In: Malley-Morrison K, editor. International perspectives on family violence and abuse: a cognitive ecological approach (Chapter 8). Mahwah: Erlbaum; 2004.
221. Yalçinkaya A, Mandracoğlu A, Turan F. Turkey: a pilot study of elder mistreatment in a convenience sample. J Elder Abuse Negl. 2006;18(2–3):105–21.
222. Yalçinkaya A, Turan F, Rapoza K. North American and Turkish young adults' attitudes toward elder abuse. Poster presented at the meeting of the American Psychological Association, Washington, DC; 2000.
223. Yalçãnkaya A, Turan F, Rapoza K. North American and Turkish young adults' attitudes toward elder abuse. Poster presented at the meeting of the American Psychological Association, Washington, DC; 2000.
224. Yan E. Abuse of older persons with dementia by family caregivers: results of a 6-month prospective study in Hong Kong. Int J Geriatr Psychiatry. 2014;29:1018–27.
225. Yan E, Tang C. Prevalence and psychological impact of Chinese elder abuse. J Interpers Violence. 2001;16:1158–74.
226. Yao C, Yu H. The impact of rural–urban migration on rural elder care system. Market and Demography. 2005;11:2 (In Chinese).
227. Yazdani E, Ghaderi A. Generation gap; sociological investigation of generation distance from Islamic revolution to the present. Islamic Revolut Stud. 2011;8:207–38.
228. Yeh KH, Bedford O. Filial belief and parent–child conflict. Int J Psychol. 2004;39:132–44.
229. Yeh KH, Yi CC, Tsao WC, Wang PS. Filial piety in contemporary Chinese societies: a comparative study of Taiwan, Hong Kong, and China. Int Sociol. 2013;28:277–96.
230. Yi CC, Lin JP. Types of relations between adult children and elderly parents in Taiwan: mechanisms accounting for various relational types. J Comp Fam Stud. 2009;40:305–24.
231. Yue X, Ng SH. Filial obligations and expectations in China: current views from young and old people in Beijing. Asian J Soc Psychol. 1999;2:215–26.
232. Yun HA. Ideology and changing family arrangements in Singapore. J Comp Fam Stud. 2004;35:375–92.
233. Zhang QF. Economic transition and new patterns of parent–adult child coresidence in urban China. J Marriage Fam. 2004;66:1231–45.
234. Zhang Z, Gu D, Luo Y. Coresidence with elderly parents in contemporary China: the role of filial piety, reciprocity, socioeconomic resources, and parental needs. J Cross Cult Gerontol. 2014;29:259–76.

23 Elder Abuse and Culture: Latino Anthropological and Ethnographic Experiences

María D. Pérez-Cárceles

At the beginning of the 1990s, the great French anthropologist Claude Levi-Strauss suggested that we need to revise our understanding of the world in light of demographics. It is increasingly evident that our near future will be influenced by the result and consequences of demographic changes. The case of population aging and the impact of changes in the age structure of the same is proof of this. A "silent revolution" that tends to invert the population pyramid is happening, especially in western societies.

It is not necessary to remind ourselves that the elderly show characteristic and differentiating changes in their last stages of their life cycle—physical, psychological, and social changes—that have to be taken into account if we are to correctly deal with the problems of this population. In the twenty-first century, this demographic transition is unavoidable and starting to manifest itself in every corner of the world, a transition in which the elderly themselves become the main players in the puzzle of an aging society. In this context and in all areas that affect social human beings, society is beginning to worry seriously about this expanding group.

Throughout history, different cultures have assigned the elderly different places in society: they have been idolized for their wisdom or persecuted because of their weakness, listened to because of their experience or shunned for their infirmity.

M.D. Pérez-Cárceles (✉)
Institute of Research into Aging, Department of Legal Medicine, Biomedical Research Institute (IMIB-Arrixaca), Regional Campus of International Excellence "Campus Mare Nostrum", School of Medicine, University of Murcia, E-30100 Murcia, Spain
e-mail: mdperez@um.es

23.1 The Elderly in Different Cultures: An Anthropological Vision

Throughout time, man has been playing the role of the elderly in society based on political, artistic, aesthetic, demographic, ethical and religious factors, as well as factors related to family and kinship. In recent decades, the elderly population has grown in number and diversity and in turn, has begun to present a greater spectrum of needs of all types.

In all societies there are different conceptions about aging, and, contrary to what some authors think, the contemporary situation is not the least propitious that this age group has suffered, but there were many other periods where the old were punished ruthlessly, scorned, and generally considered in a negative way [80].

Although modern society has taken a big step forward caring for the elderly, we should rethink what the role of the elderly is within different cultures and communities, by bringing them into daily life and not contributing to their social marginalization. For this purpose, it is necessary to develop strategies and interventions at a sociocultural level, which require an a priori reinterpretation of what the situation of the elderly has been so far, from a historic-anthropological perspective [27].

The elderly in Prehistory Prehistoric individuals lived in tribes, which was the basic social structure of coexistence and where the only objective was survival. Struggles, hunting, difficulties in adaptation to the environment and diseases made reaching old age very difficult, so elderly people were scarce during this period. Longevity was considered as special, "supernatural", with "divine protection". In fact, shamans and sorcerers were tribal elders. The elderly were considered as the depository of knowledge and transmitter of the clan memory, and reaching an advanced age was considered a privilege. Old age in Prehistory was appraised positively because of the virtue of survival; the elderly were a symbol of a divine value within the tribe [56].

X. Dong (ed.), *Elder Abuse*, DOI 10.1007/978-3-319-47504-2_23

Egyptian civilization The elderly first becomes visible in history through the writings of an elderly Egyptian scribe in a piece of self-analysis that is moving because of its antiquity and present-day relevance. Ptahhotep, Vizier of Pharaoh Tzezi of the V dynasty, written around year 2450 BC wrote: "Old age is here, old age arrives!/Exhaustion comes, weakness is made new./One lies down in discomfort all day,/ eyes are dim, ears deaf,/strength wanes, the heart is weary./ The mouth, silent, speaks not,/the heart, ended, recalls not the past,/the bones ache throughout./Good becomes evil,/all taste is gone./What age does to people/is evil in everything./ The nose clogged, breathes not,/difficult are standing and sitting."

The elderly were granted a leading role because of their experience and wisdom which came with their long life. Within Egyptian culture, the word elderly meant wisdom. There was an interesting relationship of the elderly Egyptians with their function in society as educators and guides to youth, i.e., they acted as advisors. In Egypt, the elderly were seen from a positive perspective, as a fundamental pillar in the education of young people and as a symbol of wisdom.

Old age as understood by the Greeks Ancient Greece was the cradle of western civilization and left us as a legacy our conception of the world. The naturalist perception and sense of perfection relegated the elderly to a deteriorating position. For a society that adored beauty, old age did not mean anything but an offense to the spirit; a reason for mockery in comedies which even considered it a blemish. In general, Old Age together with Death produced what the Greeks called Keres, evil spirits that must be driven away [9].

In classical Greece (eighth to second centuries BC) different ways of understanding old age existed: a negative view of the elderly shown to us in the city of Athens, where the elderly were losing power since the Archaic period. In the times of Homer (eighth century BC), the Council of Elders was merely a consultative body since decisions were made by young people, although Athenian law insisted on respect for parents. On the other hand, in the period of King Solon (sixth century BC), power was concentrated in the Areopagus, an aristocratic institution of elders enjoying great power. The increased power of the Democrats (509 BC) meant the fall of the Areopagus whose members lost their political and judicial powers, leaving them only with honorific power. All in all, Athens remained faithful to youth.

A contrary attitude was present in the city of Sparta, which had a senate, the Gerusia, formed of 28 members all of them over 60, demonstrating how Spartans respected the elderly as transmitters of wisdom.

During the Hellenistic period (third to second centuries BC) the elderly had more opportunities than in classical Greece since society was more open and cosmopolitan, and less prejudiced against age.

Old age in the Hebrew world The other great cultural source of western civilization is the Hebrew-Christian tradition. The story of this civilization is reflected in the Old Testament, which not only provides information of historical events, but also of the way of life of that time. The basics of Hebrew civilization are contained in the Ten Commandments. The fourth commandment is a rule of behavior toward parents: "Honour thy father and thy mother." Hebrews were commanded to show respect for their parents, care for them, and honor them [28]. The elderly played an important role in the leadership of Jewish people (Ex. 3, 16). God's order to Moses: "Walk out in front of the people…and call some of the elders of Israel to join you". (Ex. 17, 5). In the Book of Numbers, we find the description of the creation of the Council of Elders as a divine initiative, an entity with wide-ranging religious and judicial powers, almost unchecked in their respective cities. When the monarchy's political power was institutionalized, the Council of Elders was relegated to the role of advisers, but members continued to have great power. During the period of the Hebrew King Rehoboam, the Council lost its power and the image of the elderly began to suffer [37].

Military defeat in 586 BC and the conquest of Jerusalem by the Babylonians was attributed to the Hebrew people having distanced itself from religion, leading to revitalisation of the same and, consequently, an improvement in the position of the elderly, who once again were granted the prestige they had enjoyed during patriarchal and monarchical times. But from the fifth century onward, the elderly progressively lost their political influence.

In summary, the concept of longevity in the Hebrew world suffered extreme polarizations, swinging from positive to negative as a result of sociopolitical events.

Old age in Roman civilization Roman culture was characterized by its tolerance, adaptability, practical vision on life and its cosmopolitanism. Although Romans tended to have a pessimistic view of old age, the elderly were highly considered in texts of this period, and problems related with the same were raised in almost every aspect: political, social, psychological, demographic, and medical. The number of elderly people in Roman society was far greater than in Greek society, and there were significantly more males than females due to the high mortality rate of childbirth. This aging of the population was especially relevant in Italia during the second century.

Roman law gave authority to the elderly in the figure of the Pater Familias, who held great power over the family and slaves, which frequently led to them becoming hated and feared. This concentration of power established an asymmetrical intergenerational relationship that created major conflicts, which led to true hatred of the elderly. As for women, the figure of Mater Familias remained in second place, enjoying the sympathy and tolerance of offspring.

However, it should not be forgotten that old single women were brutally despised [58].

The golden age of the elderly was during the Republic, when political power was entrusted to men of advanced age. From first century BC onward, there was an unstable period and traditional values changed. Augustus started a new period in which the arts and the economy flourished, while the power of the Senate and the elderly waned. With the loss of family and political power, the elderly who had become tyrants in their own right, fell into contempt and were left to suffer the rigors of old age. This contempt did not include the whole of all the elderly population, since, as we have said, the Romans were very tolerant and tended to judge individuals, not a life period.

The elderly are not taken into account by Christianity, which represents timeless man, although the importance given in this culture to caring for the needy, among whom there were certainly many old people, must be highlighted [58].

The elderly during the Middle Ages The so-called "Dark Ages" or "Middle Ages", from the fifth to the tenth century, was a time of brutality and the predominance of force. In such a cultural sphere, it is not difficult to imagine the fate of the weak, to which group the elderly belonged. Old people were temporarily sheltered in hospitals and monasteries, to later confront the persistent reality of their miseries. Theirs was a group of disadvantaged people, who depended on family solidarity for subsistence.

In the church as an entity, the elderly were numerous, although associated writings did not give importance to them. It is logical to think that many reached old age, since they lived within the monasteries, sheltered from the world and with a higher standard of living than the rest of individuals.

During the first centuries of Christianity, from the fifth century onward, old age became a negative symbol and its arrival was feared by all. The Church did not pay any special attention to the elderly. An example of this can be found when studying monastic rules. In the "Rule of the Master", a set of monastic rules from the ninth century, the old are given work as gatekeepers or made to do small chores.

In the area of morality, authors used old age as an allegorical image of sin, assuming a pessimistic view of old age as a divine punishment for the sins of man. With this in mind, the only interest for old age in Christianity is the image of ugliness and decrepitude, which was used to represent sin and its consequences.

But there were differences between old men and old women. Le Roy Ladurie explores both situations in his work "Montaillou, village occitan". On the one hand, old men in this community do not live well. The head of the family is the son and he treats his elderly parents quite tyrannically, and they, in turn, do not dare do anything without consultation. On the other hand, "old age in women is not the same as in of men. A woman, oppressed as a young wife, is later loved by her children when reaching old age and respected as matriarch" [48].

According to Georges Minois, the limit to activity is physical disability. While the elderly can continue with their chores, they are not seen as such. When they reach the time of incapacity, the nobility can take care of their elders in their castles, while the monasteries welcome those who can afford such retirement. Peasants are in the worst situation, and they are left at the mercy of their children, the only thing remaining being the memory of the group. If there are no children, especially if the old person is a single woman, the situation is doubly unfortunate.

The Black Death was a catastrophe that affected all of Europe. In 1348 it entered Europe through Genoa from Central Asia, killing more than one-third of Europeans. It affected children and young adults especially, so that from 1350 to 1450, the number of elderly people showed a considerable increase. The elderly would become patriarchs and their maintenance was assured [54]. It is paradoxical that the plague helped this group socially, politically, and economically.

Longevity during the Renaissance During the fifteenth century, people became enthusiastic with the discovery of the hidden beauty of the Greco-Roman world, which had lain buried. Western Europe was attracted to Ancient Greece, the cultivators of beauty, youth, and perfection. The cultural horizon was amplified and reborn. This nascent individualistic spirit that flourished rejected old age and everything that represented ugliness, inevitable decrepitude, melancholy, and decadence. This was an almost aggressive blow against the elderly; especially if you were an old woman.

Contempt for old age was manifested in the arts and literature. Italian painters ignored old age, Flemish and Germans showed no mercy to them, especially old women, who were represented as wrinkled and decrepit, the very image of the witches who enraged the Inquisition so much. From 1480 onward, society was quite literarily rejuvenated. The increase in the numbers of young people simply pushed the elderly aside, while the printing press and systematization of parish records took from them their last remaining function as the memory of the group.

The human archetypes of the Renaissance are Courtesans and Humanists. Both rejected the elderly, because they represented everything that they wanted to suppress [28].

Lower levels of violence during the sixteenth century allowed males to reach more advanced ages, while the same happened with women in aristocratic circles, thanks to better hygiene in childbirth in this social environment. However, the attitude of the courtesans and humanists toward the elderly was probably a mere literary stance, and in daily life the relationship was more benevolent.

The Early Modern Period The state of the early modern world was impersonal, highly regulated and characterized by power being representative, i.e., based on the wishes of the people. This system led to gradual depersonalisation and the growing predominance of officials working for this new organization, who could "retire". This phenomenon involves a specialized economistic vision of caring for the elderly, which, for centuries had been carried out by family members without any remuneration and since it was considered a family duty. With the arrival of the Industrial Revolution in the eighteenth century, human beings became valued for the work they did and, in the case of the elderly, for the work they had done in the service of a public or private institution, etc., and the State, on behalf of society, felt obliged to reward them [41].

At present, a very significant milestone in the biography of every citizen is retirement. Interestingly, in Spanish, the word "jubilarse" (to retire) comes from the Latin word "*jubilare*" (to release screams of joy). Originally, it was a reward for workers older than 50 years. According to Simone de Beauvoir, this was the recommendation that Tom Paine made in 1796. A pension to government officials is known of in the Netherlands in 1844. In France, the first to obtain a pension were soldiers and civil servants; then miners and other professions considered dangerous. From an economic point of view, it moved from a benevolent gratification to an acquired right. This led to the creation of systems of social insurance and studies of the probability of survival. The system remains in place, although the age of retirement is postponed.

However, at this early time the elderly were still cared for by the family. The incorporation of women into the workforce happened gradually and, in general, it was still considered that they should do housework, which included caring for the elderly in their family. In countries such as Spain, most people inhabited rural areas, and the State would only become involved much later. At the end of the nineteenth century, old age began to distance itself from disease and Gerontology was born along with Geriatric care.

Contemporary world: The elderly in our society Our present day technoscientific culture has probably had the greatest influence ever on the lives of the elderly. Not only are they not the keepers of wisdom any more, but, quite the contrary, they are the further from knowledge than ever, because they no longer learn any more. We are in an era where the concept of experience is in decline, even work experience. Experience is no longer appreciated because it represents the past. Added to this, both physically and aesthetically, the elderly have been left an undesirable role in society.

The new living conditions created by technoscience has not only has aged the population, but now the fastest growing age group of the population is the over 85 s. Furthermore, the longer postretirement times mean growing impoverishment, aggravated by the increased need for socio-health care. At the same time, the percentage of children under 15 years is decreasing. Fertility and birth rates continue to decline in most of the developed world.

The design of current cities, consisting of small habitable spaces and nuclear families with loose ties, condemns the elderly to live alone. In the European Union, the percentage of old people living alone exceeds 30 %, and continues to rise.

The debate about aging is recent in Spain, but the whole of society is now concerned about the aging of the population structure and the growing needs of the elderly. Currently, it is the State that assumes this responsibility, which has traditionally been the task of the families. The increase in the number of elderly people and has coincided with a reduction in family size and the size of homes themselves, accompanied by other important cultural and social changes. Both the physical and social spaces of the elderly in the family have been reduced, and their ability to contribute to the family is also reduced. The feeling of any obligation toward the elderly weakens in an urban context, while the reduction in the number of children and increased employment rates among women has reduced the number of potential care providers. Professional and middle-class families have started to abandon the task of caring for their elderly themselves, although working class families, with less physical space and money at their disposal, still tend to care for their old. At the same time, another growing problem is: who will look after those who at the moment provide care? [62].

Georges Minois, in his "History of old age", establishes three factors that define the social status of the elderly. First, physical fragility: the condition of the elderly is worse in less civilized societies, based on the law of the strongest or survival of the fittest. The same applies to more anarchical periods, such as the Merovingian era or the Early Middle Ages in general. More orderly periods, with a legal structure, were more favorable to the elderly, as occurred during the Roman Empire and during the absolute monarchies of the sixteenth century. The second factor is the knowledge and experience derived from a long life. In this respect, the most favorable civilizations are those which are based on oral tradition and custom, where the elderly constituted a link between generations and collective memory. Writing and the keeping of archives—and now the use of computers—have rendered this function of the elderly unnecessary. The acceleration of History has led to old age becoming synonymous with old fashioned. The third factor is the changing of physical features. Old age was displeasing during periods in which society worshipped physical beauty, such as in Classical Greece and during the Renaissance. Patriarchal societies favored the elderly with access to wealth.

Transition periods were less favorable than, stable "classical" ones. If we compare these factors, expressed throughout history, with those applicable to our time, it is clear that the so-called "old" adults of today do not enjoy the most favorable of circumstances.

According to authors such as Butler and Lewis [13], the characteristics of the elderly today are: (a) a desire to leave a legacy: not wanting to be forgotten and influencing others after death, (b) share experience with youths and establish generational contacts, (c) attachment to familiar objects that have accompanied them during life (home, animals, family, memories, etc.) gives them a sense of continuity in time, (d) a change in the perception of time: they live in the present, (e) full consciousness of the life cycle: they value life as a whole, (f) creativity, curiosity, and surprise, (g) sense of self-accomplishment when a conflict has been resolved.

23.2 Aging from a Biopsychological Perspective

The progressive physical and psychological deterioration that accompanies the human life cycle can not be associated with any specific age as there are large interindividual differences which blur the border between being old and not being old.

To age is not to become ill, and organic deterioration does not necessarily imply cognitive impairment or a decrease in the psychological response of the subject. The most important factor is how the subject faces their deficiency, because the same alteration does not produce the same impact in different individuals.

Aging is a multifactorial process characterized by the progressive decrease in functional capacity in all bodily tissues and organs, and the consequent ability to adjust to environmental stimulus. Harman defines aging as "the progressive accumulation of changes with time that are associated with or responsible for the ever-increasing susceptibility to disease and death which accompanies advancing age" [35]. Strehler [84] points to four characteristics that refine the concept: (1) Aging is universal: a phenomenon associated with the process of aging must occur in different degrees in all individuals of a species. (2) Aging must be intrinsic: the causes that are the origin of aging must be endogenous; they must not depend on extrinsic factors. (3) Aging must be progressive: changes that lead to aging must occur progressively throughout the life span (they must also occur in young individuals, albeit in a small proportion). 4. Aging must be deleterious, i.e., a phenomenon associated with aging will only be considered as part of the aging process if it is "bad" for the individual.

A biopsychosocial consideration of the elderly leads us to consider that the changes associated with the process of aging occur from three perspectives: (1) Biological: Organic changes that affect physical capacities. (2) Psychological: Changes in behavior, self-perception, values, and beliefs; and (3) Social: Changes in the role of the elderly in the community.

Biological changes affect all organs and tissues of the individual. We shall only highlight that the level of dependency of the elderly increases as their physical capabilities decrease, which has important implications for the issue that concerns us. In relation to psychological changes, the aging of intellectual abilities involves a decrease in the ability to solve problems and a lack of spontaneity in thought processes. Language ability and expression may be altered, while creativity and capacity of the imagination are preserved. There are alterations in memory, and the elderly often suffer from time-focused amnesia. On the other hand, personality is not usually altered, unless pathological changes occur. Adaptability is often diminished through the fear of unfamiliar situations.

Social changes acquire particular importance at this stage of life. **Individual role changes** can be looked at from three viewpoints:

The elderly as an individual People in their last stage of life are aware that death is near. One of the aspects of development of the individual is the acceptance of the reality of death. This is regarded by the elderly as a liberation, as the end of a life of struggle, worries, and problems; for others, it is a more acceptable alternative to impairment or disease. Other old age people reject the idea of dying and are engulfed by fear and anxiety.

The elderly as a member of the family group Family life can offer the elderly something and give meaning to their lives, letting them assume their role in the transmission of life and family values, and allowing them to know that when they disappear from the world, there will be people who will carry their name and will carry their values into the future.

The family is one of the institutions that has most changed in recent years and at different levels: in conception, in legal aspects, in relationships, in relations between parents and children and between generations, in family dynamics and the different roles assumed by each individual.

In another time, the whole family (parents, grandparents and children) lived under the same roof, which fostered a feeling of cohesion and solidarity between its members, and respect and defense for the elderly. In this model, the male's role was as sustainer of the family while women were in charge of the household, raising children and caring for the elderly.

This traditional model is changing; the elderly do not usually live together under the same roof as their children and their grandchildren, and there are many reasons to explain this separation between the generations of each family:

- The sense of family cohesion and solidarity, which is being transformed, giving way to a break up of the family and greater individual independence.
- The changes in family dynamics, the roles of each member and relations between family members.
- The problems of space within dwellings, especially in big cities.

Increasingly, the close family environment is disappearing and there is more distance between its different members. Within the family network, there are relations that can be regarded as reciprocal; the family helps the elderly and the elderly helps the family. When there is no reciprocity, some families stop taking responsibility for the care of the elderly, which has to be done by a health or social institutions. The most influential key factors in these reciprocal relationships are often the physical and economic capacity of the elderly. As their health, and the ability to carry out daily activities and functional capabilities of the elderly get worse, it becomes more difficult to maintain this reciprocity with the family.

Relations between the elderly, their children, and their grandchildren fundamentally go through two stages. The first stage is when the elderly are independent and have no health problems; they dedicate themselves to helping their children, performing small domestic tasks and taking care of their grandchildren. The second stage begins when the first health problems appear, and family relationships are inverted. The elderly no longer have the same weight within the family, and may begin to feel rejection and abandonment. The stereotype of an old person with a family that does not care for them, is that of a useless person. However, the elderly have a greater need to be accepted and loved by the family, receiving affection at the moment in which their physical and mental abilities are diminished. The family, or some of its members, may fail to understand and accept the situation of the elderly, and fall into conflict about whether to allow them to continue living with them.

In this last stage, the life cycle varies according to family composition, subsystems, limits, and the rules that differentiate, in each one of its members, their role, functions, and tasks, giving rise to a new structure where the elderly may or may not be involved.

Thus, in close-knit families, the elderly occasionally live with their grandchildren and take on voluntary or imposed functions that no longer correspond to them, such as the role of surrogate parent, a situation that occurs most often in extended families where parental tasks seems to have no set end. In difficult economic situations, there is a need to coexist, and, in this case, it is necessary to set clear boundaries whereby the parents' function is preserved and they receive support from the grandparents, each assuming responsibilities that are appropriate for the proper family functioning.

With the increase in life expectancy, especially in the case of women, they will spend more time caring for elderly parents than their own children, especially when they leave home early or other causes such as education or the need to work; when an old woman lives in the house of her son, there is a completion for authority between her and her daughter-in-law, and if she lives with her daughter, she shares authority with her.

Another frequent family situation in the last stage of the life cycle is the woman who is head of the family because of widowhood, separation, or old age, where she maintains her status when she is the owner of the house and provides care to all family members who require it.

Also of note within family types, is the disunited family, where only one child assumes care for the living parent, which corresponds to a family where solidarity, sharing, and mutual aid did not exist or was not inculcated in all its members, a attitude that becomes even more evident when sharing any inheritance. Another alternative available to this family is to send the old to an institution, regardless the state of their health, so that the children may continue their life without interference. Institutionalization is an alternative that most elderly people do not want and most times the family does it against their will, a very different situation from when it is the elderly themselves who take the decision.

One-parent or reconstituted families are those when the offspring return home, either because they are single, widowed, or have a new marriage and children; they go back not only in the search for shelter, food, and affection, but also for someone to care for their children. In this case, the elderly pass from playing the role of grandparent to one foster parent, meaning they must also conform to new customs and ways of life.

There are many times, too, when this role is actively sought by the grandparents, who, in an effort to continue the overprotection of their children, offer such an alternative and effective measure to ensure their return and to bring them once again into their care and protection. They never let their children grow and assume their autonomy and independence, preventing them from making decisions and assuming logical consequences from their behavior. They always play the role of saviors but quickly assume the role of victims to perpetuate these dependency relationships. The most frequently observed situation is widowed grandmothers because of the increase in life expectancy and the need to compensate loneliness with the company of one of her children.

In extended families, due to the presence of children and grandchildren that return home, the "empty nest" and lonely couple stages of life do not happen, and this way of life becomes a natural way of living out the final years.

A balanced family is one where the couple assumes that commitment is for both: giving and receiving, perpetuating family life through continued work for individual growth and as a couple, with the singularity that each one recognizes their own space, that of their partner and shared space, with functions and very clear limits, sharing support, respect, and solidarity.

Some families may agree to receive a grandparent in the house, but conflict may arise in the relationships because customs, beliefs, standards, lifestyles, and communication systems are different and, although everyone tries to adapt and make adjustments, they do not succeed. Coexistence is not easy for the families or for the elderly, but both must talk, make adjustments, agreements, and try to establish a harmonious relationship.

Structural changes in a family in the presence of an elderly person cover many different areas. The physical environment of the house should include spaces and safety measures to prevent accidents, facilitating movement without major difficulties and promoting independence and privacy. A proper and comfortable environment is needed for the whole family in accordance with their economic capacity.

In the area of children, the limits must be very well defined, to avoid friction and interference in bringing them up and in their; the couple must have keep their own space and their own life, and resist the temptation to make alliances with the grandparent, which would affect the family relationship.

The elderly as a person facing losses Old age is a stage characterized by losses (physical, psychological, affective, economic, role-related). The emotional losses characterized by the death of a spouse or a friend are accompanied by great emotional tension and feeling of loneliness.

23.2.1 Change of Role in the Community

Today's society only values active persons, who are able to work and gain wealth. The elderly person is often retired and is a "nonactive" person, although they have the possibility to contribute knowledge and perform new tasks for the community. The act of aging changes the role that has been developed during the working life, but not the individual.

The role expected from the elderly has much to do with social stereotypes about older people and the expectations that are expected from a person after retirement, which has been marked, paradoxically, by what has been called "the role without a role". Society expects nothing from the nonproductive, who may be rewarded with a life pension for the services provided in the past. Within the role that we give to the elderly would be the relationship with other people, which is marked by a rejection in our society of what is old, because old age is associated with something decrepit, ugly, and useless; aging is a trauma, a disease, a disability involving physical pain and dependence, apart of an existential terror toward the proximity of death.

Old age reunites the greatest taboos of western society: pain, decrepitude, madness, and death. Western man has turned his back on such being and unconsciously rejects them and turns away from them.

One of the most important changes for actively working people is the change in role. At this stage of life, the greatest change is retirement, but the elderly should use alternatives to avoid the most negative consequences. For the individual, leaving behind what they are used to has important implications, and adaptation is difficult because life and values revolve around work and activity. Social relations decrease when you leave the workplace, as do economic resources. The elderly must prepare themselves before retirement, know the consequences of retirement to prevent its negative effects. In some cases, it will be necessary to search for extra hobbies for retirement so that, rather than assuming a fall in the quality of life, the pensioner should perhaps assume an increase in the quality of the same [8].

23.3 Demographics of the Older Population in Spain and Latin American

The aging of the population is a tangible reality in our society, and is the result of the major demographic changes that have occurred in Spain in recent decades. Since the end of the 1970s, there has been a sharp decline in fertility that has meant that the percentage of older people has grown. The birth rate stands at 1.2 children per woman, which is far from the natural replenishment rate of 2.1.

The increase in life expectancy has meant an increase in the number of survivors in all groups over 65 years of age. The elderly are the fastest growing age group throughout the world. The average life expectancy in Spain in 1900 was around 34 years for men and 36 for women. These numbers, a century later have multiplied by two and a half; something similar has happened in the rest of European countries. Different factors have contributed to this such as technological advances in health and nutrition, but especially hygiene and other measures related to prevention [87]. At the beginning of the twentieth century, only 26 out of every 100 births reached the age of 65, and in 1990, it was 84. In Spain, the population pyramid is inverted, although, at the same time, the strong migration movements of recent years of people of working age has allowed the aging "process" to slow down. However, the tendency of many immigrants to return home in recent years, due to the economic crisis, may well accelerate the process again.

The main consequence of these demographic changes is the restructuring of the age pyramid. For the first time in

Spanish history, there has been a demographic inversion and there are now more older people (65 years and over) than children (0–14 years). In 1996 there were over 6 million people older than 65 years, approximately 16 % of the population, while only a few years later it will soon be 20 %. In addition to this increase in the percentage of older people, these old people are living longer. In the last decade, the group of people over 80 years old has grown more than other age groups. Between 1991 and 2005 the number of people over 80 years old has increased by 66 %, while the population as a whole has increased by 13 %. And we should not forget another population segment that has also gained greater relevance lately, people who reach 100 years. The projections of the Spanish Institute of Statistics estimate that their numbers will reach about 55,240 by 2050.

The population projections of the United Nations for 2050 estimate that Spain will be the third oldest country in the world, with 34.1 % of the population older than 65, second only to Japan and Italy (with 35.9 and 35.5 %, respectively). In a previous projection in 2002, the United Nations foresaw that Spain would be the most aged country in the world in 2050, but, as several different indicators have evolved, in subsequent revisions, this has changed, giving top positions to the aforementioned countries.

Latin America has had the highest life expectancy among major areas in the less developed regions. From 51.4 years in 1950–1955, life expectancy in Latin America increased to 71.5 years in 2000–2005. In 2005 people older than 65 years were approximately 6 % of the population, while the projections estimate that their number will reach 18 % [87].

This strong aging process will contribute to the change in relationships between generations and in the mid-twenty-first century. Also, as the elderly population increases, the resources and possibilities for the elderly to end their lives with their families, cared for by those bound to them by affection and/or family ties, will also decrease.

23.4 Global Review of Elder Abuse in Latin Culture

Modern day society favors the practice, transmission, and development of certain types of behavior, which, influenced by family ties, culture and social interaction, promotes—consciously or not—a series of social, economic, cultural, and gender-related inequalities that directly affect the weakest and most vulnerable.

Maltreatment toward the elderly is a recent typology within the most generic study field concerning family violence. In Spain, as in other Latin European countries, interest in the ill-treatment of the elderly arose after interest into other forms of ill-treatment—of children and spouses, for example, which seem not to surprise society so much as the idea that the old may also suffer at the hands of their family.

Although it is not a new phenomenon, it has only recently captured the attention of society, particularly of health professionals and those involved in the social sciences. The gravity of the situation is compounded by the fact that it remains a mostly hidden phenomenon. Politicians rarely mention it and the media give little space to it, while professionals have just woken to the problem. Reports come to light of very few cases, thus prolonging and widening the short-, medium-, and long-term suffering of an extremely vulnerable group.

However, the great interest in elderly abuse is closely connected with the fact that we live in an aging society, which contrasts with the fact that the elderly are relegated in the scheme of things, suffering situations of inequality and discrimination, denominated by some authors as ageism [13, 14, 66]. However, ageism is a hidden problem because its manifestations are subtle and may pass unnoticed, almost making it more acceptable.

The combination of ageism and aging society generates the worrying reality of elder abuse.

A person's dignity does not diminish with the passing of the years or with a deterioration of physical and psychological health, although this may be difficult to accept in the framework of a culture that does not look beyond given social stereotypes and which associates a person's value with youth, efficiency, physical vitality, and good health. In this situation, it is easy to marginalize the old and condemn them to "social death" before biological death intervenes, while maltreatment is manifestation of this discrimination and denigration.

Both within the family and institutions, elder abuse is a complex question that is related with demography, social position, the role of the family and social services, social policy, the welfare state in general, bioethics and justice.

The reports of the countries that took part in the World Assembly on Ageing held in Madrid (Spain) in 2002 coincide in the view that violence against the elderly is widespread, hardly denounced, and involves substantial economic and human costs (Report of the Second World Assembly on Ageing [76]).

The problem has received more attention since the 1980s due to greater preoccupation for human rights, which establishes a legal framework for responding to elder abuse and discrimination, helping, among other aspects, to combat economic abuses that this group suffers. Of great help in this respect is the International Network for the Prevention of Elder Abuse (INPEA) and the contribution of the World Health Organization (WHO). The Toronto Declaration on the Global prevention of Elder abuse was a call to action on the part of the WHO in 2002, awakening awareness of the problem worldwide. The declaration mentioned the lack of any legal framework, encouraged a multidisciplinary approach and the involvement of health professionals, political intervention, and education. However, Latin European countries and Latino countries do not seem to have taken much heed in this respect.

23.4.1 Social Changes and the Emergence of New Situations

In recent years, especially since the above-mentioned World Assembly on Ageing held in Madrid (Spain) in 2002, analysis of and reflection on the condition of old people have become more evident. The reality of this group seems to have become more visible and society as a whole is more interested in looking into their needs and demands, so that they recover a more active social role, be recognized as a group with certain rights, be provided with adequate social resources, receive attention and respect—until now not always guaranteed.

The importance of the old is not only based on demographics, but society should take more pains in involving them in social, cultural, and political activities, not forgetting their value as a consumer group.

Nobody doubts that old age is the antithesis of modern ideals. The gap between the generations is growing and giving rise to increasing social and cultural discrimination. The fact that the elderly are the fastest growing age group will have a significant effect on production, consumption, the provision of social and health services and public expenditure, generating new areas of conflict. Old age is still seen as a burden rather than a positive outcome of social advance.

Study and analysis of population aging, especially in the more developed countries, point to the great changes that have taken place as a consequence of improved health, the level and quality of life, consumption, education, etc., but also reveal the great risks, vulnerability, lack of protection and care provision that is urgently needed.

Problems of loneliness, abuse, emotional, physical, and economic maltreatment—in institutions, the family environment and society as a whole—are beginning to ring alarm bells in health and social services circles.

23.4.2 Interest of Elder Abuse in Latin European Countries

While we know that it has been a problem since ancient times, until the advent of initiatives to confront the maltreatment of children and domestic violence in the last quarter of the twentieth century, the way in which old people are treated was considered a private matter and not one to be aired in wider society. Initially considered as a problem of social well-being and subsequently one related with an aging society, elder abuse has become intertwined with public health and legal justice. These two disciplines largely determine the way in which we regard the topic in hand and how it should be dealt with.

During the inevitable process of aging, the morphological and functional changes that take place, along with the increasing risk of developing chronic and invalidating illnesses, may lead to an older person, despite their strong ability to adapt to changing circumstances, becoming dependent on others, whether a family member or social and/or health services. However, risk factors increase at the same time as such dependence increases, meaning that dependent people need more help and attention than they perhaps receive.

Interest in the topic hardly dates from 10 years ago in Spain, despite its wide recognition by doctors and social organizations. Internationally, the first bibliographical references of this phenomenon appear in 1975 [5, 11, 12]. Subsequent contributions emphasize the important role of health professionals, who are often the first to see elderly victims in their respective work places. However, in contrast to children and women who have been the object of ill-treatment, older people are reluctant to denounce such treatment on the part of their family. Health professionals therefore frequently find it difficult to recognize and attribute signs and symptoms of abuse and to report the same to the relevant organisms.

In Europe, the British Geriatrics Society organized the first multidisciplinary conference on elder abuse in 1988, and the following year edited a guide containing a series of proposals and recommendations [85], while in France a declaration of the rights and freedom of people of a dependent age was promulgated by the National Foundation of Gerontology towards the end of the 1980's in an attempt to raise awareness of the problem and to prevent cases of abuse and maltreatment, both in the family and institutions.

In 1994, the European Commission published the White paper on European Social Policy in Europe, which recognized that the interests of the elderly go beyond the traditional theme of pensions and the provision of services. The main challenge is to maintain the level of social integration of the most vulnerable. Maltreatment and abuse of the elderly, especially the most fragile and incapacitated, is recognized as being one of the main obstacles to such integration [88]. The report from the Third European Conference on Family Law held in Strasbourg (France) in 1995 included the maltreatment of elderly people. In Spain, Marín et al. were the first to make a public declaration on the syndrome of elder abuse in the National Congress of the Spanish Society of Geriatrics and Gerontology held in Las Palmas (Spain) [57].

In 1994, the research carried out by Larrión et al. led to publication of the article "Elder abuse Syndrome" [47]. In light of the information available, the lack of agreement between professionals and the daily appearance of problems related with elder abuse (most with little possibility of being solved) the First National Conference on Maltreatment of the Elderly (Primera Conferencia Nacional de Consenso sobre el Anciano Maltratado) was held in Almeria (Spain) in 1996. The resulting Almeria Declaration (Declaración de Almería) was published to bring to the attention of the national and regional governments the need for funding to promote education, information, and multidisciplinary research into the problem. The declaration stated that the lack of knowledge and hidden nature of elder abuse hindered prevention and intervention, and underlined the scarcity of specific training programs. The consequence was that health professionals began to look at the problem with greater rigor in their daily practice. However, epidemiological data remain scarce.

In this context, the multidisciplinary approach fomented in the USA has been decisive in increasing our knowledge. The report "Missing Voices: views of older persons on elder abuse" has become a reference for putting into practice processes of investigation-action in many countries, including Latin European and Latino countries. The same document made a series of recommendations concerning the overall strategies that should be followed to confront the problem.

23.4.3 Views of the Elderly

In Spain the first research effort was into the perceptions of maltreatment on the part of the elderly themselves and professionals in primary healthcare centers. This was a qualitative investigation carried out in other European countries taking into consideration the views of the protagonists closest to the problem. The project was the first step in a wider framework to develop an overall strategy for the prevention of elder abuse that could help put into practice political measures, research, and specific actions [40].

Notwithstanding the similarities of the views of the subjects from the different countries, it became clear that the cultural and social context was important in the analysis of what was considered by maltreatment, and what measures were considered acceptable to reduce or prevent the same, and what professionals should be given responsibility in this respect. Among the conclusions was the recommendation to carry out studies in national contexts, so that the information obtained was the closest to the reality of each community where policies were to be decided.

The elderly people taking part in Spain identified six areas which were considered critical for a good quality of life in old age. The balance between these factors would give rise to different degrees of well-being. If any area was infringed, this would hint at possible situations of maltreatment and the information would at least help explain why such was considered important.

The first area was the economic situation of the elderly. The association between pensions and quality of life was immediate and unalterable. Its importance was not only due to the conditions for survival, but also to the respect and social value that old people felt they deserved. Great emphasis was put into preventing themselves from being regarded as passive members of society and on the rights they have accumulated during a long life of work. The position they were assigned in the world was especially important. They belong to a generation in which elders were considered with respect and even granted a degree of authority and to which was attributed wisdom accumulated through experience. However, the opinion was that things had swung to the opposite extreme and what old people could offer society was being devalued. They were aware that old people were looked down upon, considered a passive population, with obsolete views and who lived on the backs of society without contributing and therefore without the right to demand more than the vague right to be considered for what they were rather for what they are. While they were viewed by others as people with no interests or desires and not belonging to the modern world, the elderly viewed themselves as active people with the capacity to lead interesting lives and have valuable ideas.

Another fundamental area for old people was the existence or not of a community or group of reference to be able to lead a good life. Clearly, the advantage of taking part in a community was the ability to socialize and share interests. This feeling of belonging provided the elderly with affective security, other than that provided by the family, especially children whom they almost always considered to be occupied and busy with their own affairs. Forming part of a community ensured a degree of reciprocity that was considered more symmetrical than that offered by the family—there would always be someone to turn to without suggesting a lack of personal autonomy or the need to disturb. In many cases the idea of community is quite literal and refers to the fellow inhabitants of the village or town that they belong to in a more urban setting, it may mean the neighbors they have known for a long time, or those who belong to the same association, social center or club for senior citizens. Such a sense of belonging encourages people to get out of their house and relate with others, which, from the point of view of the elderly, is essential for their quality of life.

The affective sphere is considered crucial by old people for their well-being when the preoccupations of working life (in and outside the home) and child raising lose weight in the face of an increased private life doing what they want, rather than what other people want.

As regards sons and grandchildren, the elderly hold the idea that modern day life is responsible for the breakdown in generational relations, whereas in "their day" the duties and rights of both parts were clear, with a tacit agreement that each successive generation would be responsible for the new generation and the previous one. As children, they would have benefited from this system and expected to enjoy the same when old. They recognize that this unspoken contract has been broken and that one generation is only prepared to look after its children and young.

However, for the elderly, this intergenerational contract seems to remain fully in force regarding their responsibilities: they agree that it is their duty to support their children as much as possible (although they are not sure about the reciprocity of this obligation) and ensure that their elders, in many cases still alive and in a dependent situation due to the increase in life expectancy. This same phenomenon of increased life expectancy means that they often have the additional task of caring for an equally old spouse with impaired autonomy. This role as caregivers, ingrained in their identity, especially among women, is at the same time a source of satisfaction and gives them a sense of personal fulfillment—although it may be a disproportionate burden for those who do not have the personal, physical, or economic resources that allow them to deal with such a situation, especially in the case of those who might be described as working class, when pain, frustration, and impotence are the predominant feelings.

An unwavering aspiration for the elderly is to live safely/with peace of mind, since they consider that they have worked all their life to achieve this status. Remaining in their own physical and emotional environment seems to be this key to security. In many cases, their own experience as primary caregivers for an elderly dependent relative makes them fear the worst for themselves if they find themselves in a similar situation of dependence toward the end of their life. They are aware of the enormous physical and mental cost to carer and the distortion that occurs in a family taking care of the elderly in these conditions, and, consequently, they do not want to put their family in a situation that would be as painful as that which they themselves experienced. They believe that their children are not ready to shoulder the burden as they were, that the role of caregiver does not fit into the lifestyles of young people.

23.4.4 Conceptual Framework of Elder Abuse

In Spain, a recent study of the Sociological Research Centre (Centro de Investigaciones Sociológicas) [39] in which questions related to old age were formulated, 36.2 % of the Spanish population defines as elder as "those who can not fend for themselves and need care," only 6.2 % of these people associating this group with "active people, who enjoy life," suggesting that a large number of people have a distorted perception of the reality of the elderly, who are identified with fragility, shortcomings, and being a social burden. These are with social representations which generate an underestimation of the elderly as a group which makes it possible that society can live with a degree of excessive tolerance in the face of situations than in any other group of people would be unacceptable.

The reasons for which abuse occurs are many, and there are many theories that try to explain the causes, although there is no consensus. Theoretical proposals that have been made about bad treatment toward the elderly start from various points: those related to the characteristics of persons, those that analyze the interaction between people, and those that emphasize the importance of social structures, transforming violence against the elderly into a complex and multidimensional phenomenon.

Knowledge of the causes helps to identify the factors that lend themselves to an abusive situation and allows us to look into preventive strategies and the need to avoid unnecessary biases in the subsequent detection. We should not forget that, quite often, the root of elder abuse is multiple factors.

In Latin European countries and Latino culture, the most referenced causal theories for elder abuse are as follows:

- **Situational model** It is postulated that elder abuse is generated as an irrational response to stressful situations. This answer depends on various factors related with caregivers (life crisis, burnout, overload or exhaustion due to care efforts, problems of substance abuse, and previous experiences of violence), the victim (emotional and physical dependence of the elderly, bad health, impaired mental state, and the difficult personality of the elderly), and socioeconomic situations of both (economic tension, social isolation, and environmental problems). In this context, the caregiver could perceive the elder person as a source of stress. With this theory there is a risk of blaming the victim for being the source of the stress. This theory is especially associated with child abuse and less with other forms of intrafamily violence. Some authors conclude that the situational model is inappropriate.
- **Pathological model** This theory focuses on certain characteristics present in the person responsible for the abuse, for example, psychiatric problems and drug and alcohol abuse. The decrease in the ability of the caregiver to tolerate frustration and to control their behavior, for example, because of alcohol dependence, is associated with violent and abusive actions toward a person.

Economic abuse could also be a result of substance abuse, since the person responsible for the abuse may need money to pay for the consumption of alcohol or other substances. While this theory has been supported by a large number of authors, the existing data cannot endorse this perspective completely.

- **Model or social change theory** This model maintains that the dependency relation increases risk, that the imbalance of the interaction of two people lies between satisfaction and punishment, and that the feeling of lost autonomy of the elderly and the sense of power of the caregiver trigger responses of bad treatment. This theory is based on the idea that social interaction includes the exchange of rewards (reception of resources and/or services, positive feelings, etc.) and punishments (negative feelings, withdrawal of resources and services, and the exchange of punishment behavior) between people, so individuals try to maximize rewards and minimize punishment. When the exchange is balanced, the situation is perceived as fair. When this exchange is not balanced, anger, resentment, and punishment appear. However, the results of this line of thought do not completely explain elderly abuse.
- **Symbolic interaction theory** According to this model, social interaction is a process in which there is an interaction of at least two people over time, with recurring identifiable phases, interrelated and sequenced in a flexible manner and which requires negotiation and constant renegotiation to establish a consensus on this point. It refers to the symbolic interpretations of the behavior of both the victim and the person responsible for the bad treatment. It is based on social learning and suggests that those responsible for bad treatment learn to be violent by witnessing acts of violence, and that the victims learn to accept them as normal.
- **The feminist model** This defends a model based on the imbalance of power existing between men and women in a chauvinist society. However, this provides only a partial vision of the problem since elderly males are also victims of bad treatment.
- **The theory of excessive demands** The theory of excessive demands or internal stress or "exhausted caregiver" proposes that the stress of providing care to an older person increases the risk that the caregiver will behave in an abusive way. This theory has become quite popular also amongst professionals in mental health and the population in general, possibly because it is easy to create intervention strategies.
- In our context we must also highlight as a causal model of elder abuse, the theoretical perspectives of a critical economy and a political economy of aging that make reference to the image of the elderly in society and the impact of this on the lives of the elderly. Abuse would be due to marginalization of the elderly by society. This model proposes that many of the problems that the elderly have are not the result of the natural or biological processes of aging itself, but reflect the social inequalities that limit the roles and resources of the elderly.
- **Intergenerational transmission of violence** Another hypothesis identifies the importance of "learned violence" and the intergenerational transmission of violence within families. This theory assumes that violent behavior is learned as a means to express anger and frustration. Some situations of abuse include partner violence whereby individuals have grown old together and where the beginning of old age and the associated increase of contact with the healthcare and social services systems could result in the violence coming to light for the first time. It has also been hypothesized that some situations of abuse are a result of reverse violence, that is, situations where the person responsible for current abuse was in the past the possible victim of child or partner abuse at the hands of the elderly person who is being abused or whereby violence has come to be accepted as a standard within the history of the relationship. Although some data support this theory, taking into account gender-based violence and child abuse, there are still no convincing data to support the extension of this theory of bad treatment toward the elderly.
- **The ecological model** Given the complexity of the issue of abuse in old people and the fact that various relevant risk factors are related to the people who provide care or who are looked after, with the environment or the social/cultural context and the interaction between people and the environment, an ecological approach also in Latin European countries and Latin culture could be the most appropriate model to better understand abuse of the elderly, as this model provides an interpretation of intergenerational relations between the offspring (caregiver) and the elderly parent throughout the course of life as a basis for the development of prevention and intervention programs, with the aim of improving the quality of life of the elderly and their families in an aging society.

  The ecological perspective not only empowers professionals to deal with the complexity of the problem, but it also provides a framework for understanding the interrelationship and interdependence between different risk factors. The organization of risk factors enables researchers to better understand the dynamic of abuse within the context of family care.

  There seems to be no sole explanation for any form of domestic violence, including elder abuse, and different theories explain different aspects of a complex problem. Research suggests that theoretical explanations should be directed not only toward the individual characteristics of possible elderly victims and those responsible for their maltreatment but also toward the general context within which the maltreatment occurs.

23.4.5 Elder Abuse in Latino Communities

The World Health Organization ecological model is the most frequently used theoretical frame to understand violence. It considers that interpersonal violence, including elder abuse, is a complex and multifaceted phenomenon, with determinants that operate at several levels. Beyond individual features and circumstances, country and societal characteristics can help to understand the problem of elder abuse. Macroeconomic indicators and social-educational conditions, commonly used to represent contextual characteristics in cross-country comparisons, may thus contribute to a better understanding of the recognized geographical variation in the prevalence of elder abuse and provide clues to preventive measures [29].

A critical area that continues to be understudied is elder abuse in Latino families [31]. Latino culture is not monolithic and comprises cultures from multiple nations. While Latinos are the fastest growing ethnic minority in the United States, information about the prevalence of and risk factors for elder abuse in Latino families residing in the United States is scarce. There is no reason to doubt that this phenomenon will have a different profile from elder abuse in Spanish people. Among other factors, cultural identity differences, social isolation through lack of language abilities and knowledge of U.S. culture, or being undocumented [69] may lead to situations of elder abuse and neglect in such families. Moreover, neighborhood seclusion, a tradition of resolving conflicts within the family, and mistrust of authorities may impede survey research and suppress abuse reporting. All these factors will influence the model of family violence in inmigrant Latino families [20]. A recent study found that 40.4 % of Latino elders had experienced some form of abuse and/or neglect within the previous year. Nearly 25 % reported psychological abuse, 10.7 % indicated physical assault, 9 % reported sexual abuse, 16.7 % indicated financial exploitation, and 11.7 % were neglected by their caregivers. Younger age, higher education, and experiencing sexual or physical abuse before the age of 65 were significant risk factors for psychological, physical, and/or sexual abuse. The number of years lived in the United States, a younger age and prior abuse were associated with increased risk of financial exploitation. The years spent living in the U.S. was also a significant risk factor for caregiver neglect. Abuse prevalence was much higher in all mistreatment domains than findings from previous research on community-dwelling elders, suggesting that low-income Latino immigrants are highly vulnerable to elder mistreatment [20].

There is little information about the perception and issues of specific subtype of elder abuse in Latin European countries and Latino communities. In Spain, the existing information comes directly from the views of older people [40], who that within the term "abuse" two main types can be identified:

1. "Maltrato" (in Spanish), "Abuse" (in English) which is a serious infringement of rights (physical, sexual, situations of extreme neglect...) and is very rare. For the elderly, this term refers to situations of physical aggression or extreme neglect, which threatens the integrity of a totally dependent elderly person in cases, for example, of demented or immobilized individuals. In general, this refers to the scandals seen in the media about inhumane conditions in homes, or videos of caregivers who physically assault the demented person are under their care. They consider that such situations may occur in the context of a family, with physical abuse, excessive supply of sedatives or negligence in feeding the elderly, but, in their opinion, this only is conceivable in an unstructured environment, as a continuation of a previous situation of abuse. As such, they consider it very uncommon and confined to eye-catching anecdotal cases.
2. However, there is a group of situations, or minor forms of abuse "mal trato" in the Spanish study, (perhaps "unpleasant treatment" in English) that tend to go unnoticed by the public, but which they value as inadmissible or constituent of "abuse" of elderly people, although they use terms such as shame, abuse, protection, or unacceptable treatment. The difference with "maltrato" ("abuse") is in the severity of the consequences.

Elderly people seem to consider obvious that the existence of "abuse" toward old people can be explained by the social image attributed to the elderly, who are characterized as passive subjects, unproductive, and therefore "socially terminal patients". They believe that society perceives them as a medium/short term load, and that the elderly should be in debt for everything that they receive, as if they were living at the expense of society, to which they do not contribute anything but from which they demand much. Whatever they think is considered obsolete, and therefore hardly relevant to young people, whose view is one of indifference or resignation/tolerance toward the elderly.

From their point of view, the consumer society, narcissistic and individualist in nature, promotes a rejection of responsibility and behavior toward the elderly that may lead to "abuse".

The perception that the elderly have of the changes in family structure that have taken place in such a short time leads them to consider this as a major factor. In their opinion, the appearance of women in the labor market (which, in general, they value as a breakthrough) and their subsequent disappearance as permanent caregivers has provided society as a whole with a challenge yet to be resolved. A crucial figure has been lost, and there is no mechanism to replace it or support it. The consequence is that it is very difficult to assume the care of an elderly person that is not completely independent.

They are aware that the tension and the contradictions that arise from the difficulty in taking care of the needs of the elderly without any external support lead to difficult situations in which relations deteriorate and "abuse" appears daily.

They also recognize the existence of "inappropriate" attitudes by some of the elderly, who refuse to accept the limitations imposed by the new lifestyles, hampering the adoption of intermediate solutions between traditional models (where the duty of care lies exclusively with the family) and the tendency to ignore the elderly.

Forms of abuse identified by the elderly are divided into two groups, one the situations that occur privately, and the other what might be called public or institutional elder abuse. In the private aspect they distinguish a series of constituent situations which, within the gravity they give to all, show a certain degree of gradation. From lesser to higher, they are:

Exploitation of "free labor" In these situations there is a certain asymmetric relationship. In their opinion, exploitation of the elderly (initially gladly assumed by their desire to help their children and support them in their difficulties) occurs when they become trapped in a situation in which they have to bear a burden of work and concern that can exceed their physical capacities, the alternative being to stop being useful and therefore assume the role of burden to the family. When this dynamic is installed, from their point of view of the elderly, it is considered abuse. When the elderly inevitably enter a phase of dependency, where they can no longer help, but need help themselves, this form of abuse culminates: they are marginalized in the family, becoming a nuisance that overrides the previous relationship, or what seems even worse to them, are admitted into home.

Remove from family This is an attitude that some people graphically describe as "putting up with the old person", that is letting them know they are an inconvenience and that their presence is considered unwelcome. The ways in which this manifests itself are, according to the elderly, varied and with varying degrees of subtlety, ranging from systematically refusing to let them watch the television programs they like to the most extreme case in their opinion, which it consists of forcing them to spend long periods of time out of the house with the excuse that they should walk alone.

Uprooting In this category, we consider any scenario in which the elderly, against their will, are forced to leave what they consider their home. The most evident for them seems to be the circumstances in which an elderly person cannot live alone, rote by the homes of their children. This situation, as much as they understand it, seems frankly regrettable and, in their opinion, encourages a feeling of being a "piece of junk or old thing", of being of hindrance. The natural consequence is social withdrawal that is for them a prelude to death. Another circumstance described in this category is to force an elderly person who has not lost their cognitive faculties to enter a residence, either through moral pressure or deceit or deception on the part of their children. Such situations inevitably lead to deep bitterness and rapid physical and mental deterioration.

Economic exploitation of affection This modality involves making the elderly believe that they are loved or appreciated in order to convince them to put their economic resources—pension, savings, or real estate—at the disposal of the family member, who, in turn, offers to be an unconditional caregiver.

Abandonment This refers to situations in which an elderly person who lives alone is abandoned to their fate, without direct relatives caring for the conditions in which they live, whether through indifference or overtly conflicting relationships, or where they live far away, limiting their contact to sporadic phone calls or occasional visits. The elderly faces solitude and daily tasks that become high risk situations that are very difficult to deal with.

There is still another type of situation that they classify as abuse attributable to the family, although in this case it proves to be a source of suffering for those who receive it as well as for those who, according to the elderly, often unintentionally, inflict it: the lack of training of informal caregivers. This refers to situations in which the care of the dependent elderly person is inappropriate, such as incorrect physical manipulation or lack of relational or psychological skills on the part of the caregiver. This arises mainly in the case of the disabled or demented. They also express fear of situations of abuse that may occur with paid caregivers who, on occasions, can economically exploit or neglect their elderly dependants.

To date very little information on elder abuse is available for Latino countries and more is known about abuse in Spain, although no specific study at national level has been carried out.

Elder abuse is expressed in specific behavior patterns, but all are based on structural variables. For example, in Spain, it is estimated that 33 % of old people are poor and 43 % are on the threshold of being so. Furthermore, it is women, frequently widows, of a low educational level and surviving on widows' pensions or state aid, who are most likely to live in precarious conditions. This should be borne in mind since although elder abuse is common to all social classes, situations of social exclusion are a breeding ground for the phenomenon. However, it is perhaps the dependence of the elderly that should concern us most. In Spain more than a million old people are in a serious dependent situation, and the social/sanitary resources available to face the situation are clearly insufficient.

There are documents and protocols on elder abuse in Spain but hard research is scarce. Despite this, a report by the State Public General Prosecutor [86] made special mention of the vulnerability of the old to maltreatment. Most such maltreatment, it is known, is committed by descendents (children and grandchildren), the violence of children being of especial concern since there is little possibility of abuse being reported to the social services when the aggression is carried out by the person supposedly providing care. The elderly very rarely report ill-treatment, and the physical and emotional dependence on the aggressor or aggressors is maintained. Impunity is the norm since the offense is committed without witnesses and with little evidence. For justice to be done, such behavior hidden within the family itself must be exposed. Mention should also be made of the cases of domestic violence between partners (of either sex) when both mental and physical health may be failing, malefactor in this case acting because he or she cannot face the situation of having to provide care any longer.

Epidemiological data on elder abuse are scarce. In Spain, one of the first papers in this respect was that of Bazo [7]. This study presented the first results of a research on elder abuse and neglect at home. The study was carried out on a sample of persons receiving home help services. Home care assistants caring for 2351 persons from different Spanish regions were interviewed. Hundred and four cases of elder abuse were detected, which amounts to 4.7 % of the total population. It was also noticed that abuse was committed by biological and sons and daughters-in-law in 55 % of the cases and in 12 % by husbands. The rate of abandonment and neglect was higher (physical and/or psychological neglect) than abuse as such. In addition, males suffered more neglect proportionally than women, whereas women suffered more abuse (physical, psychological, and financial). The author emphasized that social and health policies need to achieve the aim of identifying existing cases of abandonment and abuse, as well as detecting those persons and groups who may be at higher risk of suffering abuse. Similarly, measures should be adopted (such as setting up protocols) so that, by making victims visible, both victims and their families can be cared for adequately.

In another study carried out in an urban health district in 307 patients over 70 years old the prevalence or suspicion of elder abuse was 11.9 % (95 % CI 7.6–16.2), breaking down into 6 physically ill-treated, 20 psychologically, 1 sexually, 3 by negligence, and 3 by neglect. Nine people suffered more than one kind of ill-treatment. Significant associated variables were: being a woman (18 %), receiving social assistance (46 %), being a widow/widower (21 %), not having had paid employment 20 % and having a rotating residence (28 %). On application of multivariate analysis, being a woman (OR: 4.99) and receiving social assistance (OR: 7.55) maintained their significance. The presumed perpetrators were son/daughter (57 %), spouse (8 %), son/daughter-in-law (23 %). Of these 19 % were drug-dependent and 15 % suffered psychiatric disorders. With these results the authors managed to alert doctors to a previously underrated health problem [79].

In 2003 the Spanish government approved a comprehensive Action Plan for Older People (2003–2007), aimed at improving quality of life and increasing resources for the elderly. It included 135 specific measures based on the principles of independence, self-fulfillment, participation, and care. Central to the plan was the detection and eradication of violence against older people both at home and in nursing homes. To achieve this goal, the government intended to define violence against the elderly as a legal entity distinct from violence against women and children. Protocols to identify such violence in health centers and nursing homes were to be implemented. In 2003, the violence against older people in Spain had increased by 14 % in the previous 5 years. Risk factors for being abused included dementia, high levels of dependence, poverty, and female sex [10].

Risco Romero et al. [78] included a total of 209 patients over 72 years of age without cognitive deterioration. The questionnaire of suspicion of elder abuse used was one recommended by the Canadian Task Force and the American Medical Association consisting of nine questions, the presence of one positive answer being considered indicative of suspicion of abuse. The prevalence of suspicion of elder abuse was 52.6 % (at least one positive answer to the questionnaire). 8.6 % responded affirmatively to two questions and 2 % to three. Female gender, widowhood, deficiency of studies, living alone or in institutions and not having exerted remunerated work were the associated variables in the bivariant analysis with regard to the suspicion of abuse. In the logistic regression model, there was a significant association with the civil status and the coexistence of the family nucleus, with a greater risk of elder abuse in unmarried and/or widowers and in those living alone. The results confirmed a high prevalence of suspicion of elder abuse in the old population.

In 2009 Pérez-Cárceles et al. ascertained the extent of suspicion of elder abuse and the different types of abuse. The authors designed a cross-sectional survey including 460 patients over 65 years at different health centers (Southeast

Spain). A face-to-face interview and a physical examination were carried out. The extent of suspected abuse was 44.6 %, while the different types of suspected abuse can be listed in decreasing order as follows: withholding care (31.1 %), psychological abuse (20.7 %), physical negligence (17 %), financial abuse (7.2 %), emotional negligence (7 %), and physical abuse (2.4 %) and, lastly, sexual abuse (1.3 %). Female sex, over 75 years, widowhood, living alone or with children, accommodation in house of relatives and income lower than 300 euros/month were the associated sociodemographic variables. The risk factors associated were recent worsening of health, living with a mentally ill person, excessive consumption of alcohol or illegal drugs, arguing frequently with relatives or the dependence on someone to carry out a daily activity. In the physical examination, the associated signs were dehydration/malnutrition, pressure ulcers, and poor body and/or mouth hygiene. Again, in Spain these results confirmed a high extent of suspicion of elder abuse.

Also in 2009, Garre-Olmo et al. mentioned an overall prevalence of elder abuse of 29.3 % in 676 subjects aged 75 and older. The prevalence of suspected neglect abuse was 16.0 % (95 % CI 13.2–18.9), of psychosocial abuse 15.2 % (95 % CI 12.8–18.2), of financial abuse 4.7 % (95 % CI 3.0–6.4), and the prevalence of physical abuse was 0.1 %.

Pérez-Rojo et al. [73] estimated the prevalence of suspicion of elder abuse in 340 old persons without cognitive impairment, dwelling in community, who were attended in primary healthcare or social services centers. They found a 12.1 % prevalence of suspicion of elder abuse. Psychological abuse suspicion was the most frequent type (11.5 %) and it was very common the simultaneous presence of different types of abuse (psychological and physical and sexual, 22.5 %). The suspicion of elder abuse was more frequent in women (15.2 %) and spouses were responsible at a high great frequency (51.2 %).

Spanish researches also developed the project conducted by the Spanish Geriatrics and Gerontology Society (SEGG) and the Institute for the Elderly and Social Services (IMSERSO) and under the auspices of the World Health Organization and Geneva University, called "Global response to abuse and neglect of the elderly: Building Primary Health Care Services capacity to deal with a worldwide problem" (Sociedad Española de Geriatría y Gerontología 2004). The following project was the validation of the tool for detecting suspected elder abuse, called Elder Abuse Suspicion Index (EASI) as well as the Social Worker Evaluation Form (FETS) which is used for the confirmation of suspected abuse cases [74].

From January 2009 to July 2009, the first cross-sectional community-based European study was carried out: "Abuse of the elderly in the European region" (ABUEL). This study was carried out in seven cities in Europe (including Spain) using different sampling and administration methods. The ABUEL study was designed with the general objective of assessing elder abuse in different European countries, using a standardized methodology [52, 51, 55] to overcome some of the previously identified caveats. Although not unequivocal, there seemed to be signs that it is increasingly difficult to obtain high response rates in studies in Europe [52]. The response rates ranged from 18.9 % in Germany to 87.4 % in Portugal. The total prevalence of elder abuse (elders who report being victims of any type of abuse at least once during the past year) showed large variations across countries. The lowest prevalence of psychological abuse occurred in Italy (for females, 6.9 %; for males, 16.9 %) and the highest in Sweden (for females, 24.9 %; for males, 35.6 %). In Portugal, the prevalence of financial abuse was 7.8 %, representing the highest proportion of such abuse among the study countries. Greece presented the highest proportion of combined physical, sexual abuse, and injury. In Spain, the prevalence of abuse was 14.5 % (psychological abuse 11.5 %, financial abuse 4.7 %, and physical and sexual abuse and injury 1.5 %).

One finding in this project was that men tended to be underrepresented in all countries. Several studies on elder abuse indicate that a large number of victims are women, but others report that men in later life are also significantly abused, especially when they show symptoms of disability and poor health, and require help for their daily activities as a result. For example, one study focused on the prevalence of different types of abuse experienced by men and on a comparison of male victims and nonvictims concerning demographic/socioeconomic characteristics, lifestyle/health variables, social support, and quality of life. Additionally, the study identified factors associated with different types of abuse experienced by men and characteristics associated with the victims. The data were collected by means of interviews from a sample of 4467 not demented individuals aged between 60 and 84 years. Multivariate analyses showed that older men educated to higher levels, blue-collar workers, and men living in rented accommodation were more often victims than the less well educated, low-rank white-collar workers and home owners, respectively. In addition, high scores for factors such as somatic and anxiety symptoms seemed linked with an increased probability of being abused. Conversely, factors such as increased age, worries about daily expenses (financial strain) and greater social support seemed linked with a decreased probability of being abused. The study confirmed the fact that male elder abuse exists but is still underrecognized. The study also confirmed what the previous literature had already highlighted [44, 81], namely that the usual socially constructed meaning of gender, which considers males as violent and women as pacific, seems to be anachronistic. Thus, we can with confidence that men may be as exposed to abuse just as women are. These results destroy the erroneous belief that elder abuse is a female question [60].

Another study carried out as part of the same project focused on the associations between social support, demographics/socioeconomics, health variables, and elder mistreatment. Multivariate analyses showed that women and persons living in large households and with a spouse/partner or other persons were more likely to experience high levels of social support. Moreover, frequent use of healthcare services and low scores on depression or discomfort due to physical complaints were indicators of high social support. Low levels of social support were related to older age and abuse, particularly psychological abuse.

With regard to geographical differences in the level of perceived social support, some authors [45], observed cross-national/cultural variations. Other studies [53] reported a strong family culture tradition in Mediterranean countries, and a greater support from nonfamily networks in the non-Mediterranean ones. However, in some Mediterranean countries they found a negative association with the level of perceived social support. The authors argued that these two typical Mediterranean contexts, with a strong "family-oriented" connotation, have been negatively influenced by recent demographic/socioeconomic changes (e.g., low fertility rates, smaller households, increasing presence of women in the labor market, urbanization, and increasing individualization). These changes, according to some authors, could possibly account for a dramatic reduction of the traditional resilience of family networks as primary welfare providers for older people in these areas [59].

Recent revisions [82] show a variation in overall abuse prevalence between countries, ranging from the extreme of 1.1 % in the United States [30] to 44.6 % in Spain [72] in developed countries. Variations also existed between European countries, the lowest overall abuse prevalence being in Italy (12.7 %) and the highest in Sweden (30.8 %) [59]. The elderly self-report high rates of elder abuse in China [24, 22], even higher than their counterparts in Western countries with a reported prevalence of 36.2 % [90]. This may seem surprising given people's belief that elder mistreatment is not common in China because of strong family ties in that culture. There are indeed variations across countries in terms of norms influencing behaviors, attitudes, and relationships in society, and within the family [44]. The idea of abuse as a "contextual phenomenon" [61] provides further evidence for the relevance of different historical, geographical, cultural, political, and economic contexts for understanding the phenomenon itself.

Different reviews suggest that the experience of elder abuse is not unusual in many cultures. As regards subtypes of abuse, it appears that psychological abuse accounts for 1.1 % of elder abuse in the United States compared with 41.8 % in Thailand. In other countries such neglect ranged from 0.2 % in the Netherlands to 31.1 % in Spain, financial abuse from 1.3 % in Ireland to 20.59 % in Thailand, and physical abuse from 0.1 % in Spain to 11.7 % in Israel. Sexual abuse is the least commonly encountered, ranging from 0.6 % in the United States to 1.3 % in Spain [82]. The results of different investigations point to a prevalence of elder abuse that depends on a country's economic level of development. Countries belonging to high-income groups generally have a lower prevalence, with the exception of Spain, than upper middle- or lower middle-income group countries. The Northern American continent appears to have the lowest prevalence of overall elder abuse, while Asia has the highest range, most being in the 20th percentile, along with Europe, where a vast range could be observed, from 5 % in Finland and the Netherlands to more than 40 % in Spain [32, 72]. Mention should also be made of the results of recent ABUEL study in seven countries of European countries, which showed an overall prevalence of abuse of 30 % in Germany and Sweden, the populations of both countries enjoying high-level incomes.

One of the subtypes of abuse that needs special attention is self-neglect, when an elderly person endangers or threatens their own health or safety. Self-neglect is characterized by poor hygiene, unsanitary living conditions, and inattention to basic healthcare needs. It may arise from cognitive deterioration and an inadequate level of support [1]. Generally, self-neglect does not form part of the open research lines in the United Kingdom, not only because of the difficulties involved, but also because of the definition of the same; however, the problem does form part of the research lines of American investigators.

Despite the probable magnitude of the problem in Latino communities, research into elder self-neglect has lagged behind other forms of mistreatment, mainly due to difficulties in detecting and assessing the problem. Epidemiological research about self-neglect among Hispanic populations is almost nonexistent. A lack of systematic studies has led to various definitions being postulated for the syndrome of elder self-neglect. In European countries, situations in which the elderly person decides, consciously or voluntarily, to act in a way that is dangerous for their own health or safety is not included in the definition of elder abuse. However, there are some data available on Hispanic elders in the USA (Texas). Among 16,677 Hispanic elders living in the community who were abused between 1991 and 1995, self-neglect was the most commonly identified form of abuse (63.2 %) [65].

Self-neglect, which is the most common form of elder mistreatment seen by Adult Protective Service Agencies across the United States, is an often unrecognized geriatric syndrome characterized by squalor and unsafe living circumstances. It is a result of medical, neurological, or psychiatric disorders coupled to a lack of capacity for self-care and self-protection in the absence of necessary services or medical care, and leads to increased morbidity and mortality [77]. Older adults with lower levels of cognitive, physical, and psychological health were more likely to report self-neglect and its phenotypes [23].

23.5 Role of Community Organization and Faith-Based Communities

The elderly in western society, at least, have achieved considerable advances in their quality of life; in general, they are better informed and educated, they are more integrated in social terms and enjoy a better economic status than the old of previous generations, although not enough in all cases. They also have greater independence, have more time to enjoy pursuits of their choice, and have better access to health and social services.

However, as a counterweight to these undeniable gains, the elderly have also suffered losses and are exposed to new situations or, at least, classic ones which manifest themselves differently: loss of authority and social recognition, differences within the age group, whose origins lie within the social condition or class, gender-based differences and differences that depend on where they live—social and health services tend to be concentrated in cities or large towns, whereas old people who live in villages or the countryside have very limited access to the same services and the possibility of enjoying their leisure time or of taking part in social and entertainment activities.

Both the advances and positive changes achieved and the risks associated with old age point to the great diversity of situations faced by the elderly and the way in which they may be included (or not) in the social dynamics. To have postponed the time that old age begins and to have gained more years of life are the result of enormous advances, achievements, and social victories, although the result has not been able to protect the "environment" of the old or to guarantee them adequate juridical and social protection. They may still be subject to abuse, negligence, abandonment, and maltreatment, both on the part of their own family members and professionals who have dealings with them. This is especially true when age limits the capacity and autonomy of people, rendering them more fragile and vulnerable.

Consequently, what can be said with all certainty is that the aging of the population represents a challenge to politicians and welfare systems alike, so that old people can continue to participate in society and have the services they need. For old age brings with it the growing need for care, especially in those who can no longer live independently.

The changes in social and economic habits and the gradual loss of autonomy and the consequent need for personal attention have led to old people being considered a burden, exposing them to violent behavior and ill-treatment. They may become victims of exploitation or abuse, especially when they still may be useful for given tasks, perhaps because of their possessions or wealth or because of the service they themselves can still offer to relatives.

The care and attention that old people need may represent an added stress to those families which have to provide the same. And such stress may lead to maltreatment.

In Latin European countries cultures, it is the family that traditionally looks after the old, especially when they are dependent on others. This continues to be the case, because, among other reasons, there is a generalized feeling that this is a family duty and the care that the family can offer is the best. The invisible army offering care is mainly composed of women (83 % of nonprofessional care providers are female) with a low sociocultural and economic profile, who, moreover, have other family duties. This inevitably causes stress among those who dedicate on average 8 to 10 years of their lives looking after the aged, and may be responsible cases of undesirable behavior, while making up for the deficit of professional carers. However, the traditional family model has changed and the continuity of informal care provision is ever less stable. Social policy orientated toward community care maintains that the family is the ideal place for looking after the old, although such discourse is not accompanied by real support for the families concerned. The result in many cases is an overworked care provider and the ideal breeding ground for potential elder abuse.

Providing care to a family member is a life-altering experience. Being a caregiver involves changes and sacrifices in order to meet the needs of the dependent older adult. This situation makes caregivers a vulnerable population [26]. Many studies in recent years have documented the physical and psychological consequences and negative impact on the quality of life of acting as family caregiver in a variety of situations [71]. This role increases the possibility of developing emotional stress, anxiety, and depression [18, 19], while one of the principal objectives of health professionals and social policy is "Caring for the caregiver".

According to some authors, the way in which caregivers react to and cope with situations of stress may change with the way in which the problem is regarded and with the personal resources of the provider. Those with greater personal resources (e.g., greater self sufficiency, more social support) will tend to view the stress factors involved as less troublesome and therefore be less vulnerable to the physical and psychological consequences of providing care. This underlines the importance of assessing the influence of personal resources of carers on their attitude.

Although the number of studies that analyze the stress of care providers has increased exponentially since the 1990s, some factors of influence merit more attention than they have received, among them the religiosity or spirituality of carers. For example, among the different personal resources of carers who may influence the stress they feel some authors [49] consider that religion may have a moderating effect on feelings. There is now a demand for more research on the beneficial aspects of caregiving to better understand the possible antecedents that facilitate caregivers' adaptation to the caregiver role among ethnic populations.

Religiosity studies commonly use the following classifications: (a) intrinsic, entailing internalization of basic faith principles on a day-to-day basis; (b) organized, entailing the public practice of both basic and significant religious rituals; and (c) nonorganized, entailing the private practice of religious rituals [70]. The aspects of religion and spirituality that have received most attention in this respect range from the merely descriptive (e.g., following a given religion) and behavioral (e.g., the frequency that an individual prays) to more internalized and personal aspects (e.g., the importance of religion to the subject), coping strategies (using religion to face down difficulties) or religious well-being (a sensation of oneness with a superior power).

Religion and spirituality may affect overall well-being by (1) providing a framework for understanding why bad things happen and (2) offering the prospect of an afterlife for followers. Previous research findings demonstrate that caregivers may use their religiosity and spirituality as a way of coping with stress and coming to terms with their circumstances [16, 70, 83]. While it is true that most research along these lines emphasize the beneficial effects of religiosity and spirituality [49], the effect may also be negative if such feelings generate a sense of guilt, self-blame, shame low esteem, obsessively scrupulous, or having the idea that one is being punished by one's god [68]. According to the conceptual framework of Herrera et al. [38], religious beliefs have a bidirectional relationship with cultural factors and instrumental support. Contextual and socioeconomic factors, such as the caregiving environment and the functional status of the care recipient, have a direct impact on caregiver well-being, but may be moderated by cultural perceptions and the availability of formal and informal support. This recent study explores the association of religious and spiritual coping with multiple measures of well-being in Latinos (population along the California/Mexico border) caring for older relatives. Caregivers reporting higher levels of intrinsic and organizational religiosity were less likely to perceive their caregiving role as burden some, while those exhibiting greater levels of nonorganizational religiosity reported worse mental health.

In the sociocultural context of southern European countries most carers consider themselves believers mainly referring to being Roman Catholic. Although only about one-third of the population is not practicing Catholics, religious belief is still used as an argument by carers. Indeed, it has been Baines [4] suggested that almost three-quarters (74 %) of the carers studied considered prayer as their principal arm for doping.

Religious or spiritual sentiments appear to help families to find purpose and sense in adversity, acting as something to clutch to as a sign of identity and a basis for facing up to the change, loss, uncertainty involved in the impossibility of controlling things. Further investigation is warranted regarding how knowledge of the positive and negative associations between religiosity and caregiving may assist healthcare providers in supporting Latino caregivers.

Some studies suggest that religiosity and spirituality, especially the social support of religious communities, may act as a tool for alleviating and palliating the feelings of caregivers [63].

From the results of such research, it can be deduced that religion may act as protector against elder abuse, since decreasing the level of anger will diminish the probability of maltreatment. Such evidence points to the need for health professionals to have regular contact with carers and provide them with the ways of managing the difficulties they feel in the task they have.

Studies into interventions designed to prevent situations of elder abuse are scarce and none have been carried out in Latin communities in Europe. A recent systematic review and meta-analysis of such interventions identified 24 studies about this area and authors report specific areas that are still lacking evidence at the present time are interventions that target (1) elder neglect, (2) public awareness, (3) older adults who experience maltreatment, (4) professionals responsible for preventing maltreatment, (5) family caregivers who abuse, and (6) carers who abuse [3].

23.6 What Do We Know, What Do not We Know, What We Need to Know

Elder abuse, the most hidden forms of violence, is a growing problem in Western and developed countries, and will probably increase as the population grows older [89]. Several articles have been published in a variety of countries describing different aspects of such abuse.

Most Spanish authors consider maltreatment to be increasing and that it is an underreported problem since the perpetrators belong to the same family of the victim, with all the issues of affective ambivalence and emotional dependence that such a situation implies, favoring denial and hindering prevention and intervention [72].

The subject of abuse and neglectful behavior is increasingly a topic in social media, schools, and scientific publications. The fact that it is only now being discussed is due to a number of reasons-not because it did not formerly exist in private relationships in our society, but rather because we were not aware of its existence.

One of the many reasons why abuse and neglect is such a concern is the growing cohort of older adults. The size of the group of elderly people, especially octogenarians, has and will increasingly have a severe impact on health and social services, as loneliness, incapacity, and dependence increase. It is also likely that the prevalence and incidence of abuse and neglect will increase. While some studies have been carried out in different geographical areas and environments, there are no studies which reflect reality at a national scale. Moreover, from the studies made, it is difficult to accurately state in Spain whether or not there has been an increase or decrease in mistreatment, prevalence, or incidence rates. As mentioned above, all the authors involved emphasize the importance of healthcare professionals in their respective places of work, since they represent the first point of contact with the suspected victims.

Although our epidemiological knowledge of the problem is limited, most data accepted in international circles establishes an overall extent of elder abuse in the family at 3–12 % in those aged 60 and over, although many authors suggest that the real number of cases is greater. It is estimated that less than one in five cases of elder abuse is reported, due to denial or minimization of the problem by the victim, abuser, or health professional [42]. In Spain figures between 4.7 and 12 % have been suggested with a prevalence of around 6 % [79]. The high overall extent of suspected abuse found in the study by Pérez-Cárceles et al. (44.6 %) is similar to the 52.6 % found in another study carried out in Spain [78].

The detection of cases of maltreatment of the elderly is important but a series of barriers hinder the process. One such barrier is the fact that there is no single and widely accepted definition of the phenomenon. For professionals to be able to identify and detect whether an elderly person is suffering maltreatment and/or negligence, it is first necessary to clearly define the term so that all those concerned use the same concept. However, reaching a consensus on the term has been plagued by problems in both research and clinical practice, especially where the line between such treatment and care, between the victim and the perpetrator or between acts that diminish an old person's quality of life and those that do not, is finely drawn [33].

Several authors have attempted to define and classify elder abuse and, while all may have some aspects in common, they cover different questions. This may have consequences for the very people that need help since two professionals may arrive at different conclusions based on different definitions. Among the reasons that may help explain this situation in Latino communities are, first of all, the different values, attitudes and individual beliefs involved. Second, the concept of maltreatment has been developed from the professionals' point of view without considering the views of the elderly themselves [67]. Third, the lack of willingness on the part of society, institutions, and professionals to recognize the situation as a sociosanitary problem. Fourth, there is a lack of discussion and cooperation between different organisms and institutions in which health and social workers are employed. And lastly, the perspectives from which investigators have approached the matter differ, among them, that of the victim, care provider, professional (doctor, nurse, social worker), or institutions themselves. Among this confusion, several definitions have been proposed; indeed, the words maltreatment and negligence themselves are interchanged, leading to more confusion and detracting from any comparisons made between studies. This situation not surprisingly hinders the task of professionals when identifying maltreatment when it occurs and may even confuse maltreatment with normal family conflict in situations of stress. All this lends weight to the fact that consideration must be given to a given behavior within a cultural context.

Given the great diversity of the definitions provided for maltreatment, abuse, or negligence of the elderly, it may be interesting to show the results of a study carried out in Spain for IMSERSO and published in 2004, "Old age, negligence, abuse and maltreatment. Views of the elderly and professionals", which presented a series of views and perceptions held by old people and professionals on the matter in hand. The novelty of this study was that it based definitions on an analysis of the situations that both the old and professionals identified as negligence, abuse, or maltreatment.

The recent recognition of the existence of maltreatment toward the old led to the publication in Spain of "Maltreatment of the elderly. A guide on how to act" [6], intended for consultation by health and social professionals to intervene in and act upon such situations and, if possible, prevent them.

Too little information is available on the problem to serve as a base to understand it sufficiently. However, there is a certain consensus in admitting that elder abuse is an "iceberg phenomenon" (between five and seven of every eight cases are probably not even detected), since many cases are hidden by the victims themselves. Frequently, the result of the overload of caregivers and domestic violence in general, the different forms of dependence result in negligence and abandonment and the victim frequently suffers more than one type of maltreatment.

Nor should it be forgotten that the terms in Spanish and English do not always overlap. The term "elder abuse" is frequently rendered as "malos tratos", with no differentiation of the type. The term "abuso", widely found in the corresponding literature should not be used in Spanish. The nuances of the word "abuse" in English differ from those of the Spanish word, which implies intentionality. In general, Spanish research is based on the presumption that, while the contrary is not demonstrated, an old person is sufficiently competent to take decisions concerning their own life, and the tem self-neglect is not widely used.

Recent validation of the tool for detecting suspected elder abuse, called (Elder Abuse Suspicion Index, EASI) as well as the Social Worker Evaluation Form (FETS), which is used for the confirmation of suspected abuse cases, should help unify the procedures for evaluating ill-treatment of the old. The use of the same methodology will allow results to be compared when the instrument is used in different countries, throwing light on the different form of ill-treatment that are prevalent throughout Europe.

Risk factors and some of the consequences of the maltreatment of old people have been identified in some countries carried out in Latin European and American countries, where they have been seen to be similar to that identified in other communities, several authors associating the suspicion of abuse and sociodemographic variables such as being female or widowed [15, 78, 79]. One of the most important factors has been described is living alone or in an institution [78] or alternating the family member with whom the old person lives [79]. Access to limited resources and economic problems within the family have also been described as being associated with abuse. As regards risk factors have been identified that associate the suspicion of abuse and a recent worsening of health (72.2 %), living with a mentally ill person (83.3 %) or with family members considered by the interviewee to consume drugs or alcohol in excess. Several authors have emphasized that one of the most important risk factors in abuse, is alcohol consumption on the part of the aggressor [34, 75]. In physical examinations, there is a significant relation between signs of dehydration/malnutrition (87.5 %), pressure ulcers (84.6 %), poor body/mouth hygiene (84.6 %), and suspected abuse [72]. Similar results were found by other authors [21, 36, 50].

There have been several recent interventions that attempt to prevent elder abuse. The elderly, particularly in later life or near its end are at risk of becoming frail. Increasingly, dependency and vulnerability to maltreatment are leading people to need long-term nursing care. The MILCEA project (Monitoring Elder Abuse in Long-term Care—Pilot project on elder abuse), which was funded by the European Commission and conducted between December 2009 and the end of March 2012, aimed to contribute to the prevention of elder abuse (EA) in long-term care (LTC). The subordinate aim was to develop a monitoring system that allows the assessment of elder abuse in long-term care as a precondition for prevention. In the course of the project, the LTC systems in different Member States of the EU were systematically analyzed for elder abuse, using a mixture of scientific methods (focus groups, stakeholder analysis, literature analysis, interviews, etc.). The main thrust of the MILCEA project was to provide a framework for EU Member States on how to put in place the structures needed to monitor elder abuse. The framework has been developed for use in all EU Member States. Prevention includes the recognition of elder abuse and the risk of elder abuse. The MILCEA project focuses on long-term care because people who are in need of care are permanently dependent on the help of others. The care relationship is usually not reciprocal and thus very vulnerable to abuse in its widest sense. As dependence on care and attention by others increases, so does the risk of becoming a victim or an offender of elder abuse. To protect the older person in need of care as well as the caregiver a special and comprehensive approach is needed—one that, to date, has not been put into effect on a sufficiently large scale.

23.7 Challenges in Doing Research on Elder Abuse in Latino Communities

A literature review of elder abuse in Spain shows that some progress has been made, although there is still no consensus regarding definitions and indicators of abuse, which hinders the effectiveness of national research studies. Therefore, one of the first challenges is to unify such definition. Most studies to date are of the overall prevalence of elder abuse and different types of risk factors in given populations of old people. However, studies are still few and there are no studies at national level.

It is essential that future studies focus on elder abuse in both genders, in order to raise awareness of existing mistreatment of older men. There are indeed still strong social/cultural norms which prevent men acknowledging victimization, although aging and ageism can expose older persons in general to episodes of violence and neglect, especially when the persons in later life are disabled and depend on others for assistance in carrying out daily activities.

Future research should also explore in more depth men and women as both victims and perpetrators, in addition to exploring the perception of support from family and social relationships.

Recent screening tools have also been validated in Spain and should be used more systematically across the country, thus enabling more victims of abuse to be discovered and receive help. Only one elder abuse tool has been designed in Spain (EDMA). This is an observational tool applied by a professional to assess elder abuse and self-neglect. Screening tools are necessary to detect elder abuse, and there is a gap in Spain surrounding them. It is necessary to develop new tools or to conduct validation of the existing tools in Spain.

Research into the isolation of the elderly, especially in large cities, as a result of negligence or abandonment on the part of carers is situation that needs to be remedied. Social isolation in its maximum manifestation of self-neglect and abandonment, while relatively uncommon, deserves special attention in order to offer the help that is needed. The joining of several factors such as health problems or the absence of social support make the elderly extremely vulnerable to loneliness, negligence, or social isolation, leading on occasions to death. The definition of self-neglect and the methodology for investigating it is practically absent in Latin European and South American countries.

One of the challenges is to evaluate the consequences of maltreatment. In general and paradoxically the authors of violent conduct against the elderly are those charged with their care, it is also important to know the risk factors that may be associated with mistreatment to be able to detect those at risk and to understand the possible consequences that may arise from such treatment.

Normally mistreatment does not solve itself. Such situations tend to be repetitive and to continue unless there is some important change in the environment surrounding the events. Recent research has shown that elder abuse may have a short and long-term negative impact on the victim both in terms of physical and mental health. However, information on the consequences of abuse is very scarce. More research focusing on the impact of mistreatment on health is crucially needed, as is the exploration of pathways by which community-societal level factors are linked with individual ones and their impact on elder abuse.

There is also limited information on the influence of religion and spirituality as a personal resource in care stress in Latino communities, despite the fact that they seem to play an important role. More research is necessary into the conceptualization of religiosity and spirituality; better assessment of its role in care giving; more qualitative data and longitudinal studies of "religious coping". Although initiatives to support caregivers are beginning, few programs have addressed the unmet needs, and spiritual and special concerns of ethnic minorities, including Latinos.

There is a growing body of literature pointing to the importance of preventing elder abuse, given its negative effects on the quality of life, well-being, health, and mortality of elder abuse. Another challenge, then, is the development of interventions designed to prevent or stop elder abuse in Latin countries, directed at the professionals responsible for preventing elder abuse, and interventions that target older adults who experienced maltreatment and interventions that target careers who maltreat. No such intervention program has been put in place to date.

There are significant national efforts to increase awareness to the topic of elder maltreatment and to make legislative changes to reduce or prevent elder maltreatment, but the effectiveness of these efforts has not been examined scientifically. Investment in training programs for professionals responsible for reducing elder maltreatment and in awareness campaigns is necessary, and there is an urgent need to systematically assess the effectiveness of these interventions.

In effect, there are several promising theoretical perspectives and professionals are beginning to recognize the problem of elder abuse. These could be a good start for further research studies in the area of abuse and neglect of older adults and could be interesting for practitioners to reflect upon as a base for their intervention models, prevention programs and policies.

23.8 Prevention and Implications for Social, Professional, and Policy Practice

The care provided to the elderly involves a series of problems in present day society, which affects the attention given to them. Amongst these problems are the insufficient availability of socio-health resources and the lack of coordination of health and social administrations. This lack of resources and difficulty of coordination are important barriers that can affect the ability to detect situations of possible abuse.

Elder abuse can be seen as the natural history of a "*disease*". From an ideal "*healthy*" situation with no risk of the appearance of elder abuse, we pass to a situation of risk, but with no actual abuse, and subsequently to another situation of hidden abuse or even manifest abuse, which is sometimes recurrent [6]. The existence of abuse toward elderly people has only recently been recognized in professional fields in Latin countries and social awareness of this dramatic issue has only just begun to emerge with any force.

The key recommendations of the WHO concerning a global strategy to respond to elder abuse are gradually being assumed by Latin countries, although at different paces and applying different economic and human resources. In Spain, for example, these recommendations have been assumed by the Institute of Social Services and the Elderly (Instituto de Mayores y Servicios Sociales—IMSERSO) and the Spanish Society of Geriatrics and Gerontology (SEGG) since 2002, the aims being to:

- Create and disseminate a research method to study violence against the elderly.
- Design and validate an instrument for detection and assessment for social and health professionals working at the community level.
- Develop educational materials aimed at professionals for a correct approach to the problem.

- Mobilize civil society through awareness campaigns that generate changes in attitude toward elder and especially elder abuse.

In a society in which discrimination against elderly people in many areas is a reality, we cannot expect to find scenarios in which the risk of the appearance of abuse is nonexistent. For this reason, prevention must begin with the promotion of positive social attitudes that create a "social climate" which minimizes the risks. This perspective helps to understand intervention as a process that begins with primary prevention.

Prevention must involve professionals, family members, health organizations, social and educational services, elderly people and, ultimately, the entire social structure. Primary prevention aims to prevent the emergence and consolidation of those patterns in social, economic, and cultural life that contribute to the risk of ill-treatment.

The measures proposed here are indirect and intended to influence the attitudes and moral assumptions of a society and its different groups. Experts agree that these measures have greater efficiency than is evident at first glance. A primary elder abuse prevention program must act on three fronts: information, training, and institutional policies concerning planning gerontological and geriatric care.

Information is necessary, but not sufficient, to promote changing attitudes toward old age. There are two key areas which can be used to generate positive attitudes in society toward elderly people: the media and the school system.

Several strategies have been developed through the media such as the broadcast of programs that help integrate old age with normality and acceptance, advertising campaigns with positive key messages, promoting good treatment of the elderly, etc. However, most information in the media is about violence between partners. A novel strategy would be to apply what has been learned in recent years of other family violence situations to elder abuse. But this road is still little explored in Latin countries. Experts' opinion on elder abuse is that it can be more difficult to identify than child abuse and intimate partner violence due to the presence of a variety of barriers erected by the victims themselves, caregivers, profession bodies, and society in general.

On the other hand, the training of caregivers and professionals is considered to be one of the key strategies in the prevention of elder abuse. It is very important for professionals to be aware of the specific needs of elderly people, with special attention paid to situations of dependency and care and to be able to recognize the signs and risk factors of elder abuse. In recent years, the issue of elder abuse has been included in the undergraduate and postgraduate curriculum, and in the continuing education of health, social, and law professionals.

It is also essential that caregivers acquire skills that will enable them to cope with the care of the elderly people correctly, avoiding overload in their care load, which has been confirmed as one of the main risk factors generating abuse toward elderly people.

A key point in the prevention of elder abuse is the performance of primary healthcare bodies. Primary care health professionals have contact, over the years, with virtually all the elderly who have been assigned to them. Also, in many cases, they are the only people "authorized" to enter the homes of the elderly. From this privileged position, their involvement in the prevention of abuse is essential.

People who are in need of care permanently are dependent on the help of others. The care relationship is usually not reciprocal and thus very vulnerable. As dependence on care and attention by others increases, so does the risk becoming a victim of elder abuse or an offender. To protect the older person in need of care as well as the caregiver we need a special and comprehensive approach. In addition to raising awareness in each country, appropriate and validated screening/assessment instruments and/or signal cards should be available and incorporated into an obligatory monitoring system.

From a theoretical point of view we know what the prevention measures are; however, information on the implementation of these measures and the evaluation of their results are virtually inexistent. Previous experience on child abuse and intimate partner violence has highlighted the need for the development of specific protocols and guidelines on prevention, evaluation and intervention in elder abuse.

Interventions for the prevention of elder maltreatment are scarce and, to the best of our knowledge, there are no published results for Latin European countries or Latino communities. In light of this, it is clearly necessary to develop intervention programs, as in many other countries, primarily dealing with three main categories: (a) interventions designed to improve the ability of professionals to detect or stop elder maltreatment, (b) interventions that target older adults who experience elder maltreatment, and (c) interventions that target caregivers who maltreat the elderly [3].

Significant efforts have been made to increase awareness to the topic of elder abuse and to make legislative changes to reduce or prevent such maltreatment, but the effectiveness of these efforts has not been examined scientifically. Moreover, it is necessary to evaluate the effectiveness of the limited training programs that are directed toward professionals responsible for reducing elder maltreatment and to raise awareness by campaigns directed at both professionals and the general population.

Statistics on abuse in old age are far from reality that, although, fortunately, the views on gender and human rights have added to the study of this phenomenon, bringing it into the light and demanding attention. Gender studies dealing with the exploitation and abuse of elderly women have favored a greater concern for the elderly in general, regardless of sex. In addition, the interest of civil associa tions, both public and private institutions that work in the field of violence (both theoretically and through direct action), has favored the creation of new public policies aimed at combating the phenomenon. Raising awareness and identifying the damage that is caused by abuse in all its dimensions will allow us to take more and improved steps to eliminate it.

As regards elder abuse, Spanish society is now where it was two or three decades ago regarding child abuse and intimate partner violence. Both were underreported and little studied phenomena, and therefore attracted little attention or were even considered nonexistent. However, there are no national statistics referring to the different situations of elder abuse.

Although studies about elder abuse are scarce and partial, legislation in Latin countries is slowly making progress. Each country's legislation is being developed on the basis of the regulatory global framework of, for example, the Universal Declaration of Human Rights, which establishes fundamental rights—applicable, by extension, to the elderly and of great importance for the development of freedom in old age, the International Plan of Action on Ageing and related activities, and the recommendations of the Report of the Second World Assembly on Ageing, which set targets related to the elimination of all forms of elder abuse. Since 2002 different conferences of international organizations such as the Toronto Declaration on the global prevention of elder abuse [89], the Regional Intergovernmental Conference on Ageing in Latin America and the Caribbean (2003), amongst others, have provided a frame of reference which countries are slowly adapting to their national realities in order to respond effectively to the needs and interests of the elderly, leading to the creation of conditions that favor individual and collective aging in safety and with dignity. The challenge of every country is the implementation of such agreements, which requires designing measures that contribute to their realization.

In recent years, elder abuse has been included in the national legislation of some countries, although there are still no specific laws about elder abuse in most. Also, different agencies at a national level are responsible for the design of programs against elder abuse and for funding these programs.

The Penal Code covers the abandonment of people with disabilities, punishing those who neglect those in their custody and whom they owe assistance, punishing the omission of such assistance. Most of the countries have recently included in their national laws criminal sanctions against those who abuse family members, including the elderly, and the penalization of psychological violence. Amongst other measures, adequate and effective complaint mechanisms are being developed in cases of violence toward the elderly in recognition of the need to strengthen judicial and administrative mechanisms in cases. The Civil Code regulates the guardianship of incapable subjects due to physical or psychological deterioration, and the obligation to provide food and care.

There is still no special public prosecutor for the abuse of elders, similar to that existing in Spain for the case of gender violence. And more must be done to develop community action programs.

In Spain, the Law of Promotion of Personal Autonomy (Dependency Act) and Attention for people in situations of Dependence (2006) seeks to ensure attention for people with disabilities, including elderly persons who require it. And five aspects are already being put into practice such are: (1) legal recognition of the figure of the family caregiver, (2) labor legislation to reconcile working life and caregiver tasks, (3) economic legislation to benefits people with disabilities and caregiver, (4) the incorporation of men as informal caregiver, (5) the development of a system of social services to help the caregiver (respite care units, day centers for elderly, residential places, home help service).

All these actions stem from an interest to regulate the protection of elderly people in our midst, but are perhaps still far from what should be considered appropriate, especially considering the progress made in legislations on partner abuse against women and the social awareness and support that this area has aroused in recent years. However, little has been done in the case of protection of the elderly at the same time.

In Spain, research into topics linked to the elderly is insufficiently developed. Research funds are needed to carry out projects on elder abuse and to increase the number of researchers in different areas. Elder abuse is not a priority line of research in the National Scientific Research Plan. However, the detection and attention of intimate partner violence and mistreatment at all ages is included in the portfolio of services of the Spanish National Health Service, especially in regard of the elderly, children, and persons with disabilities. Greater effort from the health sector at a national level and better coordination would make possible a nationally representative longitudinal study and enable the incidence of elder abuse subtypes to be examined, at least at primary care level.

It is necessary to know and understand the problem thoroughly, because available studies are scarce and disparate because of the lack of international consensus in carrying them out—and knowledge is necessary for prevention. A multidisciplinary approach to this issue is urgent, as the data of national studies from other countries are based on sociological and family models that are of little relevance in the context of Latin European and American countries.

In other countries such as the United States and Canada, prevention focused on the abusive caregiver has become the focus study. Several studies emphasize intervention concerning risk factors in the family context, such as a reduction of caregiver stress, promoting care by the caregiver, training in the handling of the often problematic behaviors of the elderly, and clinical intervention in the case of caregivers considered as being risks. Although progress is being made in the field of intervention, especially on the part of social workers and doctors, much remains to be done in Latin culture.

Addressing elder abuse, especially if the person is not independent, requires coordinated planning at all levels and with all kinds of abuse in mind. Such planning must take into account the multidimensional factors of the problem and tackle it in an interdisciplinary way at all levels. If this is not done, it will be difficult for current society to significantly reduce this type of behavior, powered on many occasions by patterns of behavior learned from the same society that criticizes the same. This will require multiple interventions: increasing social awareness, the training of professionals, making people aware of their own rights, the systematic application of quality criteria, evaluation services, listening to people—in short, detection, prevention, and intervention.

Everything related with domestic violence is treated in a very fragmented manner; for example, child abuse and intimate partner violence are often mentioned with special emphasis. In attempt to overcome these fragmented considerations the Plan of Action against domestic violence has been initiated, but it will still be difficult to separate all collective references to talk about abuse in general. Some experts believe that a generic and global treatment of abuse is much more suited to our social reality than breaking it down into age ranges, gender, or any other circumstance. The person who mistreats does so for many reasons, amongst them, especially, the fragility of the abuse receiver, particularly the elderly.

Prevention must begin with the promotion of positive attitudes toward the elderly that create a "social climate" which is beneficial for them. It is necessary to create the necessary conditions for the development of a healthy personality with their need for consideration, love, and recognition that leads to self-esteem satisfied. There is need for generosity and the will to accompany. In the absence of these conditions, there is maladjustment, bitterness, and frustration. Prevention involves everybody: professionals, family members, health, educational and social organizations, and the elderly themselves—ultimately, the entire social structure. In Spain, various guides promoting good treatment toward the elderly have been published to encourage these positive attitudes.

Prevention consists of minimizing or even eliminating individual, family, and social factors contributing to violent behavior, and encouraging the development and strengthening of the basics of nonviolence, while neutralizing the risk factors that predispose individuals toward violence. All preventive efforts must include direct actions against the conditions that facilitate the appearance of an abusive environment. Prevention is a key in the whole process of intervention, and the best way to prevent is by increasing social awareness, training professionals and providing the elderly and their families with sufficient resources to limit exhaustion and the feeling of helplessness and loneliness. When suspicion becomes certainty, there is an obligation to report matters to the competent judicial authorities as a form of contributing to the eradication of this serious problem which is the responsibility of us all.

International actions also have an impact in Latin countries, such as the World Elder Abuse Awareness Day (WEAAD) launched on June 15, 2006 by the International Network for the Prevention of Elder Abuse and the World Health Organization at the United Nations. The purpose of WEAAD is to provide an opportunity for communities around the world to promote a better understanding of the abuse and neglect of older persons by raising awareness of the cultural, social, economic, and demographic processes that affect the same. By this day, Latin countries and Latino communities also express their commitment to the defense and protection of human rights of the elderly in the face of this problem.

On June 15, 2015 the member states of the Organization of American States (OAS) approved the Inter-American Convention on Protecting the Human Rights of Older Persons during the General Assembly of the institution, which was immediately signed by the governments of Argentina, Brazil, Chile, Costa Rica, and Uruguay at the OAS headquarters in Washington DC. The purpose of the Convention—the first regional instrument of its kind in the world—was to promote, protect, and ensure the recognition and full enjoyment and exercise, on an equal basis, of all human rights and fundamental freedoms of older persons, in order to contribute to their full inclusion, integration, and participation in society. The starting point of the Convention was the recognition that all existing human rights and fundamental freedoms apply to older people, and that they should fully enjoy them on an equal basis with other segments of the population.

Finally, technological research may represent one step more in the care of the elderly. Robotics, a technology undergoing rapid advances in all fields is beginning to look at care of the elderly and people with dementia. According to experts, there are many advantages of this new robotic assistance, which can help supplement the lack of sufficient personnel in the labor market for certain functions, such as that which concerns us here, the care of elderly people. Increasingly, "intelligent" systems can be incorporated into these devices, which can move freely through physical spaces, interact with people and make their own decisions. Amongst their advantages may be patience and consistency when it comes to assisting the elderly; for example, they will remind people of the time to take medicines, eat or even go to bed.

23.9 Conclusion

Abuse will only be detected if there is a high index of suspicion since only that which we are conscious of can be diagnosed. To remain alert implies the need for training in evaluating situations of risk, indicators, etc., but always keeping in mind that suspicion is not the same as confirmation of abuse. Healthcare professionals may be the only people in victims' life who have the opportunity to recognize the abuse and offer help [43]. Health centers are the front door of the health service, the easiest and most accessible way to communicate health problems and the most widely used by elderly patients [17, 46, 78]. It is from this privileged point of view that their involvement in the prevention of abuse is essential. Vigilance is needed within the whole primary care team if the security of this vulnerable group is to be effected [25]. The causes of abuse are complex, and legal and ethical issues add to this complexity. On the one hand, the individual must be protected from harm, and on the other, his/her autonomy in decision-making must be respected. The Criminal Code of Spain provides the legislation necessary to deal with physical, psychological, sexual, and financial abuse. However, individuals are often reluctant to press charges against a close relative or caregiver. The keyword continues to be prevention, in order to avoid the occurrence of serious cases of maltreatment [2, 64]. But it should not be forgotten that the best way of prevention is to provide old people, families, institutions, and the professionals concerned with sufficient resources to limit exhaustion, precariousness, and lack of sensitivity, and to set to work on generating positive attitudes in society toward old age.

References

1. Ahmad M, Lachs MS. Elder abuse and neglect: what physicians can and should do. Cleve Clin J Med. 2002;69(10):801–8.
2. Akaza K, Bunai Y, Tsujinaka M, Nakamura I, Nagai A, Tsukata Y, et al. Elder abuse and neglect: social problems revealed from 15 autopsy cases. Legal Med. 2003;5:7–14.
3. Ayalon L, Lev S, Green O, Nevo U. A systematic review and meta-analysis of interventions designed to prevent or stop elder maltreatment. Age Ageing. 2016;45(2):216–27.
4. Baines E. Caregiver stress in the older adult. J Commun Health Nurs. 1984;1(4):257–63.
5. Baker AA. Granny-battering. Mod Geriatr. 1975;5:20–4.
6. Barbero J, Barrio IM, Gutiérrez B, Izal M, Martínez A, Moya A, et al. Malostratos a personas mayores: Guía de actuación. Madrid: Ministerio de Trabajo y Asuntos Sociales (IMSERSO); 2005.
7. Bazo MT. Negligencia y malos tratos a las personas mayores en España. Rev Esp Geriatr Gerontol. 2001;36:8–14.
8. Belsky J. Psicología del envejecimiento. Madrid: Paraninfo; 2001.
9. Bodley J. Victims of progress. Menlo Park, CA: Cummings; 1975.
10. Bosch X. Spain takes action to improve quality of life for the elderly. Lancet. 2003;362(9387):882.
11. Burston GR. Granny battering. Br Med J. 1975;3:592.
12. Butler RN. Warning signs of elder abuse. Geriatrics. 1999;53:3–4.
13. Butler RN, Lewis MI. Aging and mental health. St. Louis, MO: Mosby; 1973.
14. Bytheway B. Ageism. New York: McGraw-Hill; 1995.
15. Carmona-Torres JM, López-Soto PJ, Coimbra-Roca AI, Gálvez--Rioja RM, Goergen T, Rodríguez-Borrego MA. Elder abuse in a developing area in Bolivia. J Interpers Violence. 2015. doi:10.1177/0886260515608803.
16. Chang BH, Noonan AE, Tennstedt SL. The role of religion/spirituality in coping with caregiving for disabled elders. Gerontologist. 1998;38:463–70.
17. Comijs HC, Pot AM, Smit JH, Bouter LM, Jonker C. Elder abuse in the community: prevalence and consequences. J Am Geriatr Soc. 1998;46:885–8.
18. Cooper C, Balamurali TB, Livingston G. A systematic review of the prevalence and covariates of anxiety in caregivers of people with dementia. Int Psychogeriatr. 2007;19(2):175–95.
19. Crespo M, López J, Zarit SH. Depression and anxiety in primary caregivers: a comparative study of caregivers of demented and nondemented older persons. Int J Geriatr Psychiatry. 2005;20(6):591–2.
20. DeLiema M, Gassoumis ZD, Homeier DC, Wilber KH. Determining prevalence and correlates of elder abuse using promoters: low-income immigrant Latinos report high rates of abuse and neglect. J Am Geriatr Soc. 2012;60(7):1333–9.
21. Dong X. Medical implications of elder abuse and neglect. Clin Geriatr Med. 2005;21:293–313.
22. Dong X, Chang ES, Wong E, Wong B, Simon MA. How do U.S. Chinese older adults view elder mistreatment? Findings from a community-based participatory research study. J Aging Health. 2011;23(2):289–312.
23. Dong X, Simon M. Prevalence of elder self-neglect in a Chicago Chinese population: the role of cognitive physical and mental health. Geriatr Gerontol Int. 2015. doi:10.1111/ggi.12598.
24. Dong X, Simon MA, Gorbien M. Elder abuse and neglect in an urban chinese population. J Elder Abuse Negl. 2007;19(3–4):79–96.
25. Drury M, Neuberger J. Ageing Britain-challenges and opportunities for general practice. Br J Gen Pract. 2001;51:5–6.
26. Epps F. The relationship between family obligation and religiosity on caregiving. Geriatr Nurs. 2014;35(2):126–31.
27. Fericgla J. Envejecer—Una antropología de la ancianidad. Barcelona: Anthropos; 1992.
28. Fliman KM, Amillo Garayoa S. Algunos aspectos de la historia del maltrato del adulto mayor. Geriatrika. 1996;12:267–74.
29. Fraga S, Lindert J, Barros H, Torres-González F, Ioannidi-Kapolou E, Melchiorre MG, et al. Elder abuse and socioeconomic inequalities: a multilevel study in 7 European countries. Prev Med. 2014;61:42–7.

30. Fulmer T, Ramirez M, Fairchild S, Holmes D, Koren MJ, Teresi J. Prevalence of elder mistreatment as reported by social workers in a probability sample of adult day health care clients. J Elder Abuse Negl. 2000;11:25–36.
31. Garcia A. Elderly abuse in Hispanic families. Natl Center Elder Abuse Newsl. 2002;5(3):2–3.
32. Garre-Olmo J, Planas-Pujol X, López-Pousa S, Juvinyà D, Vilà A, Vilalta-Franch J, et al. Prevalence and risk factors of subtypes in people aged 75 and older. J Am Geriatr Soc. 2009;57:815–22.
33. Gordon RM, Brill D. The abuse and neglect of the elderly. Int J Law Psychiatry. 2001;24(2–3):183–97.
34. Haggard-Grann U, Hallqvist J, Langstrom N, Moller J. The role of alcohol and drugs in triggering criminal violence: a case-crossover study. Addiction. 2006;101:100–8.
35. Harman D. The aging process. Proc Natl Acad Sci. 1981;78:7124–8.
36. Harrell R, Toronjo CH, McLaughlin J, Pavlik VN, Hyman DJ, Dyer CB. How geriatricians identify elder abuse and neglect. Am J Med Sci. 2002;323:34–8.
37. Harris M. Antropología cultural. 7th ed. Madrid: Alianza; 2004.
38. Herrera AP, Lee JW, Nanyonjo RD, Laufman LE, Torres-Vigil I. Religious coping and caregiver well-being in Mexican-American families. Aging Ment Health. 2009;13(1):84–91.
39. Instituto de Mayores y Servicios Sociales (IMSERSO). Un perfil de las personas mayores en España. Madrid: Ministerio de Trabajo y Asuntos Sociales; 2009.
40. Instituto de Mayores y Servicios Sociales (IMSERSO). Vejez, negligencia, abuso y maltrato. La perspectiva de los mayores y de los profesionales. Madrid: Ministerio de Trabajo y Asuntos Sociales; 2004.
41. Jiménez L. Hombre, Historia y Cultura. Desde la ruptura innovadora de Nietzsche. Madrid: Espasa-Calpe; 1983.
42. Jogerst GJ, Daly JM, Brinig MF, Dawson JD, Schmuch GA, Ingram JG. Domestic elder abuse and the law. Am J Publ Health. 2003;93:2131–6.
43. Kahan BS, Paris BE. Why elder abuse continues to elude the health care system. Mt Sinai J Med. 2003;70:62–8.
44. Kosberg JI. Reconsidering assumptions regarding men as elder abuse perpetrators and as elder abuse victims. J Elder Abuse Negl. 2014;26(3):207–22.
45. Kumar S, Calvo R, Avendano M, Sivaramakrishnan K, Berkman LF. Social support, volunteering and health around the world: cross-national evidence from 139 countries. Soc Sci Med. 2012;74:696–706.
46. Lachs MS, Pillemer K. Recognozing elder abuse and neglect. Clin Geriatr Med. 1993;1993(9):665–8.
47. Larrión Z, De Paul JL, Ochotorena J. El síndrome del anciano maltratado. Med Clin (Bar). 1994;102:216–9.
48. Le Roy Ladurie E. Montaillou, village occitan. De 1294 à 1324. Paris: Gallimard; 1975.
49. Leblanc AJ, Driscoll AK, Pearlin LI. Religiosity and the expansion of caregiver stress. Aging Ment Health. 2004;8(5):410–21.
50. Levine JM. Elder neglect and abuse. A primer for primary care physicians. Geriatrics. 2003;58(37–40):42–4.
51. Lindert J, de Luna J, Torres-Gonzales F, Barros H, Ioannidi-Kopolou E, Melchiorre MG, et al. Abuse and neglect of older persons in seven cities in seven countries in Europe: a cross-sectional community study. Int J Public Health. 2013;58 (1):121–32.
52. Lindert J, Luna J, Torres-Gonzalez F, Barros H, Ioannidi-Kapolou E, Quattrini S, et al. Study design, sampling and assessment methods of the European study 'abuse of the elderly in the European region'. Eur J Public Health. 2012;22(5):662–6.
53. Litwin H. Social networks and well-being: a comparison of older people in Mediterranean and non-Mediterranean countries. J Gerontol B Psychol Sci Soc Sci. 2010;65B:S599–608.
54. Lévi-Strauss C, Spiro ME, Gough K, et al. Polémica sobre el origen y la universalidad de la familia. 7th ed. Barcelona: Anagrama; 1995.
55. Macassa G, Sundin O, Viitasara E, Barros H, Torres-Gonzales F, Ioannidi-Kapolou E, et al. Psychological abuse among older persons in Europe: a cross-sectional study. J Aggress Confl Peace Res. 2013;5(1):16–34.
56. ManriqueSáez P. Consideraciones sobre la vejez desde la prehistoria hasta la peste negra, Madrid. Gerokomos. 1999;10:156–60.
57. Marín N, Delgado JL, Aguilar JL, Martínez MA, Díez A, Soto JA, et al. Síndrome de maltrato y abuso en el anciano. Rev Esp Geriatr Gerontol. 1991;26:40–6.
58. Mederos A, Puente A. La Vejez. Madrid: Acento. Enciclopedia Microsoft Encarta 1996;99.
59. Melchiorre MG, Chiatti C, Lamura G, Torres-Gonzales F, Stankunas M, Lindert J, et al. Social support, socio-economic status, health and abuse among older people in seven European countries. PLoS ONE. 2013;8(1):e54856.
60. Melchiorre MG, Di Rosa M, Lamura G, Torres-Gonzales F, Lindert J, Stankunas M, et al. Abuse of older men in seven European countries: a multilevel approach in the framework of an ecological model. PLoS ONE. 2016;11(1):e0146425.
61. Merlo J, Chaix B, Yang M, Lynch J, Rastam L. A brief conceptual tutorial of multilevel analysis in social epidemiology: linking the statistical concept of clustering to the idea of contextual phenomenon. J Epidemiol Commun Health. 2005;59:443–9.
62. Murdock GP. Social structure. Nueva York: MacMillan; 1949.
63. Márquez-González M, López J, Romero-Moreno R, Losada A. Anger, spiritual meaning and support from the religious community in dementia caregiving. J Relig Health. 2012;51(1):179–86.
64. Ortman C, Fechner G, Bajanowski T, Brinkmann B. Fatal neglect of the elderly. Int J Legal Med. 2001;114:191–3.
65. Otiniano ME, Herrera CR. Abuse of Hispanic elders. Tex Med. 1999;95(3):68–71.
66. Palmore E. Ageism: negative and positive. 2nd ed. Berlin: Springer; 1999.
67. Papadopoulos A, La Fontaine J, editors. Elder abuse. Therapeutic perspectives in practice. Oxon: Winslow Press; 2000.
68. Pargament KI. The psychology of religion and coping. New York: Guilford Press; 1997.
69. Parra-Cardona JR, Meyer E, Schiamberg L. Post L Elder abuse and neglect in Latino families: an ecological and culturally relevant theoretical framework for clinical practice. Fam Process. 2007;46 (4):451–70.
70. Pearce M. A critical review of the forms and value of religious coping among informal caregivers. J Relig Health. 2005;44:81–119.
71. Pinquart M, Sörensen S. Differences between caregivers and noncaregivers in psychological health and physical health: a meta-analysis. Psychol Aging. 2003;18(2):250–67.
72. Pérez-Cárceles MD, Rubio L, Pereñiguez JE, Pérez-Flores D, Osuna E, Luna A. Suspicion of elder abuse in South Eastern Spain: the extent and risk factors. Arch Gerontol Geriatr. 2009;49(1):132–7.
73. Pérez-Rojo G, Izal M, Montorio I, Regato P, Espinosa JM. Prevalence of elder abuse in Spanish dwelling in community. Med Clin (Barc). 2013;141:522–6.
74. Pérez-Rojo G, Izal M, Sancho MT, Grupo de Investigación Trátame Bien. Linguistic and cultural adaptation of two tools for the detecting suspected elder abuse. Rev Esp Geriatr Gerontol. 2010;45(4):213–8.
75. Reay AM, Browne KD. Risk factor characteristics in carers who physically abuse or neglect their elderly dependants. Aging Ment Health. 2001;5:56–62.
76. Report of the Second World Assembly on Ageing. Madrid, United Nations Publication; 2002.

77. Reyes-Ortiz CA, Burnett J, Flores DV, Halphen JM, Dyer CB. Medical implications of elder abuse: self-neglect. Clin Geriatr Med. 2014;30(4):807–23.
78. Risco Romero C, Paniagua Vicioso Mdel C, Jiménez Mendoza G, PobladorCurtó MD, Molina Martínez L, Buitrago F. Prevalence and risk factors of suspicion abuse in elder population. Med Clin (Barc). 2005;125(2):51–5.
79. Ruiz Sanmartín A, Altet Torner J, Porta Martí N, Duaso Izquierdo P, Coma Solé M, Requesens Torrellas N. Domestic violence: prevalence of suspected ill treatment of the elderly. Aten Primaria. 2001;27(5):331–4.
80. Sendrail M. Historia cultural de la enfermedad. Madrid: Espasa-Calpe; 1983.
81. Soares JJF, Luo J, Jablonska B, Sundin Ö. Men's experiences of violence: extent, nature and determinants. Int J Soc Welf. 2007;16 (3):269–77.
82. Sooryanarayana R, Choo WY, Hairi NN. A review on the prevalence and measurement of elder abuse in the community. Trauma Violence Abuse. 2013;14(4):316–25.
83. Stolley JM, Buckwalter KC, Koenig HG. Prayer and religious coping for caregivers of persons with Alzheimer's disease and related disorder. Am J Alzheimers Dis Other Demen. 1999;14:181–91.
84. Strehler BL. Ageing: concepts and theories. In: Lectures on gerontology. London: Academic Press; 1982;1:1–57 (Part A).
85. Tomlin S. Abuse of elderly people: an unnecessary and preventable problem. London: Br Geriatr Soc; 1989.
86. Torres-Dulce E. Memoria Fiscalía General del Estado. Centro de Estudios Jurídicos. Madrid: Ministerio de Justicia; 2014.
87. United Nations. World population prospects: the 2004 revision. New York: United Nations; 2006.
88. Unspecified. European Social Policy—a way forward for the union—a white paper. Part A. COM 1994;(94):333. final, 27 July 1994.
89. WHO (World Health Organization). World report on violence and health. Switzerland: WHO; 2002.
90. Wu L, Chen H, Hu Y, Xiang H, Yu X, Zhang T, et al. Prevalence and associated factors of elder mistreatment in a rural community in People's Republic of China: a cross-sectional study. PLoS ONE. 2012;7(3):e33857.

Disrespect: Native American Elder Abuse 24

Jacqueline S. Gray

24.1 Introduction

This chapter will address what we know about elder abuse among the Native American populations of the United States. Native American as used in this chapter refers to American Indian tribes, Alaskan Native villages, and Hawaiian homesteads. The United States has over 560 federally recognized American Indian tribes and Alaskan villages in addition to about 400 state recognized or unrecognized tribes [1]. In the 2010 Census, 5.2 million people indicated they were American Indian/Alaska Native (AI/AN) or AI/AN and some other race which accounted for about 2 % of the U.S. population [2] and about 50 % of the U.S. diversity. These groups have a special status as domestic-dependent nations within this country meaning they have the right of self-government or sovereignty [3]. As will be demonstrated in this chapter, elder abuse and maltreatment research, practice and policy in Indian Country[1] is a new and developing field that is quite complex given the multiple jurisdictions involved. This chapter highlights what is known about elder abuse with Native Americans and what is being done in indigenous communities. It also addresses the importance of understanding indigenous culture, perspective, and challenges when addressing practice and development of policy. The first section will address general information about American Indian/Alaska Native populations and the culture to orient the reader to the populations being discussed. The second part of the chapter addresses the current state of the research on elder abuse in Indian Country including the paucity of information on incidence, reporting, and intervention. Next we will address the policies that impact the issue of elder abuse in Indian Country and what current policies work and do not work, as well as, what is needed. The fourth section will address what is happening with practice in addressing elder abuse and prevention in Indian Country. Promising practices that are being utilized in Indian Country will be described demonstrating how social connections with vulnerable elders, the work of social services and law enforcement, in addition to interdisciplinary response, help to address and prevent elder abuse and maltreatment. These practices include cultural variations in the prevention of elder abuse including family conferences, Native ombudsmen, sacred and restorative justice, family mediation, and peacemaker models utilizing holistic community-healing approaches with offenders providing restitution and a part of the relationship restoration as elders are protected. Finally, this chapter examines recommendations for the future to decrease the prevalence of elder mistreatment.

24.2 Background

In 1491, prior to colonization of North America, indigenous peoples of North, South, and Central America inhabited all of the land in the Western Hemisphere with population estimates between 8.4 million and 112 million people [4]. The North American estimates were between ten and twelve million [4]. By 1776, due to disease (including measles, smallpox, tuberculosis, alcoholism, and others), warfare, and genocide from colonizers, the North American indigenous population had decreased to about 250 thousand just prior to 1900 [4]. Genocide did not become a crime under international law until 1948 when according to Article II of the U.N. Genocide Convention defined genocide as

[1]Indian country includes all land within the limits of an Indian reservation under the jurisdiction of the United States Government; all dependent Indian communities, such as the New Mexico Pueblos; and all Indian allotments still in trust, whether they are located within the reservations or not. The term includes land owned by non-Indians, as well as towns incorporated by non-Indians if they are within the boundaries of an Indian reservation. It is generally within these areas that tribal sovereignty applies and state power is limited.

J.S. Gray (✉)
Center for Rural Health, University of North Dakota School of Medicine and Health Sciences, 1301 North Columbia Rd, Stop 9037, Grand Forks, ND 58202-9037, USA
e-mail: Jacqueline.gray@med.und.edu

X. Dong (ed.), *Elder Abuse*, DOI 10.1007/978-3-319-47504-2_24

"Any of the following acts committed with the intent to destroy, in whole or in part, a national, ethnical, racial, or religious group, as such:

(a) Killing members of the group;
(b) Causing serious bodily or mental harm to members of the group;
(c) Deliberately inflicting on the group conditions of life calculated to bring about its physical destruction in whole or in part;
(d) Imposing measures intended to prevent births within the group;
(e) Forcibly transferring children of the group to another group."[2]

Among Native American people there was little war and few casualties before European contact [5]. Today, there are over 560 federally recognized American Indian tribes and Alaska Native villages in the United States and over 400 state recognized and unrecognized tribes and villages. Unrecognized tribes and villages can apply to the federal government for recognition, but must meet certain requirements before they may be recognized [6, 7]. Each tribe is a domestic, sovereign nation in that they govern themselves, "as always declare by the tribes—and confirmed by congress, the Executive, and the Supreme Court—the present rights of Indian nations to govern their members and remaining territories derive from sovereignty that predates European arrival" [8]. Each tribe is able to make and enforce its own laws subject to limitations by the U.S. Government.

A common misconception about the indigenous people of the United States is that they are an ethnic minority group, when in actuality, they are a political group of domestic nations that were established within the United States by treaties between the United States government and the governments of the tribes [8, 9]. Although the 2010 U.S. Census reports 5.2 million or 1.7 % of the total population of the United States [10], this differs from actual tribal membership/enrollment in that the census includes people who self-identify as American Indian/Alaska Native (AI/AN) where tribal membership is based upon requirements established by each tribe and approved by the Bureau of Indian Affairs (BIA) [8, 11]. AI/AN are the only group of citizens in the United States required to document they are a member of that group, the Certified Degree of Indian Blood (CDIB) card [8]. This documentation also indicates if they are eligible for services provided by the U.S. government due to treaties established with tribes in exchange for land. The 2010 U.S. Census indicated 78 % of the AI/AN population lived outside of AI/AN lands or reservations [12]. Only 9.4 % of AI/AN Americans compared to 17.8 % White, non-Hispanic Americans are age 65 and over [13].

Elder Abuse in Indian country has become a growing concern. A culture that holds elders in high regard is also facing the same epidemic as other older adults throughout the world. Some connect the incidents of elder abuse, neglect, and exploitation to poverty in Indian country, but until recent years, despite the poverty, elder abuse was a rare occurrence [14]. Many households in Indian Country consist of children, adults, and elders living under the same roof. Sometimes these conditions are favorable for the family, and other times these living conditions may be burdensome. There are various reasons for these living situations such as culture, economics, and housing opportunities. Often times, family members who have limited means may need to live with an elder or vice versa because they do not have adequate income or shelter. Under these circumstances, families see it as their responsibility to take care of each other even if it means they need to give up their own resources. Some homes will have multiple families living with an elder. These living situations in Indian country open the elder up to exploitation such as taking an elders' monthly income or medication and using it for their own advantage. While tribes are continuously trying to battle poverty and the social impacts it brings, some tribes are attempting to also combat the incidences of elder abuse through the adoption of elder abuse, neglect, and exploitation provisions in their tribal codes. Other tribes have looked toward traditional methods of combating elder abuse, whereas some tribes do not have the means, education, or resources available to create a formal program against elder abuse. Tribal Governments have a special trust relationship with the Federal Government of the United States. The elder abuse policies passed by the federal government often have provisions that outline how the policy will apply to tribes within the United States.

Some research has shown that Native Americans see more types of behaviors as abusive when compared with elders of other demographic backgrounds. However, identifying more behaviors as abusive does not mean that abuse is reported [14–16].

24.2.1 Native American Elders

Native American elders are estimated to increase in number from 266,000 in 2012 to 1.2 million by 2060, an increase of 450 % [17], see Fig. 24.1. With this increase in population, currently, 78 % live outside traditional Indian land areas and in primarily urban areas [12]. This brings into question the jurisdictional issues and rights of AI/AN outside Indian Country compared to those on tribal lands and within Indian Country. The complexity inside Indian Country with various

[2] The complete text is available at the United Nations website http://www.un.org/millenium/law.iv-1.htm.

jurisdictional issues and lack of resources is a conundrum and requires extensive work to sort out the issues.

24.3 Research

24.3.1 Paucity of Research

At this date, there are no large-scale, population-based studies of the prevalence or incidence of elder abuse among Native Americans. A complication for this type of study are the numerous governmental bodies throughout Indian Country with over 560 federally recognized tribes and Alaskan villages that, through sovereignty, decide if their group will participate in a study and processes for approval should someone try to undertake this project. It is further complicated by the diversity within this population.

The National Indian Council on Aging (NICOA), created by the National Tribal Chairmen's Association in 1976, received a grant from the National Center on Elder Abuse in 2002 to gather basic information regarding Elder Abuse in Indian Country. NICOA found that there is a lack of information, awareness, and data on Elder Abuse in Indian Country [16]. NICOA conducted a small survey of Title VI directors and hosted a focus group. Based upon their findings, many tribal leaders and advocates agreed, despite the lack of data and research, elder abuse is a serious and pervasive problem [14]. They also feel that American Indian people's response and attitudes toward elder abuse are very different than that of non-Indians as the assessment suggests a need for new responses to prevention of elder abuse [16]. To date, there is still no data that reveals the prevalence or incidence of Elder Abuse in Indian country.

Of the research conducted thus far, three studies provide an indication of primarily physical abuse in some Native American populations. A survey of 110 "very traditional"[3] Navajo older adults and their families with a small random sample of participants providing detailed interviews (n = 27) found that 16 % of elders reported physical abuse [18]. Another study based upon medical record reviews, Buchwald and associates found that 10 % of 550 American Indian/Alaska Native (AI/AN) urban patients 50 years and older were definitely or probably abused in the past year [19]. Those identified as abused were significantly more likely to be younger females, experiencing depression and dependent upon others for food. Of those who were

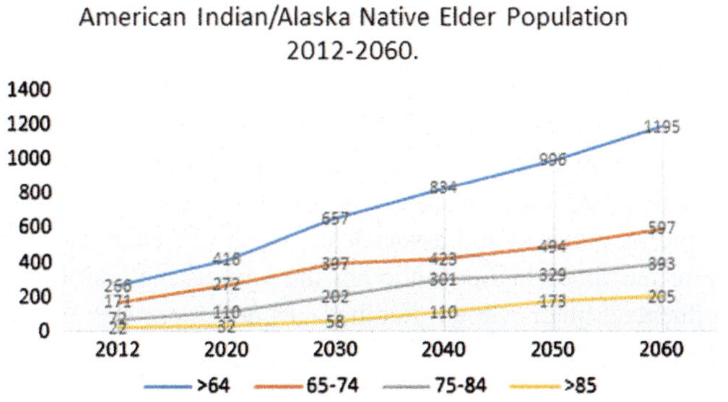

Fig. 24.1 American Indian/Alaska Native elder population projections from 2012 to 2060 by age group presented in thousands

definitely abused, only 31 % were reported to authorities. In a third study conducted by the National Resource Center on Native American Aging (NRCNAA) and Tribal Title VI program staff between 2010 and 2012, the comprehensive health and social needs assessment surveys with 18,062 American Indian/Alaska Native/Native Hawaiian (AI/AN/NH) elders (age 55 and older) from over 240 tribes, villages, and homesteads found that 0.5 % of elders currently used elder abuse prevention services and 13.4 % would use the services if they were available to them [20]. The NRCNAA Cycle V, 2012 through 2014, with 17,049 participants indicated that 1.1 % currently use elder abuse prevention services and 12.7 % would use the services if they were available [21].

Within the two studies of elder physical abuse the prevalence is estimated to be between 10 and 16 %, with an indication from the NRCNAA survey that between 12.7 and 13.4 % of Native American elders would be interested in using elder abuse services. The general population report rates of physical abuse are known to be the minimal compared to emotional abuse, financial exploitation, and neglect [22]. In this national-randomized survey of 5,777 older U.S. adults—where 2.3 % (n = 132) identified as AI/AN—11.4 % (n = 589) of the total sample reported experiencing at least one type of mistreatment in the previous year [23, 24]. When examining the type of abuse or neglect, the prevalence rates for the previous year with the total sample (n = 5777) were financial exploitation by a family member (5.2 %, n = 263), potential neglect[4] (5.1 %, n = 297), emotional mistreatment (4.6 %, n = 254), physical mistreatment (1.6 %; n = 86), and sexual mistreatment (0.6 %; n = 34) [23, 24]. The most prevalent forms of abuse reported are financial exploitation and neglect on a national basis. Jervis [25] found that financial exploitation emerged as the major

[3]"Very traditional" as described by Brown [18] is being geographically and culturally relatively isolated, primarily Navajo-speaking with little English spoken in the homes, oriented primarily to Navajo cultural traditions, and subsisting pastorally with resource and responsibilities shared among extended family and clan networks (p. 20).

[4]Potential neglect was defined as "an identified need for assistance that no one was actively addressing" (Acierno et al. [24], p. 293).

issue in a study of elder abuse indicators among 100 American Indians 60 years of age and older in a south-central metropolitan area and a rural Mountain West reservation with physical abuse discussed in very few cases.

The reported rates of physical abuse in studies of Native American communities are considerably higher than those found by Acierno and associates [24]. In one case the rates were ten times higher, although the various methodologies influenced their varied findings. Under reporting is frequently a possibility in studies that use direct questioning or interview methods due to social desirability bias and the highly sensitive nature of elder mistreatment [26].

Financial exploitation and neglect are reported more frequently in Native American populations. In one study, neglect (32.4 %) and financial exploitation (21.6 %) were the most common types of elder maltreatment reported among a sample of Navajo elders [18]. Neglect and financial exploitation were also most common among the concerns on Lone Mountain, and secondary neglect was the only form identified on Abundant Lands [3]. Baker-Demaray [27] found that emotional abuse and neglect were of greater concern to Native American elders than physical and sexual abuse, but financial exploitation was considered a moderate concern. Baker-Demaray [27] also found that Native American elders were more apt to respond when asked about "disrespect" rather than "abuse." When dealing with sensitive topics it is easy to put off possible participants by bringing up topics in a way they find offensive. There may also be difficult in acknowledging the treatment they may be receiving which is abuse or neglect and is easier to talk about in terms of "disrespect" or, in the case of sexual abuse, "bothering."

24.3.2 Risk Factors for Elder Abuse and Neglect

Brown's [18] surveys of elders and caregivers in a small Navajo community found that elder mistreatment was correlated with elder dependency (especially a sudden onset), mental health concerns among both the elders and the caregivers, and neglect due to caregiver fatigue or economic deprivation. These results were similar to Pillemer's [28] findings of risk factors for the general U.S. population. Brown [18], like Maxwell and Maxwell [3], found in reservation settings that when an elder has an income, but lives with younger family members who are unemployed, the elders were more likely to experience psychological and physical abuse while having no income made them more vulnerable to neglect. Brown also found an increased risk for elder mistreatment when there were multiple caregivers sharing responsibility [18].

Brown et al. [15] asked 152 health and social service providers, law enforcement officers, tribal officials, and community volunteers about their views of mistreatment of Navajo elders. Abused elders were described as most commonly women, very old and physically vulnerable, socially isolated in their home, and perceived by their live-in caregivers as a burden [15]. Abusers were described as family caregivers with substance abuse issues and/or mental health issues such as depression, unemployed, experiencing effects of long-term poverty, and take the role of caregiving as another burden for which there are inadequate resources [15].

24.3.3 Native American Cultural Norms Versus Disrespect

Despite the diversity among Native American groups, the majority would cite respect for elders as an important value within their culture. Elders are viewed as the teachers and keepers of the culture with each group embracing different definitions, ideals, and perceptions of appropriate eldercare and what reaches the point of maltreatment [3, 29, 30]. Actions within one cultural group may be seen as abusive, while within another group it may be seen as acceptable [31, 32]. In one study with 424 white, 318 African American, and 202 Native American adults (n = 944), 40 years of age and older in North Carolina found similarities in their perceptions of elder mistreatment. These perceptions of mistreatment included "assault; battery; threatening; coercion; unreasonable confinement, intimidation, or cruelty; sexual abuse; emotional abuse; exploitation, abandonment; and breach of fiduciary duty." Native Americans in this study were more likely to consider a single incident as abuse than the other ethnic groups [18, 31, 32].

In a study of elder abuse among 100 American Indians age 60 years and over, good and bad treatment by family members and caregivers was viewed as respectful or disrespectful. Mistreatment or disrespect was considered to be financial exploitation (primarily theft and exploitive childcare), neglected, or generally disrespects while good treatment included elders being taken care of, having their needs met, and being treated respectfully within their families and communities [29, 33]. Some gray areas included elders feeling disrespected when grandchildren were left in their care without their consent [29]. Within Native American cultural values, a close grandchild–grandparent relationship includes both child care by the grandparent and eldercare by the grandchild [34, 35], but when grandchildren are left for weeks or months at a time for the grandparents to raise them without the financial resources to supplement their income, the lines between culturally accepted behavioral and exploitation are blurred. It can be unclear even to the Native

American elders to what extent they are being "disrespected" [29, 36, 33]. The lines between exploitation and culturally appropriate sharing of resources are blurred when the financial resources of the elder are used to support multiple generations in the household. Investigation as to what each member of the household is contributing in work or resources to the well-being of the family system to sort out whether it is exploitation.

24.3.4 Financial Resources

Within Native American communities and families the issue of financial exploitation is complex. Many tribal norms are based on reciprocity within the family. An elder sharing their resources with family members is historically (and remains today) a "cultural privilege and duty" for the elder [18, 37]. Caring for elders within a Native American context may be viewed as reciprocal between caregiver and elder and a source of fulfillment to both rather than a burden [37, 38]. Elders are considered teachers and holders of the language and culture so as the caregiver provides for the physical and emotional needs of the elder, the elder passes along the stories, history, culture, and language to the caregiver [39]. Traditional socioeconomic systems of reciprocity, such as giveaways, potlatch rituals, and other resource distribution customs, were a way of re-equalizing society, conferring honor to the givers, maintaining equilibrium in spiritual domains, and maintaining social structure and family and economic interdependency [39]. These as well as other community-building customs were opposed by US colonizing forces who valued individualism, land ownership, and capitalism as the pathway to being "civilized" [40]. The colonizing practices systematically overwhelmed, displaced, or disrupted traditional ways of life, gender roles, child development processes, kinship systems, marriage patterns, spiritual practices, and land usage that also altered ways that elders were treated [41]. The center of spiritual, cultural, moral, and subsistence resources once came from elders and older adults (some chiefs and healers) to the community, which (1) validated their authority; (2) enabled them to fulfill their responsibility to do the best for the community; and (3) established a firm basis for the respect that expected to and for them. Colonial policies displaced these traditional lines of authority and replaced them with individuals willing to function within the guidelines of the colonizing government [41]. This established the way for assimilation, but also stripped elders and traditional leadership of the resources, respect, and moral authority to lead. By disrupting normative age expectations, colonization effectively reduced some of the previously valuable citizens to a state of vulnerability and dependence, setting them up for disrespect and mistreatment.

Tribal elders may also be financially exploited in economic systems that value reciprocity. Research and anecdotal reports indicate that financial exploitation is an extremely common form of elder disrespect in some Native American communities, as in the general population [24]. In societies where reciprocity is the norm, an unemployed adult child or grandchild may ask an elder to provide economic support. This places the elder in a dilemma of contributing to the needs of others or meeting their own immediate needs for medicine or food. Contributing to the support of family in need is seen as generosity which is a common Native American value, and also, it is improper to neglect the needs of an extended family member, if one has resources they are shared. It is expected if the family member who was helped has resources they will help in return if it is ever needed. These values are violated more in today's society and the intergenerational reciprocity is not returned (often by children and grandchildren who were helped previously).

24.3.5 Neglect and Self-Neglect

Although common for Native elders to move in with family members such as children, grandchildren, nieces, or others as they age or lose a partner, with the majority of Native Americans living in urban areas and not necessarily close to family, this becomes more of an issue [42]. Since there are few nursing homes and long-term care facilities on reservations, many rural indigenous elderly remain in their homes or live-in multigenerational homes with children, grandchildren, or other extended family [43]. Only sixteen nursing homes are currently operating on tribal land [43]. Issues of geographic isolation, poverty, and lack of access to adequate health services in reservation areas result in AI/AN elderly seeing care at later states of disease, which lowers survival rates and increases need for a 24-hour day care [43–45]. Lack of cultural sensitivity in many facilities serving AI/AN populations might cause these elders to seek care at later stages of their disease [45].

Although it is traditionally common for Native elders to move in with family members such as children, grandchildren, nieces, or others as they age or lose a partner, this tends to happen more with men than women alone. Elderly women both in urban and reservation areas may stay in their own home when there is no family close by to check on them, tend to their needs, or with room to take them into their homes. In these cases, as the elders decline in their self-care abilities there is more risk for self-neglect, injury, and illness from which there may be no recovery. There have been no studies of neglect or self-neglect among Native American populations. This makes it difficult to address the extent and severity of the problem in this population due to low numbers included in national studies and the lack of indigenous-specific studies.

24.3.6 Spiritual Abuse

An area of abuse and exploitation that is not usually listed among legal forms of abuse, but is brought up repeatedly by Native American elders, is spiritual abuse, which is defined as "the erosion or breaking down of one's cultural or religious belief system" [46]. Spiritual abuse involves more than emotional/psychological abuse, financial exploitation, or neglect by impacting at a deeper level of who the person is. This can include being denied access to ceremonies in hospitals, traditional healing, or healers; not being allowed to attend ceremonies or cultural activities; having traditional regalia or spiritual items taken without permission for use or sale [47]. When spiritual abuse occurs, it interrupts the connection with cultural, spiritual, and language traditions which are tightly woven into the identity and soul of the individual [48]. Duran and Duran [46] called this "soul wounding." Even more so, the elders' teachings, spiritual practices, and ceremonies ensure the continuity of these values from past generations, into the present, and on to future generations [49].

24.4 Policy

24.4.1 Legal Review of Elder Abuse

While Elder Abuse in the United States and Tribes is very common, due to a variety of factors, there has not been much case law regarding elder abuse [50]. Some reasons as to why there is not much case law are because not all cases of elder abuse result in a judicial opinion and not all judicial opinions get recorded in case law reporters; this is especially true for tribal court law [50]. The available case law for tribal courts is sparse because many tribal courts may opt out of publishing their judicial opinions.

Cases that are appealed and heard before a higher court are the cases that are reported to case law books. Elder Abuse most often does not make it past the trial level, if it even makes it to trial at all. If the case does make it to the appellate process, it is not labeled as elder abuse; rather it is categorized as fraud, deed rescission, or some other factor dealing with the financial exploitation of the elder. Other forms of elder abuse such as physical abuse may have charges of assault or murder associated with them. Victims of elder abuse are also reluctant to file charges against their abusers for many reasons: (1) the elder does not realized they are being abused; (2) they want to protect their family member; (3) the elder may fear not having anywhere to go or anyone to take care of them; or (4) the elder does not have the financial means necessary to provide for their care [50]. Elder abuse within tribal communities may not be reported because of cultural values and beliefs, because there are limited resources for elders to bring charges against the perpetrator if they choose to do so, or fear of retaliation by other friends or family members if they do report abuse, neglect, or exploitation.

24.4.2 Elder Programming Funding

Elder programs within tribal communities of the United States are primarily funded through the Administration on Aging provided through Title VI of the Older Americans Act [51]. Title VI of the Older Americans Act outlines resources for American Indians. This includes funds toward elder abuse prevention, caregiver programs, nutrition services such as meals on wheels, and adult protection. The Administration on Aging is housed under the U.S. Department of Health and Human Services (DHHS; [52]). The Administration on Aging's primary focus is to carry out the Older Americans Act.

24.4.3 Older Americans Act

In the mid-twentieth century, the US Congress passed, and President Lyndon Johnson signed into law, the Older Americans Act of 1965 (OAA; [51]). Title VII of the OAA provided funds for states to create programs to provide protection for vulnerable elders. "The OAA set out specific objectives for maintaining the dignity and welfare of older individuals and created the primary vehicle for organizing, coordinating and providing community-based services and opportunities for older Americans and their families" [52]. Title VI programs were added to the OAA in 1978 [53]. Title VI (Grants for Native Americans) of the OAA specifically addressed some of the unique needs of Native American elders and provided funding for program development for their support in the areas of establishing resource centers that gather information, conduct and disseminate results of research, and provide technical assistance and training, especially in the areas of health, mental health, long-term care, elder abuse, and other concerns; nutrition services or meal programs; funding for improving or altering multipurpose senior centers; legal services; and other supports [52].

The AoA whose primary duty is to carry out the provisions of OAA contains the following offices: Office of Supportive and Caregiver Services; Office of Nutrition and

Health Promotion Programs; Office of Elder Justice and Adult Protective Services; Office of American Indian, Alaskan Native and Native Hawaiian Programs; Office of Long-Term Care Ombudsman Programs [53].

The Office of American Indian, Alaskan Native, and Native Hawaiian Programs serves as an advocate for Native elders as well as other racially diverse groups. The office works with federal, state, local, and tribal governments as well as National organizations such as Indian organizations, aging organizations, and national provider organizations. Coordination, providing services, and overseeing policies that affect Native people are their primary focus. The office also manages the Resource Centers on Native American Elders whose primary focus is to gather information, perform research, disseminate information, as well as provide technical assistance and training to providers and tribal leaders [53].

Nearly, two decades would transpire before culturally appropriate guidelines or laws were developed to define, prevent, and remediate elder mistreatment in culturally specific ways by and for tribal communities, first by the Oglala Lakota Nation in 1984; then the Yakima Nation a few years later [54]. It took several more years before research studies were conducted examining elder mistreatment in tribal communities [3, 15, 18]. Within a few years of these seminal studies on elder mistreatment in tribal communities, American Indian/Alaska Native (AI/AN) and First Nations of Canada began to assemble to address this issue within their communities [14, 55].

24.4.4 Elder Justice Act

The Elder Justice Act was a component of the Patient Protection and Affordable Care Act signed into law in 2010 [56] provided under Title VI Subtitle H. This allowed for new language in the Elder Justice provisions of the OAA to create opportunities for States and Tribal organizations. Title II and Title VII of the OAA contains new language that emphasizes multidisciplinary and collaborative approaches for addressing elder abuse as well as to develop programs and long-term care plans for elder justice activities [53]. States and Tribes will have an opportunity to work with the AoA to develop a long-term care plan to "facilitate the development, implementation, and continuous improvement of a coordinated, multidisciplinary elder justice system in the United States" [53]. The new language in Title VII of the OAA allows States and Tribal organizations to use some of the Title VII allotments for detection, assessment, intervention in, investigation of and response to elder abuse, neglect, and exploitation [53].

24.4.5 Funding to Tribes Under the OAA and EJA

In the 2015 Fiscal Year, Tribes received funding for elder programs under the Administration on Aging through the Older Americans Act. Currently, Elder Justice Programs for Indian Country are receiving new funding from amendments to current legislation.

24.4.6 Tribal Court Systems

Many Tribes receive funds to operate their tribal court systems from the Department of Interior [53, 57]. Often tribes will supplement the funding from the Department of Interior with tribal resources [57]. Traditional tribal courts differ from the western model courts. Many of the tribal courts have adopted the western model through past Indian Law policies [57]. However, there have been a few tribal courts that have been able to maintain their customary court proceedings. These courts have gained attention from other governments as a proactive approach to handling crime. The approaches of western model court systems and indigenous court systems differ in many ways. The following table has been adapted from the Victim Assistance Training Online Module [58]. See Table 24.1.

24.4.7 Tribal Law and Order Act (TLOA) and the Violence Against Women Act (VAWA)

The TLOA and the VAWA Reauthorization have had an impact on Indian Law and Policy in Indian Country. The TLOA of 2010 amends the Indian Civil Rights Act, clarifies jurisdiction within Indian country, increases coordination and communication between the federal government, states, and tribes, empowers tribal governments, and reduces violent crime [58–60]. However, 6 years after the adoption of the Tribal Law and Order Act only about 20 tribes have adopted or are in the process of adopting the provisions of the Tribal Law and Order Act [61]. The TLOA has not had a significant impact on Elder Abuse in Indian Country as the tribes overall have not actively adopted the provisions of TLOA. The TLOA, which is optional for tribes, comes with both positives and negatives. It moves toward a more regimented western court system, but allows for longer sentences within tribal courts, which are especially needed in the case of more serious crimes. Without the TLOA, tribes can only sentence offenders for less than 1 year and there is no provision for cross-jurisdictional

Table 24.1 A comparison of Western versus Indigenous Justice concepts as adapted from Harrold [58]

Western justice concepts	Indigenous justice concepts
Vertical	Holistic
Rehearsed communication	Fluid Communication
English language used	Native/Tribal Language can be use
Written statutory law learned from rules and procedure	Oral customary law learned as a way of life by example
Separation of church and state	May pray to a higher power through ceremony and prayer
Separation of powers	Law and justice system part of a whole, may have leaders rule on proceedings
Adversarial and conflict oriented	Builds trusting relationships to promote resolution and healing
Argumentive	Talk and discussion are essential
Isolates behavior, freeze frame acts	Reviews problem in its entirety; contributing factors are examined
Fragmented approach to process and solutions	Comprehensive problem solving
Time-oriented process	No time limits on the process; long silences and patience are valued
Exclusive-limit participants in the process and solutions	Inclusive of all affected individuals in the process and problem solving
Representation by strangers	Representation by extended family members
Focus on individual rights	Focus on victim and communal rights
Punitive—removes offender	Corrective offenders are accountable and responsible for change
Prescribed penalties by and for the state	Customary sanctions used to restore victim–offender relationship
Right of the accused especially against self-incrimination	Obligation of accused to verbalize accountability
Vindication to society	Reparative obligation to victims and community, apology, and forgiveness

issues. The Act permits tribes to prosecute violations that involve more than 1 year in jail. However, many tribes are not able to implement the TLOA due to inability to afford the added costs involved (e.g., providing a tribal judge that has passed the bar and a legally trained public defender).

Elder mistreatment in Indian Country has frequently gone unaddressed because of the cross-jurisdictional issues related to what charges could be filed and where they would be filed. For example, a financial exploitation case with a tribal elder who has a tribal caregiver who misappropriated funds withdrawn from a bank with a state charter creates questions as to where the offense took place, on tribal land or on state land, and hence who should prosecute. If the crime took place within the bank, should it be charged in the state or county courts, even though the victim and perpetrator were tribal members living on tribal lands? This also complicates investigation and arrest of the perpetrator since state officials do not have authority to make arrests on tribal (federal) lands. The TLOA disentangles some of this complexity by mandating that federal, state, and county officials assist, coordinate, and work with tribal officials in the investigation, arrest, and prosecution of crimes in Indian Country.

The TLOA also encourages cross-deputizing of law enforcement entities so they can enforce laws across jurisdictional boundaries. It provides the framework to establish memoranda of understanding (MOU) between tribes and counties and/or states regarding how cross-jurisdictional issues will be handled. TLOA provides that cases occurring in tribal and non-tribal jurisdictions may be prosecuted concurrently by all relevant jurisdictions (TLOA, Subtitle B, Section 401, a (2)) [59]. It also provides for the prosecution of non-Indians who commit crimes on Indian land. Other than federal offenses, this has not been allowable in the past. Thus, in a state where tribes have MOUs with the state or county regarding the investigation, arrest, and prosecution of offenders, if a non-Indian caregiver were to take money from a tribal elder's bank account, the MOU would allow the bank to cooperate with the tribal officials by providing

Table 24.2 Offender, victim, and jurisdiction are indicated for offenses on tribal land

Offender	Victim	Jurisdiction
Indian	Indian	*Federal* jurisdiction for felonies listed in Major Crimes Act 18 U.S.C. 1153; Tribal jurisdiction for misdemeanors; no jurisdiction for felonies not in 1153
Indian	Non-Indian	*Federal* jurisdiction for felonies listed in 1153; felonies and misdemeanors not listed in 1153 (including assimilative crimes) unless the tribe has already punished the defendant; Tribal jurisdiction for misdemeanors
Non-Indian	Indian	*Federal* jurisdiction for felonies and misdemeanors, including assimilative crimes
Non-Indian	Non-Indian	*State* jurisdiction applies for both felonies and misdemeanors
Indian	Victimless crime	*Tribal* jurisdiction applies in most cases; *Federal* jurisdiction applies in some cases
Non-Indian	Victimless crime	*State* jurisdiction applies in most cases; *Federal* jurisdiction applies in some cases

evidence related to the bank account and deposits and withdrawals, the tribal police to arrest the non-Indian caregiver, and the tribal courts to prosecute, see Table 24.2.

In summary, the Tribal Law and Order Act of 2010 opens the door for county, state, tribal, and federal officials to work together for enforcement of laws across jurisdictions regardless of whether the perpetrators or victims are Indian or non-Indian. It is an opportunity for tribes to use their sovereignty to work for their people rather than focusing on having no state or local regulation [62].

The Violence Against Women Reauthorization Act has allowed tribes jurisdiction over non-Indians in domestic violence situations [60]. VAWA amended the full faith and credit statute and clarified that a "court of an Indian tribe shall have full civil jurisdiction over any person" [58]. VAWA protects elders in domestic violence situations if there is a restraining order in place.

24.4.8 Tribal Elder Abuse Codes

One of the most significant challenges facing Native communities with respect to elder abuse has been the lack of a tribal legal framework in which to respond to it. A survey of over 580 American Indian tribes, Alaskan Villages, and Hawaiian Homesteads by the National Indigenous Elder Justice Initiative (NIEJI) in 2012 found that less than 10 % of American Indian tribes and Alaskan villages addressed elder abuse in their tribal codes [63–65]. This has led to issues with how to handle the elder abuse cases that previously were rare (or under-reported and under-recognized), but today are becoming more common. Many tribes address the issue of elder abuse under existing criminal codes addressing physical assault, sexual assault, theft, robbery, and other related offenses. Since 2012 other tribes have enacted codes, but many, as yet, do not have policies in place in order to enforce the codes. This is the next step in empowering tribes to address the issue of elder abuse in Indian Country.

The National Indian Council on Aging (NICOA), an advocacy organization for tribal elders, provides a number of useful guidelines for tribes and supporting agencies as they develop and implement policies and programs for preventing, intervening, and addressing elder mistreatment [16]. The basis for these guidelines is the belief that tribally specific traditional values and beliefs should inform, reflect, and provide the foundation for programs from conception through design and implementation to evaluation. Community consensus building and intergenerational dialog should determine culturally appropriate programs and policies that will

> promote family unity and cooperation; reflect traditional models of dispute resolution; employ informal community networks; [and] attempt to prevent abuse by maintaining or supporting families and preserving and restoring cultural values and traditions [16], p. 6.

Additionally, these programs and policies must recognize and respect tribal sovereignty, including the nature and extent of the tribe's involvement and control over elder mistreatment prevention and justice programs, and how the tribal and non-tribal agencies cooperate and interrelate. Programs and policies must be specifically tailored to each tribe, allowing for their own unique histories and traditions regarding interpersonal and community disruptions to be processed and addressed [14, 16, 66]. These may include multiple areas of traditional jurisdictions over the care and protection of elders, including the family and extended family, tribal elders and healers, peacemakers and mediators, tribal courts, tribal and non-tribal social and government agencies, and legal systems. It is critical that non-tribal state and federal agencies along with state and federal governments mitigate or eradicate the structural factors that increase likelihood of abuse and neglect of elders, such as high rates of youth and young adult unemployment; inadequate or non-existent funding for culturally appropriate child care and elder care; and lack of culturally appropriate nutrition assistance programs that recognize the multigenerational households commonly existing in AI communities [16].

24.5 Practice

Turning our attention to practice, when working with Native Americans it is important to understand the traditions and values of the tribe or group involved. The values and teachings of indigenous cultures in North America vary, but they have commonalities. These general concepts are important to keep in mind when working with the indigenous people of North America. All things are sacred, not religiosity, but a role in the universe that is respectful of reciprocal relationships, family, the community, environment, past, present, and future. Change occurs in cycles or patterns, not a linear process. The concept of wholeness is important in that all things are connected, interrelated, and part of a single whole. Compartmentalism misses the beauty of the whole. Events in life can best be understood as lessons for whom we are and whom we are to become. Respect and honoring are essential to true or long-lasting relationships. Relevant healing places emphasis on the social, historical, and political contexts that have shaped Indigenous experiences, lives, and perceptions. Relevant healing encourages balance and harmony within a person's life and in relationship to others; the mental, physical, spiritual, and contextual (social) are learned in a balanced manner to keep all four dimensions involved in the process. Individuality is valued by how it improves the community. Collaboration is more highly valued than autonomy. Competition should enhance collaboration. Sustainability is essential for all of us to survive and thrive. This generation is not the most important for all time. Mystery, awe, wonder, intuition, and miracles occur naturally in everyday life. The seen and the unseen [67].

The issues of justice, law enforcement, and intervention are at the forefront of practice in Indian Country. Several noteworthy community-based programs or models exist in Indian country. Some of the practice approaches involve development of codes, policies, and implementation of elder abuse protection from a legal perspective. Other programs address restorative justice, mandatory reporting multidisciplinary elder protection teams, community policing, elder councils, and family restoration. The programs may involve several disciplines, namely social services, law enforcement, medicine, jurisprudence, nursing, and tribal, state, and federal governments or utilize traditional indigenous approaches. This portion of the chapter examines some of the currently developed approaches to addressing the issues of elder abuse in indigenous communities.

24.5.1 Development of Tribal Codes

Although elder abuse model codes have been available through the Southern Plains Tribal Law Center, the Tribal Law and Policy Institute, and other organizations, only 50 tribes had elder abuse codes in their tribal law in 2012 [65]. Development of a model tribal code for elder abuse that would also be in compliance with the TLOA has been a challenging project for NIEJI. The diversity of the 567 federally recognized tribes and Alaskan Villages in the United States made the idea of regional codes complex. Review of existing codes indicated they were located in a variety of areas within the various tribal codes: some aspects were in family code, some in criminal code, and some in the health and safety portions of the tribal codes. Moreover, as information was gathered on existing tribal codes and, due to the requirements of the Tribal Law and Order Act of 2010 that was being implemented during the process, it became apparent that a model code should be framed for Public Law (PL) 280 tribes. PL 280 refers to Public Law 83-280 that transferred significant civil and criminal legal jurisdiction over tribal lands from the federal government to five—then six—US states (California, Wisconsin, Minnesota, Nebraska, Oregon, and upon statehood, Alaska) [68]. Since its enactment in 1953, other states have joined and some tribes have receded from this jurisdiction. These PL 280 tribes have agreements with the states where they reside to utilize state resources for elder abuse reporting, investigation, and prosecution.

To be in compliance with the Tribal Law and Order Act of 2010, a civil code and a criminal code were developed by NIEJI, in addition a sample resolution allowing for the adopting of the elder abuse codes was also developed [69–71]. The civil code was to address minor offenses that usually included family members and recovery of property, while the criminal code was for prosecution of severe offenses in the criminal court.

24.5.2 Mandatory Reporting

While mandatory reporting laws require that people in certain professions (e.g., health care, social work, etc.), report suspected elder abuse to an investigating authority, a lack of mandatory reporting requirements is very common within many American Indian tribes. Within Indian Health Service (IHS) some policies imply but do not explicitly state that health care professionals are required to report abuse. The IHS is currently in the process of evaluating and revising these policies, but with the lack of consistency in the existence of tribal codes and policies this is very complicated. Outside of the formal contexts requiring mandatory reporting, there is evidence that people are often very reluctant to report abuse for variety of reasons, especially among cultures that value familial and kinship cohesiveness more than the rights or health of any individual member [72]. These reasons may include the elder's dependency upon the abuser for assistance (economic, shelter, and general care) and the major disruption and heightened vulnerability that would occur in inadequate resource settings by causing harm to the abusive caregiver, as well as shame about failures to act in accordance with tribal expectations and cultural values concerning respect for elders [37, 73–75]; the elder's awareness of their geographic isolation from social services and police, who are already understaffed and yet responsible for serving large reservation and rural areas, coupled with the high likelihood of repeated contact with the perpetrator after reporting abuse; and reticence to report due to the shame and humiliation that reporting would bring upon the elder and their family; and distrust of law enforcement and federal agents [16, 29, 37, 73, 74, 76, 77]. There is also the concern that the punitive aspect of the justice system may do more harm than good in the long term. One elder remarked, "Jail doesn't help anyone. A lot of our people could have been healed a long time ago if it weren't for jail. Jail hurts them more, and then they come out really bitter. In jail all they learn is hurt and bitterness" [16], p. 30.

In summary, elders who experience mistreatment must assess the costs versus the benefits of reporting the incidents to police or agencies that may be associated with colonizing forces or contemporary ineffectiveness. For many, the results of these analyses force them to choose the lesser of "evils," which may be tolerating physical, emotional, financial, or sexual harm or neglect, rather than subjecting themselves and their families to greater harm from other unknown sources, such as deeper poverty, fewer resources, homelessness, unfamiliar environments (such as in nursing homes far away from their tribal lands and communities), and increased vulnerability and desperation [72, 78]. Very few tribes have nursing homes. If an elder's caregivers are subjected to prosecution and are barred from the home, and if the elder has no other viable means of care or residence, then a nursing home placement will likely be far from family, friends, culture, and homelands. This deeply wounds the elder's soul and their will to live.

24.5.3 Need for Training of Tribal Court Personnel

Elder abuse is not a well-known topic in America or in Indian country. Judges, prosecutors, and tribal court personnel are finding that when an elder abuse case is heard they may have no prior knowledge of what elder abuse is and the family dynamics. The American Bar Association Commission on Law and Aging and the National Center for State Courts Center for Elders and the Courts have published a number of training resources for court personnel; however, these materials have not yet been adapted for tribal court models [50, 79–82]. The resources outline what Elder Abuse is as well as effective strategies for investigating and prosecuting cases.

24.5.4 Restorative Justice Approach

"Sacred Justice" or traditional Indian justice is becoming more common place in tribal programs [83]. Sacred justice reflects tribal values and practices by focusing on the importance of restoring balance to relationships. This is viewed as an alternative to the western distributive adversarial system with its "wild-and-rough" justice focused on punishment [83]. Other terms such as restorative justice, peacemaker programs, and elder councils focus on healing with a positive outcome for all rather than the adversarial, punitive approach found in most court systems [83].

The restorative justice approach utilizes the traditional practices of tribes as opposed to the western judicial system, and utilizes talking circles to prevent or respond to elder abuse [84]. The talking circles empower the elder, the family, and the abuser to identify the reasons behind the abuse. The family, victim, and abuser are allowed to develop solutions for how they can prevent future abuse while restoring the relationship to a healthy interaction. Many feel that a restorative justice approach is more effective than a jail sentence in certain situations [84–88]. Many times, the abuser needs to seek treatment or the family needs to resolve an issue to correct the problem. Placed in a situation where a family member is not in jeopardy of incarceration or punishment, elders are more apt to report abuse or neglect. Often the elder does not want to prosecute their caregiver/family member but they do not want to be mistreated. A restorative justice approach allows the elder regain control of the situation. [84–87] seek justice and dignity for themselves [16]. Other restorative justice approaches include multidisciplinary elder protection teams, elder councils, community policing, and family restoration programs.

Restorative justice calls upon individuals within society to advocate for and commit to humane and socially just policies that ultimately provide healing to victims and restore offenders into healthy relationships within healthy societies [85]. Restorative justice models emerging in North America have come out of the First Nations of Canada and are now being adopted by various tribes in North America [89], as well as non-Native communities.

As it pertains to elder mistreatment specifically, restorative justice is a mechanism for bringing together the elder, abuser(s), caregiver(s), and other family and community members of both victim and perpetrator to look for a positive approach and long-term solution for all involved without involving the courts [85, 86, 88, 90]. There is usually a written plan that the parties agree to and what the consequences will be if not followed. This is a preferred approach when the elder abuse or neglect was perpetrated by a family member that the elder does not want to see prosecuted and sent to jail, hence making him/her reluctant to take action should there be future violations. In cases where caregiver stress is a contribution factor and where respite can be arranged, restorative justice can have a very positive result. However, in cases involving substance abuse and/or severe physical abuse, restorative justice may not be a viable alternative.

24.5.5 Elder Mediation and Peacekeeping

Elder mediation builds upon restorative justice by bringing together all parties involved and working to find a solution that all can agree to with an intensified focus on mediation. The peacemaking is a contrast to Western courtrooms and is based upon the community's culture, religion, and collective life experience [91]. Peacemaking is viewed as "sacred justice" and is based upon the importance of restoring balance to relationships [83]. It emphasizes healing instead of guilt, restitution instead of punishment, community instead of the individual, and the future instead of the past [91]. Peacemakers are called "healers" instead of judges and a peacekeeping session is a "ceremony" rather than a hearing or a trial [91]. In the Pueblos of New Mexico, a revival of the Elder Council has been utilized to restore the old ways of addressing elder issues. If there is an issue of elder abuse, neglect, or exploitation, it comes before the Elders' Council for disposition. The Council draws upon the wisdom and guidance of the elders to determine what is right and just. This is a more traditional approach than the Western court system that lets the offender know that elders in the community are watching how the offender is taking care of the elder in his/her charge. The Elder Council can admonish the caregivers as to their treatment and care of the elder in question, but, from the healing perspective, may know of supports within the community that may help caregivers and the elders. This type of model is gaining in popularity. The Native American Rights Fund now has a Peacemaker project which is based upon this model for resolving issues.

24.5.6 Family Restoration Program

The Family Care Conferences are an elder-focused, family-centered intervention for the preventing and mitigating of elder mistreatment that used trained community members as group facilitators [92, 93]. Based on a model developed by the Maori in New Zealand, this model has been used extensively by U.S. states and other nations in intervening in child maltreatment but has not been systematically applied to elder protection. The Family Care Conference consists of six stages, beginning at the time of a case's referral through the family meeting and extending to follow-up. This model was piloted in one northwestern Native American community using a community-based participatory research strategy [93], and results while the study was ongoing showed that families appreciated the Family Care Conference's emphasis on family healing, harmony, and finding solutions within the family and community [92]. Thus, this model shows promise as an alternative to prosecution in Indian country, especially in cases where abuse does not appear to be life-threatening.

The Family Restoration Program utilizes the Family Conference and adds additional resources to it. This program, established at the Tohono O'odham Adult Protective Services (APS) in Southern Arizona, focuses on addressing the issues causing the abuse or neglect to allow the family to come together in a healthier way [94]. A report comes to the tribal APS office and is investigated. When the family restoration approach is more appropriate than prosecution, a social worker meets with the family and the elder to determine what the family may need to resolve the issues and helps to facilitate engagement with the appropriate services. Sometimes it can be resolved simply, and other times more extensive counseling and intervention is required, but the families are more open to this approach than utilizing the Western legal system that may take the only provider for the family away or create other problems for the family that are considered worse than the abuse [94].

24.5.7 Multidisciplinary Team Approach to Elder Abuse

Multidisciplinary elder protection teams (MEPT) are intended to utilize the expertise and knowledge of all of the available services for elders in the community. MEPTs may include law enforcement, social services, courts, attorneys, counselors, adult protective services from tribes or states and counties, fiduciaries, caregivers, health providers, Bureau of Indian Affairs, Federal Bureau of Investigation, and other relevant programs who are involved with the elder's care and well-being. There are several types of these multidisciplinary teams including tribally based teams, PL 280 tribal and state teams, and intertribal councils (e.g., comprised all the tribes within a state), and state services teams. MEPTs all work in much the same way to assess areas of risk and needs for vulnerable adults. They bring together all the parties involved in the care of the elder and in many cases the elder is a part of that team. Resources, services, and needs are discussed to provide a safe and caring support network for the elder. There can also be subtle pressure placed on caregivers by knowing that all of these programs are paying attention to what is happening with the elder and discourage future abuse, neglect, or exploitation.

There are many barriers to collaboration in community settings that are even more difficult in tribal communities [16]. Nerenberg et al. [16] identify possible barriers to collaboration in their 2004 report as well as providing recommendations for tribes. Barriers identified in the report include the following [16]:

- Tribal, county or state APS workers may receive and investigate reports of abuse, or the responsibility may rest with tribal enforcement, court personnel or social service programs. Other tribal programs that have a role to play in elder abuse prevention include housing and health services. The extent to which tribal departments collaborate and coordinate their efforts, as well as the extent to which they collaborate and coordinate their efforts with non-tribal entities, varies widely.
- On reservations with more than one tribe, separate law enforcement or social service programs may work jointly; however, personnel from the programs may disagree on matters related to elder abuse.
- Reservations that extend across state lines must relate to multiple state and county programs [16], p. 15.

Recommendations presented in the report include the following:

- Tribes need strategies developed for improving coordination among tribal departments and non-tribal entities that play roles in elder abuse prevention. This may include developing task forces, teams, or planning councils.
- Tribal officials' active involvement and leadership are necessary for successful negotiation of interagency agreements among tribal, county, and state adult protective service systems and sensitizing all personnel involved about tribal needs.
- Coordination among law enforcement agencies is particularly important and is covered in a separate section of the report [16], p. 15.

Not all tribes have MEPT. But for those that do, tribal or organizational relationship and arrangements with the states where the tribe is located may impact how the team functions. For PL 280 tribes, the state adult protective services and state prosecutors will be involved in elder abuse investigations and complaints in addition to the tribal and federal authorities. There are some states where the tribes form an intertribal council in order to join resources for services or to provide a more comprehensive program across the tribes in the area. At times it may make sense for an intertribal council or consortium to share resources such as an ombudsman that could not be afforded by one tribe alone, especially when tribes are smaller and/or less affluent.

MEPTs are a team of professionals who conduct case reviews to address elder abuse or coordinate services for an individual; however, the primary difference in tribal teams and those from the Western system are that included in the team is the elder, him/herself. The teams have different models depending upon the resources of the community and relationship to the state resources. In this chapter, we will present three examples of these teams: (1) The Standing Rock Sioux Tribe of North and South Dakota; (2) The Confederated Tribes of Warm Springs, Oregon; and (3) the Cheyenne and Arapahoe Tribes of Western Oklahoma.

The Standing Rock tribe in North Dakota has had a multidisciplinary team for some time and it is coordinated by the Tribes' Community Health Representative (CHR). The team includes representatives from the tribal veterans program, the Indian Health Service as well as the Bureau of Indian Affairs [16]. This team works within the tribal system and resources to address the elder justice needs of the tribe. There is also a group led by the CHR to address abusers from a traditional Lakota perspective. This program has a near-zero recidivism rate [16, 95].

The Confederated Tribes of Warm Springs, Oregon has an effective MEPT that has helped the tribe coordinate and prevent elder abuse within their community [96]. The team comprised the senior wellness center, tribal police, BIA/Tribal social services, housing, Indian Health Services, Community Health Representatives, Victims of Crime office, Assisted Living, and Oregon Adult Protection Services. The tribal council has signed a memorandum of agreement with the state of Oregon to enhance abuse awareness education and improve communication, cooperation, and collaboration. The MOU allows the tribe to utilize the state powers of the APS to investigate and make recommendations to the MEPT to resolve abuse outside the boundaries of the reservation. Some of the successes of the multidisciplinary team have been successfully averting further abuse, educating tribal members about elder abuse, decreased the expense of litigation, connected elders with services, and made participating organizations or programs aware of potential needs [96].

The Cheyenne–Arapahoe Tribes of Western Oklahoma have a MEPT that served as the model for the Bureau of Indian Affairs (BIA) Adult Protective Services (APS) Handbook [97]. The Cheyenne–Arapahoe team includes service providers, law enforcement, health care, elder services, and the state adult protective services and district attorney's office as part of one combined team. This helps deal with cross-jurisdictional issues that create confusion, blaming, and inaction in many elder abuse cases. This program has served as the national BIA model for elder justice for tribes [97].

24.5.8 Community Policing Approach to Elder Justice

The BIA at the Anadarko Agency of Oklahoma has taken a unique approach to elder justice. The Operation Golden Shield Project was developed by the BIA police and social services [98]. This program identifies at risk elders and when the police are not busy with other calls they visit the elders on the list. This is just a friendly visit, a cup of coffee, a chance to check in, and make sure everything is alright with the elder. On holidays such as Thanksgiving, Christmas, and Valentine's Day, officers stop by with a prepared dinner, a small gift or card letting the elder know they are special. This project helps to build a positive, trusting relationship between the elders and the officers and it provides an opportunity for an elder to talk about how things in their lives are going. In one case, this program prevented a perpetrator from financially exploiting an estimated $45,000 from one vulnerable adult [98]. Operation Golden Shield is funded entirely by contributions of the BIA police officers and social workers and community donations. The Anadarko Agency, the bureaucratic home of over seven tribes provides other supports through Operation Golden Shield including a prepared Thanksgiving meal, the "Golden Angel Tree" at Christmas time, and "Sweethearts" on Valentine's Day. These positive outreach efforts to vulnerable adults by police and social services promote a sense of trust and connection between those providing the services and community members who may need them [98].

24.5.9 Ombudsman Program

Tribal Long-Term Care Ombudsman programs have been held out by the Administration on Aging/Administration on Community Living (AoA/ACL) as effective in managing the quality of care and life in long-term care facilities [99]. The ombudsman position enables the tribal system to comply with the Tribal Law and Order Act. An ombudsman hears and investigates complaints between parties prior to involving legal or human services for an investigation of elder abuse. Concerned parties can go to the ombudsman and request an inquiry into the issue at hand, and the ombudsman will then advise, mediate, or assist in making referrals to other services. Long-Term Care Ombudsman programs do not serve elders that reside in their own homes or those of relatives. Additional resources would be necessary for ombudsmen to address elder abuse issues in community settings outside of nursing homes [99]. Making ombudsman services available through tribal programs to elders residing in their homes or with family would provide a beneficial intermediary where other more comprehensive services are not available.

24.5.10 Elder Protection within Tribes Requires Planning

Some tribal community members feel as though elder abuse occurs as often as child abuse [16]. However, the awareness and justice system do not reflect that elder abuse occurs as often as child abuse because of the infrequency of incidences ending up in the judicial system. Some tribes are finding that updating their tribal codes is not a priority in preventing elder abuse. Various model's elder abuse codes exist that tribes may use to help develop their code; however, the codes need modification to display the tribes' jurisdiction, departments, and resources. Frequently staff is not available within the tribe that can customize the codes for the tribe's specific needs. Some tribes have created elder abuse codes, but the code did not identify funding sources or departments that will be responsible for investigation and response into elder protection [16]. By not addressing this in the code it is not functional or enforceable. NICOA has made the following recommendations when it comes to Tribes adopting policies and procedures surrounding elder abuse:

- The process of developing codes can be used as an opportunity for raising community awareness about abuse and services.
- In developing codes, advocates should work with tribal councils from the early stages and involve elders in making decisions about what to include.
- Codes must include, or be accompanied by, policies and procedures that clearly define the roles of key agencies, steps in the reporting and investigation processes, timelines, and penalties.
- Tribes need funding, sample materials, and technical assistance to develop and refine tribal elder abuse codes, policies, and procedures.
- Codes should provide for a team approach to assessing abuse. Teams may include tribal elders and representatives from the fields of substance abuse, law enforcement, domestic violence, mental health, and aging and adult services.
- In assessing abuse, attention should be paid to the following:
  - People who are significant to victims, including friends, neighbors, and family members

- People who are significant to, and who wield influence with, alleged abusers
- The interrelationships and interdependencies among these individuals (above), the extent to which they can provide support and help, and the resources they can offer
- Substance abuse by any of the parties involved and how it contributes to abuse or case resolution
- The extent to which the parties involved participate in traditional culture and adhere to traditional values and laws.

- Codes should contain provisions for alternative dispute resolution proceedings as deemed appropriate. Further exploration is needed to determine when these approaches are appropriate and do not endanger victims. This may need to be determined on a case-by-case basis.
- Codes should contain provisions for translators for elders who need them.
- Codes should contain provisions for assessing and treating offenders [16], pp. 12–13.

24.5.11 Need for Review of Existing Data

Tribes have been cautious when it comes to sharing data with outside organizations because of how it has been used in a negative way in the past [100, 101]. Many tribes have signed Memorandums of Agreement with researching organizations to conduct research within tribes but tribes have agreed to be the owner of the data [63, 102]. However, tribes themselves need to collect data for their membership to determine the prevalence of abuse within Indian communities. Because there is no systematic mechanism for gathering data on elder abuse within American Indian, Alaska Native, and Native Hawaiian communities currently exists, it is important to find a way for a trustworthy mechanism for tribal programs to collect data that could give an accurate estimate of elder abuse, neglect, and exploitation within indigenous communities [103].

24.6 Conclusion

Elder abuse in Indian Country is a hidden issue where little culturally relevant information is available. Recent funding of the National Indigenous Elder Justice Initiative (NIEJI) by the Administration on Aging Elder Justice Program and Title VI Program has started the process of an organized, focused approach to developing resources, providing technical assistance, and developing training for indigenous communities [104]. Since the prevention of elder abuse is a multidisciplinary responsibility, it may be easier to tie elder abuse prevention into other programs within tribes. Tribes have historically held elders in high regard, and it is time for them to realize that changing times have now required changing practices to the care of our elderly. Elders are living longer and requiring more care than they have in the past. Tribes need to be proactive and prepare for the growing population of elders as well as the growing need for elder programs and elder protection services. The resources are available and growing in number, but it is ultimately up to individual tribes to develop the policy to utilize those resources in a way that protects our elders.

References

1. Bureau of Indian Affairs. 2013. Retrieved May 21, 2013, from http://www.bia.gov/WhoWeAre/index.htm.
2. US Census Bureau. Population: estimates and projections by age, sex, race/ethnicity. 2012. https://www.census.gov/newsroom/releases/archives/facts_for_features_special_editions/cb12-ff22.html
3. Maxwell EK, Maxwell RJ. Insults to the body civil: mistreatment of elderly in two Plains Indian Tribes. J Cross-Cultural Gerontol. 1992;7(1):3–23.
4. Thornton R. American Indian holocaust and survival: a population history since 1492. Norman: University of Oklahoma Press; 1987.
5. Jennings F. The invasion of America: Indians, colonialism and the cant of conquest. Chapel Hill: University of North Carolina Press; 1975.
6. Bureau of Indian Affairs (BIA). How does an Indian Tribe become "Federally Recognized?": an overview of the Administrative Process for Federal Recognition. 1994. http://fcnl.org/issues/nativeam/Federal_Tribal_Recognition-Administrative.pdf.
7. BIA. Indian Entities Recognized and Eligible to Receive Services from the United States Bureau of Indian Affairs. 2016; 2016-01769.
8. Utter J. American Indians: answers to today's questions. 2nd ed. Norman: University of Oklahoma Press; 2001.
9. Dunbar-Ortiz R. An indigenous peoples' history of the United States. Boston: Beacon Press; 2014.
10. Hodgkenson HL. The demographics of American Indians: one percent of the people; fifty percent of the diversity. Washington, D.C: Institute for Educational Leadership, Inc. Center for Demographic Policy. 1990.
11. Bureau of Indian Affairs. Bureau of Indian affairs FAQ. 4/1/2016. http://www.bia.gov/FAQs/.
12. Norris T, Vines PL, Hoeffel EM. The American Indian and Alaska Native Population: 2010. 2012;C2010BR-10.
13. U.S. Census Bureau. Annual estimates of the resident population by sex, age, race alone or in combination, and hispanic origin for the United States and States: April 1, 2010 to July 1, 2013. 2014. http://www.census.gov/popest/data/counties/asrh/2013/PEPSR5H.html
14. Nerenberg L, Baldridge D, Benson WF. Elder abuse in Indian country: research, policy, and practice. Albuquerque: National Indian Council on Aging; 2004. p. 1–26.
15. Brown AS, Fernandez RC, Griffith TM. Service provider perceptions of elder abuse among the Navajo (Research Report RR-90-3). Flagstaff: Northern Arizona University Social Research Laboratory; 1990.

16. Nerenberg L, Baldridge D, Benson WF. Preventing and responding to abuse of elders in Indian country. Albuquerque: National Indian Council on Aging; 2004.
17. Ortman JM, Velkoff VA, Hogan H. An aging nation: the older population in the United States. Current Population Reports. 2014; P25-1140.
18. Brown AS. A survey on elder abuse at one native American tribe. J Elder Abuse Negl. 1989;1(2):17–38.
19. Buchwald D, Tomita S, Hartman S, Furman R, Dudden M, Manson SM. Physical abuse of urban Native Americans. J Gen Intern Med. 2000;15:562–4.
20. Walker P, Carter PM, Gray JS, Baker-Demaray TB, Davis J. Elder abuse indicators in Indian country. Paper presented at the American Psychological Association's 121st Annual Convention, Honolulu. 2013.
21. The Three Cycle Comparison of Native American Elder Abuse Indicators. American Psychological Association 2015 Convention Presentation; 2015.
22. Tatara T, Kuzmeskus LB, Duckhorn E, Bivens L, NCEA, APHSA, et al. The national elder abuse incidence study: final report. Washington, DC: DHHS: AOA and ACF. 1998.
23. Acierno R, Hernandez-Tejado MA, Muzzy W, Steve K. National Elder Mistreatment Study: final report. Washington: USDOJ; 2009.
24. Acierno R, Hernandez-Tejado MA, Amstadter AB, Resnick HS, Steve K, Muzzy W, et al. Prevalence and correlates of emotional, physical, sexual, and financial abuse and potential neglect in the United States: The National Elder Mistreatment Study. Am J Public Health. 2010;100(2):292–7.
25. Jervis LL, Fickenscher A, Beals J. Shielding American Indian Elders Project Team. Assessment of elder mistreatment in two American Indian samples: psychometric characteristics of the HS-EAST and the Native Elder Life-Financial Exploitation and -Neglect measures. J Appl Gerontol. 2014;33(3):336–56.
26. de Jong MG, de Pieters R, de Fox J. Reducing social desirability bias through item randomized response: an application to measure underreported desires. J Mark Res. 2010;47(1):14–27.
27. Baker-Demaray TB. Perceptions of elder abuse among Native American seniors (Doctoral dissertation, University of North Dakota); 2009.
28. Pillemer K. The dangers of dependency: new findings on domestic violence against the elderly. Soc Probl. 1985;33 (2):146–58.
29. Jervis LL. Native elder mistreatment. In: Paper presented at the Forum on Global Violence: Elder Abuse and Its Prevention Workshop, Washington, DC. 2014
30. Rittman M, Kuzmeskus LB, Flum MA. A synthesis of current knowledge on minority elder abuse. In: Tatara T, editor. Understanding elder abuse in minority populations. Philadelphia: Brunner/Mazel; 1999. p. 221–38.
31. Hudson MF, Armachain WD, Beasley CM, Carlson JR. Elder abuse: two Native American views. Gerontol. 1998; 38(5):538–48.
32. Hudson MF, Carlson JR. Elder abuse: its meaning to Caucasians, African Americans, and Native Americans. In: Tatara T, editor. Understanding elder abuse in minority populations. Ann Arbor: Taylor & Francis; 1999. p. 187–204.
33. Jervis LL, Sconzert-Hall W. Native Elders. American Indians at Risk [2 volumes] 2013. Oct 28, p. 307.
34. Jervis LL, Boland M, Fickenscher A. American Indian family caregivers' experiences with helping elders. J Cross-Cultural Gerontol. 2010;25(4):355–69.
35. Schweitzer MM. Otoe-Missouria grandmothers: linking past, present, and future. In: Schweitzer MM, editor. American Indian grandmothers: traditions and transitions. Albuquerque: University of New Mexico Press; 1999. p. 159–80.
36. Jervis LL, Fickenscher A, Beals J, SHIELD. Assessment of elder mistreatment in two American Indian samples: psychometric characteristics of the HS-EAST and the native elder life-financial exploitation and -neglect measures. J Appl Gerontol. 2013; 25 (4):336–356.
37. Smyer T, Clark MC. A cultural paradox: elder abuse in the native American Community. Home Health Care Manag Pract. 2011;23 (3):201–6.
38. Carson DK. American Indian elder abuse. J Elder Abuse Negl. 1995;7(1):17–39.
39. Cole D, Chaikin I. An Iron Hand upon the People: The Law against the Potlatch on the Northwest Coast. Vancouver: Douglas & McIntyre, University of Washington Press; 1990.
40. Dawes HL. Senator Dawes's Address. Annual Report of the Board of Indian Commissioners, 1885. Washington, DC: US Gov.: Board of Indian Commissioners. 1886.
41. Biolsi T. Organizing the Lakota: The Political Economy of the New Deal on the Pine Ridge and Rosebud Reservations. Tucson: University of Arizona Press; 1992.
42. Evans-Campbell T, Lindhorst T, Huang B, Walters KL. Interpersonal violence in the lives of urban American Indian and Alaska Native women: Implications for health, mental health, and help-seeking. Am J Public Health. 2006;96(8):1416–22.
43. Kaufman and Associates. LTSS Research: Nursing Home Facility Inventory. Department of Health and Human Services, Centers for Medicare and Medicaid Services 2015 March 16; 2015
44. Hamilton JW. End-of-life issues for American Indians: a commentary. J Cancer Educ. 2005;20(1):37–40.
45. Hendrix LR. Intercultural collaboration: an approach to long term care for urban American Indians. Care Manag J. 2003;4(1):46–52.
46. Duran E, Duran B. Native American postcolonial psychology. Albany: State University of New York Press; 1996.
47. Baker-Demaray TB, Gray JS, Carter PM, Davis J, Speaker K, Whitefishwoman, et al. Elder Abuse in Indian Country. LTSS Elder Abuse Webinar, Kaufman and Associates: Spokane, WA 2012.
48. Dumont-Smith C, Aboriginal Healing Foundation. Aboriginal elder abuse in Canada. Ottawa: Aboriginal Healing Foundation; 2002.
49. Crowshoe R, Manneschmidt S. Akak'stiman: a blackfoot framework for decision-making and mediation processes. 2nd ed. Calgary: University of Calgary Press; 2002.
50. Stiegel L. The changing role of the courts in elder-abuse cases. Generations. 2000 Jul 1; 24(2):59–64.
51. Fogarty JD. Older Americans Act of 1965. 1965; PL89-73
52. O'Shaughnessy C. Basics of the Older Americans Act. 2012.
53. Administration on Aging. Unofficial Compilation of the Older Amerincans Act of 1965 As Amended in 2006 (Public Law 109-365). 2006.
54. National Center on Elder Abuse. Paper presented at the Addressing Elder Abuse with American Indian Tribes. A National Teleconference, Web. 1995
55. NARCEA. Paper presented at the American Indians and Elder Abuse: Exploring the Problem. Albuquerque, NM. 1989.
56. Rangel CB. Patient Protection and Affordable Care Act. 111. 2010; 148.
57. Jones BJ. Role of Indian Tribal Courts in the Justice System. US Department of Justice, Office of Justice Programs, Office for Victims of Crime; 2000 Mar.
58. Barker Harrold D. Victim Assistance Training Online Module Tribal Justice System. 02/11/2016; https://www.ovcttac.gov/views/TrainingMaterials/dspOnline_VATOnline.cfm.
59. Law T. Order Act of 2010, Pub.

60. Berney B. The Violence Against Women Act Reauthorization of 2013: A policy analysis. California state universtity, Long Beach; 2015.
61. Folsom-Smith C. Enhanced Sentencing in Tribal Courts: Lessons Learned from Tribes. 2015. https://www.ncjrs.gov/App/Publications/abstract.aspx?ID=270721
62. Cross JA. A conversation on elder rights. Paper presented at the 2014 National Title VI Training and Technical Assistance Conference, Washington, DC. 2014.
63. Gray JS, Davis J, Carter PM. Elder abuse codes in Indian Country. 2015. https://www.nieji.org/codes.
64. BIA. What we do. Retrieved March 15, 2014, from http://bia.gov/WhatWeDo/index.htm 2014.
65. NIEJI. Elder abuse codes. Retrieved July 14, from University of North Dakota: NIEJI 2014.
66. Jackson MY, Sappier T. Elder abuse issues in Indian Country. Washington, DC. 2005.
67. Society of Indian Psychologists (SIP). Society of Indian Psychologists Commentary on The American Psychological Association's (APA) Ethnical Principles of Psychologists and Code of Conduct. Logan, UT: Society of Indian Psychologists; 2013.
68. Jimenez VJ, Song SC. Concurrent tribal and state jurisdiction under public law 280. Am Univ Law Rev. 1998;47:1627–707.
69. National Indigenous Elder Justice Initiative (NIEJI). Civil Elder Abuse Model Code. 2014.
70. National Indigenous Elder Justice Initiative (NIEJI). Criminal Elder Abuse Model Code. 2014.
71. National Indigenous Elder Justice Initiative (NIEJI). Sample Resolution for Adopting Elder Abuse Code. 2014.
72. Beaulaurier RL, Seff LR, Newman FL, Dunlop B. Internal barriers to help seeking for middle-aged and older women who experience intimate partner violence. J Elder Abuse Negl. 2005;17(3):53–74.
73. Anisko B. Elder abuse in American Indian communities. Am Indian Cult Res J. 2009;33(3):43–51.
74. Carson DK, Hand C. Dilemmas surrounding elder abuse and neglect in native american communities. In: Tatara T, editor. Understanding elder abuse in minority populations. Philadelphia: Brunner/Mazel; 1999. p. 161–86.
75. Walsh CA, Olson JL, Ploeg J, Lohfeld L, MacMillan HL. Elder abuse and oppression: voices of marginalized elders. J Elder Abuse Negl. 2010;23(1):17–42.
76. Shipler LK, Anand R, Hadi N. Cultural considerations in assisting victims of crime: report on needs and promising practices. National Multicultural Institute, Washington, DC: Department of Justice: Office for Victims of Crime. 1998.
77. Wakeling S, Jorgensen M, Michaelson S, Begay M. Policing on American Indian reservations: a report to the National Institute of Justice. National Institute of Justice, Washington, DC: US Department of Justice: National Crime Justice Reference Service. 2001.
78. Beaulaurier RL, Seff LR, Newman FL, Dunlop B. External barriers to help seeking for older women who experience intimate partner violence. J Fam Violence. 2007;22(8):747–55.
79. Bureau of Justice Assistance (BJA). Identifying and responding to elder abuse: a bench card for judges. 2008. http://www.eldersandcourts.org/Elder-Abuse/~/media/Microsites/Files/cec/Benchcard.ashx
80. Stiegel L. Legal issues related to elder abuse: a desk guide for law enforcement. 2015. http://www.americanbar.org/groups/law_aging/resources/elder_abuse/legal_issues_related_to_elder_abuse_guides.html
81. Stiegel L. Recommended guidelines for state courts handling cases involving elder abuse. 1995. http://www.americanbar.org/content/dam/aba/administrative/law_aging/2011/2011_aging_ea_rec.authcheckdam.pdf
82. Stiegel L. Elder abuse and the state courts: three curricula for judges and court staff. 1997. http://www.americanbar.org/content/dam/aba/administrative/law_aging/ElderAbuseintheStateCourts_ThreeCurriculaforJudgesandCourtStaff.authcheckdam.pdf
83. LeResche D. The reawakening of sacred justice. Clearinghouse Rev. 1993;27(8):893–9.
84. Blue AW, Blue MAR. The case for aboriginal justice and healing. In: Hadley ML, editor. The spiritual roots of restorative justice. First ed. Albany, NY: State University of New York; 2001. p. 57–79.
85. Elliott EM. Security, with care: restorative justice and healthy societies. Halifax: Fernwood Pub; 2011.
86. National Institute of Justice. Indigenous Justice Systems and Tribal Society. Restorative Justice: Perspectives on Restorative Justice; 2007. http://www.nij.gov/topics/courts/restorative-justice/perspectives/pages/indigenous-tribal.aspx
87. Hadley ML, editor. The spiritual roots of restorative justice. 1st ed. Albany: State University of New York; 2001.
88. Umbreit MS. Crime victims seeking fairness, not revenge: towards restorative justice. Federal Probation. 1989;53(3):52–7.
89. Haslip S. The (Re)Introduction of restorative justice in Kahnawake: "Beyond Indigenization". Murdoch Univ Electron J Law 2002; 9(1):1–61.
90. Ellis J. First nations justic initiatives in Canada. Totem: the University of Western Ontario. J Anthropol. 2009;17(1):36–42.
91. Wolf RV. Overlap between Public Health and Law Enforcement: Sharing Tools and Data to Foster Healthier Communities. Int Rev Law Comput Technol. 2012;26(1):97–108.
92. Holkup PA, Salois EM, Tripp-Reimer T, Weinert C. Drawing on wisdom from the past: an elder abuse intervention with tribal communities. Gerontol. 2007;47(2):248–54.
93. Salois EM, Holkup PA, Tripp-Reimer T, Weinert C. Research as spiritual covenant. West J Nurs Res. 2006;28(5):505–24.
94. Ramon A. Family preservation services. Elder Abuse Pre-Conference, National Indian Nations Conference, 2014. https://www.nieji.org/pdf/family-preservation-services-presentation-121014.pdf
95. EagleShield J. A Lakota approach to abuse prevention. 2014.
96. Wewa W. Multidisciplinary team approach on elder abuse: confederated tribes of Warm Springs, Oregon. Elder Abuse Pre-Conference, National Indian Nations Conference, 2014. https://www.nieji.org/pdf/multidisciplinary-team-approach-elder-abuse-presentation-121014.pdf
97. U.S. Department of Interior, Bureau of Indian Affairs. Adult protective services handbook: a guide to protecting vulnerable adult and elder Indians from abuse, neglect and exploitation. 2013. https://www.nieji.org/resources/files/2013-adult-protective-services-handbook.pdf
98. Allen SK, Longhat M. Community policing and social services: operation golden Shield. 2014. https://www.nieji.org/resources/files/operation-golden-shield.pdf
99. Hollister BA, Estes CL. Local long-term care ombudsman program effectiveness and the measurement of program resources. J Appl Gerontol. 2013;32(6):708–28.
100. Gray JS. The Good, the Bad, and the Ugly: Ethical Research in Indian Country. 2011. https://ruralhealth.und.edu/pdf/gray_gbu_path_ethical_research_indian_country_nursing.pdf

101. Gray JS. Trails and Traps: The path to research in Indian Country. Presentation to the University of North Dakota Indian Association, Grand Forks, ND 2010. https://ruralhealth.und.edu/presentations/pdf/041610timeout_gray.pdf
102. Gray JS, Mason G. Suicide in Indian Country: the continuing epidemic. In: D. A. Lamis N. J. Kaslow, editors. *Advancing the science of suicidal behavior: Understanding and intervention,* Hauppauge, NY, US: Nova Science Publishers; 2015. p. 321–334.
103. Litton LJ, Ybanez V. Reclaiming what is sacred: addressing harm to indigenous elders and developing a tribal response to abuse in later life. Madison, WI: National Clearinghouse on Abuse in Later Life/End Domestic Abuse Wisconsin; 2015.
104. Gray JS, NIEJI. Elder abuse in Indian Country: disrespect of our elders. Paper presented at the Title VI Administration on Aging Conference, Washington, DC. 2013.

25 Coping with Abuse Inside the Family and Out: LGBT and/or Male Victims of Elder Abuse

Loree Cook-Daniels

Basketball was at the center of Margaret Kucera's[1] life, a passion for which she paid dearly. As a kid, she would be locked in the garage by her male playmates whenever she had the temerity to beat them.

In middle school, she was barred from the Knights of Columbus Hoop Shoot because she was female. (After the competition, she took the floor and scored ten free throws in a row; the winning boy had sunk nine).

She did manage to play—and score many wins—in high school, and was recruited by multiple colleges.

She chose Gonzaga University in Spokane because their coach was a lesbian, and she thought she would be safe there. She was, until she was severely injured in a game and they refused to take her back, fearing she risked paralysis.

She fell in love with another female athlete. Her mom responded by trying to send her to the family doctor because "being with a woman is not normal."

She played a year for Montana State University, but wanted educational opportunities they didn't offer, and transferred to the University of Montana. The coach there was excited about her coming, and arranged a job for her to help her out. Two weeks after she arrived, an assistant coach called her and told her the coach didn't want "her type" on the team. The athletic director at her new job coaching high schoolers told her to turn in her keys. She said, "I finished coaching with parents sitting behind the bench making comments about me being a lesbian, and I had parents pull their girls from the team because I was the coach."

She was recruited for Eastern Montana College by a coach who had also coached her in high school. The first practice, her teammates were cold and during play one teammate smacked her hands and bellowed out, "Don't you touch me again you fucking dyke!" She notes, "Some of the members on the team were lesbians but they had to keep quiet and go along with the bullying in order for their closet doors to remain securely closed." A week later, her coach, accompanied by his closeted lesbian assistant, told her the team had had a meeting and voted her out.

Another lesbian coach told her that a coach had taken it upon himself to call all the coaches in Montana to out her as a lesbian and allege she had a drinking problem.

Let us pretend that Margaret is now 73, and her long-term partner has become emotionally and physically abusive. This is the same Margaret who was repeatedly denied the right to play a game she clearly excelled at not only by heterosexuals, but also lesbian teammates. Her own parent called her "not normal." People went out of their way to make sure doors were closed in her face. How likely is it that she will call Adult Protective Services for help, or let them in the door if someone else reports her? Which is likely to seem more self-protective to Margaret: trusting a stranger with the information she is a lesbian and is being hurt by her partner, or closing the blinds, sealing the door, and trying to lower the volume on her emotions with alcohol or drugs? If her partner were to be arrested or "just" forced out of the house, where would Margaret's support come from?

25.1 LGBT Elder Abuse

Many people question why someone's sexuality (the gender of the person(s) they partner with and/or have sex with) or their gender identity (whether they think they are male, female, both, or something else entirely) have any relevance to elder abuse. They do not. What can make elder abuse different for lesbian, gay, bisexual, and/or transgender (LGBT) elders is not their sexuality or gender identity, but how others—ranging from their closest family members to strangers thousands of miles away in buildings devoted to

[1]Margaret Kucera is a Wisconsin resident who kindly granted permission to use her name and history for this chapter. Her story was published in "Full Court Press," (2015), *Our Lives Magazine*.

L. Cook-Daniels (✉)
FORGE, Inc, P.O. Box 1272 Milwaukee, WI 53201, USA
e-mail: LoreeCD@aol.com

X. Dong (ed.), *Elder Abuse*, DOI 10.1007/978-3-319-47504-2_25

law making, law enforcement, and policy interpretation—have created the environments in which sexual and gender minorities have had to survive.

An estimated 1.5 million lesbians, gay men, and bisexual people in the U.S. are aged 65 and older, a figure that is expected to double by the year 2030 [14]. Estimates of the size of the transgender population vary widely, but are likely to be around 1 % [1]. In the first of three sections, this chapter will explore what makes LGBT elder abuse victims different from non-LGBT victims; review studies of LGBT elder abuse; and discuss LGBT-specific elder abuse tactics and reasons victims may not access or accept help. In the second section we will explore why half of LGBT elder abuse victims also face another challenge: they are male. We will discuss how male victims have been affected by the history of programs addressing domestic violence and sexual assault; what research says about them; how sexual assault has been defined so as to exclude male victims and female perpetrators; how male socialization negatively affects male victims' ability to access help; and how service systems' biases play out for male and/or transgender survivors. This section closes with recent federal efforts to make services more available to male and/or LGBT victims. The third and final section addresses research challenges and future directions, and gives advice and resources for working with LGBT elder abuse victims.

25.1.1 Life as a Gender and/or Sexual Minority

Every culture has norms (expectations) around how people will behave sexually and how they will present themselves to others. Throughout history people have had sexual relationships with people of their same gender. In some times and places, these have been considered totally unremarkable [18]. In recent Western cultures, however, same-sex relationships have been largely condemned. Countries which were colonized by Western cultures often adopted that same censure, even when they had histories that included open homosexuality [21, 28]. For example, although open homosexuality was common in precolonial Africa, currently 38 of 53 African nations criminalize homosexuality in some way [15].

Similarly, gender identity concepts have varied over time and culture. Some cultures have been more aware that humans come in a range of biological and identity configurations. Many American Indian tribes, for example, had specific titles and roles for people who chose a gender identity, role, or expression different from the one they were assigned at birth. Similar third- or fourth-gender roles have been acknowledged in Indian and Hawaiian societies, among others [12]. In Western Christian-based culture, however, the belief is that there are only two genders (male and female), that they are indistinguishable from biological structures (i.e., genital shape equals gender), and that an individual cannot change from one gender to another. Those who violate these assumptions are widely derided and discriminated against.

Obviously, many countries have made much progress in dismantling anti-LGBT prejudice over the past years. But it is critical to remember that people do not just live in the "now": they bring their whole history into their current belief sets and actions. Many people who are younger than current LGBT elders and/or are not themselves LGBT are shocked to hear just how bad legalized discrimination and violence against LGBT people in the U.S. has been over the past 60 or so years. LGBT people were part of the McCarthy period "red scare" of the 1940s and 50s, labeled "moral perverts," banned from federal employment, and blacklisted. In 1952 the American Psychiatric Association listed homosexuality as a "sociopathic personality disturbance" in its first official list of mental disorders; immigrants with a "psychopathic personality" (including homosexuality) were banned from the U.S. In 1955, 29 Sioux City, Iowa men suspected of being gay were committed to mental asylums in the wake of the murder of a boy. Two-years later, the American Civil Liberties Union approved a policy statement endorsing laws against sodomy and federal restrictions on employment of lesbians and gay men [3].

Things got measurably better in the 1960s, although gay bars were still routinely raided and their patrons shaken down and arrested by police officers, a practice that led to what is widely considered (at least in the U.S.) the start of the gay liberation movement: the Stonewall Riots, a fight against police, at a New York City bar called the Stonewall [3].

The '70s, however, saw a backlash. Backlashes are critical to keep in mind: LGBT elders have seen progress and then setbacks many, many times. They are therefore often wary of fully embracing—or at least, counting on—new legal rights and achievements. Among the setbacks in the 70s: the Supreme Court refused to hear the case of an Oregon teacher fired for lesbianism; Anita Bryant lead a highly visible anti-LGBT campaign that resulted in the repeal of a Miami law protecting lesbians, gay men, and bisexuals from discrimination; Arkansas recriminalized gay sex after 2 years without such a law; and Florida forbid lesbians and gay men from adopting children. The 80s were marked by the AIDS crisis. This was a time in which the government's attitude toward LGBT people became, many thought, crystal clear: the silence of President Reagan and the slowness with which the health crisis was addressed led many LGBT people to conclude that their government would prefer they simply dic [3].

In the '90s, more backlash resulted in Colorado voters banning state and municipal rights laws for lesbians and gay men; the suspension of the United Nations observer status of the International Lesbian and Gay Association (at U.S. insistence); and passage of the Defense of Marriage Act ensuring that any same-sex marriages legalized by a state would not be honored by the federal government. LGBT people still lack a federal law forbidding discrimination against them, although various court decisions and regulatory guidance has interpreted existing laws as providing some measure of protection. Legal discrimination, however, remains: it was only in 2014 that the U.S. government began the process of outlawing health care discrimination against transgender people [3].

That describes some of the overall environment within which LGBT elders have lived. How much impact has all that had on individual elders? The 2011 study, *The Aging and Health Report: Disparities and Resilience among Lesbian, Gay, Bisexual, and Transgender Older Adults,* surveyed 2560 U.S. LGBT older adults from ages 50 to 95. Eighty-two (82 %) of respondents had experienced at least one anti-LGBT victimization during their lifetime; 64 % had experienced three or more of such incidents. The most common type of victimization was verbal insults (68 %), followed by threats of physical violence (43 %), and being hassled by police (27 %). Nearly 1 in 5 (19 %) had been physically assaulted (punched, kicked, or beaten), 14 % had been threatened with a weapon, and 11 % had been sexually assaulted. More than half had been discriminated against in employment and/or housing [13]. Survey participants who were transgender reported much more discrimination than did their non-trans peers: On average, the transgender older adults reported 11 incidents of lifetime discrimination and victimization, almost double the average of 6 for non-transgender LGB participants.

The ebb and flow of rights and respect for LGBT people must be remembered now that so much progress is being made; elders have experienced newly won rights being rescinded time and time again. Caution remains prudent.

25.1.2 Studies of LGBT Elder Abuse

Studies of LGBT victims of elder abuse are practically nonexistent. One of the primary reasons for this void is that the U.S. (along with many other countries) has not included sexual orientation questions in its national, representative samples until very recently. The first national study that looked at violence rates as they are affected by sexual orientation was the 2013 publication, *The National Intimate Partner Sexual Violence Survey* (Centers for Disease Control and Prevention), which found that lesbians and bisexual women experience intimate partner violence at rates higher than heterosexual women. While gay and heterosexual men have lower reported intimate partner violence rates than do women of any sexual orientation, bisexual men have higher rates than heterosexual women. In the case of sexual violence other than rape (which accounts for more of the sexual violence experienced by men), there were similar findings: bisexual men, lesbians, and bisexual women are all sexually violated more often than gay and heterosexual men [31]. This study did not report out its findings broken down by age, making it impossible to determine what percentage of the crimes it documented would be considered "elder abuse."

Another potential source of LGBT elder abuse data would be reports from Adult Protective Services (APS). Unfortunately, it is unclear that any APS is asking or recording the sexual orientation and/or gender identity of their clients; if any are, they have not yet published that data.

Which leaves convenience surveys: reports from individuals who happen to come across or are referred to a specific survey or study and who agree to participate. Obviously, the results from such studies cannot be assumed to be representative of all LGBT elders, but they do provide some information.

One of the largest of such studies was published in 2011. *The Aging and Health Report: Disparities and Resilience Among Lesbian, Gay, Bisexual, and Transgender Older Adults,* as noted above, surveyed 2560 U.S. LGBT older adults from ages 50 to 95. They found that in the year prior to the study, 7 % had experienced verbal abuse by a partner, family member, or close friend, and 3 % had experienced physical abuse [13]. Rates of abuse were highest for bisexual men (9 %), bisexual women (14 %) and transgender elders (15 %). Physical abuse rates were not correlated with age, but verbal abuse decreased with age. LGBT elders with annual incomes at or below 200 % of the U.S. federal poverty level had higher rates of physical and verbal abuse.

While published studies of abuse of LGBT elders are nonexistent, we do know from anecdotal stories and from the experiences of younger LGBT domestic violence survivors that there are specific ways in which being LGBT can be used by abusers as power and control tools.

25.1.3 LGBT-Specific Elder Abuse Tactics

LGBT elders are subject to the same types of abuse as non-LGBT elders: virtually every type of abuse described in this book can and does happen to elders who are LGBT. The history of social and interpersonal discrimination, violence, and trauma that LGBT elders have experienced simply adds to the ways in which they can be threatened or manipulated by abusers. The following section outlines some of the additional tactics used by those who abuse LGBT elders.

25.1.3.1 Threats to "Out" the LGBT Elder

One of the primary ways in which LGBT people have sought to protect themselves from others' prejudices is by keeping their sexual orientation and/or gender identity a secret, at least from some. That secrecy provides an opportunity for an abuser who knows (or suspects) the elder's LGBT status and that they are trying to keep that status a secret: they can "blackmail" the elder by saying they will "out" them (reveal their sexual orientation and/or gender identity) if the elder does not comply with their demands. LGBT grandparents may be at particular risk if the abuser threatens to out them to their children, who may then cut off access to their grandchildren.

25.1.3.2 Abuser Gains Control of Finances and/or Assets

Same-sex marriage became legal in the U.S. only very recently, and not all long-term same-sex couples have taken advantage of the institution. If they have not, like other unmarried couples, it can be fairly easy for an exploitative partner to gain control of the couple's finances and/or assets, without much fear that authorities will step in to correct the injustice. Indeed, many LGBT couples have put all their assets under one name as a *protective* measure, to avoid questions that might be raised by having the names of two men or two women on a mortgage or bank account. When these exploitation cases occur, the victim may not only have little recourse to reclaim what belongs to them, but they may also lose out on monthly income that would, for example, go to someone who could draw on their spouse's Social Security account. Victims may feel they have to stay with an exploitative partner simply to keep a roof over their heads.

25.1.3.3 Victim Fears "Spending the Rest of My Life Alone"

Older LGBT adults typically have been told for decades that LGBT elders "end up alone," and ageism within the LGBT community can seem to confirm this gloomy prediction. The threat of spending the rest of one's life alone or never being touched again can be another way in which an abusive partner or caregiver keeps their victim close. This set of beliefs about what it means to grow old LGBT may also make some LGBT elders particularly vulnerable to "sweetheart scammers," people who befriend or become lovers with an elder specifically to gain access to their financial resources.

25.1.3.4 Victim May Be Easier to Isolate

Abusers often look for isolated elders to target and/or isolate their victims once a relationship established. Isolation has clear benefits for abusers: there are fewer people around to notice what is happening to the victim, and the victim becomes more dependent on the abuser because they have a dwindling number of alternatives. Isolating an LGBT elder may be easier than isolating a non-LGBT elder because family members may already be estranged and because many LGBT elders avoid settings that predominately cater to non-LGBT people such as senior centers and meal sites, in order to avoid interacting with people who may prove to be discriminatory or prejudiced. Some LGBT elders even avoid health-care professionals, preferring to cope with injuries and diseases on their own rather than risk encountering a biased provider.

25.1.3.5 Abuser Says, "This Is What It Means to Be LGBT"

Because there have been so few public models of healthy LGBT adults, it is still possible for LGBT people with limited experience in the LGBT community to be misled by abusers who claim whatever they are doing is "what LGBT people do." For example, an older person in their first same-sex relationship may believe it if their partner says that in same-sex relationships, one is expected to be sexually available to the partner at all times.

25.1.3.6 Society Says, "This Is the Best You Can Expect"

"Internalized" homophobia, biphobia, or transphobia is the label for what happens when an LGBT person believes the social messages that surround them that say being LGBT is not normal, is lesser, is a sin, or is somehow not as good as being non-LGBT. When an LGBT elder has internalized these beliefs, he or she is far more likely to put up with being abused, neglected, or exploited because they feel they do not deserve anything better. People who have been previously abused—especially as children—are also far more likely to believe that being abused is normal and to be expected and accepted as "just the way the world is."

25.1.4 Why LGBT Elder Abuse Victims May Not Ask for or Accept Help

This book explores many reasons abuse victims may not ask for help, and LGBT elders are subject to all of them. LGBT elders may also have some additional reasons to resist asking for or accepting help.

25.1.4.1 Abuser Harps on Authorities' Prejudices

As previously described, if LGBT elders haven't had direct negative experiences with law enforcement and other government officials, they know others who have. That means that when abusers tell their LGBT victims that if they report the abuse, "no one will believe you," or "they'll think you are crazy and lock you up instead," they are highly likely to be believed. This tactic can keep an LGBT elder abuse victim from reaching out for help.

25.1.4.2 Fear of Nursing Homes

Whether reality plays out this way or not, many elder abuse victims fear that if authorities intervene in their lives, they will end up in a nursing home. While few elders of any sexual orientation or gender identity look forward to moving into a nursing home, the fear appears to be elevated for LGBT elders. In the 2011 report, "LGBT Older Adults in Long-Term Care Facilities: Stories from the Field," a coalition of aging organizations found that a majority of their 769 respondents—including aging professionals and family and friends as well as LGBT elders themselves—believed that nursing home staff would discriminate against, abuse, or neglect an LGBT resident [22]. This perception can easily lead to an abused LGBT elder preferring to remain with the abuser they know rather than chance moving in with abusers who may be even worse.

25.1.4.3 Fear of Cost

In a 2011 national study of transgender people's knowledge of and willingness to access a wide variety of victim service agencies, the transgender education and advocacy organization FORGE was surprised to find that "cost" of accessing services was perceived to be a barrier even when the service was provided at no fee [20]. Professionals who are offering services need to always remember to be explicit when there is no cost involved, as the potential client they are talking to may otherwise turn down the referral out of the assumption they cannot afford it.

25.1.4.4 Victim Prides Themselves on Self-reliance

Particularly for older lesbians, developing skills that allowed them to be self-sufficient in as many ways as possible has been a key imperative and source of pride. Self-sufficiency meant not just being able to support themselves (and, possibly, a partner), but also not needing outside assistance such as plumbers, electricians, and the like. Self-sufficiency not only offered pride of mastery, but protected the elder and her loved one(s) from others' homophobia. Where it exists, a commitment to self-reliance can set an older person up for refusing all offers of help and/or self-neglecting when self-care becomes difficult.

25.1.4.5 Victim Does Not Want to Expose Abuser to Mistreatment

It is always important to remember that with intimate partner violence and family violence, the victim often feels love, responsibility, and/or protectiveness toward their abuser(s). If an LGBT elder's abuser is also LGBT, they may not be willing to expose their abuser to authorities who may in turn subject them to abuse, discrimination, or denigration.

25.2 Male Elder Abuse Victims

Half of LGBT elder abuse victims face an additional set of barriers to recognizing and getting help resolving situations of intimate partner violence and/or sexual assault: they are, or are perceived to be, male.

25.2.1 The System's Roots in Women's Consciousness-Raising Groups

Both the domestic violence and rape crisis systems grew out of women's consciousness-raising groups in the 1960s and '70s [25]. In these groups, women began to give voice to previously unspoken experiences and thereby began to recognize the pervasiveness of problems like domestic violence and sexual assault. The drawback of this discovery was that only women participated in the groups. This naturally led to the presumption that the uncovered commonalities were not based on a shared *experience* (being an assault survivor), but a shared *identity*—being female. Because the vast majority of women who participated in consciousness-raising groups were either heterosexual or, if lesbian or bisexual, closeted about their partner's identity, it also seemed that everyone who perpetrated such violence was male.

Compounding those original errors, the federally funded system that the U.S. created to offer services to domestic violence and sexual assault survivors was labeled the "Violence Against Women Act (VAWA)."[2] Services have predominately been offered only to women. They have also been designed specifically for women victimized by men. That means policies like this are widespread: domestic violence shelters have typically refused to house men and older boys with the rationale that this policy precludes perpetrators from gaining access to their victims in shelter by claiming to also be abused. Yet few shelters who knowingly serve lesbians have adopted policies to ensure that those female abusers are not also admitted.

Once established as one-sex-only, the VAWA service structure has further foreclosed opportunities for male and female victims' stories to be heard and compared with each other. Consequently, even some who are advocating for serving male victims continue to assume that male survivors' needs are very different from female survivors' needs. The system has also, paradoxically, shielded women from "being

[2]The Violence Against Women Act is U.S. legislation, but similar women-only systems were developed in Canada and the U.K.

held accountable" for their violence, as all violence by women is presumed to be in self-defense against a male aggressor.

The elder abuse field is not directly sourced in the women's movement, but it has strong ties to it. Many leaders in the elder abuse field began their work in the violence against women movement, and key organizations (like the National Clearinghouse on Abuse in Later Life) are closely tied to organizations that focus solely on violence against women. One of the ways in which one can see the influence of the "violence against women" movement on elder abuse is the nearly universal assertion that female elders are more likely to be victimized than are men [24]. There are, in fact, more female than male elder victims. However, it is not clear that women are more vulnerable. Most studies have found that the older the elder, the more likely they are to be abused [24]. Given that at every (old) age there are fewer and fewer older men due to men's earlier mortality rates, it is obvious that most victims would be female, just because there are more women in the most vulnerable age groups. But are they actually being victimized more often than are their male peers? Those calculations remain undone.

25.2.2 Research Paints Another Picture

Between April 2012 and April 2013, the journal *Partner Abuse* published the results of a huge meta-analysis of 1700 studies related to domestic violence published in peer-reviewed journals in 1990 or after. The 47 scholars from three countries who participated eventually summarized every study and organized them into tables. Seventeen lengthy analyses were completed, each looking at one or a small set of related issues. The consensus conclusion: there is little difference in the rates, motives, or consequences of intimate partner violence inflicted by women and men [7].

Despite this overwhelming evidence, some researchers allege that there have been planned as well as inadvertent efforts to downplay, in particular, women's violence against men. In his lengthy 2010 article, "Thirty Years of Denying the Evidence on Gender Symmetry in Partner Violence: Implications for Prevention and Treatment," long-time family violence researcher Murray Straus lays out seven methods by which violence by women has been "denied" by other researchers:

1. Conceal the evidence
2. Avoid obtaining evidence on female perpetration
3. Selective citation of research
4. State conclusions that contradict the data
5. Block publication of articles that report gender symmetry
6. Prevent funding of research to investigate female partner violence
7. Harass, threaten, or penalize researchers who publish evidence on gender symmetry.

It's not just academic researchers and government officials who distort or misreport the data: a 2006 AARP magazine article on domestic violence among older couples claimed that the number of elderly women abusing male partners is "negligible." However, the citation led to a study that clearly undermined that assertion: 43 % of elder domestic abuse cases were of the wife assaulting her husband [29].

25.2.3 Sexual Assault is Defined by Gender

Laws themselves have served to mask sexual assault of men. When the federal government began tracking violent crime in 1930, the rape of men was explicitly excluded [27]. Until 2012, "forcible rape" was defined as "the carnal knowledge of a female forcibly and against her will." Even the post-2012 federal definition defines rape as "the penetration, no matter how slight, of the vagina or anus with any body part or object, or oral penetration by a sex organ of another person, without the consent of the victim" [27]. This seemingly gender-neutral definition nevertheless excludes the type of sexual assault men are most subject to [26]. The 2011 *National Intimate Partner and Sexual Violence Survey* attempted to correct this bias and found that while an estimated 1,270,000 U.S. women had been raped in the previous year, nearly as many men (1,267,000) had been "made to penetrate." "…[B]oth men and women experienced 'sexual coercion' and 'unwanted sexual contact,' with women more likely than men to report the former and men slightly more likely to report the later" [27].

Many other studies have confirmed that men are sexually assaulted at nearly the same rate as women [27]. These figures have been widely ignored, even by (sometimes especially by) those who are trying to raise visibility of the issue of sexual assault. For example, the Oscar-nominated film *The Invisible War* focused on military sexual assault, but gave the majority of victims—men—less than 5 minutes of the 99 [23]. Even though the filmmakers were widely publicly criticized for ignoring male victims, they adopted a similar approach in their next film, *The Hunting Ground,* on campus-based sexual assault. Again, the film downplays how often men are sexually assaulted on campus.

Elder abuse is not exempt from the bias against seeing male sexual assault victims and/or female perpetrators. In 2008, Teaster and colleagues issued a meta-review of elder sexual abuse studies. They concluded, "this is a problem involving primarily female victims and male perpetrators with few identified male victims and female perpetrators," even though some of the same researchers participated in a study that found that fully 40 % of alleged elder sexual abuse victims were male, and 26 % of the alleged perpetrators were female [6]. Another study, of elders sexually assaulted in care facilities, concluded that even though 61 % of all the reports were made by the residents themselves, the lower rate of substantiation for male victims (12 % vs. women's 22 %) "could indicate that more erroneous reports of alleged sexual abuse were made concerning men than women." Interestingly—but noted without comment—was the fact that although 22 % of the alleged male perpetrators were ultimately listed as "confirmed," only 9 % of the female perpetrators were [6]. These researchers were not explicit about whether they were implying that men are more likely to falsely claim rape than women are, but the leader of a Milwaukee sexual assault services agency has been: she has repeatedly publicly said that 50 % of the men who call her agency requesting services are "lying." (The comparable rate for women callers, she estimates, is 2–3 %) [5]. Not surprisingly, when her agency leads advocacy efforts, they tell policymakers that there is very little demand for services for male survivors.

25.2.4 Male Socialization Takes Its Toll

In addition to the outside pressures men may feel to not admit or talk about their victimization is the problem of internalized sexism. This refers to the social stereotypes men may have internalized saying that to be masculine, they must not show fear, not be a victim, successfully defend themselves, and not show weakness. All of these qualities are damaged, if not destroyed, when a man is beaten up and/or sexually assaulted by either a man or a woman. Male victims and female victims alike feel powerlessness, terror, and the loss of human connection when assaulted. Men, in addition, may feel that their very masculinity has been stripped from them. In these cases, admitting that one has been victimized in essence means proclaiming that one is no longer fully male. This, of course, adds to the pressure on men not to admit they have been victimized and creates another loop in the spiral that helps keep the existence of male victims unacknowledged [17].

25.2.5 Service System Biases

In the lead-up to the 2013 Reauthorization of the Violence Against Women Act (VAWA), countless cases of discrimination against male and/or LGBT victims by the VAWA-funded service system were documented. A 2011 study by Emily Douglas and Denise Hines found that of 302 men aged 18–59 from 45 states who had experienced intimate partner violence and sought help from domestic violence agencies, hotlines, or online programs, 43–64 % (depending on type of agency they contacted) were told, "we only help women." More than 40 % of those who called domestic violence agencies were accused of being the batterer in their relationship, and 25 % of those who contacted an online resource were given a phone number that turned out to be the number for a batterer's program [9].

Transgender survivors—both trans men and trans women—also reported service problems. In a 2011 national study that FORGE did of more than 1000 transgender people, more than 60 % said they would not or might not use a rape crisis center or domestic violence shelter if they suffered from those crimes. Explanations for this reluctance included [20]:

- I have personal experience training this [rape crisis] group on trans issues and their responses were largely negative. They also have fired volunteers when they come out as trans.
- They are not trans-friendly. They do not allow "men" on their hotline. They kicked off a F to M[3] trans volunteer during their transition. These are not allegations. This is admitted to by the organization.
- None of the rape crisis services in my area serve male bodied or male-identified victims, none acknowledge same-sex/gender rape, none acknowledge transitioned identities.
- I know a trans woman who, just a few years ago, was turned away from a shelter like this in blizzard, state of emergency conditions and told that the shelter was for women, not men who dress like women.
- Local shelters DO NOT WELCOME US!
- I have volunteered for years at our local D[omestic] V[iolence] shelter and they do try to be "trans-inclusive" but the staff is not trained in trans issues, plus they only take people who identify as women, which leaves trans men who need help getting themselves (and sometimes kids) away from abusive transphobic ex-partners (usually men).
- Past experiences of trans survivors accessing the hotline were not positive. Past experiences of trans people volunteering with the rape crisis center were terrible.
- Not trans-friendly. Others have tried and were told that there was no way they could be rape victims.
- The major rape crisis line in my area has been reported to be transphobic.
- Not inclusive, particularly for transwomen/transfeminine folks and non-binary identified folks. Also, if perpetrator

[3] F to M means female-to-male transgender person, also known as FTM.

is not a cisgender[4] (non-trans) man, the assault is generally not seen as "real."

- They are horribly inadequate in rape crisis services to the community at large, the interactions that I have had with them with regards to the trans community have been appalling.
- Most would not serve trans people because of biology (MTF[5]) or gender (FTM). They are only set up to serve ciswomen.
- Shelters in this locale are extremely unfriendly toward trans people.
- There is only a women's shelter and I would not be allowed to use it.
- There is not one that will take a transgenders any where near me.
- The only domestic violence shelters I'm aware of in my area are for "women born women," so they are explicitly not welcoming to people of trans experience and I would not use them.
- Most [city name removed] shelters do not allow trans people.
- Many of the shelters that are available are for women and children and I have yet to hear about a shelter service for men or for transgender inclusive services.
- On "religious grounds" some of the shelters refuse to deal with TS [transsexual] people.
- Only shelter I know of around here is anti-trans/gay.
- To use any shelters provided in my community would mean I would have to go back to living in my former gender, which would cause anxiety issues again.
- NOT welcoming of transwomen/transfeminine folks, and none of the women's shelters will welcome transmasculine folks, either. There are no safe men's shelters or any that provide D[omestic] V[iolence] services.
- I know that the domestic violence shelters that exist in my area only cater to people identifying as women (i.e., non-trans women).
- None accept trans women.
- No [county name removed] domestic abuse programs accept trans persons, especially pre-op, non-op, and partial op MTFs.
- Because I do not know a single shelter that would accept a trans person.
- They do not allow transgender people.
- Services not provided to Trans persons or males.
- I do not know of anywhere that offers shelter or housing for trans people. I only know of women's agencies and they are not friendly to transwomen.
- D[omestic] V[iolence] shelter has decided not to admit transgender females.

25.2.6 Federal Nondiscrimination Provisions Strengthened

Although the Violence Against Women Act already had said men could be served under the program (before, in fact, many of the respondents in Douglas and Hines's study requested help), in its 2013 VAWA reauthorization Congress responded to the reports of anti-LGBT discrimination by strengthening that nondiscrimination provision, adding protections for survivors on the basis of actual or perceived sexual orientation and gender identity. The next year the Department of Justice's (DOJ) Office for Civil Rights issued guidance that further explained what DOJ expected of agencies funded (even in part) by VAWA funds [8]. Although the new provisions focused on LGBT survivors, the new programming requirements have the potential for radically restructuring programs that have not previously served or only minimally served (such as providing 3 days' hotel vouchers) male victims.

For example, the Frequently Asked Questions (FAQs) document DOJ issued pertaining to the new nondiscrimination provisions defined programming as sex-segregated "when males and females receive services in separate settings." Programming is sex-specific "when a recipient designs it differently for males and females." DOJ went on, "If the Department receives a complaint of sex discrimination based upon a recipient's sex-segregated or sex-specific services, the onus will be on the recipient to articulate clearly why sex-segregation or sex-specific programming was necessary to the essential operations of the program" and should include reference to "established best practices and research findings." This includes considering "the literature on the efficacy of the service being sex-segregated or sex-specific, the impact on transgender individuals seeking services, and whether similarly situated recipients providing the same services have been successful in providing services effectively in a manner that is not sex-segregated or sex-specific." DOJ continued, "A recipient should not assume that, because services have been sex-segregated or sex-specific in the past, continued sex-segregation or sex specificity is 'necessary' to its programming."

If sex-segregated or sex-specific programming is permitted, "comparable services" for those who are excluded must be provided: "A comparable service is one that is designed to confer a substantially equal benefit," taking into account such factors as nature and quality of the services provided, the relative benefits of different modalities or interventions, and characteristics of the individuals who

[4]"Cis" or "cisgender" is a term used to describe someone whose birth gender and current gender identity are in alignment. A cisgender individual is someone who is not transgender.

[5]Male-to-female transgender person.

provide the service. One of DOJ's examples is that if male clients are housed offsite, they must be provided transportation to supportive services that are made available onsite. In another example, "the therapeutic benefits of group counseling may be different than the therapeutic benefits of individual counseling, [so] the [agency] recipient should make every reasonable effort to provide comparable services through the same therapeutic modality."

Where there are sex-segregated or sex-specific programs, transgender beneficiaries should be assigned "to the group or service which corresponds to the gender with which the beneficiary identifies," with room to consider whether "a particular housing assignment would ensure the victim's health and safety." DOJ cautions, however, that an agency "may not make a determination about services for one beneficiary based on the complaints of another beneficiary when those complaints are based on gender identity." The guidance also bars agencies from "ask[ing] questions about the beneficiary's anatomy or medical history or mak[ing] burdensome demands for identity documents."

The FAQs provided a complaint mechanism that can be used by both individuals and organizations or advocates if they believe the law has been violated. Instructions and links can be found in the FAQs (http://www.justice.gov/sites/default/files/ovw/legacy/2014/06/20/faqs-ngc-vawa.pdf) and at http://www.ojp.usdoj.gov/about/ocr/complaint.htm.

The Family Violence Prevention and Services Administration (FVPSA) is another major federal source of funding for programs that address intimate partner violence, and they, too, have addressed discrimination against LGBT survivors. FVPSA now requires grantees to sign an assurance that they have taken the needs of LGBT survivors into account, that they are providing inclusive and non-stigmatizing services to them, that they have in place non-harassment policies, that staff members are trained to "prevent and respond to harassment or bullying in all forms," and that they will monitor, address, and document claims and the corrective action(s) taken [11].

These efforts, while still in their infancy, hold promise for helping reverse the current system's bias against recognizing and meeting the needs of male survivors of domestic violence and sexual assault, including elder survivors.

25.3 Research Challenges and Future Directions

Researching LGBT elder abuse is going to remain extremely challenging. We are only beginning to see federally funded nationally representative surveys ask people about their sexual orientation, and questions on gender identity are still being formulated. Even where such questions are asked, many elders—for all the reasons listed in the first part of the chapter—are not going to answer truthfully, believing that even if the survey promises anonymity, it is dangerous to tell the government one is LGBT. Nationally representative studies may also not be large enough to give us the data we need: the first violence study (2013) that asked about sexual orientation, *the National Intimate Partner Sexual Violence Study,* did not have sufficient respondents to perform a number of analyses of interest, including breaking down responses by age and sexual orientation. These issues are going to continue to plague representative studies.

Nonrepresentative studies are also going to face ongoing problems. Existing studies of LGBT elders tend to show higher levels of isolation, poverty, poor health, and service needs [19]. However, such surveys are almost universally distributed by LGBT service organizations; it is highly likely that elders who have strong personal and financial support resources are not engaged with these organizations and so are not being exposed to the surveys. How do we reach LGBT elders who are completely "mainstreamed," i.e., not attached to the LGBT community?

Adult protective services are the best-situated to shed light on what abuse looks like among LGBT elders. However, they do not generally inquire about or report their clients' sexual orientation and/or gender identity, nor are their clients likely to be honest if asked.

There are also definitional issues when researching LGBT communities. The federal government learned this when it began more nuanced studies related to the transmission of HIV. That was when the designation of MSM—men who have sex with men—was developed; many of the men others presumed were gay did not define themselves as such. If educational materials or presentations were addressed to gay men, these men ignored them. In other words, there can be differences between identity and behavior. Which is the most important when it comes to elder abuse? Whether someone calls themselves a lesbian or is in a committed relationship with another woman? Does it matter if one has been transgender for 50 years or only 5? Those kinds of definitional dilemmas are always going to plague research that attempts to divide humanity into different categories.

Until very recently, there has been strong opposition in the elder abuse/aging field to discussing LGBT elder abuse issues: this author has experienced multiple incidents of professional discrimination and censorship because of my work on these issues, and others similarly were told by their employers to drop their LGBT work. Perhaps observing these responses, other high-level LGBT researchers have not come out and/or have not been willing to publish or present on LGBT elder abuse issues. Since the topic was first raised in the 1980s, we have made little progress. We are still at the speculation stage: taking what we know about elder abuse in general and LGBT elders in general, and speculating on how the two knowledge bases may fit together.

We need to start where all new fields start: with case studies. Case studies are in-depth reports of an individual (or a few) cases addressing a particular subject, such as abuse of LGBT elders. Only when we have dozens of detailed stories to discuss with each other will we be able to begin formulating more in-depth research questions. What is needed now is for elder abuse and aging organizations to finally step up and declare that it is time to begin talking about this long-ignored population, and begin soliciting and publishing case studies.

25.3.1 Working with LGBT Elder Abuse Victims

This chapter opened with Margaret Kucera's backstory because it is exactly that backstory that makes LGBT people different from non-LGBT people: we have a history of being abused, betrayed, denied our rights, forced into unwanted treatment, discriminated against, denied the right to build and protect our families, and so much more [10, 16]. The wounds have been inflicted not just by strangers, but also by our parents, our coaches and teachers, our LGBT peers, our religious homes and, especially, our government. These experiences have not only taught us that you cannot count on other people for help—even if they are also LGBT—but that abuse is normal for LGBT people. Many of us have heard variations of the phrase, "if you insist on being LGBT, you are going to end your life alone and miserable." Wrap all of these experiences together, and you end up with LGBT elders who believe they have few, if any, options if their loved ones start abusing them.

Approaching an elder abuse victim you suspect may be LGBT therefore calls for extraordinary care and listening skills. It is *not* necessary to determine whether the elder is, in fact, LGBT. It may even be counterproductive to bring the question up, as it may start the elder wondering what they did or said that tipped you off. What is called for includes the following:

25.3.1.1 Follow Your Client's Lead

Ask people to tell you about "the people you live with," or "the people who are important in your life." Many LGBT elders describe their partners by a neutral and vague term such as "roommate," or "friend," in order to protect both of them from prejudice and discrimination. Follow their linguistic lead. If you suspect the elder is LGBT, do *not* ask, "who is your partner?" or "is that your partner?" You do not need to know the exact nature of their relationship in order to discern and meet their needs. If the elder is transgender, always call them by the name they introduced themselves by. If you are not clear about which pronouns the person uses, ask them: "My name is Anne and I use 'she and her' pronouns. What pronouns do you use?"

25.3.1.2 Spread a Wide Net

If you ask an LGBT person only about their "partner" and "family members," you are liable to miss out on a huge portion of the picture. LGBT people often develop relationships that are far deeper than usual friendships, taking on more of the flavor of family relationships, including strong expectations of mutual care. Here too, "tell me about the people who are important in your life" is a good start.

25.3.1.3 Signal—but Don't Overemphasize—the Diversity of Your Clients

It may take a role-play or two before you can do it smoothly, but make a point of figuring out how you can bring up the diversity of people you serve when you talk to clients. One way to do this is to include an explicitly LGBT resource in a list of resources, such as the "LGBT community center's older adults group" as a socialization option. If a client (LGBT or not) expresses confusion or concern about the referral, simply say, "we serve the whole community, so we talk about many different options; just ignore any resource that doesn't appeal to you." Practice inclusion as a matter of course, since at least some of the time, you will not suspect a client is, in fact, LGBT.

25.3.1.4 Listen for and Respond to Concerns and Fears

This recommendation, while basic and applicable to all clients, deserves repetition when it comes to LGBT clients. You may need to do gentle probing to unearth the real reasons why a victim might be resisting one or more recommendations.

25.3.1.5 Know (and Use) LGBT Resources

In order to better respond to concerns and fears, know what LGBT-specific resources are available. For example, be familiar with the new laws and guidance that provide LGBT people protection from discrimination in housing, health care, and other settings (see Sect. 25.3.2). Many LGBT elders have not kept up with all the recent changes and may be reassured to know that the law is now on their side in most cases. Also learn where discrimination complaints can be filed, and provide support to your clients in filing complaints; many of these new protections are only invoked when complaints are filed. Even if a complaint would not result in your client being served (perhaps because you have to find them another resource in the interim), future LGBT clients will be helped.

25.3.1.6 Respect Privacy

Get your client's permission before you "out" them as LGBT to other service providers. Again, it is *not* necessary for people to know if an elder is LGBT to serve them well. Some LGBT elders do want to be sure ahead of time that the people coming into their lives know and accept their LGBT status, and would welcome a sensitive discussion beforehand about who will say what to whom. Others would prefer to do the coming out themselves, or want to continue to stay private about their sexual orientation and/or gender identity. Respecting privacy is particularly important for transgender elders. Many professionals falsely believe that colleagues should be "warned" someone is transgender, particularly if they have not had surgery to realign their genitals. This is not only not true, but such conversations are likely to violate HIPAA and other laws. A document that was prepared with frontline nursing home workers in mind, "I Have a New Transgender Client…Now What?," may be helpful for any service provider who has concerns about caring for a transgender client (see Sect. 25.3.2).

25.3.1.7 Be Sensitive to LGBT-Specific Wounds

When the U.S. began looking at elder abuse involving racial minorities in the 1990s, we learned that cultural differences can affect whether a given practice was considered abuse or not [30]. In a 2007 survey of transgender people, FORGE found that trans people sometimes applied standard elder abuse terms to situations that would not be covered under state or federal law. Examples of "abandonment" included family and friends who quit speaking to the transgender person once they came out. Examples of "abuse" included incidents in which trans people were refused access to a public restroom [4]. While officials must, obviously, follow the law's definitions of what is legal and illegal, it is important to recognize the depth of pain an elder may be feeling when they talk about such anti-LGBT actions.

25.3.1.8 Problem-Solve to Keep Connections Alive

Remember the advice above to "spread the net wide" and ask about the people important to the elder? When it's care-planning time, check this list again and keep it handy. Even more than non-LGBT clients, abused LGBT elders need to have care plans that explicitly keep them linked to their LGBT support network. Remember that most LGBT elders will enter or use mainstream agencies, such as home care agencies, day care programs, or residential living with even more trepidations than non-LGBT elders, because they will be worried about how to handle their LGBT identity and whether others will be prejudiced. Make especially sure they are connected with at least one individual staff person before they go through any new doors, and that they know they will have an opportunity to "de-brief" with an LGBT loved one soon after a new experience. Don't do what one adult protective worker did early on: she moved her gay male client out of a "dangerous" neighborhood to "nice senior housing." Problem was, all of this man's friends and social contacts were young gay male hustlers who were unwilling to follow him to his new neighborhood and navigate the "secure" building. So she left him secure—and alone [2].

25.3.1.9 Consider Changing the World

This recommendation is only a little tongue-in-cheek. The extra problems LGBT and/or male elder abuse clients face are not of their own making; it is totally society's stereotypes and prejudices and the actions that stem from them that create the extra hurdles LGBT and/or male elder abuse victims must cross. If we are to eliminate the sort of disparities we are seeing in various minority groups' health, income, education levels, exposure to violence, etc., we are going to have to eliminate stereotypes and prejudices altogether. While this may sound impossible, it is not: each of us can check ourselves every time we think or say something that is based not on the individual in front of us, but on what we believe about one or more categories we have assigned them to. "Person-first" service is becoming better known as a service philosophy; it also works in the broader world: learn who is in front of you directly from them instead of relying on assumptions that you carried into the interaction.

25.3.2 Resources

25.3.2.1 National Organizations

The National Resource Center on LGBT Aging
https://www.lgbtagingcenter.org/
This federally funded resource center offers multiple training curricula put together by a committee of the most experienced LGBT elder trainers in the country. The website hosts the most comprehensive compilation of resources specific to LGBT aging, categorized by topics that include elder abuse, transgender aging, and housing and long-term care.

FORGE Transgender Aging Network (TAN)
http://www.forge-forward.org/aging
TAN offers a peer support listserv for transgender people age 50+ and their close loved ones, and a listserv for professionals. The website also contains an archive of publications and training webinars specific to trans and/or LGBT elders.

National Center for Transgender Equality (NCTE)
http://www.transequality.org/

NCTE is the leading transgender policy advocacy group. Check here for plain-English "Know Your Rights" documents.

Movement Advancement Project (MAP)

http://www.lgbtmap.org/

MAP tracks LGBT policy changes on a wide range of federal and state issues.

CenterLink

http://www.lgbtcenters.org/

Includes directory to U.S. LGBT community centers.

25.3.2.2 Federal Rights and Policies

Employment nondiscrimination

What You Should Know About the Equal Employment Opportunity Commission and the Enforcement Protections for LGBT Workers

http://www.eeoc.gov/eeoc/newsroom/wysk/enforcement_protections_lgbt_workers.cfm

Health care discrimination protections

http://healthcarebillofrights.org/

Social Security Administration and married couples

http://www.ssa.gov/people/same-sexcouples/

Housing discrimination protections

http://portal.hud.gov/hudportal/HUD?src=/program_offices/fair_housing_equal_opp/LGBT_Housing_Discrimination

Veterans Administration LGBT protections and programs

http://www.diversity.va.gov/programs/lgbt.aspx

Violence Against Women Act non-discrimination Frequently Asked Questions

http://www.justice.gov/sites/default/files/ovw/legacy/2014/06/20/faqs-ngc-vawa.pdf

25.3.2.3 Publications

A Self-Help Guide for LGBT Older Adults and their Caregivers and Loved Ones: Preventing, Recognizing, and Addressing Elder Abuse

http://www.lgbtagingcenter.org/resources/pdfs/SELF-HELP_elderAbuse_Guide.pdf

Residents' Rights and the LGBT Community: Know YOUR Rights as a Nursing Home Resident

http://www.lgbtagingcenter.org/resources/pdfs/LGBTRRFactSheet-FINAL.pdf

Creating Equal Access to Quality Health Care for Transgender Patients: Transgender-Affirming Hospital Policies

http://www.lgbtagingcenter.org/resources/pdfs/fs_transgender-affirming-hospital-policies.pdf

I Have a New Transgender Client…Now What?

http://www.lgbtagingcenter.org/resources/pdfs/newTransClientFactSheet.pdf

Legal Developments and Practical Considerations: Improving the Quality of Care for Older LGBT Adults in the Long-Term Care Setting

http://www.lgbtagingcenter.org/resources/pdfs/AHLA_ConnectionsMagazine_olderadultsLongterm.pdf

25.3.2.4 Trainings

Advocating for LGBT Long-Term Care Consumers: Resources for Long-Term Care Ombudsmen (Training Webinar)

http://www.lgbtagingcenter.org/resources/resource.cfm?r=586#sthash.wN8Z8NzV.dpuf

Building Respect for Older LGBT Adults (DHHS training video for long-term care personnel)

http://www.lgbtagingcenter.org/training/buildingrespect/index.cfm.

References

1. Conway L. How frequently does transsexualism occur? 2002. http://ai.eecs.umich.edu/people/conway/TS/TSprevalence.html. Accessed 15 Sept 2015.
2. Cook-Daniels L. Lesbian, gay male, bisexual and transgendered elders: elder abuse and neglect issues. 2002. http://forge-forward.org/wp-content/docs/LGBT-Elder-abuse.pdf.
3. Cook-Daniels L. Living memory LGBT history timeline. 2007a. http://forge-forward.org/wp-content/docs/LGBT_elder_timeline_FINAL.pdf.
4. Cook-Daniels L. Abuse and violence directed at transgender elders. 2007b. http://forge-forward.org/wp-content/docs/Abuse-and-Violence-Directed-at-Transgender-Elders.pdf.
5. Cook-Daniels L. Seeing past the "L": addressing anti-male bias in sexual assault services for the "LGBT" community. 2008. http://forge-forward.org/wp-content/docs/Anti-Male_Bias_SeeingpasttheL.pdf.
6. Cook-Daniels L. "Atypical" sexual abuse survivors and perpetrators: Where are the male victims and female perpetrators? (Part Two of Two). In: Victimization of the elderly and disabled. vol. 11, no. 5. Civic Research Institute; 2009.
7. Cook-Daniels L. The partner abuse state of knowledge project. In: Victimization of the elderly and disabled, vol. 16, no. 3. Civic Research Institute; 2013.
8. Department of Justice. Frequently asked questions: Nondiscrimination grant condition in the Violence Against Women Reauthorization Act of 2013. 2014. http://www.justice.gov/sites/default/files/ovw/legacy/2014/06/20/faqs-ngc-vawa.pdf. Accessed 15 Sept 2015.
9. Douglas E, Hines D. The helpseeking experiences of men who sustain intimate partner violence: an overlooked population and implications for practice. J Fam Violence. 2011;26(6):473–85.
10. Duberman M, Vicinus M, Chauncey G, editors. Hidden from history: reclaiming the gay and lesbian past. New York: New American Library; 1989.
11. Family Violence Prevention and Services Administration. LGBTQ (Also known as "Two-Spirited") accessibility policy. 2014. http://docs.regulations.justia.com/entries/2014-07-01/2014-15384.pdf. Accessed 15 Sept 2015.

12. Feinberg L. Transgender warriors: making history from Joan of Arc to RuPaul. Boston: Beacon Press; 1996.
13. Fredriksen-Goldsen K, et al. The aging and health report: disparities and resilience among lesbian, gay, bisexual and transgender older adults. 2011. http://caringandaging.org/wordpress/wp-content/uploads/2011/05/Full-Report-FINAL-11-16-11.pdf. Accessed 15 Sept 2015.
14. Gates G. How many people are lesbian, gay, bisexual and transgender? Williams Institute. 2011. http://williamsinstitute.law.ucla.edu/wp-content/uploads/Gates-How-Many-People-LGBT-Apr-2011.pdf. Accessed 15 Sept 2015.
15. International Lesbian, Gay, Bisexual, Trans and Intersex Association (ILGA). The lesbian, gay, and bisexual map of world laws. 2015. http://old.ilga.org/Statehomophobia/ILGA_WorldMap_2015_ENG.pdf. Accessed 15 Sept 2015.
16. Katz J. Gay American history: lesbians and gay men in the USA. New York: Thomas Y. Crowell Company; 1976.
17. Lew M. Victims no longer: the classic guide for men recovering from sexual child abuse. 2nd ed. New York: Harper; 2004.
18. Miller N. Out of the past: gay and lesbian history from 1869 to the present. New York: Advocate Books; 2008.
19. Movement Advancement Project, SAGE and Center for American Progress. LGBT older adults: facts at a glance. 2010. http://www.lgbtagingcenter.org/resources/pdfs/LGBTOlderAdultsFactsataGlance.pdf. Accessed 15 Sept 2015.
20. Munson M, Cook-Daniels L. Transgender individuals' knowledge of and willingness to use sexual assault programs, a survey approved by the Morehouse School of Medicine's Institutional Review Board. Unpublished manuscript. Milwaukee, WI; 2011.
21. Murray S, Roscoe W. Boy wives and female husbands: studies of African homosexualities. New York: St. Martin's Press; 1998.
22. National Senior Citizens Law Center. LGBT older adults in long-term care facilities: Stories from the field. 2011. https://www.lgbtagingcenter.org/resources/pdfs/NSCLC_LGBT_report.pdf. Accessed 15 Sept 2015.
23. NBC News. "Betrayed": male rape victims slam Oscar-nominated filmmakers over focus on women. 2013. http://usnews.nbcnews.com/_news/2013/02/08/16890167-betrayed-male-rape-victims-slam-oscar-nominated-filmmakers-over-focus-on-women. Accessed 15 Sept 2015.
24. Otto J, editor. Abuse and neglect of vulnerable populations. New Jersey: Civic Research Institute; 2005.
25. Pizzey E. This way to the revolution: a memoir. London: Peter Owen Publishers; 2011.
26. Rosin H. When men are raped: a new study reveals that men are often the victims of sexual assault, and women are often the perpetrators. Slate. 2014. http://www.slate.com/articles/double_x/doublex/2014/04/male_rape_in_america_a_new_study_reveals_that_men_are_sexually_assaulted.html. Accessed 15 Sept 2015.
27. Stemple L, Meyer I. The sexual victimization of men in America: new data challenge old assumptions. Am J Public Health. 2014;104:e1–8.
28. Stern K. Queers in history: the comprehensive encyclopedia of historical gays, lesbians, and bisexuals. Dallas: Ben Bella Books; 2009.
29. Straus M. Thirty years of denying the evidence on gender symmetry in partner violence: implications for prevention and treatment. Partner Abuse. 2010;1(3):332–62.
30. Tatara T, editor. Understanding elder abuse in minority populations. London: Taylor and Francis; 1999.
31. Walters M, Chen J, Breiding M. The national intimate partner and sexual violence survey (NISVS): 2010 findings on victimization by sexual orientation. Atlanta: National Center for Injury Prevention and Control, Centers for Disease Control and Prevention; 2013.

Role of the Community and Community-Based Participatory Research in Elder Abuse

26

E-Shien Chang and XinQi Dong

If a person merely learns without reflection, he will learn in vein.
If a person merely thinks but does not reflect, he will face trouble.
Confucius, The Analects of Confucius, 475-221 BC

26.1 Introduction

26.1.1 Minority Health and Health Disparities Research

Understanding health disparities across life span is a major initiative of the public health research establishment in the U.S. [1] and around the world [2]. In particular, health disparities in marginalized older adults are ever-increasing public health concerns. Older adults and racial/ethnic minorities are currently two of the fastest growing demographic groups in North America [3, 4]. It is estimated that by 2050, older adults aged 60 and above will comprise nearly 26 % of the total population [5]. The trend of minority aging is even more salient. Compared to a projected increase of 77 % in the U.S. native population aged 65 and above between 2014 and 2060, the U.S. foreign-born population aged 65 and above is projected to increase over 300 %, from 6 million in 2014 to 25 million in 2060 [6]. In only about a decade's time, by 2030, approximately 1 out of 3 (28.5 %) older adults will be from racial and ethnic minority backgrounds [7].

This pronounced demographic shift exposes the urgency in achieving equality in health. Broadly speaking, health disparities are considered to be population differences in (1) environmental exposures, (2) health care access, utilization, or quality, (3) health status, (4) health outcomes [8]. However, the causes of health disparities are immensely intricate. Racial and ethnic differences in socio-demographics or socioeconomic variations alone may no longer adequately address disparities in health [9]. In its 2002 report *Unequal Treatment: Confronting Racial and Ethnic Disparities in Health Care*, the Institute of Medicine (IOM) reviewed disparities and further raised the consciousness of this issue in the policy arena. This landmark report has shown that even after controlling for socioeconomic status, insurance status, site of care, stage of disease, comorbidity, and age, among other potential confounders, racial and ethnic disparities in health outcome continue to persist in the diagnosis and treatment of various conditions [10]. The complex interactions of multiple factors including individual, biological, social, and environmental risk factors as well as pervasive structural inequalities may all play a role in the cause of health disparities. While some scholars have documented various individual, provider, and system-level factors that have contributed to health and health care disparities [11], others have garnered equally compelling evidence in suggesting how individuals' highly culturally and socially imbedded health beliefs and values may be manifested as amongst the root causes of health disparities [12, 13].

During the past two decades, concerted academic and regulatory interventions have been made to better address the contexts of health disparities beyond the dimensions of racial and ethnic parameters. On a national level, health promotion efforts such as the Healthy People initiatives—a program of the National Institutes of Health (NIH) intended to improve public health in the U.S., have continued to prioritize *reducing* health disparities in 2000, evolved into *eliminating* health disparities in 2010. However, the perplexing relationships underlining the barriers and facilitators of health equality may be aptly defined by Healthy People 2020. In this initiative, health disparities pertain to "a particular type of health difference that is closely linked with social, economic, and/or environmental disadvantage. Health disparities adversely affect groups of people who have systematically experienced greater obstacles to health based on their racial or ethnic group; religion; socioeconomic status; gender; age; mental health; cognitive, sensory, or physical disability;

E.-S. Chang
Department of Chronic Disease Epidemiology, Yale School of Public Health, Yale University, 60 College Street, New Haven, CT 06510, USA

E.-S. Chang (✉) · X. Dong
Rush Institute for Healthy Aging, Rush University Medical Center, 1645 W. Jackson Blvd, Suite 675, Chicago, IL 60612, USA
e-mail: e-shien.chang@yale.edu

X. Dong (ed.), *Elder Abuse*, DOI 10.1007/978-3-319-47504-2_26

sexual orientation or gender identity; geographic location; or other characteristics historically linked to discrimination or exclusion" [14]. Therefore, efforts to ameliorate health disparities must address the intersection of multiple factors beyond the simple cause–effect model. It is within this racial–ethnic, social–cultural, physical environmental, and structural framework of disparities that we wish to systematically explore the community's critical role in reducing differences in health, in particular, pertaining to elder abuse.

26.1.2 Rationales to Engage Community in Health Disparities Research

To date, our ability to assess health disparities is hampered by the peripheral participation of members from these disadvantaged communities. The need to increase community participation in health disparities research is scientifically driven. From a life-span perspective, older adults are systematically excluded from many research studies by overt age cut-offs or covert exclusions based on comorbidity and frailty [15]. However, exclusion of older adults from ongoing public health research projects is problematic because older adults carry the greatest health burdens compared to other age groups [16]. Older adults also have the highest prevalence of various chronic conditions, greatest health care expenditure costs, yet at the same time most likely to suffer from the psychological or social consequences of agism [17]. Equitable participation of older community members becomes necessary to advance public health knowledge as well as medical treatments that may be generalizable to aging populations.

From a racial and ethnic diversity viewpoint, the demographic composition of U.S. is increasingly pluralistic, with the racial/ethnic minorities reaching a numerical majority of 54 % by 2050 [18]. Adequate minority representation is called for in all research, including drawing samples from geographic areas in which substantial numbers of one or more minority group reside. Such efforts must be made to further ensure that findings apply to a diverse population, and to allow sufficient sample size for racial/ethnic-specific analyses and data representation [9]. However, it is important to be wary of race as a persistent social-political marker, not as a biological descriptor. As aforementioned, race has been postulated as a robust indicator of health outcome in the U.S. largely due to the social values and structured opportunities or barriers assigned to the collective interpretations of one's physical appearance [19]. Therefore, attention should be directed in ways to engage community participation in capturing the social classification of people beyond race as a proxy for socioeconomic status, culture, or genes.

From the viewpoints of social and economic inequalities, the lack of community inclusiveness may often undermine study effects. Major health disparities prevail along the three main dimensions of socioeconomic status (SES) characteristics: education, employment, and wealth. SES disparities in health status do not merely stem from a "threshold effect" of poverty or illiteracy [20]. Rather, there is a gradient effect in health across SES such that higher levels of education, properties, occupational ranking are associated with lower risks of adverse health outcomes. On the one hand, disadvantaged members' low SES status may intuitively place them at "risks of risks"; i.e., limited or no resources contributing to high risks of disease or illness exposure. On the one hand, for members of socio-economically advantaged backgrounds, while it is true that they may possess greater social capital, better access to resources, they may also experience ceiling effects, i.e., having a diminished capacity to benefit from preventive interventions [21]. However, it is not feasible to isolate SES factors that contribute to health disparities because social systems are active and ongoing. Given SES status is strongly correlated with insurance status, healthcare access, and health services utilizations, the role of community in facilitating health-seeking behaviors is even more critical in understanding health disparities both on the micro and macro levels. Community-integrated health needs assessment would also benefit minority members along the lines of faith, gender identity, or sexual orientations.

Finally, perhaps one of the most commonly discussed rationales in involving the community in research activities pertains to its inherent strength in addressing culture. The concept of culture as distinct from race and ethnicity has been proposed as a better explanation for differences in health behavior and health outcomes [22]. Often perceived as the underlying cause of the undue burden of disparities by minority communities, culture is nonetheless difficult to measure or operationalize [23]. Scientifically, culture is a complex, integrated, and dynamic conceptual framework. To properly address community's needs, researchers need close collaboration with the culture of the community, regardless of which race or ethnicity involved. Health disparities research can greatly benefit from community input in better conceptualizing research agenda as well as collecting relevant data to address "deep culture" (i.e., beliefs, values, and behaviors), as opposed to only the "surface culture" (i.e., language, food, music) [24]. As a critical response to the poorly defined and inadequately operationalized concept of culture, a panel of experts supported by the NIH office of Behavioral and Social Science Research recently released a comprehensive report on the Cultural Framework of Health [25]. Calling for a flow-map approach, this processual framework recommends six checkpoints to facilitate a more thorough account for cultural process in health, all of which may only be thoroughly accomplished via interdisciplinary collaboration with equitable community input. Application of this dynamic framework could increase the likelihood for research findings that truly reflect the contextual underpinnings of health disparities across populations.

26.2 Special Research Challenges in Minority Populations

There has been an increased regulatory effort to encourage the representation of underserved racial/ethnic groups in epidemiological research. As a whole, federal requests for applications for studies in diverse populations have increased. NIH-led Revitalization Act of 1993 has formally requested minority recruitment plans or scientific justification for their exclusion [26]. Similarly, the Food and Drug Administration (FDA) formally issued guidance in 2005 to call for the collection of race and ethnicity data in clinical trials [27], in addition to the existing offices dedicated to improving the health of vulnerable populations in the Centers for Medicare & Medicaid Services (CMS) and several operating divisions at the U.S. Department of Health and Human Services (HHS), including the Centers for Disease Control (CDC) and the Agency for Healthcare Research and Quality (AHRQ). Furthermore, a recent NIH-led nationally representative study argued that minority population might have equal willingness to participate in the biomedical or epidemiological study, as their Non-Hispanic White counterparts [28]. This report, among others [29, 30], argued that minority communities may be as willing to enroll in health research as mainstream groups if they were prioritized and offered the opportunity to participate.

Despite a series of national-level initiatives calling for increasing community participation in research, evidence suggested that racial and ethnic minority populations continue to participate less frequently than Non-Hispanic Whites. While currently racial/ethnic minorities constitute more than 30 % of the U.S. population, reports from nationally representative studies revealed minority group members represented less than 20 % in the ongoing clinical trials [31]. The discrepancy in participation rate may be starker in older adults of color compared to their White counterparts across study various types, e.g., clinical trials [32], interventions [33], as well as studies on chronic conditions, including Alzheimer's disease [34], cardiovascular diseases [35], arthritis [36], or mental health research [37]. Similarly, gender and sexual minorities such as women or members of LGBT groups are also largely neglected in many ongoing health research studies [35, 38]. A review paper published in the early 2000s reported that despite LGBT persons likely constitute between 1 and 10 % of the total population, only 0.1 % equivalent of the medical database has focused on LGBT persons over the past 20 years [39]. In short, lack of diversity in ongoing epidemiological research will run the great risks of extrapolating data from a study population that no longer resembles the general population.

26.2.1 Historical Context of Research in Minority Populations

From a historical perspective, research was traditionally carried out by investigators of majority backgrounds, i.e., White researchers targeting mostly majority membership; most research maintained the "gold standards" which tended to include erroneous stereotypes about research content areas or methods when transferred to minority populations [31]. For examine, investigators' use of recruitment, study retention, or finding dissemination strategies among racial and ethnic minority groups that were developed for majority memberships have been noted concerns [33].

As one of the most egregiously unethical conduct in contemporary health research, the case of Tuskegee Study of untreated syphilis in African Americans in Alabama has continued to shape public attitudes toward research participation, particularly among racial/ethnic members [40, 41]. Such reservations are particularly prominent in older Americans because some may have personally witnessed or experienced medical research abuses. Some minority older adults may therefore feel uncomfortable in traditional research settings [42]. However, as many scholars argued [43–45], minority members' negative sentiment in medical research participation may be rooted in their experience extending back to the slavery times. This dark history of medical and science abuse toward adults of color has been extensive and pervasive over the last four centuries [46]. In aggregate, these historic events highlight how inequity can pervade public health and medical research even when researchers and federal government acknowledge the needs to protect participants from potential harm from research participation [47]. For many minority groups, the deep suspicion in medical and public health research go beyond slavery and Tuskegee to the present day.

26.2.2 Racism and Racial Discrimination

The literature on minority participation in clinical, medical, and epidemiological research has burgeoned over the past decade [29, 31, 38]. Most of this scholarship has systematically focused on the impact of racism and racial discrimination in light of the historical abuses associated with the Tuskegee Study. Several studies have raised questions about both overt and covert forms of racism and discrimination at multiple levels that may lead to the under-representation of minority populations in health research [44, 45]. Barriers to minority participation in research resulting from such racism can occur at different levels, from institutional, to interpersonal, to internalized racism [19].

The Chinese Exclusion Act of 1882 symbolizes to date the most infamous systematic, institutionalized racism in barring minority members' participation in all civil activities. The Exclusion Act outlawed all Chinese immigration to the U.S. and denied citizenship to those already settled in the U.S., making Chinese immigrants the first group to be legally barred from becoming naturalized citizens in the U.S. Although the Exclusion Act was repealed in 1943 and decades later in 2012, the Congress issued a formal apology for the Chinese Exclusion Act with the passage of Senate and House resolution, harsh discrimination and racial tension have instilled long-lasting distrust among the Chinese community, especially among older generations. Persistent effects of colonization or slavery at an institutionalized level also have manifested in ongoing health inequalities. Another example of a dark history of systematic abuse pertains to U.S. Public Health Services' misconduct on minority groups. Decades after slavery, Indian American, and Puerto Rican women were encouraged to be sterilized as a method of population control [48, 49]. Consequently, overcoming the perception of systematic discrimination continues to be a formidable research challenge in these populations.

Interpersonal racism is often manifested in prejudicial and discriminatory acts resulting in poor health care experiences and health outcomes for racial/ethnic minorities. Patients with such experiences are also less likely to participate in health research [50]. Finally, at the level of internalized racism, stigmatized populations accept negative messages and stereotypes about their own abilities and worth, resulting in lower psychological health and self-esteem, which can in turn pose a negative effect on health practices and outcomes. The same stereotypes and negative messages internalized by minorities may also shape health care providers' and organizations' interactions with minorities. For instance, in the case of Chinese Americans, they are often perceived as "the model minority" which then may decrease the visibility of Asian Americans as a racial/ethnic minority group experiencing chronic disease health disparities and deserving of health-related resources and consideration [51]. These deleterious effects of internalized racism on the provider–patient relationships may negatively affect decisions of minorities to participate in health research.

26.2.3 Mistrust

As a result of system-level discrimination, mistrust of academic institutions and investigators is the most significant attitudinal barrier to research participation. Its etiology may stem from historic events and minority discrimination, but may also exacerbate by contemporary avenues, including socioeconomic and healthcare system inequities.

There are also racial and ethnic disparities in the different dimensions of trust [52]; i.e., interpersonal distrust in clinical research may be based on personal experiences and interactions of individuals within health care or research settings. In contrast, societal distrust is characterized by a negative global outlook on clinical research based on perceptions of collective research entities or life experiences in society at large. The societal-level trust also depends largely on the construct of health advocacy, the belief that persons and institutions will act in a manner consistent with our interests. On an interpersonal level, compared to Non-Hispanic Whites, Corbie-Smith et al. [45] found that African Americans were less likely to trust that their physicians would fully explain research participation, and stated that their physicians may expose them to unnecessary risks. Beliefs about physician mistrust among African American patients are then reinforced through differential treatment in comparison with Whites [53]. Moreover, previous research indicates that a lack of cultural diversity and competence among physicians is a major contributor to minority members' mistrust of physicians [54]. Ethnic minority patients receive less information, empathy, and attention from their physicians regarding their medical care than their White counterparts. Despite these concerns, other research showed that there were no differences in interpersonal distrust in clinical or medical research, but rather significant variations existed in societal distrust among African Americans compared with Whites [55]. Similarly, another national-representative survey of U.S. population suggested that in general, distrust of the health care system was relatively high, with between 20 and 80 % of respondents reported distrust, and that the distrust of the health care system was strongly associated with self-reported poor health [56].

Distrust of healthcare professionals and the healthcare system is rooted in a legacy of discrimination in the healthcare system. The notion of "mistrust" may not best illustrate the widespread reluctance of the minority community in research participation. When *mistrust* is replaced with *accountability* as an expectation on the part of the minority community from the investigators, the responsibility for action no longer lies with the community but with the investigator and research organizations [34]. This change of langauge often requires a markedly new set of activities to engage the community in research.

26.2.4 Stigma

Stigma occurs when labeling, stereotyping, separation, status loss, and discrimination co-occur in the context of an unequal power situation. In the social cognitive model, signals of symptoms or appearance are translated into stereotypes, which resulted in behavioral responses or discriminatory behaviors [57]. Stigma is often related to the health condition of interest in the research study such as mental burden or HIV research. Ethnic minority groups, who already confront prejudice and discrimination because of their membership affiliation, suffer double stigma when faced with the burdens of mental illness [58]. In HIV-related research, there exists the fear of the social repercussions of disclosing HIV status [59]. Stigma is also coupled with privacy and confidentiality concerns related to the participant's medical condition, personal health history, and genetics. The lack of acceptance and support from family members that may manifest itself in judgment for participating in a study also contributed to stigma. The fear of stigmatization often prevents minority groups from research participation.

Beyond prominent psychosocial and attitudinal barriers, minority communities also experience structural barriers in study participation such as transportation barriers, time constraint, competing demands, or lack of access to information [31]. As a result, many national surveys including the National Research Study, National Health and Nutrition Examination Survey, the National Health Interview Survey, often oversampled racial and ethnic minority groups in order to support cross-group comparisons by race and ethnicity, [60]. However, as aforementioned, the evidence is mixed as whether there is significant variance in survey participation by race and ethnicity. In addition, less likely to participate does not equate to less willing to participate. Re-examining the effectiveness of past and current approaches to reach minorities will be crucial to increasing and maintaining sufficient research enrollment and retention rates [61].

26.3 Community-Based Participatory Research Principles, Techniques, Practice

The notion of community-engaged research activities in reducing mistrust, discrimination as well as stigma is well-established. Although community-engaged approach offers a novel road map for epidemiologists who seek to strengthen the link between research and practice, there is a wide range of research endeavors and levels of community engagement within this orientation. Among its variations, community-based participatory research (CBPR) places most emphasis in engaging the community as a full equitable partner throughout research initiation, implementation, and dissemination [62]. As opposed to community-placed research which community only serves as a physical venue of research conduct, CBPR recognizes community as a holistic unit of identity, and that research should be built and developed based on the strengths and resources of the collective community. Another important feature that differentiates CBPR from other community-engaged research lies within its emphasis on the participatory nature. Different from conventional orientation toward research, participatory methodologies shares the location of power with all equitable members in the projects. As Cornwall and Jewkes described [63], what is distinctive about CBPR is "the attitudes of researchers, which in turn determine how, by and for whom research is conceptualized and conducted [and] the corresponding location of power at every stage of the research process."

In other words, participatory, action, and research elements are given full and equal consideration and executions within the CBPR orientation [64, 65]. With its attention to action as the central tenant of research progress, CBPR encourages researchers to pursue a data-minded approach to improving health and well-being. By equitably engaging both community and academic partners in this action-driven investigation, CBPR approach enhances the quality and quantity of research by developing trusting relationships in partnerships and avoiding "parachute" or "helicopter" drive-by research [66]. Furthermore, CBPR brings in a diverse group of stakeholders to co-own a solution that makes sense to them. Therefore, implementation will more likely be sustained.

26.3.1 CBPR Origins and Historical Roots

It is important to note that CBPR should not be interpreted as a research method per se, but rather a systematic orientation toward research and an in-depth understanding of the co-learning, long-term and social change oriented relationships between academic and community partners. The roots of CBPR appeared to be influenced by two separate traditions [64]. The earlier northern action research school developed by the social psychologist Kurt Lewin in the 1940s placed great emphasis on the process of change and action research as a means to overcoming social inequalities [67]. Later writings in the 1970s by a Brazilian educator, Paulo Freire, highlighted the social benefits of having communities identify their own problems and solutions [68]. His calling was followed by other emerging southern participatory research activists from developing communities in America, Asia, and Africa. These scholars, along feminists and post-colonialist scholars in the 1980s, persistently questioned the oppressive nature of research in which the most affected communities were also those who were highly subjected and isolated in the decision-making process [69, 70]. Another key tenant of participatory action research points to the process as highly political in nature, one that is committed to creating social change and establishing a self-critical community [71].

26.3.2 Principles

Drawing upon over two decades of work, Barbara Israel and her colleagues have identified eight key principles of CBPR that support successful research partnerships [72]. These widely cited principles are as follow:

- Recognizes community as a unit of identity
- Builds on strengths and resources within the community
- Facilitates collaborative partnerships in all phases of the research
- Integrates knowledge and action for mutual benefit of all partners
- Promotes a co-learning and empowering process that attends to social inequalities
- Involves a cyclical and iterative process
- Addresses health from both positive and ecological perspectives
- Disseminates findings and knowledge gained to all partners.

The key words in these principles are "collaborative", "equitable", "partnership", "affects social change". Successful CBPR partnerships demonstrate tangible benefits to all members involved. First, broadly speaking, the nature of community health and health disparities is often multi-faceted and thus its solutions requires interdisciplinary collaborative work which transcends the capacity of one single academic perspective [72]. Therefore, the solutions require diverse knowledge and cultural sensitivity rather than the traditional expert-led public health research approach. Second, CBPR honors community participation and self-determination. Belief in community's rightful place in planning and sustaining its health was deemed as the right thing to do. Third, CBPR is considered to be seen as the kind of health intervention in and of itself. Engaging community in each step of the scientific inquiry not only contributes in orchestrating positive community changes [66]; furthermore, it enhances members' co-ownership in sustaining change. Hence, CBPR orientation presents a unique synergistic framework to increase the likelihood of program success [73–75].

26.3.3 Putting Principles into Practice

The movement toward CBPR research has gained national attention and is now recognized by health policy makers, managed care administrators, researchers and service providers as a strategy to eliminate racial and ethnic disparities in health and health care. While CBPR brings rewarding outcomes, its practice could be challenging. In particular, employing CBPR approach with minority older adults demands extra culturally sensitive measures. While many health equity researchers across all disciplines have synthesized strategies employed in translating CBPR principles into practice on health behavior change, results suggest that the level of true community participation still varies across the research phase. For instance, a recent systematic review study of eight completed CBPR projects reported that the proportion of community participation appeared greatest during the selection of research questions, recruitment and retention. Community was involved the least, however, in financial responsibility or proposal development [76]. Apart from disproportional input in the research phase, community partners also had less power in the scientific integrity interpretation [77]; project visions, expectations, or data interpretation [78]. Overall, the inherent challenge in CBPR research is to manage and resolve the conflicts that may arise between contrasting goals, values, or priorities between scientists and community partners [79].

There are a few useful strategies to address power inequity in CBPR partnerships. One common establishment is the community advisor board (CAB), which provides a window into the context in which many participants live, helps define the consent process, and creates trusting relationships between partners [80]. Many large research centers have created these Boards to co-develop the project design, review study procedures, and identify and address modifiable community-specific barriers to participation. Besides establishing a Community Advisory Board, many CBPR practitioners also believe that the key to conflict resolutions is to reduce negative stereotypes regarding research. Historical distrust coupled with contemporary structural and systematic inequities often leave community members with the feeling of being treated as guinea pigs [81]. After research is completed, local community is often left with no resources, data, or infrastructure to advance their own needs. While many CBPR groups have different action plans in addressing the deleterious perception toward research, a few common strategies include recruiting staff who have diverse and extensive experiences working with the local communities [82]; educating investigators and faculty members on the importance of eliciting community partners' perspectives and attending cultural competency trainings [83]; among others. Overall, CBPR research in many ways has reshaped and improved scientific enterprise itself. Community input in CBPR resembles a strategic focus that further strengthens the rigor, relevance, and reach of the science. In the next section, we will examine how violence preventions and interventions can benefit from the multi-level orientations of CBPR approach.

26.4 Translating CBPR into Violence Preventions and Interventions

26.4.1 History of Violence as a Public Health Issue

Violence is now widely recognized as a public health crisis worldwide. In the past 30 years in the U.S., violent acts have occurred with greater intensity, frequency, and detrimental health consequences. Not only homicide and suicide have been among the top leading causes of death, but the risks of self-inflicted or interpersonal violence were particularly elevated in members of minority groups, notably young men, women, children, or the poor [84]. In addition to the epidemic trends, another important development that has gained traction within the public health community was the understanding of social-behavioral factors in the etiology and prevention of violence. For instance, the emergence of child mistreatment and intimate partner violence as recognized social problems in the 1960–1970s demonstrated the need to move beyond law enforcement or judicial system which remains mainly reactive to the scope of violence. Greater interdisciplinary collaboration and cultural competency must be integrated in our understanding of the behavioral, social, cultural, environmental factors that give rise to violent acts.

Living in a violence-free environment is a fundamental human rights issue that transcends age, gender, race, socio-economic status, or country borders. Violence was placed on the global agenda in 1996 when the World Health Assembly declared violence as a leading worldwide public health problem. The World Health Organization defines violence as: "The intentional use of physical force or power, threatened or actual, against oneself, another person, or against a group or community, that either result in or has a high likelihood of resulting in injury, death, psychological harm, mal-development or deprivation" [85]. Faced with this alarming human rights violation, the public health community is cautious of violent acts not just because of its strong association with detrimental health outcomes, but also because of the significant contributions that could, and should be done, by public health practitioners in violence preventions [86].

26.4.2 Role of Community in Violence Preventions and Interventions

Adopting community-based approach in understanding violence prevention and intervention strategies has gained much momentum in the past decade. The public health approach in violence involves three elements: a focus on violence prevention, a focus on scientific methodology to identify risk and patterns of violence and multi-disciplinary and multi-dimensional collaboration to address the problem of violence as well as assuring the availability of services for violence survivors [87]. This public health framework of violence further emphasizes on the role of community as central to the success of all three components, including prevention, understanding risk factors, and intervention.

Researchers have documented the complex cultural and societal influences that intersect with the causes of violence [88–90]. For instance, traditional gender roles of male dominance and female submission, the influence of "familismo" and the inter-generational transmission of violence compounded by immigration and acculturation stress have all contributed to Hispanic cultural aspects that linked to domestic violence [91]. In a CBPR needs assessment of domestic violence preventions among Hispanics community in Miami, Gonzalez-Guarda et al. [91] described how community-engaged and participatory-orientation project design contributed in dissecting culture as a double-edged sword. Many of the family-oriented cultural factors perceived by community members may both serve as risk or protective factors of violence and only the meaningful understanding of these cultural-societal contexts from community perspectives would contribute to advance prevention strategies.

CBPR also plays an important role in understanding violence survivors' help-seeking behaviors and health care access that are linked to better delivery of appropriate interventions. Violence victims are extremely vulnerable and many fear that their experiences would not be validated. For example, victims of family violence often believed that it was their responsibility to keep the family intact at all costs. In this context, victims often shared that an additional reason for not reporting the abuse to the police was their fear that their family member perpetrator might be incarcerated and the family income would be adversely affected. Not only victims may be fearful, but their families may also be intimidated by the consequences of reporting the abuse to the police and entering the judicial system. As Latino family violence survivors expressed, they opted to "keep things inside" ("Guardarse Las Cosas Adentro") to avoid shame and stigma [92]. Adopting a community-based approach provides a roadmap to develop trust between communities and survivors in order to support the process of disclosing interpersonal violent acts. Furthermore, CBPR allows survivors to be an integral part of study design and findings interpretations, which contributes to enhancing culturally appropriate interventions [93].

26.4.3 Lessons Learned from Adopting CBPR in IPV or Child Abuse

Researchers have adopted CBPR approach in a wide array of violence prevention and intervention studies across difference age groups, including child abuse [94], adolescent violence prevention initiatives [95, 96], or intimate partner violence prevention and interventions [97, 98]. In aggregate, these evidence-based programs in interpersonal violence such as child abuse and intimate partner violence (IPV) have provided useful insights in advancing the field of elder abuse research which is relatively still in its infancy.

Defined as "any behavior within an intimate relationship that causes physical, psychological or sexual harm to those in the relationship" [99], IPV prevalence varied by country as well as by the methodology used. Population-based studies from various countries indicate that between 10 and 69 % of women reported that an intimate partner has physically abused them at least once in their lifetime [100]. Given its global scope and magnitude, WHO endorsed community-based prevention as an essential strategy to increase the visibility of violence against women and particularly in settings where resources are likely limited [99]. These strategic meeting reports persuasively pointed to the barriers and facilitators in adopting community-based approaches in IPV prevention and interventions. From the participants' level, participatory methods are well-received in engaging victims, as well as engaging their male or female family members who could have been the perpetrators. In addition, CBPR allows researchers and communities to co-identify existing norms and to recognize the optimal messages and channels to reach the target audience, allowing a far-reaching impact on those vulnerable victims or who are stigmatized by their experiences. On a macro level, CBPR maximizes the impact of findings by connecting individual-level intervention initiatives with broader violence advocacy activities.

There are a few caveats for CBPR approach to be successful in effectively preventing IPV [99, 101]. First, similar to the key challenge facing all CBPR projects, community must be involved enough to take ownership of the research process. Repeated exposure to ideas through multiple channels will be necessary in the community settings. Second, CBPR approach is typically a labor-intensive and time-consuming project; ensuring community and individual involvement overtime is the key to partnership satisfaction. Third, given a supportive social environment will greatly increase the likelihood of sustainable positive change, efforts need to be made in mobilizing and fostering such social environment. However, an ongoing challenge is perhaps linked to program efficacy; how do we conceptualize and measure beyond individual behavior change to consider a violence-free social change at the community levels? How does CBPR partnership measure the long-term effects of this collaboration? Despite ongoing challenges may confront CBPR partnership, it is important to recognize and celebrate any short-term accomplishments of the partnership as a whole. The celebration of partnership in a trust-building manner will in turn motivate all members to continue to achieve mid-term and long-term goals. The more closely a community change addresses a perceived need from the part of community partners, the more likely the change is to be sustained.

26.5 Applying CBPR to Aging and Elder Abuse Research

26.5.1 Minority Aging

The older population is becoming more socio-economically and racially diverse as the overall minority population grows and experience greater longevity. However, minority older adults often suffer a double disadvantage in health due to the interactive effects of age, race and ethnicity, and social standing [102]. As discriminated against by minority membership and by being identified as aged in an agist society, racial/ethnic minority older adults are faced with unique challenges in health and aging. Furthermore, researchers in minority aging have come to reject the notion of ethnocentric use of Euro-American standard model from which other populations deviate. Rather, diversity in aging discourse has proposed a multi-ethnic perspective to encompass the biological, behavioral, socio-cultural and environmental factors that influence population-level health differences in aging [103]. The social structures of inequality along lines of race, gender, and class impact older adults and that minority subgroups experience aging differently. This research has used CBPR approach to address a host of health issues among diverse older adults of socioeconomic, religious, racial/ethnic or sexual orientations, including community needs assessment [104], disease management [105], health behavior change [106], or intervention research [104, 107], to name a few. However, social-behavioral violence prevention or intervention research that embedded a CBPR framework continues to be scarce. In spite of the potential that CBPR approach holds in reducing health inequities, its implementation in violence research demands additional culturally and linguistically sensitive measures.

26.5.2 Elder Abuse and Subtypes

Elder abuse, sometimes referred to as elder mistreatment or elder maltreatment, is an important global health issue. Elder abuse manifests in various forms including physical abuse, sexual abuse, psychological abuse, caregiver neglect and financial exploitation [108]. The World Health Organization reports the prevalence of elder abuse in developed countries ranges from 1 to 10 % [109]. The U.S. National Elder Mistreatment Study reported that 11.4 % of older adults suffered from elder mistreatment in the previous year [110]. As detrimental to one's health and well-being, elder abuse has been linked to increased risks of morbidity and mortality [111–113]. In addition, older adults victimized by abuse are at higher risks of increased nursing home placement, emergency department utilization and premature mortality [114, 115]. Despite the accessibility of Adult Protective Services in all fifty states, an overwhelming number of abused older adults may pass through healthcare system undiagnosed and overlooked.

Elder abuse affects all older adults across socio-economic and cultural backgrounds. Given its public health significance, the Institute of Medicine gathered experts in the field of elder abuse to discuss prevention programs in April 2013 [116]. In addition, U.S. Preventive Services Task Force (USPSTF) recommended elder abuse as a priority research topic in it is report to US Congress. Despite the growing attention, researchers still have rudimentary understanding of the issue of elder abuse in diverse minority populations.

26.5.3 Barriers in Elder Abuse Research

Like child abuse, elder abuse interventions have predominantly arisen from agency or community-based initiatives. Existing approaches to elder abuse intervention focus primarily on some overlapping goals and strategies, including legislative, community services, and educational outreach. Modeled after domestic violence interventions module, community services are based on integrated models to provide coordinated services spanning from legal, medical, and psychosocial needs of at-risk seniors. Derived from the aging network, education and prevention initiatives include advocacy and empowerment for older adults [108]. However, very few elder abuse intervention programs were crafted according to CBPR modalities. In addition, for those existing interventions, recent review studies reported that they had no significant effects on improving the social and psychological well-being of older victims [117, 118].

Furthermore, compared to their younger counterparts, elder abuse victims face more pronounced structural, cultural, and social barriers when seeking for help. For elder abuse victims, barriers to obtaining services may include physical frailty, cognitive impairment, and dependence on the abusers [119]. At the same time, victims may also serve in a caregiving or support capacity to their dependents or abusive family members, which in turn create different but equally challenging barriers to the victims' willingness and acceptance of needed services for themselves [120].

The issue of cultural diversity surrounding elder abuse further exemplifies a major complexity in advancing the field of elder abuse intervention [121]. Major knowledge gaps remain in understanding the cultural complexities of effective psychological well-being care supporting victims of elder abuse, particularly for minority older adults including African, Hispanic, American Indian, and Asian populations [122]. In light of the inherent vulnerabilities and complexities in abuse in older age, it is of paramount importance to develop and sustain a CBPR partnership in elder abuse research.

26.5.4 CBPR in Elder Abuse: Behavioral Intervention Stage Model

Focused on participation and action, CBPR is well-suited to address elder abuse. Not only does CBPR approach firmly accounts for the culture and the diversity of the population when developing and conducting elder abuse research, furthermore, CBPR also ensures that the research directly responds to community-driven concerns in elder abuse interventions, such as providing community-based interventions in respite programs, social support and informal networks in supporting caregiving, or other community-based caregiving training programs.

As interest in CBPR grows, there is also a growing demand for strategies that help advance the knowledge and skills needed to translate CBPR principles in elder abuse research. However, CBPR principles by and large are meant to serve as a guideline that allows partners to develop community-specific content and structures. Based on NIH Behavioral Intervention Stage Model, we created a summary table to detail the application of CBPR principles in elder abuse research (Table 26.1). Created by the Division of Behavioral and Social Research at National Institutes of

Table 26.1 Translating NIH behavioral intervention stage model into CBPR-based elder abuse research

Research phase based on NIH stage model	Traditional approach	CBPR principles	Applying CBPR to elder abuse intervention
Stage 0—Basic science			
0A: Formative stage	Researchers plan project and assemble research team, including researchers, staff, clinicians	Recognize, distinguish, and respect the community as a unique and vital partner in the research process	Define who the community in elder abuse intervention is; ensure community input is horizontally integrated in each of the research step. Start building community-based research infrastructure
0B: Study design	Researchers choose topic and design based on scientific theory, academic interest, evidence, data, and methodological feasibility	Partners incorporate community voices, priorities, and assets, emphasizing rigor and accountability	Partners co-design effective quantitative or qualitative measures that can emphasize the cultural, environmental, and contextual reasons that give rise to elder abuse and local knowledge on family violence and older adults' help-seeking behaviors
0C: Funding	Grant written by researchers; funds go to researchers	Partners co-develop grant and equitable division of funds based on contributions to project	Partners commit to reducing violence and evolving relationships with all federal or private funders. Start sustainability planning beyond funding availabilities
0D: Implement study	Researchers responsible for study conduct	Partners collaborate on all efforts and propose community-driven questions and ensure local relevance of findings	Community advisory board members co-lead study operations with researchers and community members to maximize language and cultural sensitivity surrounding violence
0E: Analyze, interpret data	Researchers responsible for data analysis and interpretation based on literature	Ensure community's input in interpretation of the data based on cultural and contextual understandings	Joint input on data interpretation and recognize the need to strengthen community-level sensitive data on elder abuse
Stage 1—Intervention generation/refinement	Researchers responsible for identify promising findings relevant to develop interventions and plan feasibility and pilot testing	Emphasize local relevance of public health problems and interdisciplinary perspectives that recognize and attend to the multiple determinants of health	Continue to ensure community buy-in in the proposed elder abuse intervention and reinforce the preferred intervention component is integrated and assure that in this bottom-up approach, community continues to be a key stakeholder in shaping elder abuse intervention
Stage 2—Efficacy-research clinics	Researchers test promising behavioral interventions in research settings	Testing efficacy may primary takes place in research settings, both partners co-evaluate promising strategies	Community participation as well as input is critical to ultimately interpret benefits and harms (e.g., to whom—Victims? Perpetrators? Family members? Community members?) associated with proposed interventions in a controlled setting
Stage 3—Efficacy-community clinics	Researchers test interventions to be implementable and community-friendly	In highly controlled community clinics, strengthen the structured feedback loop to partners	
Stage 4—Effectiveness	Intervention with efficacy may not show effectiveness. Researchers examine the mechanism of the actions of interventions; ensure external validity	Community plays critical role in effectiveness research; critically centered to ensure success of effectiveness due to variability of study participants, providers, or settings	Partners should continue to understand the perception of intervention effectiveness from community perspectives; which will help both partners to further identify strategies to culturally adapt other evidence-based violence intervention programs. Accounting for community input will help understand effectiveness at the external victim-, perpetrator-, provider- and society-level influences

(continued)

Table 26.1 (continued)

Research phase based on NIH stage model	Traditional approach	CBPR principles	Applying CBPR to elder abuse intervention
Stage 5—Implementation and dissemination			
5A: Disseminate findings	Disseminate to academic audiences	Share findings and lessons learned with all members in meaningful ways to meet all partners' goals	Organize elder abuse prevention and intervention educational forums and research training opportunities to equip community members with analytical and dissemination skills. Disseminate information back to all members involved
5B: Translate research into practice and policy	Ends with publication of results	Partners mobilize the community to use findings to advocate for policy change, enhance local resources, and improve practices	Work towards a balance between research and action so that all partners benefit meaningfully from elder abuse research; continue to empower community members from practice and policy feedbacks
5C: Sustain team, benefits, and resources	When grant ends, researchers often move to new project	Sustainability built into work from inception; partners honor initial commitment to continue partnership and work beyond funding cycle	Routinely check in with the community to see how their needs may continue to evolve and what strategies will better address the next set of challenges

Aging, the Stage Model is a model of behavioral intervention development composed of six stages: basic science (Stage 0), intervention generation, refinement, modification, and adaptation and pilot testing (Stage I); traditional efficacy testing (Stage II); efficacy testing with real-world providers (Stage III); effectiveness research (Stage IV) and; dissemination and implementation research (Stage V). Based on this conceptualization of research activity development, we first identify conventional research approach, potential CBPR approach, and propose strategies to translate CBPR principles in elder abuse research. Broadly speaking, community engagement can already play a critical role prior to building intervention; i.e., in better understanding the mechanisms of change during the study formative stage, study design and implementation, as well as during the data interpretation stage. Community-based settings can also serve as an important testing site for the theoretical and real-world efficacy as well as effectiveness of elder abuse interventions.

26.6 CBPR in Elder Abuse: A Case Study

Drawing upon our CBPR work with the Chinese American community in Chicago in the past 10 years, in this next section, we would like to illustrate how elder abuse research can benefit from CBPR orientation in different stages of the research process based on the Behavioral Intervention Stage Model.

26.6.1 Background and Context

As one of the fastest growing subpopulation, the health status of Chinese older adults in the U.S. remains poorly understood. Among Asian American population, Chinese is the oldest and largest subgroup with an estimate of 3.6 million people [123]. One in four Asian Americans is of Chinese descent. Compared to other immigrant groups, U.S. Chinese community is older in average age and less acculturated [124]. It is reported that more than 80 % of Chinese older adults are foreign born and more than 30 % of Chinese older adults immigrated to the U.S. after the age of 60 years old [125]. With the majority of Chinese American older adults foreign-born, they also experience a pronounced migratory and psychosocial distress accompanied by vastly different cultural and linguistic barriers. Prior health disparities literature indicated that Chinese older adults were especially vulnerable due to the impact of aging and acculturation stress, and exhibited low utilization of health services as well as low levels of health literacy [126]. In addition, evidence suggested that Chinese older adults had the highest suicide rate than any other racial groups nationwide. Specifically, suicide rate among older Chinese women was a higher leading cause of death compared with the general population [127, 128].

To a large extent, culture determines and shapes social and psychological distress as well as its symptoms, treatment, and help-seeking behavior. Heavily influenced by

Confucianism, Chinese older adults perceived the balanced interconnection between mental outlook and physical health as a successful model for aging. Confucian traditions, which greatly emphasized filial piety, further provided guidelines regarding obligatory roles and responsibilities of each person in the family. Failure to meet such expectations may be a root cause for conflict and distress [129, 130]. However, migration, acculturation, access to health care as well as linguistic and cultural barriers has posed great challenges to traditional values in Chinese American families. Meanwhile, immigrant families are faced with enormous challenges as the aging population rapidly increases. These challenges may fundamentally threaten the support system of frail older adults, which further exacerbate vulnerability, physical dependency and psychological distress, and reflect conditions that strongly contribute to the increased risk for elder abuse [131].

Despite these prior reports have demonstrated a number of alarming health disparities, systematic health data on Chinese older adults remain limited. Chinese older adults have not been fully engaged in the conduct and content of research. Vast subgroup diversity in cultures and languages, in addition to recruitment difficulties, has resulted in the scarcity of data [132]. Most federal level health data collection often aggregates diverse Asian groups under the same racial category, masking the specific health disparities facing the Chinese aging population. In addition, Chinese population in the U.S. is inherently heterogeneous. Owing to the history and development of immigration trajectories, the Chinese community comprises at least five generations of Chinese Americans, of varying acculturation degrees, settling in from mainland China, Taiwan, Hong Kong, Vietnam as well as refuges of Chinese descent in Southeast Asia, Latin America and Caribbean countries. Immigrants' diverse experiences of aging in different social, political and historical contexts call for culturally sensitive research design.

26.6.2 Study Formative Stage

The lack of representative population-based surveys about the health of Chinese older adults has left researchers with incomplete knowledge about the mechanisms behind these health disparities and the impact of these challenges on individuals, families, communities and health care systems. As a response, guided by CBPR principles back in 2008, we initiated a community-academic partnership in Chicago is a synergetic effort between Rush University Medical Center, Northwestern University Feinberg School of Medicine, Chinese American Service League (CASL) and Xilin Asian American Community Center. The formation and conduct of the community-academic partnership allow us to develop appropriate research methodology in accordance with Chinese cultural context, in which community advisory board (CAB) played a pivotal role in provided useful community perspectives and research strategies. Board members worked extensively with the investigative team to review findings and examine study instrument to ensure cultural sensitivity and appropriateness. With support from National Institute on Aging, we first aimed to build a sustainable partnership through establishing collaborations and the aforementioned community advisory board. Prior to the formation of this partnership, academic and community partners have long-standing collaborations in health outreach programs and education forums. The informal partnership has helped laid the groundwork to foster expertise exchange and commitment to empower the community.

Consistent with prior studies that assembling a team of co-researchers who share the same ethnic culture as the studied community may help build trust [133], our bicultural and bilingual investigators' cultural insights contributed in fostering a mutual understanding of common goals. However, our experience demonstrates that research team's strong commitment and humble attitude in mutual learning is perhaps more instrumental in building a sustainable relationship. With the acknowledgment of the inherent power imbalance between researchers and the community, we have learned that a humble approach towards partnership building is critical. For example, research scientists organized series of mock-focus group training workshops for CASL and other community stakeholders. Whereas community partner gained useful skills in research facilitation and instruments, researchers also learned more insights of the Chinese culture, such as respect and honor for seniors. During our training, culturally specific issues as such were given particular emphasis. For instance, how to encourage Chinese older adults to speak up without being authoritative or making them feel "losing-face" which is a taboo in Chinese culture. The humble exchange of knowledge and experiences deepened trust among the partners from the outset.

26.6.3 Study Design and Procedure

The goal of our pilot needs assessment was to understand health issues in the Chinese community through conducting focus group and survey methodology. However, in working towards focus group recruitment, we came across challenges that some Chinese community members were unwilling to participate in research due to language concern, confidentiality issue, and unfamiliarity with research protocols and processes. To address these concerns, we fist drew upon the strengths and resources available in the Chinese community. We approached eligible candidates (60 years and above, residing in Chicago) after their attendance in CASL-sponsored cultural activities, such as calligraphy, Chinese painting classes, and social activities. Our bilingual project assistant and project-affiliated CASL staff explained details of the research project to Chinese older adults in both Mandarin and Cantonese. We also asked older adults to consult with their family members regarding participation, owing to the fact that collective decision-making remains a core value of Chinese family life.

Additionally, we learned to utilize the positive impact of word-of-mouth of community opinion leaders on the perception of research. In order to appreciate the time and efforts of participants, we not only delivered gift cards compensation for each participant, but also a customized bilingual Certificate of Appreciation. For Chinese participants, this red-cardstock-certificate, or "gan-xie-zhuang" in Chinese, symbolized a traditional token of honor. This gesture was well-received and was spread through word-of-mouth that, Chinese older adults, too, could make an impact to community health by working alongside with research scientists.

26.6.4 Study Implementation and Findings

Congregating community resources also contributed to the quality of focus group discussions and retention. We organized focus group discussions in community centers, where participants felt most comfortable and had easy access to. CASL staffers, who were trained and experienced in guiding interviews, took turns leading twelve focus groups. The arrangement helped facilitated open conversations, as Chinese older adults were more expressive among familiar and trusted CASL staff.

In the community that needs assessment study co-designed by the Community Advisory Board, elder abuse was a frequently expressed concern that emerged from our data. Our quantitative and qualitative data further suggested elder abuse was common and considered unacceptable in Chinese culture [104]. During focus group discussion, Chinese older adults mostly characterized elder abuse in terms of caregiver neglect, and identified psychological abuse as the most serious form of abuse, preceding the severity of financial exploitation, physical abuse, and abandonment. In addition, our community needs assessment revealed that Chinese older adult had limited knowledge of help-seeking resources other than seeking assistance from local community service centers [134]. The locally relevant findings further underscore the urgent needs to advance research in elder abuse and educational initiatives with culturally and linguistically appropriate measures.

26.6.5 Findings Dissemination

CBPR principles encourage the dissemination of knowledge as a crucial part to translate research findings into action. Furthermore, we learned that the action-oriented approach to partnership building is vital in our collaboration with the Chinese community. After completing data collection, we organized an Appreciation Dinner for project participants and their family members. The dinner provided the participants with an opportunity to learn about how they contributed in advancing science. Moreover, the occasion permitted community and academic partners to witness the well-received impact of this partnership at the grassroots level. We learned that dissemination of research findings and health knowledge has helped raised health awareness of Chinese older adults, who were passive in seeking medical intervention due to traditional cultural beliefs. Whereas translating research findings into public policy changes may be time-consuming, conducting CBPR study with Chinese older adults highlighted the urgency to improving community research capacity.

Furthermore, in order to further raise community awareness on elder abuse, we organized a World Elder Abuse Awareness Day commemoration for the first time in the Chinese community in 2011. During the commemoration, older adults were able to gather information regarding the issue of elder abuse in the Chinese community with respect to recent research findings and learn about the concerted community and academic efforts to deal with this alarming health issue. Older adults were also invited to join follow-up focus group discussions regarding their views on abuse interventions. Results from the qualitative data further helped the investigative team to understand community's perception of the barriers, facilitators and the effectiveness of elder abuse interventions and preferred intervention domains in order to design culturally adapted interventions. Our findings suggest that older adults not only viewed many benefits of intervention programs but voiced important facilitators to implement interventions such as efforts to increase education and public health awareness, integrating social support with existing community social services, as well as establish and sustain an interdisciplinary team. Perceived social support, empowerment, and community-based interventions design were viewed as most effective to promote the psychological well-being of victims [135].

26.6.6 The PINE Study

From our ongoing collaborations in research initiatives and community health workshops, the CBPR partnership continued to struggle with the lack of systematic community-level sensitive data that longitudinally depict health trajectories over time. To date, federal level health data collection aggregates diverse Asian groups under the same racial category, masking the specific health issues in the Chinese aging population. Despite a number of national investigations that examined the health of Asian-American communities, including the Honolulu Heart Program (HHP), Honolulu-Asia Aging Study (HAAS), Multi-Ethnic Study of Atherosclerosis (MESA), and National Latino and Asian American Study (NLAAS); these studies primarily focused on specific diseases, such as cardiovascular and neurodegenerative disease of Japanese–American men examined in the HHP and HAAS studies, in which the sample did not enroll any Chinese Americans [136, 137]. In addition, existing studies that sampled U.S. Chinese population tended to collect a small cohort of older Chinese Americans. For instance, the MESA study enrolled 307 Chinese Americans aged 65 and older in which the primary aim of the study was to examine clinical cardiovascular disease [138, 139]. In the NLAAS study, [139] which the primary outcome of interest was accessing mental disorders and mental health service utilization in minority populations, a national representative sample of 150 Chinese Americans aged 51 and older were surveyed [140]. To our knowledge, there were no population-based investigations that specifically focused on elder abuse epidemiology among Chinese American older adults.

Building upon the existing CBPR infrastructure, our partnership expanded beyond the original set-up and further invited over twenty community-based organizations and social services agencies in the greater Chicago area. With the goal to collect a population sample of Chinese older adults in the Greater Chicago Area, the PINE study (Population-Based Study of Chinese Elderly in Chicago) partnership developed up-to-date community-based sampling strategies to increase resource efficiency and cost-effectiveness [141]. Out of 3542 eligible participants who were approached in baseline in 2011, a total of 3159 agreed to participate in the study, yielding a response rate of 91.9 % [142]. Currently in its third wave of data collection, PINE study collects comprehensive epidemiological data in elder abuse extent, subtypes, frequency, intensity, and self-perceived seriousness of the program. With detailed information on elder abuse prevalence, incidence and adverse health consequences in Chinese aging population [143–145], our community members can benefit from local context-specific interventions and community organizations can also pursue program advancement needs based on quality data [146].

In our experience, we believe an important indicator of the success of the PINE partnership is the community's changed opinion on research participation. The CBPR approach in implementing the PINE study has given Chinese older adults a voice that was otherwise unheard and deepened their trust in federally funded research projects. In addition, CBPR approach also enables us to build and enhance community research infrastructure. The PINE study was operationalized on a multi-lingual and multi-cultural infrastructure, ranging from interviewer training, study materials, to data collection hardware and software Infrastructure building in a community-academic research partnership contributes to bridging the current knowledge level with a long-term vision [147]. Each step of the field implementation is designed for serving the needs of linguistically and culturally diverse Chinese community. Whereas conventional infrastructure building may be essential, through our community-academic partnership in designing the PINE study, we learned that utilizing creative measures to address the bilingual and bicultural needs concerning Chinese community are equally critical in the maximizing recruitment effort. For instance, when organizing bilingual community health workshops on elder abuse to empower the community, our CBPR partnership also aimed to enhance community research capacity and leverage minority aging research to practice and policy implications [83].

Last, benefits of such community-academic collaboration extend to increased interactions between the Chinese community and academic institutions, health care professionals, aging networks, and other community organizations [148]. Increased community participation not only improves the quality of data collected, but the invested interests gathered from the community-academic partnership further increases the practical relevance of epidemiological research.

26.7 Challenges Faced and Lessons Learned in Elder Abuse Research with CBPR Approach

Over the past two decades, we have seen a steadily increased number of CBPR-invested research teams in addressing elder abuse research in diverse communities including minority ethnic/racial groups [149–151], socio-economically disadvantaged groups [152, 153], to faith-based or LGBT communities [154]. Broadly speaking, CBPR not only facilitates the recruitment and retention of potential and existing participants from marginalized communities, but also enables researchers to comprehend the highly culturally unique contextualized perceptions on elder abuse. Integrating the collaborative efforts of diverse community stakeholders, culturally appropriate research methodology can contribute to the salience of preventions and interventions.

26.7.1 Reframing Elder Abuse

Recent research has expanded our knowledge about elder abuse in African American, Latino, Korean, Indian, Native American, and Chinese populations. However, we need more studies to fill in large knowledge gaps. A few quantitative and qualitative studies have started to better define the concept and cultural variations in the construct, definition, and understanding of elder abuse [134, 151], and its results show that elder abuse cannot be separated from the cultural context in which it occurs. While researchers urge systematic cultural explorations to better study the barriers to reporting elder abuse and help-seeking behaviors on the specific socio-cultural contexts, the role of the community would be best situated to address such knowledge gaps.

For example, in the global Asian communities, studies reported that younger Asian generations, influenced by social changes brought about by modernization and industrialization, may be less likely to adhere to traditional Confucianism cultural values and practices. In addition, guided by the value of collectivism that encourages conformity and cohesiveness, older adults may be less likely to disclose abuse and seek professional help. A prior study on Chinese older adults' perceptions of abuse suggested that older adults tended to tolerate elder abuse so as to protect family reputation [134]. Another study among Asian American older adults further demonstrated that such tolerance for abuse may be associated with not favoring reporting and outside intervention [155]. Similarly, in the tribal communities, Baker-Demaray [156] also found that Native American older adults were more apt to respond when asked about "disrespect" rather than "abuse." Older adults in this tribal community struggled in acknowledging that the treatment they may be receiving is abuse or neglect, and shared that it would be more comfortable to report in terms of "disrespect" or, in the case of sexual abuse, "bothering." Working alongside with community not only helps researchers to refine the conceptual framework of elder abuse, but also ensures elder abuse intervention achieve salient relevancy to the local contexts and notions.

26.7.2 Improved Elder Abuse Screening and Treatment Strategies for Subtypes of Abuse

Special efforts should be given into developing culturally sensitive approach to screen and treat elder abuse victims [157]. Moreover, community-based social services organizations should increase efforts on improving knowledge in relation to elder abuse in minority older adults. Given that the majority of older adults may lack knowledge on help-seeking channels, considerable efforts should be made in creating a linkage between available social services and the aging populations. In addition, support groups that incorporate efforts from family members should be created.

In the African American community, researchers have proposed that elder abuse screening and its untoward effects need to be modeled after successful prevention strategies in the African American community. Because responses to interpersonal violence are influenced by cultural norms and African Americans are less likely to seek help from institutions that have historically contributed to their oppression, culturally competent screening and treatment strategies need to be developed and implemented for abused older adults. These violence prevention programs have used barber shops, beauty salons, and local churches as a focus of prevention strategies. Researchers also emphasized on the importance of including victims of physical and psychological abuse in the development of interventions and pointed out that this collaborative progress was likely to be empowering and a healing progress [158].

Other opportunities for community-based interventions may also be available to address elder abuse and in particular caregiver neglect. Conflict resolution for families at risk has been shown to be effective in the African American and tribal communities. Strategies that provide a safe, stable forum to discuss areas of family conflict may be essential for restoring family harmony. Extending these services, especially in minority communities, may be an essential resource component to prevent elder abuse. For financial abuse, strategies to protect older adults may include guardianship services or bilingual fraud prevention workshops. The local chapters of Chamber of Commerce may be recruited to develop targeted programs for their constituents.

26.7.3 Community Empowerment with Participatory Education

In addition to the cultural complexities in how to operationalize elder abuse in diverse communities, minority older adults may remain skeptical towards the implementation of research outcomes. While most epidemiological studies depend heavily on surveys for quantitative data, the instruments are typically developed under the direction of academic researchers with limited community collaboration. However, in the case of elder abuse research in minority groups, it may be challenging to document and evaluate how the research questions de facto documents the health and well-being needs of the community. In addition, it may be challenging to document and evaluate how the research collaboration de facto meets community's health, and well-being needs. This challenge further resonates with the experiences of other CBPR projects that increasing community's capacity to understand the tangible advantages of research is instrumental to project sustainability [159]. In response to the challenge, researchers who adopted a CBPR approach created community health forums combined with educational training to individuals and their family members [134]. Their progress-to-date has shown that these truly equitable insights from both community and academic partners on elder abuse can contribute to enriching the understanding of elder abuse, and further helped refine the culturally adequate screening tools in detecting elder abuse as well as the preferred intervention modalities [135, 160].

26.7.4 Horizontal and Vertical Integration of Cultural Sensitivity Measures

Cultural sensitivity embodies more than matching languages and geographic locations preferred by the targeted community. Incorporating the cultural, social, and environmental forces that affect health behavior in the community contributes to the salience of policy impact [24, 161, 162]. Through implementing the CBPR approach with culturally sensitive measures, elder abuse intervention programs could build on strengths and resources in the community. One example of horizontally integrating CBPR in elder abuse prevention pertains to the family-oriented approach in the Native American community. Developed in a northwestern tribal community, the Family Care Conference was created to bring family members' attention to the problem of elder abuse and to incorporate their efforts into intervention [163]. The CBPR approach in elder abuse research empowers older adults and their family members to take part in investing in their own health and well-being. In addition, benefits of community-academic collaboration extends to increased interactions between the community and academic institutions, health care professionals, aging networks, and other community organizations [164].

Vertically integrating culture in elder abuse research pertains to cultural competency trainings at the community level as well as in the healthcare professional work force. In our experience working with Chinese American families in Chicago, our CBPR partnership has collaborated with American Psychiatric Foundation and Albert Schweitzer Foundation to assess health interventions with Chinese older adults in Chinatown elderly apartments. With the help of skilled medical student volunteers, this "Saturday with Seniors" program gathered feedbacks from Chinese older adults on cultural sensitive measures applicable for long-term health promotion. The program in turn provided hands-on training to healthcare professionals to better understand Chinese family and community dynamics in culturally appropriate settings. Given the intrinsic diversity among Chinese immigrants in the U.S., we acknowledge our findings may not be generalizable to other Chinese populations including Chinese minority groups and suburban and rural Chinese populations, as they may be subjected to varying degrees of social and economic influence. Therefore, it is imperative to branch out to other Chinese communities in the country. We are currently spearheading outreach efforts to the Chinese Immigrant Services Agency Network International (CISANI) which is an international social services agency network serving Chinese immigrants around the world. The genuine understanding and practice of culturally sensitive research are critical for advancing social change in minority aging.

26.7.5 Planning Program Sustainability

Sustainability planning is indeed central to the management of successful community health initiatives. From an evaluation standpoint, sustainability may be difficult to conceptualize, given that it often refers to a future stage [165]. Public health literature examines sustainability mostly in the forms of maintaining specific health programs, such as sustaining health initiatives, or in retaining knowledge, capacity, and values generated from the collaboration [166, 167]. Although sustainability is a key indicator for partnership success, it raises challenges for many organizations. Much literature showcased the strong structural challenges facing community-university partnerships. Some have noted that partnership building is a cultural exchange in progress [72]. When combining two different systems together, it inevitably results in a series of compromises in order to achieve a valued goal. In addition, it may be challenging to document and evaluate how the research collaboration de facto meets community's health and well-being needs [168].

Sustainability in CBPR partnership is more than just funding. A thriving partnership requires broad community participation. When it comes to critically considering partnership impact, making institutional and governmental policy changes may be the most powerful approach to sustainability. To begin with, an engaging community in research offers the opportunity for academic researchers to conduct practice-based research that translates findings into effective clinical practice in improved elder abuse prevention and reporting mechanisms [169].

Furthermore, envisioning long-term goals as well as its realizations perhaps carry more significance to moving the partnership forward. The CBPR partnership also needs to decide which efforts to continue in elder abuse research, as well as preparation to weather potential changes beyond funding years; i.e., what are the probable potential of this collaboration—what do academic and community partners envision this partnership into the next 5–10 years? What would be the critical elements to sustain this partnership? Through the exchange of expertise between diverse partners,

CBPR contributes to the organizational capacity building, and furthermore creates a research-practice interface that elevates public policy changes in elder abuse [170]. Whereas sustaining partnerships may imply the continuity of specific infrastructure, programs or initiatives, the collective goal of long-term policy-actionable impact would help sustain this CBPR partnership into the future.

26.8 Practice and Policy Implications

26.8.1 Health Professions Education: QIAN-Cultural Humility

We cannot emphasize enough that the humble exchange of engaging dialogues between researchers and community members is critical in CBPR longitudinal epidemiological research operations. Whereas health research was traditionally set in the community without community's active engagement in framing the research phases, the lack of cultural insights and sensitivity in approaching community often renders research results inapplicable to health care services. Furthermore, the community is left without infrastructure to address its own needs. Therefore, the humble exchange of knowledge and experiences deepened trust among the community partners, researchers, and study participants from the outset in addressing social and behavior health of older adults. A committed attitude to mutual learning will enable both community partners and researchers to better explore, comprehend and appreciate each other's standpoint. Ultimately, the truly equitable partnership will contribute to the well-being of underserved populations and immigrant communities in the U.S. [171].

Based on the conceptualization of cultural humility, we propose a conceptual model to address the urgent needs in enhancing mutual understanding between physicians and patient. The virtues of humility have been an integral part of Chinese philosophy, and it remains the Dao (way) to a peaceful coexistence among diverse cultures. Inspired by Chinese ancient thinkers, these core values are summarized in the acronym **QIAN** 謙, or "humbleness" in Chinese—the importance of self-Questioning and critique, bi-directional Cultural Immersion, mutually Active-listening, and the flexibility of Negotiation (see Fig. 26.1) [172].

26.8.1.1 Questioning

True understanding requires curiosity. Self-questioning can heavily impact the way researchers approach community partners. Traditionally, researchers approached community members with a list of questions. Yet, here we encourage healthcare practitioners and researchers to first and foremost ask oneself in relations to others: what are the specifics that constitute your background? What are the assumptions you

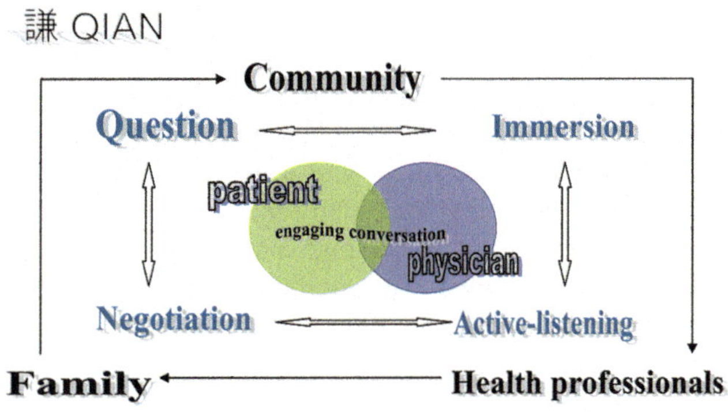

Fig. 26.1 The framework of QIAN model

make about the community? From what sources and based on what facts do these assumptions come from? We invite researchers to constantly undergo the process of self-questioning and self-critique, and maintain the curiosity to understand the unique stance of communities. This holistic approach takes into account that social determinants other than cultural factor, such as education, religion and gender, play a pivotal role in forming one's health beliefs and practices.

26.8.1.2 Immersion

One avenue to humility is through cultural immersion. By cultural immersion, we do not imply seeking for exposures in a foreign milieu. It is the cultural difference between healthcare professionals and that of the community partners that warrant more attention. As Brody and Hunt described in a clinical encounter, "Every physician-patient encounter is a cross-cultural exercise—even if the physician grew up on the same street in the same small town" [173]. Cultural humility is a bi-directional process, which requires equal investment from healthcare professionals and patients. Lack of understanding in research language and its long-term aspects may leave community partners unsatisfied or even dissuaded from research participation. Likewise, at the core of CBPR approach lies within the promise to break the inherent power imbalance that exists in the academic-community or physician–patient relationships. Perhaps researchers could first attempt to tackle the hierarchy by seeking answers to the following questions: How would I like to be treated today if I were the patient being studied? What could I do to foster respect in exchange? Mutual understanding is the starting point.

26.8.1.3 Active-Listening

Listening is often regarded as a form of art. Despite healthcare professional's legitimate role to actively seek for treatments for their patients, the quality of conversation as well as the quantity has not kept pace with the holistic care. Researchers have pointed out the technique of patient-oriented interviews can facilitate increased understanding of their patients' stories. Other equally valid efforts include actively listening out to patients, families and colleagues with the help of body (gestures and body languages), mind (stories and narratives) and soul (feelings and emotions) [174]. Allowing community members, stakeholders, and leaders as well as academic researchers to serve as each other's informants, one may often find that the similarities between both parties on priorities, goals, and capacities often outweigh differences.

26.8.1.4 Negotiation

The wiliness to negotiate mutually acceptable alternatives carries equal weight as learning each other's preferences. Both researchers and community partners are encouraged to be flexible enough to comprehend each other's particular belief system. The willingness to find mutually acceptable alternatives, not only in terms of treatment, but also in the course of communication, would further engage community members in each step of the scientific inquiry. In other words, the ongoing negotiation brings an equal information exchange that transforms the partnership encounter into a "therapeutic alliance" [174]. When cultural inquiry begins to move into the domain of humility, both parties may gain a better understanding of health issues.

Overall, we believe that the principles of the QIAN model could help enhance the exploration, comprehension, and appreciation of the cultural orientations between researchers and community partners which ultimately sustain community engagement and the reduction of health disparities. QIAN model is highly adaptable to other cultural and ethnic groups in multicultural societies around the globe.

When socio-cultural differences between researchers and community partners are explored, understood, and appreciated, the result is improved participant satisfaction. Outstanding community-academic partnerships are not only approaching challenging health disparities from their minds, but hearts.

Overall, it is imperative to vertically integrate cultural sensitivity training into the current healthcare professional training and education. Such curriculum should encourage health professionals to become better listeners and humble students of the older adults, which are essential steps to comprehend the cultural variations of health, aging, and elder abuse issues. Culturally appropriate training and resources for the Adult Protective Services and other frontline workers will also be critical to alleviating factors exacerbating abusive situations in the Chinese communities, and to prevent elder abuse recidivism. True community-academic collaboration is to be fostered over time through a humble exchange of engaging dialogues between researchers and community members.

26.8.2 Policy Implications

Advocacy for older adults' health is integral to the field of public health and gerontology [175]. Driving policy changes in lights of community needs should emerge as a long-term goal of CBPR projects. However, a major gap in the field of health inequalities identified through our CBPR research project in elder abuse is in the realm of public policy. We need to work with policy makers on relevant national policies (e.g., Older Americans Act, Elder Justice Act, Violence Against Women Act, among others) to ensure that linguistically and culturally appropriate services are provided to protect vulnerable older adults [176]. The Older Americans Act of 1965 was designed to improve the independence of older adults. It included many specific provisions to address the well-being of community-dwelling older adults, including minority populations. However, the act has not been reauthorized since 2011. Its reauthorization should be a policy priority to ensure the health, security and well-being of older adults.

In addition, the Elder Justice Act may be another potential opportunity to address health disparities, as it is responsible for sponsoring and supporting training, services, reporting, and evaluation of elder justice programs in community and long-term care settings. The Elder Justice Act is the most comprehensive federal legislation to address elder abuse. Enacted as a part of the Patient Protection and Affordable Care Act, the Elder Justice Act makes significant contributions to elder abuse investigation by authorizing $100 million for state and local Adult Protective Service programs (APS). The APS is responsible for receiving and investigating reports of abuse, neglect and financial exploitation and by matching the needs of potential victims with community partners. As the EJA is being implemented, policy makers partnering with community stakeholders should pay special attention to cultural issues surrounding elder abuse definitions in estimating the prevalence of elder abuse. At the state level, government should provide culturally appropriate resources and education to APS and other frontline workers to manage cases involving minority older adults [121]. The full appropriation of the Elder Justice Act is critically needed to address the major gaps in funding, policy, research, and education.

Finally, the Violence Against Women Act is one of the most pertinent programs to the well-being of victimized women. This Act authorizes the attorney general to formulate grants in order to enhance training and services to end violence against women. Furthermore, we need to work with the Department of Health and Human Services (Administration for Community Living, Centers for Medicare and Medicaid Services, Substance Abuse and Mental Health Services Administration) to examine relevant existing programs that can potentially impact the health and well-being of the diverse populations.

26.9 Global Implications on Elder Abuse and Health Disparities

The world population is aging rapidly. With the post-World War II baby boom generation in the U.S. and Europe joining the older ranks in recent years and with the accelerated growth of older populations in Asia and Latin America, the next 10 years will witness an increase of about 236 million people aged 65 and older throughout the world [177]. It is projected that from 2025 to 2050, the older population will grow to almost double to 1.6 billion globally, whereas the total population will grow by roughly only 34 % over the same period. There is also great variation in the demographic phenomenon of population aging. Europe currently remains the oldest region and is further along in the demographic transition. However, by 2050, almost two-thirds (62.3 %) of the world's older adults, or an equivalent of 975.3 million older adults will live in Asia.

While population aging reflects the medical success in increased longevity, what remains unknown is the quality of these prolonged years. As life expectancy increases in most nations, so do the likelihood that several generations are alive at the same time. In developed countries, this is manifested as a "beanpole family," a vertical extension of family structure characterized by more but smaller generations. However, while the number of surviving generations in a family may have increased, today these generations are more likely to live separately. In many countries, the shape of the family unit reflects changing social norms; economic security; rising rates of migration, divorce, and remarriage; and blended and stepfamily relations [178]. The changing roles of family, caregiving, as well as the evolving family structure, may likely predispose older adults to greater challenges in health management or caregiving arrangement leading to greater levels of distress [129]. The aging of the global population warrants our timely attention as it implies a higher number of older adults who may be victimized by elder abuse.

Consequently, the understanding of how CBPR processes impact health disparities in aging needs to be strengthened in response to the rapidly growing population aging phenomenon. First identified by British gerontologists in 1975 [179], it is not until recently that researchers have rigorously examined the issue and its health impact nationally, and internationally. A recent global review reveals that elder abuse, including psychological, physical, sexual abuse, neglect, and financial exploitation was common among community-dwelling older adults and especially prevalent among minority older adults around the world [177]. Learning how the added value of participatory processes works can improve our capacity to reduce elder abuse. With these recommendations, the upward trend to engage community members, public health professionals, and researchers can support the reciprocal learning needed to alleviate elder abuse health disparities on a global scale.

In addition, we call for an expanded global collaborative research agenda to shed more light on the biological, behavioral, social, and cultural factors that predispose global populations to health burdens brought about by elder abuse. In order to design effective prevention strategies, we need to conduct longitudinal studies to examine how the health status of these older adults changes over time in order to better understand the risk and protective factors associated with elder abuse globally. Future CBPR research should also extend to assessing caregiving experiences and viewpoints of adult children and key family members with cross-cultural study design. Due to the vast diversities within the global populations, we need national and international studies on diverse populations in order to provide in-depth information useful for generating meaningful comparative analyses in elder abuse.

26.10 Summary

Community's critical participation in reducing elder abuse is centrally situated within the multi-level racial–ethnic, social–cultural, physical environmental and structural framework of health disparities. As with any participatory process, CBPR may take extensive time and labor in the process. With proper preparation, however, participatory action research will yield highly valid and reliable data to advance elder abuse research, and bring tremendous benefits for community empowerment and social change. We call for concerted interdisciplinary efforts from research scientists, public health practitioners, and healthcare professionals to work collaboratively with community members to end health disparities and achieve global health equity.

References

1. LaVeist T. Minority populations and health: an introduction to health disparities in the U.S. San Francisco: Wiley; 2005.
2. WHO. Closing the gap in a generation: health equity through action on the social determinants of health. Final Report of the Commission on Social Determinants of Health. Geneva; 2008.
3. Statistics Canada. Canadian demographics at a glance. Ottawa, Canada; 2008.
4. Cherlin A. Demographic trends in the United States: a review of research in the 2000s. J Marriage Fam. 2010;72:403–19.
5. Bureau USC. Table 12 Projections of the population by age and sex for the United States: 2010–2050. 2008. Report No.: NP2008-T12.

6. Colby S, Ortman J. Projections of the size and composition of the U.S. population: 2014 to 2060. Current Population Report. Washington, DC; 2014.
7. AoA. A profile of older Americans: 2014. Washington, DC; 2014.
8. Carter-Pokras O, Baquet C. What is a "health disparity"? Public Health Rep. 2002;117:426–34.
9. Yancey A, Ortega A, Kumanyika S. Effective recruitment and retention of minority research participants. Ann Rev Public Health. 2006;27:1–28.
10. Io Medicine. Unequal treatment: confronting racial and ethnic disparities in health care. Washington, DC: Institute of Medicine; 2002.
11. Chin M, Walters A, Cook S, Huang E. Interventions to reduce racial and ethnic disparities in health care. Med Care Res Rev. 2007;64:7S–28S.
12. Betancourt J, Green A, Carillo J, Ananen-firempong O. Defining cultural competence: a practical framework for addressing racial/ethnic disparities. Public Health Rep. 2003;118:293–302.
13. Giger J, Davidhizar R, Purnell L, Harden J, Phillips J, Strickland O. American academy of nursing expert panel report. J Transcult Nurse. 2007;18:95–102.
14. U.S. Department of Health and Human Services SAaMHSA. The Secretary's Advisory Committee on National Health Promotion and Disease Prevention Objectives for 2020. Phase I report: recommendations for the framework and format of Healthy People 2020. Washington, DC; 2010.
15. Witham MD, McMurdo ME. How to get older people included in clinical studies. Drugs Aging. 2007;24:187–96.
16. Townsley CA, Selby R, Siu LL. Systematic review of barriers to the recruitment of older patients with cancer onto clinical trials. J Clin Oncol. 2005;23:3112–24.
17. Centers for Disease Control and Prevention, Administration on Aging, Agency for Healthcare Research and Quality, and Centers for Medicare and Medicaid Services. Enhancing use of clinical preventive services among older adults. Washington, DC: AARP; 2011.
18. Bureau USC. Table 4 Projections of the population by sex, race, and hispanic origin for the United States: 2010–2015. 2008. Report No.: NP2008-T4.
19. Jones C. Levels of racism: a theoretic framework and a gardner's tale. Am J Public Health. 2000;90:1212–5.
20. Glymour M, Avendano M, Kawachi I. Socioeconomic status and health. In: Berkman LF, Kawachi I, Glymour MM, editors. Social epidemiology. Oxford: University Press; 2015. p. 17–62.
21. Britton A, McKee M, Black M, McPherson K, Sanderson C, Bain C. Threats to applicability of randomised trials: exclusions and selective participation. J Health Serv Res Policy. 1999;4:112–21.
22. Pasick R. Socioeconomic and cultural factors in the development and use of theory. In: Glanz K, Rimer BK, Viswanath K, editors. Health behavior and health education—theory, research and practice. San Francisco: Josse-Bass Inc; 2008.
23. Kagawa Singer M. Applying the concept of culture to reduce health disparities through health behavior research. Prev Med. 2012;55:356–61.
24. Resnicow K, Braranowski T, Ahluwalia J, Braithwaite R. Cultural sensitivity in public health: defined and demystified. Ethn Dis. 1999;9:10–21.
25. Kagawa-Singer M, Dressler WW, George S, Elwood WN. The cultural framework for health. Washington, DC: National Institutes of Health; 2015.
26. NIH Policy and guidelines on the inclusion of women and minorities as subjects in clinical research—Amended, Oct, 2001. Retrieved from https://grants.nih.gov/grants/funding/women_min/guidelines_amended_10_2001.htm.
27. Administration FaD. U.S. Department of Health and Human Services Food and Drug Administration. Guidance for industry—collection of race and ethnicity data in clinical trials. Sep, 2005. Retrieved from http://www.fda.gov/downloads/RegulatoryInformation/Guidances/ucm126396.pdf.
28. Wendler D, Kington R, Madans J, et al. Are racial and ethnic minorities less willing to participate in health research? PLoS Med. 2009;3:e19.
29. Brown D, Topcu M. Willingnes to participate in clinical treatment research among older African Americans and Whites. Gerontologist. 2003;43:62–72.
30. Wallington S, Luto G, Noone A, et al. Assessing the awareness of and willingness to participate in cancer clinical trials among immigrant Latinos. J Community Health. 2012;37:335–43.
31. George S, Duran N, Norris K. A systematic review of barriers and facilitators to minority research participation among African Americans, Latinos, Asian Americans and Pacific Islanders. Am J Public Health. 2014;104:e16–31.
32. Herrara A, Snipes S, King D, Torres-Vigil I, Goldberg D, Weinberg A. Disparate inclusion of older adults in clinical trials: priorities and opportunities for policy and practice change. Am J Public Health. 2010;100:S105–12.
33. Fuentes D, Aranda MP. Depression interventions among racial and ethnic minority older adults: a systematic review across 20 years. Am J Geriatr Psychiatry. 2012;20:915–31.
34. Ballard E, Gwyther L, Edmonds H. Challenges and opportunities: recruitment and retention of African Americans for Alzheimer's disease research: lessons learned. Alzheimer Dis Assoc Disord. 2010;24:S19–23.
35. Heiat A, Gross C, Krumholz H. Representation of the elderly, women, and minorities in heart failure clinical trials. JAMA Intern Med. 2002;162:1682–8.
36. Elley C, Robertson M, Kerse N, et al. Falls assessment clinical trial (FACT):design, interventions, recruitment strategies and participant characteristics. BMC Public Health. 2007;29:185.
37. Woodall A, Morgan C, Sloan C, Howard L. Barriers to participate in mental health research: are there specific gender, ethnicity, and age related barriers? BMC Psychiatry. 2010;10:1–10.
38. Kwiatkowski K, Coe K, Bailar J, Swanson G. Inclusion of minorities and women in cancer clinical trials, a decade later: have we improved. Cancer. 2013;119:2956–63.
39. Boehmer U. Twenty years of public health research: including of lesbian, gay, bisexual and transgender populations. Am J Public Health. 2002;92:1125–30.
40. Shavers VL, Lynch CF, Burmeister LF. Knowledge of the Tuskegee study and its impact on the willingness to participate in medical research studies. J Natl Med Assoc. 2000;92:563–72.
41. McCallum J, Arekere D, Green B, Katz R, Rivers B. Awareness and knowledge of the U.S. Public Health Service syphilis study at Tuskegee: implications for biomedical research. J Health Care Poor Underserved. 2006;17:716–33.
42. Earl C, Penny P. The significance of trust in the research consent process with African Americans. West J Nurs Res. 2001;23: 753–62.
43. Scharff D, Mathews K, Jackson P, Hoffsuemmer J, Martin E, Edwards D. More than Tuskegee: understanding mistrust about research participation. J Health Care Poor Underserved. 2010;21:879–97.
44. Gamble V. A legacy of distrust: African Americans and medical research. J Prev Med. 1993;9:35–8.
45. Corbie-Smith G, Thomas S, George D. Distrust, race and research. Arch Intern Med. 2002;162:2458–63.

46. Washington H. Medical Apartheid: the dark history of the medical experimentation on Black Americans from colonial times to the present. New York: Random House Digital Inc; 2006.
47. Heitman E, Wells AL. Ethical issues and unethical conduct: race, racism and the abuse of human subjects in research. In: Beech BM, editor. Race & research: perspectives on minority participation in health studies. Washington, DC: American Public Health Association; 2004.
48. Lawrence J. The Indian Health Service and the sterilization of native American women. Am Indian Q. 2000;24:400–19.
49. Carpio M. The lost generation: American Indian and sterilized abuse. Soc Justice. 2004;31:50.
50. Murthy VH, Krumholz HM, Gross CP. Participation in cancer clinical trials: race-, sex-, and age-based disparities. JAMA. 2004;291:2720–6.
51. Yi SS, Kwon SC, Sacks R, Trinh-Shevrin C. Commentary: persistence and health-related consequences of the model minority stereotype for Asian Americans. Ethn Dis. 2016;26:133–8.
52. Shoff C, Yang TC. Untangling the associations among distrust, race, and neighborhood social environment: a social disorganization perspective. Soc Sci Med. 1982;2012(74):1342–52.
53. Harris LM. Academic/community-based collaboration: benefits academic institutions, senior centers and elders. Gerontol. 2012;52:127.
54. Jacobs EA, Rolle I, Ferrans CE, Whitaker EE, Warnecke RB. Understanding African Americans' views of the trustworthiness of physicians. J Gen Intern Med. 2006;21:642–7.
55. Durant R, Legedza A, Marcantonio E, Freeman M, Landon B. Different types of distrust in clinical research among Whites and African Americans. J Natl Med Assoc. 2011;103:123–30.
56. Armstrong K, Rose A, Peters N, Long JA, McMurphy S, Shea JA. Distrust of the health care system and self-reported health in the United States. J Gen Intern Med. 2006;21:292–7.
57. Corrigan PW. Mental health stigma as social attribution: implications for research methods and attitude change. Clin Psychol Sci Pract. 2000;7:48–67.
58. Gary FA. Stigma: barrier to mental health care among ethnic minorities. Issues Ment Health Nurs. 2005;26:979–99.
59. Cargill VA, Stone VE. HIV/AIDS: a minority health issue. Med Clin N Am. 2005;89:895–912.
60. Ofstedal MB, Weir DR. Recruitment and retention of minority participants in the health and retirement study. Gerontol. 2011;51 (Suppl 1):S8–20.
61. Epstein S. The rise of 'recruitmentology': clinical research, racial knowledge, and the politics of inclusion and difference. Soc Stud Sci. 2008;38:801–32.
62. Minkler M, Wallerstein N. Community-based participatory research for health. San Francisco: Jossey Bass; 2003.
63. Cornwall A, Jewkes R. What is participatory research? Soc Sci Med. 1982;1995(41):1667–76.
64. Wallerstein N, Duran B. Using community-based participatory research to address health disparities. Health Promot Pract. 2006;7:312–23.
65. Leung M, Yen I, Minkler M. Community based participatory research: a promising approach for increasing epidemiology's relevance in the 21st century. Int J Epidemiol. 2004;33:499–506.
66. Green L, Mercer S. Can public health researchers and agencies reconcile the push from funding bodies and the pull from communities? Am J Public Health. 2001;91:1926–9.
67. Lewin K. Action research and minority problems. J Soc Issues. 1946;2:34–46.
68. Freire P. Pedagogy of the oppressed. New York: Seabury Press; 1970.
69. Maguire P. Participatory research: a feminist approach. Amherst: Center for International Education; 1987.
70. Duran E, Duran B. Native American postcolonial psychology. Albany, NY: State University of New York Press; 1995.
71. McTaggart R. Sixteen tenets of participatory action research. In: Wadsworth Y, editor. Everyday evaluation on the run. Sydney: Allen & Unwin; 1997. p. 79.
72. Israel BA, Schulz AJ, Paker EA, Becker AM. Review of community based research: assessing partnership approaches to improve public health. Annu Rev Public Health. 1998;19:173–202.
73. Knight EK. Shifting public health practice to advance health equity: recommendations from experts and community leaders. J Public Health Manag Pract. 2014;20:188–96.
74. Martinez IL, Carter-Pokras O, Brown PB. Addressing the challenges of Latino health research: participatory approaches in an emergent urban community. J Natl Med Assoc. 2009;101:908–14.
75. Minkler M. Community-based research partnerships: challenges and opportunities. J Urban Health. 2005;82:ii3–12.
76. Salimi Y, Shahandeh K, Malekafzali H, et al. Is community-based participatory research (CBPR) useful? A systematic review on papers in a decade. Int J Prev Med. 2012;3:386–93.
77. Diaz AEK, Johnson CRS, Arcury TA. Variation in the interpretation of scientific integrity in community-based participatory health research. Soc Sci Med. 1982;2013(97):134–42.
78. Flicker S, Travers R, Guta A, McDonald S, Meagher A. Ethical dilemmas in community-based participatory research: recommendations for institutional review boards. J Urban Health. 2007;84:478–93.
79. Resnik DB, Kennedy CE. Balancing scientific and community interests in community-based participatory research. Account Res. 2010;17:198–210.
80. Ashing-Giwa KT. Can a culturally responsive model for research design bring us closer to addressing participation disparities? Lessons learned from cancer survivorship studies. Ethn Dis. 2005;15:130–7.
81. Deloria Y. God is red: a native view of religion. Golden: North American Press; 1992.
82. Chau T, Islam N, Tandon D, Ho-Asjoe H, Rey M. Using community-based participatory research as a guiding framework for health disparities research centers. Prog Community Health Partnersh. 2007;1:195–205.
83. Dong X, Chang E, Wong E, Simon M. Working with culture: lessons learned from a community-engaged project in a Chinese aging population. Aging Health. 2011;7:529–37.
84. Dahlberg LL, Mercy JA. History of violence as a public health issue. AMA Virtual Mentor. 2009;11(2):167–72.
85. Krug EG, Mercy JA, Dahlberg LL, Zwi AB. The world report on violence and health. Lancet. 2002;360:1083–8.
86. Krug EG, Dahlberg LL, Mercy JA, Zwi AB, Lozano R. World report on violence and health. Geneva: World Health Organization. 2002.
87. Dahlberg LL, Krug EG. Violence: a global public health problem. In: Krug E, Dahlberg LL, Mercy JA, Zwi AB, Lozano R, editors. World Report on Violence and Health. Geneva, Switzerland: World Health Organization. 2002:1–56.
88. Lee YS, Hadeed L. Intimate partner violence among Asian immigrant communities: health/mental health consequences, help-seeking behaviors, and service utilization. Trauma Violence Abuse. 2009;10:143–70.
89. Bent-Goodley TB. Health disparities and violence against women: why and how cultural and societal influences matter. Trauma Violence Abuse. 2007;8:90–104.
90. Ferrari AM. The impact of culture upon child rearing practices and definitions of maltreatment. Child Abuse Negl. 2002;26:793–813.

91. Gonzalez-Guarda RM, Cummings AM, Becerra M, Fernandez MC, Mesa I. Needs and preferences for the prevention of intimate partner violence among Hispanics: a community's perspective. J Prim Prev. 2013;34:221–35.
92. Nicolaidis C, Perez M, Mejia A, et al. "Guardarse las cosas adentro" (keeping things inside): Latina violence survivors' perceptions of depression. J Gen Intern Med. 2011;26:1131–7.
93. Poleshuck E, Mazzotta C, Resch K, et al. Development of an innovative treatment paradigm for intimate partner violence victims with depression and pain using community-based participatory research. J Interpers Violence. 2016. Published online before print 12 Feb, 2016. doi:10.1177/0886260516628810.
94. Gewirtz A. Promoting children's mental health in family supportive housing: a community-university partnership for formerly homeless children and families. J Prim Prev. 2007;28:359–74.
95. Leff S, Thomas D, Vaughn N, Thomas N, MacEvoy J. Using community-based participatory research to develop the PARTNERS youth violence prevention program. Prog Community Health Partnersh. 2010;4:207–16.
96. Merves M, Rodgers C, Silver E, Sclafane J, Bauman L. Engaging and sustaining adolescents in community-based participatory research: structuring a youth-friendly CBPR environment. Fam Community Health. 2015;38:22–32.
97. Sullivan M, Bhuyan R, Senturia K, Shiu-Thornton S, Ciske S. Participatory action research in practice: a case study in addressing domestic violence in nine cultural communities. J Interpers Violence. 2005;20:977–95.
98. White J, Yuan N, Cook S, Abbey A. Ethnic minority women's experiences with intimate partner violence: using community-based participatory research to ask the right questions. Sex Roles. 2013;69:226–36.
99. Harvey A, Garcia-Moreno, C, Butchart, A. Primary prevention of intimate-partner violence and sexual violence: background paper for WHO expert meeting, May 2–3, 2007.
100. Watts C, Zimmerman C. Violence against women: global scope and magnitude. Lancet. 2002;359:1232–7.
101. Shea B, Nahwegahbow A, Anderson N. Reduction of family violence in aboriginal communities: a systematic review of interventions and approaches. Pimatisiwin. 2010;8:35–60.
102. Carreon D, Noymer A. Health-related quality of life in older adults: testing the double jeopardy hypothesis. J Aging Stud. 2011;25:371–9.
103. Hill C, Perez-Stable E, Anderson N, Bernard M. The national institute on aging health disparities research framework. Ethn Dis. 2015;25:245–54.
104. Dong X, Chang E, Wong E, Wong B, Skarupski KA, Simon MA. Assessing the health needs of Chinese older adults: findings from a community-based participatory research study in Chicago's Chinatown. J Aging Res. 2010;2010, Article ID 124246:12 pages http://dx.doi.org/10.4061/2010/124246.
105. Horowitz C, Robinson M, Seifer S. Community-based participatory research from the margin to the mainstream. Circulation. 2009;119:2633–42.
106. Yen I, Michael Y, Perdue L. Neighborhood enviroment in studies of health of older adults. Am J Prev Med. 2010;37:455–63.
107. Campbell M, Hudson M, Resnicow K, Blakeney N, Paxton A, Baskin M. Church-based health promotion interventions: evidence and lessons learned. Annu Rev Public Health. 2006;26:213–34.
108. National Academies of Sciences. Elder abuse: abuse, neglect, and exploitation in an aging America. Washington DC: National Academy Press; 2003.
109. World Health Organization. Facts: abuse of the elderly. 2002.
110. Acierno R, Hernandez M, Amstadter A, Resnick HS, Steve K, Muzzy W. Prevalence and correlates of emotional, physical, sexual, and financial abuse and potential neglect in the United States: the National Elder Mistreatment Study. Am J Public Health. 2010;100:292–7.
111. Burnett JP, Jackson SLP, Sinha AKM, et al. Five-year all-cause mortality rates across five categories of substantiated elder abuse occurring in the community. J Elder Abuse Negl. 2016;28(2):1–17.
112. Dong X, Simon M. Association between elder abuse and metabolic syndromes: findings from the Chicago health and aging project. Gerontology. 2015;61:389–98.
113. Dong X, Simon M, Mendes de Leon C, et al. Elder self-neglect and abuse and mortality risk in a community-dwelling population. J Am Med Assoc. 2009;302:517–26.
114. Dong X, Simon M. Elder abuse as a risk factor for hospitalization in older persons. JAMA Intern Med. 2013;173:911–7.
115. Lachs MS, Williams CS, O'Brien S, Pillemer KA. Adult protective service use and nursing home placement. Gerontol. 2002;42:734–9.
116. Institute of Medicine. Elder abuse and its prevention—workshop summary. Washington, DC; 2013.
117. Daly JM, Merchant MI, Jogerst G. Elder abuse research: a systematic review. J Elder Abuse Negl. 2011;23:348–65.
118. Ploeg J, Fear J, Hutchison B, MacMillan H, Bolan G. A systematic review of interventions for elder abuse. J Elder Abuse Negl. 2009;21:187–210.
119. Brownell P, Heiser D. Psycho-educational support groups for older women victims of family mistreatment. J Gerontol Soc Work. 2006;46:145–60.
120. Brownell P, Berman J, Salamone A. Mental health and criminal justice issues among perpetrators of elder abuse. J Elder Abuse Negl. 1999;11:81–94.
121. Dong X, Simon MA. Enhancing national policy and programs to address elder abuse. J Am Med Assoc. 2011;305:2460–1.
122. Miranda J, Bernal G, Lau A, Kohn L, Hwang W, LaFromboise T. State of the science on psychosocial interventions for ethnic minorities. Annu Rev Clin Psychol. 2005;1:113–42.
123. Barnes L, Mendes de Leon C, Wilson R, Bienias J, Bennett D, Evans D. Racial differences in perceived discrimination in a community population of older blacks and whites. J Aging Health. 2004;16:315–7.
124. Shinagawa L. A portrait of Chinese Americans. Maryland: Asian American Studies Program at the University of Maryland. 2008.
125. Mui AC, Shibusawa T. Asian American elders in the twenty-first century. New York: Columbia University Press; 2008.
126. Aroian KJ, Wu B, Tran TV. Health care and social service use among Chinese immigrant elders. Res Nurs Health. 2005;28:95–105.
127. Dong X, Chang E, Zeng P, Simon M. Suicide in the global chinese aging population: a review of risk and protective factors, consequences, and interventions. Aging Dis. 2015;6:121–30.
128. Simon Chang E, Zeng P, Dong X. Prevalence of suicidal ideation, attempts, and completed suicide rate in Chinese aging populations: a systematic review. Arch Gerontol Geriatr. 2013;57:250–6.
129. Dong X, Chang E. Lost in translation: to our Chinese patient, Alzheimer's meant 'crazy and catatonic'. Health affairs (Project Hope). 2014;33:712–5.
130. Dong X, Chang ES, Wong E, Simon M. Perception and negative effect of loneliness in a Chicago Chinese population of older adults. Arch Gerontol Geriatr. 2012;54:151–9.
131. Dong X, Chang ES, Wong E, Simon M. The perceptions, social determinants, and negative health outcomes associated with depressive symptoms among U.S. Chinese older adults. Gerontol. 2012;52:650–63.
132. Moreno-John G, Gachi A, Fleming C, Napoles-Springer A, Mutran E. Ethnic minority older adults participating in clinical research: developing trust. J Aging Health. 2004;16:123.

133. Suh EE, Kagan S, Strumpf N. Cultural competence in qualitative interview methods with Asian immigrants. J Transcult Nurs. 2009;20:194–201.
134. Dong X, Chang E, Wong E, Wong B, Simon M. How do U.S. Chinese older adults view elder mistreatment? Findings from a community-based participatory research study. J Aging Health. 2011;23:289–312.
135. Dong X, Chang E, Wong E, Simon M. Perceived effectiveness of elder abuse interventions in psychological distress and the design of culturally adapted interventions: a qualitative study in the chinese community in chicago. J Aging Res. 2013;2013:845425.
136. Harada N, Takeshita J, Ahmed I, et al. Does cultural assimilation influence prevalence and presentation of depressive symptoms in older Japanese American men? The Honolulu-Asia aging study. Am J Geriatr Psychiatry. 2012;20:337–45.
137. Stewart R, Masaki K, Xue QL, et al. A 32-year prospective study of change in body weight and incident dementia: the Honolulu-Asia Aging Study. Arch Neurol. 2005;62:55–60.
138. Bild DE, Bluemke DA, Burke GL, et al. Multi-ethnic study of atherosclerosis: objectives and design. Am J Epidemiol. 2002;156:871–81.
139. Bild DE, Detrano R, Peterson D, et al. Ethnic differences in coronary calcification—the multi-ethnic study of atherosclerosis (MESA). Circulation 2005;111(10):1313–20.
140. Alegria M, Takeuchi D, Canino G, et al. Considering context, place, and culture: the National Latino and Asian American Study. Int J Methods Psychiatr Res. 2004;13:208–20.
141. Dong X, Wong E, Simon MA. Study design and implementation of the PINE study. J Aging Health. 2014;26:1085–99.
142. Simon MA, Chang ES, Rajan KB, Welch MJ, Dong X. Demographic characteristics of U.S. Chinese older adults in the Greater Chicago area: assessing the representativeness of the PINE study. J Aging Health. 2014;26:1100–15.
143. Dong X. Do the definitions of elder mistreatment subtypes matter? Findings from the PINE Study. J Gerontol Ser A Biol Sci Med Sci. 2014;69(Suppl 2):S68–75.
144. Dong X, Chen R, Simon MA. Elder mistreatment in U.S. community-dwelling Chinese older women. Violence Against Women. 2016;22(9):1097–112.
145. Dong X, Chen R, Fulmer T, Simon MA. Prevalence and correlates of elder mistreatment in a community-dwelling population of U.S. Chinese older adults. J Aging Health. 2014;26:1209–24.
146. Chang E, Dong X. Understanding elder abuse in the Chinese community: the role of cultural, social, and community factors. In: Prevention FoGV, editor. Elder abuse and its prevention. Washington DC: Institute of Medicine; 2014.
147. Wolff M, Maurana CA. Building effective community-academic partnerships to improve health: a qualitative study of perspectives from communities. Acad Med. 2001;76:166–72.
148. Dong X, Chang E, Wong E, Simon M. Sustaining community-university partnerships: lessons learned from a participatory research project with elderly Chinese. Gatew Int J Community Res Engagem. 2011;4:31–47.
149. Holkup PA, Tripp-Reimer T, Salois EM, Weinert C. Community-based participatory research—an approach to intervention research with a Native American community. Adv Nurs Sci. 2004;27:162–75.
150. Sapra K, Jubinski S, Tanaka M, Gershon R. Family and partner interpersonal violence among American Indians/Alaska Natives. Inj Epidemiol. 2014:1–7.
151. Dong X, Wong E, Simon M. Study design and implementation of the PINE study. J Aging Health. 2014;26(7):1085–99.
152. Roberto K, Brossoie N, McPherson M. Violence against rural older women: promoting community awareness and action. Australas J Ageing. 2013;32:2–7.
153. Brossoie N, Roberto K. Community professionals' response to intimate partner violence against rural older women. J Elder Abuse Negl. 2015;27:470–88.
154. Cook-Daniels L. Lesbian, gay male, bisexual and transgendered elders: elder abuse and neglect issues. J Elder Abuse Negl. 2008;9:35–49.
155. Moon A, Williams O. Perceptions of elder abuse and help-seeking patterns among African-American, Caucasian American, and Korean-American elderly women. Gerontol. 1993;33:386–95.
156. Baker-Demaray TB. Perceptions of elder abuse among native american seniors. 2009.
157. Fulmer T, Guadagno L, Bitondo Dyer C, Connolly M. Progress in elder abuse screening and assessment instruments. J Am Geriatr Soc. 2004;52:297–304.
158. Interpersonal violence in the African-American Community. Springer; 2006.
159. Kobetz E, Menard J, Diem J, Barton B, Blanco J, Pierre L, Auguste PD, Etienne M, Brewster C. Community-based participatory research in little Haiti: challenges and lessons learned. Prog Community Health Partnersh Res Educ Action. 2009;3:133–7.
160. Dong XC, Chang ES, Wong E, Simon M. Perceived barriers and facilitators to implement elder abuse intervention for victims and perpetrators: views from US Chinese older adults. J Adult Prot. 2014;16:307–21.
161. Kreuter MW, McClure SM. The role of culture in health communication. Annu Rev Public Health. 2004;25:439–55.
162. Fisher TL, Burnet DL, Huang ES, Chin MH, Cagney KA. Cultural leverage: interventions using culture to narrow racial disparities in health care. Med Care Res Rev. 2007;64:243S–83S.
163. Holkup PA, Salois EM, Tripp-Reimer T, Weinert C. Drawing on wisdom from the past: an elder abuse intervention with tribal communities. Gerontol. 2007;47:248–54.
164. Dong X. Advancing the field of elder abuse: future directions and policy implications. J Am Geriatr Soc. 2012;60:2151–6.
165. Alexander JA, Weiner BJ, Metzger ME, et al. Sustainability of collaborative capacity in community health partnerships. Med Care Res Rev. 2003;60:130S–60S.
166. Bryant E. Sustaining comprehensive community initiatives: key elements for success. Washington DC; 2002.
167. Paine-Andrews A, Fisher JL, Campuzano MK, Fawcett SB, Berkeley-Patton J. Promoting sustainability of community health initiatives: an empirical case study. Health Promot Pract. 2000;1 (3):248–258.
168. Kreuter MW, Lezin NA, Young LA. Evaluation community-based collaborative mechanisms: implications for practioners. Health Promot Pract. 2000;1:49–63.
169. Westfall JM, Mold J, Fagnan L. Practice-based research—"Blue highways" on the NIH roadmap. J Am Med Assoc. 2007;297:24–31.
170. Davis S, Nolan M. Nurturing research partnerships with older people and their carers: learning from experience. Qual Ageing. 2003;4:2–23.
171. Simon MA, Chang ES, Dong X. Partnership, reflection and patient focus: advancing cultural competency training relevance. Med Educ. 2010;44:540–2.
172. Chang E, Simon M, Dong X. Integrating cultural humility into health care professional education and training. Adv Health Sci Educ Theory Pract. 2012;17:269–78.
173. Brody H, Hunt L. Moving beyond cultural stereotypes in end-of-life decision making. Am Fam Physician. 2005;71:429.

174. Austerlic S. Cultural humility and compassionate presence at the end of life. http://www.scu.edu/ethics/practicing/focusareas/medical/culturally-competent-care/chronic-to-critical-austerlic.html. Santa Clara University; 2009.
175. Hinrichsen GA, Kietzman KG, Alkema GE, et al. Influencing public policy to improve the lives of older Americans. Gerontol. 2010.
176. Dong X. Cultural diversity and elder abuse: implication for research, education, and policy. Gener J Am Soc Aging. Generations, Number 3/Fall 2012;36:40–2.
177. Dong X. Elder abuse: systematic review and implications for practice. J Am Geriatr Soc. 2015;63:1214–38.
178. Global health and aging. National Institute on Aging National Institutes of Health NIH Publication no.11-7737. 2011.
179. Burston GR. Letter: Granny-battering. Br Med J 1975;3:592.

Part VI

Policy Issues Surrounding Elder Abuse

History of the Elder Justice Movement

27

Robert B. Blancato and Meaghan McMahon

27.1 Understanding Elder Justice

Elder justice is defined by statute as "… efforts to prevent, detect, treat, intervene in and prosecute elder abuse, neglect and exploitation, and protect elders with diminished capacity while maximizing their autonomy; and from an individual perspective, the recognition of an elder's rights, including the right to be free from abuse, neglect, and exploitation." The elder justice movement has evolved over the time period of 1978 to the present. Elder justice is best accomplished through the prevention of elder abuse.

Elder abuse can occur in many different ways, including mistreatment of an older adult by a single individual, a group of people or an institution [1]. More than one type of abuse can occur at a time and the mistreatment can be repetitive [2]. Studies have shown that elder abuse may result in increased risk of disease and premature death for the victim [3]. For those individuals living with mental and physical disabilities, as well as those experiencing cognitive impairment and social isolation, an increased risk of elder abuse has been documented [2].

The most commonly referred to forms of abuse are physical, psychological, sexual, financial and neglect [4]. Any actions or statements that harm or threaten the physical or psychological health of an older adult can be considered abuse [5]. If an older adult's possessions or money are mistreated or stolen, authorities can report the situation as financial abuse [5]. Unlike deliberate threats and harmful actions against an older adult, neglect is a failure to take action that results in the older person being vulnerable and at risk [5].

Unfortunately, the majority of elder abuse is committed by family members, including adult children, spouses and partners. According to one national study, 76 % of physical mistreatment abusers were family members [6]. Of those perpetrators, 57 % were partners or spouses, 10 % were children or grandchildren and 9 % were other relatives [6]. Although elder abuse is predominant in community settings, it also occurs in institutions such as nursing homes [7]. In 2012, abuse, gross neglect, and exploitation reports represented 7.1 % of all nursing home complaints received by the National Long-Term Care Ombudsman Program [8]. According to the Department of Justice, in the United States there are more than six million victims of elder abuse, or roughly one of every 10 persons over age 60. In 2009, it was estimated that victims of elder financial abuse lose an estimated $2.9 billion a year [9].

27.2 Elder Justice Public Policy Chronology

In 1962, the Public Welfare Amendments to the Social Security Act passed and authorized payments to states for establishing protective services to those with physical and mental limitations [10]. When discussing elder abuse, an important population to consider is people with lifelong disabilities who are aging and face abuse, neglect and exploitation, many of whom are living in the community with their aging parents in a "two-generation geriatric context" [11]. Today, approximately 14 million seniors in the United States over the age of 65 are living with a disability [12]. The Americans with Disabilities Act (ADA) was signed into law on July 26, 1990, by President George H.W. Bush. The ADA of 1990, including changes made by the ADA Amendments Act of 2008, defines disability in Section 12102 as a physical or mental impairment that severely limits one or more major life activities of such an individual; a record of such impairment; or being regarded as having such an impairment (P.L. 110-325). Studies have found that all types of health care experts struggle to accurately and routinely report maltreatment they witness of persons with developmental disabilities [11].

R.B. Blancato (✉)
Elder Justice Coalition, 1612 K Street N.W, Washington, DC 20006, USA
e-mail: bob@elderjusticecoalition.com

M. McMahon
1348 Florida Ave NW, Washington, DC 20009, USA
e-mail: meaghmcm@umich.edu

X. Dong (ed.), *Elder Abuse*, DOI 10.1007/978-3-319-47504-2_27

The Older Americans Act (OAA) became law in 1965 as a result of the first White House Conference on Aging (WHCOA), which was held in May 1961 [13]. The White House has held a Conference on Aging every decade since the 1960s to recognize and move forward actions to improve the quality of life of aging Americans. The OAA established the Administration on Aging (AoA) within the Department of Health and Human Services (HHS) and this organization is considered the primary federal agency for providing national leadership in the field of elder justice [14].

In 1974, protective services were authorized under Title XX of the Social Security Act for all adults 18 years and older regardless of income with a focus on abuse, neglect and exploitation [10]. This title also allowed states to create Adult Protective Services (APS) units by statute or regulation. States can prioritize this funding for either older adults or younger people based on perceived state needs [10]. The eligibility for those wanting to receive APS services is determined by state law and it is the state APS program that is responsible for receiving reports of alleged abuse, investigating such reports and determining if the abuse should be substantiated so that they can arrange services to protect the older adult's well being [2]. In 1981, when Title XX was converted to Social Services Block Grant, the mandate to fund APS was removed leading to the uneven, uncoordinated APS system of today [7]. Since APS programs are the primary responsibility of the state, each state has developed its own data collection system in the absence of a national data tool [2].

In the 1970s, the federal government began to recognize violence against women as a national problem and introduced legislation in 1990 that proposed a possible response. Congressional action to combat violence resulted in the Violence Against Women Act (VAWA), which is Title IV of the Violent Crime Control and Law Enforcement Act of 1994 [15]. In 2000, the language of the Special Training Officers and Prosecutors (STOP) grants, which are administered by the Attorney General to help state, tribal and local government protect women against violent crime, were amended in the VAWA to provide funds to increase protection of older adults and individuals living with disabilities against abuse, neglect, and exploitation [15].

The Child Abuse Prevention and Treatment Act (CAPTA) was passed in 1974 (Public Law 93-247) [10]. According to the U.S. Department of Health and Human Services, CAPTA is the key Federal legislation that addresses child abuse and neglect by "...providing Federal funding to States in support of prevention, assessment, investigation, prosecution, and treatment activities and also provides grants to public agencies and nonprofit organizations, including Indian Tribes and Tribal organizations, for demonstration programs and project" [16]. CAPTA was amended numerous times throughout the 1980s and 1990s and the act was reauthorized on December 20, 2010 [16]. In contrast to this generous funding, currently only 2 % of federal funds for abuse prevention are spent on elders, compared to children and women, and no single person in the federal government worked on elder abuse specifically before the Elder Justice Act became law in 2010 [17].

In 1987, the Federal government first described elder abuse, neglect and exploitation under the amendments to the Older Americans Act (OAA) [10]. Today, certain Titles of the OAA, including Titles II, III, IV and VII, include provisions that relate to elder abuse, neglect and exploitation [3]. The amendments [Pub. L. No.100-175, §144, 101 Stat. 926, 948-50 (1987)], require state agencies on aging to assess the need for elder abuse prevention services and create a plan to prevent elder abuse within the state [5].

In 1988, the National Center on Elder Abuse (NCEA) was authorized under Title II of the OAA and became a national resource center for the elimination of elder abuse [13]. The first director of the NCEA was Toshio Tatara, Ph. D [10]. The NCEA is directed by the AOA and administered as a grant program which aims to be an information clearinghouse demonstration project on abuse, neglect, and exploitation [18]. The center operates as an association of partners which from 1985 to today have included, the American Public Welfare Association (APWA), the National Association of State Units on Aging and Disabilities (NASUAD), the University of Delaware, the National Citizen's Coalition for Nursing Home Reform (NCCNHR), the American Bar Association (ABA), the National Institute on Aging (NIA), the National Committee for Prevention of Elder Abuse (NCPEA), the National Adult Protective Services Association (NAPSA), and the University of California Irvine's Center of Excellence on Elder Abuse [19].

In the OAA amendments of 1992, Title VII, entitled Vulnerable Elder Rights Protection Activities, included "... all elder rights protection activities..." which included the establishment of the Long-Term Care Ombudsman program which now operates in every state, Washington DC, Guam, and Puerto Rico [8]. The purpose of a state Long-Term Care Ombudsman agency is to investigate any alleged cases of elder abuse that take place in licensed long-term care institutions such as skilled nursing facilities [3]. The OAA stipulates that the Administration for Community Living (ACL) must establish and lead a National Ombudsman Resource Center, which is supervised by the Director of the Office of Long-Term Care [3].

In September 2002, Sen. John Breaux (D-LA) first introduced the Elder Justice Act (S. 2933) to the 107th Congress. The goal of the act was to bring together federal systems cohesively to respond to elder abuse by laying the groundwork for important training, services, and demonstration programs [3]. The Elder Justice Act (EJA) was then reintroduced in the 108th, 109th, and 110th Congresses and in the 111th Congress Sen. Orrin Hatch (R-UT) introduced the Elder Justice Act of 2009 [4]. The Senate Finance Committee took action on the EJA on three different occasions, in the 108th, 109th, and 110th Congresses.

When the EJA was first introduced, it included what is now the Elder Abuse Victims Act (EAVA), which aims to train law enforcement personnel to help detect elder abuse and allows funding for special prosecutor units in localities that specialize in elder abuse. One version of this bill, H.R. 2564, the Elder Abuse Victims Act of 2011 was introduced July 15, 2011 by Rep. Peter King but ultimately was not enacted [4].

Another version of the bill was introduced on February 27, 2013 in the 113th Congress by Rep. Peter King (R-NY) as H.R. 861 or the Elder Abuse Victims Act of 2013. Cosponsors on the bill were Rep. Janice Schakowsky (D-IL), Rep. Alcee Hastings (D-FL), Rep. Raul Grijalva (D-AZ), Rep. William Owens (D-NY), Rep. Keith Ellison (D-MN), and Rep. Juan Vargas (D-CA). The full title of H. R. 861 is, "To better protect, serve, and advance the rights of victims of elder abuse and exploitation by establishing a program to encourage States and other qualified entities to create jobs designed to hold offenders accountable, enhance the capacity of the justice system to investigate, pursue, and prosecute elder abuse cases, identify existing resources to leverage to the extent possible, and assure data collection, research, and evaluation to promote the efficacy and efficiency of the activities described in this Act" [4].

According to the Elder Justice Coalition, the EAVA would establish an Office of Elder Justice in the Department of Justice (DOJ) whose job it would be to provide information, training, and technical assistance to help state and local governments to prevent, investigate, and prosecute elder abuse and mistreatment. The act would also improve data collection, allow for opportunities for states to receive grants and develop a compensated victims program within the DOJ. As of August 1, 2014, it has 10 cosponsors, 8 Democrats and 2 Republicans [4].

The EJA became law in 2010, not including the EAVA provisions, as part of the Patient Protection and Affordable Care Act (ACA, P.L. 11-148, as amended) and introduced the term "elder justice." The EJA provides a coordinated federal response by focusing on certain public health and social service approaches to the prevention, detection and treatment of elder abuse [4].

27.3 Challenges of the Elder Justice Act

There was a combination of challenges throughout the 7-year legislative odyssey of the Elder Justice Act. As a start, the issue was viewed as a new one. There had been scant legislative history on elder abuse prevention over the years and it was the author of the first bill who wished to use the phrase elder justice. The term while relevant and laudable did confuse people on the Hill.

The EJA was always a Senate driven process with one important exception, described later in this section. Thanks to the legislative wizardry of Senator Breaux, when the bill was introduced in the Senate, it managed to be referred to only one committee, the Senate Finance Committee on which he served as a high ranking member. There was resistance that developed from the Senate Judiciary Committee who felt those provisions in the original S. 333 that related to law enforcement belonged under their jurisdiction, and that resistance always lurked near the surface as the process moved forward. On the House side—the identical bill to S. 333 ended up being referred to four Committees—Ways and Means, Energy and Commerce, Judiciary and Education and the Workforce, almost guaranteeing that it would never get serious consideration in that body.

The exception to the Senate driven process occurred in 2008 with the introduction of H.R. 5352, the "Elder Abuse Victims Act of 2008" sponsored by Rep. Sestak of Pennsylvania, which focused on enforcement strategies for prosecuting abusers. Together, with H.R. 1783, "The Elder Justice Act" these bills created a comprehensive strategy for preventing and fighting elder abuse, neglect and exploitation. A decision was made by the House Democratic Leadership to separate out the law enforcement provisions of the EJA and allow them to be introduced as a separate bill. This was to help the politically endangered freshman House member Rep. Joe Sestak of Pennsylvania. The Elder Justice Coalition was consulted about the decision and while in agreement we did see where it might pose later problems with the bill. The positive response in the House was immediate. Within weeks of there were introduction hearings held in both the Crime Subcommittee and full House Judiciary Committee and soon thereafter the bill passed the full House of Representatives in September 2008. When the House checked with the Senate about the prospect of moving the House passed bill they encountered resistance and no action was ever taken on the Sestak bill.

Meanwhile, the Elder Justice Act, which had not initially been broken up in the Senate, continued to move through the process. Several hearings were held on elder justice including in the Senate Finance Committee. At the time the bill was to be 'marked' up in the Committee—the Judiciary Committee provisions were removed from the bill. The Senate Finance Committee passed the EJA by unanimous vote on three occasions.

On each occasion the Finance Committee waited very late into the session of Congress to consider the EJA. As a result the only way to gain Senate passage of the bill was to have it considered under the process called unanimous consent. It is a very literal process. All 100 Senate members must sign off before the bill can pass. The first time Senator Bob Graham of Florida put a temporary 'hold' on the bill seeking to have an unrelated provision added. By the time he lifted the hold it was too late for the Senate to pass.

On the second occasion an unnamed Senator put a hold on the bill citing the Bush Administration opposition to the EJA. This had been one of the major challenges to the bill over its history. Their position was that the EJA was "duplicative" and that much of what it called for was already being done within the Department of Health and Human Services. This hold was never lifted and forced the EJA to die awaiting action on Senate floor.

When the new Congress convened in 2009 and the Obama Administration took office it was determined by the bipartisan authors of the bill that the EJA would never pass as a freestanding bill. Therefore, for it to advance further, it was attached to a moving vehicle out of the Senate Finance Committee. As it turned out that vehicle proved to be the Affordable Care Act (ACA).

This was initially bipartisan legislation but by the time the final bill emerged from the Senate Finance Committee and included the Elder Justice Act it was entirely partisan to the extent that no Republican ended up voting for the ACA. This meant that the primary author of the bill Senator Hatch of Utah had to abandon his work on the EJA and shift to it the top cosponsor Senator Blanche Lincoln who guided the bill through Committee and to Senate floor. Senator Lincoln was greatly aided with support from the Obama Administration. President Obama's chief of staff at the time was former Congressman Rahm Emanuel who had authored the EJA in the House. He steered the EJA onto one of the President's signature bills.

The net result was a mixed victory. The bill became law however this historically bipartisan bill ended up in the Affordable Care Act which was reviled by Republicans, thus making the ability to properly fund the EJA very difficult in the future.

Opponents of the bill were known and unknown. Known opponents included the Bush Administration and fiscal conservatives who wanted no new programs. The opponents not as obvious but evident included some in the domestic violence world who felt that funding elder abuse might compete with resources dedicated to their cause. In addition there was some opposition registered about the EJA's emphasis on a dedicated funding stream for Adult Protective Services especially from those in Congress who came from weak APS states.

The reality is passage of any new legislation in the political environment between 2003 and 2010 would be difficult. We were entering a recession with deep deficits and the idea of new funds being provided was even more difficult. In the end consistent national and grass roots advocacy combined with great Congressional champions and the Obama Administration made it happen and the Elder Justice Act became the law of the land in March 2010.

Some elder abuse activities are funded through the Affordable Care Act Prevention and Public Health Fund (PPHF). In FY 2012, the Department of Health and Human Services transferred $6 million to the Administration for Community Living (ACL) from the PPHF for new grants focused on elder abuse prevention strategies. Following that, a transfer of $2 million in FY 2013, no funds transferred in FY 2014 and a presidential budget request in FY 2015 for $25 million in discretionary funds for an Elder Justice Initiative [4]. The $2 million transferred to ACL from PPHF in FY 2013 was used for the National Adult Protective Services (APS) Data Reporting System Project, which lasted two years [4].

The enactment of the EJA put elder abuse on the same level as the Child Abuse Prevention and Treatment Act and Violence Against Women Act [4]. As mentioned earlier, elder abuse awareness received more attention when The Department of Justice Reauthorization Act of 2005 amended the VAWA of 1994 to authorize grants for programs that supported those over the age of 50 who had experienced elder abuse, neglect, and/or exploitation [14].

However, funding of elder mistreatment continues to fall far behind child and domestic violence protections [10]. In a Government Accountability Office (GAO) report issued in 2011, statistics from 2010 indicate that average expenditures per child resident for Child Protective Services (CPS) was $45.03 while the average expense for Adult Protective Services was $3.90 [2]. In March 2011, the GAO reported on funding given to elder abuse research in 2009 and found little being expended [20]. For instance, the National Institute on Aging (NIA) spent $1.1 million that year which was just 1/1000th of its total budget. Similarly, the Centers for Disease Control and Prevention (CDC), spent $50,000 total representing just 0.0008 % of its budget compared to the millions spent on child abuse and domestic violence that same year [20]. Finally, the Office of Victims of Crimes (OVC) spent 0.5 % of its budget on older adult abuse victims [20].

On October 11, 2012, the Department of Health and Human Services Secretary initiated the first meeting of the Elder Justice Coordinating Council. The EJA mandated the creation of a Federal Elder Justice Coordinating Council to include the heads of key government agencies [4]. The Council includes members of the Department of Health and Human Services, the Justice Department and other federal agencies that lead efforts to combat elder abuse [14]. The Administration for Community Living (ACL) is responsible for implementing the Council [4].

At the inaugural meeting of the Council in October 2012, there were four topics identified as primary action areas including financial exploitation, public policy and awareness, enhancing response and advancing research [14]. Since then, the Council has convened three meetings. At the May 2014 meeting, the Council agreed to a set of eight recommendations for increased federal involvement [4]. According to the Administration on Aging the first four recommendations were trying to accomplish an improved response to elder abuse and the last four recommendations aimed to improve awareness and prevention. The recommendations were [21]:

- *Support the Investigation and Prosecution of Elder Abuse Cases* by disseminating training and resource materials to local, state and federal investigators and prosecutors.
- *Enhance Services to Elder Abuse Victims* by increasing identification of elder abuse and improving response and outreach to those afflicted.
- *Develop a National Adult Protect Services (APS) System* established through standardized data collection and a primary set of service provision standards and essential practices
- *Develop a Federal Elder Justice Research Agenda* that spans across federal agencies in order to seek out best practices for protecting elders against abuse and financial exploitation
- *Develop a Broad-Based Public Awareness Campaign* that is both comprehensive and strategic to clearly communicate about awareness and understanding of elder abuse, neglect, and exploitation to the general public
- *Cross-disciplinary Training on Elder Abuse* created to educate multidisciplinary stakeholders on preventing, identifying, intervening in and reacting to elder abuse, neglect, and exploitation
- *Combat Elder Financial Exploitation, including Abuse by Fiduciaries* through federal enforcement, public policy changes, coordination, regulation, and education by working industry to improve fraud detection and provide resource support to victims
- *Improve Screening for Dementia and Cognitive Capacity, Financial Capacity, and Financial Exploitation* by equipping APS and first responders with the skills necessary to identify impairment, diminished financial capacity, and susceptibility to or experience of financial exploitation.

The Elder Justice Act authorization expired at the end of FY 2014. In February 2015, representative Peter King (R-NY) and eight cosponsors introduced H.R. 988, the Elder Justice Reauthorization Act. The Act amends the Patient Protection and Affordable Care Act to reauthorize the following through FY2019: (1) the National Training Institute for Federal and State Surveyors, and (2) grants by the Secretary of Health and Human Services to state agencies that perform surveys of skilled nursing facilities or nursing facilities [22]. As of today, the Elder Justice Act has received $4 million in direct appropriation, of the $25 million requested, in funding through the FY 2015 Appropriations Bill under President Barack Obama.

In 2011, a National Adult Protection Services (NAPSRC) Resource Center was created through a discretionary grant award given to the National Adult Protective Services Association (NAPSA) by the AoA. Adult Protective Services (APS) is the only entity that is statutorily authorized and responsible for investigating elder and vulnerable adult abuse [23]. The goal of APS is to offer a system for reporting and investigating abuse and assisting victims with finding social services [4]. Federal policy established APS with the 1975 enactment of Title XX of Social Security Act [4]. Currently, APS relies solely on state funding decisions and has no national standards and little research on national APS practices [7]. The NAPSRC works with the National Association of States United for Aging and Disabilities (NASUAD) to research APS programs nationally [7]. There are two primary federal funding sources for elder abuse research: the National Institute of Justice and the National Institute on Aging [1].

In April 2012, the Department of Health and Human Services (HHS) created the Administration for Community Living (ACL) which brought together the Office on Disability and the Administration on Developmental Disabilities in order "...to better align the federal programs that address the community living service and support needs of both the aging and disability populations..." [14]. The mission of the ACL is to serve individuals living with disabilities and older adults by supporting their right to live where they feel most comfortable and can actively engage in their communities. Within the ACL, there is the Office of Elder Justice and Adult Protective Services which, "...manages the operation, administration, and assessment of elder abuse prevention, legal assistance development, and pension counseling programs funded through the OAA and leads the development and implementation of comprehensive Adult Protective Service systems in order to provide a coordinated and seamless response for helping adult victims of abuse and to prevent abuse before it happens" [24]. This office also supports the Elder Justice Coordinating Council mandated by the EJA.

In late 2014, President Obama signed the FY2015 spending bill which included record funding for the Victims of Crime Act (VOCA). Funding was increased from $700 million to $2.36 billion in order to support crime victim services and compensation nationwide [25]. The Victims of Crime Act was passed in 1984 to fund victim services fines and fees that are paid by the offenders. During the 2015

White House Conference on Aging, a final VOCA assistance rule was announced by the U.S. Department of Justice (DOJ) that will be released by the end of 2015 to revise current guidelines so that VOCA funds can be used to support services for underserved victims such as older adults who have suffered from abuse, financial exploitation, fraud, and neglect.

27.4 Elder Justice Advocacy Chronology

In 1978 the Subcommittee on the House Select Committee on Aging held its first hearing on elder abuse [26]. The hearing that year was chaired by Rep. Mario Biaggi (D-NY) [10]. Other public hearings in the 1970s were initiated by Rep. Claude Pepper (D-FL) [10]. According to the National Adult Protective Services Association, Rep. Claude Pepper suggested in 1985 that, "Congress should act immediately to assist the states in preventing, identifying and assisting our nation's elder abuse victims." By that point in time, there were a total of 46 states in America that had a state office responsible for leading Adult Protective Services [27].

Since the 1980s, Dr. Rosalie S. Wolf was considered a pioneer in the elder abuse field and in 1988 Dr. Wolf founded the National Committee for the Prevention of Elder Abuse. Dr. Wolf launched the Journal of Elder Abuse and Neglect in 1989, as the official publication of the National Committee for Prevention of Elder Abuse [1]. The Journal of Elder Abuse and Neglect is widely considered the primary source of scholarly information on elder abuse [28].

The White House Conference on Aging (WHCOA) in 1995, entitled "The Road to an Aging Policy for the 21th Century," was led by Executive Director Robert Blancato and focused on elder abuse as an important topic of discussion. According to the National Academy on an Aging Society, resolution 20 of this WHCOA was preventing elder abuse, exploitation and neglect [29]. According to the administration at the time in response to this resolution, the White House would support policies that fully fund the Older Americans Act, create a national public awareness campaign, require states to pick a single agency to address elder abuse, implement training and education of professionals working with older adults about abuse, increase authority of the Long-Term Care Ombudsman program and encourage public/private partnerships to conduct research on elder abuse and mistreatment [29].

In 1997, the International Network for the Prevention of Elder Abuse (INPEA) was founded [30]. The INPEA created its mission statement and objectives in 1998. The objectives of INPEA are to (a) promote education and training of professionals and para-professionals in identification, treatment, and prevention, (b) further advocacy on behalf of abused and neglected elders, and (c) stimulate research into the cause, consequences, prevalence, treatment, and prevention of elder abuse and neglect [20]. The organization was incorporated by Dr. Wolf in 1998 and went on to achieve nonprofit, non-governmental organization (NGO) status with the United Nations in 2003 [30]. This status with the UN allows INPEA to have 2 or 3 min at every other UN session to speak [20]. The INPEA continues to present the Rosalie Wolf Memorial award each year to a person that has demonstrated a dedication to preventing elder abuse through policy, practice, research or education [30].

The first National Summit on Elder Abuse took place in December 2001 and was organized by the National Center on Elder Abuse. It was tasked with recommending a national policy agenda for protecting America's most at risk elders. Ten essential priorities were identified and adopted [31]:

Priority 1 *Support a National Elder Abuse Act* to be enacted by Congress in order to accomplish a clear national policy on elder victimization. The law would build a national communication and funding structure to better coordinate elder protection, provide training for technical assistance for the government and business sectors, and develop a grant program to create a database on elder abuse to be used to influence future policy making.

Priority 2 *Mount a National Education and Awareness Effort* in order to achieve widespread public understanding of the crimes committed against older adults. Some actions toward fulfilling this goal include creation of a National Elder Abuse Awareness Month, a national toll-free 800 assistance phone number, and the establishment of a national archive of stories cataloguing experiences of elder abuse.

Priority 3 *Improve the Legal Landscape by Strengthening Elder Abuse Laws* so that the justice system clearly understands the unique situation of the vulnerable victims of elder abuse as well as the types of crimes committed by the abusers. With this fresh framework in mind, old laws should be amended and new laws created that better serve to protect victims and increase effectiveness of investigations and prosecutions.

Priority 4 *Develop and Implement a National Elder Abuse Training Curriculum* in order to better equip professionals and first responders with the tools they need to achieve the best outcomes for victims of elder abuse. The curriculum should include teaching modules and be developed with the input of key stakeholders and funds made available to create coalitions for these individuals to collaborate and share best practices nationally, regardless of geographic location.

Priority 5 *Ensure Age-appropriate, Specialized Mental Health Services are Available and Accessible* so that older adults vulnerable to abuse and those who have experienced it, can receive the crisis care and support they need to protect their health and well being. This goal can be achieved by increasing team-based specialized clinicians providing care, creating rehabilitation programs for abusers, establishing process for accurate treatment, and diagnosis of dementia and investing in crisis intervention resources.

Priority 6 *Commission a General Accounting Office (GAO) Study* in order to best assess how well federal programs are fighting elder abuse and how this can inform future public policy and budget decisions. The study would ascertain areas of weakness and in so doing identify opportunities for new research. It would track the use of federal funds like the Social Services Block Grant and review the effectiveness of statutes and regulations.

Priority 7 *Increase Awareness within Justice System* so that victims of elder abuse are fully protected and abusers face punishment that dissuades them from attempting future crimes against this vulnerable population. This can be achieved by raising awareness in the justice system about the needs of victims and creating a comprehensive system of policies and procedures that results in a coordinated response by all parties involved.

Priority 8 *Establish a National Institute on Aging (NIA) Research and Program Innovation Institute* in order to accomplish the establishment of a comprehensive database that identifies the current scope of elder abuse nationally and the obstacles faced by APS in responding timely and effectively.

Priority 9 *Invest in a National Resource Center on Adult Protective Services (APS)* to better support the direct care workers advocating for elders on the front lines through increased capacity and more effective service support. This can be accomplished with the establishment of a national certification system for APS workers as well as a training system that educates staff on best practices.

Priority 10 *Seek Presidential Executive Order* which would instruct all federal organizations, and encourage governors, to take a closer look at the strengths and weaknesses of current government wide policies in place to protect victims of elder abuse. The order would involve the creation of a report outlining the findings from this analysis and suggestions for improvement.

It is worth noting that priorities 1, 6, and 9 were specifically achieved and several more of these recommendations saw important progress made since the summit.

The Senate Special Committee on Aging has held many hearings on elder abuse dating back to the early 2000s and it was the culmination of these hearings that formed the basis for the introduction of the Elder Justice Act. Although the committee does not have legislative authority it can study issues, conduct oversight programs, and investigate reports of fraud and waste [32].

The hearings on elder abuse by the committee include:

- Elder Fraud and Abuse: New Challenges in the Digital Economy, Portland OR (2000)
- Saving Our Seniors: Preventing Elder Abuse, Neglect, and Exploitation (2001)
- Safeguarding Our Seniors: Protecting the Elderly from Physical and Sexual Abuse in Nursing Homes (2002)
- Shattering the Silence: Confronting the Perils of Family Elder Abuse (2003)
- Old Scams-New Victims: Breaking the Cycle of Victimization (2005)
- Abuse of our Elders: How We Can Stop It (2007).

On March 2, 2011, the Senate Special Committee on Aging convened a hearing on elder abuse entitled "Justice for All: Ending Elder Abuse, Neglect and Exploitation" [3]. The opening statement at the hearing was given by Senator Herb Kohl (D-WI), which outlined the importance of federal, state and local agencies coming together to work cohesively and prevent elder abuse. The late actor Mickey Rooney testified at this hearing as a victim of elder abuse and The Elder Abuse Victims Act was reintroduced, though ultimately it did not get enacted [33].

In addition, hearings on elder abuse were held by the Senate Finance Committee, the Senate Health Education Labor and Pensions Committee, as well as the House Judiciary Committees.

27.5 Elder Justice Coalition (EJC)

In February 2003, the Elder Justice Coalition (EJC) was founded, to coincide with the introduction of the Elder Justice Act (S.333), as a non-partisan coalition of 3,000 members. The Coalition has five founding organizational members: The National Committee for the Prevention of

Elder Abuse (NCPEA), the National Academy of Elder Law Attorneys (NAELA), the National Association of State Units on Aging (NASUA), the National Association of Adult Protect Service Administrators (NAAPSA), and the National Association of State Long-Term Care Ombudsman Programs (NASOP). According to the EJC's statement of principles, the organization was created based on the belief that, "Victims of elder abuse need to have their voices heard and issues addressed. An adequate public–private infrastructure and resources need to be in place to prevent detect, treat, understand, intervene in and, where appropriate, prosecute elder abuse, neglect, and exploitation" [34].

The EJC has become a critical resource to Congress, the administration and media organizations. They have done this by focusing on specific goals and activities including [34]:

- Increase public awareness of the tragedy of elder abuse, neglect and exploitation at the local, state, and national levels
- Increase awareness, support, and funding for the Elder Justice Act in the Senate and House of Representatives as a comprehensive approach to addressing elder justice issues
- Monitor and appropriately influence other relevant legislation and regulations that pertain to the prevention of elder abuse, neglect and financial exploitation.

One main accomplishment of the EJC has been its work in advancing The Elder Justice Act with a particular focus from 2003 until the act became law in 2010. During that time, the EJC's National Coordinator, Robert Blancato, testified on several occasions before Congress on behalf of elder justice. The EJC helped secure not only the passage of the EJA into law but also the Elder Abuse Victims act in the House of Representatives. The advocacy of the EJC included testimony before the Elder Justice Coordinating Council, The Institute of Medicine and in 2015 at the first Summit on Elder Abuse held by the SEC. The EJC's work led to the establishment of The Office of Older Americans in the bill creating the Consumer Financial Protection Bureau. Additionally, their work involved being a resource to members of Congress on a bipartisan basis to introduce legislation related to elder justice and elder abuse prevention.

Elder abuse received further visibility in December 2005 at the WHCOA program in Washington D.C. entitled "The Booming Dynamics of Aging-From Awareness to Action" [10]. There were 1200 appointed delegates who attended the conference and more than 130,000 American citizens who assisted in the planning and execution of the gathering [35]. The first goal of the program was to reexamine local, state and federal budgets in a way that fosters innovation and outlines priorities that allow our country to strategically and effectively serve our growing population of elders. The second objective was to recognize that services and supports to older adults must be undertaken in a collaborative manner across the public and private sector by identifying what is working nationally and building on those successes [35]. The fifteenth resolution of the fifty adopted by conference delegates was "Protection from Abuse and Neglect" which, according to the report to the President, would mean that the country, "Create a national strategy for promoting elder justice through the prevention and prosecution of elder abuse." In the remainder of the Report to the President and the Congress about the proceedings elder abuse and justice figured prominently in the implementation strategies outlined [35].

In 2006, elder justice language provisions were incorporated in the Older Americans Act (OAA) reauthorization [4]. Under the OAA, the Administration on Aging (AoA) has primary federal responsibility for carrying out elder justice activities. The AoA has provided more than forty years of support and leadership on strengthening elder justice programming nationally [36].

World Elder Abuse Awareness Day (WEAAD) was created out of the International Network for the Prevention of Elder Abuse's (INPEA) desire to have one full day dedicated to support and respect for older adults and their human right to live in abuse free communities [36]. In New York City on June 15, 2006, the inaugural WEAAD was initiated as more than 150 people gathered at the United Nations [36]. The first official White House recognition of World Elder Abuse Awareness Day occurred in June 2012 [28]. The first global summit of WEADD took place on June 15, 2015 at the U.S. Securities and Exchange Commission to celebrate the 10th anniversary of WEADD. The event was led by the National Adult Protective Services Association, the National Center for Victims of Crime, and the International Network for the Prevention of Elder Abuse.

As elder abuse and justice became a part of our national dialogue, more opportunities to advocate for the importance of protecting older adults arose in both the policy and research fields. In June 2010, the National Institute on Aging (NIA) and the National Academy of Sciences (NAS) led a state-of-science conference about elder abuse and neglect that aimed to focus on significant research conducted and the need for new analysis and investigation [3]. Advocacy against elder abuse received further support when the UN General Assembly, on December 19, 2011, officially recognized elder abuse as a global social issue affecting the well being and human rights of millions of older adults [20].

Several years later, on April 17 and 18, 2013, the Institute of Medicine's (IOM) Forum on Global Violence Prevention held a two-day workshop on the state of elder abuse globally and strategies for its prevention [20]. The IOM was established in 1970 by the National Academy of Sciences and the organization acts as an advisor to the federal government on issues relating to medical care, research, and education. The goal of the workshop according to the summary report was to "...determine the global and multi-sectoral evidence-based approaches to preventing elder mistreatment" [20]. Speakers during the workshop addressed the prevalence of elder abuse globally by focusing on how elder mistreatment, such as physical, sexual, emotional and financial abuse, affects individuals, families, communities and society at large [20].

With the support of the Department of Justice (DOJ) and the Department of Health and Human Services (HHS), the Elder Justice Roadmap framework was announced on July 8, 2014.

The Roadmap was created as a call to action for the public to understand the most immediate needs in the fight against elder abuse. The necessary domains of action identified in the Roadmap are direct services, policy, education, and research. In addition to the domains, the framework outlined its top five priorities for understanding and reducing elder abuse which include awareness, brain health, caregiving, economics and resources. The authors of the document conclude that, "*The Elder Justice Roadmap*" is a groundbreaking partnership-among those who work primarily to address elder abuse and critical allies in related field to apply a wider lens to elder abuse in drafting this first national strategic plan for elder justice. This document reflects priorities that hundreds of practitioners identified as important and leading experts deemed critical and attainable [37].

On January 28, 2015, the Senate Health, Education, Labor and Pensions (HELP) Committee approved a three-year reauthorization of the Older Americans Act. The Senate passed S.192, Older Americans Act Reauthorization Act of 2015 on July 16, 2015 without opposition. This effort was led by Chairman Alexander (R-TN) with support from Ranking Member Murray (D-WA) and Sen. Sanders (I-VT) and Sen. Burr (R-NC). Several key components of the bill are provisions for modernizing multipurpose senior centers, addressing economic needs, promoting evidence-based health promotion and disease prevention and support for chronic disease self-management and falls prevention. Importantly, the bill includes strong elder justice and legal services provisions to protect older adults [38].

On July 13, 2015, President Barack Obama was the first president to mention elder abuse in his address at the White House Conference on Aging (WHCOA), and elder justice was one of four primary focus areas during the conference proceedings. The other key discussion topics were retirement security, technology and healthy aging. Typically, the OAA mandates that the WHCOA happens every 10 years but because the OAA hasn't been reauthorized since 2011 the White House decided to proceed with the gathering but without funding from Congress to do so. In the past, thousands of delegates from across the country would descend on the nation's capital for several days of policy debate and discussion whereas the 2015 WHCOA was held for one day with only 200 invited guests. Executive Director of the conference, Nora Super, tried to broaden the audience and opportunities for discussion by holding five regional forums leading up to the conference. These forums took place in Tampa, Florida, Phoenix, Arizona, Seattle, Washington, Cleveland, Ohio and Boston, Massachusetts.

The topic of elder justice during the conference was addressed during the "Elder Justice in the Twenty-First Century" panel moderated by Assistant Secretary for Aging and Administrator at the Administration for Community Living, Kathy Greenlee. Several policy initiatives were announced in relation to elder mistreatment including, the National Institute of Health's (NIH) convening of an elder abuse workshop with research and clinicians to take place in the fall of 2015, the Department of Justice (DOJ) funding of a multiyear pilot project to evaluate current strategies for responding to and avoiding elder abuse and the Consumer Financial Protect Bureau's (CFPB) commitment to assisting financial institutions in recognizing, preventing, and reporting elder financial abuse.

The Administration for Community Living (ACL) also announced important policy initiatives in conjunction with the 2015 WHCOA. For instance, the ACL has funded an Elder Abuse Prevention Interventions Program that tests the effectiveness of current programs combating elder abuse. They also plan to complete the National Adult Maltreatment Reporting System by September 2015 and the Department of Health and Human Services will then award 10 states up to $3 million to test the new platform. Finally, the ACL is committed to creating evidence-based national standards for improving Adult Protective Services (APS) organizations and plans to complete its final guidelines in December 2015 for the National Voluntary APS System Guidelines Development Project [39].

27.6 Elder Justice Triumphs and Struggles

The elder justice movement to date has seen some important triumphs while also encountering certain setbacks toward reaching its full potential. The greatest accomplishment thus far is the Elder Justice Act (EJA) being signed into law by President Barack Obama in March 2010. This capped a seven-year legislative journey involving both the House and the Senate. The support of the Obama Administration was crucial as was the persistent advocacy work done at the national, state and grass roots level led by the bipartisan Elder Justice Coalition.

Since the enactment of EJA other accomplishments have been achieved, some related to the legislation and others separate from it. Among these successes are the creation and convening of the Elder Justice Coordinating Council that makes recommendations to the Secretary of Health and Human Services, the establishment of a first time Office of Elder Justice in the Department of Health and Human Services as well as this being the first time federal home for Adult Protective Services (APS). Another accomplishment to note includes the creation of an APS Resource Center and Elder Abuse Resource Center, the Department of Justice Roadmap project and the work done by the Institute of Medicine toward global acknowledgement of elder abuse and justice. The Centers for Medicare and Medicaid services have also incorporated a measurement of maltreatment within the Physician Quality Reporting System (PQRS).

President Obama's elevation of World Elder Abuse Awareness Day (WEAAD) to being the subject of a Presidential proclamation was an important accomplishment for focusing attention on the global nature of this issue.

Furthermore, in 2000 the Violence Against Women Act (VAWA) language was amended to provide funds to increase protection of older adults and individuals living with disabilities against abuse, neglect, and exploitation resulting in another victory for the elder justice movement.

More recently, the 2015 White House Conference on Aging made elder justice one of only four priority issues to illustrate the growing importance of this topic as a policy concern. A number of important initiatives were announced that day and their implementation in the remaining time of the current Administration will add to the triumphs of the elder justice movement.

Another critically important success was a call by the President for the Department of Justice to issue a final rule by the end of 2015 to revise current Victims of Crime Act (VOCA) Victim Assistance Guidelines to clarify that victim assistance funds may be used to support legal services for crime victims and to emphasize the needs to use VOCA funds to support social and legal services to underserved victims including elder victims of abuse, financial exploitation, fraud and neglect (Fig. 27.1). The significance of this rests with the fact that in late 2014 Congress voted to add $1.6 billion in new funds for VOCA.

Finally the work of both advocates and the media in getting more national attention focused on federal actions started around elder abuse prevention is another important success. The fact that elder justice is and has always been bipartisan is vitally important.

For all that has been accomplished in the elder justice national space, we are still far from where we should be. First, in order to move forward in combating elder abuse on a national scale and providing critical resources and programs to victims, we must renew the Older Americans Act (OAA) as well as the Elder Justice Act (EJA). In addition to renewing the EJA, it is crucial that all provisions of the law are implemented as well. Furthermore, the cause would be advanced greatly if the Elder Abuse Victims Act (EAVA) passed the Senate.

Despite advances in research and data collection focused on elder abuse and justice, we still lack a coordinated and national system for reporting and cataloguing abuse. The research that has been done is frequently not translated into programs and practices that can be applied in the field.

Although the amended language of the VAWA showed support for protecting older adults against abuse, there is still a failure to gain widespread support for this issue from the domestic violence community. The justice system is also lagging in its support as we have failed to gain resources to expand the criminal justice system to combat elder abuse. This issue is perpetuated by the fact that states are not responding appropriately to criminal background checks of those caring for older adults.

The best example of the struggles faced by the elder justice movement relates to funding of the Elder Justice Act and especially the failure to get dedicated funding stream for APS. The EJA became law 36 years after the Child Abuse Prevention and Treatment Act (CAPTA) became law. CAPTA has received billions of dollars in funding during that time. The EJA after 5 years has seen just over $10 million in funds provided including a first time Congressional appropriation of $4 million in 2014. At the time the EJA was first introduced one of the rationales was that all of the funds we were spending on abuse prevention a decade or so ago, less than 2 % was dedicated to elder abuse. We have many millions of dollars to go for sure. The EJA will be most fulfilled when a dedicated funding stream for APS is accomplished.

The reality that the EJA must be renewed has to be addressed, and a more concerted effort must be undertaken by both the House and Senate during this Congress (Table 27.1).

The national elder justice movement has come a long way over the past dozen years. Yet there is no one associated with the movement that believes that we have done enough. Elder justice in America will not be achieved until we genuinely prevent elder abuse. It will take better use of existing resources but also an infusion of new funding at all levels. The protection of older adults from the ravages of abuse must be a stronger national policy and political priority.

27.7 Future of the Elder Justice Movement

As we close 2015 we note that the state of the elder justice movement is somewhere between making further advancements and being stalled when it comes to achieving more progress. The future of the elder justice movement does depend on a number of short and longer term factors.

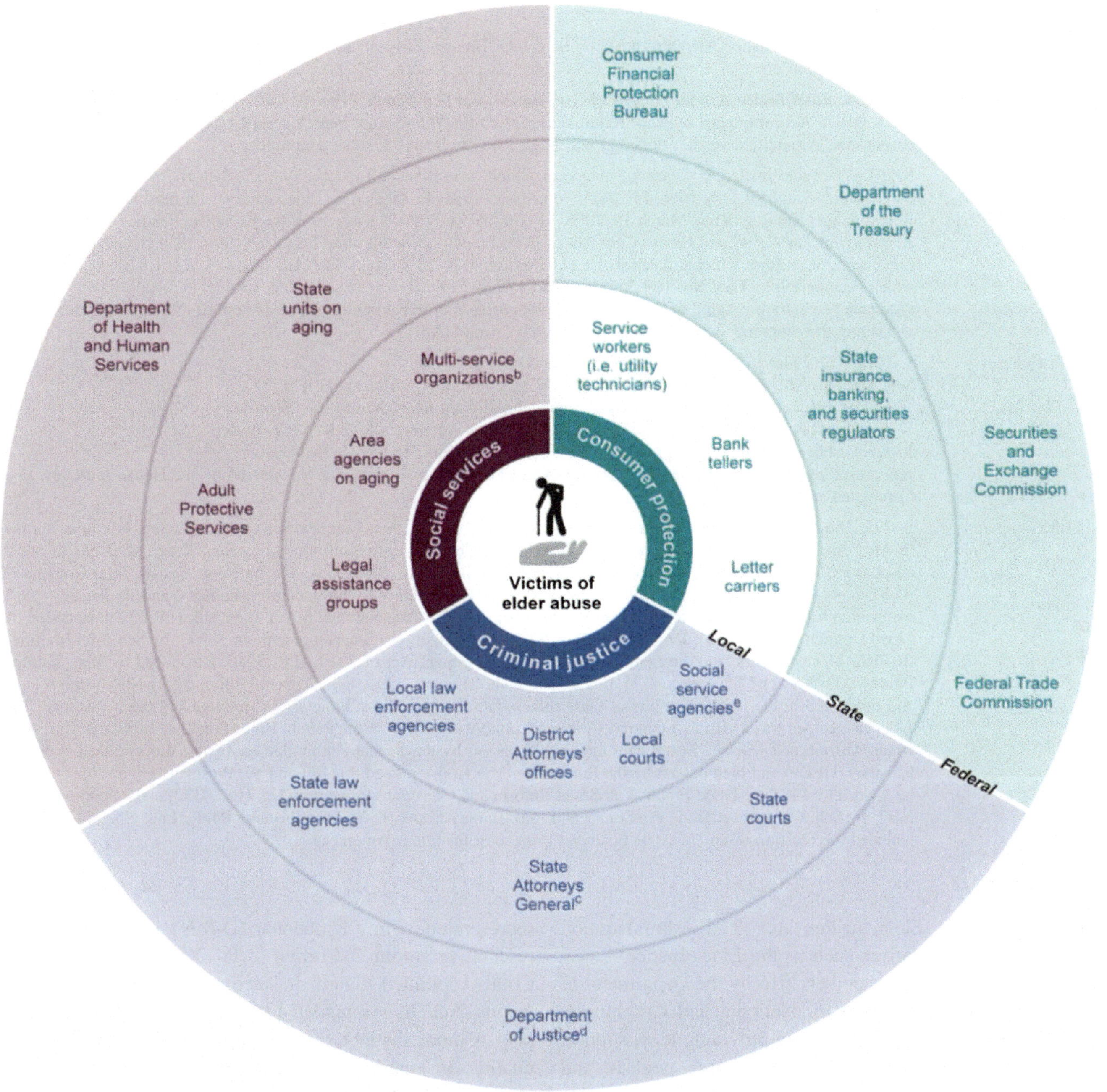

Fig. 27.1 Federal agencies with missions that involve combating elder financial exploitation [14]

The first factor is getting as much from the Obama Administration as possible in its last year. The majority of progress made in the movement has occurred during this Administration and there is much more it can do. The release of new rules on use of Victims of Crime Act funds by the end of the year could be the most significant action that can be taken. This could authorize the use of more funds for victim and legal services for elder abuse victims and if it is accompanied by new resources it will be that much more significant.

The President in his final budget to Congress should dramatically increase his request for funding an Elder Justice Initiative and then make it a priority to fight for its approval by Congress. His highest request to date has been $25 million. A request of $100 million would be most appropriate.

The Administration should move where it can on the recommendations of both the Elder Justice Coordinating Council and the Roadmap project of the Department of Justice. In addition, by executive order it should name and convene the civilian based Advisory Board on elder abuse

Table 27.1 Elder Justice Act Legislative Timeline [41]

107th Congress	S.2933 The Elder Justice Act, introduced by Sen. John Breaux (D-La.) and Sen. Orrin Hatch (R-Utah), September 12, 2002, 17 cosponsors
108th Congress	S.333 The Elder Justice Act, introduced by Sen. Breaux and Sen. Hatch, Feb. 10, 2003, 43 cosponsors; H.R. 2490, The Elder Justice Act introduced by Rep. Rahm Emanuel (D-Ill.-5) and Rep. Peter King (R-N.Y.-3), June 17, 2003, 91 cosponsors. A modified version of S.333 was passed by the Senate Finance Committee
109th Congress	S. 2010 The Elder Justice Act, introduced by Sen. Hatch, Sen. Blanche Lincoln (D-Ark.), Sen. Herb Kohl (D-Wis.), and Sen. Gordon Smith (R-Or.), Nov. 15, 2005, 30 cosponsors; H.R. 4993, The Elder Justice Act, introduced by Rep. Emanuel and Rep. King, March 16, 2006, 51 cosponsors. S. 2010 was passed by the Senate Finance Committee. H. R. 6111, the Tax Relief and Health Care Act of 2006, which became Public Law No. 109-432, included a study on establishing a uniform national database on elder abuse. H.R. 6197, the Older Americans Act Amendments of 2006, which became Public Law No. 109-365, included several provisions related to elder justice, including directing the Assistant Secretary on Aging to develop a comprehensive plan for an elder justice system in the United States, and expanding the programs on elder abuse in Title VII of the OAA
110th Congress	S. 1070, The Elder Justice Act of 2008, introduced by Sen. Hatch Sen. Lincoln, Sen. Kohl, and Sen. Smith, March 29, 2007, 33 cosponsors; H.R. 1783 The Elder Justice Act, introduced by Rep. Emanuel and Rep. King, March 29, 2007, 122 cosponsors. Also introduced was the Elder Abuse Victims Act of 2008, H.R. 5352 by Rep Joseph Sestak (D-Pa.-7) on February 12, 2008, four cosponsors. The Elder Justice Act was passed by the Senate Finance Committee. The Elder Abuse Victims Act was passed by the House Judiciary Committee and the full House
111th Congress	S. 795, The Elder Justice Act of 2009, introduced by Sen. Hatch, Sen. Lincoln, Sen. Kohl, and Sen. Olympia Snowe (R-Me.) April 2, 2009, 16 cosponsors; H.R. 2006, The Elder Justice Act, introduced by Rep. King, April 21, 2009, 73 cosponsors. Also introduced were the: Elder Abuse Victims Act of 2008, H.R. 448 by Reps. Sestak, John Conyers (D-Mich.-14), King, and Robert "Bobby" Scott (D-Va.-3) on January 9, 2009, four cosponsors, and its Senate companion bill by Sen. Kohl, four cosponsors, October 21, 2009; the National Silver Alert bill, H.R.632, introduced by Lloyd Doggett (D-Texas-25), January 22, 2009, 22 cosponsors, and its Senate companion S. 557, by Sen. Mel Martinez (R-Fla.), 11 cosponsors, and the Senior Financial Empowerment Act of 2010, H.R. 3040, introduced by Rep. Tammy Baldwin (D-Wis.-2) 17 cosponsors, and its Senate companion, S. 3494, Sen. Kirsten Gillibrand (D-N.Y.), one cosponsor. All of the House versions of these three bills were passed by Judiciary Committee and the full House. The Elder Justice Act was added to the Senate Finance Committee version of the Patient Protection and Affordable Care Act, which was merged with the health care reform bill passed by the Senate Committee on Health, Education, Labor and Pensions (HELP) and then passed by the full Senate. The House passed this bill and the President signed it into Public Law No. 111-148. The Dodd-Frank Wall Street Reform and Consumer Protection Act, H.R. 4173, and its companion S. 3217, by Sen. Christopher Dodd (D-Conn.) and Rep. Barney Frank (D-Mass.-4) became Public Law No. 111-203, and included the creation of an Office of Financial Protection for Older Americans

called for in the Elder Justice Act. The Administration should build on initiatives such as the Elder Justice AmeriCorps, announced in September 2015 by the Department of Justice and the Corporation for National and Community Service (CNCS), as a grant program providing legal support and services to victims of elder abuse, neglect and exploitation [40]. They must look for other interagency initiatives that can be activated to help promote elder justice.

In Congress, more champions of elder justice need to emerge. A variety of important bills have been introduced in this 114th session of Congress. These include the Elder Justice Reauthorization Act (H.R.988) sponsored by representative Peter King (R-NY) and the Robert Matava Elder Abuse Victims Act of 2015 (S.1663) sponsored by senator Richard Blumenthal (D-CT).

The future of elder justice must also include a deeper involvement in the issue of guardianship. While often thought of as a state issue, the introduction of bipartisan legislation in each of the past three sessions of Congress changes this dynamic. The bill S. 975 sponsored by representative Amy Klobuchar (D-MN) and cosponsor representative John Cornyn (R-TX) is entitled the Court-Appointed Guardian Accountability and Senior Protection Act. It is intended to have the federal government play a more distinct role in improving access to and the quality of guardianships across the country. This is an important issue for the future.

Finally, the future of elder justice is about linkages. Elder abuse must be viewed as the public health crisis it is. Elder abuse prevention must be seen as a key element in long-term services and supports. Elder abuse prevention activities should be 'scored' to demonstrate how much they might save Medicare and to a lesser extent Medicaid. We should link elder abuse with issues like malnutrition and hunger because of its impact on those who are self neglecting.

If demographics are destiny then we are destined to have a grave elder abuse crisis in the future. Today, the average victim of elder abuse is an older woman living alone between the age of 75 and 80. In the United States, half of all women 75 years and older live alone. The amount that victims of elder financial abuse lose each year has jumped from close to $3 billion to close to $35 billion according to one recent report. This movement needs to grow. It must be driven by the reality that elder justice is not achieved until elder abuse is prevented.

The future of elder justice must involve more systematic collaboration with the domestic violence community. As with the child abuse community, the elder justice advocates can learn from their policy successes over the years. At the same time better communication and understanding can benefit both communities. It is time to move away from concerns about competing for similar resources and instead work to increase those resources to help all.

The future of elder justice will be judged to some degree by how much better advocacy can be done. It will be about the need to have a sharper edge, a unified message, and deeper resources. Elder justice is a special interest movement. It just needs to start acting like one. We need to advocate at all levels —and complement it with political action. Any progress that has or can be made will be hard earned.

References

1. Anetzberger G. An update on the nature and scope of elder abuse. Gener Elder Abuse Elder Justice Mov Am. 2012;36(3):12–20.
2. Government Accountability Office. Elder justice: stronger federal leadership could enhance national response to elder abuse. Washington, DC: K. Brown; 2011.
3. Dong X. Elder abuse: research, practice, and policy. The 2012 GSA Maxwell Pollack award lecture. Gerontologist. 2013;54 (2):153–62.
4. Congressional Research Service. The elder justice act: background and issues for congress. Washington, DC: K. Colello; 2014.
5. Frolik L, Whitton S. Everyday law for seniors. Boulder, CO: Paradigm; 2012.
6. Acierno R, Hernandez-Tejada M, Muzzy W, Steve K. National elder mistreatment study. U.S. Department of Justice Grant Report, NCJ 226456. 2009. https://www.ncjrs.gov/pdffiles1/nij/grants/226456.pdf. Accessed 18 Oct 2015.
7. Ramsey-Klawsnik H, Teaster P. Sexual abuse happens in healthcare facilities—what can be done to prevent it? Gener Elder Abuse Elder Justice Mov Am. 2012;36(3):53–9.
8. Miller M. Ombudsmen on the front line: improving quality of care and preventing abuse in nursing homes. Gener Elder Abuse Elder Justice Mov Am. 2012;36(3):60–3.
9. MetLife Mature Market Institute. The metlife study of elder financial abuse: crimes of occasion, desperation, and predation against America's elders. 2011. Retrieved from https://www.metlife.com/assets/cao/mmi/publications/studies/2011/mmi-elder-financial-abuse.pdf. Accessed 18 Oct 2015.
10. Anetzberger G, Teaster P, Wangmo T. A glass half full: the dubious history of elder abuse policy. J Elder Abuse Negl. 2010;22 (1–2):6–15.
11. Ansello EF, O'Neill. Aging with lifelong disabilities. J Elder Abuse Negl. 2010;22(1–2):105–22.
12. National Association of States United for Aging and Disabilities. 2015. Retrieved from http://www.nasuad.org/policy/key-issues/elder-abuse. Accessed 18 Oct 2015.
13. Niles-Yokum K, Wagner DL. The aging networks: a guide to programs and services. New York, NY: Springer Publishing Company; 2011.
14. Government Accountability Office. Elder justice: more federal coordination and public awareness needed. Washington, DC: K. Brown; 2013.
15. Laney, G. Violence against women act: history and federal funding. CRS Report for Congress. RL30871; 2005.
16. Gateway Child Welfare Information. About CAPTA: a legislative history. Washington, DC: U.S. Department of Health and Human Services, Children's Bureau; 2011.
17. Blancato R. Foreword. J Elder Abuse Negl. 2010;22(1–2):1–2.
18. Chen E, Twomey M, Eliason S. In pursuit of a useful framework to champion elder justice. Gener Elder Abuse Elder Justice Mov Am. 2012;36(3):103–5.
19. National Center on Elder Abuse. 2015. Retrieved from http://www.ncea.aoa.gov/About/NCEA/History.aspx. Accessed 18 Oct 2015.
20. National Academies Press. Elder abuse and its prevention: workshop summary. Washington, DC: R.M. Taylor. 2014. Retrieved from http://www.nap.edu/catalog.php?record_id=18518. Accessed 18 Oct 2015.
21. Administration on Aging. 2015. Retrieved from http://www.aoa.acl.gov/AoA_Programs/Elder_Rights/EJCC/docs/Eight_Recommendations_for_Increased_Federal_Involvement.pdf. Accessed 18 Oct 2015.
22. GovTrack. Summaries for the elder justice reauthorization. 2015. Retrieved from https://www.govtrack.us/congress/bills/114/hr988/summary#/. Accessed 18 Oct 2015.
23. Benson M. Elder abuse and the elder justice movement. Gener Elder Abuse Elder Justice Mov Am. 2012;36(3):66–7.
24. Administration for Community Living. 2015. Retrieved from http://www.acl.gov/About_ACL/Organization/oc_explained.aspx. Accessed 18 Oct 2015.
25. National Center for Victims of Crime. 2015. Retrieved from http://www.victimsofcrime.org/Our-programs/public-policy. Accessed 18 Oct 2015.
26. Hood A. Elder abuse: it's (not) only words. Gener Elder Abuse Elder Justice Mov Am. 2012;36(3):4–5.
27. National Adult Protective Services. 2015. Retrieved from http://www.napsa-now.org/about-napsa/history/history-of-adult-protective-services. Accessed 18 Oct 2015.
28. Blancato R. Elder abuse and the elder justice movement. Gener Elder Abuse Elder Justice Mov Am. 2012;36(3):9–11.
29. National Academy on an Aging Society. White house conference on aging 1995. Resolutions. Preventing elder abuse, exploitation, and neglect. 1995. Retrieved from http://www.agingsociety.org/agingsociety/1995%20WHCOA%20Resolutions/resolution20.pdf. Accessed 18 Oct 2015.
30. Podnieks E, et al. Elder mistreatment: an international narrative. J Elder Abuse Negl. 2010;22(1–2):131–7.
31. National Center on Elder Abuse. 2002. Retrieved from http://www.ncea.aoa.gov/Resources/Publication/docs/agenda2002.pdf. Accessed 18 Oct 2015.
32. Special Committee on Aging. History. 2015. Retrieved from http://www.aging.senate.gov/about/history. Accessed 18 Oct 2015.
33. Special Committee on Aging. Justice for all: ending elder abuse, neglect and financial exploitation. 2015. Retrieved from http://www.aging.senate.gov/imo/media/doc/hr230hk.pdf. Accessed 18 Oct 2015.
34. The Elder Justice Coalition. 2015. Retrieved from: http://www.elderjusticecoalition.com/statement-of-principals. Accessed 18 Oct 2015.
35. The National Indian Council on Aging. Report to the president and the congress: the booming dynamics of aging, from action to awareness. 2005. Retrieved from: http://nicoa.org/wpcontent/

uploads/2014/05/2005-WHCOA-Final-Report.pdf. Accessed 18 Oct 2015.
36. Greenlee K. Take a stand against elder abuse. Gener Elder Abuse Elder Justice Mov Am. 2012;36(3):6–8.
37. The United States Department of Justice. 2015. Retrieved from http://www.justice.gov/Elderjustice/research/resources/EJRP_Roadmap.pdf. Accessed 18 Oct 2015.
38. National Council on Aging. 2015. Retrieved from http://www.ncoa.org/pbulic-policy-action/older-americans-act/senate/s-192. Accessed 18 Oct 2015.
39. Administration for Community Living. 2015. Retrieved from http://www.acl.gov/NewsRoom/NewsInfo/2015/2015_07_30.aspx. Accessed 18 Oct 2015.
40. Department of Justice. 2015. Retrieved from: http://www.justice.gov/opa/pr/justice-department-and-corporation-national-and-community-service-expand-their-partnership. Accessed 18 Oct 2015.
41. Lindberg B, Sabatino C, Blancato R. Bringing national action to a national disgrace: the history of the elder justice act. Natl Acad Elder Law Attorneys J. 2011;7(1).

Senate Special Committee on Aging Hearings and GAO Reports 28

Shelly L. Jackson

28.1 Senate Special Committee on Aging Hearings and GAO Reports

Some scholars assert that the federal government has not played a substantial role—financial or otherwise—in elder abuse [28, 56, 70]. Historically, elder abuse has been a state issue, with ambivalence characterizing the federal government's role in it [60]. As one relevant and meaningful pipeline to federal legislation on elder abuse [44], this chapter assesses the role and impact of the Senate Special Committee on Aging (referred to hereafter as the Committee) and commissioned reports generated by the General Accounting Office (GAO), and where appropriate, describes the social, political, and economic context in which the Committee hearings emerged.

28.2 Creation and Purpose of the Senate Special Committee on Aging

In 1958, Congressman Patrick McNamara (D-Mich) sent a letter to the Committee on Labor and Public Welfare proposing the creation of a Subcommittee on Aging and the Aged.[1] In that letter, McNamara briefly described the plight of older Americans during the recession concerning their employment, housing, and medical care among other issues, writing "These problems, and their solutions, are the proper business of the Congress…." In 1959, Senator McNamara was appointed Chairman of the newly created Subcommittee and was authorized to conduct a complete study of any and all matters pertaining to the problems of the aging. Initially, hearings were held in Washington, DC, and then throughout the country in an attempt to learn about the plight of older Americans and how the federal government might respond to those needs. Senator McNamara introduced several bills based on the 1959 report summarizing the hearings' findings.

In 1961, Senator McNamara requested that the Subcommittee be replaced by the Senate Special Committee on Aging to expand the work of the Subcommittee and to engage in studies and investigations in many areas affecting retirement and old age. The request was bolstered by noting that the 1961 White House Conference on Aging had raised more issues than it had resolved. As it was conceived, the Committee would produce recommendations for legislative action which would be referred to regular standing Senate committees having proper legislative jurisdiction. Thus, formally created in 1961, the Senate Special Committee on Aging set to work, holding hearings, producing reports, and introducing legislation for Congressional consideration. McNamara chaired the Committee from 1961 to 1962.

The Committee continued its important work for well over a decade before the Committee became a permanent Senate Committee in 1977, comprised of 19 members, including a chairperson. The legislation carefully instructs the Committee on its activities:

> It shall be the duty of the special committee to conduct a continuing study of any and all matters pertaining to problems and opportunities of older people, including, but not limited to, problems and opportunities of maintaining health, of assuring adequate income, of finding employment, of engaging in productive and rewarding activity, of securing proper housing, and when necessary, of obtaining care or assistance. No proposed legislation shall be referred to such committee, and such committee shall not have power to report by bill, or otherwise have legislative jurisdiction (http://www.aging.senate.gov/about/rules).

Because of the fact-finding nature of the Committee, the Chairperson frequently begins a hearing with "We want to know about the …" [124, p. 109], or "We are here to find out what is going on with the people, how they are living, and to find out what can be done to correct the problems that are

[1]Information in this section was obtained from http://www.aging.senate.gov/.

S.L. Jackson (✉)
Institute of Law, Psychiatry and Public Policy, Department of Psychiatry and Neurobehavioral Sciences, University of Virginia, 1230 Cedars Court, Suite B, Charlottesville, VA 22903, USA
e-mail: slj4u@virginia.edu

X. Dong (ed.), *Elder Abuse*, DOI 10.1007/978-3-319-47504-2_28

facing many of the people here" [123, p. 134], or "Before we proceed, I want to make it clear that this is a Senate hearing and not a court of law" [119, p. 288].

28.3 History and Purpose of the Government Accountability Office

Founded in 1921, the U.S. Government Accountability Office (GAO) is an independent, nonpartisan agency that works for Congress [44], in part by investigating how the federal government spends taxpayer dollars and making recommendations to improve government operations (http://www.gao.gov/about/index.html). Of relevance here, the Committee requests reports from the GAO on a range of topics. For example, after the 1987 reauthorization of the Older Americans Act (OAA) requiring states receiving federal elder abuse prevention funds to enact mandatory reporting laws [107], Wolf urged Congress to undertake an examination of mandatory reporting laws before inserting such requirements into federal legislation [60]. With this recommendation in mind, the Committee commissioned a report from the GAO on mandatory reporting. Based on reviews and interviews with the field, the GAO [33] concluded that mandatory reporting was not an effective strategy in combatting elder abuse, opining presciently, however, that the practice was unlikely to change. Indeed, with the exception of New York, all states have some form of mandatory reporting law [43]. In a 1994 hearing on the abuse of older women, Gretel Weiss (Older Women's League Board member) recalls the first legislation to mandate reporting in New York (in 1980), noting that it was not successful because of concerns about the state's ability to respond: "We lacked the ability to assure the appropriate referral and to secure services" [98, p. 69].

Although the Committee at times requests reports on isolated topics, the Committee also commissions reports in conjunction with an impending hearing. For example, in preparations for a hearing, the Committee has requested reports on guardianship [32, 86], elder abuse [28, 81], and financial exploitation [26, 78], to name but a few.

28.4 The Nature of Committee Hearings

A review of the Committee hearings since 1961 finds that hearings can be categorized according to: (1) recurring topics, (2) topics that reflect historical time periods, and (3) isolated topics. Isolated topics, for example (none of which concern elder abuse), includes a hearing on the involuntary relocation of older adults due to highway construction [128], mental health and the elderly in the context of deinstitutionalization [120], and music and aging [101], to name a few.

Relevant topics that reflect a historical time period (none of which concern elder abuse exclusively) includes a series of hearings on crimes against the elderly in the decade beginning in 1980 [73, 105, 112, 114, 117]. At that time, crime rates were soaring and drug-related crime was of major concern to society (e.g., [11]). Social psychologists at the time were identifying high rates of fear of crime, particularly among older adults (e.g., [14]). A 1990 hearing entitled *Crimes against the Elderly: Let's Fight Back* [104] was in reality, a hearing on elder abuse. Held in Reno, Nevada, and chaired by Senator Reid, the Committee invited the same set of professionals that would appear at subsequent hearings explicitly on elder abuse. For example, testimony was provided by Tina Neuneker, a social worker; Arnold H. Greenhouse, a physician; as well as victims of mail fraud (Max Goodman) and financial exploitation (Mike Errea); Jack E. Swagerty, a regional chief postal inspector; Gail Bishop, a representative of the American Association of Retired Persons; Don Cavallo, with a public guardianship program; and Charles D. Shepherd, with the Federal Bureau of Investigation. However, 1990 was the last hearing on "crimes" against the elderly as crime rates plunged in the 1990s [50].

As another example, reflecting the progress made by the women's movement to raise awareness of women's issues, in 1984 the Committee held a hearing on the plight of older women which included a discussion on the abuse of older women [111]. To this point, there had been only one other hearing that made specific reference to women, but did not concern abuse of older women [115]. Women's issues continued to be heard periodically. In 1986 and 1991, the Committee held a hearing on employment opportunities for older women as more women were entering the workforce [102, 109], but later concerned itself with income security for older women [79, 84, 90, 94, 99] and long-term care [91]. However, the only other hearing (actually a Roundtable Discussion) exclusively on the abuse of older women occurred in 1994 entitled *Elder Abuse and Violence against Midlife and Older Women* [98], just prior to the passage of the Violence against Women Act of 1994. Joan Kuriansky, Executive Director of Older Women's League, reminds the discussants that "While we could talk a long time about the differences between the battered women's movement and the aging network, we must remember that for the woman who is experiencing the abuse, it doesn't quite matter what the philosophy is that underlies the availability of services to help her" (p. 4). Advice that is still relevant today.

In addition to isolated topics, and topics reflecting particular time periods, from its inception, the Committee regularly and consistently held hearings and recommended legislation related to housing, retirement, employment, health and health insurance, consumer protection, and the system of long-term care (nursing homes, staffing issues, abuse and neglect) in our country.

Consumer protection hearings. Of relevance to this chapter, the Committee has regularly held hearings on consumer protection (e.g., fraud). Whether violations in the consumer context constitute a form of elder abuse (i.e., financial exploitation) remains undecided [34, 41]. There currently exists no generally accepted boundaries around these concepts. However, this chapter differentiates between elder abuse, which includes financial exploitation, and financial crimes/consumer protection.

Consistent with the Committee's mandate, consumer protection was clearly on the Committee's agenda early after its inception (see Table 28.1). For example, in 1963 the newly formed Committee held a hearing entitled *Frauds and Quackery Affecting the Older Citizen* [127, p. 1]. McNamara writes:

> Ladies and Gentlemen, consumer protection has always been a matter of deep concern to many in the Congress, who believe that the Government has a duty to help the people protect themselves from fraud and deception. The need for such assistance was never greater than it is today. We live in the "Era of the Hard Sell."

The Committee continued to hold hearings on consumer protection throughout the coming decades. Topics such as interstate mail order land sales [126] and "frauds and quackery" of all kinds [125] concerned the Committee. In a 1971 hearing entitled *Evaluation of the Administration on Aging and Conduct of White House Conference on Aging* it was said in testimony that the elderly as a group are "…still the most exploited, most abused, most helpless minority-of-status, in our youth health and work-oriented society. Your committee is almost the only resource to which they may turn for exposing fraud and abuse directed at them" [122, p. 260]. However, consumer protection hearings took a 10 year hiatus.

In 1981, the Committee held a hearing entitled *Frauds against the Elderly*, asserting that $21 billion is lost on fraud annually and that the prime targets for these schemes are senior citizens [116]. Later in the report it is noted that 60 % of mail fraud involves the elderly, a type of fraud for which the United States Postal Inspection Service was later authorized to respond. In a 1983 hearing on combatting fraud against the elderly, the 10 most harmful frauds against the elderly were identified, a list remarkably similar to current observations: medical cures, home repair/improvement, bunco schemes, insurance, social cons, house sales/rental, business/investment, nursing home, automobile sales/repairs, and funeral sales [113, p. 2].

As presented in Table 28.1, with one exception in 1996 in which a hearing was held on telescams [96], consumer protection hearings again ceased, reemerging with significance in 1999 and continuing unabashedly to the present (with the exception of 2010 and 2011). In some years, up to five hearings were held on various fraud-related topics. The frequency of these consumer protection hearings likely reflects the changing economy [82, 92] and certainly reflected the changing technology within which the economy functioned such as the internet [87]. As with long-term care, Congress responded to these financial insults against the elderly with legislation, for example, the White-Collar Crime Penalty Enhancement Act of 2002, Mail Fraud and other Fraud Offenses (18 U.S. Code Chapter 63), and the Senior Citizens against Marketing Scams Act (SCAMS), adding 10 years to an offender's sentence if the victim is 65 or older [46]. The effectiveness of federal financial crimes legislation generally, however, has been questioned [21].

Long-term care hearings. The Committee began holding hearings on the care of vulnerable and needy residents in long-term care facilities in the 1960s [10, 35, 129], and since that time has regularly held hearings on the topic [59]. In fact, reports of elder abuse beginning in the 1960s focused only on victimization by formal caregivers such as those in long-term care facilities as family mediated abuse was a taboo subject at the time [67]. The Committee produced reports that were shocking to the public regarding the care of long-term care residents, but not to the lawyers and advocates working in the field [36]. In the War on Poverty era and expansive social programming of the 1960s and early 1970s, the Committee immediately recommended legislation to address these issues. The Committee's finding that Medicaid fraud was an epidemic also spurred Congress to action, requiring that states establish Medicaid Fraud Control Units (http://www.namfcu.net/about-us/namfcu-history) to investigate fraud and prosecute abuse and neglect in institutional settings receiving Medicaid funds [23, 39]. Continuing the robust response to abuses in long-term care facilities, in 2002 the US Department of Justice introduced the Elder Justice Nursing Home Initiative in which Congress appropriated funds for the Department of Justice to prosecute harms against residents of long-term care facilities [10, 17]. Congress may have felt compelled to act in this context because residents of long-term care facilities are by definition vulnerable [38], whereas Congress may be reluctant to act as aggressively in the context of elder abuse, neglect, and exploitation because intrusion into the lives of community-residing older adults is more controversial [47, 48].

Table 28.1 Comparison of consumer protection versus elder abuse hearings

Year	Title of report: consumer protection/financial exploitation[a]	Title of report: elder abuse
1961	–	–
1962	–	–
1963	Frauds and Quackery Affecting the Older Citizen: Part 1 01/15/63 Part 2 01/16/63 Part 3 01/17/63	–
1964	Interstate Mail Order Land Sales: Part 1 05/18/64 Part 2 05/19/64 Part 3 05/20/64	–
1965	–	–
1966	–	–
1967	Consumer Interests of the Elderly: Part 1 01/17/67 Part 2 02/03/67	–
1968	–	–
1969	–	–
1970	–	–
1971	–	–
1972	–	–
1973	–	–
1974	–	–
1975	–	–
1976	–	–
1977	–	–
1978	Condominiums and the Older Purchaser: Part 1, Hallandale, FL 11/28/78 Part 2, West Palm Beach, FL 11/29/78	–
1979	–	–
1980	–	Elder Abuse 06/11/80[b]
1981	Frauds Against the Elderly, Harrisburg, PA 08/04/81	–[c]
1982	–	–[d]
1983	Combating Frauds Against the Elderly 03/01/83	–[e]
1984	–	–[f]
1985	–	–[g]
1986	–	–
1987	–	–
1988	–	–[h]
1989	–	–[i]
1990	–	–[j]
1991	–	Elder Abuse and Neglect: Prevention and Intervention, Birmingham, AL 06/29/91
1992	–	–[k]
1993	–	–
1994	–	Elder Abuse and Violence Against Midlife and Older Women 05/04/94
1995	–	–
1996	Telescams Exposed: How Telemarketers Target the Elderly 03/06/96	–[l]
1997	–	–
1998	–	–[m]
1999	Funerals, Burials and Consumers, Clinton, IA and Cedar Rapids, IA 12/14/99	–

(continued)

Table 28.1 (continued)

Year	Title of report: consumer protection/financial exploitation[a]	Title of report: elder abuse
2000	Long-Term Care Insurance: Protecting Consumers from Hidden Rate Hikes 09/13/00	–
	Protecting Seniors From Fraud, Indianapolis, IN 08/10/00	
	Inviting Fraud: Has the Social Security Administration Allowed Some Payees to Deceive the Elderly and Disabled? 05/02/00	
	Funerals and Burials: Protecting Consumers from Bad Practices 04/10/00	
	Elder Fraud and Abuse: New Challenges in the Digital Economy, Portland, OR 03/15/00	
2001	Swindlers, Hucksters and Snake Oil Salesmen: The Hype and Hope of Marketing Antiaging Products to Seniors 09/10/01	Saving Our Seniors: Preventing Elder Abuse, Neglect and Exploitation 06/14/01
2002	Identity Theft: The Nation's Fastest Growing Crime Wave Hits Seniors 07/18/02	–
	Schemers, Scammers and Sweetheart Deals: Financial Predators of the Elderly 05/20/02	
2003	Ensuring the Integrity of Social Security Programs: Protecting Seniors from Representative Payee Fraud 09/09/03	Shattering The Silence: Confronting the Perils of Family Elder Abuse 10/20/03[n]
2004	Internet Fraud Hits Seniors: As Seniors Venture Into the Web, the Financial Predators Lurk and Take Aim 03/23/04	–[o,p]
	Predatory Lending: Are Federal Agencies Protecting Older Americans From Financial Heartbreak? 02/24/04	
2005	Old Scams—New Victims: Breaking the Cycle of Victimization 07/27/05	–
2006	Not Born Yesterday: How Seniors Can Stop Investment Fraud 03/29/06[q]	–
2007	Reverse Mortgages: Polishing Not Tarnishing The Golden Years[r] 12/12/07	Abuse Of Our Elders: How We Can Stop It 07/18/07
	Advising Seniors About Their Money: Who Is Qualified—and Who Is Not? 09/05/07	
2008	Foreclosure Aftermath: Preying on Senior Homeowners 02/13/08	–
2009	Reverse Mortgages: Leaving Seniors and Taxpayers on the Hook? 06/29/09	–
2010	–	–
2011	–	Justice for All: Ending Elder Abuse, Neglect and Financial Exploitation 03/02/11
2012	Pension Poachers: Preventing Fraud and Protecting America's Veterans 06/06/12	–[s]
	America's Invisible Epidemic: Preventing Elder Financial Abuse 11/15/12	
2013	876-SCAM: Jamaican Phone Fraud Targeting Seniors 03/13/13	–
	Tax-Related Identity Theft: An Epidemic Facing Seniors and Taxpayers 04/10/13	
	Social Security Payments Go Paperless: Protecting Seniors from Fraud and Confusion 06/19/13	
2014	Hanging Up on Phone Scams: Progress and Potential Solutions to this Scourge 07/16/14	–
	Trust Your Instincts? Tools to Empower Seniors to Identify Scams and Fraud Indiana State Fairgrounds, Farm Bureau Building Banquet Hall 08/05/14	
	Private Industry's Role in Stemming the Tide of Phone Scams 11/19/14	
2015	Catch Me If You Can: The IRS Impersonation Scam and The Government's Response 04/15/15	–
	Broken Trust: Combating Financial Exploitation of Vulnerable Seniors 02/04/15	

[a]Analysis excludes Medicaid and Medicare Fraud hearings
[b]Crime and the Elderly: What Your Community Can Do, Albuquerque, NM 06/23/80 (discussing crime generally, not elder abuse)
[c]Older Americans Fighting the Fear of Crime 09/22/81 (discussing crime generally, not elder abuse)
[d]Impact of the Federal Budget on the Future of Services for Older Americans 04/01/82 (mentions elder abuse in one place)
[e]Crime Against the Elderly, Los Angeles, CA 07/06/83 (discusses crime generally, not elder abuse)
[f]Women in Our Aging Society, Columbus, OH 10/08/84 (mentions elder abuse in the context of family caregiving)
[g]Challenges for Women: Taking Charge, Taking Care, Cincinnati, OH 11/18/85 (mentions elder abuse once in the context of caregiving)
[h]The American Indian Elderly: The Forgotten Population, Pine Ridge, SD 07/21/88 (many references to elder abuse)

[i]Our Nation's Elderly: Hidden Victims of the Drug War? 11/15/89 (Including abuse by family members who are drug addicted)
[j]Crimes Against the Elderly: Let's Fight Back, Las Vegas, NV and Reno, NV 08/21/90 (primarily about elder abuse)
[k]Roundtable Discussion on Guardianship 06/02/92
[l]Suicide and the Elderly: A Population At Risk 07/30/96 (family dysfunction, violence, emotional, physical and sexual abuse can be associated with suicide)
[m]Forum: Can We Rest In Peace? The Anxiety of Elderly Parents Caring for Baby Boomers with Disabilities 09/18/98 (does not mention elder abuse)
[n]Guardianships Over the Elderly: Security Provided or Freedom Denied 02/11/03
[o]Forum: Protecting Older Americans Under Guardianship: Who is Watching the Guardian? 07/22/04
[p]Crime Without Criminals? Seniors, Dementia and the Aftermath 03/22/04 (discussing whether those with dementia who commit crimes are criminals)
[q]Exploitation of Seniors: America's Ailing Guardianship System 09/07/06
[r]Ironically, the US Senate Special Committee on Aging (1982) held a hearing entitled Opportunities in Home Equity Conversion for the Elderly, generally optimistic about the prospect of converting home equity into a loan (now referred to as a reverse mortgage), although the Committee did express some concern about potential problems with the new instrument. The 1981 White House Conference on Aging and the President's Commission on Housing endorsed the concept
[s]Keeping Our Promises to West Virginia's Seniors: Strengthening the Aging Network 02/13/12 (mentioning elder abuse prevention via AAAs)

28.5 The First Hearing on Elder Abuse Occurring in Domestic Settings

Oddly, a review of the Committee hearings finds that the topic of elder abuse does not fit neatly into any of the above three categories. There has been continued interest in and hearings on elder abuse throughout the life of the Committee, but not as consistent as long-term care or consumer protection (see Fig. 28.1 providing a depiction of consumer protection versus elder abuse hearings across the tenure of the Committee), but it certainly cannot be described as a topic reflecting the times or an isolated topic.

The Committee's interest in elder abuse occurring in domestic settings was likely paved by the early and consistent attention paid to the abuse and neglect of long-term care residents beginning in the 1970s [35], in addition to the discovery of child abuse in the 1960s and intimate partner violence in the 1970s [42, 62]. Congressional hearings on the subject were prompted by Congress' increasing receipt of reports from the general public on the abuse of older adults by family members [130], as well as the publication of several small studies in the 1970s [3, 65], for example, Steinmetz [68]. Physicians are credited with first identifying elder abuse, focusing primarily on physical abuse, coined "granny bashing" by Burston [12]. However, the Committee recognized that elder abuse encompassed far more than granny bashing that first made headlines in the 1970s [37].

In 1980, the Committee held its first hearing devoted exclusively to elder abuse (see Table 28.1), simply titled *Elder Abuse* [118]. This was a joint hearing between the Senate and the House, focusing on the abuse, neglect, and financial exploitation of older adults at the hands of their

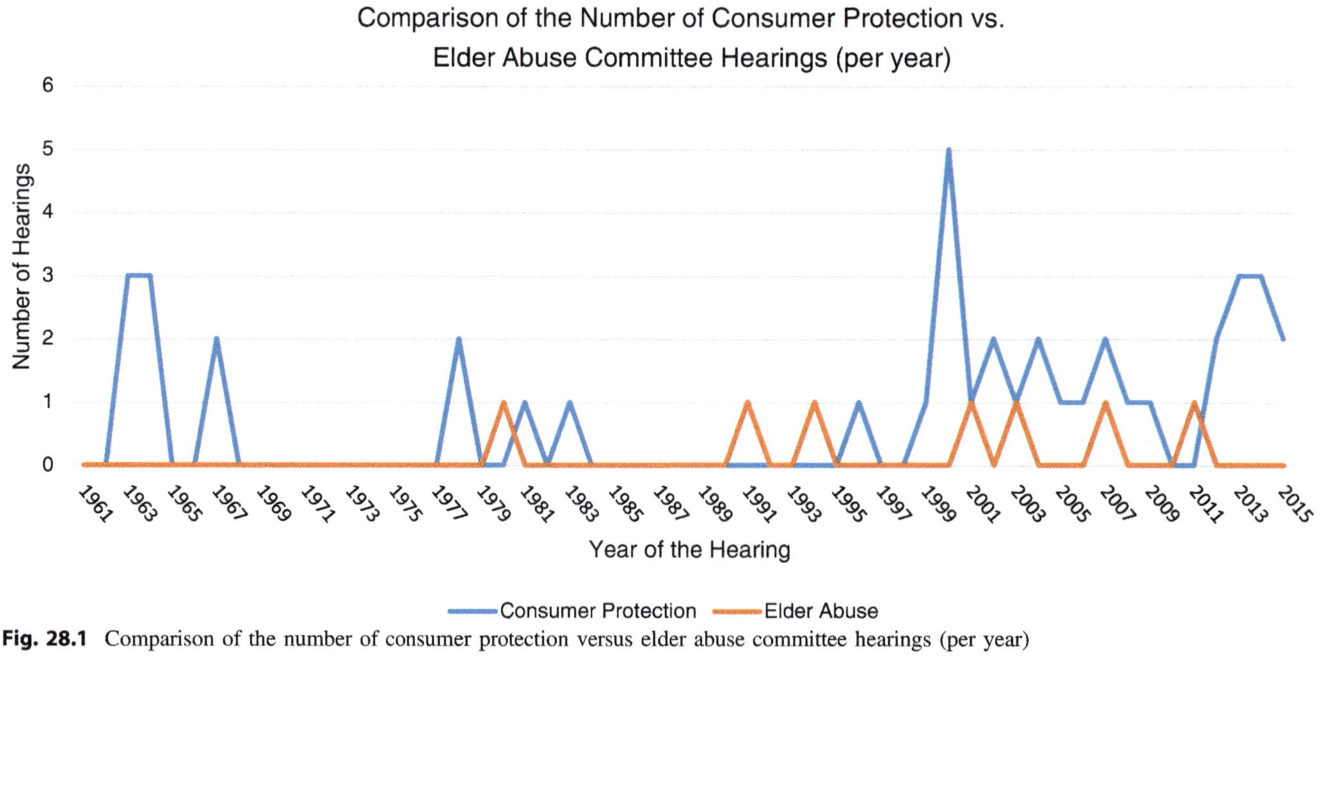

Fig. 28.1 Comparison of the number of consumer protection versus elder abuse committee hearings (per year)

family members. In addition to APS caseworkers accompanying victims, those providing testimony included representatives from Legal Research and Services for the Elderly (see [4]), Professors Suzanne Steinmetz, describing preliminary results of her research, and John J. Regan, of Hofstra Law School, providing suggestions for federal legal actions, noting that Title XX of the SSA and Title III of the OOA have "…already put the Federal Government into the business of providing protective services, …" (p. 54). Representatives from other state agencies also provided testimony.

The hearing became part of a 1981 report entitled *Elder Abuse: Examination of a Hidden Problem* [75], so titled because the report concluded that most cases of elder abuse are not reported [60]. However, little federal action followed the 1981 report [46].

Explaining the lack of federal action. The 1980 joint hearing and the 1981 report recommended that states enact mandatory reporting laws similar to child abuse mandatory reporting laws (observing the swift federal response to child abuse with the passage of the Child Abuse Protection and Treatment Act of 1974) and encouraged Congress to enact legislation to provide "financial assistance" to the states to support protective services programs [23, 46, 132]. Many states, confident that Congress would enact such legislation, passed elder abuse statutes containing mandatory reporting provisions based on the expectation that they imminently would be receiving federal funding. By 1985, anticipating federal financial assistance, at least 44 states had enacted legislation [46, 74, 66]. However, federal legislation failed to materialize.

Although states began passing legislation in anticipation of federal assistance, in the absence of a federal model, states developed their own unique elder abuse response [57, 58, 66, 131], albeit modeled on standard social work principles [57]. Mixson [54] astutely observes that APS programs have been developing independently across the country for the past 40 years. Ironically, the "unsynchronized effort" across states [55, p. 10] is often asserted to have stymied progress in the federal government's response to elder abuse, citing the lack of consistency across states as hindering the ability of the federal government to develop legislation [28, 51, 54, 60], a situation that resulted from their own inaction.

Looking at need alone cannot explain why federal legislation failed to materialize [44]. Scholars opine that federal legislation in the early 1980s was severely hampered by the economic and political climate that began to radically change in the late 1970s.

Prior to the late 1970s, Binstock [5] observes that social policy at the federal level was perceived to be a cure for any social problem that could be well articulated, especially those affecting older adults. From the 1935 Social Security Act (SAA) to the mid-1970s, society perceived all older adults as alike and deserving of assistance from the federal government. Clark [13] writes that the statement of purpose in the OAA of 1965 connotes the sentiment that society owes older adults a debt of gratitude, not only for their economic contribution to our country (social, political, technology, war efforts), but for life itself, and for this we owe them a decent retirement (p. 122). Binstock [5] reports that the 1960s and 1970s were particularly beneficial for older adults, finding that by the mid-1970s (using loose criteria) there were 134 federal programs benefiting older citizens, overseen by 49 committees and subcommittees of the Congress.

The expansive social policy characterizing the 1960s (e.g., War on Poverty, passage of the OAA of 1965) in which any social program for older adults was encouraged, came to an end in the late 1970s when the economy crashed [5, 13, 108, 110]. Consequently, there was a sea change in the way society viewed expenditures for older adults by the late 1970s. In this new economic reality, federal resources were perceived as "scarce" [13]. Older adults were increasingly viewed as selfish, not needy or deserving, and particularly overbenefitting from federal spending, especially in comparison to federal spending on children at the time. For example, Clark [13] calculates that in 1978, 58 % of the federal $46.5 billion allocated to health care was consumed by adults age 65 and older, although as a group they comprised only 11 % of the population, whereas those under age 19 comprised 33 % of the population while using only 8 % of the healthcare budget. Likewise, Binstock [5] calculated that older adults comprised 12 % of population and received one third of social benefits at a time when children were hurting. With the public's shifting perception of the elderly as wealthy and recipients of numerous social programs [40, 42, 53], older adults were perceived as receiving more than their fair share of the proverbial pie. The public became increasingly hostile to older people [5], viewing older adults as unproductive and underserving of federal benefits [13]. Throughout the 1980s and into the 1990s, a new set of images–as inaccurate as were the earlier stereotypes–depicted older adults as prosperous, hedonistic, politically powerful, and selfish [5, 61].

In the 1960s, an infusion of federal funds initially incentivized the development of state protective services programs [3, 37]. However, Title XX of the SSA of 1974 provided funding to the states for the development of *adult* protective services programs. However, in the more conservative era of the 1980s [4], this funding mechanism shifted to Social Services Block Grants (SSBG), providing social services grants to states for all citizens (young and old) on the basis of population, and giving the states even greater discretion in the allocation of funds [3, 55, 62], that is, using all or part of those funds specifically for APS [28, 60]. The total amount of funding allocated to SSBG also decreased dramatically in the 1980s [46, 73]. Even worse, fewer states were allocating those limited funds to APS [37], the sole source of federal funds for the delivery of APS, based in part on the criticism that APS was costly and ineffective and potentially infringed on civil rights [46].

There still is no comprehensive federal funding stream dedicated to elder abuse [70]. Consequently, state level elder abuse programming has been piecemealed together from a variety of federal agencies, each with its own limitations [16, 19, 58, 70]. For example, VAWA focuses on domestic violence, but excludes males. VOCA has historically been available only to victims of crime, but not those whose offense fails to reach the threshold of a crime. OAA provides assistance to states' Area Agencies on Aging efforts related to elder abuse, but not explicitly APS. As observed, little progress in elder abuse was made in the 1980s.

It should be noted that there have been no hearings, past or present, focused on the abuse of older minority populations. However, a hearing held in 1988, entitled *The American Indian Elderly: The Forgotten Population* [106], repeatedly makes reference to the abuse of older Native Americans, although this was not the focus of the hearing.

28.6 Two Decades: Two Hearings

In 1991, Olinger [60] laments that "After 10 years, the sum of these [federal] programs hardly represents a strong commitment on the part of the federal government." He goes on to write that the early promise of the hearings and reports has "…not been borne out" (p. 46). Action at the state level clearly outpaced that of the federal government. Without a doubt, "State statutes have been the primary engine for combating elder abuse" [46]. Given the political and economic climate of the 1980s inhibiting federal legislation, it is not surprising that the next hearing on elder abuse did not occur until 1991 [103]. In that hearing, Williamson, with the Alabama Department of Public Health, presciently asserts that "A coordinated effort on the local, State, and national level will be needed to combat elder abuse…" (p. 5). In testimony, R. Steven Daniels, a political science professor at the University of Alabama at Birmingham, quips that "Federal action and coordination is needed, but only if it does not repeat the organizational and funding mistakes of the States." He then goes on to say "Only if elder mistreatment is dealt with in a unified fashion will any significant steps be taken to eradicate the problem" (p. 24). Unfortunately, with the exception of the 1994 hearing described earlier on the abuse of older women, another elder abuse hearing would not occur for another 10 years, although the Committee engaged in other relevant activities during the 1990s [10].

28.7 Ushering in a New Era in Congressional Hearings and Accompanying GAO Reports

In the first decade of the new Millennium, three hearings on elder abuse were held. In 2001, a hearing entitled *Saving Our Seniors: Preventing Elder Abuse, Neglect and Exploitation* [93] featured a variety of prominent witnesses that in some ways harkened back to the 1980 joint hearing. Witnesses included Riker Hamilton, a Protective Services Program Administrator from Maine; Laura Mosqueda, a geriatrician from Orange County, CA; Sara Aravanis, administrator for the National Center on Elder Abuse; and a victim, Joanne Hopper from Fruitland, ID. However, reflecting the changing view of elder abuse, and the federal government's emerging role in it, witnesses also included Paul Greenwood, Deputy District Attorney in San Diego, CA, and Stuart Schiffer, Acting Assistant Attorney General at the U.S. Department of Justice (USDOJ). This cast of characters is important because it signals a fundamental change in the conceptualization of elder abuse. In addition to APS, victims, and geriatricians, which had historically made up the cast of witnesses, prosecutors and USDOJ personnel were also included in the hearing, signaling a shift to a more criminal justice orientation to elder abuse.

In his opening remarks, Senator Craig bemoans that "Our investigations have revealed that State efforts to address these situations are often ineffective" [93, p. 3]. Continuing to define elder abuse occurring in domestic settings as those within the family, Senator Craig exemplifies the shift in thinking at the federal level:

> Today, we seek to determine how existing state and federal efforts might be enhanced to promote collaborative and multi-disciplinary approaches in resolving these very complex cases. … Existing federal resources can and should be targeted toward providing more technical training and assistance in the collaborative identification, investigation, and prosecution of crimes perpetrated against the elderly (p. 3).

With these words, no longer was the role of the federal government in question—or was it? An exchange between Senator Craig and Mr. Schiffer exemplify the tension that exists between the legislative and executive branches of government and the role of the federal government (see [44]):

> Senator Craig asks of Mr. Schiffer: "If…I want to talk to the person who is the chief protector of seniors in this country… whom would I talk to?" In response, Mr. Schiffer describes the various divisions within the US Department of Justice. Senator Craig clarifies: "…but what I'm trying to figure out is if there is not a better way to coordinate this kind of activity…". Mr. Schiffer replies "No, each division is an expert in that type of abuse as it should be…". The Chairman then inquires of

Mr. Schiffer: "Is the major responsibility in this country for dealing with senior abuse and fraud a State matter or a Federal matter?" Mr. Schiffer responds "...the State and local government officials will always have the leadership role. ..." Senator Craig rebuts this assertion by explaining that in his state of Idaho, prosecutors are ill-trained for this type of case and goes on to say "And we could not go to the Justice Department for that training." He explains that prosecutors had to go to another state for elder abuse training, adding that if prosecutors cannot be secure in what they are doing and have a base of knowledge from which to work, "Then they will walk away from those kinds of things [elder abuse cases]" (p. 24).

The use of multidisciplinary teams was not a new idea, but such teams had not been widely utilized by the elder abuse field [2]. However, for the first time those providing testimony emphasize the need for the field to take a multidisciplinary approach, an appeal that would be relentless throughout future hearings. Testimony by Laura Mosqueda described the recently developed Vulnerable Adult Specialist Team (VAST) and Paul Greenwood emphasized how multidisciplinary teams enhanced his ability to prosecute these cases.

The caregiver stress model widely adopted by the late 1970s (e.g., [62, 107] was still prominent in this hearing. This position was exemplified by Senator Breaux who stated "...long-term care...is not provided by institutions but by families...and the...sense of burden that it puts on families...,...family caregivers are so overwhelmed..." [93], pp. 1–2).

Energized by the 2001 hearing, the following year was active for the field of elder abuse. Senator Breaux first introduced the Elder Justice Act of 2002 [9]. That same year, the Elder Justice Coalition was formed [58] to facilitate passage of the Elder Justice Act. However, although introduced multiple times and in various forms [15, 51], the legislation would not pass until 2009.

In 2003, the National Research Council released a report that had been commissioned by the National Institute on Aging (established in 1974; see [121]) to assess the state of the elder abuse field and to develop a research agenda based on the findings [7]. Sadly, the report concluded "However, so little is known about elder mistreatment that it would be premature to draw up a detailed research agenda for this nascent field" (p. xiv). However, the report defined elder mistreatment as "...(a) intentional actions that cause harm or create a serious risk of harm (whether or not harm is intended) to a vulnerable elder by a caregiver or other person who stands in a trust relationship to the elder or (b) failure by a caregiver to satisfy the elder's basic needs or to protect the elder from harm" (p. 1). This more narrow definition of elder abuse as a family (or trusted other) issue is consistent with the first 1980 hearing held over 20 years prior [118].

It is within this context that the Committee held another hearing on elder abuse in 2003 entitled *Shattering the Silence: Confronting the Perils of Family Elder Abuse* [88]. Providing testimony were Joe Snyder, representing the National Association of Adult Protective Services Administrators; Holly Ramsey-Klawsnik, a clinician and advocate; Ken Connor formerly with the Family Research Council; Joseph Lofy, a police officer; Robert Stein, Deputy District Attorney in San Diego, CA; and Leanna Watts, a victim of financial exploitation perpetrated by her son and daughter-in-law. Thus, a similar cast of witnesses appeared as in the 2001 hearing with two exceptions: No federal agencies were represented and no one was representing the medical community.

New and emerging perspectives on elder abuse were evident in the testimony, however. For example, the caregiver stress model, so prominent for decades, was publically denounced. For the first time a witness (Snyder) asserts that "We know that caregiver stress is not a valid cause [of abuse]..." (p. 44) (see [131]). During the discussion, Ramsey-Klawsnik further explains why the caregiver stress model is no longer applicable (pp. 50–51). Ramsey-Klawsnik also emphasized the need for multidisciplinary teams stating "The greatest lesson [from serving on the Board of NCPEA] has been the critical need for interdisciplinary collaboration in responding to elder abuse" (p. 41).

Although in his 2001 testimony, Greenwood discussed the need for prosecution, this hearing exemplified a change in the Committee's view of prosecution. For the first time, the Committee members queried witnesses about whether the abusers described in these cases were actually prosecuted. Deputy District Attorney Stein confesses that many cases are not prosecuted. However, creeping into this hearing is a more aggressive criminal justice stance.

On the heels of fresh defeat of the Elder Justice Act that had been reintroduced once again in 2006, the Committee held another hearing on elder abuse in 2007 entitled *Abuse of Our Elders: How We Can Stop It* [83]. Those testifying exemplify the emerging perspective on elder abuse, in particular, a social services *and* a criminal justice perspective and still vying for federal involvement. For the first time, there is simultaneous representation from the US Department of Justice (Daniel Fridman, Senior Counsel to the Deputy Attorney General) and the US Department of Health and Human Services (Gregory Demske, Assistant Inspector for Legal Affairs, Office of Inspector). Recognizing the need to acknowledge elder abuse in both domestic settings and institutional setting, also providing testimony are Ralph Tortora, Special Assistant Attorney General, Office of the Attorney General, New York City Medicaid Fraud Unit, and Beverley Laubert, Ohio Long Term Care Ombudsman and

President of the National Association of State Long Term Care Ombudsman. Paul Greenwood again represents the state's criminal justice perspective. However, this hearing also features Robert Blancato, National Coordinator of the Elder Justice Coalition, taking the lead on encouraging Congress to pass the Elder Justice Act. Daniel Reingold, President and CEO of The Hebrew Home for the Aged at Riverdale, provides a description of a possible intervention for elder abuse in the form of placing elder abuse victims in shelters located within long-term care facilities (as opposed to institutionalization). Finally, Jennifer Coldren of Rome, New York, provides testimony from the perspective of a victim.

Reflecting the shift in approach to elder abuse is testimony by Joy Solomon asserting that many cases of elder abuse involve family members and that prosecution alone may not be the answer. Solomon explains that a grandmother does not want to call the police or prosecutor about her son, "But if, as a community, we create these partnerships together to provide support, then that grandmother could get some support and her grandson could get some support, too" (p. 88–89). This perspective was also echoed in the testimony of District Attorney Greenwood. Although still not widely practiced, a multidisciplinary team approach was now considered "best practice" [8].

With the Elder Justice Coalition in operation for the past 5 years, and the Elder Justice Act continuing to be defeated, a frustrated Blancato chastises the Committee when he says "The federal commitment is piecemeal in approach and minimal in substance" (see also [6]). He asserts "It will be 30 years next year when Congress first addressed elder abuse in hearings of the old House Select Committee on Aging." … "But with all due respect to all of this work, the Nation has waited long enough" (pp. 65–66).

28.8 Complementary Committee Hearings and GAO Reports

Elder abuse. Lindberg et al. [51] eloquently explain the factors that facilitated the passage of the Elder Justice Act 2 years after the 2007 hearing. While a moral victory, the Elder Justice Act was largely a symbolic victory as Congress chose not to appropriate funding [19]. However, it did establish the Elder Justice Coordinating Council to coordinate activities related to elder abuse, neglect, and exploitation across the Federal government, as advocated nearly 30 years earlier in the 1981 report [10]. With momentum in the right direction, Senator Kohl quickly commissioned the GAO to develop a report on the state of APS and elder abuse generally and the federal role in these issues. The report [28] was released just prior to the 2011 hearing on elder abuse [81]. With the exception of the 1991 GAO report on elder abuse mandatory reporting, the 2011 report was the first GAO report on elder abuse.

The GAO [28] provided a bleak but honest picture of the field of elder abuse. For example, the report confirmed that "…no federal funding is currently dedicated exclusively to APS programs." The report found that although current public policies encourage older adults to remain in their homes as they age, the system in place to protect them [APS] may not be able to meet the demands (p. 34). Furthermore, no national policy priorities currently exist aside from the 2001 Office for Victims of Crime National Elder Abuse Policy Agenda position paper (see USDOJ [72]). Finally, most poignant, the report concluded that although federal elder justice activities have provided some financial support to APS, federal leadership is lacking. Several recommendations were offered: (1) feasibility of establishing a national resource center for APS-dedicated information (currently established); (2) nationwide APS data collection system (currently under development); and (3) a periodic national study of the extent of elder abuse to track the prevalence over time (p. 36).

With the GAO [28] report in hand, in 2011 another hearing on elder abuse was held entitled *Justice for All: Ending Elder Abuse, Neglect and Financial Exploitation* [81]. In his opening remarks, Senator Kohl asserts that "Elder abuse doesn't get the attention it deserves" (p. 1) and described three bills he was introducing (none of which pass; see also [65]). Notably, however, the federal government's ambivalent role in elder abuse was dissipating as evidenced by Kohl's statement "To begin, we must ensure that Federal, State, and local agencies work cohesively to combat elder abuse" (p. 1).

In this hearing, testimony is provided by famed film star Mickey Rooney, a victim of financial exploitation at the hands of his family; Kathleen Quinn, Executive Director of the National Adult Protective Services Association; Kay Brown, author of the 2011 GAO report; Mark Lachs, a practicing geriatrician and researcher from Weill Cornell Medical College; Bonnie Brandl, Executive Director of the National Clearinghouse on Abuse in Later Life; and Marie-Therese Connolly, Woodrow Wilson International Center for Scholars.

In an attempt to gain greater notoriety for the issue of elder abuse, a new theme running throughout the field and reflected in the testimony of Brown, Quinn and Lachs, is the appeal to society's financial conscience. For the first time, testimony described the cost of elder abuse to society, noting an expansive number of agencies that might need to respond to elder abuse in addition to APS, placing a financial burden on society. Beyond this, the four key points that emanated from the hearing included the need for federal leadership, multidisciplinary teams, training for frontline workers and research, the latter two being new elements to elder abuse hearings.

The testimony of Kay Brown, based on her GAO [28] report, was scathing of the federal government's response to elder abuse. She notes that the federal responsibility for elder abuse arises through two pieces of legislation: the Older American's Act of 1965 (PL 89-73, 73 Stat. 218) and the Elder Justice Act of 2009 (PL No. 111-148 tit. VI, sutit. H, 124 Stat. 119, 782-804 (p. 2). However, she observes that in 2009 only $11.9 m of federal funds were spent on elder abuse projects (p. 9). She concludes that the federal efforts are "scattered" (p. 6) and that "lack of strong leadership" characterizes the field of elder abuse (p. 11), echoing Blancato's 2007 testimony.

In Kathleen Quinn's testimony, she astutely observes that this "…is the first congressional hearing addressing APS" (p. 11). With the emphasis on a criminal justice response to elder abuse observed in previous hearings (and elsewhere), Quinn reminds the Committee that APS in many states responds to a broader array of cases than just criminal, including self-neglect. Upon describing a number of issues the field of elder abuse is facing, Quinn pleads "…and we would really appreciate some help…" (p. 13). For example, during the open discussion later in the hearing, Quinn asserts that a problem with mandatory reporting is "…we haven't had the resources to develop the core trainings that could be sent out across the country…" (p. 19). Observing that not all states even require training for APS caseworkers, Quinn incredulously adds that "Starbucks employees have to go through 40 h of training, but not an APS caseworker who is making "life-and-death decisions" about elder abuse victims" (p. 23).

Multidisciplinary teams are highly endorsed by Mark Lachs, who recently developed the celebrated New York City Elder Abuse Center. He further observes in astonishment that "…as a geriatrician, I had to take child abuse training…there is no such requirement for older people" (pp. 18–19). Bonnie Brandl describes and advocates for a coordinated community response to abuse in later life, later reminding the Committee of how important leadership by the federal government is to the field: "What happens here in D.C., what happens in government, this committee hearing, in and of itself, raising awareness is hugely important" (p. 21). And finally, Marie Therese Connolly made a plea for more research. Although lack of data was a recurring theme throughout the hearings, this is perhaps the first hearing to make such an impassioned plea while asserting "We don't know what works and we don't know what successful interventions even look like" (p. 21).

This is the last hearing focusing exclusively on elder abuse. It was uniquely important because many of those providing testimony appeared the following year at the inaugural Elder Justice Coordinating Council meeting (October 11, 2012) and submitting white papers. These papers formed the basis for the recommendations presented to the Elder Justice Coordinating Council in September 2013, recommendations that were ultimately adopted by the Council (ACL [1]).

Also noteworthy, to update the 2011 GAO report, Senator Kohl requested another GAO report. The title of the GAO [25] report portents the conclusion: *Elder Justice: More Federal Coordination and Public Awareness Needed.* The report finds that the elder justice programs across 12 federal agencies (most of which are concerned with primarily financial exploitation) are fragmented but minimally overlapping, thus reducing risk of duplication. However, the report concluded that "…less progress has been made in articulating and tracking common goals for federal elder justice activities" (p. 23), especially in light of the establishment of the Elder Justice Coordinating Council purportedly to model and facilitate collaborative behavior. With few exceptions (i.e., in 2010 the National Institute on Aging research program held a conference to evaluate the progress of research supported by grants awarded), "…formal evaluation of federal elder justice programs is limited" (p. 26). Given the limited federal funding available, the report urges greater efficiently by coordinating activities and strengthening their collaboration by establishing joint strategies (p. 29). The recommendations specifically included: (1) identifying common objectives and defining common outcomes and (2) developing a national campaign to increase awareness of elder abuse.

Financial exploitation. Whether financial exploitation is an elder abuse or a consumer protection issue, or both, remains undecided. Financial exploitation in one way or another has been incorporated into hearings on both elder abuse and consumer protection from the inception of the Committee. However, following the release of the commissioned GAO [26] report on financial exploitation (defined in the report as the illegal or improper use of an older adult's funds, property, or assets), the Committee held its first hearing exclusively devoted to the subject in 2012, defined broadly, however, to include consumer protection issues [78]. Financial exploitation was thought to be a prevalent form of elder abuse (e.g., [49]) and one that was receiving considerable media attention (e.g., [52]).

The opening statement of the GAO [26] report reflects the multidisciplinary approach to elder abuse now dominant in the field (if not in practice): "Because elder financial exploitation can take many forms, combating it involves state and local agencies, and their federal counterparts, across social services, criminal justice, and consumer protection systems" (p. 1). The report asserts that although states have primary responsibility for combatting elder financial exploitation, there are seven federal agencies involved in financial exploitation that have a role to play in supporting state and local efforts (p. 2) (of these seven, only the Consumer Financial Protection Bureau's Office for Older Americans has as its mission combatting financial exploitation). For example, the report suggests that the federal government could disseminate model power of attorney legislation (see [69]).

Over the years, training had become a focal point of need for the field. The report asserted that many professionals responding to elder abuse lack the skills needed to adequately respond to elder abuse (APS caseworkers, law enforcement officers, prosecutors). The report applauded the construction of the Department of Justice's elder justice website designed for among others, prosecutors (going live September 2014). The report also finds that although the National Center on Elder Abuse "...has compiled a list of elder abuse training materials from a variety of sources [as mandated by statute], ...we could find no quick and clear way to identify which trainings cover financial exploitation" (p. 24). Reflecting the fact that a multidisciplinary approach to elder abuse was now considered best practice [8], the report finds that APS focuses on protecting and supporting the victim, and the criminal justice system focuses on prosecuting and convicting exploiters. However, working together and including other partners, they could "...more easily accomplish both of these goals" (p. 25), as opined by Solomon in her 2007 testimony. Chastising the government for failing to include banks in the federal response to financial exploitation, the report asserts that "While the federal government generally requires banks to train employees on a variety of issues...we could find no similar requirements for banks to train employees to recognize and report elder financial exploitation" (p. 33). The report also finds a need for increased public awareness of financial exploitation to better understand and prevent it (more recently expressed by Riggs and Podrazik [65]). The report continues, "Each of the seven federal agencies we reviewed independently produces and disseminates public information on elder financial exploitation that is tailored to its own mission" and that the "...seven agencies we reviewed do not conduct these activities as part of a broader coordinated approach" (p. 22). The report encourages the Elder Justice Coordinating Council to "...develop a national strategy for combating this problem" (p. 40). Some assert that this call has been answered by the release of the Elder Justice Roadmap [71].

The purpose of the complementary Committee hearing, entitled *America's Invisible Epidemic: Preventing Elder Financial Abuse* [78], was to learn of financial exploitation prevention programs being implemented at the federal, state and local level. As opposed to elder abuse, which typically was defined in the context of the family, Senator Kohl describes financial exploitation perpetrated by family members, home care providers, scammers, and others. Therefore, a range of witnesses were invited. In this hearing, testimony is provided by Frank Abagnale, author and consultant; Kay Brown, author of the 2012a GAO report; Hubert "Skip" Humphrey, III, Assistant Director of the Office of Older Americans within the newly created Consumer Financial Protection Bureau (CFPB); Paul Smocer, President of BITS Financial Services Roundtable; and Paul Greenwood, Deputy District Attorney in San Diego, CA.

Testimony is offered reflecting the witness's profession. For example, Paul Smocer declared "It is also important to note that financial institutions are often the first line of defense against this financial exploitation" (p. 1) and Skip Humphrey described the varied activities of the CFPB. However, Paul Greenwood once again touts the importance of a multidisciplinary response: "I am convinced that collaboration of prosecutors with multiple agencies—where the local prosecutor's office takes the initiative—is the key to making an impact on the escalating financial crimes being committed against seniors" (p. 3). Offering a different perspective, however, Frank Abagnale (who testified first) proclaims that the Federal government can disseminate public service announcements, but that protecting one's identity is an individual responsibility. He goes on to say that if the older adult cannot do so, others around them must step in, everyone has to step in, but government regulation is not the answer.

By this point, the Elder Justice Act has been enacted and now, rather than urging Congress to pass the Act, there are pleas for Congress to fund the Act. Greenwood asks rhetorically, What is needed? Funding the Elder Justice Act. "Much has been achieved at the grassroots level in recent years but we need some leadership and responsibility from the Federal branch of government in tackling financial elder abuse" (p. 4).

Little derived from this hearing except another hearing in February 2015 [77]. However, this hearing takes a more narrow view of financial exploitation, focusing on financial exploitation by family members and trusted others consistent with a definition proposed by Bonnie and Wallace [7] a decade earlier, arguably placing this hearing more in the context of elder abuse than consumer protection. Providing testimony were Philip Marshall, grandson of legendary New York socialite Brooke Aster who was financially exploited by her son; Judith Shaw, State of Maine Office of Securities; Kathleen Quinn, Executive Director of the National Adult Protective Services Association; and Page Ulrey, Senior Deputy Prosecuting Attorney, King County, Washington.

Senator Collins remarks that "Throughout its history, the Aging Committee has spurred Congress to action on issues important to older Americans through its hearings, investigations and reports...." Collins unequivocally offers that "The federal government also plays an important role in providing leadership to combat this [financial exploitation] problem."

Following the testimony of Marshall and Shaw, Kathleen Quinn strongly admonished the federal government: "But although the first congressional hearings on elder abuse were held in the 1970's, the federal government has decided to essentially ignore this problem for half a century, although there has been some progress on this in the past few years thanks to the Elder Justice Coalition, the Elder Justice Act, and the leadership of Assistant Secretary Greenlee at the ACL [Administration on Community Living]" (p. 3). She goes on "Yet there remains no dedicated federal funding for the only nationally available, statutorily authorized, services system for the most vulnerable victims—those who cannot protect themselves—APS" (p. 3).

Ulrey's testimony reflects knowledge being generated in the field of neuroscience and for the first time the issues of dementia (for a review see [18]) and capacity (for a review see [24]) are raised. Ulrey observes that "Knowledge of these concepts is essential to properly investigating and prosecuting cases with financial dimensions, yet few in the criminal justice system are familiar with them all" (p. 2). She adds, "APS often lacks the tools, resources and training to screen for cognitive impairment...As a result, APS often unwittingly screens out cases involving victims who lack the cognitive capacity to handle complex financial transactions, thereby allowing the exploitation to continue" (p. 3).

Later that year, the GAO [27] released a report just prior to a related Committee hearing on the subject of protecting veteran's benefits entitled *Pension Poachers: Preventing Fraud and Protecting America's Veterans* [80]. The Committee observed that veterans are being encouraged to place their money in instruments that are inaccessible or that charge exorbitant fees. Once again, both the GAO report and those providing testimony at the hearing concurred that the federal government could do more to protect the assets of federal beneficiaries.

28.9 Guardianship: Distinct but Related to Elder Abuse

This chapter would be remiss if it did not address the issue of guardianship, which appears to have had an even more difficult time capturing the attention of the Committee than elder abuse. Guardianship is sometimes distinct from elder abuse, but at times, guardianship results from elder mistreatment (as a remedy) and at times guardians/conservators are the perpetrators of elder abuse [63]. The Committee, however, appears to treat guardianship as a separate issue from elder abuse. Although the Committee has held hearings on the topic, guardianship cannot be characterized as a sustaining topic for the Committee. In 1992, the Committee held a Roundtable Discussion on Guardianship [100], considering the role the federal government might play in an area that is typically a state issue, with little emanating from the hearing. The Committee again addressed this issue in 2003, 2004, and 2006 [85, 86, 89], with one accompanying GAO [32] report. The GAO was requested to review federal representative payee programs and how the state and federal governments might better ensure that guardians were being good stewards of federal funds paid to beneficiaries under guardianship. The report concluded that although the state and federal governments may be working with the same individual, the two systems lacked any systematic coordination, increasing the risk of abuse. In a 2006 hearing entitled *Exploitation of Seniors: America's Ailing Guardianship System*, Barbara Bovbjerg, author of the 2004 GAO report, noted little progress in ensuring protection for incapacitated elderly people [31]. Bovbjerg asserted that "Since the time of the 2004 GAO report on guardianship, little progress has been made" (p. 2), indeed, stressing that as none of the recommendations had been adopted, the GAO was not going to make any new recommendations.

The Committee subsequently commissioned a report specifically on elder abuse and neglect by guardians/conservators. The GAO [30] report concluded that it could not be determined whether financial exploitation by a guardian/conservator was a "widespread" problem because state requirements differ by state, (e.g., certification requirements, oversight, tracking, definitions) and that no federal, state, or local entity compiles comprehensive information on this issue (p. 5). Little space was allotted for other forms of elder abuse. However, they confirmed that financial exploitation does occur. For example, guardians stole $5.4 m from 158 incapacitated victims, many of whom were older. There was no accompanying hearing.

In 2011, the GAO [29] issued a related report regarding financial exploitation by representative payees (a person, agency, organization, or institution the federal government selects to manage someone's federal benefits when it is determined that an individual is unable to do so). The report found that the "...federal government is well-positioned and has an opportunity to lead in protecting the rights of incapacitated adults (receiving federal benefits) with court-appointed guardians, in particular by supporting evaluations of promising court guardianship monitoring practices" (p. 7) (see [45]). The report recommended that the Social Security Administration determine how to share information with states and that the Department of Health and Human Services should direct the Administration on Aging to support pilot projects related to monitoring guardianships.

28.10 Self-Neglect

Whether self-neglect is subsumed under the rubric of elder abuse remains controversial. There is evidence that self-neglect is related to forms of elder abuse [20]. However, elder abuse is typically characterized by the presence of a victim *and* a perpetrator thereby excluding self-neglect [34]. Nonetheless, the consequences associated with self-neglect (e.g., [64]) warrant the Committee's attention, and yet the Committee has failed to hold any hearings on self-neglect.

28.11 Conclusions and Future Directions

And with that, 35 years of investigations, reports, hearings, and testimony on elder abuse (and financial exploitation) is summarized. Reviewing hearing transcripts is more like reading a history book, documenting the shifting conceptualization of elder abuse over the decades, than a blueprint for achieving some goal. It is noteworthy that the question posed by the Committee has shifted over time from *What can the federal government do?* to *What is the federal government doing?* a much more active and affirmative inquiry. And yet relatively little federal legislation has resulted from the Committee's efforts. In spite of calls for federal leadership dating back to the 1970s, the federal government has not played a substantial role in structuring or funding adult protective services (APS) agencies, providing leadership for the field [28, 56, 70], or providing comprehensive federal legislation related to elder abuse. In 2003, Breaux and Hatch [10] observed that the recommendations proffered in the 1981 report are "hauntingly familiar" to recommendations made by advocates today (p. 213), suggesting little progress in the fight against elder abuse. A similar claim that could be made a decade later. Consistent with the incremental approach favored by our political system generally [44], until 2010 Congress seemed to prefer amending existing legislation to address elder abuse, e.g., reauthorization of OAA or amendments to the SSA. Capturing the attention (and pocketbook) of Congress has been challenging, with the Committee's ability to move Congress to action on this topic relatively negligible.

Unequivocally, significant good has emerged from the Committee's efforts. The Committee and commissioned GAO reports have contributed to the progress made in elder abuse over the past 35 years, although their work unequivocally is not finished. Although their actions have provided momentum in the right direction, elder abuse has yet to be recognized as a "social problem." The Committee must—and will—remain tenacious in compelling the federal government to provide leadership in elevating elder abuse to a social problem worthy of federal funding and leadership. The hearings and reports reviewed in this chapter provide guidance to the Committee on how to enhance elder abuse policy, practice, and research at the federal level.

There are five ways in which the federal government might positively impact policy. First, the need for greater federal coordination continues [25]. The federal body designed to accomplish this goal, the Elder Justice Coordinating Council, has convened and adopted eight recommendations to enhance the elder justice field [1]. However, the GAO [26] observed that there are seven federal agencies working on financial exploitation, for example, each in their own way and consistent with their own mission, but not in support of an overall goal. Through the Elder Justice Coordinating Council, the federal government still needs to develop a national strategy for combatting elder abuse by identifying common objectives, defining common outcomes [25], and developing a cohesive set of national policy priorities [28]. A process similar to that of the federal initiative on human trafficking[2] provides an excellent example for accomplishing this goal.

Second, surveillance remains an aspiration. The GAO [28] emphasized that although a few national prevalence studies had been completed, the ability to track prevalence over time has not been achieved. Periodically collecting complete and consistent data permits tracking the extent and form of elder abuse over time necessary for assessing progress, a task most aptly undertaken by the Centers for Disease Control and Prevention.

Improvements in other federal data collection activities are warranted. Fortunately, tremendous achievements have been made in the realm of data. For example, the Administration on Community Living is undertaking the development of a nationwide APS data collection system as recommended by the GAO [28]. However, there are a number of federal agencies that collect data of some type, each with their own challenge. The Federal Trade Commission, for example, receives voluntary financial fraud reports from only 12 states, potentially distorting the portrayal of fraud in the United States.

Third, the Elder Justice Coordinating Council has adopted Recommendation #5, *Develop a Broad-based Public Awareness Campaign*, as recommended by the GAO [25, 26]. However, little movement has been observed since its adoption.

Fourth, extensive training needs persist. It is essential that front line responders receive basic and professional development training. In addition, allied professionals and

[2]http://www.ovc.gov/pubs/FederalHumanTraffickingStrategicPlan.pdf.

gatekeepers need training in recognizing the signs of elder abuse and how to report it [28]. Some modest achievements have been made in this realm. Federal funding was used to develop a six-module online training for civil legal attorneys,[3] and federal funds were used to develop eight of the 23 core curriculum for adult protective services.[4] However, a national training strategy with full access for all awaits development [25, 26].

And fifth, funding. Simply put, "…no federal funding is currently dedicated exclusively to APS programs" [28], p. 27), the only statutorily dedicated agency in each state to respond to reports of elder abuse. Dedicated funding for APS is urgently needed and clearly warranted.

There are three ways in which the Committee might steer the federal government to constructively affect practice. First, too little coordination at the state and local level implicates the need for systems change. An excellent example is the Abuse in Later Life Program out of the Office on Violence against Women [81]. This program provides training on identifying and responding to abuse in later life, cross training, coordinated community response, and victim services. This model could be easily adapted to the broader context of elder abuse.

Second, the need for innovations in practice endures. For example, the utilization of multidisciplinary teams is considered best practice, but has not been widely adopted [26, 28]. The field must embrace technology, for example, by developing technologically creative approaches (e.g., virtual cognitive assessment, transmitting financial documents electronically) for accessing professionals (e.g., geriatricians, neuropsychologists, and forensic accountants) who are not readily available in many communities. Other innovations include creating elder abuse advocate positions to serve in the courts and the adoption of specialized elder abuse units in the criminal justice system [77]. Demonstration projects of the kind described here would serve to generate the development and adoption of innovative practices.

And third, a range of services for victims of elder abuse, such as emergency housing and legal services, are unavailable for many older victims [25]. The Weinberg Center for Elder Abuse Prevention is a nonprofit long-term care facility that provides emergency housing for victims of elder abuse while ensuring their receipt of wrap around services [83]. While the model garners considerable attention, the expansion of the intervention has been slow. In contrast, respite care as a service for family caregivers has received considerable federal attention and resources [22]. However, record numbers of older adults are providing care for their disabled adult children [95], some of whom commit forms of elder abuse. Equipping older parents with the supports and services they need to care for their adult children, while maintaining their safety, is highly desirable. Federal incentives could facilitate the development and expansion of these and other services.

Published elder abuse research agendas proliferate. However, populating the field with actual research to winnow down the agenda has not followed suit. The National Institute of Justice is the primary federal funding agency for elder abuse research. However, given its limited funding and narrow scope, without other federal agencies committing funds, progress will continue to be slow.

In the realm of basic research, the field has focused on victim risk factors. Little effort has been devoted to understanding the etiology of elder abuse and the contours of abuse over time, with an egregious absence of victim's voices. Ironically, elder abuse research has focused primarily on victims, to the near exclusion of perpetrators, and yet without an understanding of the interpersonal dynamics and underlying causes for the abusive situation, our ability to respond and intervene will continue to be limited. Also lacking but urgently needed is forensic research. In addition, the consequences of elder abuse have been alluded to over the years, including suicide [97, p. 78], but little quality research is available that might persuade the public of the serious consequences associated with elder abuse.

Unequivocally, the majority of research on elder abuse has been applied, although significant gaps remain. The GAO [28] identified the need for information specifically targeting APS, for example, recommended caseload sizes, investigating financial exploitation, and appropriate outcomes for APS cases. However, this information has yet to materialize.

Relatedly, the practice of APS continues to be based on experience rather than research, with limited efforts at resolving complex cases [28]. Testimony provided in 1990 describing an elder abuse case [104, p. 5] is so disturbingly similar to cases described in 2015, with the same "deer-in-the-headlights" frustration. Research into the development of interventions to promote long-term change, particularly for high-risk victims, has been palpably lacking until quite recently and should be actively encouraged.

Neuroscience is growing exponentially and is increasingly being implicated in cases of financial exploitation. And yet, APS lacks proper screening tools and at times screens out cases that should be in the system [77]. Consistent with the Elder Justice Coordinating Council's Recommendation #8, the development of psychometrically sound cognitive screening tools remains warranted in spite of a plethora of existing tools.

Education of seniors has been touted as the preferable method for preventing financial exploitation [78, 83].

[3]Available at https://www.ovcttac.gov/views/dspLegalAssistance.cfm?tab=1#onlinetraining.

[4]http://www.napsa-now.org/resource-center/training/core-aps-competencies/.

However, after concluding that educating seniors does not work, Attorney General Sorrel passionately recommended that the federal government "…support research into, and development of, evidence-based, effective programs that go beyond consumer education, to change consumer behavior" (US House Energy Subcommittee [76]. This targeted recommendation has yet to be adopted.

APS and other victim and senior serving organizations are in the field daily dispensing services, and yet the extent of unmet (or met) needs for services remains largely unknown [28]. Confidence that resources are being targeted effectively and judiciously is impossible without this type of research, but must be elicited from victims.

Social policy in this country lies at the whims of Congress [13], but is underlined by our values and perceptions of the elderly at the historical time and context in which policies are developed. Clearly society's perceptions have shifted over time. This review resolves that our lack of federal attention to the plight of older victims of abuse cannot be described as disgraceful, as it was 30 years ago [74], and yet much remains. The Committee's commitment to shepherd the recommendations outlined in this chapter has the potential to propel progress and to right some historical wrongs.

References

1. Administration for Community Living [ACL]. Elder justice coordinating council. Retrieved 1 September 2015, http://www.aoa.gov/AoA_programs/Elder_Rights/EJCC/index.aspx.
2. Anetzberger G. The evolution of a multidisciplinary response to elder abuse. Marquette Elder's Advis. 2011;13(1):107–28.
3. Anetzberger GJ. The reality of elder abuse. Clin Gerontol. 2005;28(1–2):1–25.
4. Baker JU. Elder abuse: problem in search of a policy. Praxis Where Reflect Pract Meet. 2003;3:15–22.
5. Binstock RH. From the Great Society to the Aging Society–25 Years of the Older Americans Act. Generations. 1991;15 (3):11–8.
6. Blancato RB. The elder justice act: a landmark policy initiative. J Elder Abuse Negl. 2004;14(2–3):181–3.
7. Bonnie RJ, Wallace RB, editors. Elder mistreatment: abuse, neglect, and exploitation in an aging America. Washington, DC: National Academies Press; 2003.
8. Brandl B, Dyer CB, Heisler CJ, Otto JM, Stiegel LA, Thomas RW. Elder abuse detection and intervention: a collaborative approach. New York, NY: Springer; 2007.
9. Breaux SJ, Hatch SO. S 333 IS–108th congress, 1st session: to promote elder justice, and for other purposes. J Elder Abuse Negl. 2004;14(2–3):87–179.
10. Breaux JB, Hatch OG. Confronting elder abuse, neglect, and exploitation: the need for elder justice legislation. Elder Law J. 2003;11:207–71.
11. Brownstein HH. The social reality of violence and violent crime. Boston: Allyn and Bacon; 2000.
12. Burston GR. Granny Battering. Br Med J. 1975;3:592.
13. Clark PG. The social allocation of health care resources: ethical dilemmas in age-group competition. Gerontologist. 1985;25 (2):119–25.
14. Clememte F, Kleiman MB. Fear of crime among the aged. Gerontologist. 1976;16(3):207–10.
15. Colello KJ. The elder justice act: background and issues for congress. Washington, DC: Congressional Research Service. 2014. Retrieved 31 July 2015, from https://fas.org/sgp/crs/misc/R43707.pdf.
16. Congressional Research Services. A compendium of statutory authorities that address the prevention, intervention, or treatment of elder abuse. 2010. Retrieved 29 May 2015, http://www.preventelderabuse.org/about/documents/CRSMemorandum_CompendiumofElderAbuseActivities_2011.pdf.
17. Connolly MT. Policy update: how change happens. Temple Polit Civil Rights Law Rev. 2012;21:329–36.
18. Dong X, Chen R, Simon MA. Elder abuse and dementia: a review of the research and health policy. Health Aff. 2014;33:642–9. doi:10.1377/hlthaff.2013.1261.
19. Dong X, Simon MA. Enhancing national policy and programs to address elder abuse. JAMA. 2011;305(23):2460–1.
20. Dong X, Simon M, Evans D. Elder self-neglect is associated with increased risk for elder abuse in a community-dwelling population findings from the Chicago Health and Aging Project. J Aging Health. 2013;25(1):80–96. doi:10.1177/0898264312467373.
21. Dooley DV Sr, Radke M. Does severe punishment deter financial crimes. Charlest Law Rev. 2009;4:619–59.
22. Doty P. The evolving balance of formal and informal, institutional and non-institutional long-term care for older Americans: a thirty-year perspective. Public Policy Aging Rep. 2010;20(1):3–9.
23. Dubble C. A policy perspective on elder justice through APS and law enforcement collaboration. J Gerontol Soc Work. 2006;46(3–4):35–55.
24. Falk E, Hoffman N. The role of capacity assessments in elder abuse investigations and guardianships. Clin Geriatr Med. 2014;30(4):851–68.
25. GAO. Elder justice: more federal coordination and public awareness needed (GAO-13-498). Washington, DC: General Accounting Office. 2013. http://gao.gov/assets/660/655820.pdf.
26. GAO. Elder justice: National strategy needed to effectively combat elder financial exploitation (GAO-13-110). Washington, DC: General Accounting Office. 2012a. Retrieved 10 July 2015, http://www.gao.gov/assets/660/650074.pdf.
27. GAO. Veterans' pension benefits: improvements needed to ensure only qualified veterans and survivors receive benefits (GAO-12-540). Washington, DC: General Accounting Office. 2012b. Retrieved 31 July 2015, http://www.gao.gov/assets/600/590847.pdf.
28. GAO. Elder justice: stronger federal leadership could enhance national response to elder abuse (GAO-11-208). Washington, DC: General Accounting Office. 2011a. Retrieved 3 July 2015, http://www.gao.gov/assets/320/316224.pdf.
29. GAO. Incapacitated adults: Oversight of federal fiduciaries and court-appointed guardians needs improvement (GAO-11-678). Washington, DC: General Accounting Office. 2011b. Retrieved 3 July 2015, http://www.gao.gov/assets/330/321761.pdf.
30. GAO. Guardianships: cases of financial exploitation, neglect, and abuse of seniors (GAO-10-1046). Washington, DC: General Accounting Office. 2010. Retrieved 3 July 2015, http://www.gao.gov/assets/320/310741.pdf.
31. GAO. Guardianships: little progress in ensuring protection for incapacitated elderly people (GAO-06-1086T; testimony). 2006. Retrieved 22 June 2015, http://www.gao.gov/assets/120/114716.pdf.

32. GAO. Guardianships: collaboration needed to protect incapacitated elderly people (GAO-04-655). 2004. Retrieved 22 June 2015, http://www.gao.gov/assets/250/243297.pdf.
33. GAO. Elder abuse: effectiveness of reporting laws and other factors (HRD-91-74). Washington, DC: General Accounting Office. 1991. Retrieved 10 July 2015, http://www.gao.gov/assets/220/214127.pdf.
34. Goergen T, Beaulieu M. Critical concepts in elder abuse research. Int Psychogeriatr. 2013;25(8):1217–28.
35. Gorbien MJ, Eisenstein AR. Elder abuse and neglect: an overview. Clin Geriatr Med. 2005;21(2):279–92.
36. Gordon RM, Brill D. The abuse and neglect of the elderly. Int J Law Psychiatry. 2001;24(2):183–97.
37. Gottlich V. Beyond granny bashing: elder abuse in the 1990's. Clgh Rev. 1994;28(4):371–87.
38. Hawes C. Elder abuse in residential long-term care settings: what is known and what information is needed? In: Bonnie RJ, Wallace R, editors. Elder mistreatment: abuse, neglect, and exploitation in an aging America. Washington, DC: National Academies Press; 2003. p. 446–500.
39. Hodge PD. National law enforcement programs to prevent, detect, investigate, and prosecute elder abuse and neglect in health care facilities. J Elder Abuse Negl. 1999;9(4):23–41.
40. Hooyman NR, Kiyak HA. Social geronotology: a multidisciplinary perspective. Boston: Allyn & Bacon; 1988.
41. Jackson SL. The vexing problem of defining financial exploitation occurring in domestic settings. J Financ Crime. 2015;21(1):63–78. doi:10.1108/JFC-05-2014-0026.
42. Jackson SL. The shifting conceptualization of elder abuse from social services, to criminal justice, and beyond. Int Psychogeriatr. 2016;28(1):1–8. doi:10.1017/S1041610215001271.
43. Jirik S, Sanders S. Analysis of elder abuse statutes across the United States, 2011–2012. J Gerontol Soc Work. 2014;57:478–97. doi:10.1080/01634372.2014.884514.
44. Jones BD, Baumgartner FR. The politics of attention: how government prioritizes problems. Chicago, IL: The University of Chicago Press; 2005.
45. Karp N, Wood N. Guarding the guardians: promising practices for court monitoring (#2007-21). Washington, DC: AARP Public Policy Institute; 2007.
46. Koenig RJ, DeGuerre CR. The legal and governmental response to domestic elder abuse. Clin Geriatr Med. 2005;21(2):383–98.
47. Kohn NA. Rethinking the constitutionality of age discrimination: a challenge to a decades-old consensus. UC Davis Law Rev. 2010;44:213.
48. Kohn NA. Outliving civil rights. Wash Univ Law Rev. 2009;86(5):1053–1115.
49. Lachs MS, Berman J. Under the radar: New York State Elder Abuse Prevalence Study. William B. Hoyt Memorial New York State Children, Family Trust Fund, New York State Office of Children and Family Services; 2011.
50. Levitt SD. Understanding why crime fell in the 1990s: four factors that explain the decline and six that do not. J Econ Perspect. 2004;18(1):163–190.
51. Lindberg B, Sabatino C, Blancato R. Bringing national action to a national disgrace: the history of the Elder Justice Act. NAELA J. 2011;7(1):105–22.
52. MetLife. The MetLife study of elder financial abuse crimes of occasion, desperation, and predation against America's elders. 2011. Retrieved https://www.metlife.com/assets/cao/mmi/publications/studies/2011/mmi-elder-financial-abuse.pdf.
53. Meyer MH, Bellas ML. The US old-age welfare state. In: Blieszner RH, Bedford VH, editors. Aging and the family: Theory and research. Westport, CT: Greenwood Publishing Group; 1996. p. 263–283.
54. Mixson PM. National Committee for the Prevention of Elder Abuse 2011–2012 Rosalie S. Wolf memorial award lecture: toward a more perfect union. J Elder Abuse Negl. 2015;27(3):169–73. doi:10.1080/08946566.2015.1021500.
55. Mixson PM. Public policy, elder abuse, and adult protective services: the struggle for coherence. J Elder Abuse Negl. 2010;22(1–2):16–36.
56. Mixson PM. Counterparts across time: comparing the National Elder Abuse Incidence Study and the National Incidence Study of Child Abuse and Neglect; 2000.
57. Mixson PM. Chapter five: an adult protective services perspective. J Elder Abuse Negl. 1995;7(2–3):69–87.
58. Nerenberg L. Communities respond to elder abuse. J Gerontol Soc Work. 2006;46(3–4):5–33.
59. O'Brien JG, Lansing M, Sanders MD. Diagnostic and treatment guidelines on elder abuse and neglect. Arch Fam Med. 1993;2:371–88.
60. Olinger JP. Elder abuse: the outlook for federal legislation. J Elder Abuse Negl. 1991;3(1):43–52.
61. Ory M, Hoffman MK, Hawkins M, Sanner B, Mockenhaupt R. Challenging aging stereotypes: strategies for creating a more active society. Am J Prev Med. 2003;25(3):164–71.
62. Palincsar J, Crouse Cobb D. The physician's role in detecting and reporting elder abuse. J Leg Med. 1982;3(3):413–41.
63. Quinn MJ. Guardianship of adults: achieving justice, autonomy, and safety. Berlin: Springer Publishing Company; 2005.
64. Reyes-Ortiz CA, Burnett J, Flores DV, Halphen JM, Dyer CB. Medical implications of elder abuse: self-neglect. Clin Geriatr Med. 2014;30(4):807–23.
65. Riggs AT, Podrazik PM. Financial exploitation of the elderly: review of the epidemic—its victims, national impact, and legislative solutions. In: Factora RM, editor, Aging and money. New York: Springer; 2014, pp. 1–18.
66. Salend E, Kane RA, Satz M, Pynoos J. Elder abuse reporting: limitations of statutes. Gerontologist. 1984;24(1):61–9.
67. Sayles-Cross S. Profile of familial elder abuse: a selected review of the literature. J Community Health Nurs. 1988;5(4):209–19.
68. Steinmetz SK. Battered parents. Society. 1978;15(5):54–5.
69. Stiegel L, Klem EM. Power of attorney abuse: what states can do about it. Washington, DC: AARP Public Policy Institute. 2008. http://assets.aarp.org/rgcenter/consume/2008_17_poa.pdf.
70. Teaster PB, Wangmo T, Anetzberger GJ. A glass half full: the dubious history of elder abuse policy. J Elder Abuse Negl. 2010;22(1–2):6–15.
71. US Department of Justice [USDOJ]. The elder justice roadmap. 2014. Retrieved 31 July 2015, http://ncea.acl.gov/Library/Gov_Report/docs/EJRP_Roadmap_and_Appendices.pdf.
72. US Department of Justice [USDOJ]. Our aging population: promoting empowerment, preventing victimization, and implementing coordinated interventions. Washington, DC: Office of Justice Programs (No. 186256), December 2000. http://ojp.gov/docs/ncj_186256.pdf.
73. US House Select Committee on Aging. Elder abuse: a decade of shame and inaction (H.R. REP. NO. 101-752). A Report by the Chairman of the Subcommittee on Health and Long-Term Care of the Select Committee on Aging, House of Representatives, One Hundred First Congress, Second Session. 1990.
74. US House Select Committee on Aging. Elder abuse: a national disgrace. Washington, DC: U.S. Government Printing Office; 1985.
75. US House Select Committee on Aging. Elder abuse: examination of a hidden problem. Washington, DC: U.S. Government Printing Office; 1981.
76. US House Subcommittee on Commerce, Manufacturing, and Trade. Fraud on the Elderly: a Growing Concern for a Growing

Population. Retrieved June, 2013, http://energycommerce.house.gov/press-release/commerce-manufacturing-and-trade-subcommittee-highlights-efforts-combat-fraud-america-on-americas-elderly#sthash.9jzA9PuT.dpuf.
77. US Senate Special Committee on Aging. Broken Trust: Combating financial exploitation of vulnerable seniors. Washington, DC: US Government Printing Office. Retrieved 22 June 2015, http://www.aging.senate.gov/hearings/broken-trust_combating-financial-exploitation-of-vulnerable-seniors.
78. US Senate Special Committee on Aging. America's Invisible Epidemic: Preventing Elder Financial Abuse. Washington, DC: US Government Printing Office. Retrieved 22 June 2015, testimony. 2012. http://www.aging.senate.gov/hearings/americas-invisible-epidemic-preventing-elder-financial-abuse.
79. US Senate Special Committee on Aging. Enhancing Women's Retirement Security. Washington, DC: US Government Printing Office. 2012. Retrieved 22 June 2015, http://www.aging.senate.gov/imo/media/doc/07252012.pdf.
80. US Senate Special Committee on Aging. Pension Poachers: Preventing Fraud and Protecting America's Veterans. Washington, DC: US Government Printing Office. 2012. Retrieved 22 June 2015, http://www.aging.senate.gov/imo/media/doc/06062012.pdf.
81. US Senate Special Committee on Aging. Justice for All: Ending Elder Abuse, Neglect and Financial Exploitation. Washington, DC: US Government Printing Office. 2011. Retrieved 22 June 2015, http://www.aging.senate.gov/imo/media/doc/322011.pdf.
82. US Senate Special Committee on Aging. Boomers and the Budget: What Does it Mean for America's Seniors? Washington, DC: US Government Printing Office. 2007. Retrieved 22 June 2015, http://www.aging.senate.gov/imo/media/doc/2152007.pdf.
83. US Senate Special Committee on Aging. Abuse of our elders: how we can stop it. Washington, DC: US Government Printing Office. 2007. Retrieved 22 June 2015, http://www.aging.senate.gov/imo/media/doc/7182007.pdf.
84. US Senate Special Committee on Aging. Bridging the Gender Gap: Eliminating Retirement Income Disparity for Women. Washington, DC: US Government Printing Office. 2006. Retrieved 22 June 2015, http://www.aging.senate.gov/imo/media/doc/3152006.pdf.
85. US Senate Special Committee on Aging. Exploitation of Seniors: America's Ailing Guardianship System. Washington, DC: US Government Printing Office. 2006. Retrieved 22 June 2015, http://www.aging.senate.gov/imo/media/doc/972006.pdf.
86. US Senate Special Committee on Aging. Forum: Protecting Older Americans Under Guardianship: Who is Watching the Guardian?. Washington, DC: US Government Printing Office. 2004. Retrieved 22 June 2015, http://www.aging.senate.gov/imo/media/doc/72220041.pdf.
87. US Senate Special Committee on Aging. Internet fraud hits seniors: as seniors venture into the web, the financial predators lurk and take aim. Washington, DC: US Government Printing Office. 2004. Retrieved 22 June 2015, http://www.aging.senate.gov/imo/media/doc/3232004.pdf.
88. US Senate Special Committee on Aging. Shattering the Silence: confronting the perils of family elder abuse. Washington, DC: US Government Printing Office. 2003. Retrieved 22 June 2015, http://www.aging.senate.gov/imo/media/doc/10202003.pdf.
89. US Senate Special Committee on Aging. Guardianships over the elderly: security provided or freedom denied. Washington, DC: US Government Printing Office. 2003. Retrieved 22 June 2015, http://www.aging.senate.gov/imo/media/doc/2112003.pdf.
90. US Senate Special Committee on Aging. Settling for silver in the golden years: the special challenges of women in retirement planning and security. Washington, DC: US Government Printing Office. 2002. Retrieved 22 June 2015, http://www.aging.senate.gov/imo/media/doc/5232002.pdf.
91. US Senate Special Committee on Aging. Women and aging: bearing the burden of long-term care. Washington, DC: US Government Printing Office. 2002. Retrieved 22 June 2015, http://www.aging.senate.gov/imo/media/doc/2620021.pdf.
92. US Senate Special Committee on Aging. The economic downturn and its impact on seniors: stretching limited dollars in Medicaid, Health and Senior Services. Washington, DC: US Government Printing Office. 2002. Retrieved 22 June 2015, http://www.aging.senate.gov/imo/media/doc/31420021.pdf.
93. US Senate Special Committee on Aging. Saving our seniors: preventing elder abuse, neglect and exploitation. Washington, DC: US Government Printing Office. 2001. Retrieved 22 June 2015, http://www.aging.senate.gov/imo/media/doc/61420011.pdf.
94. US Senate Special Committee on Aging. Women and social security reform: are individual accounts the answer? Washington, DC: US Government Printing Office. 1999. Retrieved 22 June 2015, http://www.aging.senate.gov/imo/media/doc/publications/2221999.pdf.
95. US Senate Special Committee on Aging. Forum: Can we rest in peace? The anxiety of elderly parents caring for baby boomers with disabilities. 1998. Retrieved 3 October 2015, http://www.aging.senate.gov/imo/media/doc/publications/9181998.pdf.
96. US Senate Special Committee on Aging. Telescams exposed: how telemarketers target the elderly. Washington, DC: US Government Printing Office. 1996. Retrieved 22 June 2015, http://www.aging.senate.gov/imo/media/doc/publications/361996.pdf.
97. US Senate Special Committee on Aging. Suicide and the elderly: a population at risk. 1996. Retrieved 3 October 2015, http://www.aging.senate.gov/imo/media/doc/publications/7301996.pdf.
98. US Senate Special Committee on Aging. Elder Abuse and Violence against Midlife and Older Women. Washington, DC: US Government Printing Office.1994. Retrieved 22 June 2015, http://www.aging.senate.gov/imo/media/doc/publications/541994.pdf.
99. US Senate Special Committee on Aging. Improving income security for older women in retirement: current issues and legislative reform proposals. Washington, DC: US Government Printing Office. 1993. Retrieved 22 June 2015, http://www.aging.senate.gov/imo/media/doc/publications/9231993.pdf.
100. US Senate Special Committee on Aging. Roundtable discussion on guardianship. Washington, DC: US Government Printing Office. 1992. Retrieved 22 June 2015, http://www.aging.senate.gov/imo/media/doc/publications/621992.pdf.
101. US Senate Special Committee on Aging. Forever young: music and aging. Washington, DC: US Government Printing Office. 1991. Retrieved 22 June 2015, http://www.aging.senate.gov/imo/media/doc/publications/811991.pdf.
102. US Senate Special Committee on Aging. Older women and employment: facts and myths. Washington, DC: US Government Printing Office. 1991. Retrieved 22 June 2015, http://www.aging.senate.gov/imo/media/doc/publications/821991.pdf.
103. US Senate Special Committee on Aging. Elder abuse and neglect: prevention and intervention, Birmingham, AL. Washington, DC: US Government Printing Office. 1991. Retrieved 22 June 2015, http://www.aging.senate.gov/imo/media/doc/publications/6291991.pdf.
104. US Senate Special Committee on Aging. Crimes against the elderly: let's fight back, Las Vegas, NV and Reno, NV. Washington, DC: US Government Printing Office. 1990. Retrieved 22 June 2015, http://www.aging.senate.gov/imo/media/doc/publications/8211990.pdf.
105. US Senate Special Committee on Aging. Our nation's elderly: hidden victims of the drug war? Washington, DC: US Government Printing Office. 1989. Retrieved 22 June 2015, http://www.aging.senate.gov/imo/media/doc/publications/11151989.pdf.

106. US Senate Special Committee on Aging. The American Indian elderly: the forgotten population, Pine Ridge, SD. 1988. Retrieved 8 August 2015, http://www.aging.senate.gov/imo/media/doc/publications/7211988.pdf.
107. US Senate Special Committee on Aging. Reauthorization of the Older Americans Act, Casselberry, FL. Washington, DC: US Government Printing Office. 1987. Retrieved 22 June 2015, http://www.aging.senate.gov/imo/media/doc/publications/721987.pdf.
108. US Senate Special Committee on Aging. Proposed fiscal year 1988 budget: what it means to older Americans. Washington, DC: US Government Printing Office. 1987. Retrieved 22 June 2015, http://www.aging.senate.gov/imo/media/doc/publications/3131987.pdf.
109. US Senate Special Committee on Aging. Employment opportunities for women: today and tomorrow, Cleveland, OH. Washington, DC: US Government Printing Office. 1986. Retrieved 22 June 2015, http://www.aging.senate.gov/imo/media/doc/publications/4211986.pdf.
110. US Senate Special Committee on Aging. Gramm-Rudman-Hollings: the impact on the elderly. Washington, DC: US Government Printing Office. 1986. Retrieved 22 June 2015, http://www.aging.senate.gov/imo/media/doc/publications/2211986.pdf.
111. US Senate Special Committee on Aging. Women in our aging society, Columbus, OH. Washington, DC: US Government Printing Office. 1984. Retrieved 22 June 2015, http://www.aging.senate.gov/imo/media/doc/publications/1081984.pdf.
112. US Senate Special Committee on Aging. Crime against the elderly, Los Angeles, CA. Washington, DC: US Government Printing Office. 1983. Retrieved 22 June 2015, http://www.aging.senate.gov/imo/media/doc/publications/761983.pdf.
113. US Senate Special Committee on Aging. Combating frauds against the elderly. Washington, DC: US Government Printing Office. 1983. Retrieved 22 June 2015, http://www.aging.senate.gov/imo/media/doc/publications/311983.pdf.
114. US Senate Special Committee on Aging. Older Americans fighting the fear of crime. Washington, DC: US Government Printing Office. 1981. Retrieved 22 June 2015, http://www.aging.senate.gov/imo/media/doc/publications/9221981.pdf.
115. US Senate Special Committee on Aging. Impact of federal estate tax policies on rural women. 1981. Retrieved 2 August 2015, http://www.aging.senate.gov/imo/media/doc/publications/241981.pdf.
116. US Senate Special Committee on Aging. Frauds against the elderly, Harrisburg, PA. Washington, DC: US Government Printing Office. 1981. Retrieved 22 June 2015, http://www.aging.senate.gov/imo/media/doc/publications/841981.pdf.
117. US Senate Special Committee on Aging. Crime and the elderly: what your community can do, Albuquerque, NM. Washington, DC: US Government Printing Office. 1980. Retrieved 22 June 2015, http://www.aging.senate.gov/imo/media/doc/publications/6231980.pdf.
118. US Senate Special Committee on Aging. Elder abuse. Washington, DC: US Government Printing Office. 1980. Retrieved 22 June 2015, http://www.aging.senate.gov/imo/media/doc/publications/6111980.pdf.
119. US Senate Special Committee on Aging. Medicare and medicaid frauds: part 3. Washington, DC: US Government Printing Office. 1975. Retrieved 22 June 2015, http://www.aging.senate.gov/imo/media/doc/publications/1251975.pdf.
120. US Senate Special Committee on Aging. Mental health and the elderly. Washington, DC: US Government Printing Office. 1975. Retrieved 22 June 2015, http://www.aging.senate.gov/imo/media/doc/publications/9291975.pdf.
121. US Senate Special Committee on Aging. Establishing a national institute on aging. 1974. Retrieved 2 August 2015, (NIA signed into law 5/31/74) http://www.aging.senate.gov/imo/media/doc/publications/811974.pdf.
122. US Senate Special Committee on Aging. Evaluation of administration on aging and conduct of White House Conference on Aging, Joint Hearings: Part 4—Washington, DC. March 31, 1971. Washington, DC: US Government Printing Office. 1971. Retrieved 22 June 2015, http://www.aging.senate.gov/imo/media/doc/publications/3311971.pdf.
123. US Senate Special Committee on Aging. Older Americans in rural areas: part 2, majestic-freeburn, KY. Washington, DC: US Government Printing Office. 1969. Retrieved 22 June 2015, http://www.aging.senate.gov/imo/media/doc/publications/9121969.pdf.
124. US Senate Special Committee on Aging. Availability and usefulness offederal programs and services to elderly Mexican-Americans: Part 2, El Paso, TX. Washington, DC: US Government Printing Office. 1968. Retrieved 22 June 2015, http://www.aging.senate.gov/imo/media/doc/publications/12181968.pdf.
125. US Senate Special Committee on Aging. Consumer interests of the elderly: part 1. Washington, DC: US Government Printing Office. 1967. Retrieved 22 June 2015, http://www.aging.senate.gov/imo/media/doc/publications/1171967.pdf.
126. US Senate Special Committee on Aging. Interstate mail order land sales: part 3. Washington, DC: US Government Printing Office. 1964. Retrieved 22 June 2015, http://www.aging.senate.gov/imo/media/doc/publications/5201964.pdf.
127. US Senate Special Committee on Aging. Frauds and quackery affecting the older citizen: part 3. Washington, DC: US Government Printing Office. 1963. Retrieved 22 June 2015, http://www.aging.senate.gov/imo/media/doc/publications/1171963.pdf.
128. US Senate Special Committee on Aging. Relocation of elderly people: part 4, Portland, OR. Washington, DC: US Government Printing Office. 1962. Retrieved 22 June 2015, http://www.aging.senate.gov/imo/media/doc/publications/1231962.pdf.
129. US Senate Special Committee on Aging. Nursing homes: part 2, Walla Walla, WA. Washington, DC: US Government Printing Office. 1961. Retrieved 22 June 2015, http://www.aging.senate.gov/imo/media/doc/publications/11101961.pdf.
130. Wolf R. Elder abuse and neglect: history and concepts. In: Bonnie RJ, Wallace RB, editors. Elder mistreatment: abuse, neglect, and exploitation in an aging America. Washington, DC: National Academies Press; 2003. p. 238–48.
131. Wolf RS. Elder abuse and family violence: testimony presented before the US Senate Special Committee on Aging. J Elder Abuse Negl. 1996;8(1):81–96.
132. Wrosch PV. What more can congress do about the elder abuse epidemic? A proposal for national movement. Temple Polit Civil Rights Law Rev. 2013;23:1–44.

Shades of Charles Dickens: Elder Abuse Policy Past, Present, and Yet to Be

29

Brian W. Lindberg and Pamela B. Teaster

29.1 Introduction

I am here tonight to warn you that you have yet a chance and hope of escaping my fate. You will be haunted by three spirits! Without their visits you cannot hope to shun the path I tread! [7].

The path from societal definition of elder abuse as a family matter or, at best, a social problem to societal recognition of and action on elder abuse as a crime has been long and circuitous. Although elder abuse dates back to the beginning of human history, the problem has only recently gained traction as a political issue and one acknowledged by the general public. The historical lack of political will to take action to prevent and punish elder abuse is surprising [20] given the length of time that advocates have been raising awareness and the scope of the problem due to the ever increasing aging of the population. Measured against its sister problems of child abuse and intimate partner violence, attention to elder abuse comes in dead last in terms of political awareness and public and private funding for addressing the problem.

The belated arrival of elder abuse in the public conscience is emblematic of the problem itself—elder abuse is a complex, wicked problem with contributing factors running the gamut from micro to macro levels of society. The complexity and scope of the problem means that it must be addressed using a committed, interdisciplinary approach engaging the brightest and most dedicated minds possible. According to Churchman [4] and Rittle and Webber [19], "wicked problems" are those in which (1) the solution depends on how the problem is framed and vice versa (i.e., the problem definition depends on the solution), (2) stakeholders have radically different world views and frames of reference for understanding the problem, (3) constraints that the problem is subject to and resources needed to solve it change over time, and (4) the problem is never solved definitively.

In the chapter that follows, we consider elder abuse as a wicked problem and examine the past, present, and future of the most significant federal laws: the Elder Justice Act, the Older Americans Act, the Violence Against Women Act, and Social Security Block Grants. In addition, we discuss the White House Conference on Aging and the Crime Victims Fund, both of which have played a part addressing elder abuse.

29.2 Shades of the Past: National Efforts to Address Elder Abuse

The origins of the Elder Justice Act, discussed below, can be traced to the 1950s when grants for "protective service unit" demonstration projects were awarded by the Department of Health, Education and Welfare. In 1961, the first White House Conference on Aging (WHCoA) was held, an event that stimulated national discussion and congressional initiatives aimed at preventing elder abuse [8]. In 1962, Public Welfare Amendments to the Social Security Act "authorized payments to states for establishing protective services" and funded demonstration projects focused on the problem of elder abuse [20]. Building from this momentum, the 1965 Older Americans Act (OAA) represented "the watershed of...new awareness and activism" around the rights and needs of older adults [8]. The OAA provided assistance to states to develop programs to help older persons but did not specifically mention elder abuse [20]. As a result of these two pieces of federal legislation, many states mobilized to enact laws providing protective services to older adults [8].

Used with permission of the authors, for portions of this chapter, we draw upon the following article: Lindberg, B., Sabatino, C., & Blancato, R. (2011). Bringing national action to a national disgrace: the history of the elder justice act. *National Academy of Elder Law Attorneys Journal* 7(105–124).

B.W. Lindberg (✉)
Elder Justice Coalition, 1612 K Street, NW, Suite 400, Washington, DC 20006, USA
e-mail: brian@consumers.org

P.B. Teaster
Center for Gerontology (0555), ISCE, 230 Grove Lane, Virginia Tech, Blacksburg, VA 24061, USA
e-mail: pteaster@vt.edu

X. Dong (ed.), *Elder Abuse*, DOI 10.1007/978-3-319-47504-2_29

In the 1970s and 1980s, both progress and setbacks continued related to bringing elder abuse into the public consciousness. The White House hosted the second WHCoA in 1971. In 1974, the Social Security Act authorized Adult Protective Services (APS) under Title XX, which prompted some states to create their own APS units and others states to go so far as requiring mandatory reporting of elder abuse [20]. Title XX authorized funding of more demonstration projects. In 1981, Title XX was converted to the Social Services Block Grant, and the mandate to fund APS was deleted, thus leading to the under-resourced and inadequately coordinated APS system of today. Also in 1981, the third WHCoA examined the issue of elder abuse, and in the same year, a House Select Committee on Aging did the same, producing a report entitled *Elder Abuse: An Examination of a Hidden Problem* [20].

Responding to these events, Democratic Congresswoman Mary Rose Oakar of Ohio sponsored the Prevention, Identification, and Treatment of Adult Abuse Bill of 1981, which proposed funding incentives to states for the provision of APS. Although the legislation was not enacted, one observer noted: "Absent federal direction on this issue, many states continued to adopt their own statutes providing adult protective services which were usually delivered by state or local social service agencies" [18].

In 1984, Congress passed the Victims of Crime Act, which provided financial compensation to victims to cover such costs as health care and lost wages resulting from crime. The law applied to crime victims in all age groups but helped boost services to victims of elder abuse [8]. Significantly, it established the Crime Victims Fund. Today, some monies from that fund are used to address elder abuse.

In 1985, U.S. Representative Claude Pepper, D-Fla., a tenacious champion of older adults for more than a decade who had hosted public hearings on the issue of elder abuse for years, issued *Elder Abuse: A National Disgrace,* acting in his capacity as Chairman of the Subcommittee on Health and Long-Term Care of the House Select Committee on Aging [20]. Congress moved the elder justice agenda forward for older adults living in nursing homes with the Omnibus Budget Reconciliation Act (OBRA) of 1987. OBRA "mandated that nursing homes protect and preserve the quality of life of the residents." OBRA resulted in regulations that specifically defined elder abuse in the context of long-term care (LTC) facilities, mandated that it was the state's responsibility to investigate abuse allegations against facilities, and instructed facilities to train staff to prevent elder abuse [20].

Also in 1987, the reauthorization of the OAA made a strong national foray into elder abuse prevention by defining it and providing for Elder Abuse Prevention Services to "address elder abuse through public education, identification of abuse, and methods for receiving reports of abuse" [8, 20]. The Congress did not appropriate funds for those services, however. Sadly, for several decades, lack of funding for elder abuse prevention has been the primary barrier to establishing and expanding elder justice services. To date, the majority of funding for APS comes from Social Services Block Grants (SSBGs) and in steadily declining amounts since the early 1980s [18]. The reauthorization also saw significant strengthening of the Long-Term Care Ombudsman Programs designed to improve their ability to address a range of abuses found in nursing homes across the nation.

Not until 1990 did Congress provide funding specifically for elder abuse prevention and, even then, the sum was meager, totaling just \$2.9 million divided among 50 states, the District of Columbia, and the U.S. territories. Compared to other victims of abuse, older victims continued to receive short shrift. "States were spending an average of \$45.03 per child and only \$3.80 per adult on protective services (U.S. Congress 1990)," [14]. Despite low funding, however, the then Administration on Aging (AoA) laid the groundwork for continued action. In 1988, the AoA launched the national center on elder abuse (NCEA), which was made permanent in the 1992 reauthorization of the OAA. Title VII of that legislation entitled Allotments for Vulnerable Elder Rights Protection Activities, thus strengthening three programs: the Long-Term Care Ombudsman Program, Programs for the Prevention of Abuse and Exploitation, and State Legal Assistance Development Programs [12]. Also in the early 1990s, the Congressional House Select Committee on Aging's Subcommittee on Health and Long-Term Care issued two back-to-back reports: *Elder Abuse: A Decade of Shame and Inaction* (1990) and *Protecting America's Abused Elderly: The Need For Congressional Action* (1991). In 1992, The Family Violence Prevention Services Act funded a major study, the National Elder Abuse Incidence Study (NEAIS), conducted by the Administration for Children and Families and AoA. Data from the study are "the political benchmark for data on elder victimization" and validated the belief that only a very few cases of elder abuse are ever reported to APS or local authorities [8]. In 1995, President Clinton announced a fourth White House Conference on Aging, the first in 14 years. Under the leadership of Executive Director Robert Blancato, the 1995 WHCoA devoted unprecedented attention to elder abuse, with two resolutions the conference produced devoted solely to the protection of vulnerable older adults.

29.3 The Elder Justice Act

Past On March 23, 2010, President Obama signed the Elder Justice Act into law as part of his landmark health care reform bill, the Patient Protection and Affordable Care Act (ACA). The Elder Justice Act (EJA) was the first federal law to specifically state that "it is the right of older adults to be free of abuse, neglect, and exploitation" [20]. Its passage was the result of tireless and lengthy negotiation and advocacy that had spanned a decade and where the issue reached across the aisle. Although Republicans in Congress opposed the ACA, a number supported inclusion of the EJA in the ACA and worked with Democrats to make it happen.

In September 2002, the Elder Justice Act (EJA) was first introduced by Senator John Breaux (D-LA) and Senator Orrin Hatch (R-UT) as part of the 107th Congress (S.2933). They reintroduced the EJA in several subsequent Congresses, each presenting unique and viable opportunities for passage. Over the years, at each of four congressional hearings on the bill, advocates, congressional staff, and bill sponsors, presented testimony and held press conferences to build support and draw attention to the issue. Advocates also highlighted the bill in conference presentations, op-ed pieces, and action alerts. A steady flow of news articles on abuse cases from around the country, including coverage of the high profile cases of the son of philanthropist and socialite Brooke Astor, who was accused of abuse and exploitation in 2007–2008, and the rising recognition of the exploitation of actor Mickey Rooney ($\sim$2010) provided public ammunition for bill supporters. Although there was never any public opposition to the bill, it took 8 years before the EJA became law. In at least two Congresses, individual senators put holds on the bill to keep it from coming to the floor for a vote, either to leverage consideration of other legislation or because of concerns about the potential cost of the bill. The Bush Administration raised objections late in the 109th Congress, killing the bill's momentum toward passage. Another year, Senator Bob Graham of Florida added an amendment that was opposed by other senators, which also derailed the bill. With the bill referred to several different committees with jurisdiction for various sections and provisions, passage became difficult and required redrafting. In the 108th (S.333, H.R.2490), 109th (S.2010, H.R.4993), and 110th (S.1070, H.R.1783) Congresses, the Senate Finance Committee passed the bill and sent it to the full Senate for votes, but to no avail. In the 110th Congress, the EJA was included in the Senate version of the must-pass Tax Relief and Health Care Act of 2006 (P.L 109-432). All of the EJA, except a study to establish a uniform database on elder abuse, was deleted in conference negotiations on the insistence of the House, which had not devoted any time to the issue.

In the 111th (S.795, H.R.2006) Congress, the Senate Finance Committee incorporated the EJA into the ACA, which was merged with the Senate Committee on Health, Education, Labor, and Pensions (HELP) version of health care reform and was passed by the full Senate.

Non-political factors also help explain why the EJA was slow to gain traction. Historically, elder abuse and neglect had been considered a "private matter" to be handled within families. This perspective discouraged public focus on prevention and prosecution. Although there is significant evidence that long-term care facilities have been a home for abuse, experts sometimes blamed a lack of action on the perception that the health care system is overregulated, making legislators loathe to add additional reporting and training requirements to long-term care facility administration. It is also likely that ageism is also a contributing factor. Further, a national focus on terrorism/security concerns and foreign affairs may have trumped the domestic issue of elder abuse, in part by competing for available resources for domestic spending in very tight budget times. Opposition also came from various administration officials who alleged that sufficient programs and provisions were already in place to deal with elder abuse and that no further mandates were necessary.

In the end, the passage of the EJA was achieved due to many forums, hearings, reports, analyses, and press accounts of elder abuse and exploitation that accumulated over decades and the dedication of myriad stakeholders, especially the Elder Justice Coalition (EJC), established by Robert Blancato, National Coordinator. Founding members of the EJC were the National Academy of Elder Law Attorneys (NAELA), National Adult Protective Services Association (NAPSA), National Association of State and Long-Term Care Ombudsman Programs (NASOP), National Association of State Units on Aging (NASUA), and the National Committee for the Prevention of Elder Abuse (NCPEA). Finally, President Obama supported the EJA and it became law, as part of the Affordable Care Act, on March 23, 2010. Once the law was passed, supporters quickly turned their attention to obtaining funding so that implementation of the act's provisions would guarantee that elder abuse and neglect could finally be addressed with gravity and urgency.

It should be noted that the original Senate bill included provisions that were dropped either in the Finance Committee negotiations or were referred to other committees (Judiciary and HELP) that did not act on the provisions. In the 110th Congress, the provisions that fell under the Judiciary Committee were introduced separately as the Elder Abuse Victims Act of 2008 (H.R.5352) by Representative Joe Sestak (D-PA). This bill was passed by the House Judiciary Committee and the full House, but was not passed by the Senate. In the 111th Congress, The Elder Abuse Victims Act of 2008 (H.R.448) was introduced by

Representative Sestak in the House and its companion S.1821 was introduced by Senator Herb Kohl (D-WI). Again, the House passed the bill, but the Senate did not.

29.4 The Present Elder Justice Act

The EJA created a new subtitle to Title XX of the Social Security Act (Codified at 42 USC §1397j to §1397m) and authorized a total of $757 million from 2011 to 2014 for its provisions. The President's annual budget requests for the EJA have been inconsistent over the years. For FY 2011, the budget proposal included $16.5 million for state adult protective services (APS) and $5 million for the state Long-Term Care Ombudsman Programs. After 2 years, the budget dropped the EJA ombudsman funding proposal (it supported other funding for ombudsmen under the OAA). It took Congress until FY 2015 to appropriate any discretionary funds to implement its provisions, although funding from the Prevention and Public Health Fund, also established by the ACA, has been used by HHS to implement some of the ACA's provisions. For example, in FY 2012, HHS used $6 million in PPHF funding for EJA activities, in FY 2013 it used $2 million. In FY 2014, no funds were transferred or appropriated for the EJA. In FY 2015 and FY 2016, the President requested $25 million for his "Elder Justice Initiative," and Congress appropriated $4 million and $8 million, respectively. The President's budget request for FY 2017 dropped to $10 million and at this writing, only the Senate Appropriations Committee has acted, providing all $10 million, but with no guarantee that amount will hold up in the final bill.

An overview of the status of implementation of its core provisions follows.

Enhancing National Coordination The EJA established an Elder Justice Coordinating Council (EJCC), made up of designees of the Secretary of HHS, the Attorney General and other federal agencies. The EJCC is charged with fostering coordination throughout the federal government on elder abuse topics. Supplementing the Coordinating Council is a 27-member Advisory Board made up of experts on elder abuse, neglect, and exploitation appointed by the Secretary. To bring uniformity to research on elder abuse protections in the field, the EJA requires the Secretary to promulgate regulations to guide researchers in the field of elder abuse.

Action on some provisions has been encouraging. From October 2012 through April 2014, the EJCC conducted five meetings. The meetings included expert testimony, public comments, presentation of white papers, and deliberation by EJCC members. The work of the EJCC is supported by a pre-existing Elder Justice Interagency Working Group. In June 2015, the EJCC issued a report to Congress that included strong recommendations for increased federal action on elder abuse. In July 2010, federal regulations were published establishing the public Advisory Board, however, no further action has been taken to establish it [9].

Establishing Forensic Centers Section 2031 (42 U.S.C. 1397l) of the EJA authorizes a total of ten centers to develop forensic expertise pertaining to elder abuse, neglect and exploitation, provide services in local communities, and make data available to develop the capacity of geriatric health care professionals and law enforcement to collect forensic evidence. Although the EJA authorizes $26 million over 4 years for this purpose, to date Congress has not provided the needed funding (appropriations).

29.5 Strengthening Adult Protective Services

Section 2042 of the act (42 U.S.C. 1397m^{-1}.) requires the Secretary of HHS to accomplish five tasks:

1. Provide funding to state and local APS offices. The act authorizes $100 million a year—$400 million total—for this purpose, the largest amount authorized for any component of the act. The Secretary must apportion funds according to a formula based on a state's population over age 60. Since inadequate funding and staffing chronically plague APS programs nationwide, this provision has the potential to enhance significantly APS capacity. An additional $100 million is authorized to fund demonstration programs by state and municipal governments for training in methods of detection or prevention.
2. Coordinate with the Department of Justice to collect and disseminate on an annual basis data relating to abuse, neglect, and exploitation of elders.
3. Develop and disseminate information and conduct training on best practices in carrying out adult protective services.
4. Conduct research related to the quality of APS programs.
5. Provide technical assistance to states and other entities that provide APS.

The act authorizes $15 million to the Secretary to carry out these functions. Congress has provided limited funding (mentioned above) in addition to the HHS funds from the PPHF for elder justice activities. The $6 million in PPHF funds were used for five awards to states for Elder Abuse Prevention Intervention Programs. Further, in FY 2015, ACL received a $4 million appropriation for demonstration grants to states to enhance their APS systems. With FY 2016 funds, the ACL announced funding opportunities under its Elder Justice Innovation Grants program which included the areas of self-neglect, abuse in guardianship, elder abuser forensic centers, and elder abuse in Indian Country.

Enhancing the Capacity of Long-Term Care Settings

The EJA authorizes several initiatives to enhance the capacity to prevent and respond to elder abuse, neglect, and exploitation in long-term care settings. Section 2041 (42 U.S.C. 1397m) requires the Secretary of HHS, in coordination with the Secretary of Labor, to provide grants to long-term care facilities and community-based long-term care entities to create incentives for direct care workers to seek, train for, and maintain employment in long-term care facilities. The Secretary must also adopt electronic standards for the exchange of clinical data by long-term care facilities and develop procedures to accept electronic submission of clinical data from long-term care entities. A total of $67.5 million is authorized for these purposes; however, to date, Congress has not appropriated funds for these activities.

Section 2043 (42 U.S.C. 1397m^{-2}) provides grants to improve the capacity of long-term care ombudsmen to respond to elder abuse and neglect, conduct pilot programs and provide support. The EJA authorizes $32.5 million for this purpose. An additional $40 million is authorized for ombudsman training with respect to elder abuse, neglect, and exploitation. Although the President's FY 2011 and FY 2012 budget proposals included $5 million in funding for the LTCOP, which was not provided by Congress, subsequent budget proposals did not include that proposal. Section 2046 of the act lumps together a number of mandates to accomplish the above objectives. The EJA:

- Creates a National Training Institute (42 U.S.C. 13951-3a) to provide and improve the training of surveyors to investigate allegations of abuse and neglect and misappropriation of property in programs and facilities that receive payments under medicare or medicaid. In addition, the institute is to evaluate specified capacities, provide technical assistance, identify best practices, assess the performance of and provide back-up to state complaint intake systems, and report annually on several parameters. The act authorizes $12 million for the institute. An additional $20 million in grants is authorized for state agencies that oversee skilled nursing facilities to design and implement effective complaint investigation systems.
- Requires long-term care facilities to report a crime or the reasonable suspicion of a criminal act against a resident to law enforcement within 2 hours in the case of serious bodily injury, or otherwise within 24 h (42 U.S.C. 1320b-25). Failure to comply with this regulation or retaliation against any reporter will trigger substantial civil monetary penalties.
- Requires the Secretary to study the need to establish a national nurse aide registry and to report its findings to the Elder Justice Coordinating Council and specified congressional committees by September 2011.

Overall, Congress has generally not appropriated funds for these activities; however, HHS has taken action to implement requirements for reporting crimes that occur in long-term care facilities. In June 2011, the centers for medicare and medicaid services, an agency within HHS, issued guidance to state regulators on Reporting Reasonable Suspicion of a Crime in a Long-Term Care Facility (LTC): Section 1150B of the Social Security Act.

Finally, two related provisions in the ACA not technically part of the EJA deserve mention. Section 6121 amends the initial training requirements for nursing facility staff to include training in dementia management and patient abuse prevention. Section 6201 requires the Secretary of HHS to establish a program to identify efficient, effective, and economical procedures for long-term care facilities to conduct background checks on prospective direct patient access employees on a nationwide basis. Note that Section 307 of the Medicare Prescription Drug, Improvement, and Modernization Act of 2003 (42 U.S.C. 1395aa.) previously created a pilot program for national and state background checks. The ACA provision expands the program nationwide and makes it permanent; however, Congress has not appropriated funds for these purposes to date, and action has not been taken to implement it.

29.6 The Elder Justice Act Yet to Be

Like most enacted legislation, the final provisions of the EJA were the product of compromise. Several important provisions of the original EJA were cut out along the way to enable passage of the overall package. Important original provisions that did not make it into the final law carry the potential for future policy action and include the following:

(1) Establishment of Offices of Elder Justice at the Department of Health and Human Services (HHS) and Department of Justice (DOJ) and an Office of Adult Protective Services at HHS. Although some of the responsibilities to be carried out by these offices were incorporated into tasks assigned to the Elder Justice Coordinating Council, failure to establish dedicated offices is significant. Establishing dedicated offices gives the issue recognition and ensures that the issue will continue to receive the attention it needs;

(2) Amendment of the federal criminal code to provide for a cause of action for elder abuse and neglect;
(3) Collection of uniform national data on elder abuse and neglect through the Centers for Disease Control and Prevention. Elimination of this provision is regrettable because the lack of reliable nationwide data on the incidence of elder abuse plagues a lack of public awareness and creates difficulty with defining the scope of the problem and the concomitant political will to address it. Absent this provision, ACL, in partnership with the HHS Office of Assistant Secretary for Planning and Evaluation, has taken action to move forward with the institution of national data collection, as detailed below.
(4) Study of and recommendations for model state laws and practices relating to elder abuse, neglect, and exploitation through the Department of Justice. Noted above, currently, state laws, and practices related to elder abuse vary significantly from state to state.
(5) As mentioned previously, the Elder Abuse Victims Act of 2008 (H.R.448/S.1821) was never passed by the Senate, and some of its provisions remain important to the field including: grants to support police, sheriffs, detectives, public safety officers, corrections personnel, and others who handle elder justice matters as first responders; creation of designated elder justice positions in state prosecutors' offices; training coordination funds; victim grant programs; creation of emergency crisis response teams; and support for counseling and shelter.

As noted previously, one key accomplishment of the EJA was establishment of the EJCC. The Department of Health and Human Services (DHHS) Elder Justice Coordinating Council 2012–2014 Report to Congress, as required by the EJA, provides an excellent overview of current federal efforts to address elder abuse and helps set the course for action on this issue. The report includes eight recommendations focused on preventing and improving response to elder abuse, neglect, and exploitation:

Recommendation 1: Support the Investigation and Prosecution of Elder Abuse Cases
Recommendation 2: Enhance Services to Elder Abuse Victims
Recommendation 3: Develop a National Adult Protective Services System
Recommendation 4: Develop a Federal Elder Justice Research Agenda
Recommendation 5: Develop a Broad-Based Public Awareness Campaign
Recommendation 6: Promote Cross-disciplinary Training on Elder Abuse
Recommendation 7: Combat Elder Financial Exploitation, including Abuse by Fiduciaries
Recommendation 8: Improve Screening for Dementia and Cognitive Capacity, Financial Capacity, and Financial Exploitation

The report also details work done on elder justice across a broad spectrum of federal agencies since the EJA became law. Although, as noted above, most EJA provisions have not been funded or implemented, some of the activities described below and in the report incorporate parts of initiatives contained in the EJA. Activities of particular note include these:

(1) A grant by the Administration on Aging and the Administration for Community Living to provide a National Adult Protective Resource Center from 2011 to 2015
(2) A 2-year pilot by ACL and the HHS Office of the Assistant Secretary for Planning and Evaluation to design and test a National Adult Mistreatment Reporting System. In FY 2013, HHS transferred $2 million from the PPHF to ACL for this purpose.
(3) Elder Abuse Prevention Intervention Grants made by ACL in FY 2012—FY 2015. The project evaluated replicable best practices in support of the development of secondary and tertiary prevention and intervention strategies. Using the results, AoA/ACL developed a resource for APS programs to use to improve their programs.
(4) AoA/ACL collaboration with SAMHSA, CDC, and NIH/NIA to incorporate elder abuse screening into the CMS proposed rule on annual wellness visits.
(5) In March 2013, CMS convened an Elder Mistreatment Symposium to revise existing elder abuse measures and to make recommendations for elder abuse screening, screening tools, and protocols for handling suspicions of elder abuse.
(6) The Department of Justice's Elder Justice Initiative (EJI) established the Elder Justice Web site as a resource for elder abuse prosecutors, researchers, practitioners, and for victims of elder abuse and their families, as well as a forum for law enforcement and elder justice policy communities to share information and enhance public awareness on the subject matter. Also, the EJI collaborated with DOJ's Access to Justice Initiative and the Office of Victims of Crime to support the development of an online training for legal aid offices to detect and address elder abuse, neglect, and exploitation.

(7) In July 2014, the Federal Trade Commission launched a new fraud education campaign aimed at active older people. The "Pass It On" campaign is based on the theory that older adults are part of the solution, not simply the victims of scammers. It gives older adults tools to start conversations with friends, neighbors, or relatives about scams, identify theft, fundraising fraud, and paying too much.
(8) DOJ, with support from AoA/ACL, created an Elder Justice Roadmap, to set strategic priorities to advance elder justice by collecting information from 750 stakeholders across the country.

Going forward, sustained advocacy will be needed in order to ensure implementation of the EJCC's recommendations and continued action by federal government agencies to address elder abuse. Perhaps the most pressing task at hand for advocates is to work with congressional supporters to pass legislation reauthorizing the EJA. In February 2015, Representative Peter King (R-NY-2) introduced the Elder Justice Reauthorization Act (H.R. 988), which reauthorizes the EJA and funding for its programs through FY2019. It is currently under consideration by four separate committees in the House of Representatives. At the time of this writing, no action on the bill had been taken.

The Elder Justice Coalition has been working during the 114th Congress with key Senators and their offices to secure a Senate sponsor. Obvious choices have included Senator Hatch (R-UT), who sponsored the EJA that became law, and Senator Grassley, who has a long history of supporting the EJA and work to prevent elder abuse. Others have shown interest, including staff of Senators Casey and Blumenthal. Although Senator Hatch has personally shown interest in the reauthorization bill, his staff is less enthusiastic and has been working on a separate proposal that would end the Social Services Block Grant program, but would possibly shift some of those SSBG funds to some of the provisions of the EJA. Advocacy groups have not been supportive of such a proposal, given the uncertainty of ensuring those funds would get to APS programs which rely on SSBG to exist. And one of the goals of the EJA was to supplement SSBG funds with funds under the EJA for real growth in the APS program, not simply to rename current inadequate funding. Further, there are numerous other programs (and stakeholders) that could be hurt if SSBG was ended.

Progress on elder justice in the ensuing years will be influenced by the presidential election season currently underway and the installation of a new presidential administration in early 2017. The election and new leadership provide advocates an opportunity to highlight elder justice as an issue of importance to voters in the November 2016 presidential and congressional elections. Also, in a year in which legislative activity will be slower due to the upcoming elections, advocates have an opportunity to conduct extensive outreach and education of congressional staff about the need for sustained action and support.

Two other bills of note in the current Congress are the following:

(1) The Court-Appointed Guardian Accountability and Senior Protection Act (S.1614), introduced by Senator Amy Klobuchar (D-MN) and Senator John Cornyn (R-TX), which would award grants for demonstration programs to assess adult guardianship and conservatorship proceedings and implement changes deemed necessary as a result of the assessments.
(2) The Robert Matava Elder Abuse Victims Act of 2015 (S.1633), introduced by Senator Richard Blumenthal (D-CT) and Senator Kelly Ayotte (R-NH), encourages states and other qualified entities to hold abusers and exploiters of elders accountable, and includes provisions to enhance the capacity of the justice system to investigate, pursue, and prosecute elder abuse cases. Robert Matava was a victim of financial exploitation in Connecticut.

Funding for existing programs related to elder abuse, neglect, and exploitation is also important. In his FY17 budget request, President Obama requested level funding for several related programs such as the long-term care ombudsman program ($16 million), the Prevention of Elder Abuse and Neglect Program ($5 million), and the Senior Medicare Patrol program ($9 million) and designated $10 million for ACLs Elder Rights Support Activities. Intensive advocacy is needed throughout the congressional appropriations process to make the requests for additional funds a reality.

29.7 The Older Americans Act

Past The Older Americans Act (1965) (OAA) was the first federal law to provide comprehensive services for older adults without means testing. Its passage was a triumph for the newly developing fields of gerontology and geriatrics. Based on a model of active aging [3] the OAA created the National Aging Network, which is composed of the Administration on Aging, (incorporated in 2012 into the then newly formed umbrella agency, the Administration for Community Living) (federal level), State Units on Aging (state level), and Area Agencies on Aging (local level). The OAA must be continually reauthorized by Congress, which has consistently failed to allocate funding commensurate with the OAA's lofty aspirations and considerable mandate. Although services are supposed to be provided based on age of the recipients (generally, 60 years of age and older), they have become more specifically targeted due to historically flat or slight increases in funding.

Notably, the OAA funds nutrition and supportive home and community-based services, disease prevention/health promotion services, training for employment, the National Family Caregiver Support Program and the Native American Caregiver Support Program, and elder rights programs (Title VII or the Vulnerable Elder Rights Protection Title) [1]. The purpose of Title VII is to strengthen and coordinate the Long-Term Care Ombudsman Program; Programs for the Prevention of Abuse, Neglect and Exploitation; State Elder Rights and Legal Assistance Development Programs; and Insurance/Benefits Outreach, Counseling and Assistance Programs. Two OAA programs most relevant to elder justice are discussed below in greater detail: the National Center on Elder Abuse and the Long-Term Care Ombudsman Program, which is carried out by the Office of the State Long-Term Care Ombudsman Program and in local programs housed in Area Agencies on Aging (Administration on Aging, n.d.).

Present In 2015, the Aging Network celebrated the 50th Anniversary of the OAA. The anniversary provided an opportunity to celebrate the accomplishments of OAA programs and to raise awareness about its importance and effectiveness. Although its programs receive meager funding in terms of its broad mandate, the OAA continues to undergird a vibrant nationwide network of essential services for older Americans in all of the areas delineated above. From 2009–2016, under the leadership of Kathy Greenlee, Assistant Secretary of Aging and Administrator of ACL, the Administration on Aging was merged with the Administration on Intellectual and Developmental Disabilities and the HHS Office on Disability in 2012. ACL continues to be focused on implementation of the OAA, while capitalizing on common causes and efficiencies with the other ACL divisions. Suffice it to say, all titles of the Act address elder abuse in one way or another.

In January 2015, AoA published historic final federal regulations for the long-term care ombudsman (LTCO) program. Since its establishment in the 1970s, the LTCO program has functioned without federal regulations to implement the provisions of the OAA pertaining to the program, leading to significant variation in the interpretation and implementation of the provisions among states. LTCO play a major role in identifying and addressing abuse, neglect, and exploitation of residents of nursing homes, board and care, and assisted living facilities. LTCO are advocates for residents of nursing homes, board and care homes, and assisted living facilities. They educate consumers about making informed choices and how to obtain quality care, as well as assist consumers with resolving complaints. Under the OAA, every state is required to have a LTCO program. However the programs have varied significantly from state to state. Nationwide, the program includes the provision of services by 8155 volunteers certified to handle complaints and 1293 paid staff. In 2014, long-term care ombudsmen investigated over 191,553 complaints on behalf of 125,642 individuals and provided information to an additional 370,310 people. The final rule provides guidance to states and is intended to promote equity in LTCO program services across states and greater adherence to the purpose of the program, as defined by the statute. Also through the OAA, ACL supports the National Center on Elder Abuse (NCEA), which subcontracts with partner organizations to implement its mission. The NCEA serves as a national resource center dedicated to the prevention of elder abuse. It also offers a resource database of research and training materials related to elder abuse.

In July 2015, in conjunction with the White House Conference on Aging, ACL released Draft Voluntary Consensus Guidelines for State APS Programs and asked for public comments. The comment period was reopened from January 25 through February 8, 2016. Once finalized, ACL intends to update the guidelines every 2 years. Although the guidelines do not constitute federal regulations or any new legal obligation for states, they aim to promote an effective, equitable APS response across the country. The draft guidelines were developed by subject matter experts in the fields of adult protective services and abuse, neglect, and exploitation of older adults and adults with disabilities.

Future The OAA was due to be reauthorized in 2011. Unfortunately, efforts by supporters and committees of jurisdiction to craft and pass a bipartisan reauthorization bill failed in the 112th and 113th Congresses. In the 114th Congress, the U.S. Senate passed the Older Americans Act Reauthorization Act of 2015 (S. 192) with unanimous bipartisan support on July 17, 2015. The bill was then referred to the House Committee on Education and the Workforce, where no further action was taken in 2015. In February 2016, 65 representatives wrote to the committee urging advancement of the bill. Successful House passage of S. 192 occurred on March 21, 2016 when the House agreed to a motion to suspend the rules and pass the bill as amended by voice vote. Subsequently, the Senate took up the amended S. 192 on April 7, 2016 and passed the bill by voice vote. The President signed S. 192 into law on April 19, 2016

(P.L. 114-144). The House Committee on Education and Workforce included the following in its summary of the OAA:

"This legislation reauthorizes the Older Americans Act of 1965, a federal law with longstanding bipartisan support. The law provides for the organization and delivery of social and nutrition services to older Americans and their caregivers, and increases the authorization levels for these programs 6.77 % cumulatively over FY2017 to FY2019 from current appropriated amounts. This bill reauthorizes programs and includes provisions that aim to protect vulnerable elders by strengthening the Long-Term Care Ombudsman program and existing elder abuse screening and prevention efforts."

29.8 Elder Abuse

- To be consistent with current law, updates definitions of "adult protective services," "abuse," "exploitation and financial exploitation," and "elder justice"
- Improves coordination of activities between the state and local aging offices
- Promotes best practices related to responding to elder abuse, neglect, and exploitation in long-term care facilities through the Administration on Aging
- Promotes states' submission of data concerning elder abuse
- Directs the Administration on Aging to include, as appropriate, training for states, area agencies on aging, and service providers on elder abuse prevention and screening.

29.9 Long-Term Care Ombudsman Program

- Allows ombudsmen to serve all residents of long-term care facilities, regardless of age
- Ensures private, unimpeded access to the ombudsman for all residents of long-term care facilities
- Provides for identification and resolution of potential individual and organizational conflicts of interest
- Clarifies the role of ombudsman program in advocating for residents unable to communicate their wishes
- Clarifies that ombudsman may continue to serve residents transitioning from a long-term care facility to a home care setting
- Clarifies that the ombudsman office is a "health oversight agency" for purposes of HIPAA.

A number of additional elder justice provisions was included in earlier versions of the OAA reauthorizations bill drafted by Senator Bernie Sanders (I-VT) but was cut during the negotiation process with Republican Senators on the Committee. One of those provisions would have added being a victim of elder abuse to the definition of those with the "greatest social need."

Moving forward, the aging services network is adapting to shifts in the healthcare system toward managed care and meeting the challenge of educating policymakers and health care providers about the value of the supports and services the network provides. Due to the decades-long difficulty of securing adequate appropriations for OAA programs, Assistant Secretary Greenlee has encouraged the aging network to think more broadly about sources of funding [2]. She believes that Medicaid, Medicare, private payers, and the Veterans Administration are all potentially viable funding partners.

29.10 Violence Against Women Act

Past In 1994, Congress passed the Violence Against Women Act (VAWA) in recognition of the severity of crimes associated with domestic violence, sexual assault, and stalking. Passage of VAWA occurred due to broad, grassroots coalitions of advocates, and survivors who informed the work of Congress. In the 20 years prior to its passage, a U.S. movement evolved to respond swiftly and appropriately to violent crimes against both younger and older women. Thus, it was that rape crisis centers and battered women's shelters sprang up in localities, and state and local laws changed to improve the investigation and prosecution of violent crimes against women, albeit unevenly [22]. Although crime victimization of older women is generally declining [16], older adults are less likely to report crime and more likely to sustain lasting (and sometimes fatal) injuries than their younger counterparts.

The Office on Violence Against Women (OVW) was created specifically to implement (VAWA) and subsequent legislation. In 2002, legislation made the Office of Violence Against Women (OVW) a permanent part of the Department of Justice with a presidentially appointed, senate-confirmed Director. Created in 1995, the Office of Violence Against Women (OVW) administers financial and technical assistance to communities across the country that are developing programs, policies, and practices aimed at ending domestic violence, dating violence, sexual assault, and stalking. Currently, OVW administers four formula-based and 20 discretionary grant programs that originated under VAWA and subsequent legislation. The four formula programs include the following: STOP (Services, Training, Officers, Prosecutors), SASP (Sexual Assault Services Program), State Coalitions, and Tribal Coalitions. The aim of the programs is to support victims and hold perpetrators accountable by promoting a coordinated community response. Funding is provided to local and state and tribal governments, courts, nonprofit organizations, community-based organizations, secondary schools, institutions of higher education, and state and tribal coalitions. These entities develop effective responses to violence against women through activities that include direct services, crisis intervention, transitional housing, legal assistance to victims, court improvement, and training for law enforcement and courts. They also work with specific populations (e.g., older adults, persons with disabilities, college students, teens, culturally and linguistically specific populations). When possible, OVW funds special initiatives in response to areas of special need, the purpose of which are to enhance services in areas requiring particular attention or in communities facing particularly acute challenges [22]. The 2000 VAWA reauthorization improved protections for battered immigrants, sexual assault survivors, and victims of dating violence. In addition, it improved the enforcement of protection orders across state and tribal lines. VAWA 2005 built upon these laws by providing an increased focus on the access to services for underserved populations. Since its inception, OVW has awarded over $6 billion in grants and cooperative agreements and has launched a multifaceted approach to implementing VAWA. By forging state, local, and tribal partnerships among police, prosecutors, judges, victim advocates, health care providers, faith leaders, and others, OVW grant programs help provide victims with the necessary protections and services required for the pursuit of safe and healthy lives, while simultaneously enabling communities to hold offenders accountable for their violence.

Present VAWA was last reauthorized in March 2013. The reauthorization addresses gaps in the law, including making services available to Native women, immigrants, LGBT victims, college students and youth, and public housing residents. The Violence Against Women Act (VAWA) Renewal passes the House and Senate and signed into law [21]. The following quote from the February 13, 2013 Elder Justice Coalition newsletter describes the important changes in VAWA in the reauthorization: On February 12, 2013, the United States Senate passed the Violence Against Women Reauthorization Act of 2013 (S. 47) on a vote of 78–22. The bill expands and strengthens VAWA and extends funding for various programs including investigation and prosecution of violent crimes against women.

The Elder Justice Coalition is pleased to have supported the bill including its provisions that address the scourge of violence against older women. The VAWA includes subtitle H, "Enhancing Training and Services to End Abuse Later in Life," which enables the Attorney General to make grants to entities for the purpose of training, providing services, multidisciplinary community responses, and outreach activities and awareness campaigns around elder abuse and exploitation. Organizations that would be eligible for such funding include law enforcement agencies, victim service providers, local courts, state, tribal and local governments, and others.

In addition, the section of VAWA that addresses strengthening the health care system's response to domestic violence includes grants for elder abuse and to develop training modules and policies that address the overlap of elder abuse, domestic violence, child abuse, and other violence.

This legislation faced some significant obstacles last Congress and its success this year depends on what occurs in the House of Representatives, where there has been opposition to several elements of the bill, including a provision that would allow Native American courts to try non-Native American individuals accused of domestic violence on Indian lands.

The bill passed the House on February 28, 2013 and on March 7, 2013 was signed by the President and became Public Law 113–114.

Future With VAWA operating under current authorization, the main challenge for advocates going forward is to continue to press for adequate funding for implementation of its programs, and to collaborate with providers of services to victims of domestic violence to ensure that they are equipped to meet the particular needs of victims of late-life domestic violence [11].

29.11 Family Violence Prevention and Services Act

Past The Family Violence Prevention and Services Act (FVPSA), first authorized in 1984, is the only federal funding source dedicated directly to domestic violence (DV) shelters and programs [10]. Although often regarded as the purview of younger DV victims, shelters are critical for older adults who are escaping DV. Far fewer shelters are available for older victims than for their younger counterparts. FVPSA-funded programs help more than 2000 local domestic violence agencies respond to adult and child victims of domestic violence. FVPSA, administered by DHHS, funds essential services related to domestic violence: emergency shelters, hotlines, counseling and advocacy, and primary and secondary prevention. Highlights of FVPSA include the following: funding included formula grants to states to provide shelter and supportive services; national and specialized training and technical assistance resource centers; the National Domestic Violence Hotline; grants to State Domestic Violence Coalitions; and a tribal formula grant program.

29.12 Social Services Block Grants

Past The Social Services Block Grant (SSBG) is permanently authorized by Title XX, Subtitle A, of the Social Security Act as a "capped" entitlement to states [13]. At the federal level, the SSBG is administered by DHHS. Under this arrangement and as determined by a formula, states are entitled to their share of funds out of an amount of money that is capped in statute by a funding ceiling. Although social services for certain welfare recipients have been authorized under various titles of the Social Security Act since 1956, the current SSBG was created in 1981 (P.L. 9735). Under this funding scheme, block grant funds are allocated to states to promote a wide range of social policy goals established by federal law and linked to one or more of five goals: achieving or maintaining economic self-support to prevent, reduce, or eliminate dependency; achieving or maintaining self-sufficiency, including reduction or prevention of dependency; preventing or remedying neglect, abuse, or exploitation of children and adults unable to protect their own interests, or preserving, rehabilitating, or reuniting families; preventing or reducing inappropriate institutional care by providing for community-based care, home-based care, or other forms of less intensive care; and securing referral or admission for institutional care when other forms of care are not appropriate, or providing services to individuals in institutions [13].

Although states typically have broad discretion for uses of SSBG funds have often been accompanied with rider provisions. For example, in 2001, annual appropriations for the SSBG were accompanied by a provision stipulating that states transfer up to 10 % of their Temporary Assistance for Needy Families (TANF) block grants to the SSBG. The SSBG has, from time to time, received supplemental appropriations, including appropriations for expenses related to natural disasters (2006 and 2009). The ACA health reform legislation enacted into law (P.L. 111-148) in March 2010 amended Title XX of the Social Security Act to include a subtitle on elder justice and to establish several other programs.

29.13 Present and Future

Support for the SSBG remains tenuous with annual attempts by some Republicans to cut funding. Recent appropriations levels have remained at $1.7 billion. The program is critical to keeping APS programs functioning around the country, and has many aging and children's advocates fighting to keep it alive, making it a more difficult target. At the time of this writing, the Senate Appropriations Committee in a bipartisan vote passed the Labor, Health and Human Services, Education, and Related Agencies Appropriations bill, which funded the SSBG at its current level of $1.7 billion. As mentioned earlier, Senator Hatch's staff proposal to end SSBG has, for the time being, been ignored.

29.14 White House Conference on Aging

Past In order to consider the policy ramifications of the growing number of older adults living longer in older age, in 1950, President Harry S. Truman ordered that the Federal Security Agency hold a national conference on aging. Congressman John E. Fogarty introduced legislation calling for a White House Conference on Aging (WHCOA) in 1958, which resulted in the White House Conference on Aging Act. The act, Public Law 85-908, called for a national forum to address conundrums of older Americans and to make recommendations concerning improving the economic security of older adults [23]. The first conference, held in 1961, drew more than 3000 people representing nearly 300 organizations. The conference was instrumental in the passage of the 1961 Social Security amendments, the Senior Citizens Housing Act of 1962, the Community Health Services and Facilities Act, Medicare, Medicaid and the Older Americans Act (1965). The next WHCOA, held in 1971 involved 4000 attendees who recommended more than 193 actions, some helping to establish the Senate Special Committee on Aging and the Federal Council on Aging. Ten years later, the 1981 conference (2000 delegates) used a quota system to ensure that various segments of the population (e.g., women, minorities, and persons with disabilities) were sufficiently represented. The subsequent WHCOA, held in 1995, involved over 125,000 people who participated in over 1000 mini-conferences around the country. Although few new initiatives resulted, there was broad support for existing programs. Importantly, delegates argued for many policies having to do with prevention and addressing victims of elder abuse, neglect, and exploitation. For the 2005 WHCOA (2200 delegates), nearly 50 recommendations resulted, many of which concerned older adults' transportation needs, mental health, and the medicare prescription drug benefit [23].

Present In July 2015, the Obama Administration hosted the sixth White House Conference on Aging. The 2015 conference did not establish a formal delegate process in part because the OAA had not been reauthorized and there was no funding appropriated to support the conference or bringing hundreds of delegates to DC. Instead, WHCoA organizers used technology and listening sessions and regional forums in the months leading up to the national event to allow broad participation (Department of Health and Human Services, DHHS, n.d.),. Attended by representatives of a diverse group of older Americans, caregivers, advocates, community leaders, and experts from across the country, the WHCOA produced a final report that covered public input, public and private initiatives on each of four key issue areas: retirement security, long-term services and supports, healthy aging, and elder justice. Initiatives related to elder justice grew out of the 2015 WHCOA, including the following:

- The Department of Justice announced a commitment to finalize a proposed rule that revises the current VOCA (Victims of Crime Act) Victim Assistance Guidelines, such that VOCA funds may be used to support legal services for crime victims, and emphasizing the need to support social and legal services to underserved victims, including elderly victims of abuse, financial exploitation, fraud, and neglect. The final rule has not been released at this writing [15].
- The National Institutes of Health convened a State of the Science workshop on elder abuse with researchers, clinicians, and others to review the science on understanding and preventing abuse; screening tools to identify abuse victims; effective interventions and research in related areas like child abuse and domestic violence that might inform research on elder abuse; and gaps and opportunities in this field of research.
- The Consumer Financial Protection Bureau (CFPB) released an advisory to help financial institutions prevent, recognize, and report elder financial exploitation.
- ACL announced the release and request for public comments on State APS Guidelines, as mentioned above.
- The U.S. Department of Justice announced a commitment to enroll and train prosecutors from all 50 States to effectively prosecute elder abuse and financial exploitation by 2017, building on training already completed since 2013 [23].

Future Since the inaugural WHCOA in 1961, conferences have occurred approximately once every 10 years. The next WHCOA is expected in 2025. Advocates must ensure that the initiatives announced are implemented in the next several years. The attention to elder abuse generated by the WHCOA and its final report provide information is useful for advocates to highlight the issue in the upcoming elections. Representing a part of the record of the current administration; presidential candidates from both parties should be asked to comment on how they would address elder justice in the same or different ways if elected.

29.15 Crime Victims Fund

Past The Crime Victims Fund (CVF) was established by the Victims of Crime Act of 1984 (VOCA) and provides significant funding for victim services throughout the United States [17]. Each year, "millions of dollars are deposited to the fund from criminal fines, forfeited bail bonds, penalties, and special assessments on individuals convicted of misdemeanors and on corporations convicted of felonies, and gifts, donations, and bequests by private parties, as provided by the USA PATRIOT Act 2001 and collected by U.S. Attorneys" Offices, federal U.S. courts, and the Federal Bureau of Prisons" [17].

Federal, state, and tribal victim assistance programs receive formula grants, discretionary grants, and set-asides as prescribed by a carefully established annual allocation process [17]. VOCA-funded streams include state crime victim compensation program formula grants that supplement state funds for reimbursing victims of violent crimes for out-of-pocket expenses resulting from the crime. All states, the District of Columbia, Puerto Rico, and the U.S. Virgin Islands receive VOCA compensation grants. State victim assistance program formula grants support providers who supply services directly to victims. All states and most territories receive annual VOCA assistance grants consisting of a mandated base amount plus additional funds based on population [17]. Each state administers a crime victim compensation program that provides financial assistance to victims of both federal and state crimes. Under VOCA, each state compensation program receives an annual grant equal to 60 % of what the program spends in state money annually. This calculation is based on the state dollars paid out for the federal fiscal year 2 years prior to the year of the federal grant. Although each state administers its own program independently, most programs have similar eligibility requirements and offer comparable types of benefits. No more than 5 % of each year's VOCA compensation formula grant may be used for administration and training; the rest must be used for awards of compensation to crime victims. More than 4000 VOCA awards are made by states annually to public and private nonprofit organizations to provide these and other essential services to victims of crime [17].

All states, the District of Columbia, the U.S. Virgin Islands, and Puerto Rico each receive an annual VOCA victim assistance grant with a base amount of $500,000; the Northern Mariana Islands, Guam, and American Samoa each receive a base amount of $200,000 [17]. Additional funds are distributed to states and territories based on population. In each state and territory, VOCA assistance funds are awarded to local community-based organizations and public agencies that provide services directly to victims of crime. Similar to VOCA compensation formula grants, an individual state may use no more than 5 % of each VOCA assistance grant for administration and training.

Present Currently, a point of controversy is the use of VOCA funds for purposes other than those defined in the original statute. Because of the 2000 amendments to the statute as well as a number of large deposits into the fund, the fund balance has increased by 900 % between FY 2000 and FY 2015, while disbursements from the fund over the same time period increased by only 49 %. The mounting balance in the VOCA fund has been used by Congress as an "offset" for non-VOCA programs. Also, $1.5 billion was removed from the fund through the Bipartisan Budget Agreement of 2015 (Crime Victims Fund 2016). The Fairness for Victims of Crime Act (S. 1495/H.R. 3984) has been introduced and is currently under consideration in Congress. It would prohibit the use of VOCA funds for purposes other than those specifically outlined in the statute [15].

Future At the end of 2015, advocates united to resist cuts in funding for VOCA programs for FY16. They were successful in protecting and increasing the funding available. VOCA funding supports an elder abuse grant program. The president's budget proposal for FY17 includes $6.25 million for the elder abuse grant program; an amount that is dwarfed by the requests and past appropriations for addressing other types of abuse, but which is still significant.

As with other initiatives discussed above, elder justice advocates must work to ensure that victims of elder abuse receive services they deserve through VOCA-funded state victim assistance formula grants. Advocates should work with supporters in Congress to amend the VOCA statute to specifically authorize assistance to victims of elder abuse.

29.16 Conclusion

> Men's courses will foreshadow certain ends, to which, if persevered in, they must lead," said Scrooge. "But if the courses be departed from, the ends will change [7].

The brief but iconic *A Christmas Carol* by Charles Dickens, published in 1843, provides a frame apropos to our consideration of *Elder Abuse Policy Past, Present, and Yet to Be.* Like its protagonist, Ebenezer Scrooge, the past, or its uncertainties, do not necessarily portend a bleak future as concerns the issue of elder abuse. Taken together, many of the policy changes that evolved over more than 50 years and that are discussed in this chapter augur a future far brighter than in previous decades, as much of the "heavy lifting" of getting the public (and legislators) to pay attention to the issue of elder justice has occurred. Still, it is no surprise to anyone who works either inside or outside the Beltway that the policy landscape is a constantly shifting one. Policies that appear rock solid and airtight may fall out of favor of politicians and administrators, not for the issue on its face but for the riders that are attached to it and that thus imperil their funding.

A combined front of advocacy at local, state, and national levels is the best prevention and intervention to keep the issue of elder justice alive. We, the authors of this chapter, stress that a course once charted and believed by many, that the issue of elder justice was to remain in the background of public policy initiatives has, as Scrooge opines, been changed. Thus, those who work to keep the issue alive must continue to alter the past policy course so that the ends will change, and today's and tomorrow's older adults will live freer from abuse than any generation in history. For those laboring to bring justice to abused elders, we admonish the field to learn from the past and to take heed of the words of Scrooge; *I will live in the Past, the Present, and the Future. The Spirits of all Three shall strive within me. I will not shut out the lessons that they teach!*

References

1. Administration on Aging (n.d.). The Older Americans Act. Retrieved from http://www.aoa.gov/AoA_programs/OAA/Index.aspx.
2. American Society on Aging, Aging Today. Assistant Secretary of aging sees network at a crossroads—and a place of new opportunities. 2016. Retrieved from: http://acl.gov/NewsRoom/Observances/OAA50/Index.aspx.

3. Atchley RC. A continuity theory of normal aging. The Gerontologist 1989;29(2), 183–90. Retrieved from: https://gerontologist-oxfordjournals-org.ezproxy.lib.vt.edu/content/29/2/183.full.pdf+html.
4. Churchman CW. Guest Editorial. J Manag Sci. 1967;14(4).
5. Crime Victims Fund, Victims of Crime Act (VOCA), Briefing Background 2017. National Association of VOCA Assistance Administrators 2016. Retrieved from: http://www.navaa.org/budget/17/VOCA_Backgrounder%202017.pdf.
6. Department of Health and Human Services (DHHS) (n.d.). The 2015 White House Conference on Aging. Retrieved from http://www.whitehouseconferenceonaging.gov/2015-WHCOA-Final-Report.pdf.
7. Dickens C, A Christmas Carol, (copyright: 2004). Retrieved from: http://www.pagebypagebooks.com/Charles_Dickens/A_Christmas_Carol.html.
8. Dubble C. A policy perspective on elder justice through APS and law enforcement collaboration. In: Mellor MJ, Brownell P, editors. Elder abuse and mistreatment: policy, practice, and research. New York: The Haworth Press; 2006. p. 40.
9. Elder Justice Act: Background and Issues for Congress, Congressional Research Service, September 2014. Retrieved from: https://www.fas.org/sgp/crs/misc/R43707.pdf.
10. Family Violence Prevention and Services Act. National network to end domestic violence. 2010. Retrieved from: http://nnedv.org/policy/issues/fvpsa.html.
11. Late Life Domestic Violence. What the aging network needs to know, National Center on Elder Abuse (NCEA) Issue Brief. 2006. Retrieved from: http://www.ncdsv.org/images/NCEA_LateLifeDVWhatAgingNetworkNeedsKnow_2-2006.pdf.
12. Lindberg BW, Sabatino CP, Esq, Blancato RB. Bringing national action to a national disgrace: the history of the elder justice act. 2011. Retrieved from: http://www.preventelderabuse.org/library/documents/NAELAJournal.pdf.
13. Lynch KE. Social Services Block Grant: Background and funding. Congressional Research Service. 2016. Retrieved from: https://www.fas.org/sgp/crs/misc/94-953.pdf.
14. National Adult Protective Association (NAPSA). History: About Adult Protective Services from 1960 to 2000. 2016. Retrieved from: http://www.napsa-now.org/about-napsa/history/history-of-adult-protective-services/.
15. National Association of VOCA Assistance Administrators (n.d.). VOCA funding. Retrieved from: http://www.navaa.org/budget/.
16. Office of Justice Programs. Elderly crime victims: National Crime Victimization Survey. 1994. Retrieved from http://www.bjs.gov/content/pub/ascii/ecv.txt.
17. Office of Victims of Crime (n.d.). OVC fact sheet: Crime Victims Fund. Retrieved from http://ovc.gov/pubs/crimevictimsfundfs/intro.html.
18. Otto JM. The role of adult protective services in addressing abuse. 2000. Retrieved from: https://www.questia.com/read/1P3-59724426/the-role-of-adult-protective-services-in-addressing.
19. Rittel HWJ, Webber MM. Dilemmas in a general theory of planning. Policy Sci. 1973;4(2):155–69.
20. Teaster PB, Wangmo T, Anetzberger G. A glass half full: the dubious history of elder mistreatment policy. J Elder Abuse Negl. 2010;22(1/2):6–15.
21. Violence Against Women Act. National Network to End Domestic Violence. 2013. Retrieved from: http://nnedv.org/policy/issues/vawa.html.
22. Violence Against Women Act. US Department of Justice. 2016. Retrieved from: https://www.justice.gov/sites/default/files/ovw/legacy/2011/07/08/about-ovw-factsheet.pdf.
23. White House Conference on Aging. Wikipedia. 2016. Retrieved from https://en.wikipedia.org/wiki/White_House_Conference_on_Aging.

30 The Elder Justice Act: Bridging the Gap Between Health and Public Policy

Kathy Greenlee

30.1 Introduction

Elder abuse, neglect, and exploitation are significant and under-recognized public health and human rights issues in the United States and globally. Research has demonstrated that elder abuse has significant consequences for the health, well-being, and independence of older adults. Available data suggests that each year at least 10 % (or 5 million) older adults are subjected to abuse, neglect, and/or exploitation [1]. Further, only 1 in approximately 25 cases is ever reported to social service agencies [2]. The problem is further exacerbated by the lack of standardized practice, public awareness, and public policy guidelines at the national level.

The Elder Justice Act (EJA) is a public policy approach to address the public health problem of abuse, neglect, and exploitation. This chapter provides an overview of the EJA and its major components, as well as the Administration for Community Living and its activities in implementing the EJA to demonstrate the importance of the health field in driving public policy at the federal level.

30.2 The Administration for Community Living

The U.S. Department of Health and Human Services (HHS) created the Administration for Community Living (ACL) in 2012 by combining a number of federal operating divisions and offices with purview over aging services or disability programs. By combining various efforts under one administrative umbrella, HHS sought to achieve several objectives:

- Reduce the fragmentation that currently exists in federal programs addressing the community living service and support needs of both the aging and disability populations;
- Enhance access to quality health care and long-term services and supports for all individuals;
- Promote consistency in community living policy across other areas of the federal government; and
- Complement the community infrastructure, as supported by both Medicaid and other federal programs, in order to better respond to the full spectrum of needs of seniors and persons with disabilities.

ACL is the principal agency designated to lead federal aging and disability programs. ACL provides national leadership and direction to plan, manage, develop, and raise awareness of comprehensive and coordinated systems of long-term services and supports that enable older Americans and individuals with disabilities, including intellectual, developmental, and physical disabilities, to maintain their health and independence in their homes and communities. ACL programs support strong state, tribal, and local community networks designed to respond to the needs of persons with disabilities, older Americans, and their families, through advocacy, systems change, and capacity building, to ensure access to needed community services, individualized supports, and other forms of assistance that promote self-determination, independence, productivity, and integration, and inclusion in all facets of community life.

ACL is organized as follows: ACL is headed by an Administrator, who reports directly to the HHS Secretary. The Administrator is also the Assistant Secretary for Aging, a Presidentially appointed and Senate-confirmed position. In addition to the Administrator, ACL consists of the Principal Deputy Administrator, who also serves as the senior advisor to the HHS Secretary on disability policy. Staff and program offices carry out aging and disability programs authorized under various statutes, including: the Administration on Aging, the Administration on Disabilities, the Center for Integrated Programs, and the National Institute on Disability, Independent Living, and Rehabilitation Research.

K. Greenlee (✉)
Administration for Community Living, U.S. Department of Health and Human Services, Washington, DC 20201, USA
e-mail: Kathy.Greenlee@acl.hhs.gov

X. Dong (ed.), *Elder Abuse*, DOI 10.1007/978-3-319-47504-2_30

Specifically, the provisions of the Older Americans Act (OAA) of 1965 are carried out by its subcomponent, the Administration on Aging. The provisions of the Developmental Disabilities Assistance and Bill of Rights Act (DD Act) of 2000 and Title VII of the Rehabilitation Act of 1973 are carried out by its subcomponent, the Administration on Disabilities. The provisions of Title II of the Rehabilitation Act of 1973 are carried out by its subcomponent, the Nation Institute on Disability, Independent Living, and Rehabilitation Research. ACL also administers programs authorized under the following statutes:

- Title III and Title XXIX of the Public Health Service Act (PHSA);
- Sections 262 and 292 of the Help America Vote Act (HAVA);
- Section 119 of the Medicare Improvements for Patients and Providers Act (MIPPA) of 2008;
- Section 6021(d) of the Deficit Reduction Act (DRA) of 2005;
- Section 4360 of the Omnibus Budget Reconciliation Act (OBRA) of 1990;
- The Elder Justice Act (EJA) of 2010 (Subtitle B of Title XX of the Social Security Act), contained in the Affordable Care Act;
- The Assistive Technology Act of 1998; and
- Provides continued support for the administration of the President's Committee for People with Intellectual Disabilities pursuant to Executive Order 13652.

Within ACL and under the Administration on Aging, is the Office of Elder Justice and Adult Protective Services (OEJAPS). OEJAPS serves as the focal point for the operation, administration, and assessment of the elder abuse prevention, legal assistance development, and pension counseling programs under Titles II and VII of the OAA, and for Adult Protective Services and related activities carried out under the Elder Justice Act. The office also coordinates with the Office of the National Long-Term Care Ombudsman, which oversees the Long-Term Care Ombudsman Program and the National Ombudsman Resource Center.

The Office has a number of responsibilities to ensure the funding provided by ACL to states and communities operate consistently with national priorities. In this role, OEJAPS staff review state plans to determine eligibility for funding under the OAA. This office implements Title VII in the field, in coordination with the National Long-Term Care Ombudsman, through the provision to Regional Support Centers of guidance and information, and the development and interpretation of Title VII program regulations and policy. Activities of the office aim at ensuring the implementation of guidance and instructions concerning prevention of elder abuse, elder justice, and legal assistance development programs. Furthermore, OEJAPS provides guidance and leadership in the development of the pension counseling program and effective models for nationwide replication. A key responsibility is to implement demonstration activities under Titles II and IV of the OAA and the EJA designed to test the efficacy of new and innovative models in improving the delivery and effectiveness of elder rights activities.

OAA program activities are funded by annual, Congressional appropriations. Congress appropriates funding to ACL to carry out each of its Titles, and often includes comments and instructions for agencies in accompanying budget documents. Once ACL receives its annual appropriation, funds are then dispersed to State Units on Aging via a Congressionally prescribed population-based interstate funding formula calculated on the proportionate number of people over the age of 60. States then develop, in consultation with Area Agencies on Aging, an intrastate funding formula for distribution of funds within the state. There is considerable discretion as to how those funds will be used at the local level, but are allocated in accordance with the State Plan on Aging covering a 2, 3, or 4-year period based on a bottoms-up planning process, with input from older individuals. ACL, through the Administration on Aging, provides guidance to states on priorities for crafting those plans, and provides technical assistance on the implementation of those plans.

30.3 The Elder Justice Act

ACL also has lead responsibility for implementing the provisions of the EJA. Title XX of the Social Security Act, Subtitle B, the Elder Justice Act of 2009, was signed into law on March 23, 2010 to address weaknesses in federal and state responses to elder abuse. Originally introduced in 2002 by Senator John Breaux (D-LA) and Senator Orrin G. Hatch (R-UT), it took nearly eight years for the legislation to be finally passed and be signed into law. From the beginning, experts and advocates who were called upon by Congress to testify about the proposed EJA cited several reasons why federal legislation was needed to address the issue of elder maltreatment, including:

- Unclear and inconsistent definitions of abuse, neglect, and exploitation;
- Unclear and inadequate methods to measure the phenomenon;
- Lack of population-based data to understand the etymology of the phenomenon; and,

- Lack of systematic evaluation studies for understanding effective prevention and intervention.

Moreover, experts and advocates impressed upon Congress that the widespread threat of elder abuse as a public health crisis, the costs on the US health care and social services systems to serve those who have been abused, and the dearth of collective state or local momentum clearly compelled a federal response. Indeed, the case was made that effective responses required federal involvement just as was demonstrated when the federal government recognized child abuse and domestic violence as threats to our nation's public health and safety.

30.3.1 Significant Provisions

The EJA is an effort to coordinate a multidisciplinary federal effort by law enforcement, public health, and social services to address elder abuse, neglect, and exploitation. The EJA of 2010 provisions seek a number of objectives: to elevate elder justice issues to national attention; to improve adult protective services, the state-based programs developed to receive and respond to reports of abuse; to increase knowledge; and to develop forensic capacity in both forensic pathology and geriatrics. There are three main components of the EJA: National Coordination of Elder Justice Activities, Enhancing Adult Protective Services, and Enhancing Long-Term Care.

30.3.1.1 National Coordination of Elder Justice Activities

In this section, the Elder Justice Coordinating Council is established and tasked to make recommendations to the Secretary of HHS on the coordination of activities of federal, state, local, and private agencies and entities relating to elder abuse, neglect, and exploitation. The EJA also establishes the Advisory Board on Elder Abuse, Neglect, and Exploitation, a complementary body to the EJA that is to be comprised of experts and stakeholders. Together these entities are charged with creating short- and long-term strategic plans that are multidisciplinary for the developing field of elder justice. To improve the identification and prosecution of elder abuse, neglect, and exploitation, the EJA also creates a set of national grants to establish forensic centers and forensic expertise.

30.3.1.2 Enhancing Adult Protective Services

A major and significant component of the EJA is to focus on the development of a national system for Adult Protective Services (APS). APS has historically operated as a state-established and state-managed program. Although the Administration on Aging provided support to APS programs through its work under the OAA, APS never had a home within federal government until the passage of the EJA. The only federal funding was at the discretion of States, which dedicated a portion of their Social Services Block Grant funding to support their State APS activities. As a significant component of implementing the EJA, and in response to a General Accountability Office report calling for federal leadership, the Secretary of HHS designated ACL as the federal home for APS. The components of a national system for APS called for in the EJA included:

- Dedicated formula-grant funding to support adult protective services in all states;
- Discretionary grant programs for state demonstration grants to test a variety of methods to improve APS;
- Development and improvement of data collection and dissemination for APS;
- Development and dissemination of information related to best practices for APS; and
- Conducting research related to APS.

30.3.1.3 Enhancing Long-Term Care

The EJA also includes a number of provisions to improve detection of abuse in long-term care facilities. The EJA authorizes a grant program to enhance long-term care staffing through training and recruitment, and incentives for individuals seeking or maintaining employment in long-term care, either in a facility, or in a community-based long-term care entity. In addition, the EJA authorizes a "National Surveyors Institute" to train facility surveyors on identifying and measuring quality in long-term care facilities. To increase the likelihood that abuse in facilities is reported, the EJA includes provisions that:

- Requires the immediate reporting to law enforcement of crimes in a long-term care facility and establishes civil monetary penalties for failure to report
- Provides for penalties for long-term care facilities that retaliate against an employee for filing a complaint against or reporting a long-term care facility that violates reporting requirements, and
- Authorizes a study on establishing a national nurse aide registry.

30.3.2 Implementation

In total, the EJA authorizes over $750 million for implementing its provisions. However, the EJA is an authorizing bill, not an appropriations bill. Although Congress is authorized to appropriate funds for activities within the EJA, Congress is not required to fund the bill's provisions. As of Federal Fiscal Year 2015, the President requested

$25 million and Congress provided $4 million specifically to implement the EJA. Despite the modest Congressional appropriations, ACL has been able to implement a number of the EJA provisions related to APS, initially beginning activities prior to receipt of specific Congressional appropriations.

30.3.2.1 Elder Justice Coordinating Council

On October 11, 2012, the then HHS Secretary Kathleen Sebelius convened the inaugural meeting of the Elder Justice Coordinating Council (EJCC). The purpose of the Council is to make recommendations to the Secretary for the coordination of activities of DHHS, the Department of Justice, and other relevant federal, state, local, and private agencies and entities, relating to elder abuse, neglect, and exploitation and other crimes against elders.

Another key requirement in the EJA designed to achieve the objectives was the provision calling for the establishment of an Advisory Board on Elder Abuse, Neglect, and Exploitation to create short- and long-term multidisciplinary strategic plans and to make recommendations to the Council. The Advisory Board was to consist of 27 members of the general public and individuals with experience and expertise in elder abuse, neglect, and exploitation prevention, detection, treatment, intervention, or prosecution. While the process to establish the Advisory Board was initiated, it was not completed due to a lack of specific appropriations from the Congress to fund and support it.

The Secretary of DHHS is identified as the Chair of the Council, and the Attorney General, or a designee, is identified as a permanent member. At the initial convening, Secretary Sebelius designated Kathy Greenlee, Assistant Secretary for Aging and Administrator for Community Living, as the DHHS delegate and Chair on the Council, and ACL has remained the designated chair since. Other members of the Council are to be federal department or agency heads identified by the Chair as having responsibilities, or administering programs, relating to elder abuse, neglect, or exploitation. Each member of the Council must be an officer or employee of the federal Government. As of 2015, current agency membership included:

- Department of Health and Human Services, Chair
- Consumer Financial Protection Bureau
- Corporation for National and Community Service
- Department of Housing and Urban Development
- Department of Justice
- Department of Labor
- Department of the Treasury
- Department of Veterans Affairs
- Federal Trade Commission
- Securities and Exchange Commission
- Social Security Administration
- U.S. Postal Inspection Service.

During the inaugural meeting, a select group of experts on elder abuse, neglect, and exploitation was invited to speak on four primary topic areas: financial exploitation, public policy and awareness, enhancing response, and advancing research. These experts were also asked to submit white papers that detailed the importance of the federal government in addressing specific elder abuse issues and that provided recommendations for federal action in those areas.

The expert recommendations served as the basis for additional investigation by federal staff on the Interagency Elder Justice Working Group (EJWG) into the current state of knowledge within the field of elder justice on the particular issues raised by the experts. The EJWG compiled information on best and promising practices for primary, secondary, and tertiary prevention; empirical evidence from peer-reviewed research; approaches used in related disciplines; and information about where gaps exist in the collective knowledge about elder abuse, neglect and exploitation. The EJWG further refined the expert suggestions into nine proposals with accompanying steps for federal action. The proposals were subsequently presented at two Council meetings that took place in May and September 2013.

Following the presentation at the May 2013 Council meeting, the draft proposals were made publicly available through the website of the Administration for Community Living, along with a mechanism by which the public could provide comments and suggestions about the proposals. For the September 2013 meeting, the EJWG further refined the draft recommendations based on public input, and facilitated a discussion for the Council members on possible implementation strategies.

On November 5, 2013, the Council met in a closed, Executive Session to discuss and further refine the proposals. The Council agreed to and adopted a final set of eight recommendations for federal action to combat elder abuse, neglect, and exploitation (see Table 30.1 below). The Council believes the recommendations represent a focused, yet well-balanced, approach for establishing greater federal leadership in the area of elder justice and for improving the federal response to elder abuse, neglect, and exploitation.

The Council is required to submit, every 2 years, a report to Congress describing its activities and accomplishments, and may make recommendations for legislation, model laws, or other action as determined to be appropriate. In the spring of 2015, the Council submitted its first report to Congress summarizing the recommendations for federal action that had been developed, the process to develop them, and the

Table 30.1 Recommendations for increased federal involvement in addressing elder abuse, neglect, and exploitation

Improving response
Recommendation 1: Support the investigation and prosecution of elder abuse cases
Support the investigation and prosecution of elder abuse, neglect, and financial exploitation cases by providing training and resources to federal, state, and local investigators and prosecutors
Recommendation 2: Enhance services to elder abuse victims
Support and protect elder abuse victims by improving identification of elder abuse and enhancing response and outreach to victims
Recommendation 3: Develop a national Adult Protective Services (APS) system
Develop a national APS system based upon standardized data collection and a core set of service provision standards and best practices
Recommendation 4: Develop a federal elder justice research agenda
Establish a coordinated research agenda across federal agencies to identify best practices for prevention of and intervention in elder abuse and elder financial exploitation
Improving awareness and prevention
Recommendation 5: Develop a broad-based public awareness campaign
Develop a comprehensive, strategic, and broad-based national public awareness campaign, with clear and consistent messaging to raise awareness and understanding of elder abuse, neglect, and exploitation
Recommendation 6: Cross-disciplinary training on elder abuse
Develop training to educate stakeholders across multiple sectors and disciplines on preventing, detecting, intervening in, and responding to elder abuse, neglect, and exploitation
Recommendation 7: Combat elder financial exploitation, including abuse by fiduciaries
Prevent, detect, and respond to elder financial exploitation through federal enforcement activities, policy initiatives, coordination, oversight, and education, and by collaborating with industry to enhance fraud detection and provide resources for victims
Recommendation 8: Improve screening for dementia and cognitive capacity, financial capacity, and financial exploitation
Improve the ability of APS and first responders to screen for diminished capacity, diminished financial capacity, and vulnerability to or victimization of financial exploitation

accomplishments of the Council member agencies in addressing elder abuse and promoting elder justice.[1]

Moving forward, the Council will continue to work on implementing the adopted recommendations and on strategies to embed and institutionalize the Council's recommendations for increased federal action.

30.3.2.2 Elder Abuse Prevention Intervention Demonstration Grants

In 2012, ACL was able to provide funding to begin implementing the APS demonstration grants authorized in the EJA, utilizing funding from the Prevention and Public Health Fund, also authorized within the same legislation that contains the EJA. The Elder Abuse Prevention Interventions Program provided $5.5 million to five states and three tribes to test community-based elder abuse prevention practices. With this funding, the grantees are developing, testing, and evaluating interventions in partnership with their State Adult Protective Services agency, State Unit on Aging, and appropriate justice system entities. The grantees are also participating in a national evaluation, to determine if any of the tested interventions show promise for more rigorous evaluation studies.

30.3.2.3 National Adult Maltreatment Reporting System

In September 2013, ACL again was able to leverage the Prevention and Public Health Fund to implement a provision of the EJA, as well as begin to move forward Recommendation 3 of the EJCC cited above. In partnership with the HHS Office of the Assistant Secretary for Planning and Evaluation (ASPE), ACL launched a 2-year effort to design and test a national reporting system based on data from state adult protective services (APS) agency information systems. The goal of a future data-collection system is to provide consistent, accurate national data on the exploitation and abuse of older adults and adults with disabilities, as reported to APS agencies in all of the US jurisdictions.

The future system, currently designated as the National Adult Maltreatment Reporting System (NAMRS), is being designed to collect quantitative and qualitative data on the practices and policies of state adult protective services

[1]The EJCC Report to Congress can be viewed at: http://www.aoa.acl.gov/AoA_Programs/Elder_Rights/EJCC/docs/EJCC-2012-2014-report-to-congress.pdf.

agencies and the outcomes of investigations into the maltreatment of older adults and adults with disabilities. ACL hopes that, by collecting individual-level information about persons served by APS and the alleged perpetrators of abuse, we will learn more about the risk and protective factors of abuse and be able to design more effective and targeted interventions.

30.3.2.4 Voluntary Consensus Guidelines for State APS Systems

As noted earlier, historically there has been no federal "home" for APS, nor a designated federal appropriation for this critically important service. Instead, states and local agencies have developed a wide variety of APS practices, resulting in significant variations in practice across the country. For example, APS systems differ in the populations served, settings in which services are available, types of services provided, relationships with other service providers and the justice system, and timeliness of responses.

In order to provide a core set of principles and common expectations to encourage consistency in the policies and practices of APS across the country, as well as, to further implement the APS provisions of the EJA and Recommendation 3 of the EJCC, ACL began a process in 2014 to facilitate the development of field-driven, consensus-informed, national guidelines for state APS systems. The process for developing voluntary, consensus guidelines for APS systems included an environmental scan, convening an expert-working group to draft the initial set of guidelines, and a stakeholder engagement and outreach strategy to refine and build consensus around the guidelines. The draft guidelines build upon existing work in APS agencies and in other analogous systems throughout the United States, and have been developed based on the best science available on practices and policies believed to produce the best outcomes for individuals.

Through the guidelines, ACL seeks to help ensure that adults are afforded similar protections and service delivery, regardless of which state or jurisdiction they live. The goals of this consistent approach are for the enhancement of partnerships and effective, efficient, and culturally competent delivery both of services to victims and responses to perpetrators. Most importantly, a consistent approach for APS systems displays the value this nation places on its older adults and adults with disabilities as contributing members of society.

30.3.2.5 State Grants to Enhance Adult Protective Services

To further help in addressing the gaps and challenges in state APS systems, ACL utilized its FY 2015 appropriation for demonstration grants to states to enhance their APS systems. In implementing these grants, ACL also sought to create an opportunity to advance further provisions in the EJA. This demonstration is designed to provide funding to states to enhance APS systems statewide, to include innovations and improvements in practice, services, and data collection and reporting. As APS is a system response intended to help individuals who are victims of maltreatment, grantee projects are expected to:

- Improve the experiences, health, well-being, and outcomes of the individuals served by APS, and
- Accurately document the improvements in outcomes in a manner that is consistent with national data collection efforts, such as the National Adult Maltreatment Reporting System (NAMRS).

Grantees will use these funds to:

- collaborate more closely with social, behavioral health, medical, and legal services agencies,
- collect data on outcomes,
- develop innovative tools that assess risk and safety, and
- form multidisciplinary teams to better support those served by APS.

30.4 Bridging the Gap Between Health and Public Policy

The negative effects of abuse, neglect, and exploitation on the health and independence of older adults are extensive. Research has demonstrated that elder abuse is both lethal and expensive. Older victims of even modest forms of abuse have dramatically higher (300 %) morbidity and mortality rates than older people who have not been subjected to abuse [3, 4]. Adverse health impacts include an increased likelihood of heart attacks, dementia, depression, chronic diseases, and psychological distress. Along with women and children, older adults disproportionately bear the burden of these nonfatal consequences of abuse and neglect, which are often the most expensive for health systems [5].

It is critical to emphasize that the known health consequences of abuse, neglect, and exploitation provided the evidence on which the case is made for action. In addition to making a moral argument for addressing abuse, a practical argument is provided: experiencing abuse increases the likelihood of death and exacerbates existing medical conditions. These facts establish abuse as a public health problem, and it is already understood that unaddressed public health problems result in increased costs and consequences, both to the healthcare sector but to society, as well. Therefore, there is a practical and economical imperative to develop public policy solutions to this public health problem.

To improve efforts to address public health issues, such as abuse, neglect, and exploitation, and to enable evidence-based public policy, we need to expand the involvement of health professionals and researchers in the public policy debates. The United States government allocates significant funding to health-related research each year. For example, the National Institutes of Health spent approximately $30 billion in 2003 on biomedical research, accounting for 28 % of the funding in the US in this area [6]. These investments are intended to improve the public's health by facilitating the development of evidence-based public policy.

The EJA, and more specifically the Coordinating Council, is an approach to bridge this gap between public health and public policy. In addition to documenting the consequences of abuse on health and well-being, the medical and health fields are critical components of effective prevention strategies. Older adults have more chronic conditions and seek medical care more than younger populations, and health professionals are often one of the most trusted sources of information for older adults. In addition to the research produced from the health field that advances our understanding of the effects and impact of abuse, neglect, and exploitation, health professionals are a key component in the early identification and prevention responses developed. It is critical that health professionals engage in the public policy process, as they bring invaluable and unique information about the experience of abused older adults.

30.5 2015 White House Conference on Aging

In 2015, the sixth White House Conference on Aging in the history of the United States took place. Unlike any of the previous conferences, which take place every 10 years, this one took the form of a national conversation. Five regional forums were held with each one representing the focus areas of the Conference: Healthy Aging, Long Term Supports and Services, Retirement Security and Elder Justice. The concluding event at the White House included thousands of Americans joining via "watch parties" in every state in the country. The 2015 Conference marked the first time that there was a national focus on Elder Justice. Each focus area produced a policy brief and a number of enhanced partnerships and new programs both in and outside of government (see http://www.whitehouseconferenceonaging.gov). The deliverables produced at the Conference were highly complementary to the eight recommendations of the Elder Justice Coordinating Council. In some ways, the eight recommendations helped to shape some of the direction of the products of the Conference. The recommendation categories of *Improving Response* and *Improving Awareness and Prevention* are reflected in the White House Conference on Aging efforts described below.

The following is the list of the projects and partnerships that were planned as a result of the 2015 White House Conference on Aging:

- ***Improving the Science on Understanding and Preventing Elder Abuse***:
  - In 2015, the National Institutes of Health will convene a state of the science workshop on elder abuse with researchers, clinicians, and others to review the science on understanding and preventing abuse; screening tools to identify abuse victims; effective interventions and research in related areas like child abuse and domestic violence that might inform research on elder abuse; and gaps and opportunities in this field of research. The aim of this workshop is to bring together a diverse set of stakeholders and determine promising avenues of research that could benefit from immediate investment.
  - The U.S. Department of Justice's National Institute of Justice and its Elder Justice Initiative will fund a multi-year pilot project to evaluate potential means to avoid and respond to elder mistreatment.
  - As part of a $4 million effort, the HHS Administration for Community Living launched a stakeholder engagement project on State Adult Protective Services Guidelines (APS) that will serve as core principles for APS systems throughout the nation and is awarding State grants to test full implementation of a national elder abuse, neglect, and exploitation reporting system. HHS also released research briefs on the Elder Abuse Prevention Interventions Pilot Programs, which aim to build a stronger evidence base for elder abuse prevention interventions.
  - *Private Sector Actions*: The American Banking Association Foundation announced the release of an interactive community mapping tool that identifies innovative bank programs across the country that adopt intensive banker training to stop fraud and financial exploitation of older Americans, provide robust consumer education, and create effective partnerships with law enforcement and adult protective services.
- ***Protecting Older Americans from Financial Exploitation and Elder Abuse***:
  - The Consumer Financial Protection Bureau (CFPB) will release, by the end of 2015, an advisory to help financial institutions prevent, recognize, and report elder financial exploitation. CFPB is engaging with industry, consumer advocates, and others on the development of these promising practices and tools.

- ***Training Elder Abuse Prosecutors and Developing Online Training for Law Enforcement Officers***:
  - The U.S. Department of Justice is committing to enroll and train prosecutors from all 50 states to effectively prosecute elder abuse and financial exploitation. Since 2013, DOJ has trained state and local prosecutors from 26 states and the District of Columbia through its National Institute on Prosecuting Elder Abuse, an intensive 4-day training program that covers the essential elements of bringing an elder abuse or financial exploitation case. The Department committed to enroll prosecutors from the remaining 24 states by 2017.
  - In addition, in August 2015, DOJ funded a 3-day judicial institute for judges and magistrates from federal, tribal, state, territorial, and local courts. The training program addressed elder abuse, neglect, and exploitation, including domestic violence, sexual assault and stalking.
  - DOJ will also partner with national law enforcement organizations, including the International Association of Chiefs of Police, National Sheriffs' Association, National Association of Triads and the International Association of Directors of Law Enforcement Standards and Training to develop and disseminate web accessible training materials and resources to state and local law enforcement officers nationwide.
  - DOJ also is collaborating with a wide array of federal agencies—including the Federal Bureau of Investigation, the U.S. Postal Service, and the Internal Revenue Service—to develop and promote elder abuse and financial exploitation training for their agents.
  - Additionally, DOJ will develop tools to help domestic violence advocates, sexual assault programs, and aging services organizations to serve individuals who have experienced elder abuse—including domestic violence, sexual assault, and stalking—neglect, and financial exploitation.

These federal initiatives will also provide a basis for many more state-based training programs and private research opportunities in Elder Justice. Each of these Elder Justice initiatives from the White House Conference are integrated into medical training, practice, and provides opportunities to inform effectively change policy.

30.6 Future: Themes of Research, Practice, and Policy

Looking ahead, the US government needs to build on its Elder Justice successes both domestically and internationally. Future administrations will need to understand the dynamics of the expanding older population and address the issues of elder justice. By continuing the federal government's commitment across business lines to work on these issues through the Elder Justice Coordinating Council and building additional funds to support further elder justice work, the federal government can provide leadership for state and local governments. As other federal agencies join with the 12 original EJCC members, the initial recommendations will be able to be more fully implemented and to continue a comprehensive approach to addressing the research, practice, and policy needs of our older population. Most importantly, in order to keep the work moving and improving, the federal government needs to make elder justice part of its regular work and funding stream. As we look at the issues in elder justice in this country and around the world, we need to continue down the dual tracks of public health and human rights for the best research hopes and good, thoughtful policy borne of experience.

References

1. Beach SR, Schulz R, Castle NG, Rosen J. Financial exploitation and psychological mistreatment among older adults: differences between African Americans and non-African Americans in a population-based survey. Gerontologist. 2010 Dec;50(6):744–57.
2. Lifespan of Greater Rochester, Inc., Weill Cornell Medical Center of Cornell University & New York City Department for the Aging. Under the radar: New York state elder abuse prevalence study [Final Report]. New York: William B. Hoyt Memorial New York State Children and Family Trust Fund, and the New York State Office of Children and Family Services. 2011.
3. Lachs MS, Williams CS, O'Brien S, Pillemer KA, Charlson ME. The mortality of elder mistreatment. JAMA. 1998;280:428–32.
4. Baker MW. Elder mistreatment: risk, vulnerability, and early mortality. J Am Psychiatr Nurses Assoc. 2007;12(6):313–21.
5. Women and children and the elderly also suffer a host of negative health and social consequences from these acts of violence that often last a lifetime and that are not captured in official statistics. Global Status Report on Violence Prevention 2014. World Health Organization, 2014. http://www.who.int/violence_injury_prevention/violence/status_report/2014/en/.
6. www.nih.gov.

Department of Justice: Elder Maltreatment Initiatives

31

Carrie F. Mulford and Andy Mao

31.1 Introduction

The mission of the United States Department of Justice (DOJ) is "to enforce the law and defend the interests of the United States according to the law; ensure public safety against threats foreign and domestic; to provide federal leadership in preventing and controlling crime; to seek punishment for those guilty of unlawful behavior; and to ensure fair and impartial administration of justice for all Americans".[1] As part of its mission, DOJ has engaged in a wide array of activities to combat, prevent, and expand our understanding of elder abuse, neglect, and financial exploitation. In this chapter, we will provide an overview of some of DOJ's efforts in the area of elder maltreatment. First, we will highlight the range of research, statistics, and evaluation projects that have been funded by the National Institute of Justice (NIJ) and the Bureau of Justice Statistics (BJS), the research and statistics arms of DOJ, and summarize specific project findings that have been most useful to the field. Then, we will highlight some of DOJ's other policy and programmatic initiatives, including the Elder Justice Roadmap. Finally, we will briefly discuss some of DOJ's investigative and prosecutorial efforts to combat elder abuse and financial fraud targeting elderly individuals.

[1]See DOJ home page at http://www.justice.gov/about (October 2015).

C.F. Mulford (✉)
National Institute of Justice, Office of Justice Programs, United States Department of Justice, 810 7th Street NW, Washington, DC 20531, USA
e-mail: Carrie.Mulford@usdoj.gov

A. Mao
United States Department of Justice, 601 D. Street, NW, Rm. 9432, Washington, DC 20004, USA
e-mail: Andy.Mao@usdoj.gov

X. Dong (ed.), *Elder Abuse*, DOI 10.1007/978-3-319-47504-2_31

31.2 Overview

The Department of Justice is the chief enforcer of our nation's federal laws. Given its broad array of responsibilities, DOJ is divided into various divisions and offices.[2] DOJ's litigating components are organized into divisions, including the Criminal, Civil, and Civil Rights Divisions. In addition to enforcing the nation's federal laws, DOJ provides federal leadership and support to state, local, and tribal communities through a wide array of programs. DOJ's Office of Justice Programs ("OJP"), for example, provides innovative leadership through "disseminating state-of-the-art knowledge and practice across America, and providing grants for the implementation of these crime fighting strategies." In addition to supporting law enforcement efforts through research, statistics, and evaluations, OJP oversees a wide array of programs on topics ranging from juvenile justice to substance abuse. A key component within OJP is the Office for Victims of Crime (OVC), which is committed to enhancing the nation's capacity to assist crime victims and to providing leadership to change attitudes, policies, and practices to promote justice and healing for all victims of crime.[3] Along with OJP, the Office on Violence Against Women provides federal leadership in developing our nation's capacity to reduce violence against women. Since its inception in 1995, OVW has awarded over $6 billion in grants and cooperative agreements to help communities to develop programs, policies, and practices to end domestic violence, dating violence, sexual assault, and stalking, while providing services to victims of these crimes.[4] As will be discussed below, preventing and addressing elder abuse, neglect, and exploitation is a priority that cuts across many of DOJ's components.

[2]See DOJ home page at http://www.justice.gov/agencies/chart (November 2015).

[3]See OJP Homepage at http://ojp.gov/programs/victims.htm (November 2015).

[4]See OVW Homepage at http://www.justice.gov/ovw/about-office (November 2015).

31.3 Research, Evaluation, and Statistics at DOJ

NIJ is the research, development, and evaluation agency of DOJ, with a mission of "improving knowledge and understanding of crime and justice issues through science."[5] NIJ's research in the area of elder mistreatment has been organized around six research themes—research on forensic markers; evaluation of interventions; research on incidence, prevalence, and risk factors; tool development for practitioners; financial exploitation; and elder mistreatment in residential care facilities. We will conclude the research section with a discussion of future directions and gaps in our understanding across all of the research themes.

NIJ has adopted the National Research Council definition for elder mistreatment: "(a) intentional actions that cause harm or create a serious risk of harm to a vulnerable elder by a caregiver or other person who stands in a trust relationship to the elder, or (b) failure by a caregiver to satisfy the elder's basic needs or to protect the elder from harm" [18]. This definition, which appears on NIJ's elder abuse home page, includes financial exploitation, physical abuse, and neglect.

Historically, elder abuse was viewed as a social problem rather than a criminal problem, with most states not establishing adult protective services units until the mid-1980s. As recognized by the National Academies' Committee on National Statistics in 2002, there is a dearth of research on physical abuse, sexual abuse, and neglect of elderly that results in a widespread inability to effectively prevent, detect, intervene in, or prosecute the problem. Scholars in the field claim that research on elder abuse and neglect lags behind research on child maltreatment and violence against women by two decades (e.g., [20]). The results of the NIJ-funded National Elder Mistreatment Study indicated that 11 % of elders reported experiencing at least one form of mistreatment—emotional, physical, sexual or potential neglect—in the past year [1]. Financial exploitation by a family member was reported by 5 % of elders.

In the United States, the issue of elder mistreatment is garnering attention of the law enforcement, medical, and research communities as demographic trends indicate that more people are living longer than they have in any previous time in our nation's history. This trend is expected to increase, as the U.S. Census Bureau projects that more than 62 million Americans will be aged 65 years or older in 2025, an increase of 78 % from 2001. The number of Americans aged 85 years or older is expected to be over 7.4 million, an increase of nearly 68 %. These aging members of our population will likely require more care and protection than what is currently available or possible to provide. Most importantly, every individual is entitled to equal protection from neglect, abuse, and exploitation regardless of age or infirmity. For these reasons, NIJ has established a research program that specifically focuses on the issue of elder mistreatment to assist the field in its response to the current and emerging needs of the elderly population.

Many of the priorities identified in prior NIJ solicitations for research on elder mistreatment have come from the National Research Council's 2003 landmark publication *Elder Mistreatment: Abuse, Neglect, and Exploitation in an Aging America* and subsequent interdisciplinary meetings with researchers and practitioners in the field. In particular, the *NIJ Elder Abuse Workshop* in 2008 and the National Institute of Aging hosted *Meeting on Research Issues in Elder Mistreatment and Abuse and Financial Fraud* in 2010, and the DOJ-funded *Elder Justice Roadmap* project (2014) were influential in shaping NIJ's research agenda over the past several years. More recently, DOJ funded a survey of leading researchers in the field of elder abuse and financial exploitation in order to prioritize the most salient research gaps in the elder abuse field. The three most pressing research priorities identified through that survey were the need for psychometrically sound and consistent measurement of elder abuse, the need for research to identify effective interventions to prevent the reoccurrence of elder abuse, and research on the causes and consequences of the various forms of elder abuse.[6]

NIJ, in collaboration with the Civil Division of DOJ, has made grant awards in each fiscal year (FY) from 2005 to 2015 (except for FY 2012) in response to the needs identified in the field. Since 2005, NIJ has funded over 30 projects across 6 different areas—research on forensic markers; evaluation of interventions; research on incidence, prevalence, and risk factors; tool development for researchers and practitioners; financial exploitation; and elder mistreatment in residential care facilities. These projects are examining diverse elder mistreatment issues, including the identification of victimization risk factors; measurement of incidence and prevalence of abuse, including resident-on-resident abuse; exploration of residential care systems' mechanisms for responding to abuse; examination of bruising and pressure ulcers as they relate to abuse, neglect, and care; examination of forensic technologies in the detection of elder abuse; exploration of the factors that contribute to or are associated with the financial abuse of the elderly as well as the factors that promote reporting and facilitate investigation

[5] From the NIJ Hebpage http://www.nij.gov/about/pages/welcome.aspx (October 2015).

[6] See *Building Consensus on Research Priorities in Elder Mistreatment* (at http://www.justice.gov/elderjustice/research/resources/Building_Consensus_On_Research_Priorities_In_Elder_Mistreatment.pdf).

of such abuse; evaluation of the forensic center model; and production of screening and assessment tools for financial exploitation and abuse of the elderly. See Table 31.1 for a listing of all NIJ-funded grants from 2005 to 2015.

BJS is the statistics arm of DOJ and its mission is "to collect, analyze, publish, and disseminate information on crime, criminal offenders, victims of crime, and the operation of justice systems at all levels of government".[7] BJS has supported a number of data collection projects to help document information on crimes against the elderly. BJS collects and analyzes statistics on criminal offending and criminal victimization, including crimes that are committed against elderly individuals. Statistics on crimes against the elderly are also relevant to the issue of elder abuse, although some forms of elder abuse are not criminal and some crimes against the elderly would not fit common definitions of elder abuse.

31.4 BJS Elder Abuse Statistics and Projects

A special report on crimes against the elderly [13] provides statistics about violent and nonviolent criminal activities committed against adults ages 65 and older over the decade between 2003 and 2013. Overall, the rate of nonfatal criminal victimization among the elderly is the lowest of any age group (3.6 victimizations per 1000 persons age 65 or older). However, the number of victimizations reported in the National Crime Victimization Survey (NCVS) should not be expected to align with other measures of elder abuse victimization. The NCVS is designed to measure nonfatal personal and property crimes, but does not include many of the experiences typically reported in elder abuse estimates, such as verbal and psychological abuse, some forms of mild physical abuse, or the misappropriation of financial resources [12]. Some key findings relevant to elder abuse from the report on crimes against the elderly include: (1) Elderly crime victims (59.3 %) are far more likely than all other victims to report being victimized at or near their homes; (2) Elderly individuals (5 %) were no more likely to experience identity theft than persons ages 25–49 (7.9 %) or ages 50–64 (7.8 %); (3) Domestic violence (including violence committed by an intimate partner or other family member) made up a smaller percentage of violent crimes committed against elderly individuals (14.3 %) than against individuals ages 25–49 (26.0 %) or ages 50–64 (19.9 %); and (4) Violent crime rates for elderly individuals with a disability (3.9 per 1000 persons) were similar to elderly individuals without a disability (4.1 per 1000 persons). Other factors that were associate with higher rates of criminal victimization for elderly individuals include living in urban areas, being divorced or separated (as compared to never married, married, or widowed), and being unemployed or retired.

BJS is funding the Assessment of Administrative Data on Elder Abuse, Mistreatment and Neglect project to assess the feasibility of using administrative data collected by Adult Protective Services (APS) agencies for examining cases of abuse, mistreatment, and neglect of the elderly and adults with disabilities reported to APS. The first task was to develop a taxonomy of elder abuse definitions to help guide the assessment of whether APS agencies are collecting key indicator statistics that are consistent with the definitions of specific types of elder abuse. BJS expects to make the resulting research brief, *What is Elder Abuse? A Taxonomy for Collecting Criminal Justice Research and Statistical Data* [12], available in 2016. The report presents a taxonomy of elder abuse along three dimensions—the elder abuse acts, the characteristics of the victim, and the relationship between the perpetrator and the victims. They also include a discussion of how criminal and noncriminal acts can be distinguished. The next task is to develop a survey to measure the capacity of APS data systems to generate key indicators of victimization and criminal victimization consistent with the taxonomy developed in the first stage of the project. One of the key goals of the data collection effort is to determine whether APS data can be used to distinguish between criminal and noncriminal acts. An effort will also be made to document the capacity of APS data systems to record criminal justice referrals and outcomes or link to criminal justice databases. In the third stage of the project, an on-line survey will be administered to approximately 140 state and local APS data collection entities. Results from this project will be used to assess the suitability of using administrative data from APS as the basis for a statistical system to generate national estimates of victimization and criminal victimization of elderly individuals and adults with disabilities. The final product is anticipated to be completed in 2016.

The Criminal Victimization of Persons with Disabilities Residing in Group Quarters (CVGQ) was designed by BJS to measure victimization of persons with disabilities residing in group quarters, such as skilled nursing facilities, group homes for adults, other board and care facilities, and domestic violence shelters. The project will identify the challenges associated with surveying noninstitutional group quarters populations on a routine basis as part of BJS' ongoing National Crime Victimization Survey.

31.5 Findings from Key NIJ Studies

In this section we present key research findings from NIJ funded research across the six areas mentioned above—research on incidence, prevalence, and risk factors; research

[7]From the BJS webpage http://www.bjs.gov/index.cfm?ty=abu (October 2015).

Table 31.1 List of NIJ awards by area of research

Grant #	Grantee	Title	Principal investigator	Amount	Status
Forensic research					
2005-IJ-CX-0048	University of California, Irvine	Bruising as a Forensic Marker of Elder Abuse	Laura Mosqueda	$375,655	Complete
2006-IJ-CX-0029	University of California, Irvine	A Multi-site Study to Characterize Pressure Ulcers in Long-term Care under Best Practices	Solomon Liao	$561,718	Complete
2007-DN-BX-0007	University of Maryland, Baltimore	Utility of Whole-Body Computed Tomography Imaging in Post Mortem Detection of Elder Abuse and Neglect: Comparison with and Potential Substitution for Standard Autoposy	Barry Daly	$292,341	Complete
2007-MU-MU-0002	University of California, Irvine	People with Dementia as Witnesses to Emotional Events	Laura Mosqueda	$441,017	Complete
2008-MU-MU-0021	University of California, Irvine	Coroner Investigations of Suspicious Elder Deaths	Laura Mosqueda	$526,985	Complete
2013-IJ-CX-0025	University of Southern California	Forensic Markers of Physical Elder Abuse: Establishing a Medical Characterization and Identifying the Criminal Justice Approach to Investigation and Prosecution	Diana Homeier	$518,327	Ongoing
Evaluation research					
2007-IJ-CX-0107	American Bar Association	Multi-Site Assessment of Five Court-Focused Elder Abuse Initiatives	Lori Stiegel	$219,409	Complete
2009-IJ-CX-0017	University of Southern California	Evaluating the Elder Abuse Forensic Center Model	Kate Wilber	$260,006	Complete
2011-IJ-CX-0015	University of Southern California	Evaluating the Cost-effectiveness of the Elder Abuse Forensic Center Model	Mike Nichol	$484,448	Complete
2013-MU-CX-0032	University of Denver (Colorado Seminary)	The Impact of a Forensic Collaborative for Older Adults on Criminal Justice and Victim Outcomes: A Randomized-Control Longitudinal Design	Anne DePrince	$622,283	Ongoing
Incidence/prevalence/risk factors for abuse among elders residing in the community					
2005-MU-MU-0052	University of South Florida	Florida Elder Abuse Survey	Lawrence Branch	$235,585	Complete
2005-IJ-CX-0048	University of California, Irvine	Theoretical Model Development in Elder Mistreatment	Laura Mosqueda and Kerry Burnight	$200,000	Complete
2005-WG-BX-0012	The Police Foundation	Course of Domestic Abuse among Chicago's Elderly: Risk Factors, Protective Behaviors, and Police Intervention	Karen Amendola	$438,054	Complete
2006-WG-BX-0009	Advocates for Human Potential	Statewide Profile of Abuse of Older Women and the Criminal Justice Response	Andy Klein	$118,376	Complete
2007-WG-BX-0009	Medical University of South Carolina	National Elder Mistreatment Study	Ron Acierno	$700,780	Complete
2014-MU-CX-0003	Medical University of South Carolina	National Elder Mistreatment Study: 5 Year Follow-up of Victims and Matched Non-Victims	Ron Acierno	$520,273	Ongoing
Practitioner tools for abuse assessment					
2008-IJ-CX-0025	National Council on Crime and Delinquency	Developing an Actuarial Risk Assessment to Inform Decisions Made by Adult Protective Services Workers	Kristen Johnson	$309,000	Complete
2009-IJ-CX-0202	University of Illinois	Developing End-User Criteria and a Prototype for an Elder Abuse Assessment System	Ken Conrad	$307,436	Complete
2011-IJ-CX-0014	Chestnut Health Systems	Elder Abuse Computerized Decision Support System	Ken Conrad	$731,748	Complete

(continued)

Table 31.1 (continued)

Grant #	Grantee	Title	Principal investigator	Amount	Status
2014-MU-CX-0102	University of North Texas Health Science Center	Development of a brief elder abuse and neglect screener for Emergency Medical Services: Detection of Elder abuse Through Emergency Care Technicians (DETECT)	Brad Cannell	$369,039	Ongoing
2015-IJ-CX-0022	University of North Carolina–Chapel Hill	Development and Validation of a Screening Protocol to Identify Elder Abuse in United States Emergency Departments	Timothy Platts-Mills	$968,933	Ongoing
Abuse in residential care facilities					
2005-IJ-CX-0054	Texas A&M Research Foundation	Detecting, Addressing, and Preventing Elder Abuse in Residential Care Facilities	Catherine Hawes	$208,354	Complete
2009-IJ-CX-0001	Weill Medical College of Cornell University	Documentation of Resident to Resident Elder Mistreatment in Residential Care Facilities	Mark Lachs	$626,801	Complete
2010-IJ-CX-0023	University of Pittsburgh	Examination of Resident Abuse in Assisted Living Facilities	Nick Castle	$466,441	Complete
Financial exploitation					
2006-MU-MU-0004	University of Illinois	Conceptualizing and Measuring Financial Exploitation and Psychological Abuse of Elderly Individuals	Ken Conrad	$304,300	Complete
2006-WG-BX-0010	University of Virginia	Financial Abuse of Elderly People Versus Other Forms of Elder Abuse: Assessing Their Dynamics, Risk Factors, and Society's Response	Shelly Jackson	$290,414	Complete
2010-IJ-CX-0008	Arizona State University	Financial Exploitation of the Elderly in a Consumer Context	Kristy Holtfreter	$393,174	Complete
2013-IJ-CX-0024	Arizona State University	Developing and Testing a Culturally Relevant Model to Understand Financial Maltreatment of Chinese American Elders	Fei Sun	$72,775	Ongoing
2013-IJ-CX-0026	Scripps College	Identification of Risk and Preventive Factors for Elder Financial Exploitation	Stacey Wood	$136,290	Ongoing
2013-IJ-CX-0050	University of Texas Health Science Center at Houston	Elder Financial Exploitation Victimization: Identifying Unique Risk Factors to Enhance Detection, Prevention and Intervention	Carmel Dyer	$387,736	Ongoing
2014-MU-CX-0001	Wayne State University	Integrating Improved Assessments of Financial Judgment: Conceptual and Measurement Advances	Peter Lichtenberg	$468,181	Ongoing
Other					
2015-ZD-CX-0003	University of South Maine	The Health Care Cost of Elder Abuse: An Analysis of Medicare, Medicaid, and Adult Protective Services Data in Maine, 2006 through 2014	Charles Smith	$328,940	Ongoing

Areas of research are not mutually exclusive. Grants are listed only once under the area where they fit best

on forensic markers; evaluation of interventions; tool development for researchers and practitioners; financial exploitation; and elder mistreatment in residential care facilities—keeping in mind that many studies do not fit cleanly in one category. At the end of each section, we will also discuss some of the research challenges associated with each category.

31.5.1 Research on Incidence, Prevalence, and Risk Factors for Elder Abuse

The largest, most comprehensive and most commonly cited statistics on the prevalence of elder mistreatment experienced by elderly individuals living in the community comes from the NIJ-funded National Elder Mistreatment Study (NEMS), a nationally representative study of 5777 U.S. residents ages 60 and older. Participants who were determined to have either little or no cognitive impairment were interviewed on the phone in either English or Spanish about physical, sexual, emotional abuse, neglect, and financial exploitation. Proxy interviews were also conducted with a sample of participants with more severe cognitive impairment. The proxy interviews were determined to be unreliable for identifying most forms of abuse. Among the community dwelling elders who answered the questions for themselves, the researchers reported past-year prevalence of 5.1 % for emotional mistreatment, 1.6 % for physical mistreatment, 0.6 % for sexual mistreatment, 5.2 % for financial exploitation by a family member, and 5.1 % for potential neglect [1]. In addition to questions about abuse, participants were asked a number of questions about health, social support, and demographics. Risk factors for elder mistreatment in this sample were low household income, unemployment or retirement, self-reported poor health, experience of a prior traumatic event, and low levels of social support [1].

In 2014, NIJ funded a 5 year follow-up of the original victims identified in the 2009 NEMS study, plus a matched sample of participants who did not report any past-year victimization in the original NEMS study. The follow-up study will provide the field with the most comprehensive national longitudinal data on a sample of identified victims of elder abuse. Understanding the physical health, mental health, social service utilization, and criminal justice outcomes for victims of elder abuse has long been an area of needed research in elder abuse. This study will begin to answer some of these questions and will specifically look at the relationship between mental health outcomes and criminal justice system participation.

There does seem to be consensus developing around the extent of victimization experienced by elderly individuals who are not cognitively impaired and who reside in the community. However, it has not been possible to include residents of long-term care facilities or individuals who are not able to respond to telephone surveys in the national prevalence numbers. NIJ has funded some research on the extent of abuse in residential care facilities (see section below) and others have funded smaller scale studies to estimate the extent of abuse experienced by elderly individuals with cognitive impairment. Although it would be ideal, at this point, coming up with a national estimate of elder abuse prevalence that includes all elderly individuals is not possible.

Data on the prevalence of elder abuse, neglect, and financial exploitation perpetration does not exist. In other areas of family and community violence, research participants are often asked about their experiences as victims and as perpetrators. This is not the standard in elder abuse research. Therefore, we know very little about perpetrators, with the exception of their characteristics as reported by the victims. We also know very little about the overlap between perpetration and victimization experiences among elderly individuals.

31.5.2 Research on Forensic Markers of Elder Abuse

Research to assist law enforcement, geriatricians, social service workers, and medical examiners to identify cases of elder abuse is a critical need in the field. This is also an area where NIJ has devoted a considerable amount of resources in large part because of the importance of forensic marker research to practitioners in the criminal justice system. Early NIJ-funded research on forensic markers documented normal bruising patterns among the elderly population and found that: (1) accidental bruises occur in a predictable pattern; (2) most accidental large bruises are on the extremities; (3) the initial color and appearance of bruises changes over time and is less predictable than previously thought; and (4) individuals who are on medications known to make bruising more severe and those with compromised functional ability are more likely to have multiple bruises [14]. The study included 101 participants with an average age of 83. Nurses examined any bruises that developed during the 2 weeks study window and documented the progression of the bruises for up to 6 weeks. In addition to collecting data on the color, location, and size of each bruise, demographic information along with medical conditions, medication, and functional and cognitive status was collected. Participants were also asked what caused the bruise.

A follow-up study designed to characterize bruising patters in elderly individuals who are confirmed victims of elder abuse found that: (1) abused elders were far more likely to be able to explain the cause of their bruises than nonabused elders; (2) over half of the abused elders had a large bruise (>5 cm), which is much higher than the percent of nonabused elders from the previous study with a large bruise (7 %); and (3) abused older adults were more likely than nonabused elders to have bruises on the head, neck or torso [19]. Participants included 67 adults aged 65 and older who were reported to APS for suspected physical abuse. An expert panel was used to confirm that the participants in the study were physically abused. A total of 155 bruises were documented on the bodies of participants and the measures used were similar to those in the previous bruising study.

In addition to bruises, medical and criminal justice practitioners are often called upon to determine when a pressure ulcer is a forensic marker of neglect, especially in long-term care settings. Scientific evidence is needed to assist practitioners in making these determinations. In a study supported by NIJ, investigators explored the question of whether full-thickness pressure ulcers developed in long-term care patients who were receiving high quality care. The investigators had cooperation from 63 top-performing skilled nursing facilities in three large urban areas, yet there were only 24 elderly residents who were confirmed to have received excellent or very good care and developed full-thickness pressure ulcers that began at the facility. Based on examination of the 24 pressure ulcers, Liao et al. [11] determined that a single full-thickness pressure ulcer can occur under conditions of excellent care. Although limited by a very small sample size, it is worth noting that multiple full-thickness pressure ulcers were not found on any participating patients receiving high quality care.

Another NIJ-funded forensic marker project is underway that will compare 100–120 adults aged 65 or older who are reported to APS as victims of physical abuse to a matched sample of nonabused older adults to document a broader spectrum of injuries, including but not limited to bruising and pressure ulcers, seen in physical elder abuse cases and will identify which forensic markers of physical abuse are most associated with prosecution.

Multiple challenges have impeded the progress of research on forensic markers of elder abuse. First, most of this research is focused on elder physical abuse, which is one of the least common types of elder mistreatment. Therefore, recruitment of participants in these types of studies has been extremely slow and many studies do not end up recruiting the number of participants that they had originally intended. Another challenge is access to residential care facilities for this type of research. Typically, only the facilities that provide the highest quality care have allowed investigators to conduct research in their facilities. Unfortunately, but understandably, in facilities where there is the greatest chance of finding elders who are suffering from abuse and neglect, there is resistance to participation in research. At NIJ, research on forensic markers of neglect has been limited to a single study of pressure ulcers. There is a need for research that looks at other forensic markers of elder neglect, such as malnutrition, dehydration, and environmental markers (e.g., living conditions).

31.5.3 Elder Abuse Evaluation Research

Over the past decade, NIJ has repeatedly solicited for rigorous research to test the effectiveness of elder abuse preventive interventions. Although NIJ has funded over 30 research projects related to elder abuse, neglect, and financial exploitation during this time period, only two involved intervention research. And, none of the 30+ funded projects has tested the effectiveness of a preventive intervention. In both of the NIJ-supported intervention evaluation studies, the research was designed to determine the effectiveness of an intervention model—elder abuse multidisciplinary teams—for addressing the needs of victims of elder abuse. By design, these are challenging cases where elder abuse has already been identified. No rigorous research has been done to determine the effectiveness of a program designed to prevent elder abuse either in the general population of elders (universal or primary prevention) or among an at-risk population of elders (selected or secondary prevention).

Despite the proliferation of elder abuse multidisciplinary teams, there has been little research evaluating the effectiveness of this approach on case outcomes. NIJ has funded two elder Forensic Center evaluations, one of which is still ongoing. The completed evaluation of the Los Angeles Forensic Center (FC) examined outcomes related to prosecution of financial elder abuse cases and protection of vulnerable older adults. Using propensity score matching, the researchers compared outcomes of two groups: those who received the usual APS care *plus* assistance from the FC and those who received only the usual APS care. They found that significantly more cases reviewed by the FC were submitted to the District Attorney's Office (22.0 %) compared with APS-only cases (3.0 %) and that significantly more FC cases were referred to the Office of the Public Guardian (30.6 %) compared with APS-only cases (5.9 %) [6, 16]. The second evaluation study is an ongoing randomized-control trial of a new Forensic Collaborative in Denver.

NIJ funded a team of scientists, which included some of the evaluators from the original Los Angeles FC study, to examine the cost-effectiveness of the model [17]. Using a quasi-experimental design, the researchers compared the estimated average costs of pursuing a case at the FC with the estimated average costs of a case in the usual care APS system. They found that cases heard by the FC took on longer average (just over 10 h) than usual care APS cases (just under 4 h). Factoring in staff and team member costs of \$674.25 and a facility cost of \$306.77 per case, the mean FC case processing cost was significantly higher than the mean case processing cost for usual care APS cases (\$1408.58 vs. \$153.30).

When the FC model is adopted, the investigators estimated the average additional cost per case submitted to the district attorney's office with criminal charges filed to be \$7346. Additional costs for successful prosecution (\$8731.40), referral to the Public Guardian (\$4485.97), and referral to the Public Guardian resulting in conservatorship (\$6691.93) were also estimated. The FC may be considered cost effective if society is willing to pay these additional costs per case, which is a value judgment, rather than a scientific question.

One major impediment to conducting intervention research in elder abuse is the limited theoretical work available in the field. Good preventive interventions rely on a solid understanding of why elder abuse occurs. More research on the typologies of offenders and situations that lead to elder mistreatment would be beneficial in the development of preventive interventions. In addition, conducting high quality outcome evaluations of interventions is a very expensive endeavor. One of the primary challenges that has prevented NIJ from funding many evaluation research projects is that the cost of doing them likely would exceed the total budget that NIJ allocates to elder abuse research per year. Even if the research could be done for the approximately $1 million that NIJ spends on elder abuse research each year, investigators are hesitant to submit proposals for the full amount of funding available because they expect the funds to be split over 2 or 3 projects each year.

31.5.4 Research on Tool Development for Practitioners

The development of tools to assist practitioners in identifying and assessing elder mistreatment has been a long-term goal of NIJ's elder mistreatment research agenda. NIJ-funded researchers have developed and tested actuarial risk assessment tools for use in APS settings, measurement instruments for financial and psychological exploitation, and a tool to assist medical examiners in deciding whether to take jurisdiction in suspicious elder death cases. More recently, NIJ has invested in research to: (1) develop and test screening tools for medical practitioners in Emergency Departments and 9-1-1 emergency service responders; and (2) develop a set of financial decision-making screening and assessment measures for criminal justice professionals and noncriminal justice professionals to aid in detecting and prosecuting financial exploitation of older adults.

One example of NIJ's early efforts in this area was the development of the Older Adult Financial Exploitation Measure (OAFEM; [5]) and the Older Adult Psychological Abuse Measure (OAPAM; [4]). Both measures were developed using a concept mapping method that organizes input from a variety of stakeholders in order to conceptualize the construct of interest—in this case elder financial and psychological abuse. Data was then collected from 227 substantiated elder abuse clients and psychometric analyses were conducted using item-response theory and traditional analyses to test for validity. Both the OAFEM and the OAPAM demonstrated high internal consistency, item reliability, and overall measure validity. The full 79-item OAFEM measure, along with a shortened 30-item version, has been validated and used in numerous research projects and by APS agencies in Illinois. The 31-item OAPAM is also available in an 18-item short form, but has not been adopted as widely as has the OAFEM.

The OAFEM and OAPAM are both part of the assessment protocol used by six APS agencies that were part of a recently completed pilot study of the Elder Abuse Decision Support System (EADSS; [3]). This pilot study compared reporting and assessment for the 948 elder abuse cases assessed using the EADSS to the pretest year results from the 1634 cases assessed using the standard APS protocol. The EADSS resulted in higher substantiation rates (60.2 %) compared with the standard protocol used by APS (46.6 %). The higher substantiation rate is likely due to APS clients getting the full assessment for all types of abuse under the EADSS regardless of the type of abuse that initiated the referral to APS.

An actuarial risk assessment instrument was another tool developed and tested for APS [9]. Although actuarial risk assessment had not been used previously in APS, child protection agencies use actuarial risk assessment instruments to prioritize clients for intervention. The tool was developed by collecting retrospective data from 763 APS clients and classifying them based on their likelihood of subsequent maltreatment within a year of the initial APS investigation. Then the tool was then tested prospectively with 1064 clients to determine the ability of the instrument to predict future mistreatment. The self-neglect index of the risk assessment accurately classified individuals by the likelihood of future self-harm. The risk of abuse/neglect distinguished low-risk individuals from those at higher risk, but did not distinguish well between high- and moderate-risk individuals.

The primary challenges for tool development research are related to adoption of new tools once they are validated. In every NIJ tool development study, the researchers worked closely with the practitioners in developing the tools to try to ensure that the tools would be used. One project involved the development and testing of an Elder Suspicious Death Field Screen (ESDFS) for medical examiners to use in helping them to decide when to take jurisdiction to investigate the suspicious death of an elderly individual [15]. The investigators were not even able to validate the tool because adoption was so poor in the pilot study. The investigators changed the scope of the project to try to get a better understanding of why coroner and medical examiners did not cooperate at two of the three sites involved in the pilot study. They concluded that CME offices lacked resources to cope with the investigation of elder suspicious deaths. Interviews with reluctant CMEs revealed that: (1) investigators had heavy workloads, so they tend to release cases from their jurisdiction if there was a likely natural cause of death; (2) the ESDFS was not well integrated with the automated system that was being used by their office; and (3) there was a lack of buy-in about the utility of the study to their work or society as a whole.

Similarly, the EADSS roll out in Illinois was plagued by technological problems and general lack of enthusiasm for using the new system among APS front line staff. And the actuarial risk assessment in New Hampshire was viewed with skepticism by APS front line staff, who indicated that the assessments had not changed practice during the study period. For the ESDFS, the EADSS, and the actuarial risk assessment the fidelity with which the instruments and/or systems were implemented varied greatly by APS agency or CME office. The resistance to instrument adoption by the elder abuse practice community clearly indicates a need for more implementation research and a greater emphasis on researcher–practitioner partnerships in the field.

31.5.5 Research on Financial Exploitation

In the early years of NIJ's involvement in elder abuse research, financial exploitation was considered to be a lower priority than other areas of research. In part, NIJ staff was under the impression that other institutions were funding research on elder financial fraud and would therefore be covering elder financial exploitation. Some research on elder financial fraud and capacity to make financial decisions has been funded by organizations such as the FINRA Investor Education Foundation and by the National Endowment for Financial Education (NEFE), but these organizations typically do not fund research on elder financial exploitation as it has been defined within the elder abuse community (e.g., [5]).

An additional impetus for NIJ's growing interest in financial exploitation was the groundbreaking research conducted by Jackson and Hafemeister [7]. This NIJ-funded study explored a statewide database of all substantiated cases of elder abuse over a 2-year period (N = 2142) to determine the differences between cases where an elderly person was the victim of financial exploitation, and those where he or she was the victim of both financial exploitation and neglect or physical abuse, a combination referred to as hybrid financial exploitation. They found that the 472 victims of financial exploitation alone had a very different set of risk factors than the 162 victims of hybrid financial exploitation. Victims of financial exploitation only tended to be more independent, less likely to be experiencing dementia or confusion, and have abusers who did not feel overburdened in providing support to the elder. Of particular note, victims of hybrid financial exploitation were 81 % more likely to experience hybrid exploitation when the abuser did not provide financial support to the victim, but the victim did provide financial support to the perpetrator. This study paved the way for additional NIJ-funded research on financial exploitation because it highlighted the link between financial exploitation and other forms of abuse.

Another NIJ-funded study is underway that will build on Jackson and Hafemeister's work to identify victim, perpetrator, and community-level and sociocultural risk factors for elder financial exploitation. Data for this study will come from in-depth investigation reports for 878 substantiated cases of elder financial exploitation in adults 65 years of age and older between 2004 and 2012. Data from the Texas APS Client Assessment and Risk Evaluation (CARE) tool will provide systematic and reliable data regarding the victim's social, mental health, physical, environmental, and financial conditions. Latent profile analysis will be used to identify distinct types of elder financial exploitation based on unique combinations and patterns of the ascertained risk factors. Another ongoing project is exploring a range of cognitive risk factors for elder abuse, such as executive functioning, memory, math calculation, and numeracy.

31.5.6 Research on Elder Abuse in Residential Care Facilities

Research on the extent of elder abuse in residential care facilities is extremely limited primarily because of the difficulty in accessing residents who live in long-term care facilities. One NIJ-funded study used surveys of administrators and direct case workers of 1500 randomly sampled assisted living facilities across the U.S. [2]. One-year prevalence rates were calculated for a number of indicators of resident abuse. The highest rates were for items in the verbal (e.g., humiliating remarks, 20.3 %) and psychological abuse (e.g., critical remarks, 16.3 %) categories. Generally, physical abuse, material exploitation, and medication abuse items were less common. Sexual abuse items were the least common. Low staffing levels, having residents with dementia or physical limitations, and having an administrator with a shorter tenure and lower education level were factors associated with higher rates of abuse.

Practitioners and researchers are increasingly recognizing resident-to-Resident Elder Mistreatment (R-REM) as a common source of abuse in residential care facilities and trying to develop institutional policies to address high rates of R-REM. The foundational research on R-REM was funded jointly by the National Institute on Aging and NIJ. Lachs and colleagues used a variety of reporting mechanisms to document the prevalence of resident-on-resident abuse in ten nursing homes. Although direct service staff reported an average of 4.3 resident-on-resident abuse incidents over a two week period, none were documented in formal incident or accident reports, indicating a need for better documentation [10].

There are a number of challenges associated with doing research on elder mistreatment in long-term care facilities, some of which have already been mentioned. The most obvious challenge is the bias associated with gaining access to conduct research, which typically leaves out the residents of facilities where care is likely to be of low quality. Another major obstacle for researchers is working through thorny human subjects' protection concerns, particularly related to privacy of health care records and appropriate and acceptable methods to include participants who may not have the physical or cognitive capacity to participate in standard research protocols. One potential way to ensure that all residents are included in research is to use administrative records. For example, all nursing homes are required to monitor and report on a wide array of patient conditions for their Medicare and Medicaid patients in the Minimum Data Set (MDS) component of the Resident Assessment Instrument. Data collected in the MDS include information regarding patient activities of daily living, mood and behavior, psychosocial well-being, disease diagnoses and health conditions. While such data are not collected for research purposes, they may nevertheless contain useful information that could be used to better understand risks and consequences of abuse among elderly residents of nursing homes.

31.6 Additional Research Activities

In addition to the investment in extramural research on elder mistreatment, NIJ has devoted resources to identifying key research gaps and to disseminating research findings to the field. In February 2008, NIJ brought together approximately 70 researchers, practitioners, and funders for a three-day elder abuse workshop to present ongoing and completed research projects and to identify short and long-term research goals.[8] In 2011–2012, NIJ also hosted a webinar expert chat series to highlight findings from emerging research studies.[9] More recently, NIJ has been emphasizing the development and testing of elder abuse theory. To that end, Jackson and Hafemeister [8] wrote an NIJ research brief titled *Understanding Elder Abuse: New Directions for Developing Theories of Elder Abuse Occurring in Domestic Settings*, which served as a starting point for a subsequent meeting focused on elder abuse theory.[10] The goals of the meeting were to: (1) underscore why it is important to conduct research that is guided by theory; (2) gain insight into barriers to the use of theory in elder abuse research; (3) discuss how to better integrate theory into research designs and proposals; and (4) explore mechanisms to encourage investigators to use theory when developing research proposals and designs.

31.7 Future Research Directions

Despite incremental progress in elder abuse research over the past decade, there remains a dearth of knowledge about many aspects of elder abuse. Particularly noteworthy is the lack of evaluation research on prevention and intervention efforts. DOJ intends to support pilot testing of interventions derived from models that have been demonstrated to be effective in related fields (e.g., child maltreatment, violence against women, falls prevention). Numerous other research gaps remain priorities for NIJ, including:

- the development of a taxonomy of elder abuse case outcomes that can be used to define success from multiple perspectives (taking into consideration victim preferences, physical and emotional well-being and autonomy, as well as criminal justice outcomes);
- research that tests proposed theories of elder mistreatment or research that proposes and tests new theories of elder mistreatment;
- longitudinal research on risk and protective factors and outcomes associated with elder mistreatment that considers a wide range of outcomes of abuse, including physical health, mental health, future victimization and contact with the justice system and that examines the links between financial abuse and other forms of abuse within individual victims over time;
- research identifying forensic markers of elder mistreatment such as fractures, pressure sores, dehydration, and signs of mediation abuse, in addition to a more expansive range of forensic markers to include behavioral, environmental, and financial indicators of elder abuse, neglect and exploitation;
- research to develop and test tools to assist law enforcement, APS, court personnel, and financial and medical professionals in identifying and investigating cases of elder abuse, including implementation research to understand how the tools are used and barriers to their use for various practitioner communities.

31.8 Department of Justice Programmatic and Policy Efforts

31.8.1 Establishing Priorities

On March 23, 2010, President Obama signed into law the Elder Justice Act (EJA or "the Act"), as part of the health care reform bill known as the Patient Protection and Affordable Care Act. The EJA provided for a wide array of federal activity to support organizations and programs that address elder maltreatment such as Adult Protective

[8]A meeting summary is available at https://www.ncjrs.gov/pdffiles1/nij/242211.pdf.

[9]All of the webinars are available by searching for "elder abuse" at http://www.innovations.harvard.edu.

[10]A meeting summary is available at http://nij.gov/topics/crime/elder-abuse/Documents/elder-mistreatment-theory-meeting-summary.pdf.

Services, Long Term Care Ombudsman Programs, and elder abuse forensic centers. One key component of the Act was the creation of the Elder Justice Coordinating Council (EJCC or "the Council"). The EJCC is chaired by the Secretary for Health and Human Services (HHS) and is responsible for making recommendations on the coordination of activities of federal, state, local and private agencies and entities relating to elder abuse, neglect, and financial exploitation.

In order to help inform the EJCC's considerations, DOJ, with support from the Department of Health and Human Services, launched the Elder Justice Roadmap project. This multiyear project solicited input from stakeholders and subject matter experts from a diverse array of disciplines, fields, and settings on what was needed in order "to understand, prevent, identify or respond to elder abuse, neglect or exploitation". As part of the information gathering process, the Roadmap organizers solicited the views of 750 stakeholders from around the country, convened facilitated discussions with experts, conducted leadership interviews with high level public officials and thought leaders, and compiled an extensive bibliography of resources. From that process, the Roadmap generated a wealth of information and recommendations for governmental and nongovernmental entities to consider when developing their efforts to address elder abuse. To help Roadmap users to prioritize those efforts, the Roadmap identified a) top five priorities that affected virtually all efforts to understand and reduce elder abuse, b) "first wave action items", that subject matter experts identified as foundational priorities, and then c) "high priorities" within four domains: direct services, education, policy, and research.

In developing the Roadmap, five priorities emerged as paramount in advancing our understanding of elder abuse and promoting the health, independence, and justice for elders. First, it is critical to raise public awareness of elder abuse as a multifaceted problem that required a holistic, coordinated response in direct services, education, policy and research. Second, it is critical to conduct research and to enhance focus on the cognitive capacity and mental health of both elder abuse victims and perpetrators. Third, better support and training are needed for the millions of paid and unpaid caregivers to play a critical role in preventing elder abuse. Fourth, it is important to quantify the costs of elder abuse to victims, their families, and society at large. Lastly, the Roadmap identified the need for the strategic investment of resources in direct services, education, and research. Many of the most pressing priorities within those domains were identified and discussed in the Roadmap.[11]

[11]The Elder Justice Roadmap and accompanying materials can be found at http://www.ncea.aoa.gov/Library/Gov_Report/index.aspx.

The EJCC considered many of the Roadmap recommendations, as well as the input of additional stakeholders and subject matter experts. Based on the information gathered, the EJCC made eight recommendations on how the federal government, as opposed to state, local, or private entities, could improve responses to elder abuse, as well as to improve awareness and prevention efforts. Those recommendations are as follows:

Recommendation 1: Support the Investigation and Prosecution of Elder Abuse Cases Support the investigation and prosecution of elder abuse, neglect, and financial exploitation cases by providing training and resources to federal, state, and local investigators and prosecutors.

Recommendation 2: Enhance Services to Elder Abuse Victims Support and protect elder abuse victims by improving identification of elder abuse and enhancing response and outreach to victims.

Recommendation 3: Develop a National Adult Protective Services System Develop a national APS system based upon standardized data collection and a core set of service provision standards and best practices.

Recommendation 4: Develop a Federal Elder Justice Research Agenda Establish a coordinated research agenda across federal agencies to identify best practices for prevention of and intervention in elder abuse and elder financial exploitation.

Recommendation 5: Develop a Broad-Based Public Awareness Campaign Develop a comprehensive, strategic, and broad-based national public awareness campaign, with clear and consistent messaging to raise awareness and understanding of elder abuse, neglect, and exploitation.

Recommendation 6: Cross-disciplinary Training on Elder Abuse Develop training to educate stakeholders across multiple sectors and disciplines on preventing, detecting, intervening in, and responding to elder abuse, neglect, and exploitation.

Recommendation 7: Combat Elder Financial Exploitation, including Abuse by Fiduciaries Prevent, detect, and respond to elder financial exploitation through federal enforcement activities, policy initiatives, coordination, oversight and education, and by collaborating with industry to enhance fraud detection and provide resources for victims.

Recommendation 8: Improve Screening for Dementia and Cognitive Capacity, Financial Capacity, and Financial Exploitation Improve the ability of APS and first responders to screen for diminished capacity, diminished financial capacity, and vulnerability to or victimization of financial exploitation.

In addition to the elder abuse research and data collection efforts described above, DOJ has a number of ongoing projects and efforts that are relevant to the EJCC's recommendations. Below, we discuss DOJ's efforts to raise public awareness and to develop training for responders to elder maltreatment.

31.8.2 Developing Training and Raising Public Awareness

Over the past decade, DOJ has invested in developing training and resources for a wide array of responders to elder abuse, including prosecutors, law enforcement, and civil legal aid attorneys.

Since 2006, the Office on Violence Against Women (OVW) has provided grant funding to over 60 communities through its Enhanced Training and Service to End Abuse in Later Life Program. Through this program, OVW has supported the development of national curricula for law enforcement, prosecutors, and courts to enhance their ability to recognize, address, investigate, and prosecute cases of elder abuse, neglect, and exploitation. To further enhance prosecution, DOJ established in 2013 the National Institute on Prosecuting Elder Abuse. This Institute puts on an intensive four day training that covers the essential elements of bringing an elder abuse or financial exploitation case, including working with older victims, capacity issues, how to work with medical and financial evidence, charging decisions, and coordinated community responses. Since 2013, DOJ has trained state and local prosecutors from 26 states and the District of Columbia. In order to ensure that every state has prosecutors trained to effectively prosecute elder abuse and financial exploitation, the Department has committed to enrolling and training prosecutors from the remaining 24 states by 2017.

Over the past decade, the Department has also supported the development of national curricula for criminal justice professional and others to enhance their ability to recognize, address, investigate, and prosecute cases of elder abuse, neglect and exploitation. Since that time, the Department has provided grant funding to 77 communities in 37 states and the District of Columbia to provide in-person training to over 8000 law enforcement officers on elder abuse and financial exploitation. Because not all law enforcement officers can attend these in-person training sessions, DOJ has committed to partnering with national law enforcement organizations such as the International Association of Chiefs of Police and the International Association of Directors of Law Enforcement Standards and Training to develop internet accessible training materials and resources that will be available to state and local law enforcement officers nationwide. Likewise, DOJ is collaborating with a wide array of federal agencies (including but not limited to the Federal Bureau of Investigation, the Drug Enforcement Agency, the Department of Veterans Affairs) to promote elder abuse and financial exploitation training for their agents.

In addition to supporting the training of law enforcement and prosecutors, DOJ has focused on enhancing the capacity of civil legal assistance programs to support victims of elder abuse. In 2014, DOJ's Office for Victims of Crime released online training modules on elder abuse for legal aid attorneys. This initial wave of training modules covered topics including: What Every Legal Services Attorney Needs to Know About Elder Abuse; Practical and Ethical Strategies; and Financial Exploitation. In January 2015, DOJ piloted a five-part webinar, developed in conjunction with the American Bar Association and the National Clearinghouse on Abuse in Later Life, for civil attorneys and legal advocates addressing the needs of older victims of domestic violence and sexual assault. Then in May 2015, DOJ hosted a Civil Legal Aid Research Workshop, including a panel that focused on innovative ways to address elder abuse and research needs to advance/support those efforts. Finally, in September 2015, OVC and the Elder Justice Initiative announced the creation of the Elder Justice AmeriCorps. This new grant program is designed to provide comprehensive legal assistance and support services to elder abuse victims while promoting pro bono capacity building in the field. The program will support approximately 60 full time AmeriCorps positions for 2 years.

31.9 Law Enforcement and Prosecutorial Efforts

In addition to its programmatic efforts, DOJ plays an active role in protecting elders through its investigative and law enforcement efforts. DOJ has brought and continues to bring both civil and criminal actions against both public and private entities that have targeted, harmed, or defrauded elders.

First, DOJ brings civil actions against nursing homes and other long-term care providers that provide grossly substandard care to Medicare and Medicaid beneficiaries. DOJ brings many of these cases under the False Claims Act, 31 U.S.C. § 3729–3733, and alleges that these providers billed the Medicare and Medicaid programs notwithstanding having failed to provide the essential services and care to which the beneficiaries were entitled. For example, in 2014, DOJ reached a civil settlement with the Extendicare nursing home chain. The settlement resolved allegations that between 2007 and 2013, certain Extendicare facilities billed Medicare and Medicaid for materially substandard nursing services. DOJ further alleged that Extendicare failed to have a sufficient number of skilled nurses to adequately care for its residents, failed to follow appropriate protocols to prevent pressure ulcers or falls, and failed to provide sufficient catheter care to certain of its residents.[12]

In addition to bringing False Claims Act civil actions, DOJ has criminally prosecuted nursing home providers for providing grossly substandard care to Medicare and Medicaid beneficiaries and then billing the government for services. In 2012, for example, DOJ successfully prosecuted a nursing home operator for billing the Medicare and Medicaid programs for "worthless services" provided to residents at three nursing homes. In that case, the court found that "a long-term pattern and practice of conditions at defendant's nursing homes that were so poor, including food shortages bordering on starvation, leaking roofs, virtually no nursing or housekeeping supplies, poor sanitary conditions, major staff shortages, and safety concerns, that, in essence, any services that defendant actually provided were of no value to the residents". The court further found that there was a "long-term pattern and practice of conditions at defendant's nursing homes that were so poor, including food shortages bordering on starvation, leaking roofs, virtually no nursing or housekeeping supplies, poor sanitary conditions, major staff shortages, and safety concerns, that, in essence, any services that defendant actually provided were of no value to the residents". Lastly, the court found that "defendant was well aware that ongoing jeopardy conditions existed at the nursing homes during this time. Rather than make a good faith effort to remedy the glaring issues impacting the residents' health and welfare, the evidence shows that defendant chose instead to divert significant nursing home funds for his real estate development ventures and for other personal expenses and that defendant intentionally attempted to cover up and conceal from the surveyors the nursing homes' issues and his diversion of funds".[13] The defendant in that case was sentenced to serve 20 years for health care fraud and tax fraud and ordered to pay over $32.9 million.

In order to ensure that the nursing home providers cure the deficiencies and problems that led to the civil or criminal action, providers frequently enter into monitoring agreements, known as "Corporate Integrity Agreements" (CIAs) with the Department of Health and Human Services Office of Inspector General. Pursuant to these CIAs, providers agree to certain obligations in exchange for HHS OIG not seeking their exclusion from participation in federal healthcare programs, including Medicare and Medicaid. While CIAs vary, most contain certain elements including a requirement to hire a compliance officer, to develop written standards and policies, and to retain an independent review organization to conduct annual reviews. These CIAs are publicly available and can be found at http://oig.hhs.gov/compliance/corporate-integrity-agreements.

While ensuring that Medicare and Medicaid beneficiaries receive the care to which they are entitled, DOJ has also pursued actions against pharmaceutical manufacturers and long-term care pharmacies that have targeted those same beneficiaries. Notably, DOJ investigated and reached global resolutions with several pharmaceutical manufacturers for having inappropriately marketed their atypical antipsychotic drugs for dementia, including Alzheimer's dementia, uses that the Food and Drug Administration (FDA) had not approved as safe and effective. For example, in 2009, Eli Lilly pled guilty and paid a $1.45 billion fine in connection with its promotion of Zyprexa. In its criminal information, DOJ alleged, among other things, that Eli Lilly had expended significant resources promoting Zyprexa in nursing homes and assisted living facilities and sought to convince doctors to prescribe Zyprexa to treat disorders such as dementia or Alzheimer's dementia, neither use which had been approved by the FDA.

Second, DOJ's Civil Rights Division also plays an active role protecting elders. The Special Litigation Section, for example, enforces the Civil Rights of Institutionalized Persons Act, 42 U.S.C. § 1997 (CRIPA) and protects residents of publicly owned or operated residential facilities, such a long-term care facilities. The Special Litigation Section investigates alleged CRIPA violations and monitors implementation of remedial measures designed to eliminate conditions that might lead to abuse, neglect, undue restraint or inadequate care. At the same time, the Civil Rights Division enforces the Americans with Disabilities Act, which requires that persons with disabilities are not needlessly segregate in institutions and instead, receive services in the most integrated setting appropriate to their needs. To that end, the Civil Rights Division works with state and local governments, disability rights groups, and other federal agencies, to end the unnecessary segregation of persons with disabilities in institutional residential settings.

Third, DOJ's Criminal Division has aggressively pursued financial schemes targeting or disproportionately affecting elders, including cases involving lottery scams, fraudulent investor schemes, and identity thefts. Likewise, DOJ has prosecuted the service providers who facilitated those schemes. In 2012, for example, DOJ prosecuted MoneyGram and 25 of its agents for fraud and money laundering related to consumer fraud schemes involving the elderly. The Company admitted to aiding and abetting fraud and forfeited $100 million. Those funds are being used to compensate victims. To date, DOJ has returned $66 million to 22,000 victims.

[12]See http://www.justice.gov/opa/pr/extendicare-health-services-inc-agrees-pay-38-million-settle-false-claims-act-allegations.

[13]See https://www.fbi.gov/atlanta/press-releases/2012/former-nursing-home-operator-sentenced-to-prison-for-20-years-for-health-care-fraud-and-tax-fraud.

31.10 Other DOJ Elder Abuse Related Resources

In addition to its research, training, and law enforcement efforts, DOJ has invested in developing resources and tools for elder abuse victims and their families, as well as front line responders to elder maltreatment. We highlight two such resources below.

First, in September 2014, DOJ launched the Elder Justice Website (www.justice.gov/elderjustice). This website is designed to complement existing federal resources, like the National Center on Elder Abuse, and serves as a resource for state and local prosecutors, victims and their families, researchers, and other responders. For prosecutors, the Elder Justice Website identifies relevant state laws and provides sample materials and pleadings. For elder abuse researchers and academics, the website provides a search tool specifically designed to help identify relevant articles and scientific literature pertaining to elder abuse, neglect and exploitation. For victims and their families, the website provides a wealth of information, including an interactive map which allows users to identify potential additional resources and assistance by zip code. Lastly, the website contains a repository of training and informational videos on elder maltreatment and financial exploitation.

Lastly, in November 2014, the Bureau of Justice Assistance in conjunction with the American Bar Association, released its Pocket Guide for Law Enforcement on Legal Issues Related to Elder Abuse (https://www.bja.gov/Publications/ABA-ElderAbuseGuide.pdf). This guide provides explanations of relevant legal concepts, documents and tools to assist law enforcement to identify potential elder abuse or financial exploitation. The Pocket Guide provides information on a wide spectrum of topics including types of elder abuse, risk factors, and considerations for community corrections officers.

31.11 Conclusion

Over the past decade, with the passage of the Elder Justice Act and the creation of the Elder Justice Coordinating Council, there have been a number of promising developments in efforts to combat, prevent and understand elder abuse. The DOJ, through its research, programmatic and law enforcement efforts, has contributed to those developments through the programs and projects described above. There remains, however, much work to be done and DOJ will continue its efforts to prevent and combat all forms of elder abuse, neglect and financial exploitation.

References

1. Acierno R, Hernandez MA, Amstadter AB, Resnick HS, Steve K, Muzzy W, Kilpatrick DG. Prevalence and correlates of emotional, physical, sexual, and financial abuse and potential neglect in the United States: the national elder mistreatment study. Am J Public Health. 2010;100(2):292.
2. Castle N, Beach S. Elder abuse in assisted living. J Appl Gerontol. 2013;32(2):248–67.
3. Conrad KJ. Elder abuse computerized decision support system. Final report to the National Institute of Justice, grant #2011-IJ-CX-0014, NCJ #249185. 2015.
4. Conrad KJ, Iris M, Ridings JW, Langley K, Anetzberger GJ. Self-report measure of psychological abuse of older adults. Gerontol. 2011;51(3):354–66.
5. Conrad KJ, Iris M, Ridings JW, Langley K, Wilber KH. Self-report measure of financial exploitation of older adults. Gerontol. 2010;50(6):758–73.
6. Gassoumis ZD, Navarro AE, Wilber KH. Protecting victims of elder financial exploitation: the role of an Elder Abuse Forensic Center in referring victims for conservatorship. Aging Ment Health. 2015;19:790–8.
7. Jackson SL, Hafemeister TL. Risk factors associated with elder abuse: the importance of differentiating by type of elder maltreatment. Violence Vict. 2011;26(6):738–57.
8. Jackson SL, Hafemeister TL. Understanding elder abuse: new directions for developing theories of elder abuse occurring in domestic settings. Research in Brief, National Institute of Justice. 2013.
9. Johnson K, Park K, Bogie A, Flasch S, Cotter J. Developing an actuarial risk assessment to inform decisions made by adult protective services workers. Final report to the National Institute of Justice, grant #2008-IJ-CX-0025, NCJ #240410. 2012.
10. Lachs M, Teresi JA, Ramirez M. Documentation of resident to resident elder mistreatment in residential care facilities. Final report to the National Institute of Justice, grant #2009-IJ-CX-0001, NCJ #246429. 2014.
11. Liao S, Baker M, Lowe J, Austin R, Whitney JD, Wiglesworth A, Mosqueda L. Multi-site study to characterize pressure ulcers in long-term care under best practices. Final report to the National Institute of Justice, grant #2006-IJ-CX-0029, NCJ #231614. 2010.
12. Mallik-Kane K, Zweig JM. What is elder abuse? A taxonomy for collecting criminal justice research and statistical data. Washington, DC: Bureau of Justice Statistics; 2015.
13. Morgan RE, Mason BJ. Crimes against the elderly, 2003–2013. Washington, DC: Bureau of Justice Statistics; 2014.
14. Mosqueda L, Burnight K, Liao S. The life cycle of bruises in older adults. J Am Geriatr Soc. 2005;53(8):1339–43.
15. Mosqueda L, Wiglesworth A. Coroner investigations of suspicious elder deaths. Final report to the National Institute of Justice, grant #2008-MU-MU-0021, NCJ #239923. 2012.

16. Navarro AE, Gassoumis ZD, Wilber KH. Holding abusers accountable: an elder abuse forensic center increases criminal prosecution of financial exploitation. The Gerontologist. 2013;53 (2):303–12.
17. Nichol MB, Wilber KH, Wu J, Gassoumis ZD. Evaluating the cost effectiveness of the elder abuse forensic center model. Grant #2011-IJ-CX-0015, NCJ #248556. 2014.
18. Wallace RB, Bonnie RJ, editors. Elder mistreatment: abuse, neglect, and exploitation in an aging America. Washington, DC: National Academies Press; 2003.
19. Wiglesworth A, Austin R, Corona M, Schneider D, Liao S, Gibbs L, Mosqueda L. Bruising as a marker of physical elder abuse. J Am Geriatr Soc. 2009;57(7):1191–6.
20. Wolfe DA. Elder abuse intervention: lessons from child abuse and domestic violence initiatives. In: Wallace RB, Bonnie RJ, editors. Elder mistreatment: abuse, neglect, and exploitation in an aging America. Washington, DC: National Academies Press; 2003.

32 Centers for Disease Control and Prevention: An Overview of Elder Abuse Prevention Initiatives

Jeffrey E. Hall

32.1 Elder Abuse as a Public Health Problem

A growing number of segments in society now acknowledge Elder Abuse (EA) as a problem with consequences for the public's health. EA is a public health problem because it affects the lives of an untold number of older adults, families, and communities each day in the United States. Its impacts span multiple levels of the social ecology and affect numerous facets of health (see Fig. 32.1 for the diagram of these impacts by ecological level). At the individual level, victims suffer injuries that can compromise physical functioning, exacerbate existing health conditions, or create stresses that increase risks for an array of illnesses, diseases, dysfunctions, and even death [1–7]. The experience of elder abuse can severely damage an older adult's self-esteem, deepen or cause depression, and induce symptoms indicative of Post-Traumatic Stress Syndrome [8–14].

At the relationship level, elder abuse limits older adults' potentials for involvement in meaningful social interactions that are essential for healthy aging [15, 16]. Perpetrators of abuse may restrict an older adult's movements and constrain their contacts [17–20]. They may even prevent an older adult from participating in activities such as informal socialization or past times that are key components of one's social identity. In some cases an older adult may choose to disengage from relationships or to remove themselves from certain social contexts. In such cases social isolation may be self-imposed due to concern about the social stigma of being identified and publically labeled as a victim of elder abuse or to a loss of a personal sense of safety and of trust in others [21–23]. In either situation, the loss of critical social connections and positions in social networks limits access to resources that are critical to maintaining one's well-being.

At the community and societal levels, EA creates environments which do not allow certain members to make contributions (thus depriving those communities of their particular benefits). The presence of EA can limit or remove access to older adults who are vital repositories of insights and lessons learned over a lifetime, deny opportunities to benefit from their perspectives, expertise, and presence, and compromise how and to what extent culture and social support are transmitted between generations. Moreover, EA has consequences that may challenge, confound, and tax the various health systems utilized by older adults who have experienced victimization [24–26]. Through these impacts EA constrains the possibilities for sustainability and growth that are available locally and nationally.

32.2 Approaching Elder Abuse: The Role of Public Health?

EA is a matter of significant concern to the Centers for Disease Control and Prevention (CDC) as a federal public health agency because of the aforementioned implications for individual and population health. While this may make sense to most, for many, describing public health's specific role in addressing EA would be quite a difficult task. In public arenas, EA is predominantly considered a concern or domain of other sectors such as criminal justice. It is intuitive that law enforcement, for example, has a direct role in stopping abuse and in dealing with its perpetrators. It may also be easily accepted that organizations such as Adult Protective Services Agencies, Long-term Care Ombudsmen, and other social service agencies can be called upon to act and intervene in cases where elder abuse has occurred or is suspected.

The reasons for the previously described difficulty are numerous. First, few persons in the public sphere are fully

J.E. Hall (✉)
Division of Violence Prevention, Centers for Disease Control and Prevention, 4770 Buford Highway NE–Mailstop K77, Atlanta, GA 30341, USA
e-mail: jhall2@cdc.gov

X. Dong (ed.), *Elder Abuse*, DOI 10.1007/978-3-319-47504-2_32

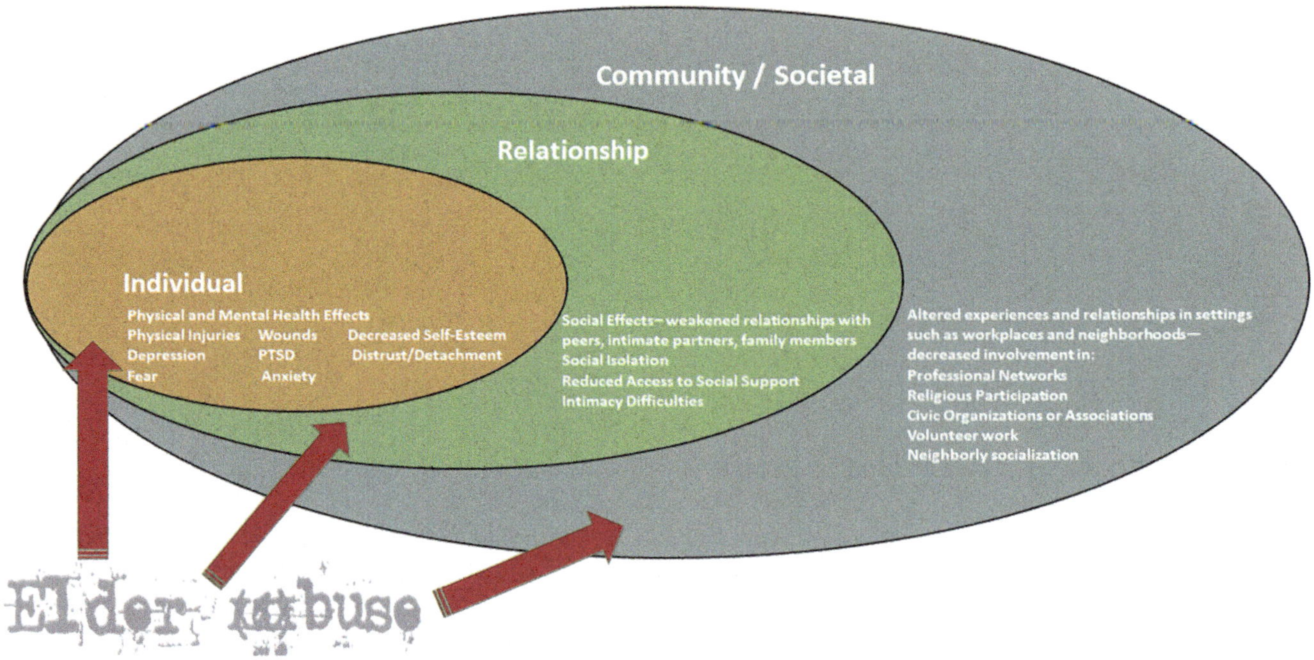

Fig. 32.1 Effects of elder abuse across the levels of the social ecology

aware of the existence of public health, of what it entails, or of how its agents act to protect and strengthen society. The relatively low awareness of public health and the functions of this sector is partly attributable to the inconspicuous way in which much public health service occurs. Generally, most persons in the U.S. general population only become aware of the existence and importance of public health and the kinds or roles played by public health servants when our society is faced with an emergent public health crisis. This happens most often when the prevalence of a given condition, typically an infectious or communicable disease, increases to levels outside of those normally expected. In the face of such occurrences the populace becomes acutely aware of the work of public health and a small selection of the extensive public health infrastructure of the nation is catapulted into the spotlight. It is rare that similar increases in awareness are stimulated explicitly by public health leadership to address conditions with overwhelmingly social in origin such as aggression, abuse, and violence.

Second, the evolution of infrastructures capable of supporting work to prevent, stop, and limit the consequences of EA perpetration within public health as a sector has been slow. Public health work originated from a largely biomedically oriented, infectious disease centered model for acting to reduce and eliminate threats to the public's health. This model and its associated approaches gradually expanded and changed to accommodate chronic disease patterns that became more prevalent with successes in reducing the impacts of infectious disease. However, concerted efforts to apply public health expertise to assist in addressing violence, neglect, and exploitation have only been embraced in earnest within the last 35 years. Public health infrastructure with the competence, capacity, and capabilities to plan, implement, and evaluate actions required to prevent and stop such problems have been developed in only a relatively small number of places. Consequently, public health-originated initiatives to address problems such as violence are rare in comparison with those created to address infectious and chronic diseases.

32.3 The Centers for Disease Control and Prevention: Addressing Violence as a Public Health Problem

CDC is considered the lead among of several public health service agencies responsible for protecting the United States from health threats. In this role, CDC is tasked with the provision of expertise and assistance in responding to Federal, State, local, and private organizations on matters and activities related to disease and injury prevention and control [27, 28]. This includes ensuring that the many state and local public health systems forming the national public health system are nurtured and shaped to grow progressively more adept and efficient in addressing public health threats such as EA and other forms of violence.

CDC pioneered the works of using public health approaches, insights, and tools to address violence and associated phenomena as significant sources of injuries, injury-related morbidity, and mortality subsequent to injury during the early 1980s (see U.S. DHHS and U.S.D.O.

J. 1986 for more specifics on Violence and Public Health [29]; see Dahlberg and Mercy [30] for a more extensive history of CDC's work on violence as a public health issue). Throughout 1980s and subsequent decades, CDC, under the leadership of staff such as Dr. James A. Mercy, successfully demonstrated that incidents of violence could be effectively examined and understood using epidemiologic methods. Moreover, CDC's leaders developed and began sharing a public health rooted framework for community action to prevent violence (see National Center for Injury Prevention and Control, 1993) [31], and initiated efforts to evaluate common approaches to violence prevention to determine what interventions and programs worked (i.e., demonstrated impacts in reducing aggressive and violent behavior), why they worked, and how their effects were achieved. These actions and achievements increased uptake and use of public health based approaches to violence prevention. They also paved the way for organizational expansions that would gradually yet steadily increase CDC's own violence prevention capacities and capabilities.

In 1993, the CDC established the Division of Violence Prevention (DVP) within its National Center for Injury Prevention and Control (NCIPC). The creation of this division transitioned CDC into an operational space where, for the first time in U.S. history, an operational component of a public health agency would be officially and permanently tasked with providing leadership in developing and implementing a national program to prevent and control violence-related injuries and deaths. DVP's initial prevention efforts continued and elaborated early work to prevent and reduce homicides and suicides among children and youth. However, the division's programmatic scope and foci eventually expanded to formally address forms of violence such as Intimate Partner Violence (IPV) and Sexual Violence (SV). CDC first formally turned its attention to the problem of EA during the late 1990s under the leadership of Dr. Rodney Hammond, who served as the director of DVP from 1996 to 2011. It was at this point that the agency's initiatives to address EA began.

32.4 Select Previously Implemented Elder Abuse Focused Initiatives

32.4.1 Funding Research Describing the Impact of State Laws and Regulations on Elder Abuse Investigations

The CDC's first EA focused initiative involved a joint venture between CDC's Division of Violence Prevention and CDC's Public Health Law Program (PHLP). A focus on public health laws, defined as any laws having important consequences for the health of defined populations [32] such as older adults, was a natural starting point for CDC's EA related work. Laws help shape public health and influence the health status of entire populations by dictating the missions pursued by public health agencies, specifying and authorizing functions expected of such agencies, and allowing funds to be allocated for specific uses in promoting, protecting, and preserving health [32]. Aspects of governmental and public bodies such as constitutions, charters, statutes, legislation, rules, regulations, and policies together determine and delimit the legal powers and duties of government officials and representatives when addressing threats to population health such as EA.

Leaders in DVP and PHLP reasoned that an improved understanding of how such legal constructs influence efforts to address EA could accelerate the development of policy-level interventions that operate more effectively. Accordingly, they funded applied research describing the impact of laws on state reported EA via a grant awarded to Gerald Jogerst, Jeanette Daily, and other scholars at the University of Iowa (Grant#: R06/CCR718677-02). The provided funds supported an important line of research that systematically and scientifically established how investigations of EA were influenced by the content and characteristics of each state's governing EA legislation, statutes, and other legal constructs. Such legal constructs were shown to directly structure how public health problems such as EA are socially constructed, categorized and responded to, as well as to dictate the specific groups that can and must take formal action to address them.

The scores of findings produced by Jogerst et al. provide important insights about how EA has been formally responded to at the state level in the United States. It is not surprising that most insights pertained to the extensive diversity in and variation across the laws enacted and the implications of this diversity for how potential EA cases are identified, formally classified, and dealt with. Because states are able to devise their own structures, processes, and systems for responding to EA their legislation, statutes, and mandates may assume many different manifestations and display an array of characteristics. Unfortunately, these differences make it difficult to distinguish the portion of the variation in the amount EA reported, investigated, and substantiated across states that is real from the portion that is caused by definitional differences [33, 34]. State by state differences in who is considered "elderly", the specific behaviors considered indicative of EA, and the number of EA subtypes acknowledged and designated formally addressable, as well as differences in the circumstances that must be operative and the types of relationships that must exist between involved persons, influence conclusions about how much EA exists, the nature of abusive experiences, and the characteristics associated with perpetration and victimization. They also determine the specific actions that may be taken to address EA and the conditions under which interventions by specific actors and agencies are authorized and mandated.

At a system level, the research by Jogerst et al. [33, 34]. suggested that nationwide improvements in efforts to address EA might be achieved through standardizing the content of state laws related to domestic elder abuse, the processes through which EA is documented, and the measures through which accountability for action are sought. EA was more likely to have been formally determined to have occurred or be occurring in states whose laws, statutes, regulations, etc., contained more comprehensive, extensive, and detailed descriptions for EA and its various subtypes. This characteristic is thought to provide more information to assist workers in making decisions about whether observed or reported behaviors or experiences truly constitute abuse as it is legally defined in a given state. Standardization of documentation would ensure that appropriate comparisons could be made across states by ensuring that data regarding EA are presenting using comparable units of analysis and measurement, and that reported data elements capture information about the same phenomena. Lastly, implementation of accountability measures such as tracking EA reports and monitoring actions taken in response to reports may increase transparency. This in turn, may promote improvements in the delivery of services by the various stakeholders that are formally responsible for recognizing, reporting, and responding to the needs of older adults.

32.4.2 Developing a Comprehensive Agenda for Public Health Activities in the Area of Elder Abuse

CDC's initial policy focused research efforts were followed with additional actions to more strategically and systematically address EA as a public health problem. The agency's next initiative was an outgrowth of work associated with the 2001 National Policy Summit on Elder Abuse [35]. Within this summit, CDC was charged with formally recognizing EA as a public health problem.

While the experience of EA had be accepted as a social problem and its health impacts long described, EA had not been officially proclaimed a threat to public health by CDC in the manner done for other conditions affecting the older adult population. It was believed that recognition of EA formally as a public health problem by the CDC would elevate the profile of EA. This recognition would confer EA with a degree of status that might increase the attention and resources desperately needed to address EA more systematically and on a greater scale. Formal recognition of EA as a public health problem would also enable public health expertise and structures to be formally leveraged to enhance the efforts of the sectors who have historically and most directly been tasked with identifying and delivering services to those who have experienced EA.

CDC not only formally acknowledged EA as a public health problem, but also moved to more firmly establish a basis from which public health based work to address EA could be launched. This was done by engaging experts and professionals most familiar with the contexts, components, and challenges that define and accompany work to prevent and stop EA. In 2002 CDC convened a panel of experts from a wide variety of backgrounds and operational settings with the goal of developing strategic recommendations for public health work to prevent EA. These recommendations would provide a "blueprint" for the agency's EA focused efforts that continues to guide CDC's investments and actions over a decade later. A high-level listing of the first five recommendations for each domain of this agenda is presented in Fig. 32.2.

A thorough description of the expert panel and the processes through which the panel carried out its charge are provided in Ingram (2003) [36]. However, it is important to provide a brief consideration of the nature of the developed EA recommendations here. The recommendations focused squarely on critical areas of need that might benefit from the application of the public health based model of a scientific approach to violence prevention developed and refined during the 1980s and 1990s. They organized work on the identified areas to reflect the four elements of this public health approach which are depicted in Fig. 32.3.

This facilitated identification of actions needed to: (1) improve the collection and use of the kinds of population level data needed to establish, monitor, and alter EA trends; (2) extend knowledge regarding factors that could be modified to decrease the likelihood of EA perpetration and victimization; (3) discover the practices, programs, and policies as well as arrangements, relationships, and environments that can be used effectively prevent and stop EA; and (4) achieve widespread adoption and successful implementation of the practices, programs, and polices that actually work.

32.4.3 Developing Uniform Definitions and Recommended Core Data Elements for Use in Elder Abuse Surveillance

Consistent with the recommendations of the expert panel, the CDC's next area of investment focused improving the collection of data about the epidemiologic characteristics of EA. Data on the incidence and prevalence of EA, its

Surveillance	Etiology	Program Development/ Evaluation	Crosscutting Issues
• Develop a surveillance system, which will accurately capture both reported and unreported cases of elder mistreatment. • Develop uniform definitions for reporting elder mistreatment. • Develop and promote the use of a common terminology within the area of elder mistreatment. • Examine the issue of measurement as it relates to elder mistreatment and seek to develop reliable and valid measurement instruments. • Develop validated screening programs to identify victims, potential victims, perpetrators, and potential perpetrators.	• Chronicle and publish research that examines the pathways to various types of elder mistreatment. • Identify risk factors for the perpetration of elder mistreatment and increase research on etiologic factors. • Promote research in elder mistreatment that includes longitudinal studies. • Conduct an analysis of the issue of caregiver accountability. • Convene and publish consensus panels on areas such as self-neglect, definitions, reporting, and measurement issues.	• Encourage all programs to include an evaluation component in order to develop a knowledge base and to enable replication and dissemination. • Conduct evaluations and assessments of screening tools. • Conduct an intensive review of communities in terms of the availability and effectiveness of elder mistreatment programs. • Seek to develop programs that address the issue of the costs of elder abuse, neglect, and exploitation. • Develop programs for caregivers.	• Include self-neglect as a part of the public health agenda. • Build the workforce in the field of elder mistreatment. • Engage in an effort to raise public awareness about elder mistreatment. • Promote cultural diversity. • The CDC is encouraged to promote the development of education programs to teach new skills and enhance existing skills of elder agency workers on how to work with the aging population and how to enhance and create multidisciplinary teams.

Fig. 32.2 Select expert panel recommendations on elder abuse

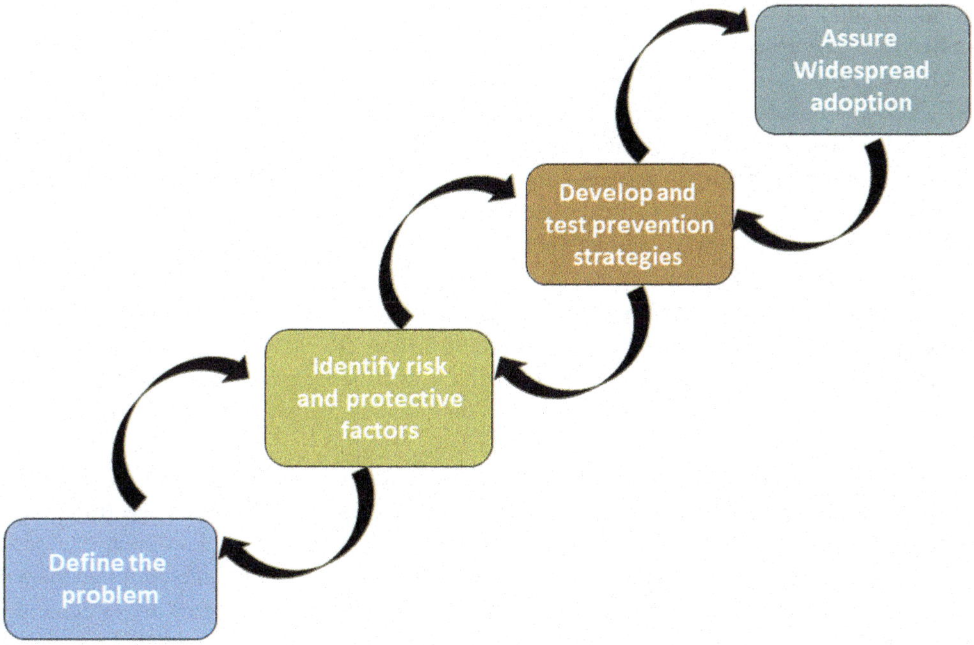

Fig. 32.3 Public health model of a scientific approach to prevention

distribution within and across population groups, and about trends in its occurrence over time were and continue to be sorely needed. Such data are accounted for and factored into decision-making regarding EA prevention and response. For example, public health surveillance[1] data can reveal patterns of occurrence suggesting relationships that should be the focus of etiologic research to clarify the determinants, correlates, and processes through which different factors create conditions that may increase or decrease the likelihood of EA. Data on individual victimization experiences when aggregated to the population level and studied over time might suggest characteristics, factors, and dynamics common to or differing across groups or settings that may reduce or increase risks for EA perpetration or victimization. These data could also shed light on how changes in such influences

[1]The term public health surveillance refers to: the ongoing and systematic collection, analysis, and interpretation of health-related data for use in setting priorities and making other decisions regarding prevention efforts.

over time may also affect experiences of EA as well as its magnitude. Such information drives decision-making regarding the types of actions and interventions that must be developed and implemented to successfully prevent and stop EA.

Accurate public health surveillance data on EA is also required to effectively raise awareness about its true burden and public health impacts. These data are the core of education and advocacy efforts designed to stimulate public movements and policy actions that can affect population level changes to eliminate EA. They are used by stakeholders to compellingly establish the urgency and importance of not just action but the right kinds of action to address EA. In the face of robust population level data on the size of EA and the span of its impacts, it becomes less possible to ignore the threat that EA poses to public health, construe it as the problem of a few individuals, or treat it as involving isolated incidents to be dealt with only on a case-by-case basis.

Lastly, data on EA collected using a public health surveillance framework also provide one indicator of how well prevention efforts are performing in keeping older adults healthy and safe at a population level. Higher level collections of surveillance data should be used in tandem with program specific evaluation data. The former can indicate whether short- or long-term changes in conditions and behaviors in target populations are noted after the implementation of strategies used to address EA (given the presence of data sufficient to allow change detection). The latter may provide answers about whether any observed changes can be plausibly attributed to the actions taken (after other non-strategy or program related factors are taken into account) and point to specific components that may be responsible for observed changes or that might be modified to achieve future changes. Both surveillance data showing evidence of change and evaluation data establishing how the changed was programmatically achieved are required to fully establish the overall effectiveness of actions to address EA.

Improvements to efforts to document EA and to collect data on EA within a public health surveillance framework were and are still needed in light of several problematic features of the EA prevention field. First, EA data are collected from multiple sources, multiple informants, and using multiple methods. Each sector with a role to play in addressing EA has its own approach to documenting and identifying EA. Each sector has its own process for determining what behaviors or experiences do or don't qualify as EA. Moreover, each sector uses specific jargon and terms to describe and communicate information about situations involving EA. These differences are, as previously stated, attributed to variations in the guidelines, regulations, policies, and legislation that dictate how and by whom EA is to be dealt with. Collectively these differences produce administrative data elements and data points that cannot be easily reconciled or harmonized. They also generate scores of records and documentation that often contain different pieces of information about the same persons and population. The noted divergences are important to attend to because they foil efforts to assemble, analyze, and employ all acquired data on experiences of EA to direct prevention and response activities.

It is important to discuss the array of informants from which EA data may be acquired because different parties offer different perspectives, knowledge, and areas of emphasis about the same behaviors, experiences, settings, and environments. Those with the most direct knowledge of behaviors and circumstances that may involve EA include those most proximal to problematic incidents or situations. They include persons who have experienced EA, alleged or established abusers/offenders/perpetrators, persons who may have witnessed actions, behaviors or incidents or their impacts, or those to whom possible and actual experiences of EA have been disclosed, reported, or otherwise revealed. Beyond this first layer of informants exist numerous other individuals, entities, and organizations with some knowledge of or data regarding incidents involving EA or where EA may be likely. These may include but not necessarily be limited to persons and units in supervisory or managerial positions who, while not directly involved in preventing or responding to EA on the "front lines" are responsible form compiling and releasing aggregate data about the occurrence and characteristics of EA. The kinds of information available to and that may be communicated by these different categories of informants is often very heterogeneous and thus extremely challenging to integrate for epidemiologic, programmatic, or evaluation purposes.

Finally, the data collection methods, materials, and approaches differ not only by sector but also according to how knowledge from various disciplines is applied in these sectors. Particular choices regarding the setting of data collection, the defining characteristics of the populations whose experiences are documented, the means through which data are obtained, and the pieces or units of information collected heavily influence how EA may be described and what conclusions might be drawn about its occurrence and consequences. Consequently, EA prevalence estimates, as just one example, based on administrative data collected in Adult Protective Services investigations may not be consistent with estimates derived using surveys. This has made conclusively determining the magnitude, scope, and nature of EA in the U.S. a goal impossible [37].

Wide variation in ideas about the nature and burden of EA is developmentally problematic. It is a source of uncertainty that has been described by some as having significantly delayed the maturation of efforts to prevent EA both nationally and locally. This uncertainty prevents the field from being properly "nourished" by causing those with the influence to authorize and/or appropriate resources to support EA prevention to hesitate to take action. The lack of widely accepted estimates of the size, severity, and degree of harm caused by EA creates challenges in assigning it an appropriate priority status, determining the precise funding amount that should be invested in agencies or initiatives that could reduce or prevent EA. This deficiency also makes it difficult to determine the specific period during which authorizations for appropriations must be active to ensure that this public health problem will be given resources sufficient to maintain as well as secure its resolution. Furthermore, without epidemiologic data to convincingly and consistently describe the nature of the threat faced, its gravity, and whether or not it is increasing, stakeholders seeking adequate support for EA prevention and response efforts are distinctly disadvantaged relative to groups who can do so for other epidemiologically well-established public health problems. Until data on EA are moved into a space that is more clear and cohesive the field of EA prevention and response will remain underdeveloped. Most importantly, an untold number of older adults will continue to suffer victimization experiences that could be halted or experience initial victimizations that may have been prevented with adequate investment, attention, and systemic action.

At the core of the described variations, discrepancies, and data collection challenges lie basic differences in how EA is conceived, defined, and interpreted. Because definitions specify behaviors indicative of EA or characteristics that may indicate heightened risk for EA they are a natural starting point for work to improve the collection and use of EA data. The 2002 expert panel explicitly recommended that CDC develop uniform definitions for reporting EA, operationalize the behaviors that constitute EA, and develop a minimum or core set of data elements that use the produced definitions to facilitate reporting [36]. CDC was exceptionally well positioned to respond to this recommendation given the agency's historical, collaborative role in developing classification systems that allow health information to categorized and presented comparably regardless of the data's origins or providers. Furthermore, CDC's DVP had successfully developed uniform definitions and recommended data elements for IPV surveillance [38], SV surveillance [39], and was developing uniform definitions and data elements for CM [40], and Self-Directed Violence [41]. Experiences with such processes could inform the planning, structuring, and implementation of tasks supporting the development of definitions and data elements for use in EA surveillance.

In 2007 CDC initiated work to create, critically review, and ultimately release uniform definitions and data elements for use in collecting EA data within a public health surveillance framework [42]. This was done by first developing critical partnerships with federal and nonfederal organizations who have historically worked with older adults and within the Aging Services Network. Two partner organizations directly and substantively involved in work to create a strong foundation for definitional activities were the National Adult Protective Services Association (NAPSA) and the Office of Elder Rights of the U.S. Administration on Aging (AOA OER).

Staff from NAPSA and AOA's OER collaborated with CDC to identify and establish relationships with two diverse groups of experts and stakeholders who would provide insights, feedback, and firsthand guidance regarding the conceptual, methodological, and practical requirements for and considerations associated with particular ways of defining and capturing information about EA. The first of these groups would constitute a multisectoral technical expert panel that would contribute to a dynamic, collaborative process addressing issues and considerations effecting the usefulness and applicability of definitions and data elements and facilitate production of a first version of a recommendations document. The second group of experts included persons sought to provide individual, independent peer review of the draft uniform definitions and recommended data elements developed in collaboration with the technical expert panel. Involvements by both groups were deemed critical given the controversial and complex nature of the task, its potential implications for the numerous sectors that serve and protect the older adult population, and CDC's desire to produce products responsive to the unique needs of a wide variety of stakeholders.

Many meetings occurred over several years as the collaborative decided how to best define EA so that data could be collected more uniformly and identified core and supplementary data elements that would be most useful to the field. Each group of contributors diligently confronted the conceptual and operational complexities described in the initial paragraphs of this section and worked collaboratively across sectors to propose content that would take important new steps towards resolving the field's definitional and measurement-related problems. Full description of the processes through which the development of the definitions and data elements occurred is beyond the scope of this chapter (please see Hall et al. [42] for more specifics). However, a high-level process summary can be reasonably offered. In brief, the development process entailed:

1. Acquiring discretionary funding and establishing logistics contracts to support each project stage;

2. Determining the specific types of EA would be the focus of the definitions process;
3. Defining points where members of the expert panel could be convened to collaboratively create draft versions of the uniform definitions that would be associated with the EA types selected for focus;
4. Iteratively reviewing, discussing, and refining subsequent versions of the draft definitions developed;
5. Identifying terms or jargon in each definition requiring sub-definition—further elaboration and description in plain language to ensure common understanding;
6. Developing new or identifying viable existing definitions for terms requiring sub-definition;
7. Selecting a pool of candidate data elements that would be recommended for use in surveillance.
8. Categorizing the selected data elements as either Core Data Elements (units of data that should be collected or documented for every case/incident) or Supplementary Data Elements (additional data that can be collected to further describe cases/incidents if resources will allow this);
9. Researching and developing descriptive documentation for each recommended data element including a:
   (a) Description/Definition of the data element;
   (b) Description of its Uses;
   (c) Discussion of conceptual or operational issues;
   d) Specification of the Data Type(and maximum allowed Field Length);
   (e) Indication of when data element Repetition may be necessary to include all answers that may apply;
   (f) Field values/coding instructions that designate recommended coding specification and valid data entries; and
   (g) where applicable, reference to one or more Data Standards or Guidelines used to define the data element and its field values, and Other References considered in developing the data element.
10. Iteratively reviewing, discussing, and refining subsequent versions of the draft recommended data elements proposed;
11. Combining the products of the previous processes into a comprehensive, formatted document including background content, reference information, and other sections typically presented in CDC uniform definitions and recommended data elements documents.
12. Redistributing the first fully formatted draft document to each member of the expert panel for an additional round of review and critique;
13. Reviewing and integrating feedback from the each expert panel member to develop a version of the document that would be distributed for peer review;
14. Identifying and recruiting an extensive group of experts (18 total) to provide independent, external peer review of the developed definitions and recommended data elements;
15. Acquiring, considering, and addressing feedback and suggestions provided by each peer reviewer to develop a version of the uniform definitions and data elements document that would be entered into CDC's scientific clearance process;
16. Completing CDC's scientific clearance process;
17. and lastly, completing graphic design, layout development, editorial, and 508 compliance processes needed to produce the document finally disseminated publically.

The initial release of *Elder Abuse Surveillance*: *Uniform Definitions and Recommended Core Data Elements*, *Version 1.0* [42] produced by the aforementioned process was intended to serve as a starting point for advancing surveillance, research, and practice aimed at preventing EA. It is CDC's hope that the proposed Uniform Definitions will assist the field in (1) further describing and delineating the core constituent elements of EA; (2) improving the classification of its behavioral manifestations and its differentiation from other, similar phenomena; (3) clarifying and explaining the practical relevance of concepts, terms, or expressions that are often esoteric and abstract; and (4) making information and vocabulary regarding EA accessible to and actionable for the widest variety of stakeholders. Through such contributions, the current effort and any ensuing work will build upon and extend the achievements of earlier definitional efforts. In addition, if the recommended data elements can be tested, refined, and at some future point uniformly recorded, then better estimates of the incidence and prevalence of EA can be obtained and problems such as data incompatibility may be eliminated.

32.5 Select Currently Active Projects and Initiatives

32.5.1 Dissemination of Supplementary Data Elements for Use in Elder Abuse Surveillance

Elder Abuse Surveillance: *Uniform Definitions and Recommended Core Data Elements*, *Version 1.0*, the document described in the prior section, only presents content for core data elements recommended for use in EA surveillance. To reiterate, the elements included in this set represent the minimum amount of information needed to establish or evaluate priorities and strategies for EA prevention and intervention. The forthcoming document, *Elder Abuse Surveillance*: *Supplementary Data Elements* will present and suggest additional data that can be collected to further describe cases/incidents if resources will allow this. The identified supplementary data will extend the information collected using the proposed core data elements. The additional data that they may provide if collected will provide more details about victimization experiences, the characteristics of perpetrated behaviors, and the individual, relational, and contextual characteristics that may have influenced EA risks. The proposed secondary data elements will also provide a more clear idea of variables and information that is seen as important to collect as communicated by professionals working in the different sectors.

32.5.2 Linking State-Level Violent Death, Adult Protective Services, and Vital Statistics Data: CDC's Fatal Elder Maltreatment Surveillance Pilot Project

CDC continues work related to a collaborative pilot project that links National Violent Death Reporting System (NVDRS) data with state Adult Protective Services (APS) data to capture details of violent deaths due to EA. The project also links "natural" death vital statistics data for older adults to assist in understanding circumstances for violent death. The project was conceived to provide information about viable strategies for linking diverse datasets, to facilitate comparisons of the kinds and quality of APS data collected across funded states, and to allow identification and pursuit of new possibilities for research made feasible by the linkage of NVDRS, APS, and vital statistics data.

NVDRS is a population-based public health surveillance system that captures information on all homicides, suicides, legal intervention deaths, unintentional firearm deaths, and deaths of undetermined intent. At the time that this project was funded NVDRS was operational in 17 states (see Fig. 32.4). This system includes information on the victims, the suspected perpetrators and their relationships to the victims, the weapons involved, and the circumstances leading up to the injury event. The underlying data sources for NVDRS include death certificates, coroner and medical examiner reports, law enforcement records, and toxicology reports. Other optional data sources that may be collected within the system include Child Fatality Review Team data, Supplemental Homicide Reports, and hospital data. The NVDRS and the nature of its data collection processes have been fully described in further detail elsewhere [43, 44].

States involved in the pilot were selected based on the presence of a Violent Death Reporting System (VDRS) operating within CDC's national system, the existence of a centralized, statewide APS system, and the possession of access to vital statistics death certificate data for all persons 18 and older. States with regionalized systems were also considered if they had the ability to consolidate the data into a single set of summary variables. A final critical requirement for involvement in the pilot was possession of a formal agreement from each of the entities providing data to participate. States who ultimately provided linked data used in the project were Kentucky, North Carolina, and South Carolina.

After data linkage, these states submitted de-identified linked datasets to CDC. Examples of victim and incident level data elements obtained from NVDRS include demographic characteristics, the reported cause and manner of death (for decedents), the specific circumstances surrounding incidents involving injuries, the type of weapon or means used to inflict injuries, and descriptions of relationships of victims to suspects. APS related data provided in the submitted datasets included but were not limited to information regarding previous contacts with APS for fatal and nonfatal incidents, the nature and results of APS investigations, as well as any information regarding victims' use of referred services, living arrangements, financial status, mental and physical disabilities, and social history. In addition, at a final project evaluation report was also submitted the end of the pilot project performance period. The evaluation reports tendered included information such as descriptions of the data sources used to provide data on EA, explanations of implemented processes for accessing and linking data, characterizations of the completeness of the final dataset, details regarding any challenges or problems encountered during linkage activities, and descriptions of how such problems were resolved.

It is CDC's hope that the insights obtained from forthcoming analyses of the provided variables will inform efforts to prevent EA by increasing and deepening knowledge about the precursors of violent death and injury as a result of elder abuse. Moreover, it is the agency's hope that the process related information provided by the participating NVDRS states will provide valuable, instrumentally useful insights regarding the considerations that must be addressed when linking diverse forms of data that may contain different pieces of information about the experiences of persons who may have suffered EA, possible strategies for successfully contending with linkage related complications, and observations that help improve the design or implementation of future attempts at integrated data use.

32.5.3 Creation of a Protocol to Inform Development of an Ongoing, Population-Based Survey of Elder Abuse and Neglect in the United States

To establish and monitor changes and trends in the prevalence and incidence of elder abuse and evaluate the effectiveness of intervention strategies, data must be collected on

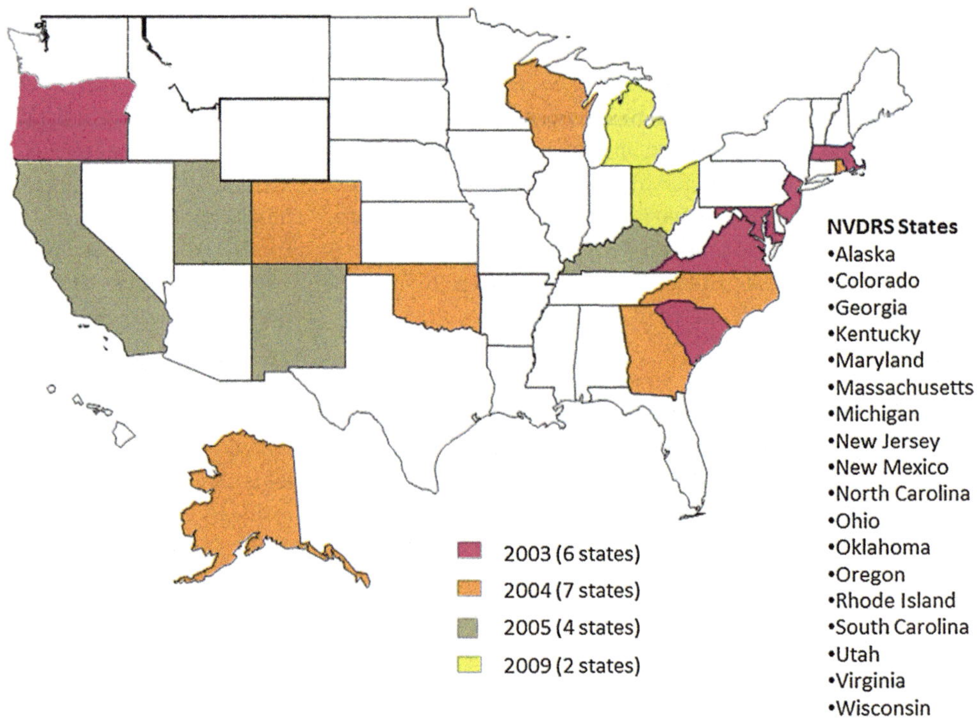

Fig. 32.4 Initial data collection year for NVDRS states operational in 2009

an ongoing basis. To do this efficiently and effectively, it is crucial that proven elder abuse data collection methods be identified, examined for strengths and weaknesses, and configured to create data collection strategies that can support continuous data collection. As a first step towards this larger goal, CDC supported work to develop a surveillance protocol to inform development of a robust ongoing, population-based survey of EA in the United States. CDC specifically worked with SciMetrika to complete essential foundational tasks to promote survey-based collection of data on elder abuse experiences. Examples of tasks completed in association with the project included:

1. completing a comprehensive, systematic literature review covering methodologies for collecting quantitative EA data (with a specific emphasis on literature related to survey research but including literature on additional complementary methodologies or research innovations);
2. produce a report summarizing information about instruments or measures that have been used to collect EA data (which should include summary information such as instrument purpose, description, application setting, length, psychometric properties, reference standards, information for use in contacting authors/developers);
3. defining content that could be considered for inclusion in an EA focused survey (e.g., indicators of various types of EA covered in the uniform definitions and core data elements recommended for use in EA surveillance) via consultations with individuals with expertise in collecting quantitative data on EA and intimate knowledge of methodological and practical considerations in collecting survey data from older adults;
4. identifying operational and sampling designs needed to assure that data collection processes are sufficiently sensitive and representative (at state and national levels and for various populations of older adults);
5. exploring if and how the current infrastructures of existing national surveys could be leveraged to add core content on EA or to host an EA survey module; and
6. production of a complete surveillance protocol containing all of the necessary specifications for implementation of a comprehensive surveillance effort specific to elder abuse and neglect.

The protocol being finalized and its accompanying series of supporting reports and resources will assist stakeholders in navigating the survey surveillance implementation process, provide comprehensive, evidence-based guidance to inform decision-making, and establish the requirements for carrying out such an endeavor, as well as the factors that may influence successful implementation and sustainability.

32.6 Select Collaborations with Other Federal Agencies

Diverse, strategic relationships and alliances are critical when attempting to deal with problems as complex and formidable as EA. To this end, many of the recommendations provided by the 2002 expert panel encouraged collaborations with other federal, state, and local entities, in pursuing the outlined agenda for protecting our nation's older adults against EA. CDC has worked closely with numerous federal agencies since the initiation of the agency's work to prevent EA and in specific compliance with these recommendations. The specific roles the agency has assumed in collaborative processes have alternated depending on the objectives of collaboration—varying beyond the convener, catalyst, and facilitator roles highlighted in this chapter's descriptions of CDC's own initiatives to include important supporting roles involving technical assistance provision, capacity development, and strategic partnership. Select examples of longstanding initiatives and contexts of collaboration are described below.

32.6.1 Elder Justice Interagency Work Group

The Elder Justice Interagency Working Group coordinates networking, cooperative, and collaborative interactions among federal officials responsible for carrying out elder justice activities, including elder abuse prevention, research, grant and program funding, and prosecution. Since 2001, members have met informally and on a regular basis to discuss emerging issues, promising practices, and ways to coordinate and align efforts. U.S. Department of Health and Human Services participants include the Administration for Community Living/Administration on Aging, the Centers for Disease Control and Prevention, the Indian Health Service, the Office of the Assistant Secretary for Planning and Evaluation, the Office on Disability, Office of Inspector General, the Office of Women's Health, and the National Institutes of Health/National Institute on Aging. U.S. Department of Justice participants include the Office of Justice Programs (including the National Institute of Justice, the Office for Victims of Crime, the Bureau of Justice Assistance, the Bureau of Justice Statistics, and the Violence Against Women Office), the Office of Legal Policy, and representatives from various offices of the Department's litigating divisions. The Consumer Financial Protection Bureau, Social Security Administration, United States Department of Housing And Urban Development, United States Department of The Treasury, United States Postal Inspection Service, and the United States Securities And Exchange Commission are also represented. CDC has worked with other work group members to: (1) develop and update documents describing "Federal Initiatives to Address Elder Abuse" for inclusion in the Elder Justice Coordinating Council Reports to Congress, (2) coordinate and sponsor federal activities for World Elder Abuse Awareness Day, and (3) identify possible areas and proposals for collaborative work in addressing provisions of the Elder Justice Act, including carrying out work to implement the eight recommendations from the Elder Justice Coordinating Council for Increased Federal Involvement in Addressing Elder Abuse, Neglect and Exploitation.

32.6.2 Assistance with the Development of Congressional Report on the Feasibility of Establishing a Uniform National Database on Elder Abuse

Staff from CDC, ACL/AOA, and NIH/NIA collaborated with staff from the Office of the Assistant Secretary for Planning and Evaluation (ASPE) in developing a report on the Feasibility of Establishing a Uniform National Database on Elder Abuse. The report describes sources of administrative data, limitations, and technical as well as resource related considerations that should be borne in mind if attempting to develop a uniform database of administrative data on elder abuse. If developed such a database could provide information on reported cases of elder abuse and used to evaluate intervention efforts and service outcomes on an iterative, ongoing basis. This report was submitted to Congress by ASPE in 2010.

32.6.3 National Adult Mistreatment Reporting System (NAMRS)

The NAMRS project was first funded in September 2013 by ACL/AOA at $1.2 million, which was received from the FY 13 Prevention and Public Health Fund (PPHF). It was initiated by ACL and ASPE, in light of the enduring need for consistent national data on adult mistreatment. Its goal is to design and pilot a national system for reporting data on adult mistreatment using data from state APS agency information systems that, while not capturing all forms of mistreatment, contain informative data and information that can help advance public awareness of and broader action to prevent and stop this most critical problem. The design of the NAMRS system has been informed by input from state agencies, as well as other stakeholders in the field of adult mistreatment including the Centers for Disease Control and Prevention and the Bureau of Justice Statistics of the Department of Justice. NAMRS not only includes data on the mistreatment of older adults but also on adults with disabilities as collected by APS agencies charged with protecting the well-being of these adults.

32.6.4 Elder Abuse Screening Related Initiatives

CDC has participated in a number of initiatives focused on the development, evaluation, implementation, and possible expanded use of EA screening tools. Two of these involved collaborations with Substance Abuse and Mental Health Services Administration (SAMHSA) and Centers for Medicare and Medicaid Services (CMS) respectively. CDC has worked in partnership with staff from the Substance Abuse and Mental Health Services Administration and ACL/AOA to provide content suggestions for the Health Risk Assessment (HRA) associated with the Affordable Care Act's (ACA) Annual Wellness Visit Benefit (AWV; authorized for Medicare beneficiaries under Section 4103). This was done to possibly seize the opportunity that the AWV provides to proactively prevent the onset of disease and disability during contacts with health care professionals to make efforts to identify, detect, and assess EA routine elements of clinical practice. The collaborative suggested, for possible inclusion in the HRA, a tool that assesses risk for elder abuse and neglect (along with supporting science), content to justify its inclusion, and important supporting implementation guidance. CDC has also worked with the Centers for Medicare and Medicaid Services, Office of Clinical Standards and Quality/Survey and Certification Group to develop an Elder Maltreatment and Care Symposium organized to explore the current state of elder maltreatment screening and elder care practices across Medicare and Medicaid beneficiary populations and care settings.

32.7 Summary and Statement of Next Steps

This chapter has provided an overview and history of a selection of CDC's public health based EA initiatives as well as information regarding the agency's participation in collaborations with other federal organizations and entities. A summary illustration of the items chronicled is presented in Fig. 32.5. CDC has worked collaboratively to make the case for the treatment of EA as a public health problem and for the use of public health approaches to help achieve its reduction and resolution. Despite lacking stable, dedicated funding to support EA initiatives, the agency has steadfastly worked with federal and nonfederal partners and stakeholders to seek surveillance, research, and policy advancements that enable older adults to live safer, healthier lives.

Admittedly, most of CDC's initiatives have sought improvements in the collection of EA data via the use of a public health surveillance framework. However, efforts implemented in this area have allowed CDC to infuse the field with insights that may someday allow all sectors to use data seamlessly in a fully integrated and interdependent fashion. The agency's next steps in relation to EA will continue to align with the agenda developed in 2002. CDC is currently taking steps to further extend its surveillance and data collection centered achievements, but it is also carefully and thoughtfully considering how it may assist the field in developing, evaluating, and implementing efforts to achieve primary prevention of EA. CDC has also included EA as an element of its strategic vision for preventing multiple forms of violence.

32.8 Extending Surveillance Achievements: Suggested Next Steps

CDC's data focused efforts have created new possibilities for unified work around EA data collection. Nevertheless, there remain a number of tasks that could not be sufficiently addressed in the highlighted initiatives, as they were beyond the scope of these efforts. These unaddressed tasks are considered key next steps that should be undertaken to help change the environments in our society to better protect us as we anticipate, enter, and occupy old age.

32.8.1 Research Strategies for Systems-Level Change in Policy and Practice

Research regarding the influences of laws and policies on the collection of EA data and on how EA cases are investigated must be complemented with additional health services and systems-level research. This additional research should focus on identifying opportunities, levers, and tactics for altering legal and administrative structures to respond to EA more consistently and uniformly. Processes that must be used to pursue change must be clearly defined, parties that must be engaged or involved to ensure the viability of change efforts must be identified, and the conditions and requirements that may enable or impede action must be itemized and appropriately taken into account. Moreover, this line of research should examine partnership, coalition-based, and movement centered strategies to support action on the scales needed to strengthen and align existing legal, administrative, or organizational structures or to, if warranted, achieve development of new more optimal structures. Future work could also seek strategies for adequately resourcing efforts to transition to new ways of operating to ensure that critical shifts occur without overtaxing stakeholders or disrupting the provision of services. In this case, examples of successful system-transitions should be identified and studied closely to glean insights on what works in leading infrastructural

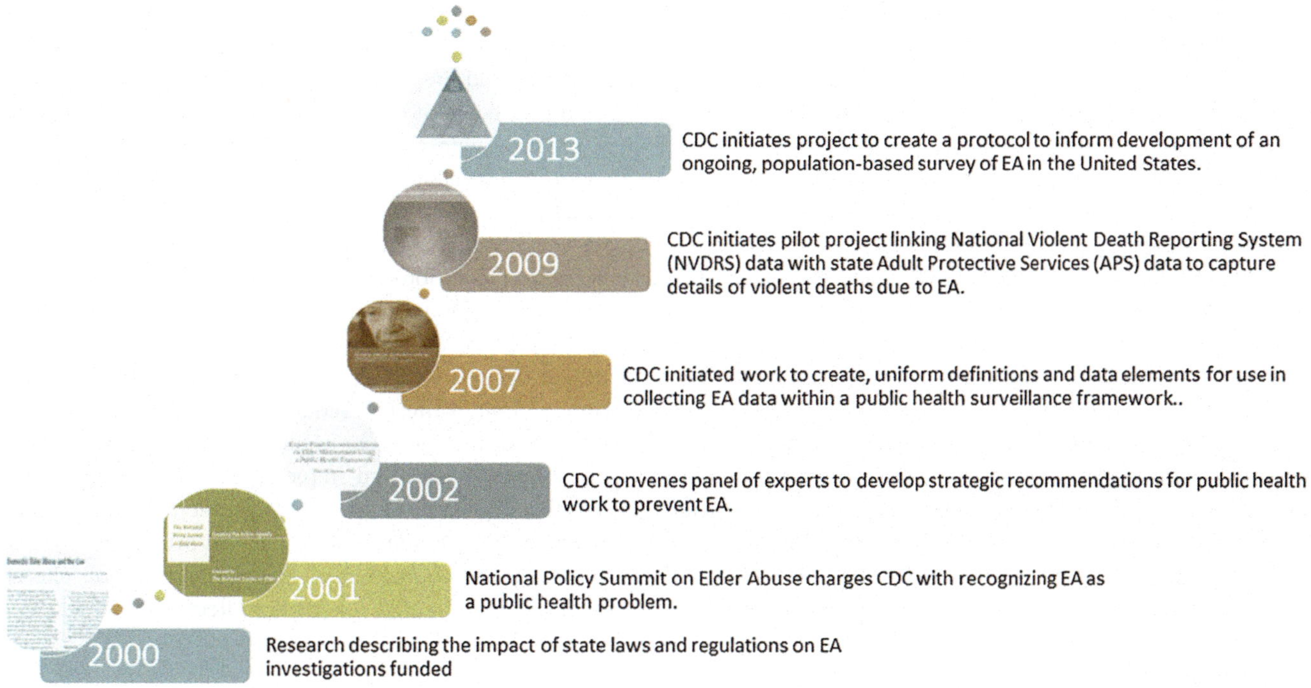

Fig. 32.5 A timeline of the centers for disease control and prevention's initiative's on elder abuse

change. Finally, information must be acquired about strategies for changing organizational culture to ensure that new ways of working are embraced and effectively implemented by professionals in every position—from those working on the frontline of service provision, to those in managerial or supervisory roles, as well as those in senior or executive level leadership positions. Insights from such research can help the field to formulate a tactical plan for restructuring programs and policies to more robustly and cohesively serve older adults.

32.8.2 Clarify Additional EA Subtypes and Distinguish Related Phenomena

The CDC's definition focused initiative did not attempt to clarify proposed EA subtypes beyond physical abuse, sexual abuse, emotional/psychological abuse, neglect, and financial abuse/exploitation. It also did not attempt to address phenomena that may have elements similar to EA or co-occur alongside EA among older adults. Examples of possible EA subtypes that could receive focused attention in subsequent definitional processes include, but could extend well beyond, abduction, abandonment, medical abuse, and abuse involving violations of fundamental freedoms and rights. These possible subtypes are difficult to frame definitively because there is considerable disagreement between those who argue that they should be lumped into other larger subtypes (e.g., medical abuse within physical abuse) and those who consider them distinct enough to warrant individual measurement and attention. Moreover, there is more variability in the definitional elements for these subtypes (e.g., what constitutes abduction, under what specific circumstances, by whom, for how long, across what distances or boundaries, whether consent must be absent and by whom—only the older adult or possibly relatives, caregivers, guardians, etc.).

Two examples of related phenomena deserving additional formal examination in a multisectoral context are Self-Neglect and Resident-to-Resident Aggression/Altercations/Mistreatment. Self-Neglect was not classified as a subtype of EA because it involves actions taken by individuals toward themselves (self-directed behaviors) versus actions inflicted by others (interpersonally oriented behaviors). Resident-to-Resident Aggression/Altercations/Mistreatment involves interpersonal violence similar to physical EA but is distinct in that it occurs between persons where there is no expectation of trust and at present appears to be exclusive to institutional settings.

Both sets of unaddressed behaviors and experiences require conceptual and operational clarification so that clear, informative data about them can be gathered and organized more systematically to inform actions to address them population wide.

32.8.3 Evaluate the Adequacy of the Developed Uniform Definitions

An additional important next step should involve pilot-testing the uniform definitions and data elements disseminated by CDC. Such testing could evaluate how the derived definitions perform when applied in different sectors and the feasibility of collecting the core data elements. Pilot-testing would capture the responses and reactions to the proposed definitions and data elements and document their experiences in attempting to use them. It could also indicate the types, combinations, and levels of resources and structural supports needed to support implementation on a broader scale. Such research could reveal important characteristics of the definitions and data elements, such as unique and shared strengths and weaknesses within and across possible end users by and between sectors. Pilot tests are essentially needed to determine what the definitions and data elements do or don't do well, for whom, and under what conditions.

The results of pilot-testing can be an impetus for additional multisectoral collaborations regarding ways to pursue definitional harmonization while supporting fulfillment of sector specific obligations. They should suggest categories of revisions that might be needed to increase the usefulness of the definitions either broadly or specifically. This information would advance consideration of the tradeoffs of gains and losses that may be required for harmonization to be realized. Pilot-testing is necessary step to establish the viability of the uniform definitions and data elements as well as the benefits of their acceptance and adoption.

32.8.4 Support Efforts to Achieve Primary Prevention of EA

Primary prevention, which at the simplest level entails efforts to modify the factors that influence risks for EA to prevent the onset of EA, is the next area of challenge and opportunity that must be mastered. It is in this domain that CDC hopes to partner within and outside of public health to make additional new advances that will substantially reduce the public health threat and burden of EA. Effective primary prevention of EA can create safer, brighter futures for older adults by making EA and its injuries problems of the past.

Foundational and ongoing research is needed to identify strategies, options, and alternatives for preventing EA from ever taking place. This research must acquire the contextual, experiential, and best research evidence required to distinguish promising and effective policies, programs, and practices that can be proactively used to prevent EA. It must also focus on (1) uncovering prevention options that reduce factors that increase risks for EA perpetration and victimization respectively (given that attributes of both perpetrator and persons at risk for victimization along with other social and environmental factors may influence whether EA occurs and it's character) and/or enhance factors that may protect against EA or make perpetration less likely; (2) rigorously evaluating policies, programs, and practices to establish how they work, the character of their effects (positive, negative, or some combination of both), the strength and duration of their effects, and the conditions, settings, and populations in which the effects are replicable; and (3) assessing the feasibility of expanding the use of any identified options to reach a greater proportion of the population without suffering reductions in effectiveness. The results of research on these aspects could be used to inform the adoption, uptake, and implementation of useful strategies, polices, programs, and practices, the enhancement and augmentation of existing options for the primary prevention of EA, or the development of new EA prevention alternatives that are configured for greater effect.

32.8.5 Connecting the Dots: Preventing Multiple Forms of Violence Experienced by Older Adults

CDC recently released a 5-year vision, *Preventing Multiple Forms of Violence: A Strategic Vision for Connecting the Dots* [45], which outlines its areas of strategic focus. This vision will help us understand, respond to, and ultimately prevent violence across the lifespan, including in older adulthood. The centerpiece of our strategic vision is that the different forms of violence are interconnected and often share the same root causes. Understanding the overlapping causes of violence and the things that can protect people and communities can help us better prevent violence in all its forms.

With regard to EA, a specific component of the effort to "connect the dots" should develop more detailed "maps" of the intersections between EA and other forms of violence. This could include violence types that may be more likely to be experienced during older adulthood, that may have been experienced earlier in life but that create or increase susceptibility to EA victimization, or that have "grown old"—first experienced before victims became older adults and that continue to be experienced into old age. Many forms of violence that overlap with EA may be experienced by younger populations. However, victimization may have more significance for health and overall well-being as one grows older because of age-related reductions in capacities for physical healing (i.e., in comparison with younger adults, older adults may be less able heal from injuries sustained, may experience longer recovery periods, and may be more likely to expire when injured), chronic diseases and other health conditions that could be severely aggravated by victimization become more prevalent, and social and economic resources to support recuperation or repositioning following victimization may less available (due to life transitions and events such as retirement and social network contractions due to the deaths of family members and friends).

It is important to determine whether and how experiences with one form of violence can affect the likelihood of experiencing others. Research could continue to explore how EA is connected to IPV, SV, and assaults by strangers as well as its relationship to violence associated with specific settings, such as Resident-to-Resident Aggression. Moreover, more extensive examinations of significance, nature, and directions of relationships among EA and self-directed behaviors such as self-harm, self-neglect, and suicide are needed to clarify whether (1) EA increases risks for self-directed behaviors, (2) experiences with, characteristics of, or factors associated with self-directed behaviors increase risks for EA, and/or (3) these phenomena should be considered co-occurring problems. Quantitative data regarding the associations amongst such forms of violence would extend insights about such overlaps in violent experiences acquired through case studies and other qualitative approaches. Data of this type could help to establish the population level prevalence of exposures to multiple forms of violence among older adults. They would also clarify the extent and kinds of needs that may require preventive and therapeutic attention among this population.

Further examination of polyvictimization in later life within frameworks such as those developed by the National Committee for the Prevention of Elder Abuse (NCPEA) is also critical. Polyvictimization in later life:

> …occurs when a person aged 60 or older is harmed through multiple co-occurring or sequential types of elder abuse by one or more perpetrators, or when an older adult experiences one type of abuse perpetrated by multiple others with whom the older adult has a personal, professional, or are recipient relationship in which there is a societal expectation of trust [46].

Beyond clarifying the ways that different types of EA may co-occur, the types of common combinations, and possible experience sequences, research on polyvictimization could examine the dynamics of relationships between EA perpetrators and victims. Studies in this domain could establish how interactions of perpetrator and victim characteristics within specific environments and relationship contexts shape patterns, histories, and trajectories of perpetration and victimization respectively and conjointly. Their results could provide more new, more specific and actionable information about risk processes and how they influence EA perpetration and victimization over time. Such information could, in turn, stimulate development of efforts that are simultaneously sufficiently comprehensive and most precisely configured to address the complexities of preventing and stopping EA.

Most importantly, scientists and practitioners should continue to partner in identifying, characterizing, and considering (1) the risk and protective factors that EA shares with other forms of violence, (2) shared risk and protective factors among the different sub-types of EA, (3) strategies known to reduce other forms of violence that may be fruitfully used to reduce EA, and (4) models illustrating how existing effective or promising strategies can be adapted to achieve crosscutting effects. Strategies to address EA that seek change in shared, modifiable risk and protective factors and that address parallel risk processes and pathways may yield wider gains in reducing the occurrence of many different forms of violence experienced by older adults throughout life. They may also reveal better options for preventing or addressing the accumulation of effects across different types and contexts of violent experiences and exposures. However, before such strategies can be implemented, much more must be learned about the kinds and degrees of etiologic commonality that may be present and about the factors and processes that must be addressed to achieve crosscutting impacts. Similarly, the benefits of exploring whether policies, programs, and practices established as promising or effective in preventing other forms of violence are considerable. Yet an even greater amount of research is required to identify proven options for prevention that are conceptually, developmentally, and practically suitable for use with older adults and in addressing the subtleties of EA. Lastly, it is highly likely that policies, programs, and practices ultimately considered viable candidates for new application in the context of EA will require adaptation. Implementation and usage studies will be necessary to determine what modifications will be needed to best fit the new use of identified candidate options, whether these changes can be carried out without compromising their core components (i.e., the critical features of the options that are deemed responsible for observed or expected changes), and whether the value of the use of these options extends appreciably beyond that of options for prevention or intervention developed specifically to address EA.

32.9 Conclusion

Elder Abuse (EA) is a problem of public health importance because of its impacts on the health and well-being of older adults throughout the U.S. population. The Centers for Disease Control and Prevention (CDC) has worked for over 15 years to safeguard older adults against this threat by helping to improve understanding of the nature, scope, and character of EA, as well as how its features and expressions may change over time. The CDC has also sought to create initiatives, relationships, infrastructures, systems, environments, etc., capable of preventing EA in all of its forms. While the agency's history has been chronicled in this chapter, the CDC's future where this crucial prevention work is concerned has yet to be written. We will continue to act more directly and meaningfully in concert with existing and new partners to use data to tell the stories of those who have suffered EA, to determine the strategies, policies, programs, and practices that can be used to stop and prevent EA, and to effectively spread word about and ensure adoption of what works in addressing this problem.

Disclaimer The findings and conclusions in this report are those of the author(s) and do not necessarily represent the official position of the Centers for Disease Control and Prevention/the Agency for Toxic Substances and Disease Registry.

References

1. Anetzberger G. The clinical management of elder abuse. New York: Hawthorne Press; 2004.
2. Lachs MS, Williams CS, O'Brien S, Pillemer KA, Charlson ME. The mortality of elder mistreatment. Jama J Am Med Assoc. 1998;280(5):428–32.
3. Lindbloom EJ, Brandt J, Hough LD, Meadows SE. Elder mistreatment in the nursing home: a systematic review. J Am Med Dir Assoc. 2007;8(9):610–6.
4. Dong XQ. Medical implications of elder abuse and neglect. Clin Geriatr Med. 2005;21(2):293–313.
5. Dong XQ, Simon M, de Leon CM, et al. Elder self-neglect and abuse and mortality risk in a community-dwelling population. Jama-J Am Med Assoc. 2009;302(5):517–26.
6. Baker MW, LaCroix AZ, Wu C, Cochrane BB, Wallace R, Woods NF. Mortality risk associated with physical and verbal abuse in women aged 50 to 79. J Am Geriatr Soc. 2009;57 (10):1799–809.
7. Schofield MJ, Powers JR, Loxton D. Mortality and disability outcomes of self-reported elder abuse: a 12-year prospective investigation. J Am Geriatr Soc. 2013;61(5):679–85.
8. Comijs HC, Penninx B, Knipscheer KPM, van Tilburg W. Psychological distress in victims of elder mistreatment: the effects of social support and coping. J Gerontol Ser B Psychol Sci Soc Sci. 1999;54(4):P240–5.
9. Pillemer K, Prescott D. Psychological effects of elder abuse: a research note. J Elder Abuse Neglect 1989;1:65–74.
10. Dyer CB, Pavlik VN, Murphy KP, Hyman DJ. The high prevalence of depression and dementia in elder abuse or neglect. J Am Geriatr Soc. 2000;48(2):205–8.
11. Begle AM, Strachan M, Cisler JM, Amstadter AB, Hernandez M, Acierno R. Elder mistreatment and emotional symptoms among older adults in a largely rural population: the South Carolina elder mistreatment study. J Interpers Violence. 2011;26(11):2321–32.
12. Cisler JM, Begle AM, Amstadter AB, Acierno R. Mistreatment and self-reported emotional symptoms: results from the National Elder Mistreatment Study. J Elder Abuse Negl. 2012;24(3):216–30.
13. Fulmer T, Rodgers RF, Pelger A. Verbal mistreatment of the elderly. J Elder Abuse Negl. 2014;26(4):351–64.
14. Dong X, Chen R, Chang ES, Simon M. Elder abuse and psychological well-being: a systematic review and implications for research and policy—a mini review. Gerontology. 2013;59 (2):132–42.
15. Spencer C. Exploring the social and economic costs of abuse in later life. Vancouver: University, Vancouver, B.C. for Health Canada, Family Violence Prevention Unit; 1999.
16. Luo Y, Waite L. Mistreatment and psychological well-being among older adults: exploring the role of psychosocial resources and deficits. J Gerontol Ser B Psychol Sci Soc Sci. 2011;66 (2):217–29.
17. Paris BEC. Violence against elderly people. Mt Sinai J Med. 1996;63(2):97–100.
18. Sijuwade PO. Cross-cultural perspectives on elder abuse as a family dilemma. Soc Behav Personal. 1995;23(3):247–51.
19. Tam S, Neysmith S. Disrespect and isolation: Elder abuse in Chinese communities. Can J Aging Revue Canadienne Du Vieillissement. 2006;25(2):141–51.
20. Von Heydrich L, Schiamberg LB, Chee G. Social-relational risk factors for predicting elder physical abuse: an ecological bi-focal model. Int J Aging Hum Dev. 2012;75(1):71–94.
21. Lantz MS. Elder abuse and neglect: help starts with recognizing the problem. Clin Geriatr. 2006;14(9):10–3.
22. Wang JJ, Lin MF, Tseng HF, Chang WY. Caregiver factors contributing to psychological elder abuse behavior in long-term care facilities: a structural equation model approach. Int Psychogeriatr. 2009;21(2):314–20.
23. Carney A. Indicators of abuse in the elderly ICU patient. Crit Care Nurs Q. 2015;38(3):293–7.
24. Lachs MS, Williams CS, Obrien S, et al. ED use by older victims of family violence. Ann Emerg Med. 1997;30(4):448–54.
25. Dong X, Simon MA. Elder abuse as a risk factor for hospitalization in older persons. JAMA Intern Med. 2013;173(10):911–7.
26. Rovi S, Chen PH, Vega M, Johnson MS, Mouton CP. Mapping the elder mistreatment Iceberg: U.S. hospitalizations with elder abuse and neglect diagnoses. J Elder Abuse Negl. 2009;21(4):346–59.
27. Etheridge EW. Sentinel for health: a history of the Centers for Disease Control. Berkeley: University of California Press; 1992.
28. Centers for Disease Control and Prevention. Centers for Disease Control and Prevention Official Mission and Functional Statement. Atlanta, GA: Centers for Disease Control and Prevention Management Analysis and Services Office; Approved 12/16/2013.
29. U.S. Department of Health & Human Services, U.S. Department of Justice. Surgeon General's workshop on violence and public health report. Washington, DC: Health Resources Service Administration; 1986.
30. Dahlberg LL, Mercy JA. History of violence as a public health problem. Virtual Mentor. 2009;11(2):167.
31. National Center for Injury Prevention and Control. The prevention of youth violence: a framework for community action. Atlanta;1993.
32. Goodman RA, Moulton A, Matthews G, et al. Law and public health at CDC. MMWR Morb Mortal Wkly Rep. 2006;55:29–33.
33. Daly JM, Jogerst G. Statute definitions of elder abuse. J Elder Abuse Negl. 2001;13(4):39–57.
34. Jogerst GJ, Daly JM, Brinig MF, Dawson JD, Schmuch GA, Ingram JG. Domestic elder abuse and the law. Am J Public Health. 2003;93(12):2131–6.
35. Nerenberg L. The national policy summit issue briefs. J Elder Abuse Negl. 2002;14(4):71–104.
36. Ingram EM. Expert panel recommendations on elder mistreatment using a public health framework. J Elder Abuse Negl. 2003;15 (2):45–65.
37. Lachs MS, Pillemer K. Elder abuse. Lancet. 2004;364 (9441):1263–72.

38. LE Saltzman, Fanslow JL, McMahon PM, Shelley GA. Intimate partner violence surveillance: uniform definitions and recommended data elements: version 1.0. Atlanta: Centers for Disease Control and Prevention, National Center for Injury Prevention and Control; 2002.
39. Basile KC, Saltzman LE. Sexual violence surveillance: uniform definitions and recommended data elements. Atlanta: Centers for Disease Control and Prevention, National Center for Injury Prevention and Control; 2002.
40. Leeb RT. Child maltreatment surveillance: uniform definitions for public health and recommended data elements. Atlanta: Centers for Disease Control and Prevention, National Center for Injury Prevention and Control; 2008.
41. Crosby AE, Ortega L, Melanson C. Self-directed violence surveillance: uniform definitions and recommended data elements. Atlanta: Centers for Disease Control and Prevention, National Center for Injury Prevention and Control; 2011.
42. Hall JE, Karch DL, Crosby AE. Elder abuse surveillance: uniform definitions and recommended core data elements, version 1.0. Atlanta: Centers for Disease Control and Prevention, National Center for Injury Prevention and Control; 2016.
43. Steenkamp M, Frazier L, Lipskiy N, et al. The National Violent Death Reporting System: an exciting new tool for public health surveillance. Inj Prev. 2006;12(suppl 2):ii3–5.
44. Blair JM, Fowler KA, Jack SPD, Crosby AE. The national violent death reporting system: overview and future directions. Inj Prev 2016;22(suppl 1):i6–i11.
45. Preventing Multiple Forms of Violence: A Strategic Vision for Connecting the Dots. Atlanta, GA: Division of Violence Prevention, National Center for Injury Prevention and Control, Centers for Disease Control and Prevention; 2016.
46. Ramsey-Klawsnik H, Heisler C. Polyvictimization in later life. Victimi Elder Disabl. 2014;17(1):3–6.

Part VII
Future Directions

33 Future Directions: Translational Research in Elder Abuse

Susan K. Roepke-Buehler and XinQi Dong

33.1 Introduction

Despite its widespread impact, research in elder abuse is in its infancy. What is particularly needed is translational research with the goals of improving older adult health, practice, and policy. The purpose of this chapter is to briefly review the translational research that has been done in elder abuse and discuss future directions for translational work that must be done in order to advance the field. In particular, we will draw from work done in various fields and discuss how these concepts can be applied in the context of elder abuse.

33.2 Definition of Translational Research

Translational research is a relatively new field of work relative to the basic sciences and clinical sciences. Indeed, the first publications using the term translational research did not appear until the early 1990s. Given that this remains a burgeoning area of research, the definition of translational research continues to evolve. The overarching goal of translational research is to bridge the gaps between various "silos" of scientific research with the ultimate goal of improving healthcare practices and public health.

Several different conceptual frameworks have been developed to characterize the nature of translational research and describe the pathways linking basic "bench" research to knowledge that improves public health, policies, and practice. The Institute of Medicine Clinical Research Roundtable initially described two "translational blocks" (T1 and T2) characterizing translational research. T1 involved the translation of knowledge of disease mechanisms gained in the laboratory setting to the development of methods of diagnosis, intervention, and prevention in humans. T2 involved transforming knowledge from clinical studies to clinical practice and health decision making [91]. A seminal paper by Woolf [101] further described translational research and broadened the scope of such work to include sciences involving populations such as epidemiology, psychology, economics, and behavioral sciences.

The National Institutes of Health (NIH) Roadmap for Medical Research focused on practice-based research and identified pathways linking "bench" research to "bedside" clinical research to research in clinical practice [99]. This model described the translation of research to humans in general, translation to patients, and translation to clinical practice in a three-stage model (T1, T2, and T3). A similar model by Dougherty and Conway [26] proposed steps necessary in transforming basic biomedical knowledge to clinical efficacy knowledge to clinical effectiveness knowledge with the ultimate goal of improving quality of health care and population health. Hommel et al. [44] built upon the framework proposed by Dougherty and Conway [26] to outline strategies for the integration of behavioral sciences at each step in the translation of basic science to improved health care and population health. Khoury et al. [55] adapted existing models of translational research and proposed a four-phase model (with T1, T2, T3, and T4 phases) describing phases the continuum of translational research in genomic medicine.

In attempts to synthesize these models, the Evaluation Committee of the Association for Clinical Research Training considered several existing working definitions of translational research and developed an operational definition of translational research [79]. The intention was to develop a framework for the design and evaluation of translational research training programs. They comprehensively defined translational research using three different stages of translational research (T1, T2, and T3) as follows:

S.K. Roepke-Buehler (✉)
Behavioral Sciences and Medicine, Rush University Medical Center, 710 S. Paulina Street, Suite 742, Chicago, IL 60612, USA
e-mail: susan_buehler@rush.edu

X. Dong
Rush Institute for Healthy Aging, Rush University Medical Center, 1645 W. Jackson Blvd, Suite 675, Chicago, IL 60612, USA

X. Dong (ed.), *Elder Abuse*, DOI 10.1007/978-3-319-47504-2_33

> Translational research fosters the multidirectional integration of basic research, patient-oriented research, and population-based research, with the long-term aim of improving the health of the public. T1 research expedites the movement between basic research and patient-oriented research that leads to new or improved scientific understanding or standards of care. T2 research facilitates the movement between patient-oriented research and population-based research that leads to better patient outcomes, the implementation of best practices, and improved health status in communities. T3 research promotes interaction between laboratory-based research and population-based research to stimulate a robust scientific understanding of human health and disease.

This operational definition of translational research is illustrated using the model presented in Fig. 33.1. The circular structure of the model symbolizes that translational research is a continuous and dynamic cycle. The bidirectional arrows reflect that not only does knowledge from the former type of research get translated or applied into the latter, but that new knowledge and hypotheses are also generated at each stage. Finally, patient-oriented research by definition addresses issues that have the potential to inform clinical practice and therefore, public health, which is why it is fully captured in this model. While some basic science research and population-based research have the ability to impact public health, not all of it does, which is why these groups are only partially included in the cycle.

T1 research can be conceptualized as the intersection between basic sciences, laboratory-based research, and patient-oriented research that is focused on improving scientific understanding of patient health and/or standards of care. In other words, T1 research reflects work that attempts to extend research done from the "bench to the bedside." Some examples of this type of translational research include, but are not limited to drug development research, human physiology research, pharmacogenomics, research examining mechanisms of disease, and genomics. T2 research is focused on the dynamic relationships between patient-oriented work and population-based research with the goal of improving patient outcomes, developing best practices, and improving health at the community level. Work in the T2 phase of translational research includes health service outcome research, clinical epidemiology, and community-based participatory research. T3 research involves the intersection between laboratory-based research and population-based research with the aim of advancing scientific understanding of human health and disease. Some examples of this type of research include epigenetic research, molecular epidemiology, and the translation of biomarkers of disease in animal models and their application to population-based models.

33.3 Review of Translational Research in Elder Abuse and What Can Be Learned from the Greater Violence Literature

Using the model proposed by Rubio et al. [79], we will briefly review some examples of work that has been published to date in the area of elder abuse.

33.3.1 T1 Research

One example of work that has been done in this area is related to identification of biomarkers of elder abuse. Much of the existing work has focused on potential biomarkers of

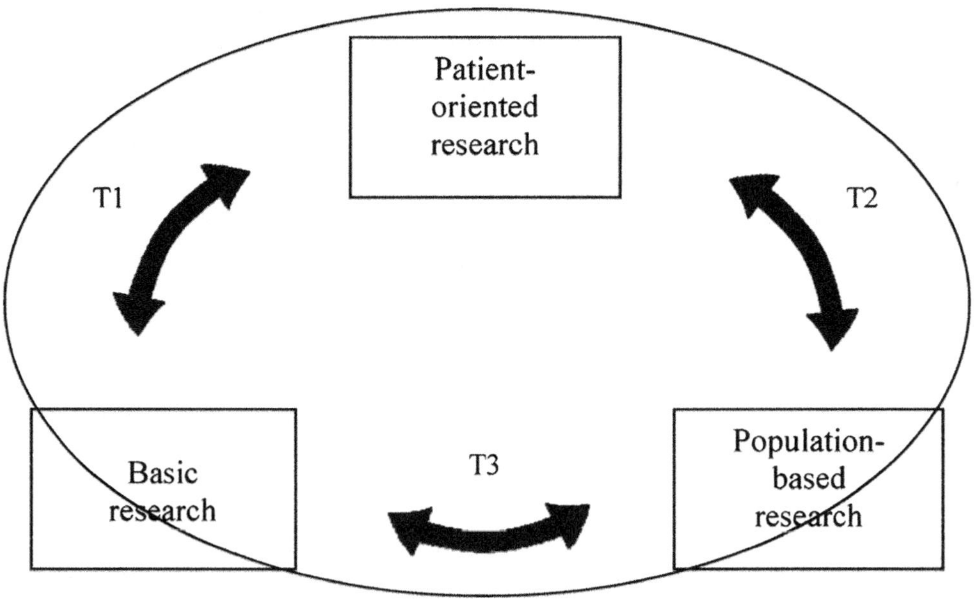

Fig. 33.1 Model for translational research, as proposed by the evaluation Committee of the Association for Clinical Research Training [79]

elder abuse in forensic pathology studies. For example, increased adrenal weight [40], as well as infiltration of "primed" neutrophils into multiple organs, and P-selectin and IL-8 in organ cells [39] can differentiate elder abuse cases from controls. Although these findings are geared towards identification of elder abuse post-mortem, conclusions drawn from these studies highlight potential physiological processes (for example, stress-induced over-production of glucocorticoid) operating in the context of elder abuse that must be explored. Clinical studies have also identified vitamin D deficiency as a potential biomarkers in self-neglecting older adults [7].

Emerging work is starting to examine potential biological consequences of elder abuse. A recent population study by Dong and Simon [21] found that elder abuse victims were more likely to have evidence of metabolic syndrome (characterized in multiple ways) compared to non-abused older adults. These findings represent a potential pathways linking elder abuse to downstream risk for cardiovascular disease-related mortality. Analyses were conducted to determine potential moderators of the relationship between elder abuse and metabolic syndrome. Findings suggested that demographic characteristics such as age, sex, and race were significant moderators, but health and psychosocial variables were not, despite research in other fields with similar findings. This research also suggests that inflammatory markers are likely important mediators in the relationship between violence and cardiovascular dysregulation. The field of elder abuse would benefit from systematic research including biomarkers of inflammation and cardiovascular disease, preferably with population-based data.

Although the research examining biological mechanisms and biomarkers of elder abuse is in its infancy, there has been a relatively larger amount of work conducted in the greater violence literature. Such studies have examined psychoneuroendocrine, neural, and epigenetic markers of violence. This research and its relevance to the field of elder abuse are reviewed in a later section.

33.3.2 T2 Research

Much of the existing work in this area of research involves studies examining outcomes related to elder abuse interventions, primarily those executed by Adult Protective Services (APS) or those done in healthcare settings. A systematic review of studies using APS data revealed a shortage of systematic research in this area, particularly for research involving the effectiveness of APS interventions [29]. The authors identified only nine studies that considered case outcomes related to APS intervention. These studies primarily reported descriptive data regarding the types of APS interventions executed and rates of APS intervention refusal. Prosecution of elder abuse perpetrators was also examined. Overall, APS interventions often involved provision of case management services, basic needs (e.g., food, shelter, healthcare), financial management services, home health services, guardianship, hospitalization (particularly when physical abuse was involved), urgent medications, and in some cases, protective court orders to arrange for safety of the victims [29, 41]. Importantly, none of these studies reported data on a national level. Equally striking is that there were no studies identified that examined the efficacy or effectiveness of any of the interventions that are often provided by APS workers. This means that interventions commonly used by APS, the primary agency entrusted to protect older adults from mistreatment are lacking empirical support and their impact is unknown.

Du Mont et al. [28] recently took a novel approach to bridge the gap between elder abuse research and development of evidence-based interventions. They conducted a systematic scoping review of literature in elder abuse to compile a comprehensive database of actionable and applicable recommendations that can directly inform the development of multidisciplinary hospital-based interventions for elder abuse. This database included recommendations and statements regarding (1) initial contact with at-risk individuals/potential victims, (2) determining capacity and consent, (3) interviewing the older adult, suspected abuser, caregiver, and or other relevant parties, (4) specific screening questions related to specific types of abuse and/or neglect, (5) assessment of physical/forensic, mental, psychosocial, and environmental/functional factors, and (6) the development and execution of a care plan. This approach is valuable in integrating research recommendations from a wide variety of sources and implementing these strategies to enhance current practices in elder abuse.

The field of elder abuse can learn a great deal from what has been done in child maltreatment and intimate partner violence with regards to interventions that are likely adaptable to elder abuse. In a recent article, Sumner et al. [90] systematically reviewed violence prevention strategies and highlighted empirically supported interventions that are likely adaptable to multiple forms of violence. The bulk of these interventions were originally developed for child abuse, however, the underlying approaches are likely applicable or modifiable for elder abuse. These approaches are as follows.

Nurse home visits to low-income families can help provide support and coaching for at risk families. Family and individual training sessions done at home or in a community setting (e.g., church, clinic, etc.) can be useful to reach a larger audience. Public policy approaches are broad in scope and include increasing alcohol prices, thereby reducing use, and minimizing alcohol abuse as a risk factor. Therapeutic approaches include cognitive behavioral therapy and other coping skills training interventions, delivered by a both mental health and non-mental health professionals. Brief primary care-based approaches can be delivered in the clinic setting by a variety of healthcare providers. Bystander training may be a community-based approach in order to increase public awareness of elder abuse and increase efficacy in reporting when abuse is suspected or observed. Income supports, such as food stamps, to at-risk groups has also been associated with decreases in violence. Finally, environmental modifications, such as increasing green space in at risk neighborhoods can also have a beneficial impact on reducing violence.

Moreover, important work has also been done to develop evidence-based interventions targeting child neglect and its consequences [5, 92]. Existing interventions are primarily family-based and many aspects of these interventions can be adapted for elder abuse and neglect. Components of these interventions have included individual- and family-based interventions that focus on coping skills acquisition, education, mentoring, social-service provision, day-treatment programs, and multi-component interventions.

Prospective work in large cohort- or population- based research has also been done to bridge the gap between various silos of research in the area of child neglect. For example, prospective work has examined the role of neighborhood crime on neglect and the development of externalizing behaviors [64]. Moreover, large scale studies have been done that suggest that race and poverty are also important in the context of child neglect and deleterious outcomes [51, 100]. Examination of neighborhood crime, violence, race, poverty, and cultural factors in the context elder abuse and neglect research is likely important to consider in the determination of how elder abuse and neglect may manifest downstream health outcomes.

33.3.3 T3 Research

Very little work focused on elder abuse has been done in this arm of translational research. However, a great deal of research has been done to examine epigenetic changes in adulthood and aging as a consequence of child adversity and abuse. Epigenetic research is an important translational step in bridging gaps in research in elder abuse. The "epigenome" refers to a second layer of information above the actual DNA sequence that regulates multiple genomic functions, particularly when and how genes are expressed. Epigenetic research focuses on the reversible regulation of genomic functions that are independent of DNA sequence and are primarily mediated through environmental and biochemical changes in DNA methylation and chromatin structure [69].

Although still in its infancy, there has been a fair amount of epigenetic research suggesting that early life events in animals and humans can impact DNA methylation [8]. Such work suggest that individuals with history of abuse as a child had higher methylation levels at specific CpG sites in the exon1_F of the promoter region of the GR gene [66]. This research mirrored previous findings in animal studies suggesting that parental care impacts epigenetic regulation of hippocampal glucocorticoid receptor expression. This type of translational research can be key in determining gene-environment interactions that may explain the link between elder abuse and health outcomes.

Similarly, there has been epigenetic work done in the area of suicide. Prior research has found that alterations in the spindle and kinetochore-associated protein 2 (SKA2) gene may pose as a useful biomarker for suicidal behavior [35]. Recent research from a large cohort study further suggest that epigenetic variation in the SKA2 gene may mediate predisposition to suicidal behaviors through a dysregulated HPA response to stress [52].

33.4 Advancing the Field of Elder Abuse Through Translational Research

Relative to the fields of child abuse and mistreatment and intimate partner violence, the field of elder abuse is in its infancy. Rather than completely "reinventing the wheel," researchers in the field of elder abuse should begin by applying lessons from what translational work has already been done in these related fields. We briefly discuss some of these concepts that have been studied in related fields. We also review an important conceptual model of elder abuse and discuss how it can be applied to translational research aimed at developing efficacious and effective practices. Finally, we discuss how community-based participatory research (CBPR) is a valuable approach that can be used to conduct translational research in elder abuse at multiple levels.

33.4.1 Recommendations for Advancing the Field of Elder Abuse Through Translational Research

33.4.1.1 Development of a Uniform National Elder Abuse Data Collection

In 2014, 750 experts and stakeholders in the field of elder abuse gathered to brainstorm priorities and recommendations in the areas of direct service, education, policy, and research in order to advance the field of elder abuse. In the resulting *Elder Justice Roadmap*, several recommendations are made in order to enhance data collection and research directions for elder abuse. In order to optimize systematic elder abuse data in this environment of limited funding availability, efforts should be focused on developing standardized data collection protocols on a national level. The child abuse and domestic violence fields have decades of data collected at the federal level. By contrast, federal law has only mandated collection of elder abuse data since 2005. This data was primary from Adult Protective Services. This is an important start, however more work must be done to ensure that these data are useful and include a wide variety of information potentially important in the context of elder abuse.

They particularly recommended developing standardized data collection methods on a national level to ensure that data can be used collectively. One issue that has impeded progress in this area is the lack of standardized data collection in Adult Protective Services databases. Although procedures and laws vary by state, common elements for data collection content and methods should be identified to allow for data analysis on a national level [20]. This data should also contain longitudinal follow-up for APS cases with agreed-upon and validated indicators of successful elder abuse outcomes. Importantly, elder abuse data collection should not stop with APS and related agencies that also have contact with elder abuse victims, such as those related to health, law enforcement, financial, Medicare/Medicaid, and long term care facilities, should also have standardized protocols for collecting such data.

Indeed, the Assistant Secretary for Planning and Evaluation (ASPE) of HHS released a Congressional Report on the Feasibility of Establishing a Uniform National Database on Elder Abuse that reviewed the current administrative data collection on elder abuse. This document also provided recommendations in service of developing a uniform national database One approach outlined involved initially starting with APS data in a few select states and incrementally increasing the type of data collected and the number of states participating.

33.4.1.2 Knowledge Translation

A great deal of attention has been focused on how to bridge the gap between research evidence to practice and policy in order to develop evidence-based practices. A recent systematic review by MacGregor et al. [63] found sixty-two articles meeting their criteria for knowledge translation work in the areas of child maltreatment and intimate partner violence. Much of the existing work has focused on training healthcare practitioners in various aspects of delivery of services related to child maltreatment and intimate partner violence. Others have focused on training teachers, social services providers, and attorneys. They found that multimodal interventions (i.e., single or multiple training sessions with multiple modes of education delivery), with and without exchange between intervention facilitators and recipients, as well as complex/multifaceted intervention approaches (i.e., more intensive, multicomponent interventions) were generally effective at improving knowledge, attitudes, and behavioral outcomes related to child maltreatment and intimate partner violence.

In attempts to develop an integrated knowledge translation partnership, the PreVAil (Preventing Violence Across the Lifespan) Research Network was recently developed [60]. This public health network was developed to be an interdisciplinary partnership between researchers and knowledge-user partners within and outside health-related fields on an international level. The primary objectives of this network are to increase knowledge of the links between mental health, substance abuse, gender, and exposure to family violence on a national and international level, develop family violence prevention and intervention strategies, and to promote knowledge translation agenda in this network of investigators and partners. A key aspect of such a knowledge translation network is the reciprocal nature of the partnerships such that it is well understood that both investigators and knowledge users learn from each other and have important contributions to the advance the field. Conceptual work for knowledge translation networks is limited; however, they represent a promising, novel approach in advancing the evidence-based knowledge and application of elder abuse prevention and intervention strategies.

33.4.1.3 Applying Knowledge from Behavior Change Literature

Although disseminating existing scientific knowledge to providers who are in the field is an important step in enhancing evidence-based practices, the work does not stop there. Once providers are equipped with the knowledge about elder abuse, steps must be taken to systematically integrate evidence-based behavior change strategies targeting practitioners as well as elder abuse victims and perpetrators. Some existing evidence-based strategies that might be applied to the area of elder abuse are motivational interviewing [67] as well as a variety of cognitive and behavioral strategies such as stimulus control, cognitive restructuring, and self-efficacy-boosting interventions. Indeed, one recent elder abuse intervention study has utilized these strategies to help at-risk older adults set goals regarding difficult life changes [68]. Results suggested that this community-based intervention was effective in reducing elder abuse risk factors and decreasing ambivalence in goal-setting. This type of a strategy may also be useful in working with healthcare and social services providers who often feel ambivalent about elder abuse reporting for various reasons (e.g., worries about loss of trust, liability, etc.).

33.4.1.4 Biomarkers and Biological Mechanisms Research

A great deal of emerging research has demonstrated that elder abuse is associated with significant medical consequences, including increased utilization of health care services [24, 25, 61] and all-cause mortality [23, 85]. What is less understood are the potential mechanisms linking elder abuse to downstream health consequences. These mechanisms are likely multifaceted and include biological, behavioral, and psychological factors. Prospective work aimed at determining potential biological pathways linking elder abuse to disease is necessary.

Biomarkers and Biological Correlates of Abuse A great deal of work has been done to examine physiological processes that link psychological stress to disease and elder abuse research can benefit from this translational work. For example, elder abuse research can benefit from prior work that has identified inflammation [9, 88], hypercoagulation [49, 54], endothelial function [12, 65], sympathoadrenal medullary axis activation [2, 31], platelet activation [6], insulin-resistance [3], and hypothalamic pituitary axis activation [4, 73] as potential mechanistic links between stress and cardiovascular outcomes. Moreover, other work has been done to explore immune dysfunction in the context of chronic stress [46, 47, 56, 57, 59]. Other potential physiological consequences of stress include telomere length [58], anemia [98], and kidney function [97, 98].

A fair amount of work has been done in humans and animals to determine potential mechanism linking child abuse, neglect, and adversity to downstream mental and physical health outcomes. Some mechanisms include HPA axis functioning [13, 14, 18, 36, 42], immune system functioning [86], and inflammation [16, 17, 74, 76, 87, 93]. Moreover, there has been a fair amount of literature suggesting that childhood adversity and mistreatment is associated with shortened telomere length [53, 58, 72, 96]; Tyrka et al. [95], a biomarker that has been implicated in cellular aging. However, more recent research has failed to find a similar relationship between history of child abuse and telomere length in older adults [82], and the existing evidence between stress and telomere length is somewhat equivocal [81].

Although relatively sparse, there has been some translational work done in the area of child neglect. For example, Sullivan and colleges [89] extended existing research in stress responsivity to determine possible psychobiological consequences of neglect. They found that neglected children had higher cortisol response to self-evaluative tasks compared to non-neglected children, suggesting heightened hypothalamic-pituitary-adrenal axis reactivity. This research suggests that child neglect may have deleterious impact to health and development.

Neural Pathways Implicated in Violence and Abuse Emerging research is also being conducted to identify neural structural and pathways implicated in violence. For example, methods such as magnetic resonance imaging (MRI) and diffusion tensor imaging (DTI) have been used to explore neural correlates of violence. Findings are somewhat mixed but suggest that the corpus callosum is altered in women with intimate partner violence [32]. MRI studies also suggest that structural impairments in the ventrolateral prefrontal cortex, dorsol prefrontal corex, and orbitofrontal cortex may be markers of suicidal behavior [19]. Another study demonstrated that history of childhood mistreatment may account for variability in limbic/prefrontal brain function and prefrontal structure in PTSD as an adult, pointing to a potential neural mechanism linking childhood mistreatment to PTSD [33].

Special attention must be paid to subtypes of elder abuse, given that there may be different processes at play. For example, prior research has suggested that financial literacy is inversely associated with susceptibility to scams in older adults [48]. Han et al. [37] conducted functional MRI research and has demonstrated that financial literacy is associated with functional connectivity between the posterior cingulate cortex and the right ventromedial prefrontal cortex, left postcentral gyrus, and the right precuneus. Interestingly, these effects are not better explained by global cognitive function, suggesting that cognition and financial literacy reflect at least partially different constructs that have differing neural bases. Identifying these pathways can help increase our understanding of the neural mechanisms that may explain vulnerability to various types of abuse in older adults.

Epigenetic Research Epigenetic research is a relatively new field, although there is a lot that can be learned from the emerging epigenetic research done in violence, in general. One approach may be to start with known epigenetic markers associated with child abuse and neglect as well as intimate partner violence and examine them in the context of elder abuse. Moreover, it would be important to consider epigenetic findings in the area of trauma and PTSD as well. Such research can also be used to determine potential factors that may be important in predicting which elder abuse victims also experience downstream health issues and those who are resilient to such consequences.

Intervention Research and Health Outcomes In addition to the identification of biological and epigenetic consequences of elder abuse, research must also circle back to these findings to determine if interventions have impact on improving such biological outcomes. Although very limited, there has been some intervention research to suggest that psychosocial interventions for maltreated children can have beneficial impact on stress-biology markers, such as cortisol [15, 27, 30]. Such research would provide further evidence for potential biological and genetic mechanisms linking elder abuse to health consequences and provide stronger rationale for treating elder abuse as a critical public health concern as well as a civil rights issue.

With regards to interventions for abuse and violence, there is some evidence suggesting that pharmacological intervention for perpetrators can be effective. A study by George et al. [34] found that fluoxetine treatment in conjunction with alcohol treatment and cognitive behavioral therapy in alcoholic perpetrators of domestic violence was successful in reducing anger and physical aggression over time. Given that elder abuse perpetrators have some overlapping characteristics to those who perpetrate intimate partner violence (e.g., psychiatric illness, alcohol and substance abuse, personality traits, etc.) [50], this type of an approach may also be useful in the context of minimizing elder abuse.

33.4.2 Efficacy and Effectiveness Research for Elder Abuse Prevention and Intervention

Recent systematic reviews in elder abuse intervention suggest that the scientific, systematic study of elder abuse interventions is extremely limited [28, 75]. Those studies including a control comparison group are even scarcer. Some work that has been done has focused on victims of elder abuse, caregivers at risk for perpetrating elder abuse, as well as training for health professionals. Intervention strategies that have been published include case management, home-based geriatric assessment, support groups, adult protective service intervention, faith-based programs, and professional education. Although there are not enough systematic studies that have reliable data and analytic approaches, some work suggests that multidisciplinary team approaches and multicomponent interventions are an effective approach. Emerging work is also being done to develop multicomponent, hospital-based interventions for elder abuse that aim to impact psychological, physical, legal, and social consequences of elder abuse [28].

Given that much of the current research in elder abuse prevention and intervention is primarily descriptive in nature, future work would benefit first from systematic study of existing strategies. In order to develop evidence-based practices in the field of elder abuse, researchers must consider both the efficacy and effectiveness of proposed interventions. That is, intervention research should follow the existing models of translational work and cover the entire continuum of highly-controlled, randomized clinical trials focused on clinical outcomes to "real-world" implementation of such intervention strategies in order to determine cost-effectiveness, compliance issues, generalizability to different populations, etc.

With regards to efficacy of elder abuse interventions, the gold-standard method in systematically determining treatment/intervention effects is the randomized controlled trial [78]. In order to advance the field of elder abuse to the level of what has been done in the fields of child abuse and intimate partner violence, work must be done to ensure the efficacy of interventions that are currently being used in the field. Only recently have there been any randomized clinical trials published in the area of elder abuse. These studies have focused on education interventions for health professionals [77, 94] and coping skills training for caregivers [38, 62].

33.4.2.1 Theory-Driven Elder Abuse Intervention Research

Importantly, translational research in elder abuse research will benefit from strong, theoretical conceptualization. Many existing theoretical models have been applied, such as the *Ecological Model, Sociocultural Model, Cycle of Violence Theory,* and *Lifecourse Perspective* Model. We describe components of the *Ecolological Model* as applied to elder abuse, as it inherently incorporates multiple levels of influence, and therefore works nicely as a guide to translational research that is multidisciplinary and is intended to intersect various silos of research.

Intervention research in other public health issues has benefited from examining the issue at multiple levels. Bronfenbrenner's *Ecological Model* (Fig. 33.2) of human development [10] is a framework that has been used in the

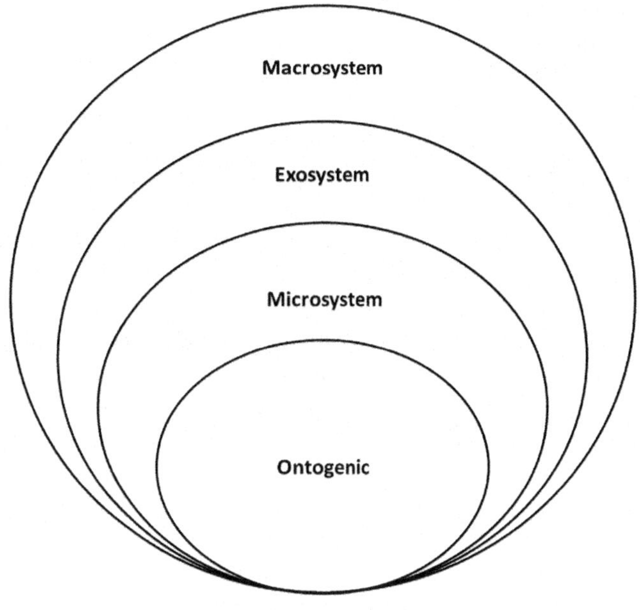

Fig. 33.2 Bronfenbrenner's Ecological Model

conceptualization of prevention and intervention for various public health issues including diabetes, smoking cessation, obesity, cardiovascular disease and various mental health issues. This multilevel model identifies nested environmental systems with which the individual interacts. Interventions can be most impactful if they address multiple levels in this framework.

The *Ecological Model* as applied to elder abuse provides an organizational schema that highlights multiple levels of potential prevention and intervention targets for impacting elder abuse, As applied to the context of elder abuse [11, 83, 84], variables in the ontogenetic system (the innermost level) might include those related to physiology, affect, and behavior such as age, sex, and mental and physical health (including medical comorbidities, cognitive status, and physical function). Therefore, prevention efforts at this level might focus on identifying vulnerable groups or individuals based on individual-level risk factors including dementia status, level of physical disability and dependence, depression and other psychiatric issues, and key demographic factors.

Indeed, [22] Dong and Simon developed a "Vulnerability Risk Index" that can be used as a tool by healthcare practitioners and social services to identifies older adults most at-risk for elder abuse based upon various risk factors including age, sex, race and ethnicity, socioeconomic status, cognitive impairment, physical disability, depressive symptoms, social network, and social participation. In addition, research should be done to examine the impact of interventions focused on reducing one's vulnerability risk index to determine if there is a future reduction in elder abuse incidence. In this vein, clinical research might focus on general health promotion as well as mental health interventions for both vulnerable older adults as well as their caregivers. Prior research has demonstrated that caregivers who participate in interventions aimed at increasing coping skills may exhibit a reduction in mood symptoms, which therefore can decrease the likelihood of resorting to abusive behavior [62].

Microsystem characteristics refer to groups and institutions that directly impact the individual, such as family, church, etc. Given that prior work suggests that elder physical abuse is most frequently perpetrated by a partner or spouse [1], family interventions are likely to be more impactful than individual interventions. Moreover, given that many elder abuse victims rely heavily on their family caregivers due to cognitive and physical disabilities, the more people who are involved, the better. At this level, elder abuse research must also consider setting. Prevention and intervention strategies would have more impact if we as researchers think "out-of-the-box" in terms of setting. Health promotion research in other areas has found success in implementing culturally-sensitive interventions in settings outside the clinic to reach a larger audience, particularly for groups who may not seek medical attention until an issue requires tertiary intervention efforts. Therefore, efforts to collaborate with community organizations with which older adults frequently interact are an important piece in making a widespread impact. For example, church-based programs may be more effective for certain racial and ethnic groups compared to clinic-based programs.

Exosystem variables include those related to the socioeconomic environment, access to social services, etc. Research at this level must focus on efficacy and effectiveness of Adult Protective Services interventions. Translational work must be done to tailor and apply efficacious intervention strategies to be implemented by APS and other social service agencies interacting with older adults. Existing APS interventions largely focus on elder abuse report investigation, risk assessment, and case management, as well as arranging for medical, social, legal, supportive, and housing services and resources [70]. Research must be done to examine the effectiveness of these services, especially within specific communities.

Also within this level includes policy-based interventions including elder abuse reporting mandates and elder abuse legislation. Prevention and intervention at this level has the potential for great impact. For example, mandates for child abuse reporting have made a significant impact on identifying children at risk for abuse. In comparison, legal responsibility in the reporting of elder abuse is often less clear and poorly understood by healthcare and social service providers. Research has been done to examine barriers at this level and future work should apply this knowledge to enhance confidence in providers to report suspected elder abuse [45, 102]. Also, population-based research must be done to strengthen the case for increased policy changes to protect older adults.

Finally, macrosystem variables refer to ethnic and cultural attitudes and contexts. In the context of elder abuse, this might involve ethnic and cultural beliefs about age and gender inequality, cultural beliefs about family responsibility and aging, and society aggression norms. Emerging research is focusing on cultural factors and cultural beliefs as they relate to aging. In particular, future research must explore how cultural beliefs and family and aging impact elder abuse and neglect in order to develop culturally-sensitive prevention and intervention approaches. The concepts studied in cultural and behavioral "bench" research are valuable in the development and implementation of elder abuse prevention and intervention efforts targeting specific sociocultural groups.

Until now, there had been no overarching theory specifically formulated to characterize elder abuse, its contributors, and its consequences. Roberto and Teaster introduce their *Contextual Theory of Elder Abuse* that builds upon the Ecological Model in that various contextual levels surrounding the elder abuse victim (in the center, as a person-centered approach). Contexts identified include the individual context, the relational context, the community context, and the societal context. This model aims to incorporate the complex nature of the intersection between aging and abuse and is designed to inform research, practice, and policy. Given that theory is intended to be an evolving process, research is needed to test components of models of elder abuse to provide confirmation or justifications for modifications to enhance our understanding of the constructs operating in elder abuse.

33.4.2.2 Community-Based Participatory Research

In recent years, community-based participatory research (CBPR) has been a fast-growing approach in translating scientific research to practice by building community engagement into research. The primary goal of CBPR is to enhance public health and minimize health disparities by collaborating with community partners in the research process. This is done by involving key stakeholders at every stage of research, including design, analysis, and communication of results [71]. Indeed, a recent systematic review demonstrated that collaboration between community members, researchers, providers, and patients is a useful research approach in lessening health disparities and improving overall health in a variety of communities [80]. This approach is a particularly useful translational approach because community partners are fully involved in the research from its infancy which means that there is a natural pipeline for research dissemination into the community. This also ensures that scientific knowledge gained from the community can best serve that very community in terms of social action and development and implementation of effective practices.

There are several strengths of using a CBRP approach in addressing public health issues. First, it enhances community buy-in and personal investment in research. Studies using a CBPR approach can benefit from improved participation rates in population-based studies given that community members feel more closely involved and directly benefit from the findings. Second, effectiveness of interventions is enhanced at an early stage because community resources can be applied in the design phase, as opposed to modifying existing work to fit the community. Third heavy involvement of community members in research phase may also help to repair longstanding perceptions and distrust of certain communities and ethnic and racial groups. Fourth, community involvement is useful in determining mutual social and health goals, rather than solely focusing on the scientific goals. Fifth, this approach is well-received by communities given that the research allows for resources to be directly poured into the community.

Holkup et al. [43] documented their work using a CPBR approach in implementing a family conference intervention for elder mistreatment in a Native American community. They described important barriers to implementing CPBR within culturally-diverse groups and offered specific suggestions for overcoming these potential challenges. In particular, it is important to recognize that flexibility is key with regards to implementing a study that involves community stakeholders and community members in collaboration with the research team. This involves making changes to the study as needed throughout the process to best meet the needs of the community while also ensuring high quality research methodology. It is also important to foster a culture for the study that places everyone involved a foundation of commitment to social justice. Discussions ensuring shared authority, responsibility and credit for the study success should be held early and often in the process. Several ethical considerations need attention throughout the study process as well. For example, issues related to gathering informed consent maintaining confidentiality, ownership of data, and protecting the public image of the community. In addition, careful attention to cultural considerations when working in a diverse team is imperative.

CBPR research in the area of elder abuse intervention is an important approach to translational research in that it can allow for cooperation between various academic, medical, social services, community stakeholders, and faith-based institutions who all have a responsibility and mission to protect elders and make efforts to enhance health. Such collaboration is particularly necessary in the field of elder abuse, given its multidisciplinary nature. CBPR also can create an infrastructure to continuously evolve its research mission as well as execute evidence based-practices that are developed from such knowledge.

33.4.3 Final Recommendations

Despite the alarming prevalence of elder abuse and its vast mental and physical health consequences, there is a paucity of research examining elder abuse prevention and intervention efforts. Translational research in elder abuse needs to begin synthesizing the current work that has been done to examine risk factors, socio-demographic correlates, cultural constructs, as well as health outcomes with the greater violence prevention research in order to develop evidence-based intervention strategies. Randomized controlled trials and CBPR represent important methodologies that must be utilized to bring the field forward. In addition to the implementation of translational intervention research in the area of elder abuse, what is needed is availability of evidence-based practices and guidelines that are presented in a user-friendly way to benefit a wide-range of practitioners who encounter individuals at risk for elder abuse.

As prevention and intervention efforts are developed and studied, researchers also should broaden their conceptualization of elder abuse to include common themes examined in the greater violence research across the lifespan, rather than focusing on abuse of older adults as a "silo" entity. Theoretical models that conceptualize processes that drive violence and victimization across the lifespan must be considered, especially given the emerging research in the areas of poly-victimization, intergenerational transmission of elder abuse, etc.

In addition to broadening our theoretical understanding of elder abuse in the broader context of violence prevention across the lifespan, it is also important to consider the importance of specific subtypes of abuse that affect older adults. Recognizing that the predisposing and maintaining factors as well as consequences can vary drastically based upon the type of abuse being examined is paramount when developing focused intervention efforts.

33.4.4 Summary

In summary, research in the field of elder abuse is in its infancy and much work must be done in order to apply principles learned from various silos of research in the areas of elder abuse and related fields to make a beneficial impact on elder abuse practice and policy. Translational research represents work that bridges the gaps between basic bench research, clinical research and practice, and population-based research. Although very little translational research has been done in the area of elder abuse, the field can learn a great deal from the disciplines of child mistreatment, intimate partner violence, trauma research, stress biology, epigenetics, knowledge translation, and CBPR research.

What is urgently needed is research to develop evidence-based practices for elder abuse. There is a lack of research demonstrating the efficacy and effectiveness of elder abuse prevention and intervention strategies. Healthcare and social services must be able to support the rationale for implementing commonly used elder abuse intervention strategies in order to justify the use of taxpayer dollars that go into these services. Translational research to develop evidence-based practices is desperately needed for these reasons. Such research should focus on population-based research, mental and physical health outcomes, mechanisms, and cultural issues.

References

1. Acierno R, Hernandez-Tejada M, Muzzy W, Steve K. National Elder Study. NCJ226456, Grant Report;2008.
2. Adler KA, Patterson TL, Mills PJ, Ziegler MG, Dimsdale JE, Grant I. Sympathoadrenalmedullary dysregulation in elderly Alzheimer caregivers with high subjective burden and low resources. Ann Behav Med. 2002;24 (Suppl):S79 (abst).
3. Ahmadi N, Arora R, Vaidya N, Yehuda R, Ebrahimi R. Posttraumatic stress disorder is associated with increased incidence of insulin resistance and metabolic syndrome. J Am Coll Cardiol. 2013;61:E1347.
4. Alevizaki M, Cimponeriu A, Lekakis J, Papamichael C, Chrousos GP. High anticipatory stress plasma cortisol levels and sensitivity to glucocorticoids predict severity of coronary artery disease in subjects undergoing coronary angiography. Metabolism. 2007;56:222–6.
5. Allin H, Wathen NC, MacMillan H. Treatment of child neglect: a systematic review. Can J Psychiatry. 2005;50:497–504.
6. Aschbacher K, von Känel R, Mills PJ, Roepke SK, Hong S, Dimsdale JE, Mausbach BT, Patterson TL, Ziegler MG, Ancoli-Israel S, Grant I. Longitudinal platelet reactivity to acute psychological stress among older men and women. Stress. 2009;12(5):426–33.
7. Aung K, Burnett J, Smith SM, Dyer CB. Vitamin D deficiency associated with self-neglect in the elderly. J Elder Abuse Neglect. 2006;18(4):63–78.
8. Bick J, Naumova O, Hunter S, Barbot B, Lee M, Luthar SS, Raefski A, Grigorendo EL. Childhood adversity and DNA methylation of genes involved in the hypothalamus-pituitary-adrenal axis and immune system: whole-genome and candidate-gene associations. Dev Psychopathol. 2012;24:1417–25.
9. Black PH, Garbutt LD. Stress, inflammation and cardiovascular disease. J Psychosom Res. 2002;52:1–23.
10. Bronfenbrenner U. The ecology of human development: experiments by nature and design. Cambridge: Harvard University Press; 1979.
11. Burnight K, Mosqueda L. Theoretical model of development in elder mistreatment. Washington: U.S Department of Justice; 2011.
12. Chumaeva N, Hintsanen M, Ravaja N, Juonala M, Raitakari OT, Keltikangas-Järvinen L. Chronic stress and the development of early atherosclerosis: moderating effect of endothelial dysfunction and impaired arterial elasticity. Int J Environ Res Public Health. 2009;6:2934–49.
13. Cicchetti D, Rogosch FA, Gunnar MR, Toth SL. The differential impacts of early physical and sexual abuse and internalizing problems on daytime cortisol rhythm in school-aged children. Child Dev. 2010;81(1):252–69.
14. Cicchetti D, Rogosch FA, Oshri A. Interactive effects of corticotropin releasing hormone receptor 1, serotonin transporter linked polymorphic region, and child maltreatment on diurnal cortisol regulation and internalizing symptomatology. Dev Psychopathol. 2011;23(4):1125–38.
15. Cicchetti D, Rogosch FA, Toth SL, Sturge-Apple M. Normalizing the development of cortisol regulation in maltreated inflants through preventive intervention. Dev Psychopathol. 2011;23:789–800.
16. Danese A, Moffit TE, Pariante CM, Ambler A, Poulton R, Caspi A. Elevated inflammation levels in depressed adults with a history of childhood maltreatment. Arch Gen Psychiatry. 2008;65 (4):409–15.

17. Danese A, Pariante CM, Caspi A, Taylor A, Poulton R. Childhood maltreatment predicts adult inflammation in a life-course study. Proc Natl Acad Sci. 2007;104:1319–24.
18. De Bellis MD, Chrousos GP, Dorn LD, Burke L, Helmers K, Kling MA, Trickett PK, Putnam FW. Hypothalamic-pituitary-adrenal axis dysregulation in sexually abused girls. J Clin Endocrinol Metab. 1994;78(2):249–55.
19. Ding Y, Lawrence N, Olie E, Cyprien F, le Bars E, Bonafe A, Phillips ML, Courtet P, Jollant F. Prefrontal cortex markers of suicidal vulnerability in mood disorders: a model-based structural neuroimaging study with a translational perspective. Transl Psychiatry. 2015;5:1–8.
20. Dong X. Elder abuse: research, practice, and health policy. The 2012 GSA Maxwell Pollack award lecture. Gerontologist. 2014;54(2):153–62. doi:10.1093/geront/gnt139.
21. Dong X, Simon M. Association between elder abuse and metabolic syndromes: findings from the Chicago Health and Aging Project. Gerontology. 2014;. doi:10.1159/000368577.
22. Dong X, Simon M. Vulnerability risk index profile for elder abuse in a community-dwelling population. J Am Geriatr Soc. 2014;62:10–5.
23. Dong X, Simon M, Mendes de Léon C, Fulmer T, Beck T, Hebert L, Dyer C, Paveza G, Evans D. Elder self-neglect and abuse and mortality in a community-dwelling population. JAMA. 2009;302(5):517–26.
24. Dong X, Simon MA. Association between elder abuse and use of ED: findings from the Chicago Health and Aging Project. Am J Emerg Med. 2013;31(4):693–8. doi:10.1016/j.ajem.2012.12.028.
25. Dong X, Simon MA. Elder abuse as a risk factor for hospitalization in older persons. JAMA Intern Med. 2013;173(10):911–7. doi:10.1001/jamainternmed.2013.238.
26. Dougherty D, Conway PH. The "3Ts" road map to transform US health care: the "how" of high-quality care. JAMA. 2008;299 (19):2319–21.
27. Dozier M, Peloso E, Lewis E, Laurenceau JP, Levine S. Effects of an attachment-based intervention on the cortisol production in infants and toddlers in foster care. Dev Psychopathol. 2008;20:845–59.
28. Du Mont J, MacDonald S, Kosa D, Elliot S, Spencer S, Yaffe M. Development of a comprehensive hospital-based elder abuse intervention: an initial systematic scoping review. PLoS One. 2015;10(5):1–21.
29. Ernst JS, Ramsey-Klawsnik H, Schillerstrom JE, Dayton C, Mixson P, Counihan M. Informing evidence-based practice: a review of research analyzing adult protective services data. J Elder Abuse Neglect. 2014;26:458–94.
30. Fisher PA, Gunnar MR, Chamberlain P, Reid JB. Preventive intervention for maltreated preschool children: impact on children's behavior, neuroendocrine activity, and foster parent functioning. J Am Acad Child Adolesc Psychiatry. 2000;39 (11):1356–64.
31. Flaa A, Eide IK, Kjeldsen SE, Rostrup M. Sympathoadrenal stress reactivity is a predictor of future blood pressure: an 18-year follow-up study. Hypertension. 2008;52:336–41.
32. Flegar SJ, Fouche JP, Jordaan E, Marais S, Spottiswoode B, Stein DJ, Vythilingum B. The neural correlates of intimate partner violence in women. Afr J Psychiatry. 2011;14:310–4.
33. Fonzo GA, Flagan TM, Sullivan S, Allard CB, Grimes EM, Simmons AN, Paulus MP, Stein MB. Neural functional and structural correlates of childhood maltreatment in women with intimate-partner violence-related posttraumatic stress disorder. Psychiatry Res. 2013;211:93–103.
34. George DT, Phillips MJ, Lifshitz M, Lionetti TA, Spero DE, Ghassemzedeh N, Doty L, Umhau JC, Rawlings RR. Fluoxetine treatment of alcoholic perpetrators of domestic violence: a 12-week, double-blind, randomized, placebo-controlled intervention study. J Clin Psychiatry. 2011;72(1):60–5.
35. Guintivano J, Brown T, Newcomer A, Jones M, Cox O, Maher BA, Eaton WW, Payne JL, Wilcox HC, Kaminsky ZA. Identification and replication of a combined epigenetic and genetic biomarker predicting suicide and suicidal behaviors. Am J Psychiatry. 2014;171(12):1287–96.
36. Gunnar MR, Donzella B. Social regulation of the cortisol levels in early human development. Psychoneuroendocrinology. 2002;27(1–2):199–220.
37. Han DS, Boyle PA, Yu L, Fleischman DA, Arfanakis K, Leurgans S, Bennett DA. Financial literacy is associated with medial brain region functional connectivity in old age. Arch Gerontol Geriatr. 2014;59:429–38.
38. Harries P, Davies M, Gihooly M, Tomlinson C. Educating novice practitioners to detect elder financial abuse: a randomised controlled trial. BMC Med Educ. 2014;14:1–9.
39. Hayashi T, Ago K, Ago M, Yamanouchi H, Bunai Y, Ogata M. The infiltration of 'primed' neutrophils into multiple organs due to physical abuse to the elderly: an immunohistochemical study. Forensic Sci Int. 2010;202(1–3):17–25.
40. Hayashi T, Bunai Y, Ago K, Ago M, Ogata M. Thymus and adrenal glands in elder abuse. Am J Forensic Med Pathol. 2011;32(4):368–71.
41. Heath JM, Kobylarz FA, Brown M, Castano S. Interventions from home-based geriatric assessments of adult protective service clients suffering elder mistreatment. J Am Geriatr Soc. 2005;53:1538–42.
42. Heim C, Newport DJ, Mletzko T, Miller AH, Nemeroff CB. The link between childhood trauma and depression: insights from HPA axis studies in humans. Psychoneuroendocrinology. 2008;33(6):693–710.
43. Holkup PA, Tripp-Reimer T, Salois EM, Weinert C. Community-based participatory research: an approach to intervention research with a native american community. ANS Adv Nurs Sci. 2004;27(3):162–75.
44. Hommel KA, Modi AC, Piazza-Waggoner C, Myers JD. Topical review: translating translational research in behavioral science. J Pediatr Psychol. 2015. doi:10.1093/jpepsy/jsv049.
45. Hoover RM, Polson M. Detective elder abuse and neglect: assessment and intervention. Am Fam Physician. 2014;89 (6):453–60.
46. Irwin M, Brown M, Patterson T, Hauger R, Mascovich A, Grant I. Neuropeptide Y and natural killer cell activity: Findings in depression and Alzheimer caregiver stress. FASEB J. 1991;5 (15):3100–7.
47. Irwin M, Patterson T, Smith TL, Caldwell C, Brown SA, Gillin JC, Grant I. Reduction of immune function in life stress and depression. Biol Psychiatry. 1990;27(1):22–30.
48. James BD, Boyle PA, Bennett DA. Correlates of susceptibility to scams in older adults without dementia. J Elder Abuse Neglect. 2014;26:107–22.
49. Jern C, Eriksson E, Tengborn L, Risberg B, Wadenvik H, Jern S. Changes of plasma coagulation and fibrinolysis in response to mental stress. Thromb Haemost. 1989;62(2):767–71.
50. Johannsen M, LoGuidice D. Elder abuse: a systematic review of risk factors in community-dwelling elders. Age Ageing. 2013;42:292–8.
51. Jonson-Reid M, Drake B, Zhou P. Neglect subtypes, race, and poverty: individual, family, and service characteristics. Child Maltreat. 2013;18(1):30–41.
52. Kaminsky Z, Wilcox HC, Eaton WW, Van Eck K, Kilaru V, Jonanovic T, Klegnel T, Bradley B, Binder EB, Ressler KJ,

Smith AK. Epigenetic and genetic variation at SKA2 predict suicidal behavior and post-traumatic stress disorder. Transl Psychiatry. 2015;5:1–7.

53. Kananen L, Surakka I, Pirkola S, Suvisaari J, Lonnqvist J, Peltonen L, Ripatti S, Hovatta I. Childhood adversities are associated with shorter telomere length at adult age both in individuals with an anxiety disorder and controls. PLoS One. 2010;25(5):e10826.
54. Rv Känel, Dimsdale JE, Patterson TL, Grant I. Acute procoagulant stress response as a dynamic measure of allostatic load in Alzheimer caregivers. Ann Behav Med. 2003;26(1):42–8.
55. Khoury MJ, Gwinn M, Yoon PW, Dowling N, Moore CA, Bradley L. The continuum of translation research in genomic medicine: how can we accelerate the appropriate integration of human genome discoveries into health care and disease prevention? Genet Med. 2007;9(10):665–74. doi:10.1097/GIM.0b013e31815699d0.
56. Kiecolt-Glaser JK, Glaser R. Psychological stress and wound healing: Kiecolt-Glaser et al. (1995). Adv Mind Body Med. 2001;17(1):15–6.
57. Kiecolt-Glaser JK, Glaser R, Gravenstein S, Malarkey WB, Sheridan J. Chronic stress alters the immune response to influenza virus vaccine in older adults. Proc Natl Acad Sci USA. 1996;93:3043–7.
58. Kiecolt-Glaser JK, Gouin JP, Weng NP, Malarkey WB, Beversdorf DQ, Glaser R. Childhood adversity heightens the impact of later-life caregiving stress on telemere length and inflammation. Psychosom Med. 2011;73:16–22.
59. Kiecolt-Glaser JK, Marucha PT, Malarkey WB, Mercado AM, Glaser R. Slowing of wound healing by psychological stress. Lancet. 1995;346(8984):1194–6.
60. Kothari A, Sibbald SL, Wathen CN. Evaluation of partnerships in a transnational family violence prevention network using an integrated knowledge translation and exchange model: a mixed methods study. Health Res Policy Syst. 2014;12:1–11.
61. Lachs M, Williams CS, O'Brien S, Pillemer K. Adult protective service use and nursing home placement. Gerontologist. 2002;42(6):734–9.
62. Livingston G, Barber J, Rapaport P, Knapp M, Griffin M, King D, Livingston D, Mummery C, Walker Z, Hoe J, Sampson EL, Cooper C. Clinical effectiveness of a manual based coping strategy programme (START, STrAtegies for RelaTives) in promoting the mental health of carers of family members with dementia: pragmatic randomised controlled trial. BMJ. 2013;347:f6276. doi:10.1136/bmj.f6276.
63. MacGregor JC, Wathen N, Kothari A, Hundal PK, Naimi A. Strategies to promote uptake and use of intimate partner violence and child maltreatment knowledge: an integrative review. BMC Public Health. 2014;14:1–16.
64. Manly JT, Oshri A, Lynch M, Herzog M, Wortel S. Child neglect and the development of externalizing behavior problems: associations with maternal drug dependence and neighborhood crime. Child Maltreat. 2013;18(1):17–29.
65. Mausbach BT, Roepke SK, Ziegler MG, Milic M, von Känel R, Dimsdale JE, Mills PJ, Patterson TL, Allison MA, Ancoli-Israel S, Grant I. Association between chronic caregiving stress and impaired endothelial function in the elderly. J Am Coll Cardiol. 2010;55(23):2599–606.
66. McGowan PO, Sasaki A, D'Alessio AC, Dymov S, Labonte B, Szyf M, Turecki G, Meaney MJ. Epigenetic regulation of hte glucocorticoid receptor in human brain associates with childhood abuse. Nat Neurosci. 2011;12:342–8.
67. Miller WR, Rollnick S. Motivational Interviewing: preparing people to change addictive behavior. New York: Guilford Press; 1991.
68. Miriam LM, McClure R, Robinson JB, Yang JA. Eliciting change in at-risk elders (ECARE): evaluation of an elder abuse intervention program. J Elder Abuse Neglect. 2015;27(1):19–33.
69. Moffit TE, Tank TK-GT. Childhood exposure to violence and lifelong-health: Clinical intervention science and stress-biology research join forces. Dev Psychopathol. 2013;25:1619–34.
70. National Center on Elder Abuse AoA. Adult protective services. http://www.ncea.aoa.gov/Stop_Abuse/Partners/APS/index.aspx. Accessed 14 Aug 2015.
71. O'Brien MJ, Whitaker RC. The role of community-based participatory research to inform local health policy: a case study. J Gen Intern Med. 2011;26(12):1498–501.
72. O'Donovan A, Epel E, Lin J, Wolkowitz O, Cohen B, Maguen S, Metzler T, Lenoci M, Blackburn E, Neylan TC. Childhood trauma assocaited with short leukocyte telomere length in posttraumatic stress disorder. Biol Psychiatry. 2011;70(5):465–71.
73. Pace TW, Heim CM. A short review on the psychoneuroimmunology of posttraumatic stress disorder: from risk factors to medical comorbidities. Brain Behav Immun. 2011;25(1):6–13. doi:10.1016/j.bbi.2010.10.003.
74. Phillips JE, Marsland AL, Flory JD, Muldoon MF, Cohen S, Manuck SB. Parental education is related to C-reactive protein among female middle-aged community volunteers. Brain Behav Immun. 2009;23(5):677–83.
75. Ploeg J, Fear J, Hutchison B, MacMillan H, Bolan G. A systematic review of interventions for elder abuse. J Elder Abuse Neglect. 2009;21(3):187–210.
76. Pollitt RA, Kaufman JS, Rose KM, Diez-Roux AV, Zeng D, Heiss G. Early-life and adult socioeconomic status and inflammatory risk markers in adulthood. Eur J Epidemiol. 2007;22(1):55–66.
77. Richardson B, Kitchen G, Livingston G. The effect of education on knowledge and management of elder abuse: a randomized controlled trial. Age Ageing. 2002;31(5):335–41.
78. Rothwell PM. External validity of randomised controlled trials: "to whom do the results of this trial apply?". Lancet. 2005;365(9453):2–93.
79. Rubio DM, Schoenbaum EE, Lee LS, Schteingart DE, Marantz PR, Anderson KE, Platt LD, Baez A, Esposito K. Defining translational research: implications for training. Acad Med. 2010;85(3):470–5. doi:10.1097/ACM.0b013e3181ccd618.
80. Salimi Y, Shahandeh K, Malekafzali H, Loori N, Kheiltash A, Jamshidi E, Frouzan AS, Majdzadeh R. Is community-based participatory research (CBPR) useful? A systematic reiview on papers in a decade. Int J Prev Med. 2012;3(6):386–93.
81. Savolainen K, Eriksson JG, Kajantie E, Lahti J, Raikkonen K. Telomere length and hypothalamic-pituitary-adrenal axis response to stress in elderly adults. Psychoneuroendocrinology. 2015;53:179–84.
82. Schaakxs R, Wielaard I, Verhoeven JE, Beekman AT, Penninx BW, Comijs HC. Early and recent psychosocial stress and telomere length in older adults. Int Psychogeriatr (In Press);28:405–13.
83. Schiamberg LB, Barboza GG, Oehmke J, Zhang Z, Griffore RJ, Weatherill RP, von Heydrich L, Post LA. Elder abuse in nursing homes: an ecological perspective. J Elder Abuse Neglect. 2011;23(2):190–211.
84. Schiamberg LB, Gans D. Elder abuse by adult children: an applied ecological framework for understanding contextual risk factors and the intergenerational character of quality of life. Int J Aging Hum Dev. 2000;50(4):329–59.
85. Schofield MJ, Powers JR, Loxton D. Mortality and disability outcomes of self-reported elder abuse: a 12-year prospective

investigation. J Am Geriatr Soc. 2013;61(5):679–85. doi:10.1111/jgs.12212.
86. Shirtcliff EA, Coe CL, Pollak SD. Early childhood stress is associated with elevated antibody levels to herpes simplex virus type 1. Proc Natl Acad Sci USA. 2009;106(8):2963–7.
87. Smith AK, Conneely KN, Kilaru V, Mercer KB, Weiss TE, Bradley B, Tang Y, Gillespie CF, Cubells JF, Ressler KJ. Differential immune system DNA methylation and cytokine regulation in post-traumatic stress disorder. Am J Med Genet B Neuropsychiatr Genet. 2011;156B(6):700–8.
88. Steptoe A, Hamer M, Chida Y. The effects of acute psychological stress on circulating inflammatory factors in humans: a review and meta-analysis. Brain Behav Immun. 2007;21(7):901–12. doi:10.1016/j.bbi.2007.03.011.
89. Sullivan MW, Bennett DS, Lewis M. Individual differences in the cortisol responses of neglected and comparison children. Child Maltreat. 2012;18(1):8–16.
90. Sumner SA, Mercy JA, Dahlberg LL, Hillis SD, Klevens J, Houry D. Violence in the United States: status, challenges, and opportunities. JAMA. 2015;314(5):478–88.
91. Sung NS, Crowley WF, Grenel M, Salber P, Sandy L, Sherwood LM, Johnson SB, Catanese V, Tilson H, Getz K, Larson EL, Scheinberg D, Reece EA, Slavkin H, Dobs A, Grebb J, Martinez RA, Korn A, Rimoin D. Central challenges facing the national clincal research enterprise. JAMA. 2003;289(10):1278–87.
92. Taussig HN, Culhane SE, Garrido E, Knudtson MD, Petrenko CLM. Does severity of physical neglext moderate the impact of an efficacious preventive intervention for maltreated children in foster care? Child Maltreat. 2012;18(1):56–64.
93. Taylor SE, Lehman BJ, Kiefe CI, Seeman TE. Relationship of early life stress and psychological functioning to adult C-reactive protein in the coronary artery risk development in young adults study. Biol Psychiatry. 2006;60(8):819–24.
94. Teresi JA, Ramirez M, Ellis J, Silver S, Boratgis G, Kong J, Eimicke JP, Pillemer K, Lachs M. A staff intervention targeting resident-to-resident elder mistreatment (R-REM) in long-term care increased staff knowledge, recognition and reporting: results from a cluster randomized trial. Int J Nurs Stud. 2013;50(5):644–56.
95. Tyrka AR, Parade SH, Price LH, Kao HT, Prorton B, Philip NS, Welch ES, Carpenter LL. Alterations of mitochondrial DNA copy number and telomere length with early adversity and psychopathology. Biol Psychiatry (In Press)
96. Tyrka AR, Price LH, Kao HT, Porton B, Marsella SA, Carpenter LL. Childhood maltreatment and telomere shortening: preliminary support for an effect of early stress on cellular aging. Biol Psychiatry. 2010;67(6):531–4.
97. von Kanel R, Mausbach BT, Dimsdale JE, Mills PJ, Patterson TL, Ancoli-Israel S, Ziegler MG, Roepke SK, Chattillion EA, Allison M, Grant I. Effect of chronic dementia caregiving and major transitions in the caregiving situation on kidney function: a longitudinal study. Psychosom Med. 2012;74(2):214–20.
98. Weisberg RB, Bruce SE, Machan JT, Kessler RC, Culpepper L, Keller MB. Nonpsychiatric illness among primary care patients with trauma histories and posttraumatic stress disorder. Psychiatric Services. 2002;53:848–54.
99. Westfall JM, Mold J, Fagnan L. Practice-based research—"Blue Highways" on the NIH roadmap. JAMA. 2007;297:403–6.
100. Widom CS, Czaja S, Wilson HW, Allwood M, Chauhan P. Do the long-term consequences of neglect differ for children of different races and ethnic backgrounds? Child Maltreat. 2013;18(1):42–55.
101. Woolf SH. The meaning of translational research and why it matters. JAMA. 2008;299(2):211–3.
102. Yaffe MJ, Tazkarji B. Understanding elder abuse in family practice. Can Fam Physician. 2012;58(12):1336–40.

Elder Abuse: Education and Training

34

James G. O'Brien

Elder abuse is a pernicious, pervasive problem, which robs victims of quality of life and results in significant morbidity and mortality in the final phase of life. Despite this fact, elder abuse remains the orphan area compared to child abuse and domestic violence judged by the amount of funding for research and for programs to combat elder abuse [1].

It is shocking to note that elder abuse first recognized in the British Medical literature in the mid-1970s, rather than declining as a result of federal and state programs where reporting abuse is almost universally mandated in fact the incidence of abuse appears to be increasing on an annual basis.

Many educational programs targeting professionals who are likely to have involvement in detection, reporting, intervention, and ongoing management have been launched with mixed success. A particular challenge exists given the nature of the topic particularly in the medical community [2] where significant barriers exist from a lack of knowledge, time pressured encounters, and frustrations when abuse is reported. Similarly, education of the public and policymakers have occurred with key researchers giving evidence to Senate hearings with the intent of recruiting champions for the cause and seeking funding support. It is evident that vast resources of educational materials exist for all who may be involved in the study or management of abuse including victims. Existing programs must be strengthened and expanded, and new initiatives that emphasize and interdisciplinary approach need to be launched.

In terms of the continuum of abuse from Child Abuse to Intimate Partner Abuse/Domestic Violence, some strategies may be applicable to the field of Elder abuse.

J.G. O'Brien (✉)
Institute on Sustainable Health and Optimal Aging, 6863 Timberlake Drive, Elk Rapids, MI 49629, USA
e-mail: jim.obrien@louisville.edu

X. Dong (ed.), *Elder Abuse*, DOI 10.1007/978-3-319-47504-2_34

Child Abuse:
In terms of recognition and generation of a response to the problem, Child Abuse has the longest history and legislation requiring mandatory reporting. Over time a variety of centers have evolved with much more funding and resources than are available for elder abuse. Pursuit of programmatic or research funding or enacting protective legislation has much more appeal when compared to elder abuse which is understandable when a helpless abused or neglected child is featured in an appeal. The National Center on Child Abuse [3] provides an array of training and educational programs. Core Principles:

1. *Competency-Based Training* Geared toward building knowledge, skills, and behaviors that are needed to provide quality family support services.
2. *Tailored Curricula* A curriculum that is specific to each organization. Initial assessment of training needs, level of knowledge, and key outcomes that organization would like to achieve.
3. *Long-Term Access* Strives to provide long-term partnerships by making staff and resources available. The first center devoted to the study and treatment of child abuse was established in 1972 by C Henry Kempe [4].

Intimate Partner Violence IPV/Domestic Violence (UK) IPV was next in the sequence of recognition and development of legislation and public policy to combat the problem. Experts in both fields would claim that there is a significant lack of funding to adequately combat the problem. The National online resource center on violence against women is a treasure trove of education and training resources [5]. A slide presentation on the chronology of domestic violence from national awareness to the present time is perhaps something that could be copied for the field of elder abuse.

The section on education and awareness has subsections devoted to:

1. Community Mobilization/Increasing Engagement.
2. Community Organizing.
3. Domestic Violence Against Men (DVAM).
4. Outreach.

Many have advocated for additional training and educational efforts, Hamberger [6] highlighted the dire need to train physicians to screen for IPV across all medical specialties and noted the lack of screening in primary care, emergency medicine and obstetrics, and gynecology. He expressed hope that the next generation of physicians may be more willing to become engaged. Yapp [7] suggested following the National Institute for Health Care Excellence (NICE) guidelines, which emphasize not only to enquire about domestic violence but also emphasizes requirement of training to understand the implications of disclosure and its impact on the patient's life, and to identify the patient's immediate and long-term needs. The guidelines also emphasize the need to understand the different cultures and their attitude toward violence. Torjesen [8] recommended training for all doctors similar to the mandatory training for child protection. He deplored the fact that training in domestic violence is absent from the curriculum in undergraduate medical education. NICE recommends four levels of response:

1. Targeting receptionists allied health professionals how to respond to disclosure.
2. Doctors, nurses, social workers to ask about IPV and refer.
3. And 4. Specialist services to address the problem and safeguard staff and domestic violence workers.

It would appear to be perhaps a model that could be duplicated in this country for elder abuse although the range of supportive/social services provided in the UK is superior to what is available in this country. Examples of training programs Integrating IPV curriculum in training program for Nurse Practitioners in response to meeting WHO objectives "A Global Campaign on Violence Prevention" [9]. Which educated nurse educators (train the trainers) to become knowledgeable regarding intimate partner violence, and to integrate this content into nursing curricula resulting in a ripple effect and impacting in a positive way new graduates. Boursnell and Prosser [10] developed a program to improve the quality of identification and response practices of emergency department nurses to domestic violence. A pre and post survey showed improvement in confidence, practice, and skills.

34.1 Target-Audience

The potential audience who can be educated and potentially play a role is vast. It is difficult to prioritize in terms of which group has the most urgent need. I suggest the elderly of this country and especially the Baby Boomers who may be able to take measures to prevent abuse occurring in the future. This group should be made aware of danger signals, available resources, and options if abuse occurs.

It is sad to note the limited education provided to Adult Protective Services (APS) caseworkers [11] with tremendous variation by state with some states providing no specific training pertaining to elder abuse. This is a potentially disastrous with the increased number of reports, increased complexity, and presence of multiple forms of abuse present in the same victim [11]. Health care providers especially physicians, nurse practitioners, physician assistants, and social workers who are most likely to encounter cases need to be educated regarding detection, intervention, and state reporting requirements. Educational programs need to reflect the context in which abuse may occur from emergency and trauma settings to primary care clinics to home care locations and long-term care settings.

Police/law enforcement officers require special training. Louisville is fortunate to have a special police unit dedicated to protection of vulnerable elderly; Crimes Against the Elderly, who are an integral part of a response team with APS and Elder Serve, a social services advocacy group.

Given the frequency with which financial abuse occurs, bankers, especially front line counter staff, lawyers, and health care providers require training in detection and intervention in abuse cases. A model program as developed by Robert Roush at Baylor [12] has done much to address this problem. Administrators, staff, and practitioners in long-term care settings who provide care to the most vulnerable and at risk population require special training [13]. Finally, policy makers at a federal and state level require education regarding the need to provide funding for adequate services to respond to suspected cases.

34.2 Minority Groups/Cultural Sensitivity

It is evident given the heterogeneity of the elderly population that one size response approach does not fit all. The challenge posed when establishing educational and training programs appropriate for minority, culturally or ethnically diverse populations is greatly magnified. Dong [14] highlights the plight of an elderly Chinese population in Chicago noting a high prevalence of abuse of 23 % with neglect being the most common type encountered. Neglect is particularly destructive in an elderly Chinese population given an implicit expectation of filial piety with continued family support. Thus, neglect violates a traditional Confucian principle. Neglect by family members may be so destructive to elderly women that it may result in suicide.

An approach to address abuse in a culturally diverse population suggested by Dong Community-Based Participatory Research Methodology (CBPRM) which requires workers to be educated regarding cultural awareness and an understanding of interventions that are likely to be successful. This approach requires learners to "become better listeners and humble students of older adults".

Another example of a minority group requiring a different approach—Native American/Alaskan native populations [15]. The challenges posed are enormous given the multiplicity of tribes many of whom have sovereign nation status. Most are underserved in terms of available resources to address abuse and neglect. Compounding factors include extreme poverty, isolation, and differences in opinion in terms of what constitutes abuse. Application of CBPRM approach as the training model has perhaps the greatest chance for success.

34.3 Training

National Center on Elder Abuse (NCEA) [16] has defined training characteristics that are most likely to be effective. Important elements include an interdisciplinary approach, which allows opportunities to understand the role of other disciplines and to respond to situations where multiple types of abuse with increasing complexity exist. This approach [17] was utilized to educate physicians in Michigan with by Sengstock utilizing experts in the field including social work, nursing, geriatrics, law, and casework. The program was offered at six different sites throughout the state. The program was well received but suffered from requiring a 6 h commitment a problem particularly for physicians and an inability to schedule a follow-up meeting to reinforce learning. It is essential with any offering that the very best trainers/teachers conduct the sessions and adapt to the specific learning styles of the audience. Case-based and problem-solving approaches are most likely to be effective and keep the audience engaged. Allowing adequate time for the participants to respond and discuss experiences and express frustrations with system failures is essential. This allows for suggestions of alternate approaches that may be more effective. A particular frustration occurs when an abuse situation is identified and the victim refuses to cooperate and corroborate the presence of abuse. Another area of frustration requiring discussion is determining capacity not that all disciplines should be capable of determining capacity but at a minimum possess a working knowledge and understand when and whom to refer for determination.

Ethical Issues Training: This is an essential area for health care providers and caseworkers to be knowledgeable when confronted with an ethical issue. Finding a balance between paternalism and respect for autonomy is at the core of the dilemma. Key elements that need to be emphasized in any educational program include the assessment of capacity with an understanding that capacity can fluctuate and should be viewed as being on a sliding scale. Capacity can be affected by a variety of factors including medications, infections, and other metabolic disturbances resulting in delirium, which may be transient in contrast with dementia, which is not reversible. A victim may lack the ability to understand and render a decision regarding a complex financial matter but retain the ability to decide to remain in an at risk situation and understand the potential consequences and express their preference. The determination of capacity is such a critical issue that intensive training is required and perhaps carried out using case studies with experts serving as teachers. Front line practitioners should understand that assessment of capacity may need to be repeated and when in doubt referral to an expert such as a psychiatrist, psychologist, or geriatrician. The mandate to report suspected abuse in most states needs to be emphasized (a particular problem for physicians [18]. The benefits of detection and intervention need to be stressed. Intervention on the part of general practitioners in Ireland [8] verified a perceived improvement in the situation for the victim. Two model programs that have proven to be particularly effective. An excellent program to educate staff in Nursing homes developed by Pillemer and Hudson [13], which targeted nursing assistants with support from administration and included eight modules addressing topics such as Identification and recognition; Understanding feelings about care giving; Abuse of staff by residents; Intervention strategies. Key strategies included case-based approaches and role-playing. Pre and post testing revealed satisfaction with the program and more importantly a decline in self-reported abusive actions by the staff. Another model program in Ireland [19] which featured an interdisciplinary training program with Public Health Nurses and Social workers primarily in response to the perceived increasing complexity of elder abuse and self-neglect cases. Topics addressed included intentional versus unintentional abuse and neglect, a critical evaluation of policies and procedures, maximizing team problem solving and collaboration, and a case-based discussion of ethical issues. The curriculum was conducted in two sessions, initially a 2 h session followed 1 week later by a 4 h session. Evaluation of the program by the participants was very positive.

34.4 Resources

A vast array of educational and training resources exists for all groups involved in some aspect of elder abuse and neglect. It is remarkable that the American Medical Association [20] published guidelines in the early 1990s to educate and assist physicians in the detection and management of elder abuse cases, despite this physicians still lag behind most other professionals in reporting [2, 21]. It is heartening to witness that major organizations such as AARP, AMA, and many professional organizations have devoted significant efforts to address the problem. The popular press, including Wall Street Journal, New York Times, local papers and a variety of TV networks have helped acquaint the public as to the existence of abuse. Unfortunately, it is the most sensational cases, which are featured at the expense of the more common but still significantly harmful cases. A recent publication of Consumer Reports [22] although with a smaller audience published a most helpful article on financial abuse and fraud in the elderly population. The article provides an excellent overview of the problem, and it first featured a variety of victims demonstrating the diversity and the vulnerability of the victims despite their level of education. Many scams specifically target older individuals because of their particular perceived vulnerability (not that all are at risk) in dealing with complex financial decisions, learning new material, perhaps being more trusting and more easily subjected to aggressive practices results in the ideal target for the scammer. Despite the fact that most are not cognitively impaired, approximately 30–50 % in their ninth decade suffers from a dementing illness making them particularly vulnerable to fraud.

Initiatives that are already in place include a program "Stop Senior Scams Acting Program" consisting of a troupe of actors in the Los Angeles area who travel to community centers, churches, dramatizing a variety of scams. Many of the actors are previous victims or near-victims thus adding credibility to the presentation.

A major emphasis highlighting fraud and scam protection requiring federal and state action is proposed:

1. Request telecom companies to offer call blocking technologies to stop "ROBOCALLS" that often result in scams.
2. Request states to pass new civil statutes to allow victims to sue perpetrators of fraud for full recovery of losses including legal fees.
3. Develop training programs to educate physicians in the recognition of fraud as developed by Roush and others with national dissemination.
4. Establish more elder abuse task forces with broad-based representation allowing for greater sharing and collaborative intervention.

An exceptional educational program developed at Baylor School of Medicine, The Elder Investment, Fraud, and Financial Exploitation (EIFFE) [12] now with a national reach utilizing experts in the involved states to teach a standardized curriculum but allowing for modification based on state laws. This is ideally taught by an interdisciplinary faculty. A product of this program has been the development of a convenient pocket guide, which highlights red flags to raise suspicion of abuse or fraud. A list of local and state resources is also included.

The NCEA houses a myriad of resources that are easily accessible to public and professionals. NCEA supported by the administration on aging serves a very broad audience including public, policy makers, social service, and health care providers, the justice system, researchers, advocates, and families. NCEA has promoted World Elder Abuse Awareness Day on June 15th 2015, an annual event with worldwide engagement and sharing of new developments in combating this problem. Leading up to this day; a weekly forum focusing on elder justice themes, which featured experts and was accessible via twitter, blogs, and included an international webinar. NCEA includes a variety of sections including definitions, warning signs, resources, preventive measures, and frequently asked questions. NCEA houses an extensive resource library housing a research database and a section on future directions of particular use to budding and established researchers in the field.

An important resource devoted to public policy, which includes congressional hearings, federal and state laws. Congressional hearings with the special committee on aging serves as the focal point to discuss elder abuse and hopefully influence more favorable legislation and increased possibility of federal funding. In 2011, during the 112th Congress the topic "Justice for All: Ending Elder Abuse, Neglect, and Financial Exploitation" was a very important opportunity to educate our legislators and recruit champions for the cause.

A section devoted to government reports, congressional reports, and testimony including the Elder Justice Roadmap Project Report a resource for strategic planning to combat abuse. Other valuable educational resources include available direct services, cultural competency, policy, and research.

Other major agencies involved in the study and development of responses to abuse include the CDC, AARP, AMA, and the National Institute of Justice to name some. Other national resources that contribute greatly to combating abuse, many based at academic medical centers such as The Center of Excellence on Elder Abuse at the University of California Irvine [23] offering a variety of educational programs and serves as a resource for victims. Faculty work with professionals in the areas of law enforcement, legal, judicial, medicine, nursing, pharmacy, social services, and the general public with a stated purpose of elder abuse prevention. A variety of programs includes a special team to respond to financial abuse. Financial Abuse Specialist Team (FAST) and an Elder Death Review team educating agencies regarding suspicious deaths. Another excellent resource includes a video featuring Dr. Laura Mosqueda on forensic markers of abuse and neglect of particular relevance to physicians and nurses and coroners.

More recently, The Keck School of Medicine at the University of Southern California with support from the Administration on Aging instituted the National Center on Elder Abuse [24], which will provide technical assistance and training to states and community-based organizations to develop effective strategies to prevent abuse and serve as a clearinghouse for resources in this area.

A major educational contribution has occurred as a result of the efforts of many of the pioneers and leaders in the field, Bitondo-Dyer, Dong, Fulmer, Lachs, Mosqueda, Pilleemer, Podnieks, Sengstock, Stahl, Tatara to name some. Clearly, there are many others who have made a major contribution to enhance understanding of the problem.

As Geriatrics/Gerontology has an increasing presence in the curriculum of most professional schools (still inadequate), elder abuse has gained an increasing presence and visibility. The Geriatrics Review Syllabus, the "Bible" [25] for fellows in training features a section on elder abuse. Another influential indispensable resource for Geriatricians, Geriatric Nurse Practitioners "Geriatrics at Your Fingertips" [26] addresses the Mistreatment of Older Adults including risk factors, assessment and treatment including issues of capacity.

A significant educational effort occurs in many professional schools with the increase in geriatrics/gerontology with elder abuse included as an element. Just as many in the field believe, geriatrics still is under-represented; it is likely that addressing the topic of abuse could be expanded. The Journal of Elder Abuse and Neglect an international publication devoted exclusively to research of abuse and neglect with an expanding audience. This has been a key resource to share a world perspective on the subject. Many other journals including major impact journals periodically publish studies of elder abuse.

National conferences in Geriatrics/Gerontology have allowed attendees with an interest to attend special interest groups creating greater dissemination of knowledge. Many of the pioneers in the field, through their tireless work have brought the phenomenon to the attention of a much wider audience from policy makers to the public, and have been key in securing funding and legislative changes.

Elder Justice Act 2002/2003 represented a significant effort to stimulate the federal government to increase funding and implement new legislation for the prevention of elder abuse. Elder abuse represents less than 2 % of the federal budget devoted to violence prevention and lacks the presence of a designated person at a federal level as an advocate on behalf of elder abuse prevention [27].

34.5 Conclusion

It would appear that all the tools to conduct effective education and training are available and accessible but the perception still exist that knowledge of abuse and more particularly intervention strategies still seem to be lacking. It appears that for many practitioners detection of abuse is delegated to a lower level when addressing the multiple medical problems that afflict older adults unless the abuse is so evident that it cannot be ignored.

Education and training to be effective need an incentive for participation whether knowledge in this area will be a requirement for licensure, specialty accreditation, a marker of quality, or a financial reward for addressing the problem. Educational and training programs need outstanding teachers who need the funding and support to effectively disseminate knowledge. Educational efforts need to be on a par with child abuse and domestic violence.

References

1. Connolly M, Trilling A. Seven policy priorities for an enhanced public health response to elder abuse. Workshop summary. Washington, D.C.: National Academies Press; 2014. www.nap.edu. Accessed 5 Sep 2016.
2. O'Brien J. A physicians perspective: elder abuse and neglect over 25 years. J Elder Abuse Negl. 2010;22(12):94–104.
3. Child Welfare Information Gateway. www.childwelfare.gov. Accessed 5 Sep 2016.
4. The Kempe Center for the Prevention and Treatment of Child Abuse and Neglect. www.kempe.org. Accessed 5 Sep 2016.
5. VAWnet, The National Online Resource Center on Violence Against Women. www.vawnet.org. Accessed 5 Sep 2016.
6. Hamberger l. Preparing the next generation of physicians: medical school and residency-based intimate partner violence curriculum and evaluation. Trauma Violence Abuse. 2007;8(2):214–25.
7. Yapp C, Training doctors to respond to domestic violence: more than just communication skills. BMJ 2014;348. p. 2203.
8. Torjesen I, Doctors need training to respond to domestic violence, NICE guidance says. BMJ 2014;348. Issue 7947, p. 1.
9. Tufts K, Clements P, Karlowicz K. Integrating intimate partner violence content across curricula: developing a new generation of Nurse Educators. Nurse Educ Today. 2009;29:40–7.
10. Boursnell M, Prosser S. Increasing identification of domestic violence in emergency departments: a collaborative contribution to increasing the quality of practice of emergency nurses. Contemp Nurse. J Aust Nurs Prof. 2010 Apr–May;35(1):35–46.
11. Quinn K. Elder neglect and the APS workforce. Institute of Medicine of the National Academies. Washington D.C. A Public Workshop of the Forum on Global Violence Prevention. 2013.
12. Roush R, Moye J, Mills W, Kuninik M, Wilson N, Taffett G, Naik A. Why physicians need to know about know about the elder

investment fraud and financial exploitation prevention program (EIFFE). Generation 2012;36(2):94–97.
13. Pillemer K, Hudson B. A model abuse prevention program for nursing assistants. Gerontologist 1993;33(1):128–1.
14. Dong Elder Abuse and Its Prevention. Forum on Global Violence prevention. IOM and National Research Council 2014.
15. Jervis L, Fickensher A, Beals J. Assessment of elder mistreatment in two american indian samples: psychometric characteristics of the HS-EAST and the native elder life financial exploitation and neglect measures. J Appl Gerontol. 2013;32(7):2–8.
16. www.ncea.gov. Accessed 5 Sep 2016.
17. Sengstock M, O'Brien, Goldynia A, Trainer T, De Spelder T, Lienhart K. Elder abuse training for health care professionals. AOA 1990.
18. O'Brien J, Collins C, Ni Riain A, Long V, O'Neill D. Elder abuse and neglect: a survey of irish general practitioners. J Elder Abuse Negl. 2014;26:291–9.
19. Day M, Bantry-White E, Glavin P. Protection of vulnerable adults: an interdisciplinary workshop. Commun Pract. 2010;83(9):29–32.
20. Physicians Obligations in Preventing, Identifying and Treating Violence and Abuse (Adopted Nov 2007) Initial Monograph 1992 www.ama-assn.org. Accessed 5 Sep 2016.
21. Clancy M, McDaid B, O'Neill D, O'Brien J. National profiling of elder abuse referrals. Age Aging 2011;40(1–6):346–352.
22. A Crying Shame. Consumer reports. 2015. www.consumerreports.org.
23. Center of Excellence on Elder Abuse and Neglect, University of California Irvine. www.centeronelderabuse.org. Accessed 5 Sep 2016.
24. The National Center on Elder Abuse at the Keck School of Medicine at University of Southern California. www.ncea.aoa.gov. Accessed 5 Sep 2016.
25. www.geriatricscareonline.org. Accessed 5 Sep 2016.
26. Geriatrics at Your Fingertips 2015, 17th Ed. AGS.
27. Blancato R, Elder abuse and its prevention workshop summary. 2014.

35 Future Directions in Public Policy Relating to Elder Abuse

Marshall B. Kapp

35.1 Introduction

As the earlier chapters of this book make abundantly clear, as the planet's population ages "[e]lder abuse is a universal phenomenon" [49]. It is present in both developed and developing [69] countries [61, 62]. Moreover, precisely defining the parameters of this multi-faceted problem, identifying specific instances of its occurrence, and devising and implementing effective preventative and corrective strategies to respond to the problem and its consequences raises an array of complicated and challenging public policy concerns. Enumerating and discussing, with an orientation toward the future, some of the most salient of these public or social policy (defined expansively as principles of government action that affect citizens individually or through group relationships [3]) concerns constitute the subject matter of the current chapter.

This chapter presents a combination of descriptive information, critical analysis, and prescriptive recommendations for public policy creators and advocates in the elder abuse arena as they attempt to navigate the often delicate boundaries between personal, interpersonal, civil society, and governmental interests [4]. Following this present brief introduction, I set the general stage by identifying some of the main relevant international proclamations, distinguishing between "hard" or real law, on one hand, and "soft" or aspirational law, on the other. In the next section, the policy landscape in the United States, which is described in depth in the previous chapters, is referenced, along with a summary of policy forays into elder abuse engaged by other nations. Ensuing after that exposition is an explication of a number of distinct but interrelated conceptual and political themes, often controversial and even contentious, that permeate the elder abuse sphere and that need to be at least properly accounted for, if not completely resolved, if we are to make meaningful progress in improving the quality of life for older persons by reducing or eliminating the threat of mistreatment. A short review of the primary lessons that may be drawn from the chapter contents serves as a conclusion.

35.2 International Statements

35.2.1 Statements

There exists no shortage of recent international pronouncements (variously labeled as declarations, proclamations, conventions, charters, statements, and other terms) pertaining to the subject of elder abuse. The Political Declaration and Madrid International Plan of Action on Ageing (Madrid Plan) adopted by the Second World Assembly on Ageing in Madrid, Spain in 2002 placed the importance of healthy aging (including as one component freedom from abuse) within the framework of the Universal Declaration on Human Rights [75]. Among its numerous other exhortations, it called on the governments of sovereign nations to "develop and fund a National comprehensive strategy and Agenda to prevent, detect and intervene in elder abuse," mainly through resource redistribution. The Madrid Plan has been endorsed by the European Commission and the 2002 Toronto Declaration on the Global Prevention of Elder Abuse and is consistent with Article 9 of the European Union's Charter of Rights [1], all of which implore individual countries to take affirmative actions to prevent elder abuse [84]. The Vienna Ministerial Declaration of 2012 referred to the need for national policies on the health and welfare of older persons to be accompanied by measures to empower older individuals and to prevent their abuse, neglect, and loneliness. The United Nations (UN) has issued a large volume of resolutions following up on the work of the Second World Assembly on Aging, for instance U.N. General Assembly Resolution 67/143 in 2013 calling upon member states to address cases of neglect, abuse, and

M.B. Kapp (✉)
Center for Innovative Collaboration in Medicine and Law, Florida State University, 1115 W. Call Street, Tallahassee, FL 32306, USA
e-mail: marshall.kapp@med.fsu.edu

X. Dong (ed.), *Elder Abuse*, DOI 10.1007/978-3-319-47504-2_35

violence against older persons by designing and implementing more effective prevention strategies and policies.

Another form of international public pronouncement is the declaration of an annual World Elder Abuse Awareness Day (WEAAD) by the self-organized International Network for Prevention of Elder Abuse (INPEA) [61]. This activity in support of the Madrid Plan is intended to raise consciousness globally and encourage individual nations to put elder abuse on their respective policy agendas. Since its inception on June 15, 2006, many civil society groups and governments around the world have joined in the exercise [49]. The 2015 edition of the WEAAD featured a First GLOBAL Summit on June 15 in Washington, DC, convened jointly by the INPEA, National Adult Protective Services Association, and National Center for Victims of Crime.

35.2.2 Soft Law Versus Hard Law

Most of the international pronouncements and activities mentioned above have been released to the public with a substantial flourish of formal pomp and circumstance. Nevertheless, these pronouncements and other exercises are hortatory in nature, "calling upon," "encouraging," and "requesting" sovereign countries to act in some particular manner or other. They emanate from organizations such as the World Health Organization (WHO), which lacks the ability to translate its rhetoric into action [25]. As such, the pronouncement and other exercises described constitute examples of "soft" law or policy that express arguably admirable aspirations but totally lack meaningful enforcement or implementation authority [5, 27]. For example, the Madrid Plan presents a list of elder rights and corresponding governmental and private duties in absolute terms, with no acknowledgement at all of costs, resource limitations, or other competing considerations; as such, it is difficult to foresee those parts of the Plan achieving anything other than aspirational status in the near future. If international frameworks and the like carried the power to actually compel concrete action by specific parties, those frameworks would amount to unfunded mandates and likely would meet resistance for that reason.

By contrast, "hard" or real law is binding on actual, named parties and is subject to enforcement by governmental agencies with legitimate authority to act. Enunciated policy frameworks may, of course, serve as the basis for subsequent hard law. In the international context, the only hard or real law is embodied in treaties that individual countries have positively chosen to ratify and thereby bind themselves to observe and be held accountable for compliance.

As described by one legal scholar,

> The challenge for lawyers, advocates and policymakers is that the human rights of older persons have not yet been well defined in international human rights law, and governments (national, regional and local) are presently developing law and policy in the absence of a specific treaty with binding obligations to respect and protect the rights of older people. ...[T]he only instruments specifically concerned with older persons reflect non-binding, soft law. ...Thus, the most pertinent instruments are cast in aspirational tones which do not always speak to older persons in terms of conferring positive "rights," but rather to their carers or those providing services to them, particularly governments. [41, p. 114]

The same scholar opines, "The consequence is that the rights of older persons are effectively marginalized under international human rights law..." [41, p. 104]. Thus, even the most idealistic proponents of soft human rights proclamations reluctantly concede, "The rights and obligations contained in international law cannot be fulfilled without robust domestic implementation through legal, policy, and economic reforms" [23, p. 71]. Stated differently, "If global health treaties fail to gain traction in the hierarchy of international law, then other regimes could effectively eviscerate their impact" [23, p. 295]. In the elder abuse context specifically, it is recognized that, "more than a decade later [after the Madrid Plan], the United Nations processes have failed to yield concrete changes in law and governance" [24, p. 115].

Various references in the text below to the policy actions of various countries show that some of those countries have attempted to turn soft law pronouncements into domestic hard law. For example, China drew significant international attention in 2013 when it amended its "Law of Protection of Rights and Interests of the Aged" to require offspring of parents older than 60 to visit their parents frequently and make certain their financial and spiritual needs are met [48]. Any particular country's response to the opportunity to convert international soft law into domestic hard law depends on a constellation of cultural and political factors that are specific to that country.

35.3 Specific National Responses

Although internationalists blame gaps in domestic elder abuse laws and the rights of older persons generally on the lack of international declarations on the subject [41], meaningful authority to make and implement social policy and law properly rests with sovereign national governments and their political subdivisions. There is enormous variation among separate governments in terms of their respective elder abuse policies or lack thereof [51]. Accordingly, it is instructive to study how specific countries have officially and unofficially responded to the challenge of elder abuse.

35.3.1 United States

In the U.S., policies related to the elder abuse situation may be, and frequently are, considered, formulated, and implemented concurrently at the federal (national), state, and local levels, unless the federal government has clearly chosen to preempt a specific portion of the subject matter [20]. Congressional authority in this sphere ordinarily emanates either from the U.S. Constitution's Article I grant of power to Congress to regulate interstate and foreign commerce or the Article I empowerment of Congress to collect taxes and then spend those revenues to promote the general welfare (usually by providing grants to the states with particular programmatic conditions or strings attached). States and local government subdivisions generally derive their authority from either their inherent police power to protect and promote the health, safety, welfare, and morals of the community or their *parens patriae* ("father of the land") power to protect individuals who are not capable of protecting themselves from potential harm.

The three main current federal statutes relevant to elder abuse are Title VII (Vulnerable Elder Rights Protection Activities) of the Older Americans Act (OAA), the Violence against Women Act, and the Elder Justice Act (EJA) portion of the Affordable Care Act (ACA) [10, 13, 15, 17]. These legislative enactments and their respective historical origins, implementation experiences, and future challenges have been discussed extensively previously in Chapters 27–31 and other literature [35]. At the time the present chapter was being written, the Elder Justice Reauthorization Act, H.R. 988, was awaiting Congressional action [11]. Also at the federal level, some commentators have criticized the Centers for Disease Control and Prevention (CDC) (examined in Chapter 32) on the grounds that "that organization has not focused scientific attention or funding on elder mistreatment, or even recognized it as a public health problem." These critics further assert that "programs funded by the Older American Act also have not placed elder mistreatment as a central priority. Much more could be done to integrate measures to reduce elder mistreatment into existing OAA initiatives, such as the aging network and caregiving programs" [59, p. 325].

Most of the hands-on programmatic activity takes place at the state level. There, elder abuse is dealt with primarily through Adult Protective Services (APS) and Long-Term Care Ombudsman programs administered by local governmental or private, not-for-profit (also termed voluntary or community) human services agencies and funded through the OAA and Social Security Title 'Adult Protective Services and the Long-term Care Ombudsman Program' block grants to the states [10, 14, 21]. The OAA was most recently reauthorized in 2015. APS professionals are represented in policy circles by their trade group, the National Adult Protective Services Association [65]. The APS network (the effectiveness of which is a hotly debated topic [56]) and Long-Term Care Ombudsman programs [50] are covered in depth in Chapter 15 of this book.

State laws on elder abuse vary significantly in terms of definitions, reporting requirements, training, and consequences for failure to report [32]. The results of state efforts thus far regarding elder abuse have been criticized [22, 81]. National reforms have been called for to increase legal accountability. Proposed reforms include a federal elder abuse court, federal private rights of action, and other federal remedial legislation [86].

In July 2015, the executive branch of the federal government sponsored a White House Conference on Aging (WHCoA), an activity that incumbent presidents have initiated every 10 years over the past half century. The 2005 WHCoA produced a recommendation on "Protection from Elder Abuse and Neglect" that stressed the creation of a national strategy for the promotion of elder justice [72]. In preparation for the 2015 event, the planners identified Elder Justice (defined to include "elder financial exploitation, abuse and neglect") as one of the four priority topical areas to receive concentrated attention at the WHCoA [34, 59]. In formulating a list of specific issues for consideration under the Elder Justice umbrella [80], WHCoA planners had available data from the Elder Justice Roadmap, an intensive joint effort of the U.S. Department of Justice and the Department of Health and Human Services designed to set strategic priorities to advance elder justice. Using a concept mapping process, this project (which is the basis for an ongoing blog maintained by the National Center on Elder Abuse) sought the perspectives of shareholders and experts in gerontology about their most critical public policy priorities [76]. Several Government Accountability Office (GAO) reports [77–79] also provided useful background information for WHCoA planners.

The 2015 White House Conference served as the opportunity for Obama Administration to announce three purportedly new initiatives. These were: an elder abuse workshop with researchers, clinicians, and others convened by the National Institutes of Health; the Department of Justice funding yet another multi-year pilot project to evaluate the means to avoid and respond to elder abuse; and the Consumer Financial Protection Bureau releasing an advisory to help financial institutions prevent, recognize, and report elder financial exploitation. On the whole, however, informed observers expressed substantial disappointment with the outcome of the White House Conference in the elder abuse sphere [73].

35.3.2 Other Countries

Some other countries, such as Australia [41], have a federal system of government like that of the U.S. In such countries, where the national government has only limited, expressly delineated powers, the hands-on policy development and implementation ordinarily occurs largely at the state and local levels. Discussion of the specific elder abuse policy initiatives undertaken by particular countries, sometimes built upon particular religious substructures [19], is woven into the thematic analysis in Sect. 35.4, below.

35.4 Issues for Policymakers

In this section, a number of distinct but interrelated conceptual and political issues that keep arising within the elder abuse sphere are enumerated and dissected. According to the report summarizing a survey of 53 countries conducted by the INPEA in response to the 2002 Madrid Plan, "An absence of consistent laws and policies was apparent at all levels of government" [61, p. 176]. However, the vague call for unspecified "better policies" [61, p. 173] is not, except perhaps in certain academic circles, a magical incantation. Participants in, and interested observers of, the public policy formulation and implementation process who are concerned with tangibly improving the quality of life for older persons by reducing or eliminating the threat of mistreatment need to confront the often challenging issues discussed below that may act as impediments to the creation and enforcement of more consistent and effective laws and policies in this arena.

35.4.1 Definitional Issues

"Elder abuse" is a shifting social construction that may be understood in a myriad of different ways [28]. Different jurisdictions have discretion to adopt their own definitions of the term. "A broad discussion about a national definition of elder abuse can be a preliminary step, although it is difficult to reach consensus in this area" [51, p. 23]. "Although efforts to standardize definitions have increased in recent years, no universally accepted definition of elder mistreatment exists in the U.S. [or elsewhere], and definitions used for research and in the agencies that respond to abuse vary" [20]. Definitions also vary significantly among policymakers and influencers. Before policymakers can effectively address the challenge of elder abuse, there must be some reasonable agreement about the working definition, and hence the parameters, scope, and resource demands encompassed within the elder abuse concept.

The World Health Organization (WHO) defines elder abuse as a "single or repeated act or lack of appropriate action, occurring within any relationship where there is an expectation of trust, which causes harm or distress to an older person" [85]. This definition, even though according to experts it "has been influential in establishing the most commonly used definition" [42], arguably is vulnerable to claims of both underinclusiveness (for example, What about self-neglect, harmful acts by strangers, or situations in which the older alleged victim does not perceive harm or distress but an objective observer would?) and overinclusiveness (for instance, Will any kind or degree of harm or distress suffice, or only certain kinds or degrees?).

There does exist rather broad consensus among researchers, service providers/practitioners, and the policy communities that the rubric of elder mistreatment or maltreatment (terms frequently used interchangeably with "elder abuse") ought to include five separate types of harm [59]: physical abuse; psychological abuse; sexual abuse; financial exploitation [63]; and neglect. These various forms of harm are not mutually exclusive and often take place simultaneously. Some groups additionally propose, and some laws include, recognition of self-neglect as part of the elder abuse definition. However, there certainly is no unanimity within the field about whether self-neglect ought to be considered a separate, unique phenomenon or it should be lumped together with neglect of the person's basic needs by others who have a duty to provide (personally or through the purchase of services) for those needs under the overall heading of elder abuse [66]. For instance, in the U.S. self-neglect ordinarily is considered a form of elder abuse, but not so in Ireland and the U.K. [58]. In an unintentionally excellent example of completely circular reasoning, one set of authors suggests that, "[W]hen addressing elder abuse policy in the U.S. it is important to include self-neglect in the discussion because self-neglect accounts for the majority of cases reported to Adult Protective Services" [20, p. 207].

There also is a possibility of definitional ambiguity regarding who qualifies as a perpetrator of elder abuse. Many verbal formulations define elder abuse as conduct (either active or by omission) done by a family member of the victim or some other party holding a position of trust relationship with the victim, but others suggest including strangers to the victim as potential elder abuse perpetrators. For example, a bill (S.B. 369) was introduced in 2015 in the Tennessee legislature to amend the state definition of elder abuse to include the expanded offense of aggravated stalking. Even if the idea of including strangers is rejected, policymakers need to decide which specific types of trust relationships qualify to make someone an elder abuse perpetrator for legal purposes.

Assuming a reasonable consensus on definitional matters can be achieved, it will be incumbent on policymakers to draft laws and policies incorporating and depending on agreed-upon definitions as clearly and unambiguously as possible. For instance, one commentator has proposed the adoption of state criminal statutes that create a permissive presumption of exploitation with regard to certain financial transfers from older persons [44]. One of the largest impediments to adequate compliance with and enforcement of current elder abuse policies is the ambiguity and consequently multiple, inconsistent possible interpretations surrounding those policies, such as interpretive questions that have been raised about the meaning of "willful neglect" in Section 44 of the United Kingdom's Mental Capacity Act (MCA) of 2005, which supplements the 1983 Mental Health Act [43].

It is understood that the different subtypes of elder abuse may implicate different kinds of policy responses. However, to keep the discussion in this chapter manageable, I do not specifically dwell on these differences here, instead analyzing policy issues and alternatives more generically.

35.4.2 Eligibility for Victim Status

Closely connected to the definitional issues is the question of criteria, particularly in the sense of chronological age, for eligibility for elder abuse victim status. In other words, which category or categories of people should public policymakers be especially concerned about protecting against elder abuse?

One approach is to classify individuals as eligible to be considered actual or potential elder abuse victims if they have reached some specific minimum chronological age. Underlying the legal use of age per se in this context is the sociological supposition that age by itself serves as a valid proxy for vulnerability, making individualized investigation of vulnerability unnecessary. It implicates "the idea of age as an overriding 'master status' *** where perceptions of all old people as frail in mind and body lead to 'an assumed need to protect the elderly' in many dimensions of their lives" [28, p. 96]. Many states in the U.S. have enacted minimum age-specific elder abuse laws. The danger of age-based policies, though, is the risk that automatically equating older age with vulnerability serious enough to merit special protection, thereby foregoing an individualized determination, promotes negative ageist stereotypes that stigmatize the very people intended to be protected by the public's benevolent intervention.

A contrasting approach is illustrated by Ireland, which has no specific elder abuse legislation, but where older persons are protected under generic Domestic Violence statutes and policies [57], reports of which trigger more individualized investigation, determination, and possible intervention. This approach is consistent with that followed by a number of U.S. states. The worldview undergirding a rejection of the per se equation between minimum age and dangerous vulnerability contemplates aging "as a lifelong process that occurs from birth to death" and focuses not on the accumulation of years of living but on protecting those particular "adults unable to protect their own interests" [52, p. 27]. This worldview has been firmly rejected by commentators who insist that using a specified age criterion is integral to the idea of elder abuse laws [60].

35.4.3 Elder Abuse as Interpersonal Failure Calling for a Criminal Justice Response

At present, the phenomenon of elder abuse is characterized in several different, but not necessarily mutually exclusive, ways in terms of its etiology. In fact, these different approaches often overlap.

How a jurisdiction perceives the etiology of elder abuse is very likely to strongly influence the main kinds of policy responses that the jurisdiction mounts in response to the phenomenon as so perceived and how well those various policy responses act synergistically. Different constituencies within a jurisdiction (for instance, legislators, social service providers, and the medical community) potentially benefit from specific policy responses and, therefore, have their own stake or interest in how elder abuse is conceptualized [58]. The prevailing vested interests may or may not coincide with the best available evidence. Thus, it is important for governments and societies to appreciate and consciously reevaluate the theoretical underpinnings of their respective elder abuse policies.

Many jurisdictions, including state governments within the U.S., theorize elder abuse as chiefly a matter involving an interpersonal dyad in which a perpetrator with power transgresses against an older vulnerable victim. This approach focuses on the faults of the perpetrator that contributed to the transgression(s). The overarching policy response to the elder abuse-*qua*-transgression-of-an-interpersonal-relationship model is to define, prosecute, and punish the abusive behavior through the jurisdiction's criminal justice system, accepting the assumption that public knowledge about possible criminal justice consequences will effectively deter other potential wrongdoers and express official moral condemnation of socially detestable behavior [29]. According to commentators representing this perspective, "This kind of [i.e., elder] maltreatment is largely preventable. Governments can enact laws and construct enforcement and implementation machinery to prevent and punish physical and emotional abuse. Law enforcement could make fraud or abuse against the elderly more of a priority" [24, p. 121]. Singapore is one nation with exceptionally strong provisions in its penal code that pertain to protecting older individuals from financial, physical, and sexual abuse [69].

The EJA enacted in the U.S. as part of the ACA is, at least in part, a good example of this policy response. One of the central prongs of the EJA is the creation and funding of a number of Elder Abuse, Neglect, and Exploitation Forensic Centers, which have as their primary mission the collection and analysis of evidence to be used in criminal prosecutions of specific elder abuse offenders. The emphasis of the EJA on these Forensic Centers reflects a "medicalization of elder abuse" that depends on the need for medical expertise to detect, assess, and treat victims. Several Forensic Centers conduct their activities with non-EJA funding [53, 54]. According to one set of scholars speculating confidently about the future, elder abuse victimization "will have a medical hue, given the Boomer obsession with health and wellness" [3, p. 212].

It should be noted that characterizing elder abuse as a breakdown of an interpersonal dyad also, but secondarily, lends itself to other potential legal and policy remedies besides criminal prosecution and punishment. Those interventions include the availability of the civil court system to impose monetary liability on abusers in individual tort actions brought by victims and statutes that make abusers ineligible to inherent property from the estates of their victims when the latter are deceased [33].

At the same time that acceptance of the interpersonal relationship breakdown theory of elder abuse can lead to policies that criminalize and punish abusive behavior or that expose wrongdoers to civil liability for monetary damages or disinheritances [30, 64], a belief in this etiology also may contribute to public policies that concentrate on improving caregiver support, so that caregivers are less likely to succumb to, and act out their frustrations and aggression in response to, the pressures of caregiver stress. Caregiver support policies may be directed to both family members and friends functioning in the caregiver role and professional caregivers working independently or as employees of residential facilities or home care agencies.

35.4.4 Objections to the Interpersonal Transgression Etiology and the Criminalization Policy Response

The criminalization policy response to elder abuse discussed in the prior section is conceptually premised on the viewpoint that many older individuals are relatively helpless and openly vulnerable to victimization by others just waiting to mistreat and exploit them. This viewpoint, arguably reflecting "Boomer self-righteousness and severity" [3, p. 212], logically supports a variety of intrusive, paternalistic interventions intended to prevent victimization from happening in the first place or to mitigate or remedy the damage once abuse does occur.

The APS model so prevalent in the U.S. and many other countries is compatible with, and indeed predicated on, a paternalistic victimization justification for external intervention into the older person's life [71]. In legal terms, states enact APS laws based on their *parens patriae* authority to protect people who cannot protect themselves.

One of the primary APS strategies flowing from the paternalistic assumption that vulnerable older individuals lack the capacity to protect themselves against danger is the enactment of laws that require the reporting of reasonably suspected cases of elder abuse by designated categories of reporters (such as health care and social service providers) to governmental offices such as law enforcement or APS agencies. "Reasonable suspicion" in this context ordinarily is interpreted very broadly to favor liberal reporting; in other words, false positive reports are preferred by policy makers over failure to report resulting in false negatives. These mandatory reporting statutes impose criminal penalties on mandated reporters for non-compliance and may serve as the basis for civil liability suits against the negligent non-reporter if the older person suffers further harm as a result of the mandatory reporter's failure to report reasonable suspicions. Additionally, mandatory reporting statutes generally contain provisions expressly granting legal immunity to anyone acting in good faith who reports suspected abuse to designated authorities. A few state statutes even guarantee that the state will pay the attorney's fees for mandated reporters if an action is brought against the reporter for making the report [33].

While other nations and the U.N. support the concept of elder abuse reporting and some have established a reporting mechanism, mandatory reporting requirements are still the exception rather than the rule. Reporting by certain categories of people is required in Scotland, Australia, Israel, and parts of Canada [33].

The criminal justice/mandatory reporting approach to elder abuse policy, and especially its inherently paternalistic inclination, has been severely criticized as a form of age discrimination by some commentators who hold a strong civil liberties orientation. Some of these misgivings draw heavily on feminist critiques of the criminal justice response to the problem of domestic violence [38]. It has been argued:

> In the United States, many state laws aimed at combating elder abuse and neglect significantly undermine older adults' civil rights. For example, mandatory elder abuse reporting statutes can deny older adults the right to engage in confidential

> communications with doctors, nurses, clergy members, attorneys, and even spouses. *** The effect is that an individual's right to privacy, even her most intimate relationships, is curtailed—I have argued unconstitutionally—simply because she has celebrated [a particular] birthday. [37, p. 323]

Besides potential personal privacy curtailment, there are other foreseeable but unfortunate collateral consequences for many of the older individuals whom the criminal justice approach purports to benefit. These consequences or costs may include imposition of involuntary guardianship [82], institutionalization of the victim in opposition to the supposedly protected person's wishes, and perpetuation of negative ageist stereotypes. Apprehension about potential criminal prosecution might compel a family caregiver to subject an older relative for whom the caregiver is caring to the attention of a professional or agency (for example, taking the relative to a physician's office or hospital, calling in a home care agency, or hiring an independent home care aide) despite the older relative's protestations that he or she prefers to be left alone. Approaches that build on the idea that older persons usually are frail, vulnerable, and dependent seem to fly in the opposite direction of "[p]olicy frameworks that support older people to age actively, allowing them to be healthy longer and to maintain independence and control over their lives [and which as a consequence] have an important preventive function against abuse" [74, p. 8].

Moreover, objections have been raised on functional grounds, namely, the questioning of whether criminalizing elder abuse actually works to incapacitate and deter future wrongdoers and mandatory reporting laws are effective and productive vis-à-vis their objectives. Older adults may be discouraged from seeking help because they are concerned that a report will be made, professionals may feel obligated to report suspected abuse even if they credibly think the report may put the apparent victim in greater danger of harm, and an excessive volume of questionable reports may overburden APS and other health and social service agencies and thereby divert finite resources into investigation and away from intervention [36]. In the UK, researchers have discovered that few prosecutions have been brought under either the willful neglect or ill-treatment offense provisions of the Mental Capacity Act or the Mental Health Act, probably because public and professional awareness of these offenses is weak or confused [43]. The same situation occurs in Italy [68]. At the least, responsible policy makers need to take heed of commentator admonitions that mandatory elder abuse reporting laws are quite unlikely to produce the desired positive impact unless the reporting requirements are accompanied by both an energetic, sustained public and professional awareness campaign and the availability of resources sufficient for the provision of relevant follow-up interventions [52].

The most piercing criticisms of the criminal justice policy approach to elder abuse flirt with indicting professionals engaged in providing supportive services to older persons for acting in bad faith by pursuing personal interests not shared by the people on whose behalf the professionals are supposed to be advocating. Professor Kohn accuses:

> The history of elder protection laws illustrates the potential consequences of such divergence of interests with regard to negative rights. Advocacy for protecting older adults from abuse and neglect has been dominated by formal service agencies and professionals. The historical dominance of aging service providers in the debate over how to respond to elder mistreatment has several major effects on policy design. *** It ***means that the nature—and at times even the very existence—of their employment will depend on the state recognizing elder abuse as a problem and funding efforts to combat it. As such, those advocating for new legislation have an interest in seeing that legislation is passed to address elder mistreatment, even when it has significant—and potentially hard to justify—consequences for older adults' freedoms. Mandatory elder abuse statutes are a prime example. Despite concerns that mandatory reporting laws are ineffective or even counterproductive, and the fact that such laws can have profound, adverse consequences for older adults' rights and liberties, they continue to be very popular within the aging services community. [39, pp. 59–60]

This skeptical critique is not just limited to the U.S. For instance, Harbison et al. [28, p. 94] observe that "In Canada the chief lobby for action on elder abuse comes from [an organization], which includes professionals, academics, community organizations (including those of seniors), and elder abuse consultants affiliated with provincial governments, as well as from other individuals and groups with similar characteristics." This group of Canadian policy analysts further asserts:

> From its beginnings as a social problem, "elder abuse and neglect" was shaped as a problem that required professional expertise because of the particular characteristics of helplessness, vulnerability and frailty assigned to the older population*** This professionalization of their problems of mistreatment and neglect placed older people in a parallel situation to children in terms both of their characterization as being "in need of protection" and the need for professional expert responses to their situations. Moreover, how older people themselves, especially those who are victims of mistreatment and neglect, view their own situations has rarely been investigated. We do know that some older people wish to maintain autonomous lives, including privacy regarding mistreatment, especially where it may lead to questions about their judgment. In addition, many older people wish to remain within their abusive families to retain a sense of positive identity and of belonging to family and culture, as well as for reasons of fear and shame. [28, pp. 91–92]

Thus, policy makers must work on reaching an acceptable accommodation, maintaining an awareness of potentially conflicting, or at least multiple, interests seeking to influence the policy outcome. In the U.S., the first step in designing an acceptable policy compromise entails assuring that the resulting policy complies with constitutional provisions intended to protect the rights of individuals affected by that policy [40]. Within applicable constitutional constraints:

> [i]t would be a mistake to abandon a criminal justice response to elder abuse altogether.*** It would also, however, be a mistake to ignore the potential costs of the current autonomy-limiting criminal justice response to elder abuse, or to assume that there are not feasible, preferable alternative approaches that could afford older adults greater agency. [38, p. 29]

As early as 1985, American law and aging pioneer John Regan discussed the dilemma posed by the tension between freedom and safety as core values. He recognized APS as an acceptable mechanism for dealing with elder abuse only if "the program is based on three fundamental principles: respect for personal autonomy, adherence to due process, and intervention based on the principle of the least restrictive alternative" [67, p. 4]. In accord is a contemporary Australian legal scholar:

> The great risk lies in avoiding a paternalistic approach to elder abuse policies. Older persons, no matter how vulnerable, disabled or dependent, are entitled to the respect and recognition of their fundamental human rights, and an older person, unlike a child, is not inherently vulnerable and in need of protection. Thus, the challenge will be in shaping law and policy in a manner that is clearly premised on the rights of all older persons to dignity, personal liberty, autonomy and self-determination. [41, p. 104]

The need for proper policy tradeoffs has also been recognized at the international level. The U.N. Economic Commission for Europe [74, p. 15] has noted:

> Protective measure should also give due weight to rights of autonomy of older persons. Especially when older people are reluctant to be placed in nursing homes, one should be careful not to force them, thereby replacing one undesired situation with another. In practice, authorities may be faced with a dilemma where a victim of abuse objects to any intervention. At the same time, leaving a person in an abusive relationship when he or she does not want to be protected is not necessarily justified in the name of autonomy. On the policy level, a trade-off has to be made between services that offer the greatest protection but are likely to restrict freedom, whereas services that maximize autonomy often involve significant risks. A good legal framework should provide guidance that is sensitive to these matters.

Put succinctly, "Care should promote autonomy while balancing risk to the older person and possible impact of such decisions on others, for example environmental hazards" [58, p. 13]. The same author expands upon this idea:

> Central… is the need to value the older person, ensure that interventions do not infringe on individual rights, guarantee full participation and engagement of older people and protect self-determination and autonomy. It is difficult when self-determination means older people choose risky environments and future debate should centre on issues of how such risks can be balanced to ensure the safety of the person [58, p. 228].

Legal commentator Jones [33, p. 321] concedes, "There are both pros and cons to mandatory reporting of any type of abuse. One must balance the individual's right to privacy and confidentiality with society's need to protect the abused. Which one a person values more can determine how she feels on the issue." How Jones [33, pp. 322–323] would weigh the competing values is clear: "There are not sufficient reasons to abandon mandatory reporting. Affronts to elder self-determination are not as important as the terrible consequences of underreporting….When victims cannot or will not protect themselves, government must step in to prevent worse abuse in the future."

One policy approach to balancing the state's legitimate interest in protecting vulnerable older people from harm against the state's equally (if not superior) interest in rights consciousness concerning older persons would be to maintain mandatory reporting requirements but apply those requirements to less expansive circumstances. The state of Wisconsin's attempt to achieve this balance is described approvingly by Professor Nina Kohn [37, p. 328] in the following language:

> Most elder abuse reporting laws in the United States mandate reporting when a would-be reporter reasonably suspects mistreatment of someone who is of a certain age, "vulnerable," or a combination of the two. By contrast, Wisconsin only requires reporters to invade victim privacy when there is a significant, current threat and reason to believe the victim will not come forward on his or her own. Specifically, unless a third party is at risk, reporting is only required where the alleged victim is: (1) at imminent risk of serious harm, and (2) cannot "make an informed judgment" about reporting. As such, Wisconsin only mandates reporting in situations in which the state has a strong interest.*** Wisconsin's mandatory reporting law underscores the fact that embracing a civil rights approach to aging policy does not mean rejecting protective policies. It simply means recognizing that protections must be balanced against the liberty interests they undermine. It means recognizing that older adults' rights should not be undermined without significant justification.

Another variation on the criminal justice model, one that deviates from its usual adversarial, confrontational character, is the idea of restorative justice. Groh and Linden [26] describe one local Canadian community's restorative justice response to elder abuse. A restorative justice approach looks on a case-by-case basis at the frayed social relationship between the victim and the perpetrator who violated a position of trust and attempts to repair the harm caused to that relationship rather than merely meting out punishment to the offender. The victim is respected as an active, autonomous participant in a therapeutic process involving the entire community, with the emphasis on reconciliation and reintegration of the parties and sustenance of a healthy and equal relationship.

Another interesting proposal has been advanced by Brank et al. [7]. They suggest replacing state mandatory reporting statutes with laws that instead place responsibility on older adults to self-report abuse. This proposal overlooks several barriers to self-reporting in the realm of perceptions of abuse and anxiety about the consequences of reporting [87].

35.4.5 The Social Climate of Ageism and Policy Responses to It

One of the main controversies surrounding the conceptualization of elder abuse as a criminal or tortious transgression of the interpersonal dyad, with perpetrators guilty of violating their particular trust relationships with vulnerable victims, involves the claim that devoting too much attention to interpersonal explanations of abuse such as caregiver stress ignores, or at least diverts valuable attention away from, important social, structural, cultural, and organizational forces within which interpersonal dyads operate [70]. XinQi Dong makes a persuasive case that, "[f]or decades, professionals and the public have viewed elder abuse and broader violence as predominantly social or family problems…[T]here has been inadequate attention to elder abuse from public health, social services, health, legal, and criminal justice professionals. [However], [t]he situation appears to be changing" [12]. A set of aging services commentators adds:

> When we continue to perceive elder abuse as primarily a family problem involving a few stressed caregivers, we focus on individual remedies rather than a social justice response. Yet current research and experience in the field do not support caregiver stress as a primary or sole reason for elder abuse. Therefore, it is not only dangerous, but also irresponsible for policy makers to continue to build and fund programmatic responses, and practitioners to provide interventions, based on the false assumption that if you address caregiver stress you attend to elder abuse victims. [6, p. 37]

The most significant of the practically universal [41] social, structural, cultural, and organizational forces contributing to the prevalence of elder abuse is the phenomenon of ageism. As expressed by the U.N. Commission for Europe [74, p. 6]:

> Social and cultural norms such as ageism *** can reinforce maltreatment in society. Stereotypes depicting older people as weaker, less worthy and a burden to society may be the breeding ground for elder abuse. Negative attitudes towards old age can also be ingrained in older peoples' own attitudes. Low self-esteem may make it seem almost natural to them to be treated with a lack of respect. This may prevent them from recognizing abusive situations.

Irish Professor of Nursing Amanda Phelan [58, p. 2] agrees, "An examination of elder abuse using an ageist lens has the advantage of incorporating structural, political and social contexts. Ageist attitudes contribute to the non-identification and non-recognition of elder maltreatment as well as the passive tolerance of abuse of older people." In the U.S. and elsewhere, ageism takes many forms [45].

For advocates of this orientation, ageism is largely responsible for deficits in public funding for elder abuse services and programs, as elder abuse struggles for priority among policy makers against the demands of other domestic concerns and national security [72]. From this perspective, policy and practice needs to emphasize forward-looking, preventive strategies to reduce the social force of ageism that subjects older people to "marginalized group" status [42, p. 1214]; policy and practice need to deemphasize the kinds of after-the-fact punitive reactions to past incidents or patterns of elder abuse that are represented by criminal prosecutions and mandatory reporting requirements [46]. "An effective approach to elder abuse requires intervention at a societal level to combat ageism and age discrimination" [18, p. 853].

Such an ecological approach [57, 58] takes aim at the source of the elder abuse phenomenon in a systemic context, purposely devoting less attention to the individual, episodic behavioral manifestations of the ageist social environment from which specific instances or patterns of elder abuse spring; the discrete individual or repeated bad acts or omissions are less concerning than the ongoing social affront to older persons posed by ageism. A social context orientation focuses on interdependencies rather than dependency, and frames population aging as a positive opportunity rather than a daunting demographic catastrophe. A 2002 WHO international survey documented "the longing by older persons for respect" [61, p. 166].

The European Reference Framework Online for the Prevention of Elder Abuse and Neglect Project (EuROPEAN) has urged as an essential elder abuse policy ingredient "formulating a positive vision of ageing and the positive power of older people in society" [51, p. 25]. Put differently, "For older people to be free of mistreatment the state should create conditions where abuse and neglect need not take place, in other words, where interpersonal relationships do not occur in the context of ageist prejudice" [4, p. 1302]. Although language such as this is too vague to be very useful, the U.N. Economic Commission for Europe [74, p. 7] gives it some substance by following up, "Positive attitudes towards older people can be encouraged by providing opportunities for meaningful interaction between older adults and young people, through intergenerational programmes, exchanging letters or e-mails, visiting local nursing homes or playing games."

Other commentators join in urging greater concentration on prevention, rather than remediation, of elder abuse by effecting changes in social attitudes. A prime rationale for this emphasis is that "[e]lder abuse combatants should focus on prevention rather than detection because elder suffer shorter life expectancies, lose indispensable life savings, and live a low quality of life after being abused" [21, p. 105]. According to the social factors school of thought, ageist social attitudes contribute to isolation of older individuals, and low levels of social support are demonstrably related to increased risk of abuse, particularly of the psychological variety, in older people. Especially "in developed nations, living alone and lack of social support contribute[s] to elder abuse" [61, p. 171]. Improving attitudes about aging and the aged is a necessary precondition of the development of intervention programs that can effectively facilitate friendships and social activities in old age [47]. In sum, "Abuse of older persons remains deeply rooted in societal attitudes towards ageing. Elder abuse can prevail as long as older people are not considered equal citizens" [74, p. 21].

35.4.6 Extent and Limits of the Role of Government and the Private Sector

In formulating and implementing public policy within the elder abuse context, a foundational task is delineating the appropriate extent of, and limits to, government's appropriate role in possible interventions. A corollary question concerns the proper role of various private sector actors in a comprehensive policy aimed at preventing, detecting, and responding to elder abuse.

One way of analyzing the respective roles of government and the private sector concerning the global phenomenon of elder abuse is to attribute the etiology of the phenomenon primarily to the risk factors of poverty, unavailability of sufficient services, lack of other resources, and additional social and economic conditions beyond the control of individuals [62]. Concentration on an inadequate socio-economic-political infrastructure (for example, not enough skilled, trained staff for agencies and facilities to deliver optimal client services) leads many international commentators to advocate a social welfare policy of intervention [74]. Advocacy of a social welfare model of elder abuse policy is based, in turn, on a philosophical and political commitment to the idea that declaring freedom from elder abuse as one of many Human Rights to which each person is categorically, automatically, and unconditionally entitled necessarily entails a binding obligation on the part of governments to positively, affirmatively generate and distribute resources in a manner and amount that assures the desired outcome to each entitled person. When "recognising that elder abuse is a violation of human rights" is a duty of "each national government," then "the role of the state in addressing elder abuse" is an expansive one indeed [51, p. 22].

Common conceptual themes found among the major international statements on elder abuse, including the Madrid Plan, are autonomy, dignity, health, poverty reduction, economic security, social inclusion, and a supportive and empowering environment. According to this thinking, whenever an older person suffers because any of these desirable infrastructure elements are not satisfactorily provided to that person, his or her Human Rights have been transgressed and the person has become a victim of elder abuse [46].

Discussing one particular facet of the question of how expansive the state's proper role ought to be, the European Reference Framework [51, pp. 9–10] has gone on record as follows:

> When elder abuse occurs within the family, the state must consider its role in this private sphere. This is especially important in situations involving vulnerable people who cannot stand up for themselves. In some countries, the influence of the state ends at the threshold of the home, while other countries allow for the protection of victims of domestic violence. The latter countries recognise that abuse is a violation of civil and human rights and therefore a matter for the state. Civil and human rights do not end at the threshold of the home. Effective efforts to combat elder abuse require the recognition that private violence is a public affair.

At the heart of the Human Rights approach is the concept of "social investment," or the spending of public monies, to enhance independence and reduce the need of older people for care provided by others. The thought is that, when governments skimp (that is, self-impose limits) on their financial investment for elder abuse prevention, independent living, and high quality care, they are in essence denying older individuals Human Rights that are not to be abused. Individuals are seen foremost as rights holders entitled to make claims that government is obligated to satisfy. As expressed by the WHO, a leader in the movement to blame elder abuse on societal risk factors and to promote Human Rights/social investment as the solution:

> Conventions and charters adopted by Member States in the European Region enshrine the principles of equity, solidarity and protecting the rights of citizens.*** The Universal Declaration of Human Rights can be interpreted as highlighting social responsibility to protect citizens, including those who are vulnerable such as older people, to provide them with appropriate support and services and promote their right to a safe environment that is free from violence. [84, pp. 8–9]

Accordingly, "Equity needs to be incorporated into all levels of government policy to address [inequity in the maltreatment of older people as] the cause of social injustice" [84, p. 10].

Australian Professor Wendy Lacey [41, p. 117] has articulated the underlying philosophy as follows:

> In the absence of specific legal obligations that protect them, there exists the potential for the elderly to be seen as a burden on the medical and welfare systems, rather than as rights-holders deserving of respect and dignified treatment. Without the

adoption of a strong rights-based approach, ageing continues to be construed as a 'problem' requiring solutions, rather than as requiring positive strategies aimed at enabling older persons to realise their inherent human rights.

In the eyes of at least one observer, China presents a tangible example of this policy approach in action. As explained by Shankardass [69, p. 1230]:

> ...the Chinese government pays attention, first to ensuring that older people have basic living allowance, second to improving their quality of life through construction and expansion of social security, and third to establishing a uniform basic old age insurance system in urban areas and a social aid system in rural areas.

In Thailand, an outline of a "minimum Standard of Housing and environment is intended to be a progressive step in reducing abuse of older persons" [69]. The U.K. and Germany, among other countries, have enunciated (albeit without necessarily actually implementing) a commitment to the Human Rights paradigm of preventing and remedying elder abuse [62].

Other schools of commentators, by contrast, appear less convinced of the salutary impact of aggressive state involvement in combatting elder abuse. "[T]he differentiation between social welfare and criminal approaches to protect [against elder abuse] ***[is] an area of some debate within the UK during the past decade" [62, p. 140]. Certainly, governments have a valid role to play in regulating institutions and individual professionals who serve older persons, in terms of institutional and professional qualifications and standards of care, since elder abuse sometimes occurs within institutional settings. According to one analysis, however:

> Although the federal government is well positioned to address issues that involve financing and regulating long-term care for the elderly, the same cannot be said for their ability to directly prevent elder abuse. While health care affordability and long-term care quality are public issues, elder abuse is private in nature as it is most often perpetrated by family members and occurs within the elder's home. [21, p. 105]

A nation's values are enshrined in its policies and laws [57]. However, as explained in Sect. 35.2. B above, the mere declaration of some desired outcome as part of a constellation of Human Rights is, by itself, merely soft, unenforceable law.

> [A]ttention has been brought to [the] propensity [of legal solutions] to distract our attention from the need for 'adequate funding for proper support services and programs in the community' in that legislation offers a very public appearance of doing something about a problems without committing many resources—a strategy that holds great attraction for governments. [28, p. 95]

Stated more succinctly, "The law is not a solution; it is a tool" [28, p. 99].

One of the several key challenges in maximizing the value of government intervention in the elder abuse arena is the need to comprehensively coordinate the many different players likely to be involved in a complicated intervention strategy. Complex federal systems in the U.S. and other countries, such as India [69] and Australia [41], introduce the challenge of "occasionally overlapping jurisdictions or a lack of cooperation between the federal and federated states, ***mak[ing] it harder to provide for the right kind of *** [policy] interventions" [9, p. 372]. Moreover, the distribution and diffusion of responsibility among various public agencies even within the same government, let alone among multiple governments, generally is complicated, presenting a significant possibility of confusion and misalignment. Just in the U.S. at the federal level, responsibility and authority regarding both distinct and overlapping aspects of elder abuse is dispersed among the Department of Health and Human Services (DHHS) (home of the AoA and other involved subdivisions), Department of Justice, Consumer Financial Protection Bureau, Federal Trade Commission, Securities and Exchange Commission, Department of the Treasury, and the Postal Inspection Service. The activities of these multiple agencies are coordinated extremely poorly or not at all [77, 79].

More clear, efficient, and effective interagency coordination (through, for example, legislative or regulatory reform and negotiated contracts and memoranda of understanding carefully delineating agencies' respective powers, limits, and chains of command) must be an important feature of elder abuse policy. "A public policy framework that regulates the roles and responsibilities of different agencies and that is conducive to interagency collaboration can enhance accountability" [74, p. 19].

Additionally, the value of government intervention will be enhanced by coordinating, combining, and leveraging public investment in elder abuse strategies with the investment made by private entities. Commentators speak of "the need for an integrated, whole-of-government strategy for preventing and responding to elder abuse, which engages the entire community" [41, p. 104]. Stated more expansively,

> A public and private partnership is required to change the standing of elder abuse and improve responses to it. On the one hand, in each country, government at every level charged with promoting human rights and the general welfare of citizens needs to establish a legal framework of elder protection along with an effective structure for its implementation, involving key public agencies and protocols for interagency collaboration. ... On the other hand, nongovernmental health and social service organizations, professional associations, and the mass media have important roles in ensuring that the legal framework and its implementation structure are widely known and understood. [61, pp. 178–179]

Involved private entities may be civil society not-for-profit agencies and organizations (nongovernmental organizations, or NGOs), including advocacy groups and professional organizations; for instance, charitable NGOs Age Concern, Help the Aged, and Action on Elder Abuse have been particularly important in influencing the UK response to elder abuse [62]. Private for-profit (proprietary or investor-owned) entities also may be involved in addressing elder abuse, particularly as service providers. The Madrid Plan assumes that governments will take the lead role regarding elder abuse, but Articles 13 and 17 also advocate robust public/private collaboration. In the U.S., there have been suggestions for new, targeted state laws that make it more advantageous and attractive (by, for instance, allowing for the recovery of attorney fees and treble damages) for individual victims of financial exploitation to civilly sue those who have fleeced them for fraud, misappropriation, breach of fiduciary duty, and other causes of action [55].

35.4.7 Cultural Factors

Culture plays an important role in defining elder abuse and envisioning and accepting policy responses to the phenomenon as defined within a particular place and time [58]. Differential effects of modernity versus tradition are on vivid display in countries that tolerate the persecution of older people thought to practice witchcraft. In many parts of the world today, discussion of elder abuse is considered strictly taboo [83]. Moreover, cultural attitudes about families, their roles, and the autonomy they should be afforded as an institutional matter also differ markedly among groups of people, sometimes imposing effective barriers to external intervention. An elder abuse policy approach that fails to take account of the globe's important cultural diversity, in terms of differing interpretations of the world and resultant differing lay and professional behaviors and practices, among different peoples inevitably will be counterproductive and disruptive. Attempts at universal, "one size fits all" policy solutions, rather than nation-specific and—sensitive approaches, are highly unlikely to succeed. "Each country must identify its own approach to and strategy for combating elder abuse. The approach taken will be influenced by cultural, economic and social aspects, demographic development and the historical response of policy to this issue" [51, pp. 22–23]. Even within individual countries, substantial cultural diversity exists among different population groups and must be acknowledged in the policy making process [16, 28].

35.4.8 The Need for Research, Education, and Training

"In order to plan and implement legal strategies to combat elder abuse, professionals and the broader community require a clear understanding of the nature of elder abuse" [46, p. 21]. Although knowledge about the taxonomy, prevalence and incidence, theoretical explanations, and consequences of elder abuse has expanded greatly in the last couple of decades [2], there is a broad international consensus about the need for an even stronger and more comprehensive research base to adequately support the development and implementation of evidence-based public policy regarding elder abuse [72]. "Much of what has occurred in response to the acknowledgement that 'elder abuse and neglect' exists has been based on value-based assumptions rather than on empirical evidence" [28, p. 100]. There is a continuing need for much better data collection and interpretation concerning the incidence and prevalence of elder abuse (however defined in a particular country), how claims are handled, what interventions have been tried, and the extent to which various trial interventions have produced the positive results sought.

The World Health Organization [84, p. 61] has joined in urging, "A more scientifically based approach is urgently needed to improve understanding of the scale of the problem, the causes and consequences." This position is echoed by the U.N. Economic Commission for Europe [74, p. 20]:

> [B]etter cross-national data collection is needed to have a better overview of development trends. Surveillance and epidemiological studies that identify risk factors and vulnerable groups are a prerequisite for targeted screening and outreach programmes. More systematic evaluation of interventions and their effectiveness in different contexts would also be desirable. Few studies have evaluated interventions with rigorous randomized control trial designs…

Deficiencies that policy makers need to address in order to stimulate and facilitate better qualitative and quantitative investigation of elder abuse topics include lack of awareness on the part of policy makers, insufficient funding, and, at least in some countries, poor academic interest [9].

Similarly, virtually everyone involved in the elder abuse arena joins in calling on policy makers to devote more attention and resources to enhance education and training opportunities for professionals (health care, human services, legal, law enforcement, and community organizations) on the recognition, reporting, and management of elder abuse, as well as supporting wider public awareness campaigns [8, 17, 51]. For instance, the Madrid Plan [75] contains several recommendations [Sections 110 (g) and 111 (d) and (e)] specifically focused on education and training. Informational challenges exist in both developed (including the U.S. [77]) and developing countries, but especially in the latter the public awareness challenges are exacerbated by illiteracy, poverty, and cultural factors [61].

35.5 Conclusion

Elder abuse is a complex and multi-faceted phenomenon presenting a panoply of difficult issues that compel multi-faceted responses. Public policy, often effectuated through "legislative teeth" [58, p. 226], is not a solution in and of itself, but it does constitute an important—indeed, imperative—tool in the quest to improve the quality of life for older persons by preventing and/or ameliorating the negative ramifications of elder abuse. This chapter has attempted to move the national and international elder abuse agendas, as addressed particularly through the lens of public policy creation and implementation initiatives, forward.

As explicated in this chapter, policy makers and implementers confront a number of basic questions, the answers to which will shape the specific details and directions of policy development and enforcement in the elder abuse sphere. Particularly, policy makers need to address: definitional conundrums (what conduct and omissions ought to constitute elder abuse, who ought to qualify as a victim or a perpetrator); whether elder abuse should be treated primarily as the breakdown of a dyadic interpersonal trust relationship, the product of societal ageist attitudes, or a matter of Human Rights calling for a social investment or welfare strategy, or some sort of combination of these paradigms; the optimum balance of personal autonomy and safety for real or potential victims of elder abuse, particularly when considering whether self-neglect represents an older adult's considered choices (the sociocultural description) or rather mental, physical, and social disturbances such as depression or cognitive impairment (the psychomedical explanation) [31]; the best allocation and coordination of public and private sector responses to elder abuse; the influence of cultural factors in framing elder abuse policy for and within specific countries; and the need for greatly expanded and improved research, education, and training opportunities involving both professionals and members of the public.

The global population profile is aging. The fate of many individuals within the burgeoning older demographic cohort around the world surely may depend on how, and how well, policy makers and implementers deal, in their own countries and collectively, with the various issues identified here.

Acknowledgments The author thanks Margaret Clark, MLS, Assistant Director for International Research at Florida State University College of Law Research Center, for her very valuable research assistance in this project.

References

1. AGE Platform Europe. European charter of the rights and responsibilities of older people in need of long-term care and assistance. 2010. http://www.age-platform.eu/images/stories/Final_European_Charter.pdf.
2. Anetzberger GJ. An update on the nature and scope of elder abuse. Generations. 2012;36(3):12–20.
3. Anetzberger GJ, Teaster PB. Future directions for social policy and elder abuse. J Elder Abuse Negl. 2010;22(3–4):207–15.
4. Biggs S, Haapala I. Elder mistreatment, ageism, and human rights. Int Psychogeriatr. 2013;25(8):1299–306.
5. Blutman L. In the trap of a legal metaphor: international soft law. Int Comp Law Q. 2010;59(3):605–24.
6. Brandl B, Raymond JA. Policy implications of recognizing that caregiver stress is not the primary cause of elder abuse. Generations. 2012;36(3):32–9.
7. Brank EM, Wylie LE, Hamm JA. Potential for self-reporting of older adult maltreatment: an empirical examination. Elder Law J. 2012;19(2):351–84.
8. Burnes D, Pillemer K, Caccamise PL, et al. Prevalence of and risk factors for elder abuse and neglect in the community: a population-based study. J Am Geriatr Soc. 2015;63:1906–12.
9. Callewaert GAG. Preventing and combating elder mistreatment in Flanders (Belgium): general overview. J Elder Abuse Negl. 2011;23(4):366–74.
10. Daly JM. Domestic and institutional elder abuse legislation. Nurs Clin N Am. 2011;46(4):477–84.
11. Dong X. Elder abuse: systematic review and implications for practice. J Am Geriatr Soc. 2015;63(6):1214–38.
12. Dong X. Screening for elder abuse in healthcare settings: why should we care, and is it a missed quality indicator? J Am Geriatr Soc. 2015;63(8):1686–92.
13. Dong X. Elder abuse: research, practice, and health policy. Gerontologist. 2014;54(2):153–62.
14. Dong X, Chen R, Simon MA. Elder abuse and dementia: a review of the research and health policy. Health Aff. 2014;33(4):642–9.
15. Dong X. Advancing the field of elder abuse: future directions and policy implications. J Am Geriatr Soc. 2012;60(11):2151–6.
16. Dong X. Cultural diversity and elder abuse: implications for research, education, and policy. Generations. 2012;36(3):40–2.
17. Dong X, Simon MA. Enhancing national policy and programs to address elder abuse. JAMA. 2011;305(23):2460–1.
18. Dow B, Joosten M. Understanding elder abuse: a social rights perspective. Int Psychogeriatr. 2012;24(6):853–5.
19. Elsaman RS, Arafa MA. The rights of the elderly in the Arab Middle East: Islamic theory versus Arabic practice. Marq. Elder's Advis. 2012;14(1):1–47.
20. Ernst JS, Brownell P. United States of America. In: Phelan A, editor. International perspectives on elder abuse. New York: Routledge; 2013. p. 206–21.
21. Fischer AR. Elder abuse: a private problem that requires private solutions. J Health Biomed Law. 2012;8(1):81–116.
22. Fowler GL. Protecting a frail generation: Georgia's need for civil protections against elder abuse. John Marshall Law J. 2012;6(1):351–98.

23. Gostin LO. Global health law. Cambridge: Harvard University Press; 2014.
24. Gostin LO, Garsia A. Governing for health as the world grows older: healthy lifespans in aging societies. Elder Law J. 2014;22 (1):111–39.
25. Gostin LO, Sridhar D, Hougendobler D. The normative authority of the World Health Organization. Public Health. 2015. http://papers.ssrn.com/sol3/papers.cfm?abstract_id=2634181.
26. Groh A, Linden R. Addressing elder abuse: the Waterloo restorative justice approach to elder abuse project. J Elder Abuse Negl. 2011;23(2):127–46.
27. Guzman AT, Meyer TL. International soft law. J Legal Anal. 2010;2(1):171–225.
28. Harbison J, Coughlan S, Beaulieu M, et al. Understanding "Elder Abuse and Neglect": a critique of assumptions underpinning responses to the mistreatment and neglect of older people. J Elder Abuse Negl. 2012;24(2):88–103.
29. Heisler CJ. Elder abuse and the criminal justice system: an uncertain future. Generations. 2012;36(3):83–8.
30. Hunt T. Disincentivizing elder abuse through disinheritance: Revamping California Probate Code § 259 and using it as a model. Brigham Young Univ Law Rev. 2014;2014(2):445–74.
31. Iris M, Ridings JW, Conrad KJ. The development of a conceptual model for understanding elder self-neglect. Gerontologist. 2010;50 (3):303–15.
32. Jirik S, Sanders S. Analysis of elder abuse statutes across the United States, 2011–2012. J Gerontolol Soc Work. 2014;57 (5):478–97.
33. Jones JTR. Abuse of elders with mental illness: generally an international and specifically a United States perspective. In: Ruebner R, Do T, Taylor A, editors. International and comparative law on the rights of older persons. Lake Mary: Vandeplas Publishing; 2015. p. 303–32.
34. Kaplan DB, Pillemer K. Fulfilling the promise of the elder justice act: priority goals for the white house conference on aging. Public Policy Aging Rep. 2015;25(2):63–6.
35. Kohl H, Sanders B, Blumenthal R. Elder abuse: what is the federal role? Generations. 2012;36(3):106–10.
36. Kohn NA. Vulnerability theory and the role of government. Yale J Law Fem. 2014;26(1):1–27.
37. Kohn NA. Elder rights: the next civil rights movement. Temple Polit Civ Rights Law Rev. 2012;21(2):321–8.
38. Kohn NA. Elder (In)justice: a critique of the criminalization of elder abuse. Am Crim Law Rev. 2012;49(1):1–29.
39. Kohn NA. The lawyer's role in fostering an elder rights movement. William Mitchell Law Rev. 2010;37(1):49–79.
40. Kohn NA. Outliving civil rights. Wash Univ Law Rev. 2009;86 (5):1053–115.
41. Lacey W. Neglectful to the point of cruelty. Syd Law Rev. 2014;36(1):99–130.
42. Lindenberg J, Westendorp RGJ, Kurrle S, et al. Elder abuse—an international perspective: exploring the context of elder abuse. Int Psychogeriatr. 2013;25(8):1213–5.
43. Manthorpe J, Samsi K. Care professionals' understanding of the new criminal offences created by the Mental Capacity Act 2005. Int J Geriatr Psychiatry. 2015;30(4):384–92.
44. McClurg AJ. Preying on the graying: a statutory presumption to presecute elder financial exploitation. Hastings Law J. 2014;65 (4):1099–143.
45. McNamara TK, Williamson JB. In: Hudson RB, editor. The new politics of old age policy. 3rd ed. Baltimore: Johns Hopkins University Press; 2014. p. 254–70.
46. McSherry B. Elder abuse and neglect: challenges and directions for legal reform. J Law Med. 2010;18(1):19–24.
47. Melchiorre MG, Chaiatti C, Lamura G, et al. Social support, socio-economic status, health and abuse among older people in seven European countries. PLoS ONE. 2013;8(1):e54856. doi:10.1371/journal.pone.0054856.
48. Meng M, Hunt K. New Chinese law: visit your parents. CNN News. 2013. http://www.cnn.com/2013/07/02/world/asia/china-elderly-law/index.html.
49. Merriman-Nai S, Stein K. World elder abuse awareness day: the concept, the reality, and the promise. J Elder Abuse Negl. 2014;26 (3):345–9.
50. Miller M. Ombudsmen on the front line: improving quality of care and preventing abuse in nursing homes. Generations. 2012;36 (3):60–3.
51. Min M. The European reference framework online for the prevention of elder abuse and neglect: background, good practices and recommendations. 2011. http://www.preventelderabuse.eu.
52. Mixon PM. Public policy, elder abuse, and adult protective services: the struggle for coherence. J Elder Abuse Negl. 2010;22 (1–2):16–36.
53. Navarro AE, Wysong J, DeLiema M et al. Inside the black box: the case review process of an elder abuse forensic center. Gerontologist. Epub. 2015;56:772–781.
54. Navarro AE, Gassoumis ZD, Wilber KH. Holding abusers accountable: an elder abuse forensic center increases criminal prosecution of financial exploitation. Gerontologist. 2013;53 (2):303–12.
55. No Author. Lies, secrets, and scams. Consum Rep. 2015;80 (11):28–37.
56. O'Brien JG. Screening for elder abuse and neglect. J Am Geriatr Soc. Epub. 2015 (August 17, 2015). doi:10.1111/jgs.1_13538
57. Phelan A. Elder abuse: a review of progress in Ireland. J Elder Abuse Negl. 2014;26(2):172–88.
58. Phelan A, editor. International perspectives on elder abuse. New York: Routledge; 2013.
59. Pillemer K, Connolly M-T, Breckman R, et al. Elder mistreatment: priorities for consideration by the White House Conference on Aging. Gerontologist. 2015;55(2):320–7.
60. Pietsch JH. Who's afraid of protecting older persons?—adressing the false illusion of having to keep "elder" out of elder abuse laws. Georget J Poverty Law Policy. 2009;16(2&3):391–411.
61. Podnieks E, Anetzberger GJ, Wilson SJ, et al. WorldView environmental scan on elder abuse. J Elder Abuse Negl. 2010;22 (1–2):164–79.
62. Podnieks E, Penhale B, Goergen T, et al. Elder mistreatment: an international narrative. J Elder Abuse Negl. 2010;22(1–2):131–63.
63. Price T, King PS, Dillard RL, et al. Elder financial exploitation: Implications for future policy and research in elder mistreatment. West J Emerg Med XI. 2011;I(3):354–6.
64. Province AG. Killing me softly: a comparative review of Chinese inheritance law to address the problem of elder abuse and neglect in the United States. Indiana Int Comp Law Rev. 2012;22(1):71–92.
65. Quinn KM, Benson WF. The states' elder abuse victim services: a system still in search of support. Generations. 2012;36(3):66–72.
66. Rathbone-McCuan E. An improved approach to treatment elder self-neglect: the self-care framework. Generations. 2014;38(3):80–5.
67. Regan JJ. Adult protective services: policy issues for the 80's. Conference on working with victims of abuse and neglect. San Antonio, TX. 1985.
68. Salsi G, Mazzotti MC, Carosielli G, et al. Elder abuse awareness in Italy: analysis of reports to the Prosecutor's Office of Bologna. Aging Clin Exp Res. 2015;27(3):359–63.

69. Sharnkardass MK. Addressing elder abuse: review of societal responses in India and selected Asian countries. Int Psychogeriatr. 2013;25(8):1229–34.
70. Stevens M, Biggs S, Dixon J, et al. Interactional perspectives on the mistreatment of older and vulnerable people in long-term care settings. Br J Sociol. 2013;64(2):267–86.
71. Strasser SM, Kerr J, King PS, et al. A survey of Georgia adult protective service staff: implications for older adult injury prevention and policy. West J Emerg Med. 2011;12(3):357–64.
72. Teaster PB, Wangmo T, Anetzberger GJ. A glass half full: the dubious history of elder abuse policy. J Elder Abuse Negl. 2010;22 (1–2):6–15.
73. Thorner NJ. White house conference on aging abuses elders by ignoring injustice. WordPress.com weblog at. 2015. https://nancyjthorner.wordpress.com/2015/07/18/thorner-white-house-conference-on-aging-abuses-elders-by-ignoring-injustice/.
74. United Nations Economic Commission for Europe. Abuse of older persons. UNECE Policy Brief on Ageing No. 14. 2013.
75. United Nations, Second World Assembly on Ageing. Political declaration and madrid international plan of action on ageing. New York. 2002. http://undesadspd.org/Portals/0/ageing/documents/Fulltext-E.pdf.
76. United States Department of Justice and United States Department of Health and Human Services. The Elder Justice Roadmap, Washington, DC. 2014. http://ncea.acl.gov/library/gov_report/docs/EJRP_roadmap.pdf.
77. United States General Accountability Office. Elder justice: More federal coordination and public awareness needed. Washington, DC. GAO-13-498. 2013.
78. United States General Accountability Office. Elder justice: National strategy needed to effectively combat elder financial exploitation. Washington, DC. GAO-13-110. 2012.
79. United States General Accountability Office. Elder justice: Stronger federal leadership could enhance national response to elder abuse. Washington, DC. GAO-11-208. 2011.
80. White House Conference on Aging. Elder Justice policy brief. 2015. http://www.whitehouseconferenceonaging.gov/blog/policy/post/elder-justice-policy-brief.
81. White W. Elder self-neglect and adult protective services: Ohio needs to do more. J Law Health. 2014;27(1):130–63.
82. Wood EF. The paradox of adult guardianship: a solution to—and a source for—elder abuse. Generations. 2012;36(3):79–82.
83. World Health Organization. Ageing and life course—elder abuse. 2015. http://who.int/ageing/projects/elder_abuse/en/.
84. World Health Organization, Regional Office for Europe. European report on preventing elder mistreatment. 2011. http://www.euro.who.int/__data/assets/pdf_file/0010/144676/e95110.pdf.
85. World Health Organization. World Report on Violence and Health, Geneva. 2002. http://www.who.int/violence_injury_prevention/violence/world_report/en/.
86. Wrosch PV. What more can congress do about the elder abuse epidemic? A proposal for national movement. Temple Polit Civ Rights Law Rev. 2013;23(1):1–44.
87. Ziminski Pickering CE, Rempusheski VF. Examining barriers to self-reporting of elder physical abuse in community-dwelling older adults. Geriatr Nurs. 2014;35(2):120–5.

Index

X. Dong (ed.), *Elder Abuse*, DOI 10.1007/978-3-319-47504-2

Printed by Printforce, the Netherlands